A Comprehensive Textbook of
MIDWIFERY AND GYNECOLOGICAL NURSING

A Comprehensive Textbook of MIDWIFERY AND GYNECOLOGICAL NURSING

Sixth Edition

Annamma Jacob MSc (N)
Former Professor-cum-Principal
Bhagawan Mahaveer Jain College of Nursing
Bengaluru, Karnataka, India

Formerly

Professor
St. Philomenas College of Nursing
Bengaluru, Karnataka, India

Principal
Graduate School for Nurses
Board of Nursing Education
South India Branch
Christian Medical Association of India
Bengaluru, Karnataka, India

Nurse Supervisor
Suburban Medical Center
Paramount, Southern California, USA

Assistant Director of Nursing
Al-Sabah Hospital, Ministry of Public Health
Kuwait, Arab, Western Asia

Sister Tutor
Leelabai Thackersey (College of Nursing)
Shreemati Nathibai Damodar Thackersey
(Women's University)
Mumbai, Maharashtra, India

Junior Tutor
College of Nursing
Christian Medical College (Hospital)
Vellore, Tamil Nadu, India

Foreword
Krishnaveni TM

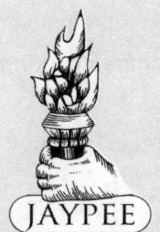

JAYPEE BROTHERS MEDICAL PUBLISHERS
The Health Sciences Publisher
New Delhi | London

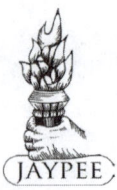

Jaypee Brothers Medical Publishers (P) Ltd

Headquarters
Jaypee Brothers Medical Publishers (P) Ltd
EMCA House
23/23-B, Ansari Road, Daryaganj
New Delhi - 110 002, India
Landline: +91-11-23272143, +91-11-23272703
+91-11-23282021, +91-11-23245672
Email: jaypee@jaypeebrothers.com

Corporate Office
Jaypee Brothers Medical Publishers (P) Ltd
4838/24, Ansari Road, Daryaganj
New Delhi 110 002, India
Phone: +91-11-43574357
Fax: +91-11-43574314
Email: jaypee@jaypeebrothers.com

Overseas Office
J.P. Medical Ltd
83 Victoria Street, London
SW1H 0HW (UK)
Phone: +44 20 3170 8910
Fax: +44 (0)20 3008 6180
Email: info@jpmedpub.com

Website: www.jaypeebrothers.com
Website: www.jaypeedigital.com

© 2023, Jaypee Brothers Medical Publishers

The views and opinions expressed in this book are solely those of the original contributor(s)/author(s) and do not necessarily represent those of editor(s) and publisher of the book.

All rights reserved. No part of this publication may be reproduced, stored or transmitted in any form or by any means, electronic, mechanical, photocopying, recording or otherwise, without the prior permission in writing of the publishers.

All brand names and product names used in this book are trade names, service marks, trademarks or registered trademarks of their respective owners. The publisher is not associated with any product or vendor mentioned in this book.

Medical knowledge and practice change constantly. This book is designed to provide accurate, authoritative information about the subject matter in question. However, readers are advised to check the most current information available on procedures included and check information from the manufacturer of each product to be administered, to verify the recommended dose, formula, method and duration of administration, adverse effects and contraindications. It is the responsibility of the practitioner to take all appropriate safety precautions. Neither the publisher nor the author(s)/editor(s) assume any liability for any injury and/or damage to persons or property arising from or related to use of material in this book.

This book is sold on the understanding that the publisher is not engaged in providing professional medical services. If such advice or services are required, the services of a competent medical professional should be sought.

Every effort has been made where necessary to contact holders of copyright to obtain permission to reproduce copyright material. If any have been inadvertently overlooked, the publisher will be pleased to make the necessary arrangements at the first opportunity.

Inquiries for bulk sales may be solicited at: jaypee@jaypeebrothers.com

A Comprehensive Textbook of Midwifery and Gynecological Nursing

First Edition: 2005
Second Edition: 2008
Third Edition: 2012
Fourth Edition: 2015
Fifth Edition: 2019
Sixth Edition: 2023
Revised Reprint: 2024

ISBN: 978-93-5696-198-2

Printed at Rajkamal Electric Press, Kundli, Haryana.

Foreword

A Comprehensive Textbook of Midwifery and Gynecological Nursing offers a unique opportunity to midwifery students as well as teachers, to assimilate an evergrowing body of scientific knowledge and to develop the technical and analytical skills necessary to apply the same into practice.

The book strives to provide the students with various aspects of midwifery to become competent and caring midwives. It includes the most accurate and clinically relevant information available, in a clearly written, visually appealing and logical format.

The book includes 12 Sections divided into 72 Chapters with an exhaustive Appendix and Glossary at the end. Each chapter is ending with a list of bibliography, which is useful to find out detailed information. In addition, a number of diagrams, tables, illustrations and nursing processes have been presented, wherever necessary. The book is in simple language.

The current concept on Community Midwifery has been included, which stresses on Preventive Obstetrics and Domiciliary Care in Maternity Nursing. A detailed discussion on Primary Health Care, the Organization of Maternal and Child Health Programs, and the Current Evolution of Reproductive and Child Health Programs is included, which is of much use to the students to deliver Community, Maternal and Child Health Services.

I hope and trust that this midwifery textbook will be of great help not only to midwifery students but also to the midwifery teachers, for study as well as for ready-reference.

With best wishes.

Krishnaveni TM PHN
Former Assistant Director
Directorate of Health and Family Welfare Services
Government of Karnataka
Bengaluru, Karnataka, India

Acknowledgments

One of the most pleasant parts of writing a book is the opportunity to thank those who have contributed to it. I am deeply appreciative of Dr Krishnaveni TM, Former Assistant Director, Directorate of Health and Family Welfare Services, Government of Karnataka, Bengaluru, Karnataka, India, for the patient and wholehearted efforts in editing the book.

Special thanks to Mr Joji George RN and Miss Aswathy Alexander BSc (N) who drew many figures in this book.

There have been many people who have touched and shaped my life and beliefs in maternal child nursing. I am indebted to Mrs Nesamoni Lazarus, my teacher at College of Nursing, Christian Medical College and Hospital, Vellore, Tamil Nadu, India, from whom I learned a lot and Mrs Phyllis Berg and Miss Chris Hamilton, Nursing Managers at Suburban Medical Center, Paramount, California, USA, who have influenced me profoundly.

I am thankful to my personal friends and professional colleagues in the institutions I had worked and with whom I shared my knowledge and aspirations. The inspiration for writing this book came as a result of my association and involvement with my former student at Leelabai Thackersey College of Nursing, Shreemati Nathibai Damodar Thackersey Women's University, St. Philomenas College of Nursing and Graduate School for Nurses, Board of Nursing Education (BNE), South India Branch (SIB), and Christian Medical Association of India (CMAI), Bengaluru, Karnataka, India.

My special thanks go to my niece Pinky Ann Thomas, nephew Pinku Cherian Thomas and brother-in-law Mr George K Cherian for their support and suggestions.

It is essential to have sustained interest and determination to keep a book updated to meet the changing needs in the field of nursing education, necessitated by the advancing trends in diagnostic and therapeutic technologies in managing health care.

Encouragement, support and cooperation of many are essential and I am deeply thankful to many who provided comments and suggestions after reviewing and using the textbook.

Management personnel of Bhagwan Mahaveer Jain College of Nursing permitted the use of the facilities of college library and laboratories for which I am extremely grateful to them.

For the many photographs and illustrations included in the book, staff of Bhagwan Mahaveer Jain Hospital, patients and their family members along with staff and students of BMJ College of Nursing offered themselves and their efforts, and I record my sincere thanks to everyone of them.

Most importantly, I thank God Almighty for giving me the physical and emotional strength required to carry out this work. Not least but most, I thank my husband Jacob AJ who encouraged me and worked with me tirelessly to complete this book and in whose honor I have decided to publish this book.

Finally, my grateful thanks to Shri Jitendar P Vij (Group Chairman), Mr Ankit Vij (Managing Director), Mr MS Mani (Group President) of M/s Jaypee Brothers Medical Publishers (P) Ltd, New Delhi, India, and Mr Venugopal Vishnumurthy (Regional Head-Business Development, DigiNerve), Bengaluru and all other staff of M/s Jaypee Brothers Medical Publishers (P) Ltd, Bengaluru, Karnataka.

Special thanks to Dr Madhu Choudhary (Director–Educational Publishing), Ms Pooja Bhandari (Production Head), Ms Sunita Katla (Executive Assistant to Group Chairman and Publishing Manager), Ms Samina Khan (Executive Assistant to Director–Educational Publishing), Ms Alisha Talwar (Development Editor), Ms Seema Dogra (Cover Visualizer), Mr Rajesh Sharma (Production Coordinator), Ms Geeta Barik (Proofreader), Mr Nitesh Jain (Graphic Designer), and Mr Kapil Dev Sharma (DTP Operator) of M/s Jaypee Brothers Medical Publishers (P) Ltd, New Delhi, India, for making my dream come true by publishing this book.

Preface to the Sixth Edition

Innovations and advances in diagnostic and therapeutic techniques have been taking place at regular and even at a faster pace in the recent years. New knowledge and inventions have made several previously used methods and techniques to become obsolete or unsafe and difficult for patients to undergo. Healthcare providers including nursing personnel, have been moving forward with the developments and participating in patient care, especially during the difficult period of the corona pandemic that affected people of all ages and stages. Women of child-bearing age group were of great concern everywhere. Indian nurses with great courage, fortitude and commitment stood up to meet the challenges and toiled to protect themselves and save their patients in all specialities including maternal-child health.

Sixth edition of the *Comprehensive Textbook of Midwifery and Gynecological Nursing* retained all the previous contents and added notes on additional diagnostic and therapeutic procedures which are based on evidence-based information. Revised National Immunization schedule and updated Nursing Diagnosis Taxonomy are added. Knowledge of special investigations and diagnostic procedures included would enable every nurse identify pregnancy-related and associated health problems and gynecological disorders in order to identify and provide need-based care, attention and support to clients in different stages of pregnancy and following child-bearing age. Nursing students of all levels and nurse educators who have well accepted the previous editions of the book are hoped to find the sixth edition a useful source for learning and teaching midwifery and gynecological nursing.

Critical comments and suggestions from nurse educators and students who have used the book always helped me to improve the contents and I thankfully welcome their encouragement and hope to receive their support in future. I thankfully acknowledge the encouragement and support of all the officials and staff of Jaypee Brothers Medical Publishers who made it possible to bring out the sixth edition of this textbook.

Annamma Jacob

Preface to the First Edition

The book is the culmination of ideas of a nurse educator who has practiced and taught maternal-neonatal nursing in India and in the United States of America. It is the fulfillment of often stated need among nurse educators and nursing students in India. Since long, teachers of midwifery have been relying on books written with an orientation for practice in the developed countries or those written by physician authors. As a midwifery educator, I became aware of the frustrations of students in trying to piece together the information from English and American midwifery texts or from physician-authored book. The former were too much in-depth and generally oriented to conditions in the developed countries, while the latter lacked nursing care aspects in order to plan, and provide comprehensive care to maternity clients and newborns.

As the concept of nursing process has been incorporated into midwifery education, a chapter on nursing process is included to familiarize midwifery students to the appropriateness of using the problem-oriented approach with their maternity and newborn clients. With a few selected topics, the nursing processes that can be carried out are included, which are hoped to serve as guidelines. In the chapter on Drugs, nursing considerations are included with a view to foster the use of nursing process in drug administration. Pertinent information from other health sciences is included throughout the book, particularly as it relates to the child-bearing and child-rearing periods in the life of the family and from preconception through the first 6 weeks' postpartum.

This book is organized into 11 Sections in logical sequence including all the units outlined in the syllabus prescribed by the Indian Nursing Council for Midwifery Course (INC syllabus, 1986). Additional information includes the chapters on Nursing Process, Childbirth Education and Preparation, and the current trends in National Reproductive and Child Health (RCH) Program. This book is written completely in the Indian context and in a simple style, and easy to understand language for the benefit of Indian nursing students. Practicing nurses will also find the content understandable and useful. Advances in the field of obstetrics and practice of midwifery in the developed countries are included wherever relevant.

Each chapter begins with a list of learning objectives. This tells the reader specifically what she/he should know after reading the chapter. The students can use this as a study aid. A large number of informative diagrams, tables and illustrations have been included and they have been designed to convey information in readily comprehensible form.

I sincerely hope that this book will greatly benefit the midwifery teachers, students and nurses practicing maternal-child nursing.

Annamma Jacob

Contents

Section I: Midwifery

1. **Historical Review** — 3
2. **Development of Maternity Services and Current Trends** — 5
   - Current Trends 6
3. **Midwife: Definition of the Term, Roles and Responsibilities** — 9
   - Development of Midwifery Education in India 10
4. **Nursing Process in Maternal-Newborn Care** — 11
   - Five Phases of Nursing Process 11
   - Assessment 11
   - Diagnosis 13
   - Planning 21
   - Implementing 25
   - Evaluating 27

Section II: Reproductive System

5. **Female Pelvis and Generative Organs** — 33
   - Pelvis 33
   - Types of Pelvis 37
   - Other Pelvic Variations 39
   - Generative Organs 41
6. **Hormonal Cycles** — 48
   - Ovarian Cycle 48
   - Menstrual Cycle 50
7. **Male Reproductive System** — 53
   - Parts of Male Reproductive System 53
   - Male Hormones 55
   - Formation of the Spermatozoa 55

Section III: Embryology and Fetology

8. **Fertilization, Implantation and Development of the Fertilized Ovum** — 59
   - Fertilization 59
   - Implantation 59
   - Development of the Fertilized Ovum 60
9. **Development of the Placenta and Fetus** — 63
   - Development of the Placenta 63
   - Circulation through the Placenta 63
   - Mature Placenta 64
   - Functions of the Placenta 65
   - Amniotic Fluid 65
   - Umbilical Cord 66
   - Variations, Anomalies and Abnormalities of Placenta 66
   - Variations, Anomalies and Abnormalities of the Umbilical Cord and its Insertion 67
   - Development of the Fetus 68
10. **Fetal Organs and Circulation** — 72
    - Fetal Anatomy 72
    - Fetal Circulation 73
11. **Fetal Skull** — 75
    - Bones of the Vault 75
    - Sutures 75
    - Fontanels 75
    - Regions of the Fetal Skull 76
    - Landmarks of the Skull 76
    - Diameters of the Fetal Skull 76
    - Molding 77

Section IV: Normal Pregnancy

12. **Physiological Changes Due to Pregnancy** — 81
    - Changes in the Reproductive System 81
    - Changes in the Cardiovascular System 83
    - Changes in the Respiratory System 84
    - Changes in the Urinary System 84
    - Changes in the Gastrointestinal System 85
    - Changes in Metabolism 85
    - Maternal Weight Changes 86
    - Skeletal Changes 86
    - Skin Changes 86
    - Breast Changes 87
    - Changes in the Endocrine System 87
    - Changes in the Nervous System 88
13. **Diagnosis of Pregnancy** — 90
    - Diagnosis of Pregnancy 90

14. Minor Disorders in Pregnancy — 94
- Digestive System 94
- Musculoskeletal System 95
- Genitourinary System 96
- Circulatory System 96
- Integumentary System 97
- Nervous System 97
- Disorders that Require Immediate Action 97

15. Antenatal Care — 98
- Meaning 98
- Objectives 98
- Antenatal Visits 98
- Initial Examination 98
- Inspection 101
- Abdominal Palpation and Leopold's Maneuvers 103
- Auscultation 103
- Other Findings 107
- Pelvic Examination 110
- Ongoing Antenatal Care 110

16. Specialized Investigations and Fetal Evaluation in the Antenatal Period — 113
- Ultrasonography 113
- Amniocentesis and Amniotic Fluid Studies 114
- Alpha-fetoprotein Testing 116
- Amnioscopy and Fetoscopy 116
- Estriol Level Determination 116
- Fetal Blood Sampling (Cordocentesis) 116
- Fetal Evaluation Procedures 116

Section V: Normal Labor

17. Physiology of the First Stage of Labor — 123
- Definition of Labor 123
- Stages of Labor 123
- Signs and Symptoms of Impending Labor 126
- Energy Spurt 127
- Causes for the Onset of Labor 127
- Physiological Processes in the First Stage of Labor 128
- Initial Assessment and Diagnosis 130
- Vaginal Examination for the Woman in Labor 132

18. Management of the First Stage of Labor — 135
- Admission to Labor and Delivery Unit 135
- Continuing Care and Evaluation 138
- Records 146
- Partograph 146
- Nursing Process During the First Stage of Labor 149

19. Physiology of the Second Stage of Labor — 151
- Physiological Processes 151
- Presumptive Signs of Second Stage and Differential Diagnosis 152
- Maternal Physiological Changes in the Second Stage 152
- Mechanism of Normal Labor 152
- Fetal Normality During the Second Stage 155
- Duration of the Second Stage 156

20. Management of the Second Stage of Labor — 157
- Evaluation of Maternal Well-Being 157
- Episiotomy 159
- Evaluation of the Fetal Well-Being 160
- Evaluation of the Progress of Labor 161
- Bodily and Supportive Care of the Woman 161
- Preparation for Delivery 162
- Conducting the Delivery 162
- Records 164
- Nursing Process During the Second Stage of Labor 164

21. Physiology and Management of the Third Stage of Labor — 166
- Physiological Processes of Placental Separation and Expulsion 166
- Management of the Third Stage of Labor 167
- Complications of the Third Stage 171
- Nursing Process During the Third Stage 174

22. Management of the Fourth Stage of Labor — 175
- Evaluation and Inspection 175
- Continuing Care and Monitoring 176
- Use of Oxytocic Drugs 179
- Summary of Postpartum Management 179
- Nursing Process During the Fourth Stage of Labor 179

Section VI: Normal Puerperium

23. Physiology and Management of the Normal Puerperium — 183
- Duration 183
- Anatomical and Physiological Changes of the Puerperium 183
- General Physiological Changes 186
- Management of Early Puerperium 187
- Continuing Physical Assessment and Daily Care 189
- Other Assessments 193
- Discomforts of the Puerperium and Relief Measures 195
- Breastfeeding Difficulties and Management 196
- Guidance and Instructions in Preparation for Home Care 197
- Nursing Process During the Puerperium 198

24. Family Planning — 200
- Magnitude of the Problem 200
- Family Planning 200

Methods of Contraception 202
- Temporary Methods of Contraception 202
- Permanent Methods (Sterilization) 212
- Postconception Methods of Birth Control (Termination of Pregnancy) 216

Section VII: Abnormalities of Pregnancy, Labor and Puerperium

25. Abnormalities of Early Pregnancy   221
- Abortion 221
- Spontaneous Abortion 221
- Induced Abortion 223
- Septic Abortion 225
- Nurses' Role with Patients Undergoing Abortion 225
- Ectopic Pregnancy/Ectopic Gestation 226
- Hydatidiform Mole 228
- Choriocarcinoma 230
- Hyperemesis Gravidarum 230
- Rh Isoimmunization and ABO Incompatibility 231
- Retroversion of the Gravid Uterus 232

26. Sexually Transmissible and Reproductive Tract Infections   234
- Extent of the Problem in India 234
- Host Factors 235
- Relevance for Women 235
- Control of STDs 236

Local Infections of the Vagina and Vulva 236
- Fungal Infections 236
- Protozoal Infections 237
- Bacterial Infections 238
- Viral Infections 240

27. Disorders of Pregnancy   246
Antepartum Hemorrhage 246
- Types 246
- Placenta Previa 246
- Abruptio Placentae 248
- Disseminated Intravascular Coagulation 251

Disorders of Amniotic Fluid 252
- Polyhydramnios 252
- Oligohydramnios 253

28. Hypertensive Disorders of Pregnancy   256
Pregnancy-induced Hypertension 256
- Pre-eclampsia 256
- Eclampsia 261
- Gestational Hypertension 264

Chronic Hypertension in Pregnancy 265
- Diagnosis 265
- Complications 265

29. Medical Disorders, Gynecological Disorders and Psychiatric Disorders Associated with Pregnancy   267
- Cardiac Disease 267
- Respiratory Disorders 271
- Diabetes Mellitus 272
- Thyroid Dysfunction in Pregnancy 275
- Anemia in Pregnancy 276
- Iron Deficiency Anemia 278
- Folic Acid Deficiency Anemia (Megaloblastic Anemia) 280
- Vitamin B_{12} Deficiency 280
- Hemoglobinopathies 281
- Sickle Cell Disorders 281
- Thalassemia Syndromes 282
- Renal Problems in Pregnancy 282
- Chronic Renal Disease 283
- Autoimmune Diseases 284
- Idiopathic Thrombocytopenic Purpura 284
- Epilepsy in Pregnancy 285
- Gynecological Disorders in Pregnancy 285
- Psychiatric Disorders During Pregnancy 290
- Adolescent Pregnancy/Teenage Pregnancy 291
- Elderly Primi 292
- Grand Multipara 293

30. Multiple Pregnancy   295
- Incidence 295
- Twin Pregnancy 295
- Triplets and Higher Order Births 302
- Disability and Bereavement 302
- Embryo Reduction/Selective Reduction 302

31. Preterm Labor, Premature Rupture of Membranes and Intrauterine Fetal Death   304
- Preterm Labor 304
- Premature Rupture of Membranes 306
- Intrauterine Fetal Death 307

32. Post-term Pregnancy, Induction of Labor, Prolonged Labor and Disorders of Uterine Action   310
- Post-term Pregnancy 310
- Induction of Labor 312
- Prolonged Labor 316
- Disorders of Uterine Action 318

33. Malpositions and Malpresentations   323
- Occipitoposterior Position 323
- Face Presentation 325
- Brow Presentation 327
- Breech Presentation 327
- Shoulder Presentation 332
- Compound Presentation 333
- Shoulder Dystocia 333
- Unstable Lie 335

34. Obstetric Operations   336
- Dilatation and Evacuation 336
- Forceps Delivery 337
- Vacuum Extraction (Ventouse Delivery) 341
- Cesarean Section 343
- Destructive Operations (Embryotomies) 346

35. Obstetric Emergencies   349
- Vasa Previa 349
- Presentation and Prolapse of the Umbilical Cord 349
- Dystocia Caused by Fetal Anomalies 351
- Amniotic Fluid Embolism 352

- Shock 353
- Rupture of Uterus 355
- Basic Life Support/Cardiopulmonary Resuscitation 356

36. Complications of Third Stage of Labor 359
- Postpartum Hemorrhage 359
- Primary Postpartum Hemorrhage 362
- Intrauterine Tamponade using Bakri Balloon 364
- Secondary Postpartum Hemorrhage 365
- Retained Placenta 366
- Placenta Accreta 367
- Inversion of the Uterus 367

37. Injuries to the Birth Canal 370
- Lacerations of Perineum 370
- Pelvic Hematomas 372
- Rupture of the Uterus 372
- Visceral Injuries 373

38. Complications of Puerperium 375
- Puerperal Pyrexia 375
- Puerperal Sepsis 375
- Subinvolution of the Uterus 378
- Breast Complications 378
- Venous Thrombosis 380
- Pulmonary Embolism 381
- Psychological Disturbances in the Puerperium 382

Section VIII: Normal Neonate

39. Baby at Birth 387
- Extrauterine Adaptation 387
- Immediate Care of the Baby at Birth 388
- Normal Characteristics and Physical Features of a Healthy Newborn 390
- Initial Assessment of the Newborn 391
- Birth Asphyxia/Asphyxia Neonatorum 395
- Resuscitation of the Newborn 395

40. Physiology, Screening, Daily Care and Observation of the Newborn 401
- Physiology 401
- Physical Examination (Screening) 406
- Gestational Age Assessment 406
- Daily Care and Observation of the Newborn 408
- Vaccination and Immunization 410

41. Infant Feeding 413
- Breasts and Lactation 413
- Properties and Components of Breast Milk 413
- Management of Breastfeeding 414
- Artificial Feeding 421
- Weaning from the Breast 422

42. High-risk Neonates—Low Birth Weight, Preterm and Intrauterine Growth Restricted Babies 423
- High-risk Neonates 423
- Low Birth Weight Babies 423
- 'Small for Gestational Age' Term Infant 424
- Preterm Baby 424
- Intrauterine Growth Restricted Babies 428
- Large for Gestational Age/Heavy for Dates Infant 429

Section IX: Ill Baby

43. Recognizing the Ill Baby 433
- Assessment of Gestational Age 433
- Warning Signs 434
- System-wise Assessment 434
- Nursing Management of the Hospitalized Newborn and the Family 438

44. Respiratory Problems of the Newborn 440
- Anatomy and Physiology of the Respiratory System 440
- Clinical Signs of Respiratory Problems 441
- Causes of Respiratory Problems 441
- Principles of Caring for a Baby with Respiratory Problem 444

45. Birth Trauma, Hemorrhage and Convulsions 446
- Dislocations 448
- Visceral Injuries 449
- Hemorrhage 449
- Prevention of Trauma in the Newborn 452
- Convulsions in the Newborn 452

46. Congenital Abnormalities, Genetic Screening and Genetic Counseling 455
- Causes of Congenital Abnormalities 455
- Common Malformations and Syndromes of Gastrointestinal Tract 456
- Abnormalities Relating to Respiratory System 458
- Congenital Cardiac Defects 459
- Central Nervous System Abnormalities 460
- Musculoskeletal Deformities 462
- Abnormalities of the Genitourinary System 464
- Genetic Disorders 465
- Chromosomal Abnormalities 467
- Genetic Screening 469
- Genetic Counseling 470
- Nursing Implications 471

47. Jaundice and Infections in the Newborn 472
Jaundice 472
- Formation of Bilirubin 472
- Excretion of Bilirubin 472
- Complications of Hyperbilirubinemia 472
- Types of Jaundice 473
- Management of Jaundice 474

- Assessment and Diagnosis 474
- Treatment 474

Hemolytic Diseases of the Newborn 476
- Rhesus Incompatibility 476
- ABO Incompatibility 477

Neonatal Infections 477
- Natural or Innate Immunity 477
- Acquired Immunity 477
- Modes of Acquiring Infection 477
- Organisms in Newborn Infection 477
- Management of Infection in the Baby 478
- Infections Acquired Before or During Birth 478
- Infections Acquired after Birth 481

48. Metabolic and Endocrine Disorders in the Newborn 483
- Inborn Errors of Metabolism 483
- Phenylketonuria 484
- Galactosemia 484
- G6PD Deficiency 484
- Cystic Fibrosis 484

Endocrine Disorders 484
- Thyroid Problems 484
- Acquired Metabolic Disorders 485

49. Neonatal Intensive Care Unit 489
- Babies Who Need Special Care in NICU 489
- Levels of NICU 489
- Goals of NICU Care 490
- Preparation of NICU 490
- History and Examination 490
- Infection Control in Neonatal Intensive Care Units 490
- Records and Reports in Neonatal Intensive Care Unit 493
- Reports 494

Section X: Community Midwifery

50. Preventive Obstetrics and Domiciliary Care in Maternity Nursing 499
- Antenatal Care 499
- Prenatal Care 499
- Intranatal Care 502
- Postnatal Care 504

51. Primary Health Care and Maternal/Child Health Services in India 506
- Health Care 506
- Maternal and Child Health Services 507
- Antenatal Care 507
- Intranatal Care 509
- Postnatal Care 510
- Neonatal Care 511
- System of Delivering MCH Services in the Country 514

Assessing Maternal and Child Health Care 515
- Maternal Mortality 515
- Mortality in Infancy and Childhood 516
- Job Functions of Health Workers for Implementing MCH Services 519

Section XI: Special Topics

52. Pain Relief and Comfort in Labor 525
- Perception of Pain 525
- Causes of Pain 526
- Analgesics 526
- Anesthesia 527
- Nonpharmaceutical Methods of Pain Relief 529
- Positioning 530
- Hygiene and Comfort 531

53. Childbirth Education and Preparation 532
- Natural Childbirth Approach 532
- Childbirth Preparation Program 532
- Role of Coach or Support Person 536
- Role of the Childbirth Educator 536

54. Special Exercises for Pregnancy, Labor and Puerperium 538
- Postural Changes in Pregnancy 538
- Posture for Comfort in Different Positions 538
- Exercises During Pregnancy 539
- Posture for Relief of Aches and Pains 539
- Antenatal Exercises 540
- Positions for Comfort During Labor 540
- Postnatal Exercises 541
- Immediate Postnatal Physical Problems 542

55. Drugs Used in Obstetrics 545
- Oxytocics 545
- Antihypertensive Drugs 547
- Diuretics 550
- Tocolytic Agents 552
- Anticonvulsants 553
- Anticoagulants 555
- Analgesics 556
- Effects of Maternal Medications on Fetus and Breastfeeding Infants 557

56. Vital Statistics in Obstetrics 560
- Registration of Vital Events 560

Maternal Vital Statistics 560
- Maternal Mortality 561
- Maternal Morbidity 562
- Perinatal Mortality 563
- Neonatal Mortality 564
- Infant Mortality Rate 564
- Record Keeping 564

57. Perinatal Loss and Grief 566
- Loss, Grief and Mourning 566
- Reproductive Loss 566
- Symptoms of Normal Grief 567

- Phases of Grieving/Mourning 568
- Pathological Grief 568
- Rights of Parents when an Infant Dies 569
- Caring for the Caregiver 569
- Record Keeping 569
- Continued Care 570
- Nursing Process for the Client Experiencing a Loss 570

58. Radiology and Ultrasonics in Obstetrics 572
- Radiology in Obstetrics 572
- Ultrasonics in Obstetrics 573
- Midwife's Responsibility Regarding Prenatal Screening 574

59. Legal and Ethical Aspects of Nursing 576
- Functions of the Law in Nursing 576
- Mechanisms of Regulation of Nursing Practice 576
- Legal Roles of Nurses 577
- Laws Related to Nursing Practice 577
- Consumer Protection Act (CPA) 579
- Areas of Potential Liability in Nursing 579
- Laws Concerning Medical and Nursing Practice 580
- Legal Issues in Midwifery Practice 580
- Practice Guidelines for Legal Protection 581
- Legal Responsibilities of Nursing Students 581
- Ethical Principles Related to Nursing Practice 581
- Ethics in Clinical Nursing Practice 582
- Nursing Codes of Ethics 582
- The International Council of Nurses Code of Ethics (2000) 583
- Indian Nursing Council Code of Ethics 584

60. National Population Policy and Family Welfare Programs 588
- National Population Policy 2000 588
- National Family Welfare Program 591
- Reproductive and Child Health Program 593
- Janani Suraksha Yojana 595
- Vande Mataram Scheme 595
- Safe Abortion Services 595
- National Rural Health Mission 595
- Integrated Child Development Services 597

61. Obstetric and Gynecological Instruments 598
- Sponge Holding Forceps 598
- Kocher's Hemostatic Forceps 598
- Hemostats (Artery Forceps) 598
- Ovum Forcep 599
- Vulsellum Forceps 599
- Green Armytage's Forceps 600
- Uterine Packing Forceps/Uterine Dressing Forceps 600
- Allis Tissue Forceps 600
- Tenaculum Forceps 601
- Laminaria Tent Introducing Forceps 601
- Laminaria Tent 601
- Dissecting Forceps 601
- Doyen's Towel Clip 601
- Doyen's Retractor 602
- Anterior Vaginal Wall Retractor 602
- Kelly's Deep Retractor 602
- Sims' Double-bladed Vaginal Speculum 602
- Cusco's Bivalved Speculum 603
- Auvard's Weighted Vaginal Speculum 603
- Sims' Double-ended Uterine Curette 603
- Das' Cervical Dilators 603
- Flushing Curette 604
- Drew Smythe Catheter Membrane Perforator 604
- Uterine Sound 604
- Scissors 604
- Bulb Syringe 605
- Mucus Sucker 605
- Cord Clamp 605
- Wrigley's Outlet Forceps 605
- Das' Long Curved Obstetric Forceps 605
- Axis Traction Forceps 606
- Kielland's Forceps 606
- Ventouse Cup with Traction Device/ Vacuum Extractor 606
- Simpson's Perforator 607
- Cranioclast 607
- Embryotomy Scissors 607
- Breech Hook and Crochet 607
- Jardine's Decapitation Hook 607
- Combined Cranioclast and Cephalotribe 607
- External Pelvimeter 608
- Pinard's Stethoscope/Fetoscope 608
- Needle Holder 608
- Female Metal Catheter 608
- Ring Pessary 608
- Hodge-Smith Pessary 609
- Babcock's Tissue Forceps 609

62. Quality Assurance and Audit in Maternity Nursing 610
- Goals of Quality Assurance 610
- Components of Quality Assurance Plan 610
- Standards in Midwifery Practice 611
- Audit in Obstetrics and Midwifery 614

Section XII: Gynecological Nursing

63. Menstrual Cycle Disorders and Abnormal Bleeding 621
- Amenorrhea 621
- Dysmenorrhea 622
- Mittelschmerz's Syndrome (Ovular Pain) 622
- Dysfunctional Uterine Bleeding 622
- Premenstrual Syndrome 623
- Menorrhagia 624
- Polymenorrhea 625
- Metrorrhagia 625
- Oligomenorrhea 625
- Hypomenorrhea 625

64. Displacement of Uterus 627
- Retroversion of Uterus 627
- Uterine Prolapse 628

- Chronic Inversion of Uterus 630
- Study Questions 631

65. Infectious Conditions of Pelvic Organs 632
- Pelvic Inflammatory Disease 632
- Endometritis 633
- Cervicitis 634
- Vulval and Vaginal Infections 634
- Nursing Process for Clients with Pelvic Infections 635

66. Benign Pelvic Conditions 636
- Fibroid Tumors 636
- Benign Ovarian Tumors 637
- Polyps 638
- Polycystic Ovary Syndrome 638

67. Gynecological Examinations and Diagnostic Procedures 640
- Examination 641
- Diagnostic Procedures 642

68. Congenital Malformations of Female Genital Organs 644
- Congenital Uterine Anomalies/Abnormalities 644
- Vaginal Malformations 646
- Abnormalities of External Genitalia 647
- Anomalies of the Ovaries 648

69. Genital Fistulae 649
- Genitourinary Fistula 649
- Vesicovaginal Fistula 649
- Urethrovaginal Fistula 651
- Ureterovaginal Fistula 651
- Rectovaginal Fistula 652

70. Perioperative Care of Gynecological Patient 653
- Types of Surgery 653
- Management in Preoperative Phase 654
- Management in Intraoperative Phase 655
- Management in Postoperative Phase 655

71. Infertility and Adoption 656
- Infertility 656
- Assisted Reproductive Technology 660
- Role of Nurses in Management of Infertility 662
- Adoption 662

72. Genital Malignancies 665
- Ovarian Cancer 665
- Uterine Cancer 668
- Gestational Trophoblastic Disease 670
- Cancer of Cervix 672
- Cancer of the Vulva 674
- Bartholin's Gland Cancer 675
- Vaginal Cancer 675
- Cancer of Fallopian Tube 676
- Breast Cancer 676
- Postmastectomy Exercises 684
- Nursing Management of Patients with Genital Malignancies 689

73. Special Gynecological Conditions 690
- Adenomyosis 690
- Endometriosis 691
- Dyspareunia 692
- Puberty 692
- Menopause 693

74. Diagnostic Procedures in Gynecology 696
- Papanicolaou Test/Pap Smear/Cervical Smear 696
- Vaginal Smear/Vaginal Wet Mount 698
- High Vaginal Swab Collection 699
- Culdoscopy 699
- Diagnostic Laparoscopy 700
- Endometrial Biopsy 702
- Hysteroscopy 703
- Tuboscopy/Salpingoscopy 704
- Hysterosalpingography 705
- Ultrasonographic Examination 706
- Culdocentesis 707
- Laser Procedures/Surgeries for Gynecological Conditions 709
- Cryosurgery/Cryotherapy 710

Bibliography 713

Appendix: Maternal Newborn Nursing Care Plans 715
- Nursing Diagnoses for Prenatal Clients 715
- Nursing Diagnoses for Labor and Delivery Clients 719
- Nursing Diagnoses for Postpartum Clients 726
- Nursing Diagnoses for Neonates 731

Annexures
- Common Abbreviations Used in Obstetrics 741
- Common Signs in Obstetrics 745
- Maneuvers Used in Obstetrics 747

Glossary 751

Index 761

PLATE 1

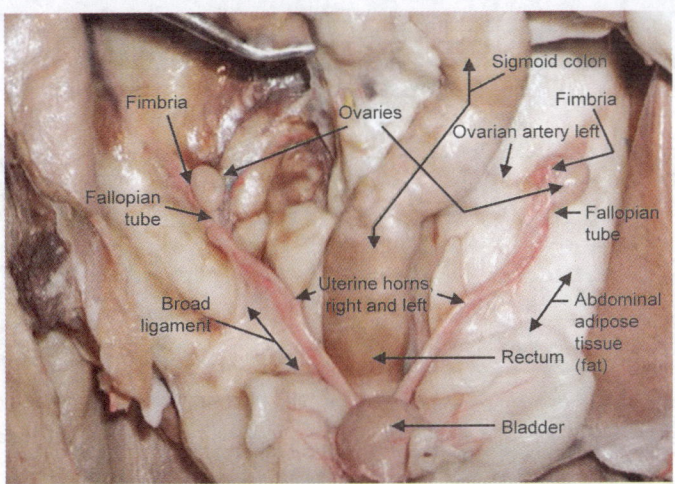

Figure 5.19: Female internal reproductive organs.

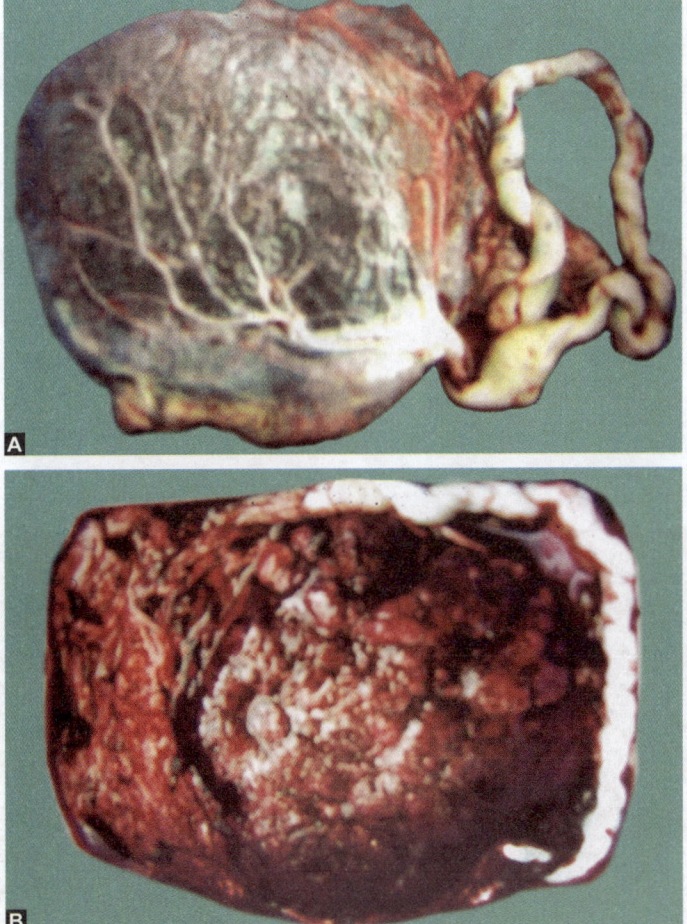

Figures 9.4A and B: Placenta at term. (A) Fetal surface of the placenta; (B) Maternal surface of the placenta.

PLATE 2

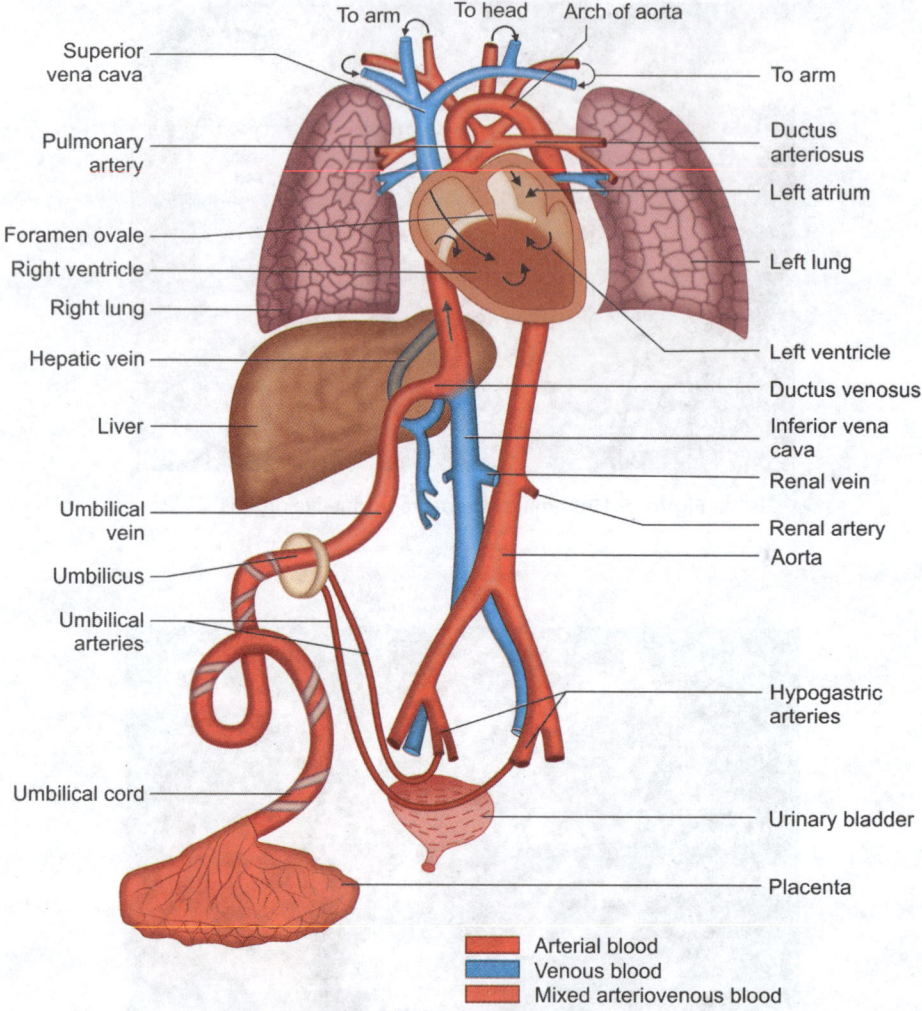

Figure 10.1: Fetal circulation.

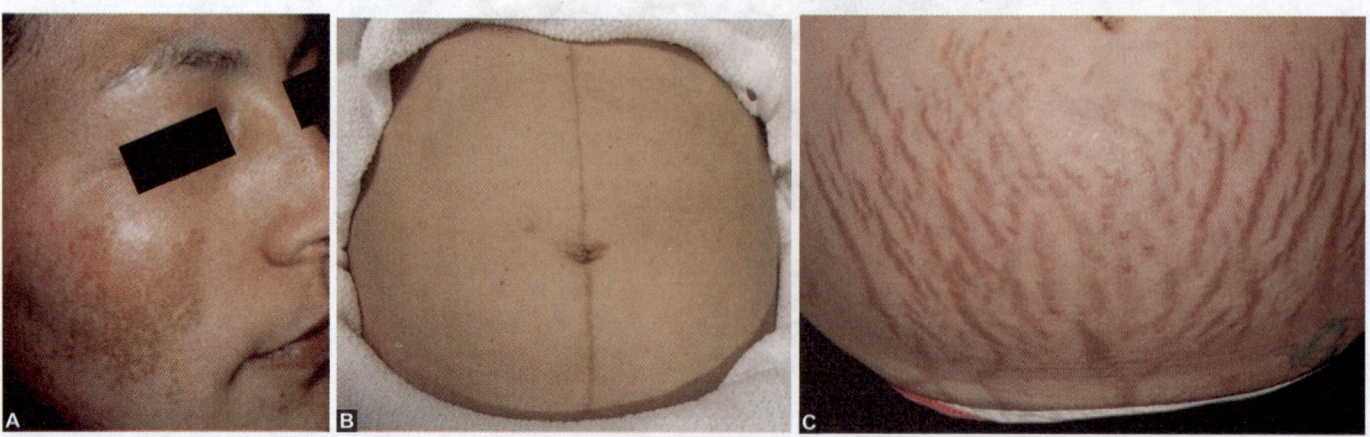

Figures 12.4A to C: (A) Chloasma gravidarum; (B) Linea nigra; and (C) Striae gravidarum.

PLATE 3

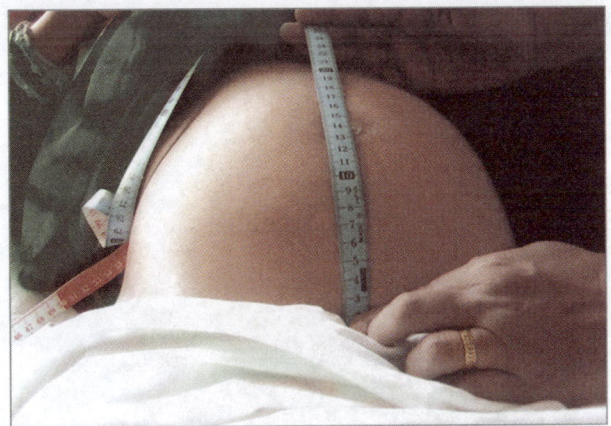

Figure 15.3: Measuring fundal height with tape measure.

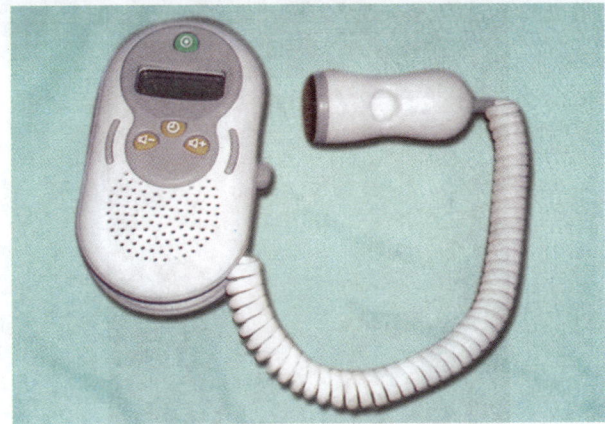

Figure 15.7: Ultrasonic Doppler device.

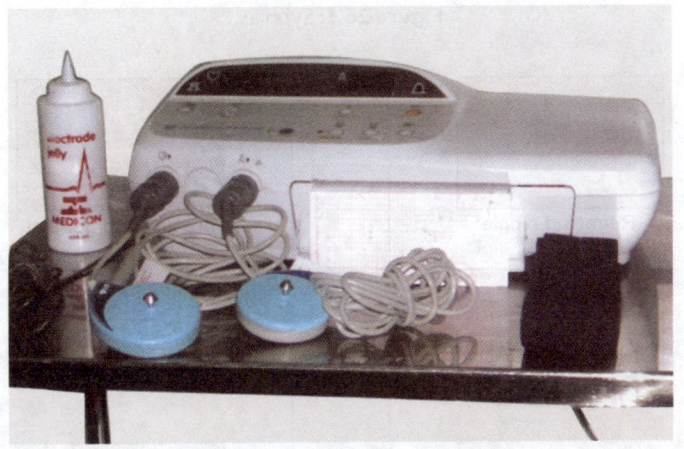

Figure 18.2: Electronic fetal monitor.

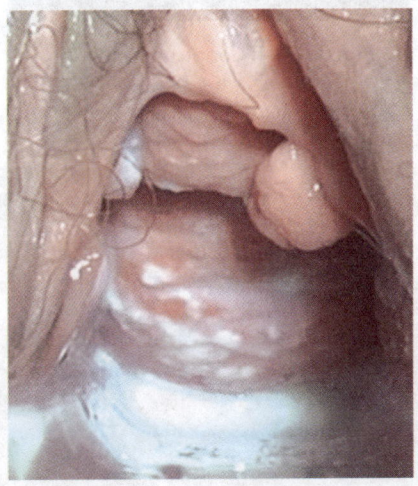

Figure 26.1: Candidia infection.

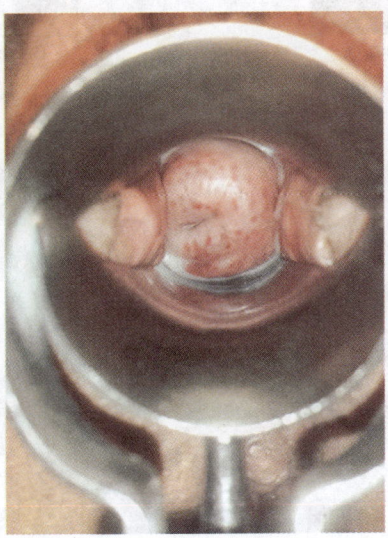

Figure 26.2: *Trichomonas vaginalis*.

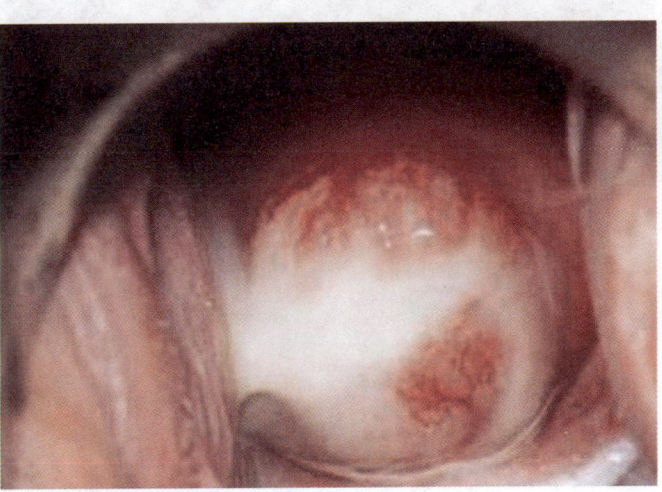

Figure 26.3: Chlamydia infection.

PLATE 4

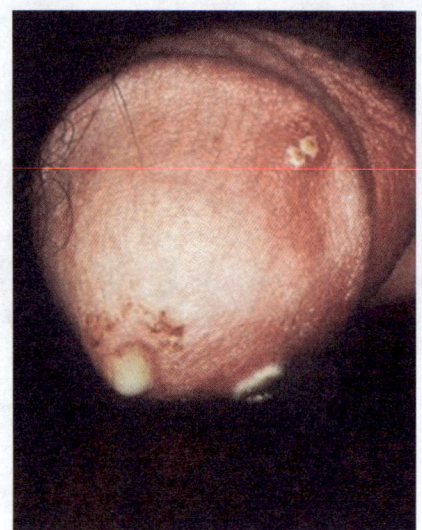

Figure 26.4: Gonorrhea infection.

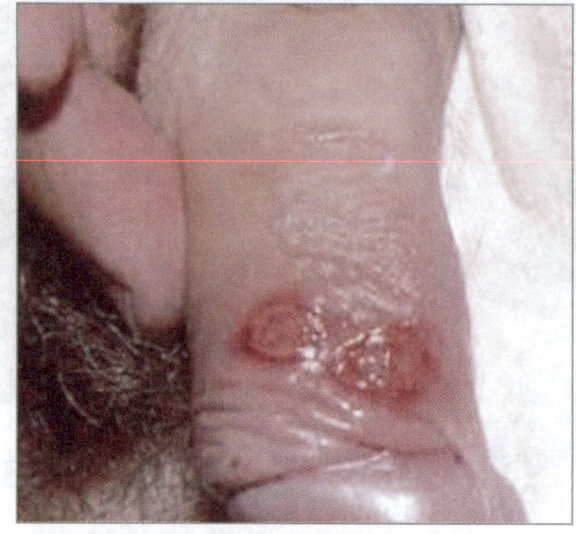

Figure 26.5: Syphilis.

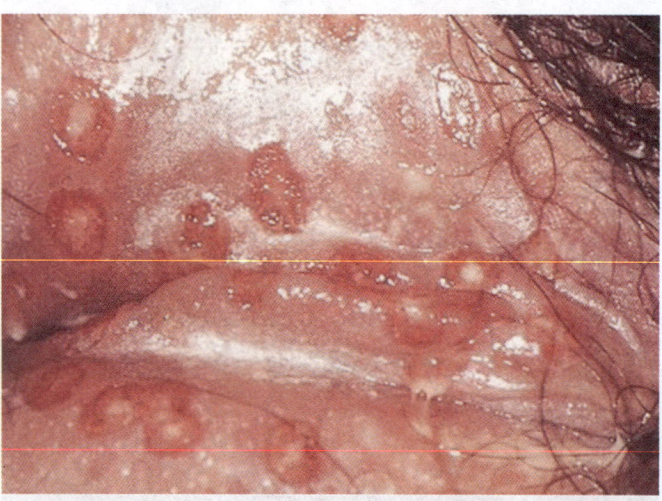

Figure 26.6: Genital herpes.

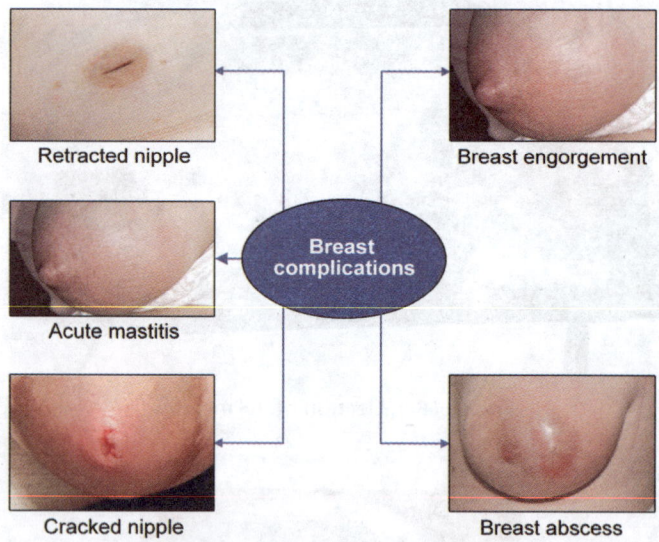

Figure 38.1: Breast complications.

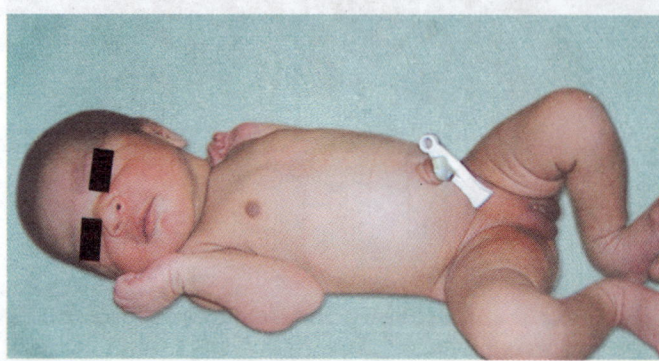

Figure 39.1: Healthy newborn.

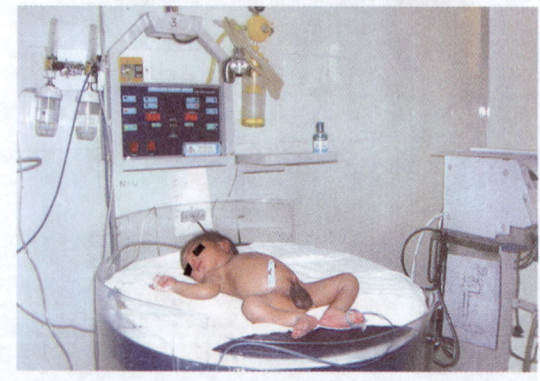

Figure 39.4: Newborn in radiant warmer.

PLATE 5

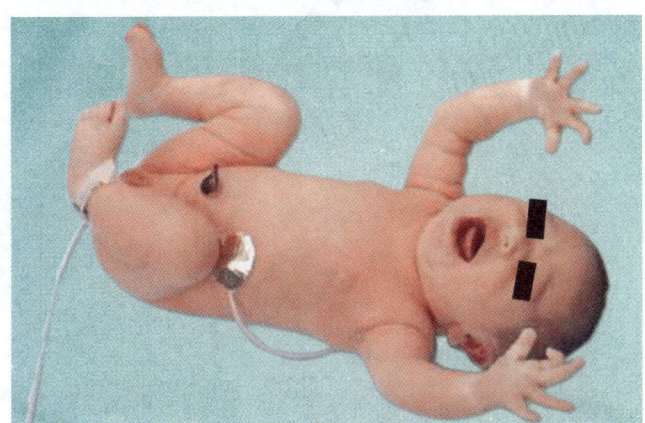

Figure 40.1: Moro reflex.

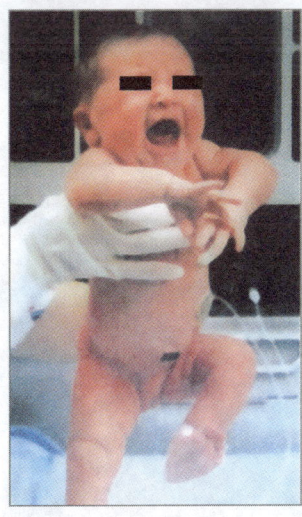

Figure 40.5: Stepping reflex.

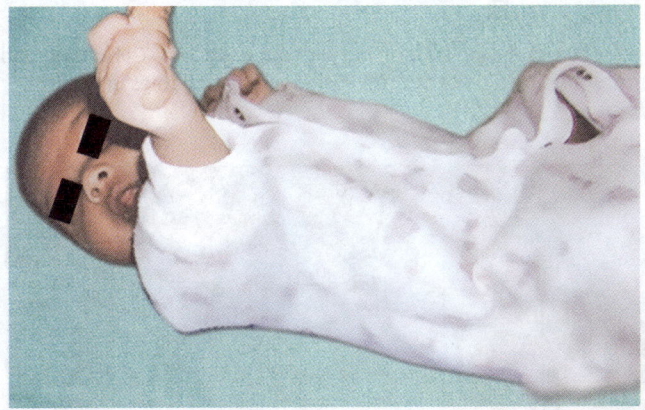

Figure 40.3: Palmar reflex.

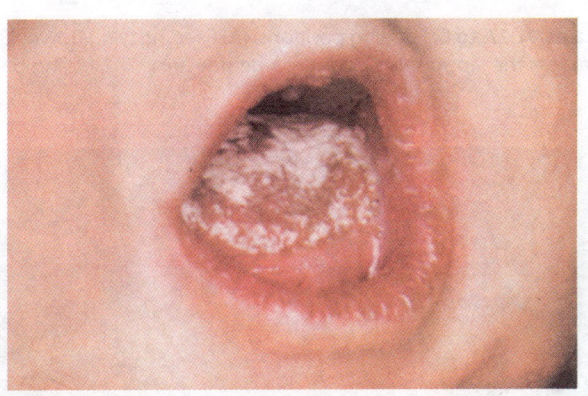

Figure 40.12: Oral thrush.

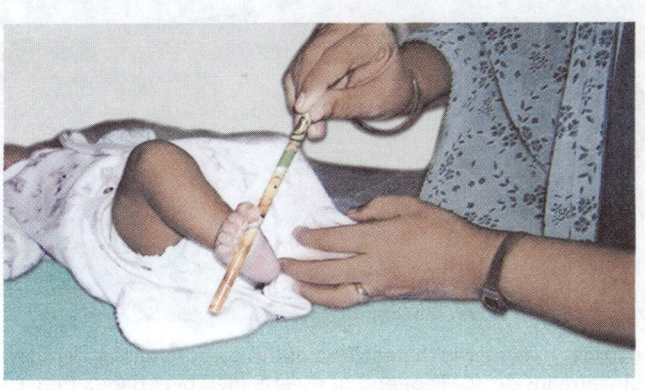

Figure 40.4: Plantar reflex.

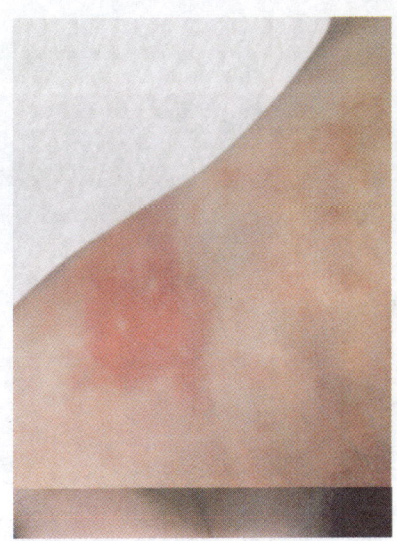

Figure 40.13: Erythema toxicum.

PLATE 6

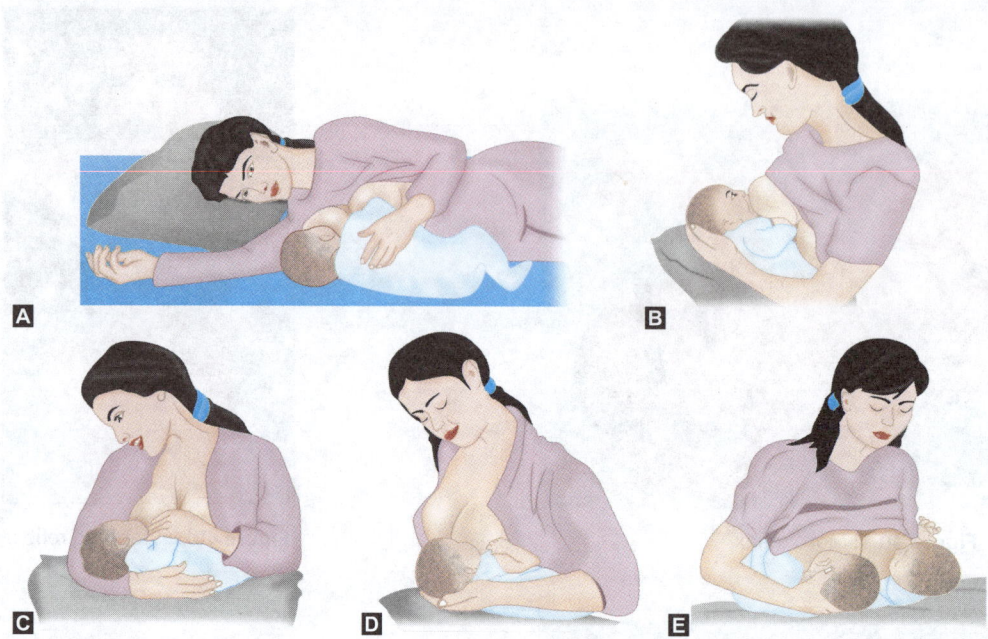

Figures 41.2A to E: Feeding positions. (A) Feeding lying down; (B) Holding baby across the lap supporting with opposite arm; (C) Holding baby across the lap supporting with same side arm; (D) Holding baby underarm, sitting on side of bed; (E) Positioning twin babies underarm.

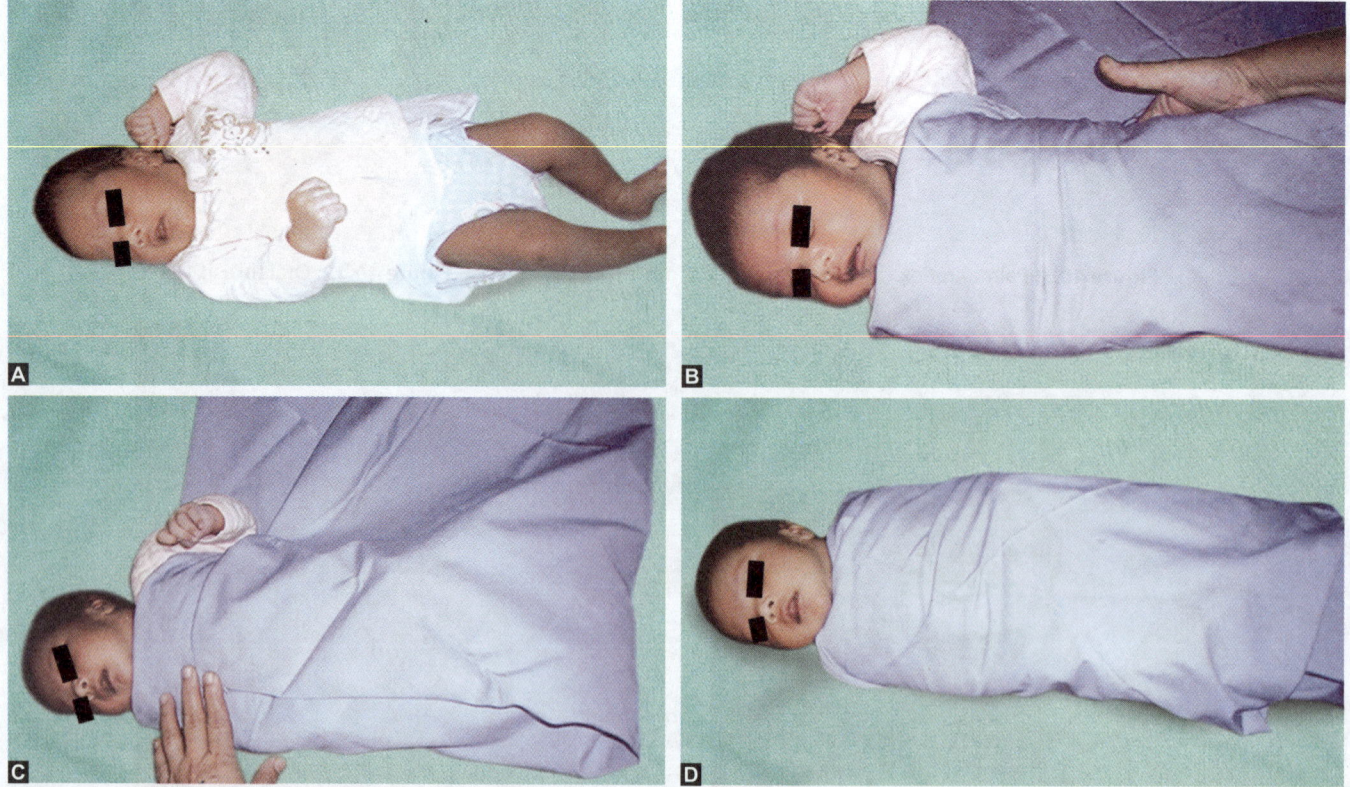

Figures 41.3A to D: Swaddle wrapping. (A) Baby placed on a baby sheet corner to corner with head end of the sheet folded at neck level; (B) One end of sheet taken over body to opposite side and tucked with one arm inside; (C) Foot end of sheet folded over baby's body; (D) Remaining end of sheet taken over body and tucked with second arm inside.

PLATE 7

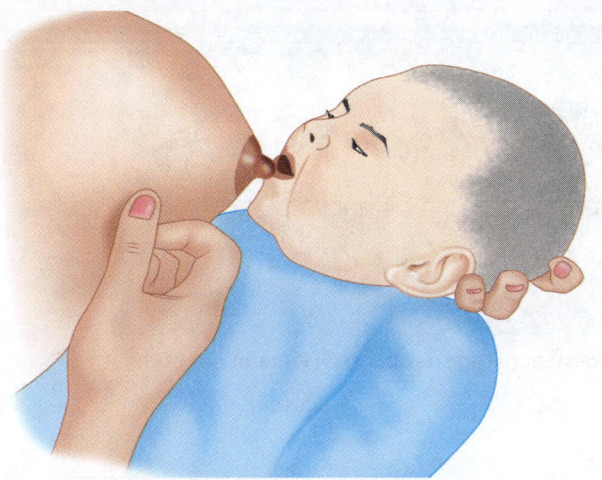

Figure 41.4: Initiating sucking.

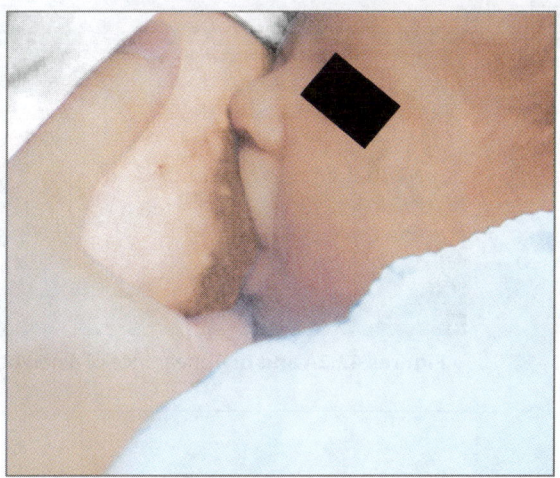

Figure 41.6: Baby's lips in contact with areola.

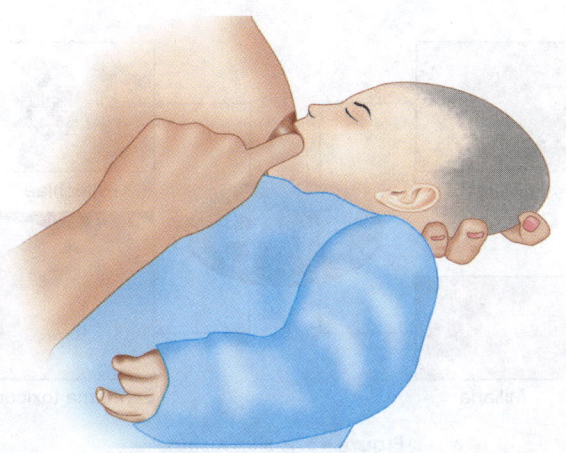

Figure 41.7: Breaking suction before removing the baby from breast.

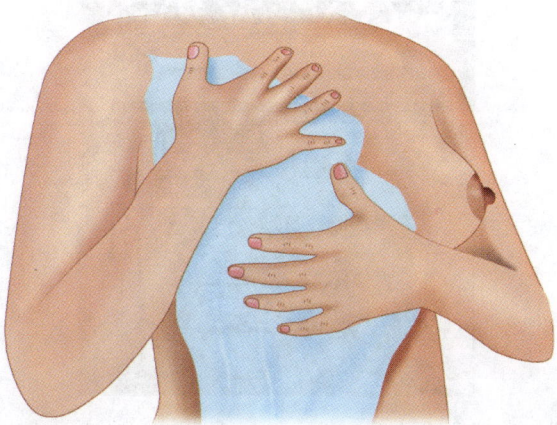

Figure 41.9: Applying warm towel to engorged breast.

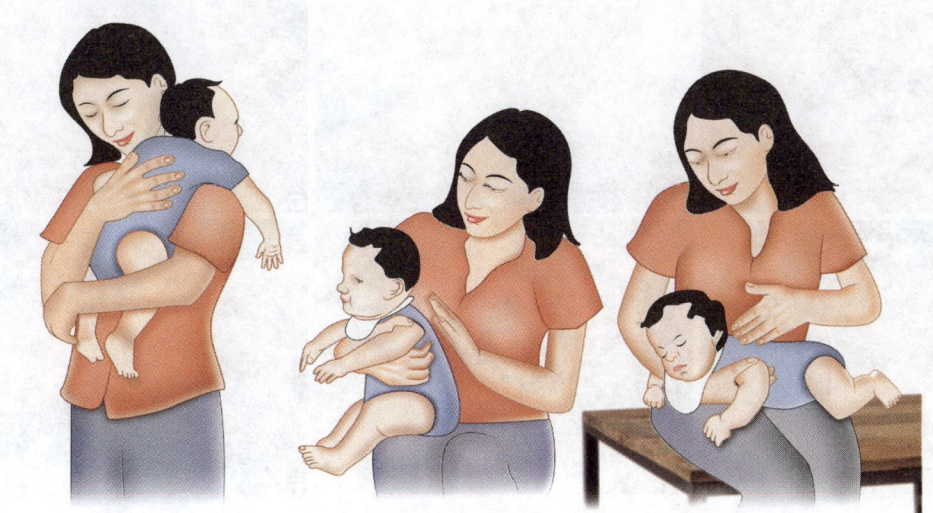

Figure 41.8: Burping positions.

PLATE 8

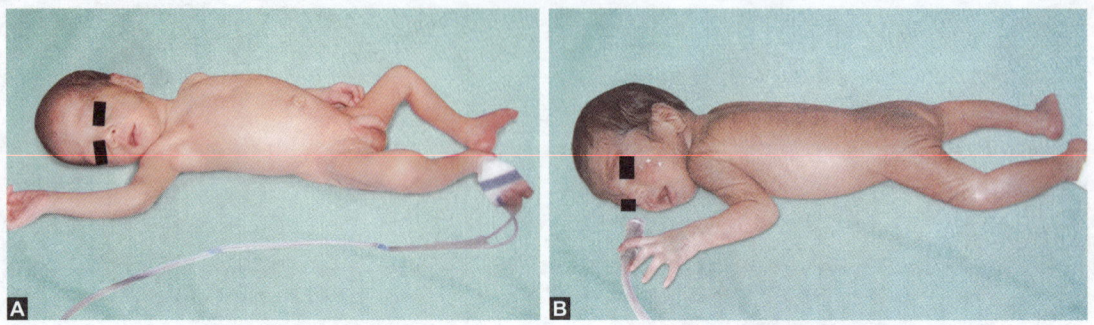

Figures 42.2A and B: Appearance of a newborn. (A) Small gestational age newborn; (B) Preterm newborn.

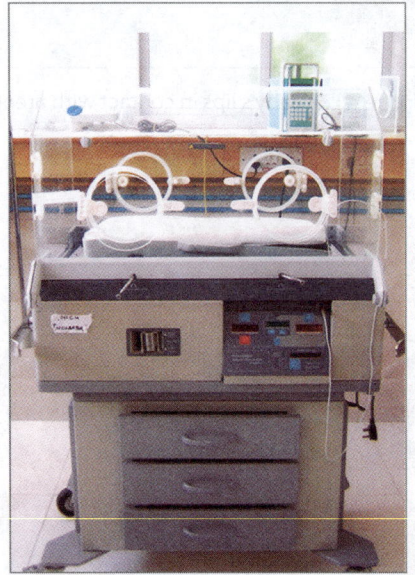

Figure 42.3: An Isolette/incubator for care of preterm baby.

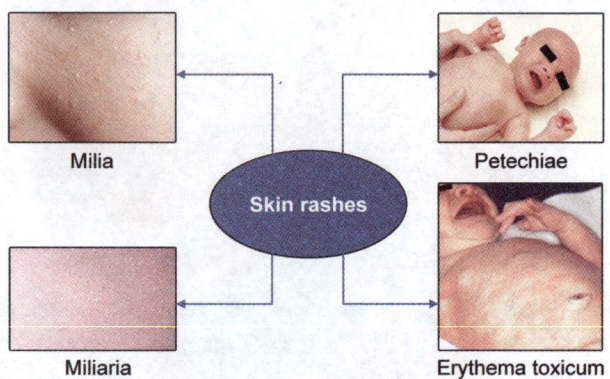

Figure 43.1: Skin rashes.

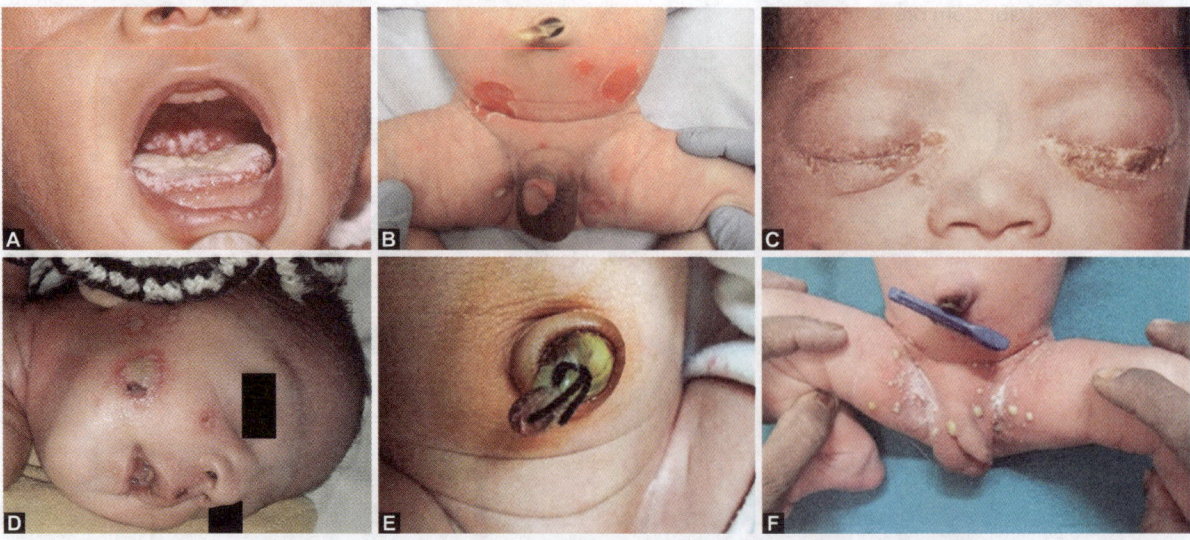

Figures 43.2A to F: Infectious lesions. (A) Oral thrush; (B) Bullous impetigo; (C) Neonatal conjunctivitis; (D) Herpes simplex virus; (E) Umbilical sepsis; (F) Pyoderma.

PLATE 9

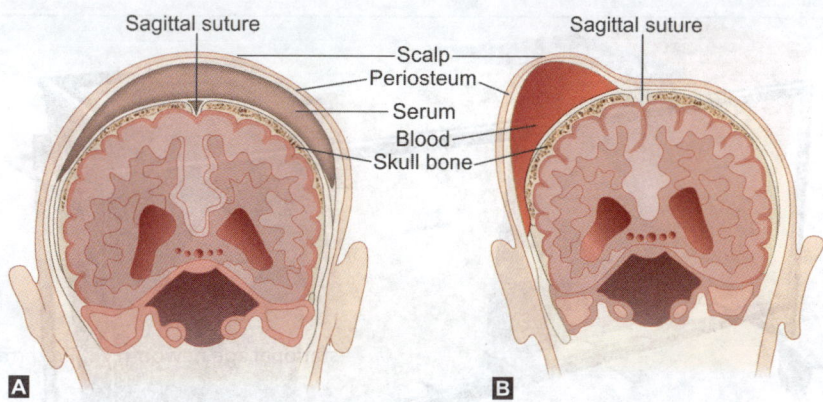

Figures 45.4A and B: Hemorrhage due to trauma. (A) Caput succedaneum; (B) Cephalohematoma.

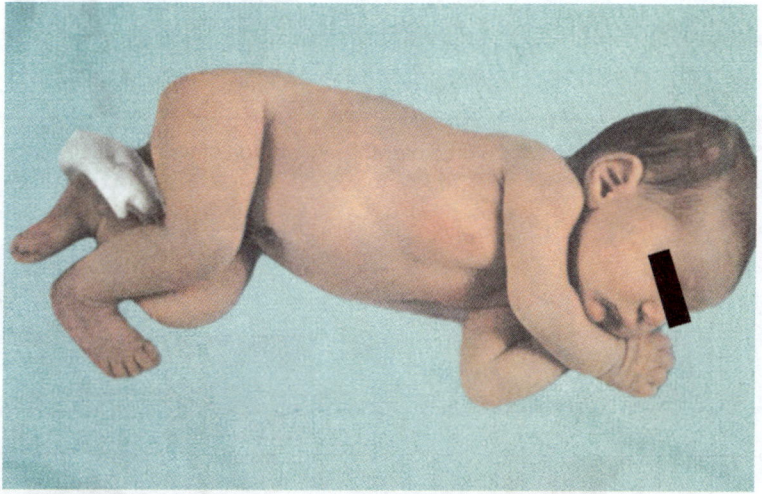

Figure 47.1: Physiological jaundice/icterus neonatorum.

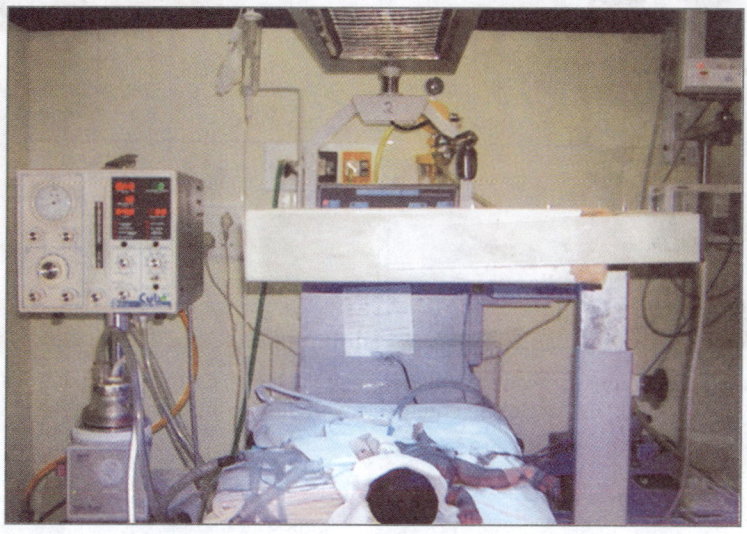

Figure 47.2: Baby undergoing phototherapy.

PLATE 10

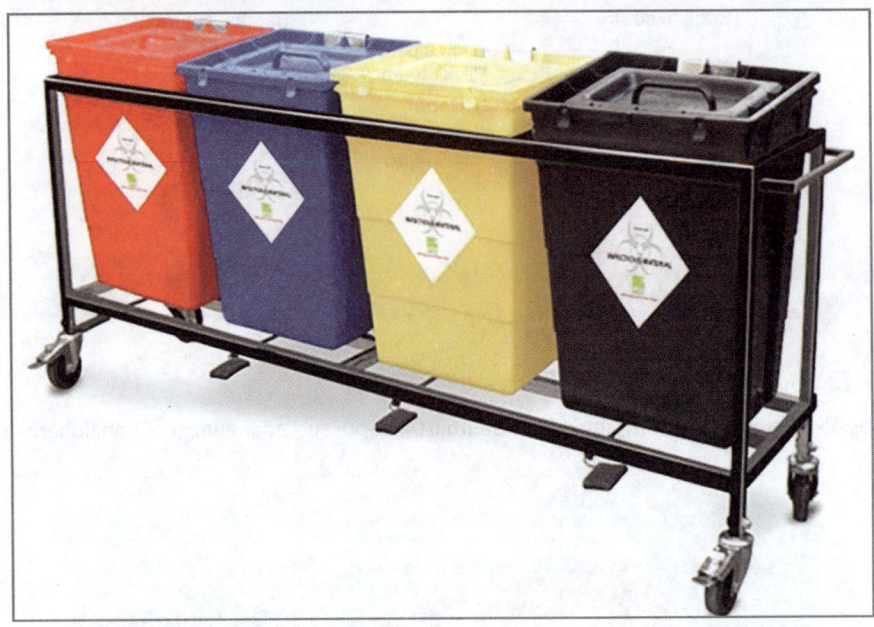

Figure 49.4: Colored bins for segregation of waste.

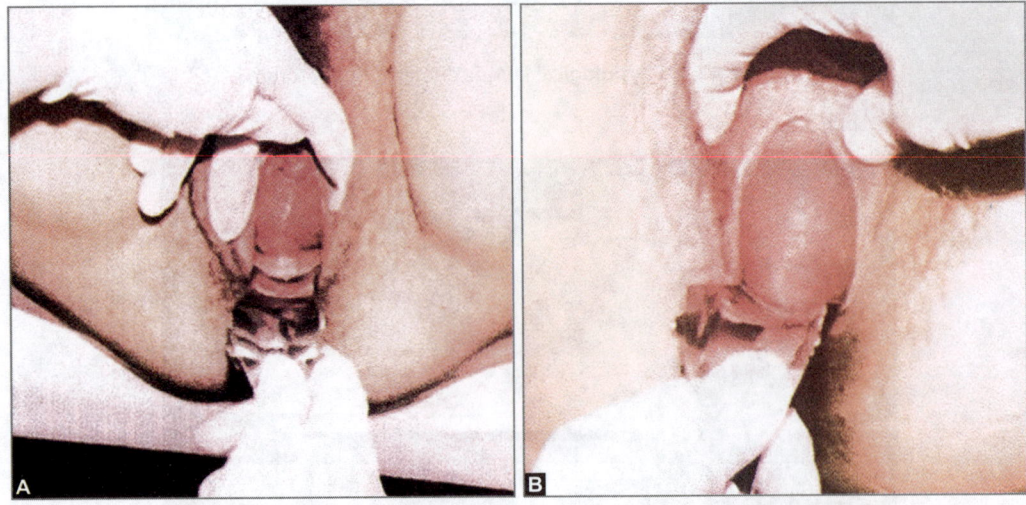

Figures 64.3A and B: Conditions associated with uterine prolapse. (A) Cystocele and uterovaginal prolapse; (B) Cystocele and enterocele with uterine prolapse.

PLATE 11

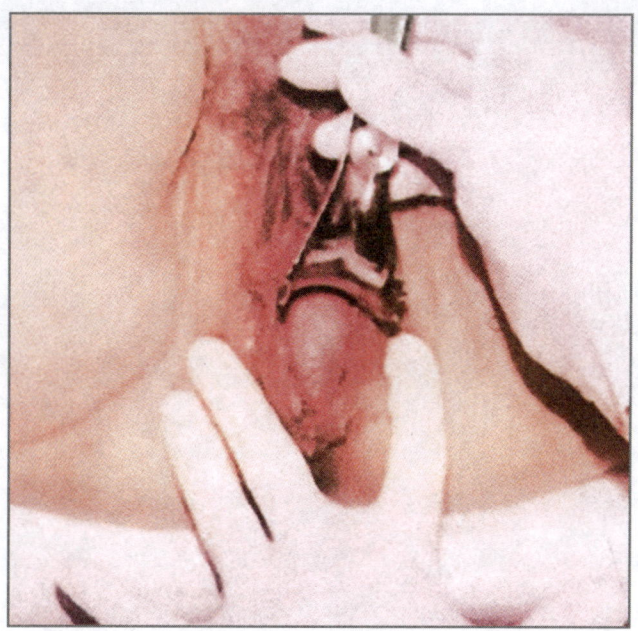

Figure 64.4: Rectocele.

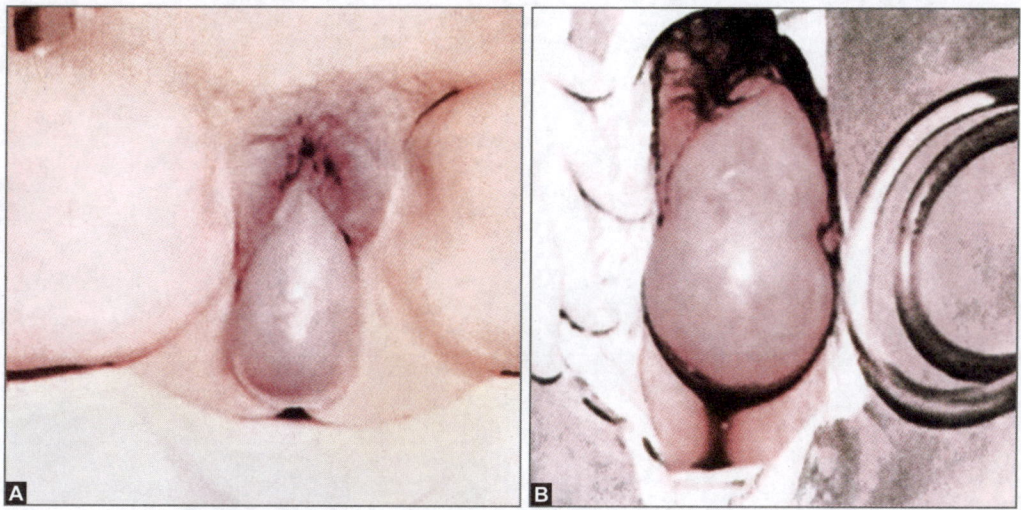

Figures 64.5A and B: Complete uterine prolapse in two different patients.

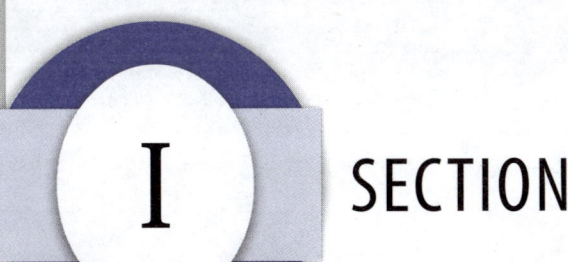

SECTION I

MIDWIFERY

Section Outline

1. Historical Review
2. Development of Maternity Services and Current Trends
3. Midwife: Definition of the Term, Roles and Responsibilities
4. Nursing Process in Maternal-newborn Care

CHAPTER 1

Historical Review

Learning Objectives

Upon completing this chapter, the learner will be able to:
- Identify the early recordings of midwifery practice.
- Appreciate the early foundations of modern midwifery.
- Appreciate the contributions to midwifery by various physicians through the centuries.

Midwifery is as old as the history of human species. Archeological evidence of a woman squatting in childbirth supported by another woman from behind demonstrates the existence of midwifery in 5000 BC. There are references to the midwives in the *Old Testament*. Genesis 35:17 "And it came to pass, when she was in hard labor that the midwife said unto her, fear not Rachel, it is another boy." In Exodus 1:15, it is recorded that the King of Egypt spoke to Shiphrah and Puah, the two midwives who helped Hebrew women when they gave birth. These two Hebrew midwives are the first midwives found in the literature. Through the centuries midwifery, the art of assisting women in childbirth has grown fulfilling its meaning 'with woman' at birth.

Hippocrates (460 BC), 'the Father of Scientific Medicine' organized trained and supervised midwives. Hippocrates believed that the fetus had to fight its way out of the womb and the membranes. The efforts of Hippocrates were not appreciated by the midwives.

Aristotle (384–322 BC), 'the Father of Embryology' described the uterus and the female pelvic organs. He also discussed the essential qualities of the midwife. Soranus, in the second century was the first to specialize in obstetrics and gynecology. His book was used for 1,500 years. He used a vaginal speculum, advised on cord care and wet nursing. From the 5th to 15th centuries, which was the period of decline of the Roman Empire, untrained midwives controlled the practice of midwifery.

Leonardo da Vinci (1452–1519) made anatomical drawings of pregnant uterus. In 1513, the first book on midwifery was printed in Germany based on the teachings of Soranus. In 1540, the book was translated into English. For a century and half it was the only book on midwifery in English. During this period, doctors were rigidly excluded from labor rooms and midwives assisted women in labor. Vesalius in 1543, opened the full-term pregnant uterus in a lower animal, extracted the fetus and demonstrated uterus as a single chamber organ.

Ambroise Paré (1510–1590) laid the foundations of modern obstetrics. He performed internal podalic version and skillfully delivered women. He was first to deliver a woman in bed instead of the birthing stool. He also sutured perineal lacerations. Ambroise Paré founded a school for midwives in Paris and France. Louise Bourgeois, a midwife trained by Pare, attended the ladies of the French court. She warned midwives against getting infected with syphilis and transmitting it to other women. She recommended induction of labor for pelvic contraction.

Julius Caesar Aranzi, wrote the first book for Italian midwives, which ran 17th edition. He advised cesarean section for contracted pelvis. William Harvey (1578–1657), 'the Father of British Midwifery', wrote the first English textbook on midwifery. He described the fetal circulation and the placenta, and was the first to deliver the placenta by massaging the uterus. He described the raw placental surface and initiated the study of uterine sepsis. Women remained largely reluctant to be delivered by men during this period. Midwives did not usually seek medical aid until the labor was hopelessly obstructed as in the case of gross pelvic deformity. The resultant death of the mother or the baby gave the physicians unwarranted reputation.

The French King Louis XIV in 1663, employed a Paris surgeon to attend one of his mistresses in labor and pleased with the result, the King honored the surgeon with the title 'accoucheur' (a person who assists women in childbirth).

The French accoucheurs built a school of midwifery, which attracted doctors from all over Europe. Mauriceau in 1668, published a treatise on midwifery. Hugh Chamberlen translated it into English, which greatly assisted the advance of midwifery in Britain.

Mauriceau was the greatest physician of the 17th century. He described the attitude of the fetus in uterus as that of one of squatting down to pass stools and lowering his head to see what he has done.

Chamberlen in 1675, designed obstetric forceps. William Smellie (1697-1763) is called 'the Father of British Midwifery'. He explained labor to be a mechanical process and described pelvimetry, cephalometry and forceps delivery of the after coming head of a breech. He devised a lock for the obstetric forceps, which permitted each blade to be introduced separately. The chair of midwifery was founded in 1726 in the University of Edinburgh. In 1772, John Leake replaced the obstetric stool by special delivery beds.

Charles White in 1773, stated that puerperal fever was infectious. He used lime as disinfectant and clean linen, isolation, adequate ventilation and sitting posture to facilitate drainage. Fielding Ould (1710-1789) described the mechanism of normal labor and performed the first episiotomy. Gordon in 1795, described puerperal sepsis as a wound contamination of the placental site.

Laennec in 1816, invented a stethoscope and Francois in 1818, first recognized fetal heart sounds in the pregnant uterus. James Young Simpson in 1847, used chloroform first in obstetrics for anesthesia. Florence Nightingale in 1862, organized a small training school in connection with King's College Hospital, where she conducted training for midwives.

Semmelweis in 1861, demonstrated the cause of puerperal sepsis and suggested preventive measures. His students practiced scrubbing their hands in chloride of lime, which reduced maternal mortality rate in the words. Louis Pasteur in 1879, wrote a thesis on puerperal sepsis, which demonstrating the presence of streptococci in the lochia, blood and in fatal cases in the peritoneal cavity. Spencer and Ballantyne promoted the concept of antenatal care for pregnant women. The first antenatal clinic was started about the time of the First World War.

The history of cesarean section dates back to 715 BC and the operation derives its name from the notification *Lex Caesarea*—a Roman law, which was followed even during Caesar's reign. The law provided for an abdominal delivery either in a dying woman with a hope to get a live baby or to perform postmortem abdominal delivery for a separate burial. The operation does not derive its name from the birth of Caesar, as his mother lived long time after his birth. The origin of the word cesarean is also related to a Latin verb *caedere,* which means 'to cut'.

A French obstetrician, François Mauriceau first reported cesarean section in 1668. In 1876, Porro performed subtotal hysterectomy. Max Sanger in 1882, first sutured the uterine walls. In 1912, Kronig introduced lower segment vertical incision and it was popularized by DeLee (1922). Munro Kerr in 1926, introduced the present technique of lower segment cesarean operation and popularized it.

STUDY QUESTIONS

Short Notes

1. The first book on midwifery.
2. Early findings on puerperal sepsis.
3. The history of cesarean section.

BIBLIOGRAPHY

1. Bullough VL, Bullough B. The Emergency of Modern Nursing. New York: Macmillan; 1969.
2. Fox CG. Toward a sound historical basis for nurse-midwifery. Bulletin of the American College of Nurse-Midwives. 1969;14:76-82.
3. Fred D. The Nursing Profession: Five Sociological Essays. New York: Wiley; 1966.
4. Parulekar SV. Textbook for Midwives, 2nd edition. Mumbai: Vora Medical Publishers; 1995.

CHAPTER 2

Development of Maternity Services and Current Trends

Learning Objectives

Upon completing this chapter, the learner will be able to:
- Identify the development of maternity services through different periods.
- Appreciate the phases of the development process of midwifery practice and midwifery education in India.
- Discuss the philosophy of family-centered maternity care.
- Discuss the technological advances in health care that have affected maternal-newborn nursing.
- Discuss the concept of mother-baby couplet care and single room maternity care.

Following reformation in the 16th century, the Church of England accepted the responsibility for issuing by the Bishops of licenses for midwives to practice. Midwifery at that time was practiced entirely by midwives, who lacked knowledge of anatomy and obstetrics. The same situation existed in India, where midwifery was practiced by traditional 'dais'. The chair of midwifery was created in Edinburgh in 1726, for giving instructions to midwives. Courses of instruction were given to midwives in various centers throughout Britain during the 18th century and a few hospitals issued certificates.

In 1756, John Douglas recommended that proper courses of instructions be given to midwives and an examination should be held before certificate to practice was given. Better midwifery practice began at this time. The Ladies' Obstetrical College, London was founded in 1864 and daughters of professional men attended lectures and became midwives. In 1902, the first English Midwives Act was passed and state registration of midwives became mandatory by law.

In 1700s and 1800s, marked a time of rapid development in medical and nursing science, discoveries and teaching pertinent to obstetric practice. These developments include the invention and refinement of obstetrical forceps, technical advances, which decreased the risks involved in cesarean section, pioneering efforts in obstetric anesthesia, conquest of puerperal fever, emergence of modern nursing and inclusion of obstetrics in medical practice. The observations and teachings of William Smellie (1697–1763), who developed teaching manikins and identified the mechanisms of labor, refuted the myths and misconceptions.

William Shippen, Junior (1736–1808), the first lecturer in obstetrics and Samuel Bard (1742–1821), author of the first American textbook on obstetrics are attributed with promoting obstetrical teaching in the United States (US). However, due to lack of educational programs for midwives, these developments, new knowledge and teachings remained inaccessible to them. The first two decades of the 20th century are notable for the recognition of inadequate maternity care and subsequent actions to improve this care in the US. The Children's Bureau in Washington, DC and Maternity Center Association in New York City were established, which contributed greatly to the development of maternal-infant health care and midwifery.

A study conducted during 1906 in New York City on maternal and infant mortality stated that approximately 3,000 incompetent and ignorant midwives attended over 40% of deliveries. While, these midwives were not solely responsible for the high maternal and infant mortality rates at that time, they received the brunt of the blame.

Progress in improving the situation was slow. It was in 1935 that the registration of births was made mandatory in all the states. In 1915, the New York City Commissioner made another study of maternal and infant mortality. The findings of this study demonstrated the connection between mortality and lack of prenatal care. Several maternity centers were established in New York City and other states followed. By 1930, obstetric care began to move out of the home into the hospital and laws were passed to regulate the practice of the indigenous midwives. Several schools were established because of the laws to regulate midwifery practice. Two of such schools to instruct the indigenous midwives in meeting the requirements for practice were the Bellevue School of Midwifery in New York City and the Preston Retreat Hospital in Philadelphia. These efforts improved the practice of midwifery and resulted in better obstetric care for mothers and babies.

During this period, nurse-midwives in European countries had proved their effectiveness and they were part of the healthcare system. The first nurse-midwives to practice in the US were British-trained nurse-midwives taken to there in 1925 by Mary Breckinridge as part of her plan to provide health care for the remote rural people in the Kentucky Mountains. Breckinridge's professional preparation as a registered nurse (RN) in the US and as a certified midwife in England suited the task she initiated and undertook. Great Britain had been the provider of midwifery education for United States registered nurses until 1939, when few schools were started in the US.

In the late 1950s and during the 1960s, nurse-midwives moved into hospitals because this was where majority of births, approximately 70% at that time were taking place. The movement of nurse-midwives into hospitals brought concepts of family-centered maternity care and a consumer advocate to childbearing women, who delivered in hospitals.

Between 1969 and 1979, several nurse-midwifery programs were established. Nurse-midwives started functioning in the full range of possible practice arenas such as clinics, federally funded programs and hospitals. Now, there are both certificate programs and higher degree programs.

In India, midwifery was practiced by traditional 'dais' without any formal training. Changes in the practice began in the early part of 20th century. The health organization in India at that time had two main branches; one was for administration of medical relief and maintenance of associated institutions and the other was for the development of preventive health services. The former was under the direction of the Director General of the Indian Medical Services at the center and Surgeon General of Civil Hospitals in the states. Preventive health services were under the direction of Public Health Commissioner at the central and Sanitation Commissioner in the States.

The British Parliament in 1921 transferred from the Central Government to the Provincial Governments, certain administrative functions, which included those relating to health, education and development of natural resources. The All India Institute of Hygiene and Public Health was established in 1930, with the aid of Rockefeller Foundation. The institution provided programs of study in maternal and child health. Maternal and infant deaths were high in all parts of the country. In 1943, the government appointed a committee called the Bhore Committee, to survey the existing health conditions and to formulate a comprehensive plan for health administration. It suggested a short-term plan and a long-term plan. The short-term plan suggested the formation of primary health centers to serve a population of about 40,000. The staff of each unit included among other members, one institutional nurse, four midwives and four trained dais. Programs for training dais and auxiliary nurse midwives (ANMs) were started based on this report.

Training programs for nurses were mainly in the mission hospitals. One of the early institutions that had nurses' training programs was the Christian Medical College Hospital, Vellore in Tamil Nadu. Nursing Superintendents of Mission Hospitals felt the need for an organization of their own by 1911. In 1931, a formal association of nurses called the Nurses Auxiliary of the Christian Medical Association of India (CMAI) was formed. The CMAI, which was registered as a non-profit charitable organization in 1926, named the Nurses' Auxiliary as Nurses League in 1964, which had two Boards of Nursing Education; the Mid India Board of Nursing Education and the Board of Nursing Education, South India Branch. Through their affiliation to the nursing schools attached to Mission Hospitals, the Boards regulated nursing education, conducted examinations and issued diplomas and certificates to those who successfully completed the general nursing and midwifery (GNM) and the auxiliary nurse midwife (ANM) programs.

With the initiative of Nursing Administration of Mission Hospitals, the Indian Nursing Council was constituted in 1949. The Indian Nursing Council formulated standards for nursing education in the country. During the last five decades, nursing education has grown and advanced. Midwifery training is incorporated into the 3 years basic general nursing program leading to diploma in nursing and midwifery. Auxiliary nurse-midwives program of 2 years leading to ANM certificate and the multipurpose health workers (MHWs) program of 18 months with midwifery training are offered in different states. Graduate programs and postgraduate specialization in maternity nursing are available in several nursing colleges. Education and practice in institutions approved by the State Nursing Council and the Indian Nursing Council followed by registration with the State Nursing Council are mandatory for practicing nursing and midwifery.

CURRENT TRENDS

Since our mothers' and grandmothers' days, enormous changes have taken place in the delivery of nursing care to the mother and the newborn. In their days, most babies were delivered at home by an untrained woman, neighbor, relative or friend or for the fortunate few by a physician or trained midwife. Surround by loved ones with her newborn brought promptly to her bed; the new mother received the attention and support of her family.

All that started changing in the second half of 20th century when parturition moved into the hospital setting. Within the 'maternity ward', priority was often given to the institution's procedures and practices, relegating the personal needs of the mother and her newborn to second place. At that point, childbearing became far from a family affair. The mother and newborn remained isolated from the family for a week to 10 days when the family had only visiting privileges. The infant separated from its mother was placed in a newborn nursery and brought to its mother only at specified times. Nursing was separated into three subspecialties; with one nurse caring for the mother during labor and delivery, another handling postpartum mothers and a third caring for the baby in the nursery.

By 1940s, the 'rooming in' concept was devised. Full-term infants were placed in a crib at their mothers' bedsides, where the mothers provided their care. Nursing care remained fragmented with the nursery nurse responsible for infant care and postpartum nurse attending to the mother. The advantages of the system included a reduction in neonatal infection from cross contamination, increased confidence and independence for the mother and greater breastfeeding success. The infant showed better weight gain and cried less. However, the downside was that the new mother evidence problems in accepting full responsibility for the baby's care.

It has been established that the new mothers experience three psychological phases such as taking-in, taking-hold and letting-go. During taking-in, new mothers are passive and dependent, requiring rest and supportive nursing care to promote bonding and attachment. With rooming-in, the mother lacked that supportive care. In taking-hold phase, where the mother is ready to learn mothering skills, had been hoisted upon her too soon. Moreover, the letting-go phase, wherein she establishes maternal role patterns and incorporates those changes into her personal and family life was almost much neglected.

In the 1960s, the focus changed from the person giving care to the recipient of that care. With that change, terminology and obstetrical care became maternity care. The broadened scope includes both prenatal and postnatal care and promotes the health and well-being of the mother, the newborn and the entire family.

The World Health Organization (WHO) offers this definition of maternity care—"The object of maternity care is to ensure that every expectant and nursing mother maintains good health, learns the art of childcare, has a normal delivery and bears healthy children. Maternity care in the narrower sense consists of the care of the pregnant woman, her safe delivery, her postnatal examination and the care of her newly born infant, and the maintenance of lactation. In the wider sense, it begins much earlier in measures aimed to promote the health and well-being of the young people who are potential parents and to help them develop the right approach to family life and to the place of family in the community. It should also include guidance to parentcraft and in problems associated with infertility and family planning."

Changing Patterns of Childbirth and their Effects on Maternal-infant Mortality Statistics

Increasing number of working women defers motherhood until they are in their 30s. As early marriage practices continue, teenage pregnancies continue to occur. At both ends of the spectrum, the older and the younger mothers face increased risks of complications during pregnancy such as preterm delivery, low-birth-weight babies; maternal, fetal neonatal and postnatal mortality.

In addition, women in increasing numbers are working outside the home during pregnancy and shortly after delivery compounding the risks to themselves and the fetus of exposure to toxic chemicals, excessive noise and other workplace stress.

Perinatal Risk Factors

The problems of society are reflected in the risks to today's neonates. Among them are acquired immunodeficiency syndrome (AIDS) in mothers and newborns and birth defects resulting from sexually transmitted diseases (STD). Low-birth-weight babies account for about 30–40% of live births in developing countries. Preterm babies constitute two-thirds of the low-birth-weight babies. In addition to maternal age, risk factors of low-birth-weight infants include the mother's medical history during past pregnancies, socioeconomic status, education level and the presence or absence of prenatal care. STD can result in infant death or in a baby born with pneumonia, cerebral palsy, epilepsy, deafness, blindness or mental retardation.

Technological Advances

Advances in technology have revolutionized the diagnosis and treatment of many health conditions. Increasingly sophisticated computers have made swifter diagnosis and continuous monitoring possible. Among those with the greatest effect on maternal and newborn nursing are the instruments available for fetal monitoring and care given by highly specialized professionals in the neonatal intensive care unit (NICU). Because of these advances, it became necessary for nursing personnel to become thorough in the procedures and protocols developed for the use of these advanced equipment and treatment. Although there is concern that the technological advances discourage the 'hands-on care' of the client, the nursing process must remain the foundation of quality nursing care.

Fetal monitoring has progressed from the use of the fetoscope to electronic fetal monitors (EFM), which allow for observation of the baby's heartbeat during pregnancy and throughout labor, even during contractions. 'Indirect' methods of EFM include ultrasound, phonocardiography and abdominal fetal electrocardiography. 'Direct' (internal) fetal monitoring used during labor and delivery is done with a spiral electrode attached to the baby's scalp. The strength of labor contractions can now be measured by means of an internally placed catheter attached to a monitor. Telemetry using radio transmission now makes it possible to monitor contractions and fetal heartbeat even when the mother is not in the same room as the monitor. This new development allows for more comfort mobility during labor. Experts predict that in the coming years births that are even more normal would utilize 'hi-tech' innovations with the result of lowering perinatal mortality and morbidity. Risk assessment and genetic counseling may begin well-before pregnancy. Risk situations may be monitored on a 24-hours basis for more active obstetric management. Fetal assessment tools will become more sophisticated and new corrective techniques will become increasingly available including in utero surgical correction and medical management of defects, direct fetal blood transfusion and drug injection and genetic diagnosis. The challenges for nurses will be enormous as they will have to provide humanistic, family-oriented care in a world of high technology.

Current Problems

Decreased Length of Hospital Stay

Our grandmothers' endured a 'confinement' of 2 weeks following childbirth. By the time our mothers' had their babies, the average postpartum hospital stay had declined to 1 week. As health care becomes increasingly ambulatory-dominant, today's new mother is up and out of the hospital or health center in 2 or 3 days.

Early discharge poses a challenge to the nurse, who must provide nursing interventions during a brief time frame and disseminate information, reinforce learning and affirm the mother's role in hours rather than days. Since, early discharge often preludes extensive patient teaching, the nurse will have to become adapt in individualizing teaching based on the unique needs of each patient.

Higher Patient Acuities

Multiple socioeconomic problems coupled with lack of knowledge about prenatal care have contributed to increasing number of women who have neglected their health during pregnancy. Many have anemia, hypertension, chronic diseases and STDs. Large numbers go into premature labor, delivering at risk low-birth-weight babies.

Lack of Facilities in the Rural Areas

About 30% of all births in India are conducted by trained dais (birth attendants), who lack scientific education. Most of the villages in India still have the traditional dais (untrained birth attendants) to help with deliveries. This results in lack of detection of prenatal problems early enough for adequate management, lack of facilities to deal with childbirth complications and inadequate reporting of morbidity.

Changes in Maternal Newborn Nursing

Social, economic, political and technological factors have contributed to the many changes that have occurred in maternal-newborn nursing within recent years. The focus is now on childbirth as a familial process with less technical interference, greater humanism and a reaffirmation of the natural birth process. In addition, recognition of the importance of mother-baby bonding in the 1st hours and days of the newborn's life has led to the encouragement of maximal mother-infant contact.

Family-centered Care

Based on the philosophy that health includes physical, social, economic and psychological dimensions. The family-centered approach assumes that family is the basic unit of society and should be viewed as a total unit with consideration given to each member. Thus, in family-centered care, the emphasis is on the delivery of professional health care that fosters family unity, while maintaining the physical safety of the childbearing unit—the mother, father and the infant. The nurse attends, educates and counsels all age groups. Integration and bonding take high priority and much anticipatory counseling is offered. In family-centered care, the nursery and postpartum staffs are combined to form one mother-baby unit.

Labor, Delivery, Recovery and Postpartum Care

Labor, delivery, recovery and postpartum care (LDRP) also called single room maternity care, was devised as a replacement for traditional maternity unit. In it, the woman labors, delivers and recovers in the same room, in the same bed and in most cases, the baby remains with the mother during her stay. The LDRP physical setup is generally circular with single birthing rooms surrounding a central area that contains all the equipment necessary for routine or emergency care. From the time of mother's admission until her discharge, a primary care nurse is assigned to the family. The LDRP system has the advantage of providing comprehensive medical care within a single setting, in more home-like environment, while maintaining all the advantages of hospitalization.

Mother-baby Couplet Care

Couplet care also known as dyad care is a system in which one-nurse cares for the postpartum mother and her newborn as single unit. It focuses and adapts to both the physical and psychosocial needs of the mother, the family and the neonate and fosters family unity, while providing a secure environment in which nurses are available for consultation, reinforcement and individual education. Nurses help both parents to assume responsibility for their baby's care and assess the family's adaptation and attachment. This system facilitates parental infant attachment, neonatal transition, lactation and involution, while supporting the taking-in and taking-hold phases of the postpartum period.

STUDY QUESTIONS

Short Answer Questions

1. Plan of health administration recommended by Bhore Committee in 1943.
2. Nursing courses incorporating midwifery training in India.
3. Rooming-in concept of newborn care.
4. Mother-baby couplet care.

BIBLIOGRAPHY

1. Bennett VR, Brown LK. Myles Textbook for Midwives, 13th edition. Edinburgh: Churchill Livingstone; 1999. pp. 49-56.
2. Cohen S Kenner, Hollingsworth AO. Maternal, Neonatal and Women's Health Nursing, 1st edition. Philadelphia: Springhouse Corporation; 1991.
3. Comeron J. The History and Development of Midwifery in the United States: Can Maternity Nursing Meet Today's Challenge? 1st edition. Columbus: Ohio: Ross Laboratories; 1967.
4. May K, Mahlmeister L. Maternal and Neonatal Nursing, 3rd edition. Philadelphia: JB Lippincott; 1994. pp. 84-126.
5. McKenzie CAM, Vestal KW. High-risk Perinatal Nursing, 1st edition. Philadelphia: WB Saunders; 1983.
6. Parulekar SV. Textbook for Midwives, 2nd edition. Mumbai: Vora Medical Publications; 1995. pp. 6-15.
7. Styles MM. Challenges for nursing in this new decade. MCN. The American Journal of Maternal Child Nursing. 1990;15(6):347-8, 350, 352.

CHAPTER 3

Midwife: Definition of the Term, Roles and Responsibilities

Learning Objectives

Upon completing this chapter, the learner will be able to:
- Describe the term 'midwife' and list her activities.
- Enumerate the skills and the responsibilities of a midwife.

The role of a midwife whether she practices in hospitals, health centers or domiciliary conditions has been recognized as one of the most rewarding jobs. Her functions carry great responsibilities and demands specific knowledge and skills.

DEFINITION

The International Confederation of Midwives (ICM) developed a definition of the term 'midwife' in 1972. The International Federation of Gynecology and Obstetrics (IFGO) and World Health Organization (WHO) adopted it in 1973. It was later amended and ratified by WHO in 1992. The international definition of a midwife and her sphere of practice are given here.

A midwife is a person, who having been regularly admitted to a midwifery educational program fully recognized in the country in which it is located, has successfully completed the prescribed course of studies in midwifery and has acquired the requisite qualifications to be registered and/or legally licensed to practice midwifery.

She must be able to give necessary supervision, care and advice to women during pregnancy, labor and postpartum period, to conduct deliveries on her own responsibility and to care for the newborn and the infant. The care includes preventive measures, the detection of abnormal conditions in mother and child, the procurement of medical assistance and the execution of emergency measures in the absence of medical help.

She has an important task in counseling and education, not only for patients but also within the family and community. The work should involve antenatal education and preparation for parenthood and extends to certain areas of gynecology, family planning and childcare. She may practice in hospitals, clinics, health units, domiciliary conditions or any other service.

Midwifery education and practice go beyond the scope of practice outlined in the definition in the European Union and the United States of America. The European Directives of 1994 outlines that the member states should ensure the midwives are at least entitled to take up and pursue the following activities:

- To provide sound family planning information and advice.
- To diagnose pregnancies and monitor normal pregnancies; to carryout examinations necessary for the monitoring of the development of normal pregnancies.
- To prescribe or advice on the examinations necessary for the earliest possible diagnosis of pregnancies at risk.
- To provide a program of parenthood preparation and a complete preparation for childbirth including advice on hygiene and nutrition.
- To care for and assist the mother during labor and to monitor the condition of the fetus in utero by appropriate clinical and technical means.
- To conduct spontaneous deliveries including where required an episiotomy and in urgent cases of breech delivery.
- To recognize the warning signs of abnormality in the mother or infant, which necessitate referral to a doctor and to assist the later where appropriate to take the necessary emergency measures in the doctor's absence, in particular, the manual removal of placenta, possibly followed by manual examination of the uterus.
- To examine and care for the newborn infant to take all initiatives, which are necessary in case of need and to carry out necessary, immediate resuscitation.
- To care for and monitor the progress of the mother in the postnatal period and to give all necessary advice to the mother on infant care to enable her to ensure the optimum progress of the newborn infant.
- To carry out the treatment prescribed by a doctor.
- To maintain all necessary records.

Nurse-midwives in the United States (US) taught a wide range of matters covering the following topics:
- Normal obstetrics, gynecology and neonatal pediatrics and their medical management.

- Knowledge, skills and judgment for the facilitation of natural process and non-intervention in these normal processes, unless indicated.
- Beliefs in continuity of care.
- Beliefs and knowledge in the promotion and implementation of family-centered maternity care.
- Beliefs, knowledge and skills in educating patients for knowledgeable participation and decision-making in their health care, and for experiencing of their bodily processes.

Midwifery also encompasses the primary focus of medicine on the diagnosis and treatment of a condition as it pertains to the essentially normal woman and neonate. Thus, nurse-midwifery is comprised of education in two disciplines that also incorporate components of a third discipline medicine. In practice, nurse-midwifery encompasses all of midwifery plus components from both nursing and medicine. Thus, it is not totally nursing or not totally midwifery, or not totally medicine. It is a unique profession in its own right and the nurse-midwife a unique professional.

DEVELOPMENT OF MIDWIFERY EDUCATION IN INDIA

India with its vast population distributed in urban and rural areas, has health problems and management problems, which are different from those in European countries or the US. In order to meet the needs of the people with varying living and economic conditions, the Government of India implemented midwifery programs of different levels. 'Dais' (untrained birth attendants) were given training to perform domiciliary midwifery. Through the rural health administration plan, their services were organized and supervised.

Another level of midwifery training was the Auxiliary Nurse Midwives (ANMs) program of 2 years. Auxiliary Nurse Midwives requires registration to practice and they function in Primary Health Centers, District Hospitals and even in certain tertiary level hospitals with supervision. General nursing program of 3 years duration includes midwifery education and practice. The graduates are registered/licensed as nurse-midwives (RN, RM) and practice in hospitals and community setups. The graduate program in nursing of 4 years duration also includes midwifery and they are registered as RN, RM by the State Registration Councils. Training programs throughout the country is regulated by the Indian Nursing Council, which prescribes the syllabus for education and training.

Textbooks written by British and American authors or physician authors are used mainly for teaching in the different programs of midwifery in undergraduate, graduate, postgraduate education. For Indian midwives, there are specific written directives for practice at the State Registration Council level and the Directives of the European Union United Kingdom Central Council [(UKCC), 1994] are used as guidelines with additional policies at the institutional level.

Skills of the Midwife

A midwife takes responsibility for her own actions, but also may initiate care by others and is able to function in a multiprofessional team. She must function within the regulations governing the profession and maintain her knowledge and skills up-to-date.

She teaches parents about healthy living both before and after the birth of the baby. The midwife must be competent to diagnose pregnancy and to carry out examinations of the woman, and the baby in order to assess their condition. The midwife is an expert in normal midwifery and in caring for the mother and newborn.

When faced with emergencies, she summons medical aid and also takes immediate steps to treat mother or baby, and continues to give care, while help is on the way. The obstetrician or the physician in-charge will be called upon to give aid when deviations from normal arise. In appropriate situations, she will utilize the assistance of neonatologists, dietitians, physiotherapists and social workers.

She is duty-bound to administer intelligently, care and treatment prescribed by obstetricians or physicians. The midwife will use her listening skills and allow her clients to voice their concern and feelings. She functions cooperatively with the multiprofessional team, which exists to care for mothers, babies and their families.

Responsibilities of the Midwife

Every midwife has a responsibility to maintain professional competence. As midwifery practice develops, she need to integrate new skills into the range of her functions. Some of these may be specific to midwives practicing in certain settings. Midwives are to keep clear, detailed records of all relevant care activities and events as required in the institution. Records must be written in an acceptable manner as they will be preserved for years for different purposes.

Midwives today ought to be able to carry out a problem-solving process in rendering care to mothers and babies. The nursing process methodology followed for the care of medical, surgical or pediatric client's needs to be implemented in maternal and newborn care as well. The process of management is elaborated in Chapter 4: Nursing Process in Meternal-Newborn Care.

STUDY QUESTIONS

Short Notes

1. Define the term midwife and list the nursing care activities that can be performed by a practicing midwife.
2. Enumerate the responsibilities of a midwife.

BIBLIOGRAPHY

1. Bennett VR, Brown LK. Myles Textbook for Midwives, 13th edition. Churchill Livingstone; 1999. pp. 3-11.
2. International Confederation of Nurse Midwives, Definition of the Midwife, ICM, London; 1992.
3. Megelen MC, Burst HV. Nurse-midwives make a difference. Nursing Outlook. 1974;22(6):386-9.
4. United Kingdom Central Council for Nursing, Midwifery and Health Visiting. The Midwife's Code of Practice, UKCC, London; 1994.
5. Warwick C. Leadership in midwifery care. British Journal of Midwives. 1996;4(5):229.

CHAPTER 4
Nursing Process in Maternal-Newborn Care

Learning Objectives

Upon completing this chapter, the learner will be able to:
- Describe the rationale for using the nursing process in mother-baby care.
- Describe the five phases of the nursing process.
- Identify appropriate nursing diagnoses for maternal newborn clients in various stages of childbearing and child-rearing experience.
- Formulate correct diagnostic statement for care of clients
- Prepare comprehensive care plans for mother and newborns.

The foundation for the practice of nursing depends upon the utilization of the nursing process in all aspects of patient care. The nursing process provides an organized and comprehensive framework for directing nursing activities. It is based on the scientific method for problem solving and follows a logical sequence, which makes it most useful to students in learning the management of care of clients. As it provides a mean of putting together isolated pieces of information, findings, judgments and skills into a meaningful whole as they perform their role of patient management, it becomes a patient-centered approach.

The term 'nursing process' was originated in 1955 by Hall and later used by Johnson (1959), Orlando (1961) and Weidenbach (1963). The purpose of the nursing process is to identify a client's health status, his/her actual or potential healthcare problems or needs to establish plans to meet the identified needs and to deliver specific nursing interventions to meet these needs. The client may be an individual, a family or a group. The use of nursing process in clinical practice gained additional legitimacy in 1973, when it was included in the American Nurses Association (ANA), *Standards of Clinical Nursing Practice*. The standards of care include the five phases of nursing process such as *assessment, diagnosis, planning, implementation* and *evaluation*. The different phases of nursing process are closely interrelated and each phase affects the others. For example, if inadequate data are obtained during assessing, the nursing diagnosis will be incomplete or incorrect and the inaccuracy will also be reflected in the planning, implementing and evaluating phases.

The nursing process is a systematic, rational method of planning and providing nursing care. The nursing process is cyclical, i.e. its components follow a logical sequence and more than one component may be involved at one time. At the end of the cycle, care may be terminated, if goals are achieved or the cycle may continue with reassessment, or the plan of care may be modified.

FIVE PHASES OF NURSING PROCESS

ASSESSMENT

Assessing is the systematic and continuous collection, organization, validation and documentation of data/information for the purpose of establishing a *database* about the client's responses to health concerns or illness and the ability to manage healthcare needs. In effect, assessing is a continuous process, carried out during all phases of the nursing process. For example, in the evaluation phase, assessment is done to determine the outcomes of the nursing strategies and to evaluate goal achievement.

There are four types of assessments: Initial assessment, problem-focused assessment, emergency assessment and time-lapsed assessment. Assessments vary according to their purpose, time available and client status:

1. *Initial assessment* is performed within specified time after admission to a healthcare agency, such as the admission assessment. The purpose is to establish a complete database for problem identification, reference and future comparison.
2. *Problem-focused assessment* is an ongoing process integrated with nursing care. It is done to determine the status of a specific problem identified in an earlier

assessment and to identify new or overlooked problems. An example for this would be the assessment of a client's ability to perform self-care, while assisting him to bathe.
3. *Emergency assessment* is done during any physiological or psychological crisis of the client. The purpose is to identify life-threatening problems. For example, rapid assessment of a person's airway, breathing status and circulation during a cardiac arrest or assessment of suicidal tendencies, or potential for violence in a psychiatric patient.
4. *Time-lapsed assessment* is done several months after initial assessment. The purpose is to compare the client's current status to baseline data previously obtained. Reassessment of a client's functional health patterns in a home care or outpatient setting, or in hospital at shift change are examples of time-lapsed assessment.

Collecting Data

Data collection is the process of gathering information about a client's health status. It must be both systematic and continuous to prevent the omission of significant data and reflect a client's changing status.

Database

Database is all the information about a client; it includes the nursing health history, physical assessment, the physician's health history and physical examination, results of laboratory and diagnostic tests and material contributed by other health personnel.

Client data should include past history as well as current problems. For example, a history of an allergic reaction to penicillin and chronic diseases are important historical data. Current data relate to present circumstances such as pain, nausea and sleep patterns.

Types of Data

Data can be subjective or objective.

Subjective data are also referred to as symptoms or *covert data*. These are apparent only to the person affected and can be reported or described only by that person or client. Pain, anxiety and fear are examples of subjective data. Client's sensation, feelings, values, beliefs, attitudes and perceptions of health status are all subjective data.

Objective data are referred to as signs or overt data, which are detectable by an observer or can be measured or tested against an acceptable standard. This can be seen, heard, felt or smelled and they are obtained by observation or physical examination. For example, a discoloration of the skin or a blood pressure reading is objective data. During physical examination, the nurse obtains objective data to validate subjective data and to complete the assessment phase of the nursing process.

A complete database of both subjective and objective data provides a baseline for comparing the client's responses to nursing and medical interventions.

Sources of Data

Sources of data are primary and secondary. The client is the primary source of data. Family members other support persons, health professionals, records, reports, laboratory and diagnostic analyses and relevant literature are secondary sources.

The best source of data is usually the client, unless *the client* is too ill, young or confused to communicate clearly. The client can provide subjective data that no one else can offer. Family members, friends and caregivers who know the client well often can supplement or verify information provided by the client. Supporting people are especially important source of data for a client, who is very young, unconscious or confused.

Client records serve as good source of data. They contain data regarding the client's occupation, religion and marital status. Type of client records includes medical records, records of therapies and laboratory records. Medical records are often a source of a client's present and past health and illness patterns. These records can provide nurses with information about the client's coping behaviors, health practices, previous illnesses and allergies.

Records of therapies provided by other health professionals such as social workers, nutritionists, dietitians or physical therapists help the nurse obtain relevant data not expressed by the client.

Laboratory records also provide pertinent health information. For example, the determination of blood glucose level allows health professionals to monitor the administration of hypoglycemic agents.

Reports from other healthcare professionals serve as other potential sources of information about a client's health. Nurses, social workers, physicians and physiotherapists may have information from either previous or current contact with the client. Both verbal and written reports of healthcare professionals add to data regarding client.

Review of nursing and related literature such as professional journals and reference texts can provide additional information for the database.

Data Collection Methods

The methods used to collect data are observing, interviewing and examining. Observation occurs whenever the nurse is in contact with the client or support persons. Interviewing is used mainly while taking the nursing health history. Examining is the major method used in the physical health assessment. In reality, the nurse uses all three methods simultaneously when assessing clients. For example, during the client interview the nurse observes, listens, asks questions and mentally retains information to explore in the physical examination.

Observing

To observe is to gather data by using the senses. Observation is a conscious, deliberate skill that is developed through effort and through an organized approach.

Although nurses observe mainly through sight, most of the senses are engaged during careful observations.

Observation has two aspects:
1. Noticing data.
2. Selecting, organizing and interpreting the data.

A nurse who observes that a client's face is flushed must relate that observation, for example, body temperature, activity, environmental temperature and blood pressure. Nursing observations must be organized so that nothing significant is missed.

Interviewing

An interview is a planned communication or a conversation with a purpose. There are two approaches to interviewing such as *directive* and *nondirective*. The directive interview is highly structured and elicits specific information. The nurse establishes the purpose of the interview and controls the interview at least at the outset. The client responds to questions, but may have limited opportunity to ask questions or discuss concerns. Nurses frequently use directive interview in emergency situations.

During a *non-directive interview* or rapport building interview by contrast, the nurse allows the client to control the purpose, subject matter and pacing. Rapport is an understanding between two or more people. A combination of directive and non-directive approach is usually appropriate during the information gathering interview.

Examining

The physical examination or physical assessment is a systematic data collection method that uses observation (i.e. the sense of sight, hearing, smell and touch) to detect health problems. To conduct the examination, the nurse uses techniques of inspection auscultation, palpation and percussion. Alternatively, the nurse may perform a screening examination. *A screening examination* also called *review of systems,* is a brief review of essential functioning of various body parts or systems. An example of a screening examination is the nursing admission assessment.

Validating Data

The information gathered during the assessment phase must be complete, factual and accurate because the nursing diagnosis and interventions are based on this information. Validation is the act of 'double checking' or verifying data to confirm that it is accurate and factual.

To build an accurate database, nurses must validate assumptions regarding the client's physical or emotional behavior. For example, a nurse seeing a man holding his arm to his chest might assume that he is experiencing chest pain, when in fact he has a painful hand.

Documenting Data

To complete the assessment phase, the nurse records client's data. Accurate documentation is essential and should include all data collected about the client's health status. Data are recorded in a factual manner and not interpreted by the nurse. In order to increase accuracy, the nurse records subjective data in the client's own words.

DIAGNOSIS

Diagnosing is the second phase of the nursing process. In this phase, nurses use critical thinking skills to interpret assessment data and identify client strengths and problems. Diagnosis is a pivotal step in the nursing process. All activities preceding this phase are directed toward formulating the *nursing diagnosis;* all the care planning activities following this phase are based on the nursing diagnoses.

The identification and development of nursing diagnoses began formally in 1973, when two faculty members of Saint Louis University, Kristine Gebbie and Mary Ann Lavin, perceived a need to identify nurses' roles in an ambulatory care setting. The first National Conference to identify nursing diagnoses was sponsored by the Saint Louis University School of Nursing in 1973. Subsequent national conferences occurred in 1975, 1980 and every 2 years thereafter.

International recognition came with the first Canadian Conference in Toronto in 1977 and the International Nursing Conference in May 1987 in Calgary, Alberta, Canada. In 1982, the conference group accepted the name 'North American Nursing Diagnosis Association (NANDA)', recognizing the participation and contributions of nurses in the United States and Canada.

The purpose of NANDA is to define, refine and promote taxonomy of nursing diagnostic terminology for general use by professional nurses. *Taxonomy* is a classification system or set of categories arranged on the basis of a single principle or set of principles. The group has currently approved more than 150 *nursing diagnosis labels* for clinical use.

Definition

The term *diagnosing* refers to the reasoning process, whereas the term *diagnosis* is a statement or conclusion regarding the nature of a phenomenon. The standardized NANDA names for the diagnoses are called *diagnostic labels* and the client's problem statement, consisting the diagnostic label plus etiology (causal relationship between a problem and its related or risk factors) is called *nursing diagnosis.*

In 1990, NANDA adopted an official working definition of nursing diagnosis "a clinical judgment about individual, family or community responses to actual and potential health problems or life processes. Nursing diagnosis provides the basis for selection of nursing interventions to achieve outcomes for which the nurse is accountable." This definition implies the following:

1. Professional nurses (registered nurses) are responsible for making nursing diagnoses, even though other nursing personnel may contribute data to the process of diagnosing and may implement specified nursing care. Nurses are accountable for this phase of the nursing process.
2. The domain of nursing diagnosis includes only those health states that nurses are educated and licensed to treat.

3. A nursing diagnosis is a judgment made only after thorough systematic data collection.
4. Nursing diagnoses describe a continuum of health states deviations from health, presence of risk factors and areas of enhanced personal growth **(Box 4.1)**.

Types of Nursing Diagnoses

The five types of nursing diagnoses are *actual, risk, wellness, possible* and *syndrome*:
1. *An actual diagnosis* is a client problem that is present at the time of the nursing assessment. Examples are *ineffective breathing pattern* and *pain*. An actual nursing diagnosis is based on the presence of associated signs and symptoms.
2. *A risk nursing diagnosis* is a clinical judgment that a problem does not exist, but the presence of *risk factors* indicates that a problem is likely to develop unless nurses intervene. For example, a client with diabetes or a compromised immune system is at *high risk* for infection than others. Therefore, the nurse would appropriately use the label *risk for* infection to describe the client's health status.
3. *A wellness diagnosis* describes human responses to levels of wellness in an individual, family or community that

BOX 4.1: The complete list of NANDA nursing diagnosis for 2018-2020 with 12 new diagnoses.

Domain 1: Health promotion
- Decreased diversional activity engagement (Nursing care plan)
- Readiness for enhanced health literacy
- Sedentary lifestyle (Nursing care plan)
- Frail elderly syndrome (Nursing care plan)
- Risk for frail elderly syndrome
- Deficient community health
- Risk-prone health behavior
- Ineffective health maintenance (Nursing care plan)
- Ineffective health management
- Readiness for enhanced health management
- Ineffective family health management
- Ineffective protection

Domain 2: Nutrition
- Imbalanced nutrition: Less than body requirements (Nursing care plan)
- Readiness for enhanced nutrition
- Insufficient breast milk production
- Ineffective breastfeeding (Nursing care plan)
- Interrupted breastfeeding (Nursing care plan)
- Readiness for enhanced breastfeeding
- Ineffective adolescent eating dynamics
- Ineffective child eating dynamics
- Ineffective infant feeding dynamics
- Ineffective infant feeding pattern (Nursing care plan)
- Obesity
- Overweight
- Risk for overweight
- Impaired swallowing (Nursing care plan)
- Risk for unstable blood glucose level (Nursing care plan)
- Neonatal hyperbilirubinemia

Contd...

Contd...
- Risk for neonatal hyperbilirubinemia
- Risk for impaired liver function
- Risk for metabolic imbalance syndrome
- Risk for electrolyte imbalance
- Risk for imbalanced fluid volume
- Deficient fluid volume (Nursing care Plan)
- Risk for deficient fluid volume
- Excess fluid volume (Nursing care Plan)

Domain 3: Elimination and exchange
- Impaired urinary elimination
- Functional urinary incontinence
- Overflow urinary incontinence
- Reflex urinary incontinence
- Stress urinary incontinence
- Urge urinary incontinence
- Risk for urge urinary incontinence
- Urinary retention
- Constipation (Nursing care Plan)
- Risk for constipation
- Perceived constipation
- Chronic functional constipation
- Risk for chronic functional constipation
- Diarrhea
- Dysfunctional gastrointestinal motility
- Risk for dysfunctional gastrointestinal motility
- Bowel incontinence
- Respiratory function
- Impaired gas exchange

Domain 4: Activity/Rest
- Insomnia
- Sleep deprivation
- Readiness for enhanced sleep
- Disturbed sleep pattern
- Risk for disuse syndrome
- Impaired bed mobility
- Impaired physical mobility
- Impaired wheelchair mobility
- Impaired sitting
- Impaired standing
- Impaired transferability
- Impaired walking
- Imbalanced energy field
- Fatigue
- Wandering
- Activity intolerance
- Risk for activity intolerance
- Ineffective breathing pattern
- Decreased cardiac output
- Risk for decreased cardiac output
- Impaired spontaneous ventilation
- Risk for unstable blood pressure
- Risk for decreased cardiac tissue perfusion
- Risk for ineffective cerebral tissue perfusion
- Ineffective peripheral tissue perfusion
- Risk for ineffective peripheral tissue perfusion
- Dysfunctional ventilatory weaning response
- Impaired home maintenance
- Bathing self-care deficit
- Dressing self-care deficit

Contd...

Contd...

- Feeding self-care deficit
- Toileting self-care deficit
- Readiness for enhanced self-care
- Self-neglect

Domain 5: Perception/Cognition
- Unilateral neglect
- Acute confusion
- Risk for acute confusion
- Chronic confusion
- Labile emotional control
- Ineffective impulse control
- Deficient knowledge
- Readiness for enhanced knowledge
- Impaired memory
- Readiness for enhanced communication
- Impaired verbal communication

Domain 6: Self-perception
- Hopelessness
- Readiness for enhanced hope
- Risk for compromised human dignity
- Disturbed personal identity
- Risk for disturbed personal identity
- Readiness for enhanced self-concept
- Chronic low self-esteem
- Risk for chronic low self-esteem
- Situational low self-esteem
- Risk for situational low self-esteem
- Disturbed body image

Domain 7: Role relationships
- Caregiver role strain
- Risk for caregiver role strain
- Impaired parenting
- Risk for impaired parenting
- Readiness for enhanced parenting
- Risk for impaired attachment
- Dysfunctional family processes
- Interrupted family processes
- Readiness for enhanced family processes
- Ineffective relationship
- Risk for ineffective relationship
- Readiness for enhanced relationship
- Parental role conflict
- Ineffective role performance
- Impaired social interaction

Domain 8: Sexuality
- Sexual dysfunction
- Ineffective sexuality pattern
- Ineffective childbearing process
- Risk for ineffective childbearing process
- Readiness for enhanced childbearing process
- Risk for disturbed maternal-fetal dyad

Domain 9: Coping/Stress tolerance
- Risk for complicated immigration transition
- Post-trauma syndrome
- Risk for post-trauma syndrome

Contd...

- Rape-trauma syndrome
- Relocation stress syndrome
- Risk for relocation stress syndrome
- Ineffective activity planning
- Risk for ineffective activity planning
- Anxiety (Nursing care plan)
- Defensive coping
- Ineffective coping
- Readiness for enhanced coping
- Ineffective community coping
- Readiness for enhanced community coping
- Compromised family coping
- Disabled family coping
- Readiness for enhanced family coping
- Death anxiety
- Ineffective denial
- Fear
- Grieving
- Complicated grieving
- Risk for complicated grieving
- Impaired mood regulation
- Powerlessness
- Risk for powerlessness
- Readiness for enhanced power
- Impaired resilience
- Risk for impaired resilience
- Readiness for enhanced resilience
- Chronic sorrow
- Stress overload
- Acute substance withdrawal syndrome
- Risk for acute substance withdrawal syndrome
- Autonomic dysreflexia
- Risk for autonomic dysreflexia
- Decreased intracranial adaptive capacity
- Neonatal abstinence syndrome
- Disorganized infant behavior
- Risk for disorganized infant behavior
- Readiness for enhanced organized infant behavior

Domain 10: Life principles
- Readiness for enhanced spiritual well-being
- Readiness for enhanced decision-making
- Decisional conflict
- Impaired emancipated decision-making
- Risk for impaired emancipated decision-making
- Readiness for enhanced emancipated decision-making
- Moral distress
- Impaired religiosity
- Risk for impaired religiosity
- Readiness for enhanced religiosity
- Spiritual distress
- Risk for spiritual distress

Domain 11: Safety/Protection
- Risk for infection
- Risk for surgical site infection
- Ineffective airway clearance
- Risk for aspiration
- Risk for bleeding (Nursing care plan)

Contd...

Contd...

- Impaired dentition
- Risk for dry eye
- Risk for dry mouth
- Risk for falls
- Risk for corneal injury
- Risk for injury
- Risk for urinary tract injury
- Risk for perioperative positioning injury
- Risk for thermal injury
- Impaired oral mucous membrane integrity
- Risk for impaired oral mucous membrane integrity
- Risk for peripheral neurovascular dysfunction
- Risk for physical trauma
- Risk for vascular trauma
- Risk for pressure ulcer
- Risk for shock
- Impaired skin integrity (Nursing care plan)
- Risk for impaired skin integrity
- Risk for sudden infant death
- Risk for suffocation
- Delayed surgical recovery
- Risk for delayed surgical recovery
- Impaired tissue integrity
- Risk for impaired tissue integrity
- Risk for venous thromboembolism
- Risk for female genital mutilation
- Risk for other-directed violence
- Risk for self-directed violence
- Self-mutilation
- Risk for self-mutilation
- Risk for suicide
- Contamination
- Risk for contamination
- Risk for occupational injury
- Risk for poisoning
- Risk for adverse reaction to iodinated contrast media
- Risk for allergy reaction
- Latex allergy reaction
- Risk for latex allergy reaction
- Hyperthermia
- Hypothermia
- Risk for hypothermia
- Risk for perioperative hypothermia
- Ineffective thermoregulation
- Risk for ineffective thermoregulation

Domain 12: Comfort
- Impaired comfort
- Readiness for enhanced comfort
- Nausea
- Acute pain
- Chronic pain
- Chronic pain syndrome
- Labor pain
- Impaired comfort
- Readiness for enhanced comfort
- Impaired comfort
- Readiness for enhanced comfort
- Risk for loneliness
- Social isolation

(*Source:* North American Nursing Diagnosis Association (NANDA), Nursing Diagnoses for 2018-2020. www.NANDA.com/nursing diagnoses).

have a readiness for enhancement. Examples of wellness diagnosis would be 'readiness for enhanced family coping' or 'readiness for enhanced spiritual well-being'.

4. *A possible nursing diagnosis* is one in which evidence about a health problem is incomplete or unclear. A possible diagnosis requires more data either to support or to refute it. For example, an elderly widow who lives alone is admitted to the hospital. The nurse notices that she has no visitors and is pleased with the attention from nursing staff. A nursing diagnosis for the client may be 'possible social isolation related to unknown etiology'.

5. *A syndrome diagnosis* is a diagnosis that is associated with a cluster of other diagnoses. Currently six syndrome diagnoses are on the NANDA international list. For example, long-term bedridden clients may experience disuse syndrome. Clusters of diagnosis associated with this syndrome include *impaired physical mobility, risk for impaired tissue integrity, risk for activity intolerance, risk for constipation, impaired gas exchange* and so on.

Nursing Diagnosis Taxonomy

Taxonomy provides a standardized language for describing the pattern of clinical judgment and is defined as a clinical judgment about the individual, family, or community responses to actual and potential health problems/life processes. Nursing Diagnosis Taxonomy list was updated on January 5, 2023 **(Box 4.2)**.

BOX 4.2: Nursing Diagnosis Taxonomy II.

Taxonomy II for nursing diagnosis contains 13 domains and 47 classes.

Domain 1: Health promotion
- Class 1: Health awareness
- Class 2: Health management

Domain 2: Nutrition
- Class 1: Ingestion
- Class 2: Digestion
- Class 3: Absorption
- Class 4: Metabolism
- Class 5: Hydration

Domain 3: Elimination and exchange
- Class 1: Urinary function
- Class 2: Gastrointestinal function
- Class 3: Integumentary function
- Class 4: Respiratory function

Domain 4: Activity/Rest
- Class 1: Sleep/Rest
- Class 2: Activity/Exercise
- Class 3: Energy balance
- Class 4: Cardiovascular/Pulmonary responses
- Class 5: Self-care

Domain 5: Perception/Cognition
- Class 1: Attention
- Class 2: Orientation

Contd...

Contd...
- Class 3: Sensation/Perception
- Class 4: Cognition
- Class 5: Communication

Domain 6: Self-perception
- Class 1: Self-concept
- Class 2: Self-esteem
- Class 3: Body image

Domain 7: Role relationship
- Class 1: Caregiving roles
- Class 2: Family relationships
- Class 3: Role performance

Domain 8: Sexuality
- Class 1: Sexual identity
- Class 2: Sexual function
- Class 3: Reproduction

Domain 9: Coping/Stress tolerance
- Class 1: Post-trauma responses
- Class 2: Coping responses
- Class 3: Neurobehavioral stress

Domain 10: Life principles
- Class 1: Values
- Class 2: Beliefs
- Class 3: Value/Belief/Action congruence

Domain 11: Safety/Protection
- Class 1: Infection
- Class 2: Physical injury
- Class 3: Violence
- Class 4: Environmental hazards
- Class 5: Defensive processes
- Class 6: Thermoregulation

Domain 12: Comfort
- Class 1: Physical comfort
- Class 2: Environmental comfort
- Class 3: Social comfort

Domain 13: Growth/Development
- Class 1: Growth
- Class 2: Development

(*Source:* NANDA Nursing Diagnosis, nurseslabs.com)

Components of a NANDA Nursing Diagnosis

A nursing diagnosis has three components:
1. The problem and its definition.
2. The etiology.
3. The defining characteristics, each component serves a specific purpose.

Problem and Definition (Diagnostic Label)

The problem statement or diagnostic label describes the client's health problem or response for which nursing therapy is given. It describes the client's health status clearly and concisely in a few words. The purpose of the diagnostic label is to direct the information of client goals and desired outcomes. It may also suggest some nursing interventions.

To be clinically useful, diagnostic labels need to be specific when the words *specify* follows a NANDA label. The nurse states the area in which the problem occurs for example, *deficient knowledge (medications)* or *deficient knowledge (dietary modifications)*.

Qualifiers

These are words that have been added to some NANDA labels to give additional meaning to the diagnostic statement. For example:
- *Deficient* (inadequate in amount, quality or degree) not sufficient; incomplete
- *Impaired* (made worse, weakened, damaged, reduced, deteriorated)
- *Decreased* (lesser in size, amount or degree)
- *Ineffective* (not producing the desired effect)
- *Compromised* (to make vulnerable or threat).

Etiology (Related Factors and Risk Factors)

The etiology component of a nursing diagnosis identifies one or more probable causes of the health problem, gives direction to the required nursing interventions and enables the nurse to individualize the client's care. For example, the probable causes of *activity intolerance* include sedentary lifestyle, generalized weakness, bedrest or immobility. Differentiating among possible causes in the nursing diagnosis is essential because each may require different nursing interventions.

Defining Characteristics

Defining characteristics are the cluster of signs and symptoms that indicate the presence of a particular diagnostic label. For *actual nursing diagnoses,* the defining characteristics are the client's *signs and symptoms.* For *risk nursing diagnoses, no subjective* and *objective* signs are present. Thus, the factors that cause the client to be more than 'normally' vulnerable to the problem form the etiology of a risk nursing diagnosis.

Differentiating Nursing Diagnoses from Medical Diagnoses

A nursing diagnosis is a statement of nursing judgment and refers to a condition that nurses are licensed to treat.

A medical diagnosis is made by physician and refers to a condition that only a physician can treat. Medical diagnoses refer to disease processes—specific pathophysiological responses that are fairly uniform from one client to another. In contrast, nursing diagnoses describe a client's physical, sociocultural, psychological and spiritual responses to an illness or a health problem.

A client's medical diagnosis remains the same for as long as the disease process is present, but nursing diagnosis changes as the client's responses change. Nurses have responsibilities related to both medical and nursing diagnoses. Nursing diagnoses relate to the nurse's *independent functions* that is, the areas of health care that are unique to nursing and separate and distinct from medical management.

Diagnostic Process

The diagnostic process uses the critical thinking skills of analysis and synthesis. Critical thinking is a cognitive process during which a person reviews data and considers explanation before forming an opinion. The diagnostic process has three steps:
1. Analyzing data.
2. Identifying health problems, risks and strengths.
3. Formulating diagnostic statement.

Formulating Diagnostic Statements

Most nursing diagnosis is written as *two parts* or *three-part statements:*
1. *Basic two-part statements include the following:*
   a. *Problem (P):* Statement of the client's response (NANDA label).
   b. *Etiology (E):* Factors contributing to or probable causes of the responses.

   The two parts are joined by the words *related* to rather than *due to*. The phrase *due to* implies that one part causes or is responsible for the other part. By contrast, the phrase *related to,* merely implies a relationship. Examples of two-part nursing diagnosis are:
   i. Constipation related to irregular defecation habits.
   ii. Ineffective breastfeeding related to breast engorgement.

   Some NANDA labels contain the word specify. For these, the nurse must add words to indicate the problem more specifically. For example, noncompliance (specify), noncompliance (diabetic diet) related to denial of having disease.

2. *Basic three-part statements:* The basic three-part nursing diagnosis statement is the **PES** *format* and includes the following:
   a. *Problem (P):* Statement of the client's response (NANDA label).
   b. *Etiology (E):* Factors contributing to or probable causes of the response.
   c. *Signs and symptoms (S):* Defining characteristics manifested by the client.

   For example:
   - Ineffective coping related to labor and delivery as evidenced by fatigue and expressed inability to cope
   - Deficient fluid volume related to postpartum hemorrhage as evidenced by decreased pulse volume and pressure.

Actual nursing diagnoses can be documented by using the three-part statement because the signs and symptoms have been identified. The format cannot be used for risk diagnoses because the client does not have signs and symptoms of the diagnosis.

In addition of using the correct format, nurses must consider the content of their diagnostic statements. The statements should for example, be accurate, concise, descriptive, and specific. The nurse must always validate the diagnostic statements with the client and compare the clients' signs and symptoms to the NANDA defining characteristics.

For risk factors, the nurse compares the client's risk factors to NANDA risk factors.

One-part statements: Some diagnostic statements such as wellness diagnosis and syndrome nursing diagnosis, consist of a NANDA label only. As the diagnostic labels are refined, they tend to become more specific, so that nursing interventions can be derived from the label itself. Therefore, an etiology may not be needed. For example, adding an etiology to the label rape-trauma syndrome does not make the label any more descriptive or useful.

The NANDA has specified that any new *wellness diagnoses* will be developed as one-part statements beginning with the words *readiness for enhanced* followed by the desired higher level wellness for example, *readiness for enhanced parenting.*

Currently, the NANDA list includes several wellness diagnoses. Some of these are *spiritual well-being, effective breastfeeding, health seeking behaviors* and *anticipatory grieving.* These are usually accepted as one-part statements, but may be made more explicit by adding a descriptor for example, *health seeking behaviors (low-fat diet)* (*refer* **Box 4.1**).

Variations of basic formats
Variations of the basic, one, two and three-part statements include the following:
- Writing the terms *unknown etiology,* when the defining characteristics are present, but the nurse does not know the cause or contributing factors. For example, *noncompliance (medication regimen) related to unknown etiology.*
- Using the phrase *complex factors,* when there are too many etiologic factors or when they are too complex to state in a brief phrase. The actual causes of chronic low self-esteem, for instance, may be long-term and complex, as in the following nursing diagnosis *chronic low self-esteem related to complex factors.*
- Using the word *possible* to describe either the problem or the etiology. When the nurse believes more data are needed about the client's problem or the etiology, the word possible is used. For example, *possible low self-esteem related to loss of job and rejection by family, and altered thought process possibly related to unfamiliar surroundings.*
- Using the word *secondary* to divide the etiology into two parts; thereby making the statement more descriptive and useful. The part following secondary to is often pathophysiologic or disease process as in *risk for impaired skin integrity related to* decreased peripheral circulation secondary to diabetes.
- Adding a secondary part to the general response or NANDA label to make it more precise. For example, the diagnosis *impaired skin integrity (left lateral ankle)* related to decreased peripheral circulation.

In writing nursing diagnosis statements, describe an individual's health status and factors that have contributed to the status. Nursing diagnoses are written as problem focused, risk diagnosis, health promotion, syndrome and possible diagnosis (**Boxes 4.3 and 4.4**).

BOX 4.3: Writing Diagnostic Statements.

Problem-focused diagnosis

(Problem/diagnostic label) + 'related to' (rt) (Related factors) + 'as evidenced by' (AEB) (Defining characteristics)

Examples of problem-focused diagnosis

- Impaired physical mobility | related to | decreased muscle control | as evidenced by | inability to control lower extremities
- Acute pain | related to | tissue ischemia | as evidenced by | Statement of 'my chest is so painful,' pain scale of 8/10

Risk diagnosis

(Risk diagnosis/diagnostic label) + 'as evidenced by' (AEB) (Risk factors)

Examples of risk diagnosis

- Risk for falls | as evidenced by | improper use of crutches
- Risk for injury | as evidenced by | altered clotting factors

Health promotion diagnosis

(Health promotion label) + 'as evidenced by' (AEB) (Defining characteristics)

Examples of health promotion diagnosis

- Readiness for enhanced family coping | as evidenced by | verbalization of desire to optimize wellness
- Readiness for enhanced nutrition | as evidenced by | patient's verbalization of desire to enhance nutrition

Syndrome diagnosis

(Syndrome diagnosis/diagnostic label)

Examples of syndrome diagnosis

- Chronic pain syndrome
- Rape-Trauma syndrome
- Disuse syndrome

Possible

'Possible' + (Diagnostic labels)

Examples of syndrome diagnosis

- Possible | Chronic low self-esteem
- Possible | Deficient knowledge
- Possible | Disturbed body image

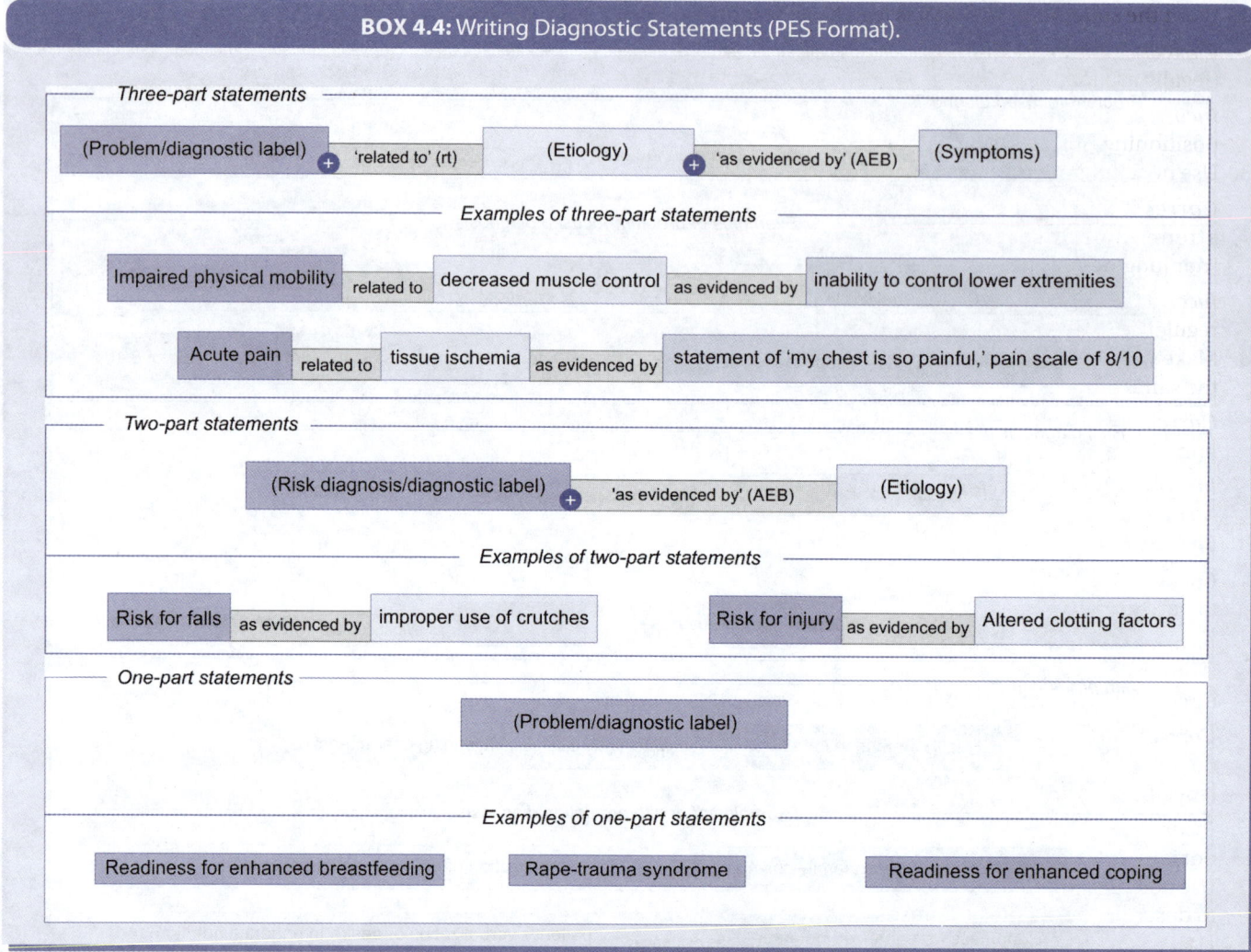

BOX 4.4: Writing Diagnostic Statements (PES Format).

Avoiding Errors in Diagnostic Reasoning

Avoiding errors is important that nurses make nursing diagnoses with a high level of accuracy. Nurses can avoid some common errors of reasoning by recognizing them and applying appropriate critical thinking skills. Errors can occur at any point in the diagnostic process, data collection, data interpretation and data clustering. The following steps help to minimize diagnostic errors:

1. *Verify*: Hypothesize possible explanations of the data, but realize that all diagnoses are tentative until they are verified. Begin and end the process by talking with the client and family. Ask them what their health problems are and what they believe the causes to be. At the end of the process have them verify your diagnoses.
2. *Build a good knowledge base and acquire clinical experience:* Nurse must apply knowledge from many different areas (applied sciences) to recognize significant cues and patterns and generate a hypothesis about the data. For example, principles from chemistry, anatomy and pharmacology each help the nurse understand client data.
3. *Have a working knowledge of what is normal*: Nurses need to know the normal physiological parameters for vital signs, laboratory tests, breath sounds and so on. In addition, she must determine what is normal for a particular person taking into accounts of his/her age, physical makeup, lifestyle and physiological changes such as pregnancy.
4. *Consult resources*: Both freshers and experienced nurses should consult appropriate resources, whenever in doubt about a diagnosis. Professional literature, nursing colleagues and nurse educators are all appropriate resources. Use of a nursing diagnosis handbook for quick reference will be useful too.
5. *Improve critical thinking skills*: These skills help the nurse to be aware of and avoid errors in thinking such as over generalizing, stereotyping and making unwarranted assumptions.

Guidelines for Writing Nursing Diagnostic Statements

1. State in terms of a problem not a need.
   Correct: Deficient fluid volume (problem) related to fever.
   Incorrect: Fluid replacement (need) related to fever.

2. Word the statement, so that it is legally acceptable.

   Correct: Impaired skin integrity related to immobility (legally acceptable).

   Incorrect: Impaired skin integrity related to improper positioning (implies legal liability).
3. Use non-judgmental statements.

   Correct: Spiritual distress related to inability to attend church services secondary to immobility (nonjudgmental).

   Incorrect: Spiritual distress related to strict rules requiring regular church attendance (judgmental).
4. Make sure that both elements of the statement do not say the same thing.

   Correct: Risk for impaired skin integrity related to immobility.

   Incorrect: Impaired skin integrity related to ulceration of sacral area (problem and probable cause are the same).
5. Be sure that problem and etiology are correctly stated.

   Correct: Pain, severe headache related to fear of addiction to narcotics.

   Incorrect: Pain related to severe headache.
6. Word the diagnosis specifically and precisely to provide direction for planning nursing interventions.

   Correct: Impaired oral mucous membrane related to decreased salivation secondary to radiation of neck (specific).

   Incorrect: Impaired oral mucous membrane related to noxious agent (vague).
7. Use nursing terminology rather than medical terminology to describe the client's response.

   Correct: Risk for ineffective airway clearance related to accumulation of secretions in lungs (nursing terminology).

   Incorrect: Risk for pneumonia (medical terminology).
8. Use nursing terminology rather than medical terminology to describe the probable cause of the client's response.

   Correct: Risk for ineffective airway clearance related to accumulation of secretions in lungs (nursing terminology).

   Incorrect: Risk for ineffective airway clearance related to emphysema (medical terminology).

Differentiating Nursing Diagnosis, Medical Diagnosis and Collaborative Problems

See **Box 4.5**.

■ PLANNING

Planning is the third phase of the nursing process in which the nurse and client develop client goals/desired outcomes and nursing interventions to prevent, reduce or alleviate the client's health problems.

> **BOX 4.5:** Nursing diagnosis, medical diagnosis, and collaborative problems.
>
> **Nursing diagnosis**
> - Ineffective airway clearance
> - Distrubed body image
> - Risk for unstable blood glucose
> - Impaired urinary elimination
> - Self-care deficit: Dressing
>
> **Medical diagnosis**
> - Pneumonia
> - Amputation
> - Type 2 diabetes mellitus
> - Postoperative prostatectomy
> - Cerebrocvascular accident
>
> **Collaborative problems**
> - Potential complication of head injury: Increased intracranial pressure
> - Potential complication of myocardial infarction: Congestive heart failure

Planning is a deliberate, systematic process that involves decision-making and problem solving. In planning, the nurse refers to the client's assessment data and diagnostic statements for direction in formulating client goals and designing the nursing interventions required to manage the client's health problems.

A *nursing intervention* is the treatment based on clinical judgment and knowledge that a nurse performs to enhance patient/client outcomes.

Although planning is basically a nurse's responsibility, input from the client and support person (family members) is essential, if a plan is to be effective. Nurses do not plan for the client, but encourage the client to participate actively to the extent possible. In a home setting, the client's family members and caregivers are the ones who implement the plan of care, thus its effectiveness depends largely on them.

Types of Planning

Planning begins with the first client contact and continues until the nurse-client relationship ends, usually when the client is discharged from the hospital.

Initial Planning

The nurse, who performs the admission assessment usually, develops the initial, plan of care. This nurse uses the client's body language as well as some intuitive kinds of information that are not solely available from written database. Planning should be initiated as soon as possible after the initial assessment.

Ongoing Planning

All nurses, who work with the client, do ongoing planning. As nurses obtain new information and evaluate the client's responses to care, they can individualize the initial care plan further. Ongoing planning also occurs at the beginning

of a shift as the nurse plans the care to be given that day/that shift. The nurse carries out the daily planning in order to:
- Determine whether the client's health status has changed
- Set priorities for the client's care during the shift
- Decide, which problems to focus on during the shift
- Coordinate nurse's activities so that more than one problem can be addressed at each client contact.

Discharge Planning

Discharge planning is the process of anticipating and planning for needs after discharge. This is a crucial part of comprehensive health care and should be addressed in each client's care plan. For patients who are discharged early, i.e. before complete recovery in such cases, care is delivered in the home. Effective discharge planning begins at first contact with client and involves comprehensive and ongoing assessment to obtain information about client's ongoing needs.

Developing Nursing Care Plans

The end product of the planning phase of the nursing process is a *formal* or *informal plan* of care.
- *An informal nursing care plan* is a strategy for action that exists in the nurse's mind. For example, the nurse may think "Mrs Ramu is very tired; I will reinforce her teaching after she is rested".
- *A formal nursing care plan* is a written or computerized guide that organizes information about the client's care. The benefit of a formal written care plan is that it provides for continuity of care.
- *A standardized care plan* is a formal plan that specifies the nursing cares for groups of clients with common needs (e.g. all clients with eclamptic fits).
- *An individualized care plan* is tailored to meet the unique needs of a specific client; those are needs that are not addressed by the standardized plan.

Nurses use the formal care plan for direction about what needs to be documented in client progress notes and as a guide for delegating and assigning staff to care for clients. *When nursing diagnoses are used to develop goals and nursing interventions, the result is a holistic, individualized plan of care that will meet the client's unique needs.*

Care plans include the actions nurses must take to address the client's nursing diagnoses and produce the desired outcome. The nurse begins the plan when the client is admitted to the hospital and constantly updates it throughout the client's stay in response to changes in the client's condition and evaluations of goal achievement.

The complete plans of care for a client is made up of several different documents are:
- Describe the routine care needed to meet basic needs such as bathing and nutrition.
- Address the client's nursing diagnoses and collaborative problems.
- Specify nursing responsibilities in carrying out the medical plan of care (e.g. scheduling laboratory tests, keeping client from eating or drinking before surgery). A complete plan of care integrates dependent and independent nursing functions.

Standardized Approaches to Care Planning

Standards of care, standardized care plans, protocols, policies and procedures are developed and accepted by nursing staff in order to ensure that minimum acceptable standards for patient care are met and to promote efficient use of nurses' time.

Standardized care plans are preprinted guides for the nursing care of a client who has a need that arises frequently in the agency (e.g. specific nursing diagnosis or all nursing diagnoses associated with a particular medical condition). They are written from the perspective of what care the client can expect.

Standardized Care Plans

- Are kept with the client's individualized care plan on the nursing unit, probably in the 'kardex'. When the client is discharged, they become part of the permanent medical record.
- Provide detailed interventions and contain additions or deletion from the standards of care of the agency.
- Are written in the nursing process format. Problem → desired outcomes/goals → nursing interventions → evaluations.

Protocols

Like standardized care plans, *protocols* are preprinted to indicate the actions commonly required for a particular group of clients. For example, a hospital may have a protocol for admitting a client to the intensive care unit, for administering magnesium sulfate to client with preeclampsia/eclampsia or for caring for a client receiving continuous epidural analgesia. Protocols may include both physician's orders and nursing interventions.

Policies and Procedures

They are developed to govern the handling of frequently occurring situations. For example, a hospital may have a policy specifying the number of visitors a patient may have. Some policies and procedures specify what is to be done for example, in the case of cardiac arrest. If a policy covers a situation pertinent to client care, it is usually entered the care plan (e.g. make social service referral according policy manual). Policies are institutional records and do not become a part of the permanent record.

Standing Order

It is a written document about policies, rules, regulations or orders regarding client care. Standing orders give nurses the authority to carry out specific actions under certain circumstances, often when a physician is not immediately available. In a hospital critical care unit, a common example is the administration of emergency antiarrhythmic medications when a client's cardiac monitoring pattern changes.

Regardless of whether care plans are handwritten, computerized or standardized, nursing care must be individualized to fit the unique needs of each client. In hospitals/healthcare settings when nursing process is followed for providing holistic care to clients, care plans usually consist of both preprinted and handwritten sections. The nurse uses standardized care plans for predictable, commonly occurring problems and handwrites an individual plan for unusual problems or problems needing special attention. For example, a standardized care plan for all 'clients with a medical diagnosis of pneumonia' would probably include a nursing diagnosis of *deficient fluid volume* and direct the nurse to assess the client's hydration status. On a respiratory or medical unit, this would be a common nursing diagnosis and the nurse may incorporate it in her care plan for the client. However, a nursing diagnosis, *risk for interrupted family process* would not be common to all patients with pneumonia, it is true only to certain clients. Therefore, the goals and nursing interventions for that diagnosis would need to be handwritten by the nurse.

Formats for Nursing Care Plan

Formats of care plan written by working nurses or practicing nurses in hospital units are often organized into four columns or categories:
1. *Nursing diagnoses.*
2. *Goals/desired outcomes.*
3. *Nursing orders interventions.*
4. *Evaluations.*

Student care plans are more lengthy and detailed as it is a learning activity as well as plan of care. They usually have an additional column for *'rationale'* after nursing orders column. To help students learn to write care plans, these are often handwritten as required by the educators. A rationale is a scientific principle given as the reason for selecting a particular nursing intervention. Students may also be required to cite supporting literature for their stated rationale.

Guidelines for Writing Nursing Care Plans

The nurse should use the following guidelines for writing care plans:
1. *Date and sign the plan:* The date and plan written is essential for evaluation. The nurse's signature demonstrates accountability to the client and to the nursing profession.
2. *Use category headings:* Different columns of the record form should have headings such as 'nursing diagnoses', 'desired outcomes/goals', 'nursing interventions' and 'evaluation', include a date for evaluation of each goal.
3. Use standardized words and symbols rather than complete sentences to communicate your ideas. For example, write 'turn and reposition q2h' rather than 'turn and reposition the client every 2 hours'.
4. *Be specific:* Write specific time or instruction for nursing interventions. For example, 'change incisional dressing q shift' may mean two dressing changes for 12-hours duty shifts and three dressing changes for 8-hours duty shifts.
5. Tailor the plan to the unique characteristics of the client by ensuring that the client's preferences and choices are considered. This reinforces the client's individuality and sense of control. For example, the written nursing intervention 'provide coffee at breakfast rather than tea' indicates that the client was given a choice for his/her breakfast drink.
6. Ensure that the nursing care plan incorporates preventive and health maintenance aspects as well as restorative ones. For example, the nursing directive 'provide active assistance for range of motion (ROM) exercises to affected limbs q2h' prevents joint contractures and maintains muscle strength and joint mobility.
7. Ensure that the plan contains interventions for ongoing assessment of the client, e.g. inspect incision q8h.
8. Include collaborative and coordination activities in the plan. For example, 'administer pain medication as indicated', arrange referral service with social worker.
9. Include plans for client's discharge and home care needs. For example, arrangements with community health nurse, social worker or specific agencies for needed equipment. Add teaching and discharge plans.
10. Refer to procedure books or other sources of information for writing selected and appropriate nursing directives.

Planning Process

The processes of developing care plans include four different activities.

Setting Priorities

Setting priorities is the process of establishing a preferential sequence for addressing nursing diagnoses and interventions. The nurse and client begin planning by deciding, which nursing diagnosis requires attention first, which is second and so on. *Life-threatening* problems such as loss of respiratory or cardiac function are designated as high priority. Health-threatening problems such as acute illness and decreased coping ability are assigned medium priority. A low-priority problem is one that arises from normal developmental needs or that requires only minimal nursing support. Nurses use Maslow's hierarchy of needs when setting priorities. In Maslow's hierarchy, physiologic needs such as air, food and water are basic to life and receive higher priority than the need for security or activity. Thus, nursing diagnoses such as *ineffective airway clearance and impaired gas exchange* would take priority over nursing diagnoses such as anxiety or ineffective coping.

It is not necessary to resolve all high-priority diagnoses before addressing others. The nurse may partially address a high-priority diagnosis and then deal with a diagnosis of lesser priority. Further, because the clients usually have several problems, the nurse often deals with more than one diagnosis at a time.

Establishing Desired Outcomes/Client Goals

After establishing priorities, the nurse and client set goals for each nursing diagnosis. The *desired outcome sentences* describe, in terms of observable client responses, what the nurse hopes to achieve by implementing the nursing interventions. The terms *desired outcomes* and *goals* are used interchangeably in this book. These are stated as specific, observable criteria and used to evaluate whether the goals have been met. For example, 'improved nutritional status as evidenced by weight gain of 5 lb by April 25'. Writing the broad general goal first, may help students to think of specific outcomes that are needed as a starting point for planning, what needs to be written on the care plan is the specific, observable, outcomes than can be used to evaluate client progress.

Purposes of Desired Outcomes/Goals

Desired outcome serve the following purposes:
- Provide direction for planning nursing interventions. Ideas for interventions come more easily, if the desired outcomes state clearly and specifically what the nurse hopes to achieve.
- Serve as criteria for judging the effectiveness of nursing interventions and client progress in the evaluation step.
- Enable the client and nurse to determine when the problem has been resolved.
- Help to motivate the client and nurse by providing a sense of achievement. As goals are met, both client and nurse can see that their efforts have been worthwhile.

Guidelines for Writing Desired Outcomes/Goals

The following guidelines can help nurses write useful goals and desired outcomes:
1. Write goals and outcomes in terms of client responses, not nurse activities. Beginning each statement with the *client, will* may help to focus the goal on client behaviors and responses. Avoid statements that start with *enable, facilitate, allow, let and permit* or similar verbs followed by the word client. These indicate what the nurse hopes to accomplish and what the client will do.
   Correct: Client will drink 100 mL of water per hour (client behavior).
   Incorrect: Maintain client hydration (nursing action).
2. Be sure that desired outcomes are realistic for the client's capabilities, limitations and designated time span, if it is indicated. Limitations refer to finances, equipment, family support, physical and mental condition and time. For example, the outcome measures insulin accurately may be unrealistic for a client who has poor vision due to cataract.
3. Ensure that the desired outcomes are compatible with the therapies of other professionals. For example, the outcome will increase the time spent out of bed by 15 minutes each day is not compatible with a physician's prescribed therapy of bedrest.
4. Use observable, measurable terms for outcomes. Avoid words that are vague and require interpretation or judgment by observer. For example, phrases such as *increase daily exercise* and *improve knowledge of nutrition* can mean differently to different people. These are not sufficiently clear and specific to guide the nurse when evaluating client responses.
5. Make sure that the client considers the desired outcomes important and values them. Some outcomes such as those problems related to self-esteem, parenting and communication involve choices that are best made by the client or in collaboration with the client.
6. The nurse must actively listen to the client to determine personal values, goals and desired outcomes in relation to current health concerns. Clients are usually motivated and expend the necessary energy to reach goals they consider important.

Computerized Care Plans

Computers are being used in recent years to create and store nursing care plans. The computer can generate both standardized and individualized care plans. Nurses access the client's stored care plan from a centrally located terminal at the nurses' station. For an individualized plan, the nurse chooses the appropriate diagnoses from a menu suggested by the computer. The computer then lists possible goals and nursing interventions for those diagnoses; the nurse chooses those appropriate for the client and types in any additional goals and interventions or nursing actions not listed on the menu. The nurse can read the plan on the computer screen or get a printout of the updated working copy.

Nursing Interventions

Nursing interventions are the actions to achieve client goals. The specific interventions chosen should focus on eliminating or reducing the etiology of the nursing diagnosis, which is the second clause of the diagnostic statement.

When it is not possible to change the etiologic factors, the nurse chooses interventions to treat the signs and symptoms or the defining characteristics in NANDA terminology. Examples of this situation would be *pain* related to surgical incision and anxiety related to unknown etiology.

Interventions for risk nursing diagnosis should focus on measures to reduce the client's risk factors, which are also found in the second clause. Correct identification of the etiology during the diagnosing phase provides the framework for choosing successful nursing interventions. For example, the diagnostic label *activity intolerance* may have several etiologies like pain, weakness, sedentary lifestyle, anxiety or cardiac arrhythmias. Interventions will vary according to the cause of the problem.

Types of Nursing Interventions

Nursing interventions are identified and written during the planning step of the nursing process. However, they are actually performed during the implementing step. Nursing interventions include both *direct and indirect care* as well as *nurse initiated, physician initiated* and *other provider-initiated* treatments. Direct care is an intervention performed through interaction with the client. Indirect care is an intervention performed away from, but on behalf of the client such as interdisciplinary collaboration or management of the care environment.

Independent Interventions

Independent interventions are those activities that nurses are licensed to initiate on the basis of their knowledge and skills. They include physical care, ongoing assessment, emotional support and comfort, teaching, counseling, environmental management, and making referrals to other healthcare professionals. In performing an autonomous activity, the nurse determines that the client requires certain nursing interventions either carries these out or delegates them to other nursing personnel and is accountable or answerable for the decisions and the actions. An example of an independent action is planning and providing special mouth care for a client after diagnosing impaired oral mucous membranes.

Dependent Interventions

Dependent interventions are activities carried out under the physician's orders or supervision, or according to specified routines. Physician's orders commonly include orders for medications, intravenous therapy, diagnostic tests, diet and activity. The nurse is responsible for explaining, assessing the need for administering the medical orders. Nursing interventions may be written to individualize the medical order based on the client's status. For example, for a medical order to 'progressive ambulation, as tolerated' a nurse might write the following:

- Dangle for 5 minutes 12 hours postoperative
- Stand at bedside 24-hours postoperative: Observe for pallor and dizziness
- Check pulse before and after ambulating
- Do not progress, if pulse rate is greater than 110/min.

Collaborative Interventions

These are actions the nurse carries out in collaboration with other health team members such as physical therapists, social workers, dietitians and physicians. Collaborative nursing activities reflect the overlapping responsibilities of and collegial relationships between health personnel. For example, the physician might order physical therapy to teach the client crutch walking. The nurse would be responsible for informing the physical therapy department and for coordinating the client's care to include the physical therapy sessions. When the client returns to nursing unit, the nurse would assist with crutch watching and collaborate with the physical therapist to evaluate the client's progress.

Writing Nursing Orders

After choosing the appropriate nursing interventions, the nurse writes them on the nursing care plan as nursing orders. Nursing orders are instructions for the specific, individualized activities and the nurse help to perform the client to meet established healthcare goals. The term order connotes a sense of accountability for the nurse, who gives the order and for the nurse who carries it out. Components of nursing orders are *date, action verb, content area, time element* and *signature*.

Example: 15/08/2007—palpate uterine fundus for firmness, for 2 hours, then q4h for 24 hours, A Jones, RN.

Date: Nursing orders are dated when they are written and reviewed regularly at intervals depending on the individual's needs. In an intensive care unit for example, the plan of care will be continually monitored and revised. In a community health clinic, weekly or biweekly reviews may be indicated.

Action verb: The action verb starts the order and must be precise. For example, explain (to the client) the actions of insulin is a more precise statement than teach (the client) about insulin. Sometimes, a modifier for the verb can make the nursing order more precise. For example, apply spiral bandage firmly to left lower leg is more precise than apply spiral bandage to left leg.

Content area: The content is, the what and where of the order. In the preceding order, spiral bandage and left leg state, the what and where of the order. The content area in this example may also clarify whether the foot or toes are to be left exposed.

Time element: The time element answers when, how long or how often the nursing action is to occur. Examples are assist client with sitz bath at 10 AM and 5 PM daily and administer analgesic 30 minutes prior to physical therapy.

Signature: The signature of the nurse prescribing the order shows the nurse's accountability and has legal significance.

IMPLEMENTING

The nursing process is client and action oriented and outcome directed. After developing a plan of care based on the assessment and diagnosing phases, the nurse implements the interventions and evaluates the desired outcomes. On the basis of this evaluation, the plan of care is continued, modified or terminated.

In the nursing process, implementing is the phase in which the nurse implements the nursing interventions. Implementing consists of *doing* and *documenting* activities that are specific nursing actions needed to carry out nursing orders. The nurse performs or delegates the nursing activities for the interventions that were developed in planning step and then conclude the implementing step by recording nursing activities and the resulting client responses. The degree of participation depends on the client's health status. For example, an unconscious person is unable to participate in his care and therefore needs to have care given to him. By contrast, an ambulatory client may require very little care from the nurse and carry out healthcare activities independently.

Relationship of Implementing to Other Phases of Nursing Process

The first three phases of nursing process are assessing, diagnosing and planning provide the basis for nursing actions performed during implementing step. In turn, the implementing phase provides the actual nursing activities and client responses that are examined in the final phase, the evaluating phase.

While implementing nursing orders, the nurse continues to assess the client at every contact, gathering data about the client's responses to the nursing activities and about any new problems that may develop. A nursing activity on the client's care plan may read 'auscultate lungs q4h'. When performing this activity, the nurse is both carrying out the intervention (implementing) and performing as assessment.

Some routine nursing activities are themselves assessments. For example, while bathing an elderly client, the nurse observes a reddened area on the client's sacrum or when emptying a urinary catheter bag, the nurse measures 200 mL of strong smelling brown urine.

Implementing Skills

To implement the care plan successfully, nurses need cognitive, interpersonal and technical skills. These skills are distinct from one another and nurses use them in various combinations and with different emphasis depending on the activity. For instance, when inserting a urinary catheter, the nurse needs cognitive knowledge of the principles and steps of the procedure, interpersonal skills to inform and reassure client and technical skills in draping the client and manipulating the articles.

Cognitive skills (intellectual skills) include problem solving, decision-making, critical thinking and creativity. They are crucial to safe intelligent nursing care.

Interpersonal skills are verbal and nonverbal activities, people use when interacting directly with one another. The effectiveness of a nursing action often depends largely on the nurse's ability to communicate with others. The nurse uses therapeutic communication to understand the client and in turn be understood. Interpersonal skills are necessary for all nursing activities; caring, comforting, advocating, referring, counseling and supporting. Before nurses can be highly skilled in interpersonal relations, they must have self-awareness and sensitivity to others.

Technical skills are 'hands on' skills such as manipulating equipment, giving injections and bandaging, moving, lifting and repositioning clients. The skills are also called tasks, procedures or psychomotor skills. Technical skills require knowledge and manual dexterity. The number of technical skills expected of a nurse has increased in the recent years because of the increased use of technology, especially in acute care hospitals.

Process of Implementing

Implementing is the process in which the nurse implements the nursing interventions and documents the care provided. The process includes:
- Reassessing the client
- Determining the nurse's need for assistance
- Implementing the nursing interventions
- Supervising the delegated care
- Documenting nursing activities.

Reassessing the Client

Before implementing an intervention, the nurse must reassess the client to make sure the intervention is still needed. Even though a nursing order is written on the care plan, the client's condition may have changed. For example, a directive-back message may be written for a nursing diagnosis of *disturbed sleep pattern,* related to anxiety and unfamiliar surroundings. During her rounds, the nurse discovers that the client is sleeping and therefore defers the back massage that had been planned as a relaxation strategy.

At times, new data may indicate a need to change the priorities of care or nursing activities.

Determining the Nurse's Need for Assistance

For implementing some nursing interventions, the nurse may require assistance for the following reasons:
- The nurse is unable to implement the nursing activity safely alone (e.g. ambulating an unsteady, obese client).
- The stress on client would be reduced, if nurse arranges for assistance for the activity (e.g. turning a client who experiences acute pain when moved).
- The nurse lacks the skills or knowledge to implement a particular nursing activity (e.g. a nurse who is not familiar with the use of an isolette needs assistance the first time it is used).

Implementing the Nursing Interventions

When implementing nursing interventions, nurses should follow certain guidelines:
- Base nursing interventions on scientific knowledge, professional standards and nursing research (evidence-based practice). The nurse must be aware of scientific rationale as well as possible side effects or complications of all interventions.
- Understand clearly the order to be implemented and any question that are not understood. The nurse is responsible for intelligent implementation of medical and nursing plans of care.
- Adapt activities to the individual client. A client's beliefs, values, age, health status and environment are factors that can affect the success of a nursing action.
- Implement safe care by following correct, steps and scientific principles.
- Provide teaching, support and comfort as required.
- View the client as whole and make the plan and implementation holistic.
- Respect the dignity of the client and enhance the client's self-esteem by providing privacy and encouraging client to make their own decisions.
- Encourage clients to participate actively in implementing the nursing interventions. Active participation enhances the client's sense of independence and control. The amount of desired involvement may be related to the severity of the illness and understanding of the intervention.

Supervising Delegated Care

If the care has been delegated to other healthcare personnel, the nurse responsible for the client's overall care must ensure that the activities have been implemented according to the care plan. Other caregivers are required to communicate their activities to the nurse by documenting them on the client's record, reporting verbally or filling out a written form. The nurse validates and responds to any adverse findings or client responses. This may involve modifying the nursing care plan.

Documenting Nursing Activities

After carrying out the nursing activities, the nurse completes the implementing phase by recording the interventions and client responses in the nursing progress notes. The nurse must record the nursing intervention immediately or as early as possible after it is implemented. The recorded data must be up-to-date, accurate and available to other nurses and healthcare professionals.

Nursing activities are communicated verbally as well as in writing. When client's health is changing rapidly, the head nurse and/or the physician may want to be kept up-to-date with verbal reports. Nurses also report client status at change if shifts or on a client's discharge to another unit, or institution in person, in writing or via a voice recording.

EVALUATING

Evaluating is the final/fifth phase of the nursing process in which the nurse determines the client's progress toward goal achievement and the effectiveness of the nursing care plan. The plan may be continued modified or terminated after the evaluation.

To evaluate means to judge or appraise. It is a planned, ongoing, purposeful activity in which clients and healthcare professionals determine:
1. The client's progress toward achievement of outcomes/goals.
2. The effectiveness of the nursing care plans.

Evaluation is an important aspect of the nursing process because conclusions drawn from the evaluation determine whether the nursing interventions should be terminated, continued or changed.

Evaluation is continuous and when carried out during or immediately after implementing a nursing order/directive, enables the nurse to make on the spot modifications in an intervention. Evaluation performed at specific intervals (e.g. once a week for a home care client) shows the extent of progress toward achievement of outcome and enables the nurse to correct any deficiencies, and modify the care plan as needed. Evaluation continues until the client achieves the health goals or is discharged from nursing care. Evaluation at discharge includes the status of goal achievement and the client's self-care abilities with regard to follow-up care.

Through evaluating, nurses demonstrate responsibility and accountability for their actions, and indicate interest in the results of the nursing activities carried out.

Relationship of Evaluating to Other Nursing Process Phases

Successful evaluation depends on the effectiveness of the steps that precede it. Assessment data must be accurate and complete so that the nurse can formulate appropriate nursing diagnoses and desired outcomes. The desired outcomes must be stated in behavioral terms, if they are to be useful for evaluating client responses and without the implementing phase in which the plan is put into action, there would be nothing to evaluate.

The evaluating and assessing phases overlap as assessment (data collection), is ongoing and continuous at every client contact. However, data are collected for different purposes at different points in the nursing process. During the assessment phase, the nurse collects data for the purpose of making diagnoses. During the evaluation step, the nurse collects data for the purpose of comparing it to preselected goals and for judging the effectiveness of the nursing care.

Process of Evaluating

Before evaluating, the nurse identifies the desired outcomes (indicators), which will be used to measure client's goal achievement. Desired outcomes serve two purposes:
1. They establish the kind of evaluative data that need to be collected.
2. Provide a standard against which the data are judged. For example, given the following expected outcomes, any nurse caring for the client would know what data to be collected:
    a. Daily fluid intake will not be less than 2,500 mL.
    b. Residual urine will be less than 100 mL.

The process of evaluation has five components:
1. Collecting data related to desired outcomes.
2. Comparing data with outcomes.
3. Relating nursing activities to outcomes.
4. Drawing conclusions about problem status.
5. Continuing, modifying or terminating the nursing care plan.

Collection of Data

Using the clearly stated, precise and measurable desired outcomes as a guide, the nurse collects data so that conclusions can be drawn about whether goals have been met. It is necessary to collect both objective and subjective data.

Comparing Data with Outcomes

Both the nurse and client play an active role in comparing the client's actual responses with the expected outcomes. For example, did the client drink 3,000 mL of fluid in 24 hours? The nurse can draw one of three of the following conclusions:
- The goal was met that is the client response is the same as the desired outcome
- The goal was partially met that is only the short-term goal was achieved and the long-term goal was not attained
- The goal was not met.

After determining whether a goal has been met, the nurse writes an evaluative statement in the nurse's notes. *An evaluative statement* consists of two parts; a conclusion and a supporting data.

The conclusion is a statement that the desired outcome was met or not. The supporting data are the list of client responses that support the conclusion.

For example, goal met: Oral intake at 300 mL more than output, skin turgor good and mucous membrane moist. In practice (in hospital units), care plans usually do not have a column for evaluation statements rather, these are recorded in the nurse's notes.

Relating Nursing Activities to Outcomes

The aspect of the evaluating process relates to determining whether the nursing activities had any relation to the outcomes. It should not be assumed that a nursing activity was the cause of or the only factor in meeting, partially meeting or not meeting a goal. For example, if the weight gain of a prenatal client meets the expected level as stated in the care plan. She must ensure that it relates to the instructions given to the mother only or due to fluid retention related to preeclamptic toxemia. It is important to establish the relationship or lack of relationship of nursing actions to the client responses.

Drawing Conclusions About Problem Status

In order to determine whether the care plan was effective in resolving, reducing or preventing client problems, the nurse uses the judgments about goal achievement. When goals have been met, the nurse can draw one of the following conclusions about the client's problem:

1. The actual problem stated in the nursing diagnosis has been resolved or the potential problem is being prevented and the risk factors no longer exist. In these circumstances, the nurse documents that the goals have been met and discontinues the care for the problem.
2. The potential problem stated in the nursing diagnosis is being prevented, but the risk factors are still present. In this case, the nurse keeps the problem on the nursing care plan.
3. The actual problem still exists even though some goals are being met. For example, a desired outcome on a client's care plan is to drink 2,500 mL fluid daily. Even though the data from intake-output record shows this outcome had been achieved, other data (dry oral mucous membrane) may indicate that there is *deficient fluid volume*. Therefore, the nursing interventions must be continued even though this goal was met.

When goals have been partially met or when goals have not been met, the nurse may conclude on one of the following:

1. The care plan needs to be revised. The revisions may need to occur during assessing, diagnosing or planning phases as well as implementing.
2. The care plan does not need revision because the client merely needs more time to achieve the goals.

Continuing, Modifying and Terminating the Nursing Care Plan

After drawing conclusions about the status of the clients' problems, the nurse modifies the care plan as indicated. Depending on policies of the hospital/agency, modifications may be made by marking portions using a highlighting pen or by drawing a line through portions of the care plan or writing 'discontinued' and the data. This requires a review of the entire care plan and a critique of the nursing process steps involved in its development.

In addition to evaluating goal achievement for individual clients, nurses are also involved in evaluating and modifying the overall quality of care given to groups of clients. This is an essential activity of professional accountability.

Utilizing the nursing process helps define and explain the unique practice of nursing. Its use encourages creative, comprehensive and systematic and client-oriented care that is more easily communicated to all healthcare team members. Its five phases such as assessment, diagnosis, planning, implementation and evaluation are founded in the scientific problem solving method that can be utilized in all settings, where nurses practice. Standardized nursing care plans, nursing diagnoses, procedures and protocols may be used to promote quality patient health care. Knowledge of and adherence to these standards and guidelines are the responsibilities of each practicing nurse.

The material in this chapter is intended to provide theoretical knowledge as background information in the pursuit of clinical management of the client. Because nursing management is a process that takes place in the clinical setting and the last two steps of the nursing process are dependent on the client and clinical situation, it is not possible to include them realistically in a textbook. However, conceptual models of nursing process for clients with different obstetrical conditions and processes are included at the end of certain chapters.

For detailed nursing care plans that could serve as guidelines for care of mothers (in prenatal, intranatal and postnatal periods) and newborns, the reader may refer to the *Appendix*.

STUDY QUESTIONS

Short Notes
1. An actual nursing diagnosis.
2. A risk nursing diagnosis.
3. A diagnostic label.
4. The domain of nursing.

Short Answer Questions
1. The primary and secondary sources of data in the assessment step of nursing process.
2. Methods of data collection in the assessment step of data collection.
3. Guidelines for writing desired outcomes in nursing care plans.

Essay Questions

1. Explain the component and qualifiers of NANDA nursing diagnosis statements.
2. Explain the two and three parts statements of nursing diagnosis.
3. List the guidelines for writing nursing diagnosis statements.
4. Discuss the process of evaluating the effectiveness of nursing interventions towards achievement of expected outcomes.

BIBLIOGRAPHY

1. Carpenito L. Nursing Diagnosis: Application to Clinical Practice. Philadelphia: Lippincott JB; 1993.
2. Christensen P, Kenny J. Nursing Process: Application of Conceptual Models, 3rd edition. St Louis: Mushy CV; 1990.
3. Doenges ME, Moorhouse MF, Murr AC. Nursing Care Plans: Guidelines for Individualizing Client Care Across Life Span, 7th edition. Philadelphia: FA Davis Company; 2006.
4. Doenges ME, Moorhouse MF. Application of Nursing Process and Nursing Diagnosis, 4th edition. Philadelphia: FA Davis Company; 2003.
5. Karpen M, Corad L, Chitwood L. Essentials of Maternal Child Nursing, 2nd edition. South Easton, MA: Western Schools Press; 1995. pp. 1-9.
6. Kozier B, Erb G, Borman A, et al. Fundamentals of Nursing: Concepts, Process and Practice, 7th edition. New Delhi, India: Dorling Kinderly Pvt Ltd; 2004.
7. The complete list of NANDA nursing diagnosis for 2012-2014 with 16 new diagnoses. [online] Philadelphia. Available from http//faculty. mu.edu. sa/public/uploads.
8. Varney H. Nurse Midwifery, 3rd edition. Boston: Jones and Barlett Publishers; 1999. pp. 43-63.
9. Vera M. NANDA Nursing Diagnosis, The Essential Guide; www://nurseslabs.com

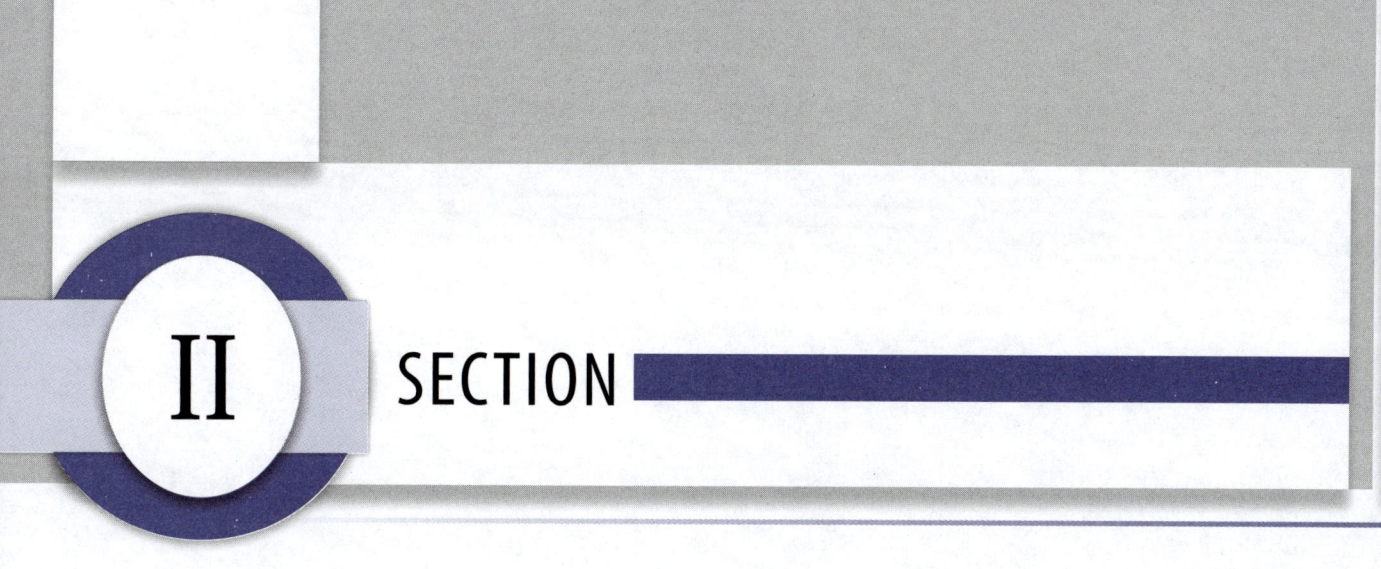

REPRODUCTIVE SYSTEM

Section Outline

5. Female Pelvis and Generative Organs
6. Hormonal Cycles
7. Male Reproductive System

CHAPTER 5

Female Pelvis and Generative Organs

Learning Objectives

Upon completing this chapter, the learner will be able to:
- List the features of a normal female pelvis.
- Discuss the different parts and measurements of gynecoid pelvis.
- Describe the female generative organs.

PELVIS

The female pelvis because of its characteristics, aids in childbirth. It is a skeletal ring formed by two innominate or hip bones, the sacrum and the coccyx **(Fig. 5.1)**.

Innominate Bone

Each innominate bone is made up of three parts; the ilium, the ischium and the pubis **(Fig. 5.2)**.

The *ilium* is the large flared out portion of the innominate bone. The upper border of ilium is termed iliac crest. When the hand is placed on the hip, it rests on this part. The prominence at the front of the iliac crest is known as the anterosuperior iliac spine. A short distance below is the anteroinferior iliac spine. At opposite end of the iliac crest similar prominences are present, which are named posterosuperior and posteroinferior iliac spines. The anterior surface of the ilium is concave in shape and termed as the iliac fossa.

The *ischium* is the thick lower part of the innominate bone. It has a large prominence known as the ischial tuberosity. In sitting position, the body rests on the ischial tuberosity. A little above and behind the tuberosity is a projection known as the ischial spine. In labor, the station (level) of the fetal head is estimated in relation to the ischial spines.

The *pubic* bones form the anterior part of the innominate bone. It has a body and two oar-like projections called superior and inferior ramus. The two pubic bones meet at the symphysis pubis. The two inferior rami form the pubic arch. The space enclosed by the body of the pubic bone, the rami and the ischium is called the obturator foramen. The innominate has a deep cup to receive the head of the femur, which is termed as acetabulum. All three bones contribute to form the acetabulum.

The two curves are found on the lower border of the innominate bone are found two curves. One extends from the posteroinferior iliac spine up to the ischial spine and is called the greater *sciatic notch*. It is wide and rounded. The

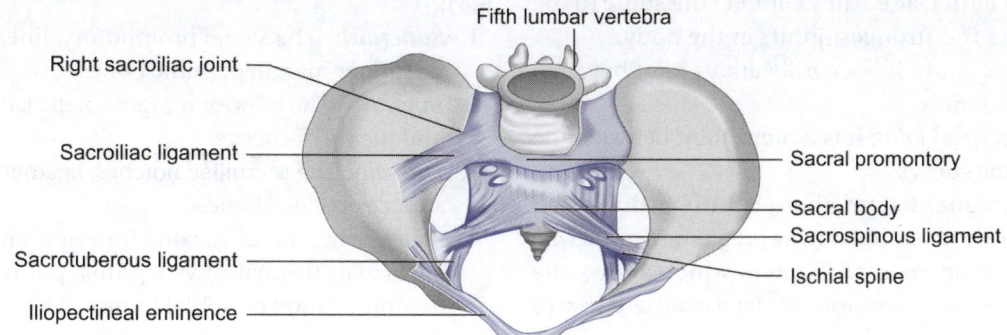

Figure 5.1: Normal female pelvis.

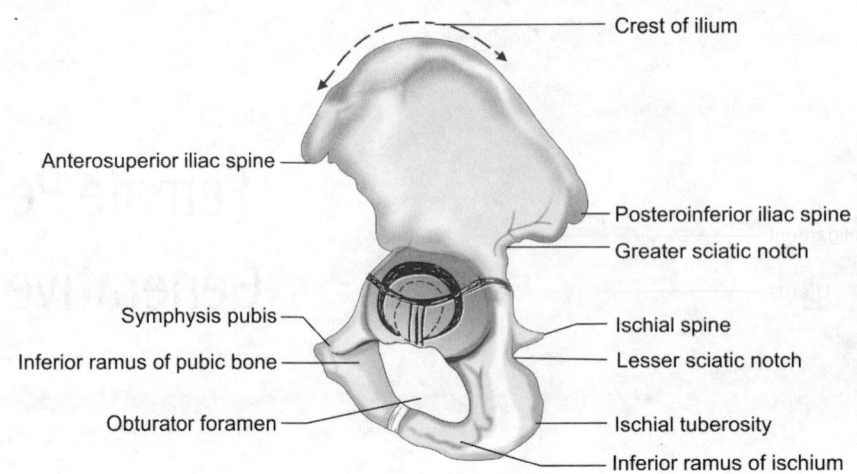

Figure 5.2: Innominate bone showing important landmarks.

other lies between ischial spine and the ischial tuberosity and is the *lesser sciatic notch*.

Sacrum

The sacrum lies between the ilia. It is a wedge-shaped bone consisting of five vertebrae fused together. The prominent upper margin of the first sacral vertebrae is called the sacral promontory. The anterior surface of the sacrum is concave and is referred to as the hollow of the sacrum. Four pairs of holes or foramina pierce the sacrum and through these the sacral nerves pass.

Coccyx

The coccyx is a small triangular bone with its base uppermost articulating with the lower end of the sacrum. During labor it moves backward, allowing more space for the delivery of the fetus.

Pelvic Joints

There are four pelvic joints:
1. *Two sacroiliac joints*: These are slightly movable joints, formed where the ilium joins the first two sacral vertebrae on either side. They connect the spine to the pelvis and are the strongest joints in the body.
2. *One symphysis pubis*: It is a cartilaginous joint between the two pubic bones.
3. *One sacrococcygeal joint*: It is a hinge joint between the sacrum and the coccyx.

In the non-pregnant state, there is little articulation (movement) in these joints, but during pregnancy endocrine activity causes the ligaments to soften, which allows the ligaments to provide more space for the fetal head as it passes through the pelvis during delivery.

Pelvic Ligaments (Fig. 5.3)

The pelvic girdle has great strength and stability in order to fulfill its functions of support. Powerful ligaments hold the pelvic joints together:
1. *Sacroiliac ligaments*: These ligaments pass in front of and behind each sacroiliac joint.
2. *Pubic ligaments*: The superior pubic ligament connects the top of the pubic bones. The arcuate (arched) pubic ligament runs under the symphysis pubis.
3. *Sacrotuberous ligaments*: One ligament runs from the sacrum to the ischial tuberosity.
4. *Sacrospinous ligament*: One ligament on each side of the sacrum and the ischial spine.
5. *Sacrococcygeal ligaments*: One ligament on each side from the sacrum to the coccyx.

True Pelvis

The true pelvis constitutes the bony passage through which the fetus must maneuver to be born vaginally. Therefore, its construction planes and diameters are of utmost interest in obstetrics.

The true pelvis has the following as its boundaries (**Fig. 5.4**):
1. *Superiorly*: The sacral promontory, linea terminalis and the upper margin of pubic bones.
2. *Inferiorly*: The inferior margins of the ischial tuberosities and the tip of coccyx.
3. *Laterally*: The sacroiliac notches, ligaments and the inner surface of ischial bones.
4. *Anteriorly*: The obturator foramen and the posterior surface of the symphysis pubis, pubic bones and the ascending rami of ischial bones.

The true pelvis has a brim, a cavity and an outlet (**Fig. 5.5**)

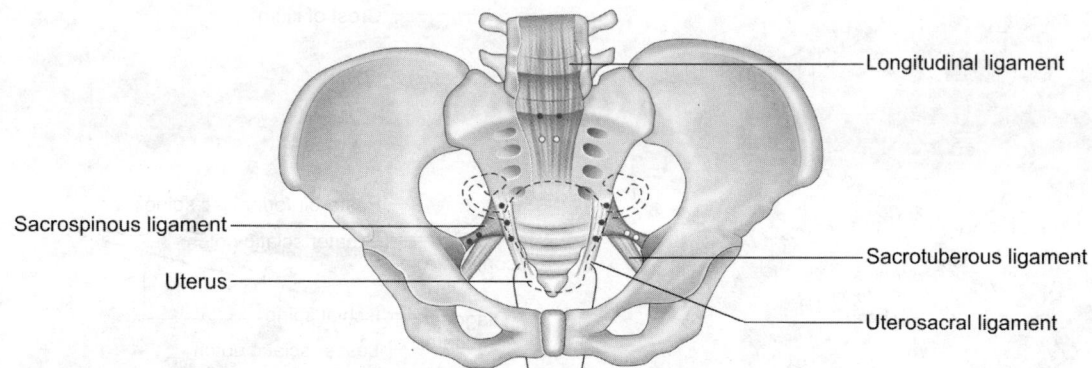

Figure 5.3: Ligaments of pelvic floor.

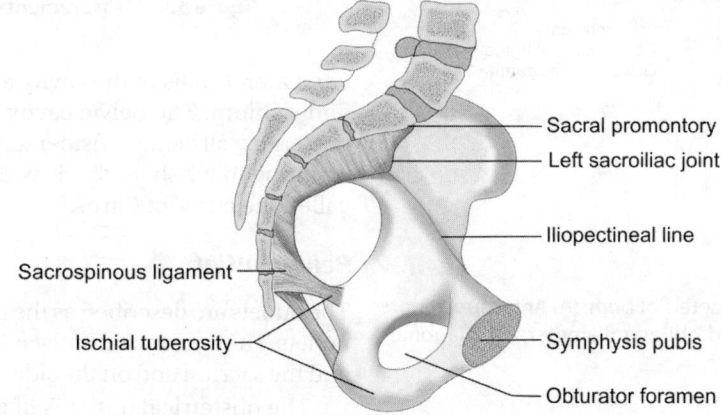

Figure 5.4: Sagittal view of bony pelvis.

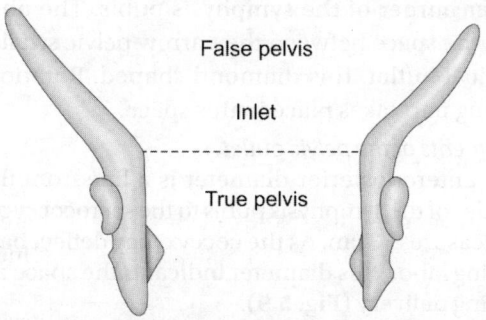

Figure 5.5: True pelvis and false pelvis.

Pelvic Brim

The brim is also termed as the inlet. Its boundaries are the sacral promontory and wings of the sacrum behind the iliac bones on the sides and the pubic bones in front.

Landmarks of the brim: These are the fixed anatomical points on the brim:
- Sacral promontory.
- Sacral ala or sacral wing.
- Sacroiliac joint.
- Iliopectineal line: The edge formed at the inward aspect of the ilium.
- Iliopectineal eminence: A roughened area, where the superior ramus of the pubic bone meets the ilium.
- Superior ramus of the pubic bone.
- Upper inner border of the body of pubic bone.
- Upper inner border of the symphysis pubis.

Diameters of the brim (Figs. 5.6 and 5.7) are of four types:
1. *The anteroposterior diameter of the brim:* It is a line from the sacral promontory to the upper border of the symphysis pubis. When the anteroposterior diameter is

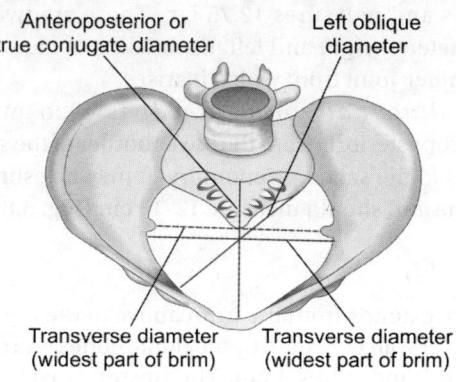

Figure 5.6: Brim of pelvis showing diameters.

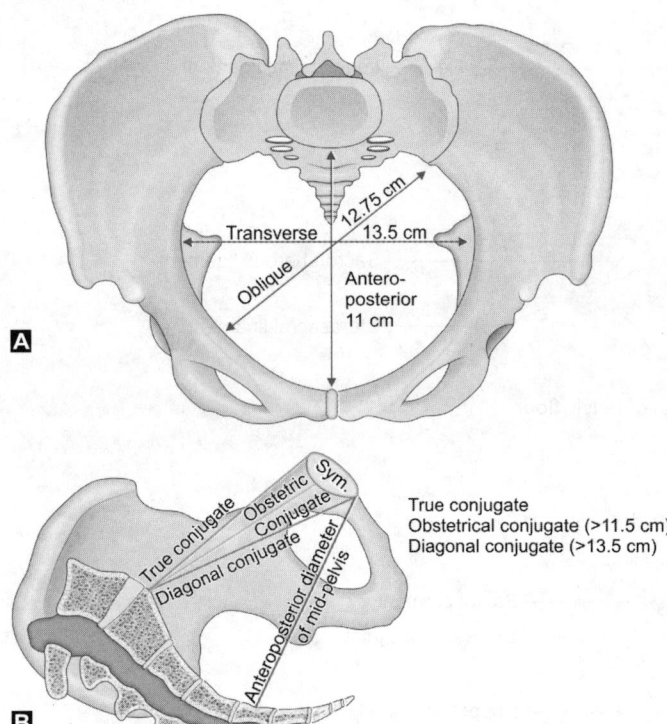

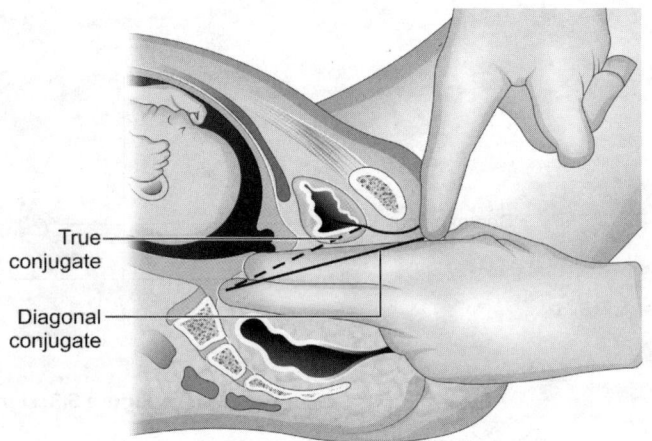

Figure 5.8: Measurement of diagonal conjugatet.

Figures 5.7A and B: Different diameters of brim: (A) Anteroposterior diameter, transverse diameter and oblique diameter; (B) Diagonal conjugate.

measured from the sacral promontory to the uppermost point of the symphysis pubis, it is called the anatomical conjugate and measures 12 cm. When it is taken to the posterior border of the upper surface, it is called the obstetrical conjugate and measures 11 cm. It is the anteroposterior diameter available for childbirth. The term *true conjugate* may be used to refer to either of these measurements.
2. *The transverse diameter of the brim of the inlet*: It is the maximum transverse diameter that can be found between similar points on opposite sides of the pelvic brim. In other words, it is a line between the furthest points on the iliopectineal lines. It measures 13.5 cm.
3. *The oblique diameter*: It is a line from one sacroiliac joint to the iliopectineal eminence on the opposite side of the pelvis and measures 12.75 cm. There are two oblique diameters—right and left. Each takes its name from the sacroiliac joint from which it arises.
4. *The diagonal conjugate*: It is also measured anteroposteriorly from the lower border of the symphysis pubis to the sacral promontory. It may be estimated per vagina and should measure 12–13 cm **(Fig. 5.8)**.

Pelvic Cavity

The cavity extends from the brim above to the outlet below. The anterior wall is formed by the pubic bones and symphysis pubis and it measures 4 cm. The posterior wall is formed by the curve of the sacrum and coccyx, which measures 12 cm. Lateral walls of the cavity are formed by the fused ilium and ischium. The pelvic cavity is short and curved with the posterior wall being considerably longer than the anterior wall resulting in a J-shaped axis with the curve directed forward called the curve of Carus.

Pelvic Outlet

The outlets are described as the anatomical and the obstetrical outlets. The anatomical outlet is indented behind by the coccyx and the sacrum and on the sides by the ischial tuberosities.

The obstetrical outlet is of greater practical significance because it includes the narrow pelvic strait through which the fetus must pass. The narrow pelvis strait (passage) lies between the sacrococcygeal joint, two ischial spines and the lower border of the symphysis pubis. The obstetrical outlet is the space between the narrow pelvic strait and the anatomical outlet. It is diamond shaped. Rotation of the presenting part takes place in this space.

Measurements of the pelvic outlet
1. The anteroposterior diameter is a line from the lower border of the symphysis pubis to the sacrococcygeal joint. It measures 13 cm. As the coccyx may deflect backwards during labor, this diameter indicates the space available during delivery **(Fig. 5.9)**.
2. The oblique diameter is the measurement between the obturator foramen and the sacrospinous ligament. The measurement is considered as 12 cm although there are no fixed points of measurement **(Fig. 5.10)**.
3. Transverse diameter is a line between the two ischial spines and measures 10–11 cm. It is the narrowest diameter of the pelvis **(Fig. 5.11)**.

False Pelvis

The pelvis is divided by the linea terminalis into the false pelvis above this demarcation and the true pelvis below it. The false pelvis is the portion above the pelvic brim. It has no obstetric significance relevant to the passage of the fetus through the pelvis.

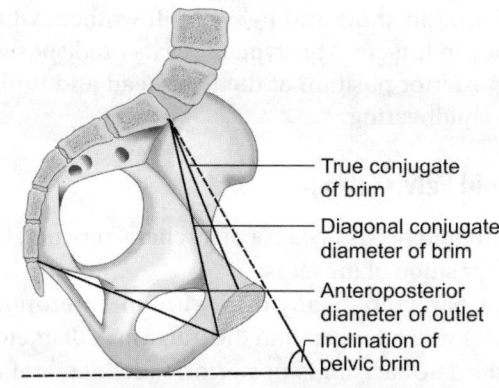

Figure 5.9: Lateral view of pelvis showing anteroposterior diameters in different plane.

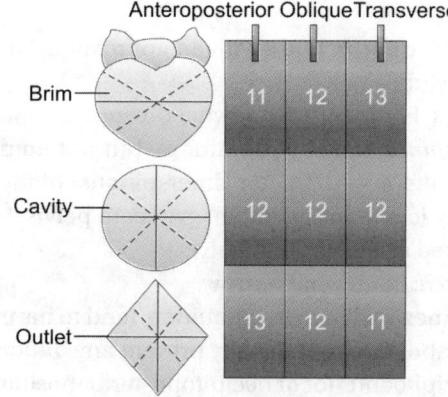

Figure 5.10: Measurements of the pelvic canal in centimeters.

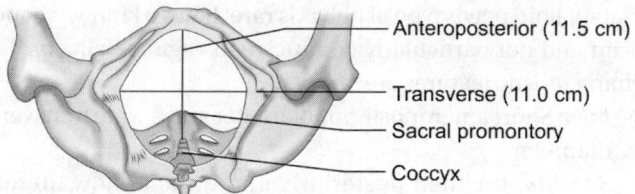

Figure 5.11: Diameters of the pelvic outlet.

Pelvic Inclination

The longitudinal axis of the symphysis pubis is normally parallel to the longitudinal axis of the sacrum. If the symphysis pubis is not parallel to the sacrum, the anteroposterior diameter of the inlet can be changed significantly. Tilting of the superior margin of the symphysis pubis towards the sacral promontory and of the inferior margin away from the sacrum is called anterior inclination. Tilting of the inferior margin of the symphysis pubis toward the sacrum and the superior margin away from the sacral promontory is called posterior inclination **(Fig. 5.12)**.

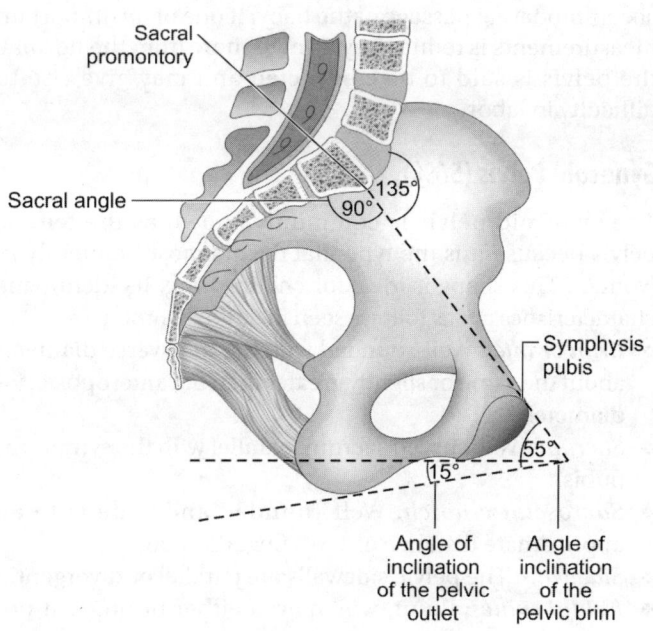

Figure 5.12: Pelvic inclination.

TYPES OF PELVIS (FIG. 5.13)

There are four basic types of pelvis according to the Caldwell-Moloy classification:
1. Gynecoid.
2. Android.
3. Anthropoid.
4. Platypelloid.

These are determined by certain characteristics of the pelvis and classified according to the shape of the brim.

Many pelvis are not pure types, but rather a mixture of types. For example, a gynecoid pelvis may be said to have an android tendency. The importance of being familiar with the pelvic types lies in the fact that many of the characteristics used in determining the pelvic types affect the obstetric capacity of the pelvis that is the adequacy of the pelvis for

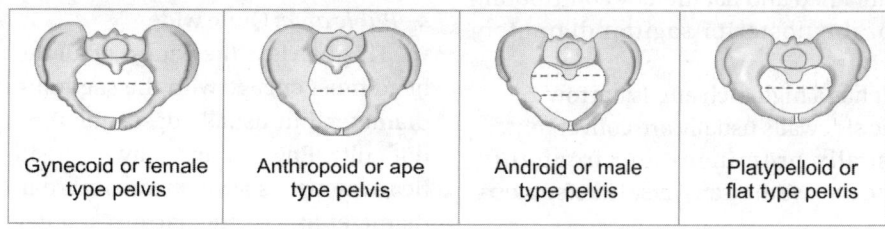

Figure 5.13: Four types of pelvis.

accommodating passage of the baby. If one of the important measurements is reduced by 1 cm or more from the normal, the pelvis is said to be contracted and may give rise to difficulty in labor.

Gynecoid Pelvis (50%)

The gynecoid pelvis is commonly known as the female pelvis because it is the type that occurs most frequently in women. This shape is ideal for childbearing. Its identifying characteristics are as follows seen in 50% of women:
* *Brim or inlet*: Well-rounded with the transverse diameter about the same or slightly greater than the anteroposterior diameter.
* *Sacrum*: Well-curved sacrum, parallel with the symphysis pubis.
* *Sacrosciatic notch*: Well-rounded and wide with an approximate distance of 2.5–3 fingerbreadths.
* *Sidewalls*: The pelvic sidewalls are parallel or divergent.
* *Ischial spines*: Blunt, which are neither prominent nor encroaching.
* *Pelvic arch*: Wide pubic arch of 90° or more.
    It is found in women of average build and height.

Justo Minor Pelvis

Justo minor pelvis is a miniature gynecoid pelvis. All diameters are reduced, but are in proportion. It is normally found in women of small stature with small hands and feet. Occasionally, this type of pelvis is seen in women of normal stature. If these women have smaller babies, normal labor and delivery will take place. However, if the fetus is large, a degree of cephalopelvic disproportion will result.

Android Pelvis (20%)

The android pelvis is commonly known as the male pelvis because it occurs more frequently in men. However, it does occur in a small percent of women. The android pelvis is a heavy pelvis that poses difficulty for vaginal delivery and increases the incidence of posterior position and transverse arrest. The midplane and outlet contracture of the android pelvis increases the incidences of fetopelvic disproportion and cesarean sections.
Characteristics of the android pelvis are:
* *Inlet*: Heart shaped with a narrow fore pelvis. Has a transverse diameter that is toward the back. The sidewalls converge making it a funnel shape.
* *Sacrum*: Anteriorly inclined and flat thereby contributing to the shortness of the posterior sagittal diameters throughout the pelvis.
* *Sacrosciatic notch*: It has a high arch and is narrow.
* *Sidewalls*: The pelvic sidewalls usually are convergent.
* *Ischial spines*: Usually prominent and frequently encroaching thereby decrease the transverse (interspinous) diameter.
* *Pubic arch*: The angle of the pubic arch is less than 90°.

It is found in short and heavy built women, who have a tendency to hirsute. This type of pelvis predisposes to an occipitoposterior position of the fetal head and is the least suited to childbearing.

Anthropoid Pelvis (20%)

The anthropoid pelvis because of its characteristics, favors a posterior position of the fetus:
* *Brim*: Characteristically oval with an anteroposterior diameter much longer than the transverse diameter.
* *Sacrum*: The sacrum is posteriorly inclined and deeply concave. Therefore, the space in the posterior portion of the pelvis is increased for accommodating the fetal head. The anthropoid pelvis has the longest sacrum of the four types of pelvis.
* *Sacrosciatic notch*: Wide with an approximate length of 4 fingerbreadth.
* *Sidewalls*: Frequently somewhat divergent.
* *Ischial spines*: Usually prominent, but not encroaching, so the transverse diameter (interspinous) of the cavity is generally less than that of the gynecoid pelvis, but not as contracted as the android pelvis.
* *Pubic arch*: Somewhat narrow.
    Tall women with narrow shoulders tend to have this type of pelvis. Labor does not usually present any difficulties, but a direct occipitoanterior or occipitoposterior position is often a feature.

Platypelloid Pelvis (5%)

Platypelloid pelvis type of pelvis is rare. It has a kidney-shaped brim and not particularly conducive to vaginal delivery. The characteristic features are:
* *Inlet*: Short anteroposterior diameter and a wide transverse diameter.
* *Sacrum*: Inclined posteriorly and quite hollow thereby presenting a short sacrum and a shallow pelvis.
* *Sacrosciatic notch*: Wide and flat with an acute angle between the ischial spines and the sacrum.
* *Sidewalls*: Slightly divergent.
* *Ischial spines*: Somewhat blunt, but because of the flattened character of the pelvis and wide transverse diameter, this prominence has no effect. The transverse diameter of the cavity of platypelloid pelvis is the widest of all the pelves.
* *Pubic arch*: Quite wide.
    This pelvis is the widest of all the pelvic types. The fetal head must engage with the sagittal suture in the transverse diameter, but usually descends through the cavity without difficulty. Engagement may necessitate lateral tilting of the head known as asynclitism, in order to allow the biparietal diameter to pass the narrowest anteroposterior diameter of brim **(Table 5.1)**.

TABLE 5.1: Anatomical features of pelvic types.

Pelvic planes and diameters	Gynecoid	Anthropoid	Android	Platypelloid
Inlet				
Configuration	Female	Ape-like	Male	Flat—female
Incidence	50%	20%	20%	5%
Shape	Well rounded	Long, oval shape	Heart shape	Transverse oval
Anteroposterior (AP) diameter	Adequate	Long	Adequate	Short
Transverse	Adequate	Adequate	Adequate	Adequate
Cavity				
AP diameter	Adequate	Long	Reduced	Short
Transverse	Adequate	Adequate	Adequate	Short
Side walls	Parallel	Straight	Funneled	Parallel
Sacrum	Wide, deep curve and slopes forward	Long and narrow	Flat, long and narrow	Wide, deep and curved
Depth	Average	Long	Long	Short
Outlet				
AP diameter	Long	Long	Short	Short
Transverse	Adequate	Adequate	Narrow	Wide
Ischial spines	Not prominent	Not prominent	Prominent	Not prominent
Subpubic arch	Wide and rounded	Normal or slightly narrow	Narrow and deep	Very wide

OTHER PELVIC VARIATIONS

High Assimilation Pelvis

High assimilation type of pelvis is seen when the fifth lumbar vertebra is fused to the sacrum and the angle of inclination of the pelvic brim is increased. Engagement of the fetal head is difficult, but once achieved, labor progresses normally.

Deformed Pelvis

Deformation of the pelvis may result from a developmental anomaly, dietary deficiency, injury or disease. Developmental anomalies are seen as Naegele's pelvis or Robert's pelvis. In the Naegele's pelvis, one sacral ala is missing and the sacrum is fused to the ilium, causing a grossly asymmetric brim. The Robert's pelvis is similar, but bilateral. In both types, the abnormal brim prevents engagement of the fetal head.

Deformities due to dietary deficiencies result from deficiency of vitamins and minerals necessary for the formation of healthy bones. Rickets in early childhood can result in gross deformity of the pelvic brim. In rachitic pelvis (caused by rickets), the sacral promontory is pushed downwards and forwards and the ilium and ischium are drawn outwards. This results in a flat pelvic brim similar to that of the platypelloid pelvis. The fetal head will attempt to enter the pelvis by asynclitism. Cesarean section is required to deliver the baby. Another pelvic deformity due to dietary deficiency is the osteomalacia pelvis. It is due to deficiency of calcium and occurs in adults. All bones of the skeleton soften and as a result of gross calcium deficiency. The pelvic canal is squashed together until the brim becomes a Y-shaped slot. Delivery impossible and a cesarean section will be performed.

Injury or disease may also cause pelvic deformities. A pelvis, which has been fractured will develop callus formation or may fail to unite correctly. This may lead to reduced measurements resulting in contraction. Fractures of pelvis or lower limbs in childhood, congenital dislocation of the hip and poliomyelitis may lead to pelvic deformity. Pelvic deformity is seen in women with spinal deformity such as kyphosis (forward angulation) and scoliosis (lateral curvature) and in women who limp. Outcome of delivery is dependent on the degree of deformity.

Muscles and Fascia

Pelvic Floor

Pelvic floor is a muscular partition, which separates the pelvic cavity from the perineum **(Fig. 5.14)**. The most important muscle supporting the pelvic organs is the levator ani, which forms the pelvic floor. The levator ani (deep layer) consists of three sets of muscles on either side:
1. The pubococcygeus muscle that passes from the pubis to the coccyx.
2. The iliococcygeus muscle that passes from the fascia covering the obturator internus muscle to the coccyx.
3. The ischiococcygeus muscle that passes from the ischial spine to the coccyx.

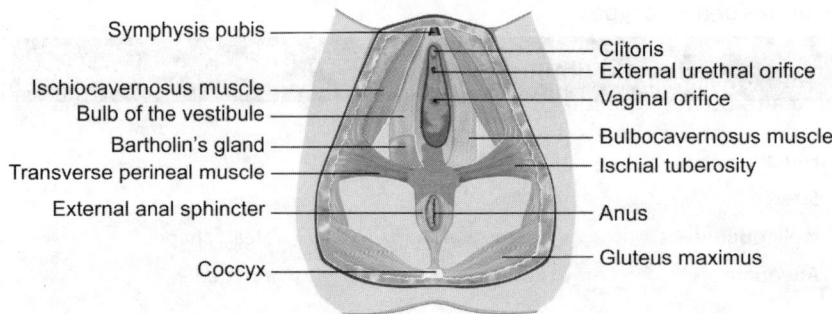

Figure 5.14: Perineum.

The superficial muscle layer of the pelvic floor is composed of five muscles:
1. The *external anal sphincter* that encircles the anus.
2. The *transverse perineal muscles* that pass from the ischial tuberosities to the center of the perineum.
3. The *bulbocavernosus muscles* that pass from the perineum forwards around the vagina and clitoris just under the pubic arch.
4. The *ischiocavernosus muscles* that pass from the ischial tuberosities along the pubic arch to the corpora cavernosa.
5. The *membranous sphincter* of the urethra is composed of muscle fibers passing about and below the urethra and attached to the pubic bones. It acts to close the urethra.

Between the muscle layers as well as above and below them, there are layers of pelvic fascia. The muscles with the covering fascia are called the pelvic diaphragm.

Functions

❖ The pelvic floor supports the weight of the abdominal and pelvic floor organs. The pubovaginalis, which forms a 'U'-shaped sling, supports the vagina, bladder and uterus. Weakness or tear of this sling during delivery is responsible for prolapse of the organs concerned **(Fig. 5.15)**.

❖ The muscles are responsible for the voluntary control of micturition and defecation, play an important role in sexual intercourse.
❖ During childbirth, it influences the passive movements of the fetus through the birth canal and relaxes to allow its exit from the birth canal (when the presenting part of the fetus presses on the pelvic floor, it facilitates anterior internal rotation).
❖ Maintains intra-abdominal pressure by reflexly responding to its changes.
❖ Steadies the perineal body.

Nerve Supply

The fourth sacral nerve, inferior rectal nerve and a perineal branch of pudendal nerve supply it.

During pregnancy, the levator ani muscle hypertrophies and becomes less rigid and more distensible. Due to water retention, it swells up and sags down.

In the second stage, the pubovaginalis and puborectalis relax and the levator ani is drawn up over the advancing presenting part. The effect of such a displacement is to elongate the birth canal.

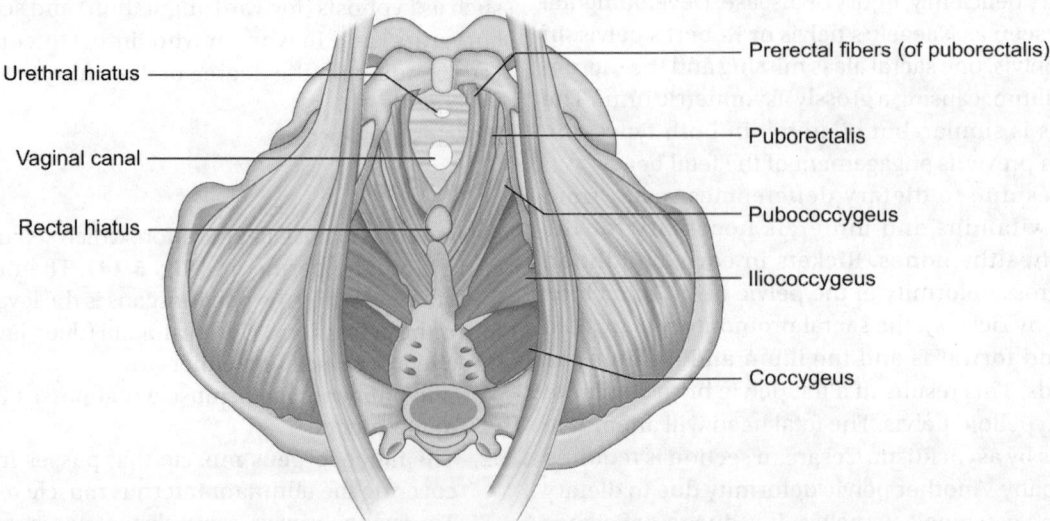

Figure 5.15: Pelvic floor muscles.

Perineal Body

Perineal body is a pyramid of muscles and fibrous tissue situated between the vagina and the rectum. It is the central point of the perineum and is called the obstetrical perineum. It measures 4 cm × 4 cm with the base covered by the perineal skin and the apex is pointed and is continuous with the rectovaginal septum. The apex is formed from the fibers of the pubococcygeus muscle; the base is formed from the transverse perineal muscles together with the bulbocavernosus in front and the external anal sphincter behind.

The perineal body helps to support the levator ani, which is placed above it. It is vulnerable to injury during childbirth. Deliberate cutting of these structures during delivery is called episiotomy.

Evaluation of Pelvis

Clinical evaluation of pelvis and pelvimetry are usually included as part of the initial antepartal examination and depending on the circumstances, repeated again either late in the third trimester or at the time of the initial intrapartum pelvic examination.

The woman needs to be prepared for this procedure as for the pelvic examination such as empty bladder, lithotomy position, proper draping and instruction about the procedure and relaxation techniques to help her cope with the examination.

Evaluation of the bony pelvis is often done as a part of the total pelvic examination. The pelvic measurements are then weighed against the estimated size of the fetus at term, the type of presenting part and its position. A determination of pelvic adequacy is made from these findings. When evaluation of the bony pelvis is done early in pregnancy, it is often evaluated as adequate for a certain size baby. For example, charting may show a summary statement such as adequate for a 2.5 kg baby. At term if the estimated fetal weight is 3 kg, one is alerted to a potential problem requiring re-evaluation of labor status with this concern in mind.

GENERATIVE ORGANS

The generative (reproductive) organs in the female are those concerned with copulation, fertilization, growth and development of the fetus, its subsequent exit into the outer world and nurture following birth. The generative organs constitute the external genitalia, the internal genital organs and the accessory reproductive organs.

External Genitalia (Vulva) (Fig. 5.16)

The external female genital organs (vulva) consist of the following structures.

Mons Pubis or Mons Veneris

Mons pubis is a pad of subcutaneous adipose connective tissue lying over the symphysis pubis. It is covered with pubic hair from the time of puberty.

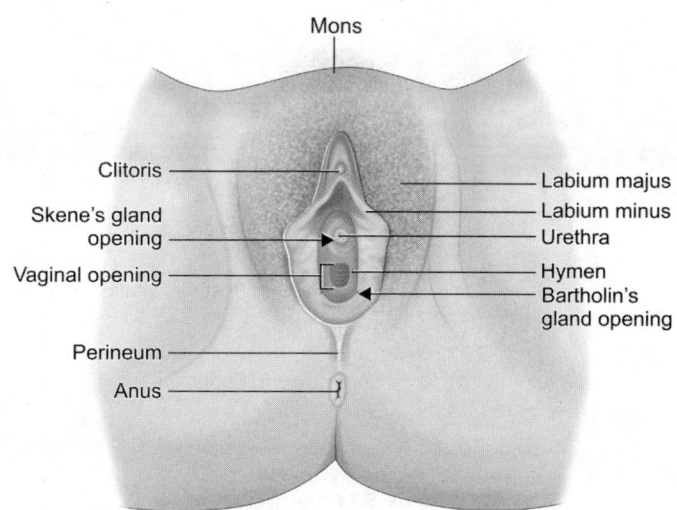

Figure 5.16: Schematic representation of female external genitalia.

Labia Majora (Greater Lips)

Labia majora are two folds of fat and areolar tissue, covered with skin and pubic hair on the outer surface. The inner surfaces of the labia majora are hairless. The labia majora are covered with squamous epithelium and contain sebaceous glands, sweat glands and hair follicles. The adipose tissue is richly supplied with venous plexus, which may produce hematoma, if injured during childbirth. The labia majora arise from the mons veneris and merge into the perineum behind. The round ligaments terminate at its upper borders.

Labia Minora (Lesser Lips)

Labia minora are two thin folds of skin lying between the labia majora. Anteriorly they divide to enclose the clitoris; posteriorly they fuse, forming the *fourchette*. It is usually lacerated during childbirth. Between the fourchette and the vaginal orifice is the *fossa navicularis*. The labia minora do not contain hair follicles. The folds contain connective tissue, numerous sebaceous glands, erectile muscle fibers and numerous vessels and nerve endings.

Clitoris

Clitoris is a small cylindrical, erectile body, measuring about 2.5 cm situated in the most anterior part of the vulva. It is a rudimentary organ corresponding to the male penis, but differs basically in being entirely separate from the urethra. It is attached to the under surface of the symphysis pubis by the suspensory ligament. It is extremely sensitive and highly vascular and plays a role in the orgasm of sexual intercourse.

Vestibule (Fig. 5.17)

Vestibule is a triangular space bounded anteriorly by the clitoris, posteriorly by the fourchette and on either side by the labia minora. There are four openings into the vestibule:

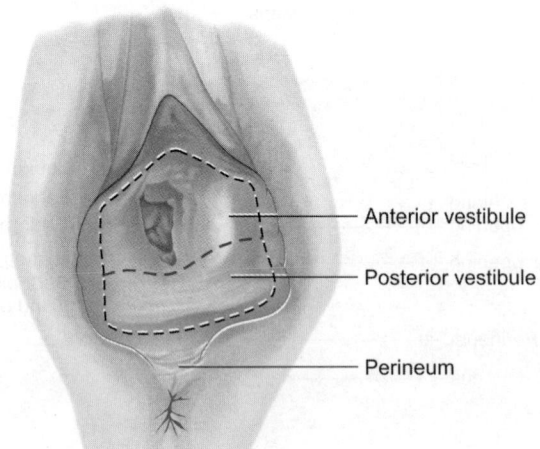

Figure 5.17: Vestibule.

1. *Urethral opening*: The opening is situated in the midline just in front of the vaginal orifice about 2.5 cm posterior to the clitoris. The *Skene's glands* open on either side of the urethral orifice.
2. *Vaginal orifice or introitus*: It occupies the posterior two-thirds of the vestibule and is of varying size and shape. In virgins and nulliparae, the opening is closed by the labia minora, but in parous women it may be exposed. It is completely closed by a septum of mucous membrane called hymen. The membrane varies in shape, but is usually circular or crescentic in virgins. The hymen is usually ruptured at the consummation of marriage. During childbirth, the hymen is extremely lacerated and is known as the *carunculae myrtiformes*. On both sides it is lined by stratified squamous epithelium.
3. *Openings of Bartholin's glands*: There are two Bartholin's glands (greater vestibular glands) one on each side. They open on either side of the vaginal orifice and lie in the posterior part of the labia majora. They are pea-shaped and yellowish white in color. During sexual excitement, it secretes abundant alkaline mucus, which helps in lubrication. Each gland has a duct, which measures about 2 cm and opens into the vestibule outside the hymen. The duct is lined by columnar epithelium.

Blood Supply

Blood supply comes from the internal and external pudendal arteries. The blood drains through the corresponding veins.

Lymphatic Drainage

Lymphatics drain into the inguinal lymph nodes and internal iliac lymph nodes.

Nerve Supply

Nerve supply is from the branches of pudendal nerve. Anterior part is supplied by the genitofemoral nerve (L1 and L2) and posteroinferior part by the pudendal branches from the posterior cutaneous nerve of thigh (S1, S2 and S3). The vulva is supplied by the labial and perineal branches of the pudendal nerve (S2, S3 and S4).

Internal Genital Organs (Figs. 5.18 and 5.19)

Vagina

Vagina is a fibromuscular membranous sheath connecting the uterine cavity with the exterior at the vulva. It is a passage, which allows the escape of menstrual flow and uterine secretions. It receives the penis and the ejected sperm during sexual intercourse and provides an exit for the fetus during delivery. The canal is directed upward and backward forming an angle of 45° with the horizontal in erect posture. The long axis of the vagina almost lies parallel to the plane of the pelvic inlet and at right angles to that of the uterus. The diameter of the canal is about 2.5 cm, being wider in the upper part and narrowest at the introitus. It has enough power of distensibility as evident during childbirth.

Vaginal walls
Vagina has an anterior, a posterior and two lateral walls. The anterior and posterior walls are opposed together, but the lateral walls are comparatively stiffer specifically at its middle, as such it looks 'H' shaped on transverse section. The length of the anterior wall is about 7 cm and that of the posterior wall is about 9 cm.

Relations
- *Anterior*: In front lie the bladder and urethra, which are closely connected to the anterior vaginal wall.
- *Behind*: The pouch of Douglas, the rectum and the perineal body each occupy approximately one-third of the posterior vaginal wall.
- *Lateral*: Beside the upper two-thirds are the pelvic fascia and ureters, while beside the lower third are the muscles of the pelvic floor.
- *Superior*: Above the vagina lies the uterus.
- *Inferior*: Below the vagina lie the external genitalia.

Structure
The posterior wall is 10 cm long, while the anterior wall is only 7 cm because the cervix projects at right angles into its upper part. The upper part of the vagina is known as the *vault*. Where the cervix projects into it, the vault forms a circular recess, which is described as its four *fornices*. The posterior fornix is the largest of these because the vagina is attached to the uterus at a higher level behind than in front. The anterior fornix lies in front of the cervix and the lateral fornices lie on either side. The vaginal walls are pink in appearance and thrown into small folds known as *rugae*. These allow the vaginal walls to stretch during intercourse and childbirth.

Layers
The lining of the vagina is made of squamous epithelium. Beneath the epithelium lies a layer of vascular connective tissue. The muscle layer has a weak inner coat of circular fibers and a stronger outer coat of longitudinal fibers. Pelvic fascia surrounds the vagina forming a layer of connective tissue.

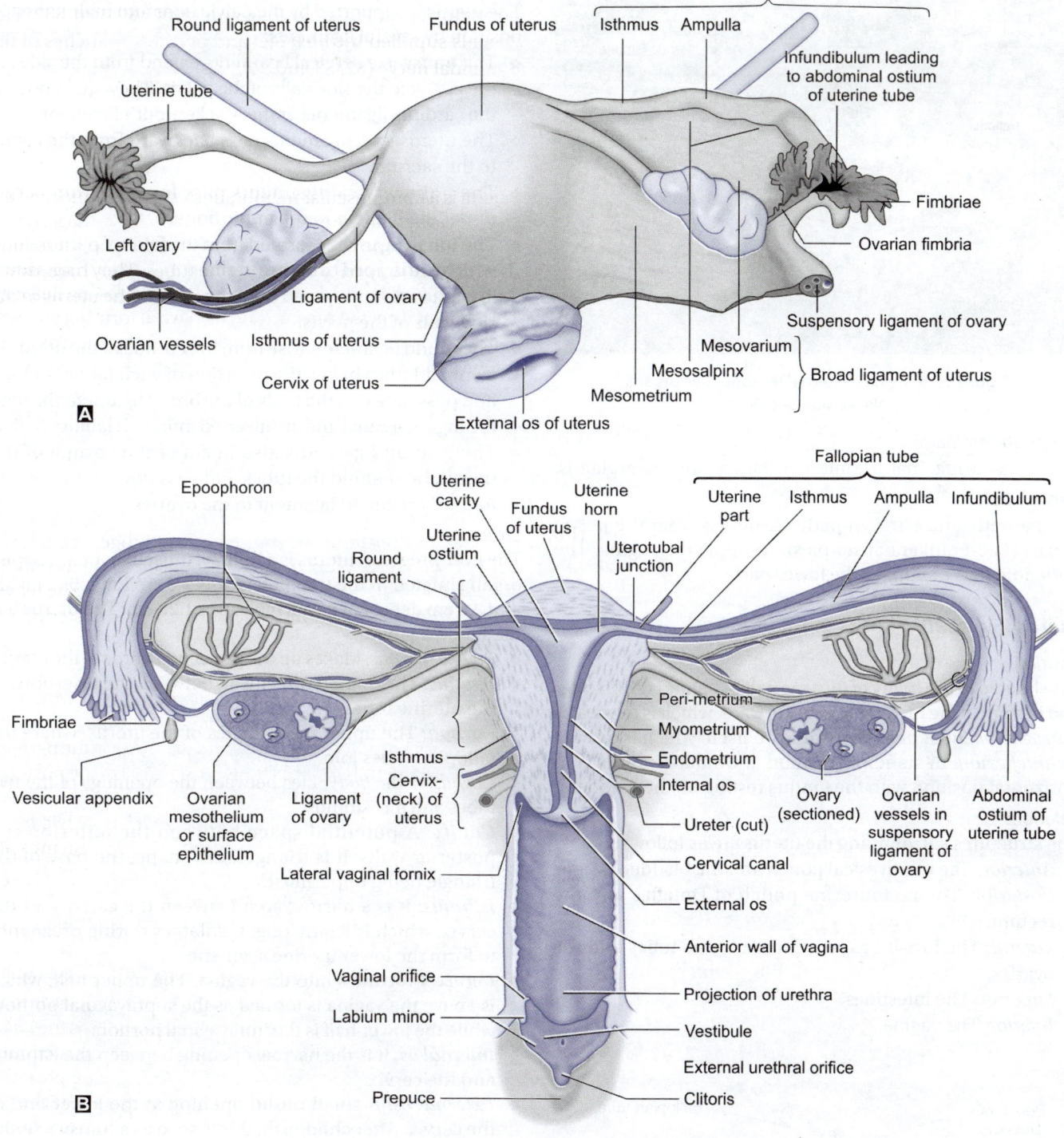

Figures 5.18A and B: Overview of female reproductive system.

Contents
There are no glands in the vagina. It is moistened by mucus from the cervix and a transudate, which seeps out from the blood vessels of the vaginal wall. The vaginal fluid is strongly acid (pH 4.5) due to the presence of lactic acid formed by the action of Doderlein's bacilli on glycogen found in the squamous epithelium of the lining. These bacilli are the normal inhabitants of the vagina. The acid deters the growth of pathogenic bacteria.

Blood supply
Blood supply comes from the branches of the internal iliac artery and includes the vaginal artery and a descending branch of the uterine artery. The blood drains through the corresponding veins.

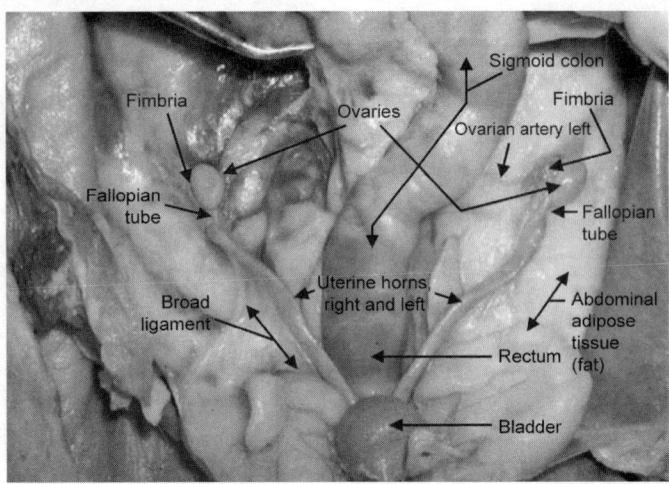

Figure 5.19: Female internal reproductive organs
(For color version, see Plate 1).

Lymphatic drainage
This is via the inguinal, the internal iliac and the sacral glands.

Nerve supply
Sympathetic and parasympathetic nerves from the pelvic plexus (Lee-Frankenhauser plexus) supply the vagina. The pudendal nerve supplies the lower part.

Uterus (Fig. 5.20)

Position
It is situated in the cavity of the true pelvis, behind the bladder and in front of the rectum. It leans forward, which is termed as *anteversion* and it bends forwards on itself, which is termed as *anteflexion*. In standing position, a woman's uterus is in horizontal position with the fundus resting on the bladder.

Relations
The structures surrounding the uterus are as follows:
- *Anterior*: The uterovesical pouch and the bladder.
- *Posterior*: The rectouterine pouch of Douglas and the rectum.
- *Lateral*: The broad ligaments, the uterine tubes and the ovaries.
- *Superior*: The intestines.
- *Inferior*: The vagina.

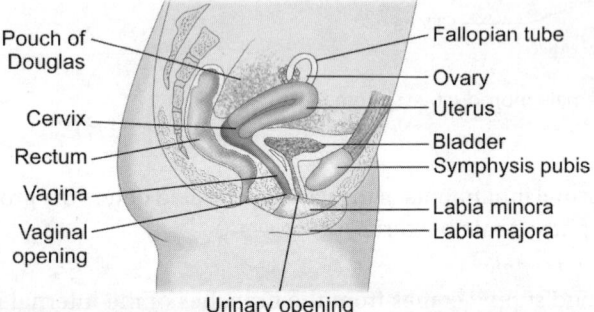

Figure 5.20: Sagittal section of the pelvis showing generative organs.

Supports
The uterus is supported by the pelvic floor and maintained in position by several ligaments:
- The transverse cervical ligaments extend from the sides of the cervix to the sidewalls of the pelvis. They are known as the cardinal ligaments or the Mackenrodt's ligaments.
- The uterosacral ligaments pass backward from the cervix to the sacrum.
- The pubocervical ligaments pass forward from cervix under the bladder to the pubic bones.
- The broad ligaments formed from the folds of peritoneum, which are draped over the uterine tubes. They hang down like a curtain and spread from the sides of the uterus to the sidewalls of the pelvis.
- The round ligaments arise from the cornua of the uterus in front and from below the insertion of each fallopian tube and pass between the folds of the broad ligament through the inguinal canal and are inserted into each labium majus.
- The ovarian ligaments also begin at the cornua of the uterus, but behind the tubes and pass down between the folds of the broad ligament to the ovaries.

Structure
The non-pregnant uterus is a hollow, muscular, pear-shaped organ situated in the true pelvis. It is 7.5 cm long, 5 cm wide and 2.5 cm deep. Each wall measures 1.25 cm. The uterus has the following parts:
- *Body or corpus:* Makes up the upper two thirds of the uterus.
- *Fundus:* The domed upper wall between the insertions of the uterine tubes.
- *Cornua:* The upper outer angles of the uterus, where the fallopian tubes join.
- *Corpus or the body:* Lies between the openings of the two tubes and the isthmus.
- *Cavity:* A potential space between the anterior and posterior walls. It is triangular in shape, the base of the triangle being uppermost.
- *Isthmus:* It is a narrow area between the cavity and the cervix, which is 7 mm long. It enlarges during pregnancy to form the lower uterine segment.
- *Cervix:* Protrudes into the vagina. The upper half, which is above the vagina is termed as the supravaginal portion, while the lower half is the infravaginal portion.
- *Internal os:* It is the narrow opening between the isthmus and the cervix.
- *External os:* A small round opening at the lower end of the cervix. After childbirth, this is seen as a transverse slit.
- *Cervical canal:* Lies between the internal os and external os. This canal is a continuation of the uterine cavity and is shaped like a spindle (slender pin), narrow at each end and wider in the middle.

Layers
The uterus has three layers of which the middle muscle layer is the thickest. The layers from inside outwards are endometrium, myometrium and perimetrium:
1. *Endometrium*: This forms a lining of ciliated epithelium (mucous membrane) on a base of

connective tissue or stroma. As there is no submucous layer, the endometrium is directly opposed to the muscle coat. In the uterine cavity, the endometrium is constantly changing in thickness through the menstrual cycle. The basal layer does not alter, but provides the foundation from which the upper layers regenerate. The surface epithelium is a single layer of ciliated columnar epithelium. The basal layer contains stromal cells, endometrial glands, vessels and nerves. The glands are simple tubular structures, which penetrate the stroma and sometimes even enter the muscle coat and secrete an alkaline muscle. The endometrium changes to decidua during pregnancy.

2. *Myometrium*: It consists of thick bundles of smooth muscle fibers held by connective tissues and are arranged in various directions. It is thick in the upper part of the uterus and is more sparse in the isthmus and cervix. Its fibers run in all directions and interface to surround the blood vessels and lymphatic, which pass to and from the endometrium. During pregnancy, however, three distinct layers can be identified as outer longitudinal, middle interlacing and the inner circular.

   In the cervix, the muscle fibers are embedded in collagen fibers, which enable it to stretch in labor.

3. *Perimetrium*: It is a double serous membrane, an extension to the peritoneum, which is draped over the uterus covering all, but a narrow strip on either side and the anterior wall of the supravaginal cervix from where it is deflected up over the bladder.

Blood supply

Blood supply to the organs is through the uterine artery and ovarian artery. The uterine artery is a branch of the internal iliac artery and enters at the level of the cervix. The ovarian artery is a branch of the abdominal aorta. It supplies the ovaries and uterine tubes. The blood drains through corresponding veins.

Lymphatic drainage

Lymph from the uterine body drains to the internal iliac glands and from the cervix to several other pelvic lymph glands. This provides an effective defense against uterine infection.

Nerve supply

This is mainly from the autonomic nervous system, the sympathetic and parasympathetic system via pelvic plexus.

Functions

The uterus serves to shelter the fetus during pregnancy. It prepares for this possibility each month. At the termination of pregnancy, it expels the uterine contents.

Uterine Tubes

Position

The uterine tubes or fallopian tubes extend laterally from the cornua of the uterus towards the sidewalls of the pelvis. They arch over the ovaries, the fringed ends hovering near the ovaries in order to receive the ovum. They are attached to the broad ligament by two layers of peritoneum called the mesosalpinx. Each tube is about 10–11.5 cm long.

Relations

- *Anterior, posterior and superior*: The peritoneal cavity and the intestines.
- *Lateral*: The sidewalls of the pelvis.
- *Inferior*: The broad ligaments and the ovaries.
- *Medial*: The uterus lies between the two uterine tubes.

Supports

The uterine tubes are held in place by their attachment to the uterus. The broad ligaments and the infundibulopelvic ligaments support them.

Structure

Length of each tube is 10 cm. The lumen of the tube provides a pathway to the peritoneal cavity. The uterine tube has four portions (**Fig. 5.21**):

1. *Interstitial portion*: It is 1.25 cm long and lies within the wall of the uterus. The lumen is 1 cm wide.
2. *Isthmus*: The narrow part that extends from the uterus and measures 2.5 cm.
3. *Ampulla*: The wider portion that is 5 cm long. Fertilization usually occurs in ampulla.
4. *Infundibulum*: The funnel shaped, fringed end of the tube, which is composed of many processes known as fimbriae. One fimbria is attached to the ovary.

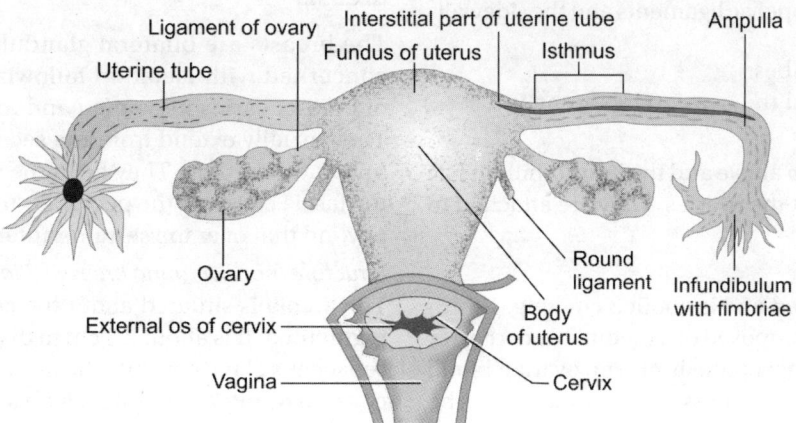

Figure 5.21: Uterus tubes and ovaries.

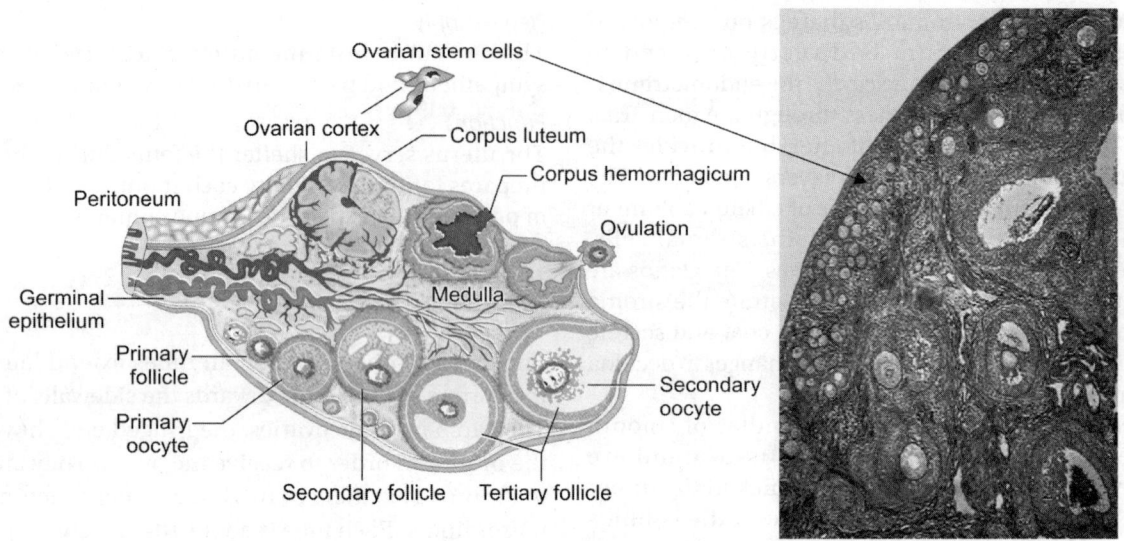

Figure 5.22: Schematic representation of human ovary.

5. *Intramural part*: It is 1 cm long and runs through the uterine wall.

Blood supply
This is via the uterine and ovarian arteries, returning by the corresponding veins.

Lymphatic drainage
This is to the lumbar glands.

Functions
The uterine tube propels the ovum towards the uterus, receives the spermatozoa as they travel upward and provide a site for fertilization.

Ovaries (Fig. 5.22)

Position
The ovaries or the female gonads are situated one on each side of the uterus and are attached to the back of the broad ligament within the peritoneal cavity (**Fig. 5.21**).

Relations
- *Anterior*: The broad ligaments.
- *Posterior*: The intestines.
- *Lateral*: The infundibulopelvic ligaments and the sidewalls of the pelvis.
- *Superior*: The uterine tubes.
- *Medial*: The uterus and the ovarian ligament.

Supports
The ovarian ligaments from above and the infundibulopelvic ligaments laterally support the ovaries. They are attached to the broad ligament.

Structure
The ovary is almond-shaped and is about 3 cm long, 1.5 cm wide and 1 cm thick. It is composed of a medulla and a cortex and is covered with germinal epithelium. The ovarian blood vessels, lymphatics and nerves pass through medulla. The hilum (opening), where the vessels enter the ovary is called the mesovarium. The cortex is the functioning part of the ovary. It contains the ovarian follicles in different stages of development surrounded by stroma (supporting framework of connective tissue). The outer layer is formed of fibrous tissue and is known as the tunica albuginea. Over this lies the germinal epithelium.

Blood supply
The blood supply is from the ovarian arteries and venous drainage through the ovarian veins. The right ovarian vein joins the inferior vena cava and the left returns its blood to the left renal vein.

Lymphatic drainage
This is to the lumbar glands.

Nerve supply
This comes from the ovarian plexus.

Functions
The ovaries produce ova and the hormones estrogen and progesterone.

Accessory Reproductive Organs

Breasts

The breasts are bilateral glandular structures, which are concerned with lactation following childbirth. The shape of breasts varies in women and in different periods of life. They usually extend from the second to the sixth rib in the midclavicular line. They lie in the subcutaneous tissue over the fascia covering the pectoralis major and in some women beyond that over the serratus anterior and external oblique.

Structure (non-lactating breasts) (Fig. 5.23)
The areola is situated about the center of the breast and is pigmented. It is about 2.5 cm in diameter and has numerous sebaceous glands over it. The nipple is a muscular projection covered by pigmented skin. It is vascular and surrounded by unstriped muscles that make it erectile. The nipple contains about 15–20 lactiferous ducts and their openings. The whole

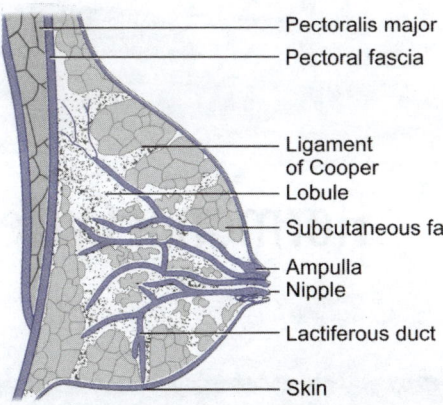

Figure 5.23: Structure of adult female breast.

breast is embedded in the subcutaneous fat. The fat is absent beneath the nipple and areola.

Each breast has 15–20 lobes, which are divided by fibrous tissue septa, which radiate from the center. The glandular tissue consists mainly of duct system and each lobe has a lactiferous duct. Each duct divides, subdivides and ultimately ends in alveoli, which number from 10 to 100. Each alveolus is lined by columnar epithelium, where milk secretion occurs. A network of longitudinal striated cells called myoepithelial cells surrounds the alveoli and smaller ducts. There is a dense network of capillaries surrounding the alveoli. Behind the nipple, the main duct (lactiferous duct) dilates to form ampulla, where the milk is stored in lactating mothers. The interlobular ducts eventually end in the openings in the nipples and muscle cells surround these ducts.

Blood supply
Blood supply to the breasts is from the branches of the internal mammary artery, the axillary artery and the intercostal arteries. Superficial veins of the breasts drain into the internal mammary veins. Veins emptying into internal mammary, axillary and intercostal veins serve deep breast tissue.

Nerve supply
The third and fourth branches of the cervical plexus provide the cutaneous nerve supply to the upper breast and thoracic intercostals nerves to the lower breast.

STUDY QUESTIONS

Short Notes

1. The ilium.
2. The sacrum.
3. The vestibule.
4. The clitoris.
5. Justo minor pelvis.

Short Answer Questions

1. The innominate bone.
2. Diameters of pelvic brim.
3. Pelvic outlet measurements.
4. The deformed pelvis.
5. Muscles of pelvic floor.

Essay Questions

1. Describe the types of pelvis and specifications of each.
2. Describe the position, relations and structure of uterus.
3. Describe the position, relations and structure of fallopian tubes.

BIBLIOGRAPHY

1. Bennett VR, Brown LK. Myles Textbook for Midwives, 13th edition. Edinburgh: Churchill Livingstone; 1999. pp. 939-95.
2. Fogel CI, Woods NF. Healthcare of Women: A Nursing Perspective. St Louis: The CV Mosby Company; 1981.
3. Marieb NE. Essentials of Human Anatomy and Physiology, 8th edition. New Delhi: Pearson Education Inc and Dorling kindersley Publishing House (P) Ltd; 2007. pp. 527-44.
4. Rutishauser S. Physiology and Anatomy: A Basis for Nursing and Health Care. Edinburgh: Churchill Livingstone; 1994.
5. Thibodeaux GA. Anatomy and Physiology. St Louis: Mosby; 1987.

CHAPTER 6

Hormonal Cycles

Learning Objectives

Upon completing of this chapter, the learner will be able to:
- Enumerate the development of Graafian follicle and ovulation.
- Describe the hormonal control of ovulation.
- Describe the endometrial changes during the different phases of menstruation.
- Explain the clinical aspects of menstruation and menopause.

The biological cycles in a woman are controlled by the hypothalamus. It governs the anterior pituitary gland by hormonal pathways. The anterior pituitary gland in turn governs the ovaries by hormones. The hormones, produced in the ovaries, control changes in the uterus. All the changes occur simultaneously and in harmony. A woman's mood may change along with the cycle and emotional influences can alter the cycle.

OVARIAN CYCLE

The ovarian cortex at birth contains about 200,000 primordial (rudimentary) follicles. From puberty onwards certain follicles enlarge and one matures each month to liberate an ovum. A mature ovarian follicle is called Graafian follicle.

Graafian Follicle (Figs. 6.1 and 6.2)

The ovum is situated at one end of the Graafian follicle and is encircled by the narrow perivitelline space. Surrounding this lies, a clump of cells called the discus proligerus, which radiate outward to form the corona radiata. The innermost cells of the corona are referred to as the zona pellucida. The whole follicle is lined with granulosa cells and contains follicular fluid. The outer coat of the follicle is the *external limiting membrane* and around this lies, an area of compressed ovarian stroma known as the theca.

Ovulation

The graafian follicle grows and matures to a size of 10–12 mm under the influence of follicle-stimulating hormone (FSH) and later luteinizing hormone (LH). It moves to the surface of the ovary and finally protrudes above it. At the same time it swells and becomes tense, finally ruptures to release the ovum into the fimbriated end of the fallopian tube, which is cupped beneath the ovary. This is ovulation and it occurs on day 14 of 28 days cycle or 14 days before menstruation in any cycle. A small loss of blood into the peritoneal cavity occurs at this time, which is termed as mittelschmerz. Some women feel pain at this time. The empty follicle is known as the corpus luteum (yellow body) **(Fig. 6.3)**.

Corpus Luteum

After ovulation, the follicle collapses. Over the next 14 days it goes through the stages of proliferation, vascularization, maturity and regression, and becomes an irregular yellow structure. If fertilization does not take place, the corpus luteum will atrophy and become the corpus albicans (white body), which is the corpus luteum of menstruation. If fertilization takes place, it develops into a corpus luteum of pregnancy due to a surge of hyperplasia. In the absence of pregnancy, the corpus albicans gets broken down into small hyaline masses, which ultimately get completely reabsorbed.

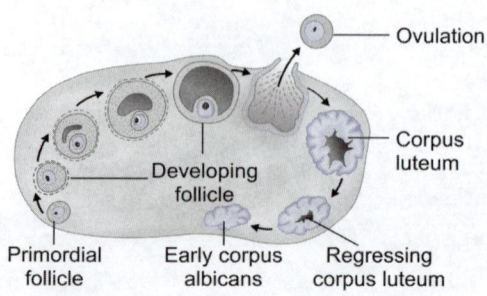

Figure 6.1: Lifecycle of a Graafian follicle.

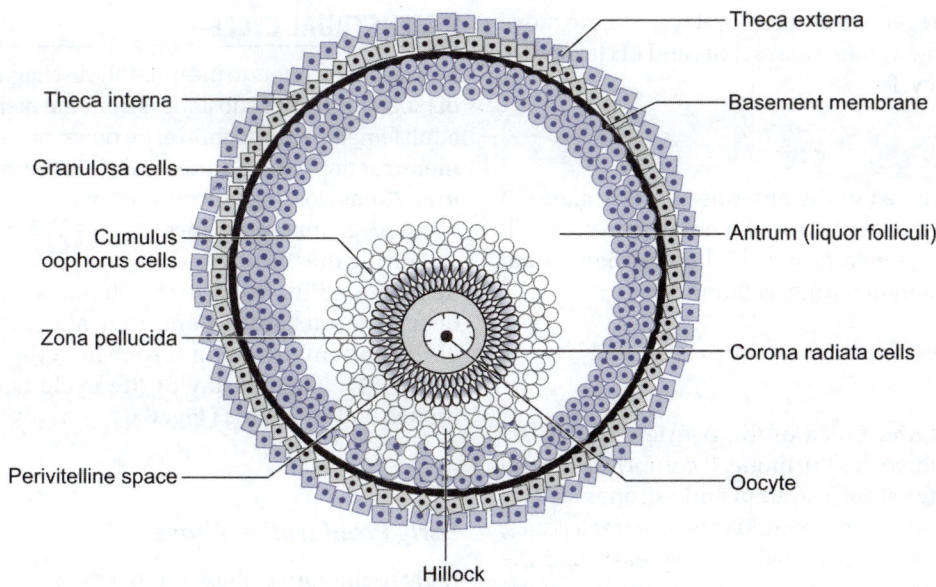

Figure 6.2: Graafian follicle.

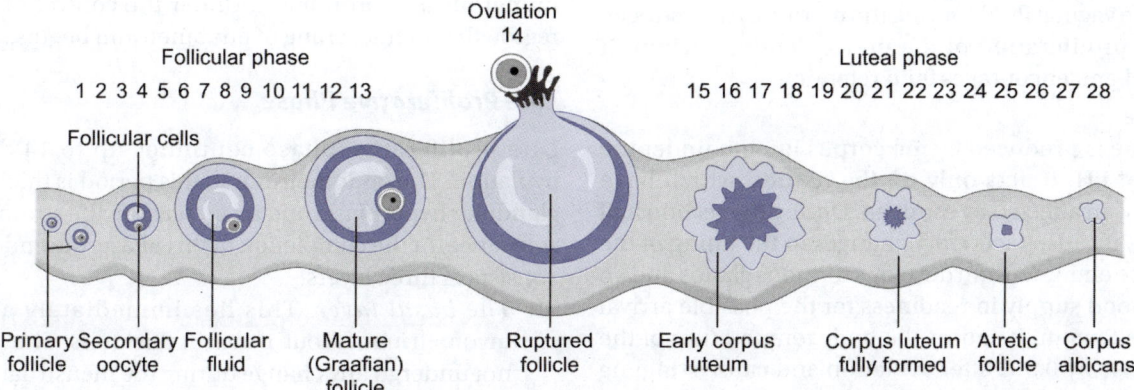

Figure 6.3: Representation of ovulation.

Hormonal Control (Fig. 6.4)

The hypothalamus synthesizes and releases gonadotropin-releasing hormone (GnRH). It reaches the pituitary through portal circulation and causes the release of FSH and LH. In other words, under the influence of GnRH, the pituitary releases FSH and LH, which are termed as gonadotropins. The gonadotropic activity of the hypothalamus and pituitary is influenced by positive and negative feedback mechanisms from the ovarian hormones.

Follicle-stimulating hormone causes Graafian follicles to develop and enlarge one of them more than all others each cycle. It stimulates the granulosa cells and theca to secrete estrogen. The level of FSH rises during the first half of the cycle and when the estrogen level reaches a certain point, its production ceases.

Luteinizing hormone production starts a few days after the anterior pituitary starts producing FSH. Rising estrogen causes a surge (an up rush) in both FSH and LH levels resulting in the rupture of a ripened follicle-ovulation. Levels of both gonadotropins then fall rapidly. If no pregnancy occurs,

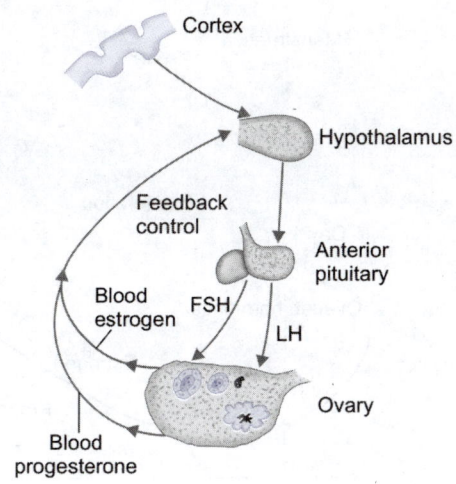

Figure 6.4: Hormonal control of ovulation and menstruation (FSH: follicle-stimulating hormone; LH: luteinizing hormone).

the corpus luteum degenerates after 14 days. The negative feedback effect of progesterone ceases; FSH and LH levels rise again to begin a new cycle.

Prolactin

The hormone is produced in the anterior pituitary gland. It does not play a role in the control of ovarian hormones. If produced in excessive amounts, it will inhibit ovulation that is the natural phenomenon during lactation.

Ovarian Hormones

Estrogen

The granulosa cells and theca of the ovaries, under the influence of FSH produce this hormone. It comprises several compounds including estriol, estradiol and estrone.

Estrogen is responsible for the secondary sex characteristics, such as the female shape, the growth of the breasts and the uterus, and the female distribution of hair. It influences the production of cervical mucus. This in turn encourages the growth of Doderlein's bacilli, which are responsible for the acidity of the vaginal fluid. During the uterine cycle, estrogen causes the proliferation of the uterine endometrium. It inhibits FSH and encourages fluid retention.

Progesterone

Progesterone is produced by the corpus luteum under the influence of LH. It acts only on the tissues, which have previously been affected by estrogen. During the second half of the cycle, it causes secretory changes in the lining of the uterus, as the endometrium develops tortuous glands and an enriched blood supply in readiness for the possible arrival of a fertilized ovum. It causes the body temperature of the woman to rise by 0.5°C after ovulation and causes tingling and a sense of fullness in the breasts prior to menstruation.

Relaxin

Relaxin is secreted in the corpus luteum and is at its maximum level, after 38 weeks of pregnancy. It relaxes the pelvic girdle, softens the cervix and suppresses uterine contractions.

MENSTRUAL CYCLE

Menstruation refers to the monthly discharge through the vagina of blood and other substances from the uterus in non-pregnant adult females. Although, every woman has an individual cycle of menstruation, which varies in length, the average cycle is taken to be 28 days long and recurs from puberty to menopause, except when pregnancy intervenes.

During the life of a woman, the endometrium is shed and degenerated no fewer than 400 times. The menstrual cycle occurs in four phases and they affect the tissue structure of the endometrium, in response to the ovarian hormones (**Fig. 6.5**). The 1st day of the cycle is the day on which menstruation begins (**Fig. 6.6**).

Phases

Early Proliferative Phase

Early proliferative phase follows menstruation and lasts up to 9 days (5–9 days). The endometrium is less than 2 cm thick. The glands are narrow and straight. The blood vessels are numerous and prominent. Under the control of estrogen, regrowth and thickening of endometrium begins.

Late Proliferative Phase

Late proliferative phase continues up to 14 days until ovulation. The endometrium in this period is thicker, due to glandular hyperplasia and an increase in the stromal ground substance. At the completion of this phase, the endometrium consists of three layers:

1. *The basal layer*: This lies immediately above the myometrium, about 1 mm in thickness. The layer does not undergo any change during the menstrual cycle and it contains the rudimentary structures for building up new endometrium.
2. *The functional layer*: This contains tubular glands of about 2.5 mm in thickness. The layer changes constantly according to the influences of ovarian hormone.

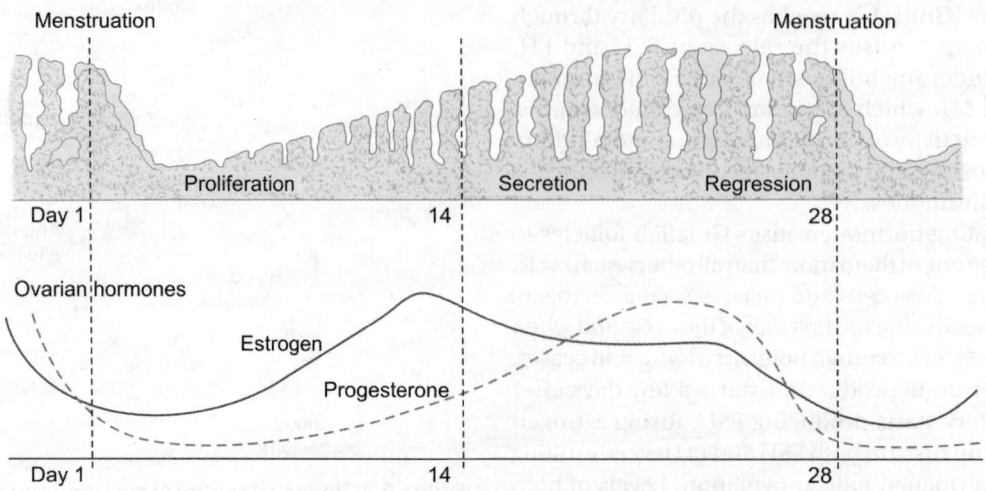

Figure 6.5: Endometrial changes related to ovulation and menstruation.

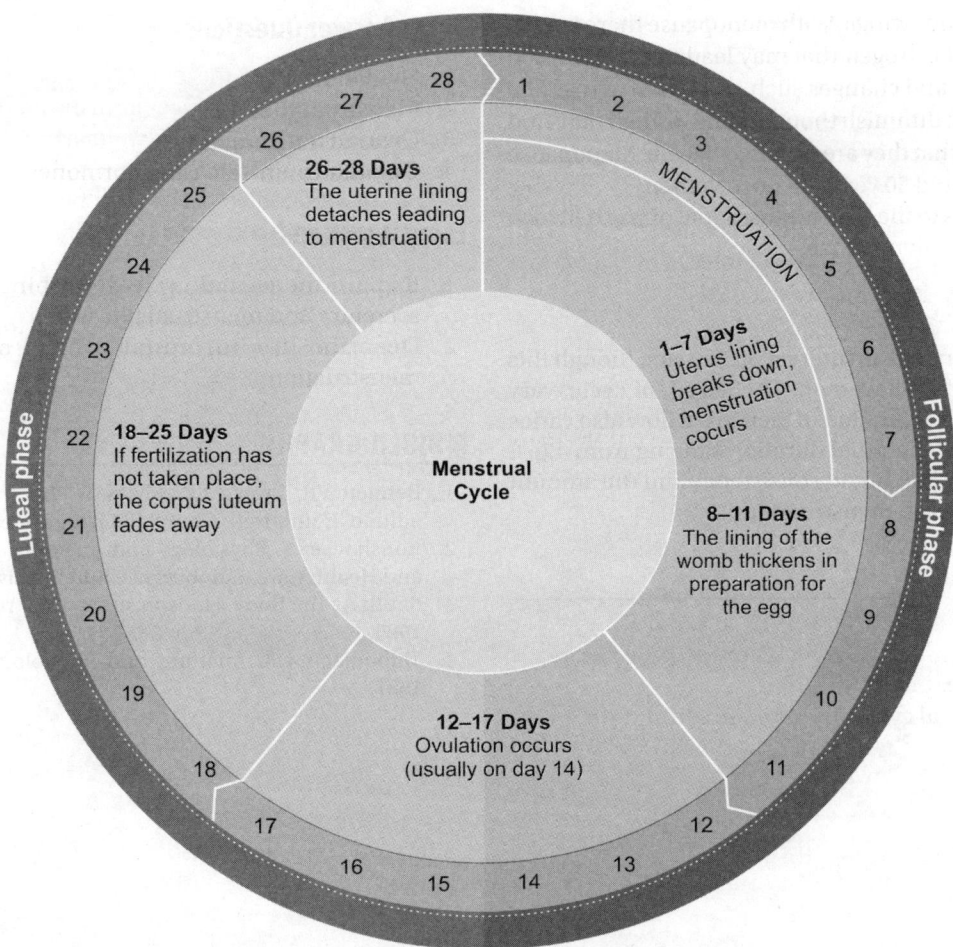

Figure 6.6: Overview of menstrual cycle.

3. *The spongy layer*: This has cuboidal ciliated epithelium and covers the functional layer.

Secretory Phase

Secretory phase follows ovulation and is under the influence of progesterone and estrogen from the corpus luteum. This phase lasts up to 26 days. The functional layer thickens to 3.5 mm and becomes spongy in appearance. The endometrium is extremely vascular and rich in glycogen in this phase. Spiral or coiled arteries develop, which become tortuous.

Premenstrual Phase

Premenstrual phase corresponds to the regression of the corpus luteum and declines in the levels of ovarian hormones and lasts from day 27 to 28.

Menstrual Phase

Menstrual phase is characterized by vaginal bleeding and lasts for 3–5 days. Physiologically, this is the last phase of the menstrual cycle. The endometrium is shed up to the basal layer along with blood from capillaries and the unfertilized ovum. Bleeding stops when the coiled arteries return to a state of constriction.

Clinical Aspects of Menstruation

Menarche and Puberty

Menarche is the first menstruation of a girl. It occurs at the age of 12 or 13 years, although it may occur as early as 10 years or as late as 16 years. Puberty refers to the period in life during which the reproductive organs develop and reach maturity, which is from childhood to sexual maturity. In females, the first signs are breast development and the appearance of pubic hair. The body grows considerably and takes on the female shape. Puberty culminates in the onset of menstruation. The first few cycles are not usually accompanied by ovulation.

Menopause and Climacteric

Menopause is the cessation of menses. Cessation of menstruation occurs gradually with the periods first becoming irregular and then stopping altogether marking the end of a woman's reproductive life. This is often accompanied by physical symptoms, such as hot flushes and emotional changes such as mood swings. With menopause there is a fall in the production of estrogen that may lead to an increased tendency to obesity and changes such as signs of aging. The sexual drive may not diminish though some women may find it difficult to accept that they are no longer fertile. Menopause occurs between 45 and 50 years in most women.

Climacteric refers to the entire transitional phase between sexual maturity and menopause.

Normal Menstrual Cycle

Menstrual cycles occur at an interval of 28 years, though this period is not same for all women. The length of cycle, vary from 22 to 35 days. The duration of menstrual flow also varies from 2 to 8 days with the usual duration ranging from 4 to 6 days. The blood flow is of liquid consistency and the amount about 25–60 mL for each menstruation.

STUDY QUESTIONS

Short Notes

1. Graafian follicle.
2. Normal menstrual cycle.
3. Prolactin.
4. Corpus luteum.
5. Menopause.

Short Answer Questions

1. Ovulation.
2. Menstruation.
3. Ovarian hormones.
4. Gonadotropin-releasing hormones.

Essay Questions

1. Explain menstrual cycle describing its proliferative, secretary and menstrual phases.
2. Describe the hormonal control of ovulation and menstruation.

BIBLIOGRAPHY

1. Bennett VR, Brown LK. Myles Textbook for Midwives, 13th edition. Edinburgh: Churchill Livingstone; 1999. pp. 963-72.
2. Rutishauser S. Physiology and Anatomy: A Basis for Nursing and Health Care. Edinburgh: Churchill Livingstone; 1994.
3. Smith A. The Body. Hudson street, New York: Penguin Books; 1985.
4. Thibodiacix GA. Anatomy and Physiology. St Louis: Mosby; 1987.

CHAPTER 7

Male Reproductive System

Learning Objectives

Upon completing this chapter, the learner will be able to:
- Name the different parts of the male reproductive system.
- Describe the process of spermatogenesis and sperm maturation.
- List and describe the male hormones.

PARTS OF MALE REPRODUCTIVE SYSTEM

The parts of male reproductive system are described in **Figure 7.1**.

Scrotum

The scrotum is a pouch of pigmented skin in which the testes are suspended outside the body. It lies below the symphysis pubis between the upper parts of the thighs behind the penis. It has two compartments, one for each testis (**Figs. 7.2 and 7.3**).

Testes

Testes are the male gonads (male reproductive gland) and produce spermatozoa and testosterone. Testosterone is the hormone responsible for the secondary sex characteristics. Along with the follicle-stimulating hormone (FSH), it promotes the production of sperm (**Fig. 7.4**).

In order to achieve their function, the testes must remain below body temperature and hence they are situated outside the body. Each testis is a rounded body measuring 4.5 cm long, 2.5 cm wide and 3 cm thick (**Figs. 7.5 and 7.6**).

It is composed of several layers of tissue:
- *Tunica vasculosa*: An inner layer of connective tissue containing a network of capillaries.
- *Tunica vaginalis*: The outer layer, which is made of peritoneum.
- *The seminiferous ('seed carrying') tubules*: The portion where spermatogenesis or production of sperms takes place. There are about three of them in each lobule. Between the tubules there are interstitial cells that secrete testosterone. The tubules join together to form a system of channels that lead to the epididymis.

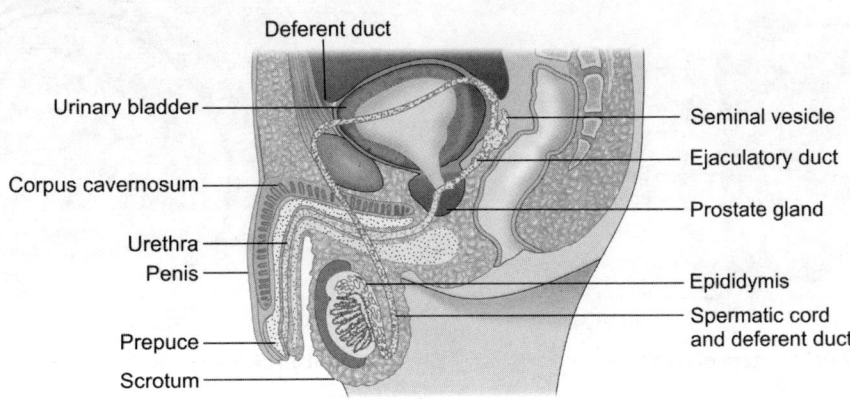

Figure 7.1: Male reproductive system.

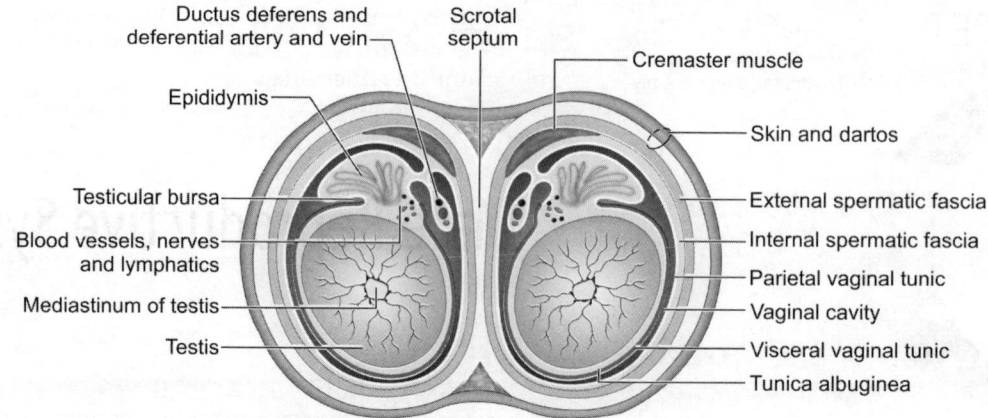

Figure 7.2: Cross-sectional overview of scrotum.

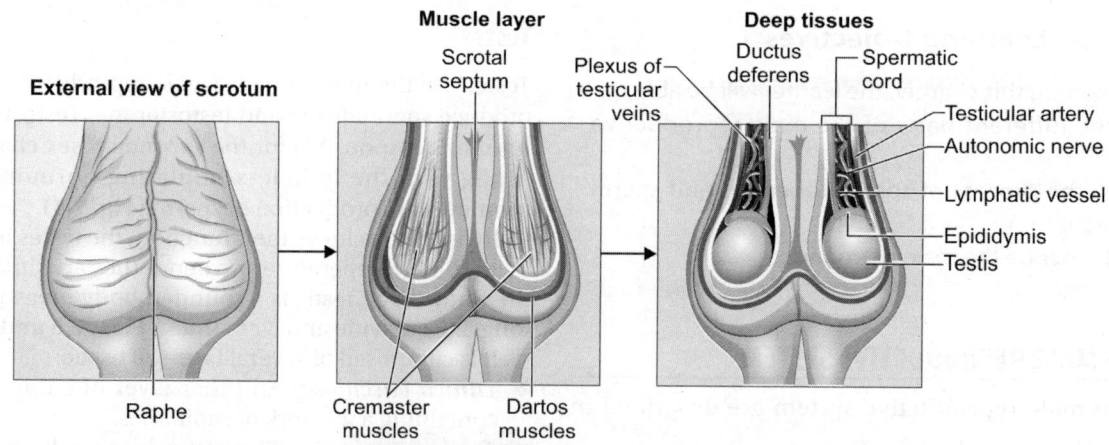

Figure 7.3: External view of scrotum.

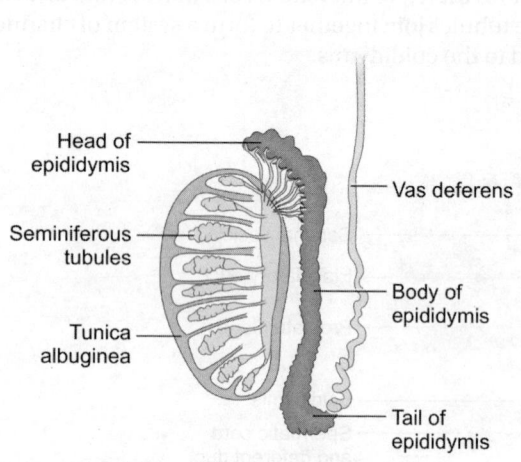

Figure 7.4: Structure of testis.

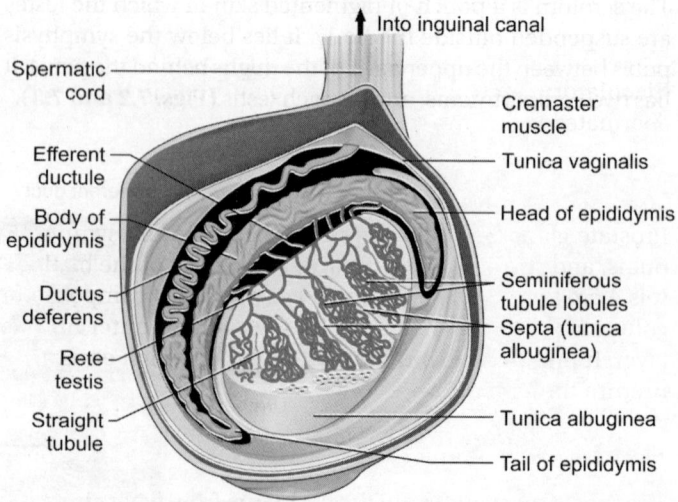

Figure 7.5: Various structure and layers comprising testis.

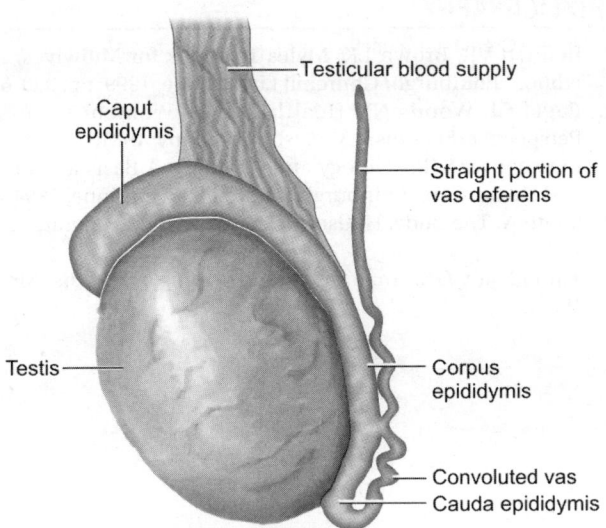

Figure 7.6: Anatomy of testis.

- *Epididymis*: A comma-shaped, coiled tube that lies on the superior surface and extends down the posterior aspect to the lower pole of testis, where it leads into the vas deferens or deferent duct.

Spermatic Cord

The spermatic cord consists of the vas deferens, the testicular blood vessels and nerves. It transmits the vas deferens with its blood vessels and nerves up into the body. The vas deferens carries the sperm to the ejaculatory duct. The cord passes upward through the inguinal canal from where the vas deferens continues upward over the symphysis pubis and arches backward beside the bladder. Behind the bladder, it merges with the duct from the seminal vesicle and passes through the prostate gland as the ejaculatory duct to join the urethra.

Ejaculatory Ducts

Ejaculatory ducts are small muscular ducts that carry the spermatozoa and the seminal fluid to the urethra.

Prostate Gland

Prostate gland lies between the rectum and the symphysis pubis, and surrounds the urethra at the base of the bladder. It is 4 cm long, 3 cm wide and 2 cm deep. It is composed of columnar epithelium, a muscle layer and an outer fibrous layer. It produces a thin lubricating fluid, which enters the urethra through ducts.

Penis

The root of the penis lies in the perineum from where it passes below the symphysis pubis. The lower two-third is outside the body in front of the scrotum.

It carries the urethra, which is a passage for both urine and semen. During sexual excitement it stiffens (an erection) in order to be able to penetrate the vagina and deposit the semen near the woman's cervix. There are three columns of erectile tissue; two are lateral columns called the corpora cavernosa, one on either side and in front of the urethra. The posterior column is termed corpus spongiosum contains the urethra. The posterior column is termed corpus spongiosum contains the urethra. The tip is expanded to form the glans penis.

The lower two-third of the penis is covered in skin. At the lower end the skin is folded back on itself above the glans penis to form the prepuce, which is a movable double fold. The penis is extremely vascular and during an erection the blood spaces fill and become distended.

MALE HORMONES

The hypothalamus produces gonadotropin-releasing factors. These stimulate the anterior pituitary gland to produce FSH and luteinizing hormone (LH). FSH acts on the seminiferous tubules to bring about the production of sperm, while LH acts on the interstitial cells that produce testosterone.

Testosterone is responsible for the secondary sex characteristics, namely deepening of the voice, growth of hair on the chest, pubis, axilla and face. The control of male hormones is similar to that of female except that it is not cyclical.

FORMATION OF THE SPERMATOZOA

Production of sperm begins at puberty and continues throughout the adult life. Spermatogenesis takes place in the seminiferous tubule under the influence of FSH and testosterone. The process of maturation requires few weeks. The mature sperm are stored in the epididymis and vas deferens until ejaculation. If ejaculation does not happen, they degenerate and get absorbed. At each ejaculation, 2–4 mL of semen is deposited in the vagina. The seminal fluid contains about 100 million sperm per mL of which 20–35% are likely to be abnormal. The normal sperm move at a speed of 2–3 mm per minute.

The individual spermatozoon (**Fig. 7.7**) has a head, a body and a long mobile tail that lashes (makes flicking movement) to propel the sperm along.

The tip of the head is covered by an acrosome, which contains enzymes to dissolve the covering of the ovum in order to penetrate it.

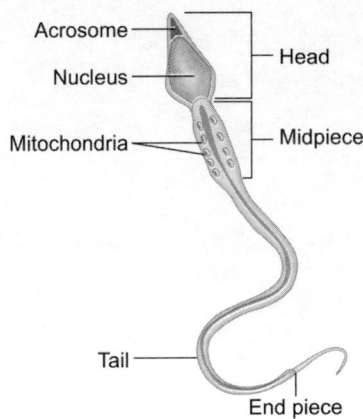

Figure 7.7: Parts of a sperm cell.

STUDY QUESTIONS

Short Notes

1. Ejaculatory ducts.
2. Scrotum.
3. Male hormones.

Short Answer Questions

1. Testes.
2. Spermatic cord.

Essay Question

1. Describe the formation of spermatozoa in the male.

BIBLIOGRAPHY

1. Bennett VR, Brown LK. Myles Textbook for Midwives, 13th edition. Edinburgh: Churchill Livingstone; 1999. pp. 939-61.
2. Fogel CI, Woods NF. Health Care of Women. A Nursing Perspective. St Louis: CV Mosby Company; 1981.
3. Rutishauser S. Physiology and Anatomy: A Basis for Nursing and Health Care. Edinburgh: Churchill Livingstone; 1994.
4. Smith A. The Body, Hudson street, New York: Penguin Books; 1985.
5. Thibodeaux GA. Anatomy and Physiology. St Louis: Mosby; 1987.

SECTION III

EMBRYOLOGY AND FETOLOGY

Section Outline

8. Fertilization, Implantation and Development of the Fertilized Ovum
9. Development of the Placenta and Fetus
10. Fetal Organs and Circulation
11. Fetal Skull

SECTION 3

EMBRYOLOGY AND FETOLOGY

CHAPTER 8

Fertilization, Implantation and Development of the Fertilized Ovum

Learning Objectives

Upon completing this chapter, the learner will be able to:
- Describe the process of fertilization and the development of the fertilized ovum.
- Describe the process of implantation and the postimplantation changes in the uterus.

FERTILIZATION

The ovum, which is about 0.15 mm in diameter, passes into the uterine tube and moves towards the uterus after ovulation. Transport of the ovum through the tube is brought about by the cilia and the peristaltic muscular contraction of the tube. At this time the cervix under the influence of estrogen, secrets a flow of alkaline mucus that attracts the spermatozoa. At an intercourse about 60–120 million sperm are deposited in the posterior fornix of the vagina. Those that reach the loose cervical mucus, survive to propel (drive forward) themselves towards the uterine tubes, while the remainder are destroyed by the acid medium of the vagina. During the journey through the uterus, more sperm die, only thousands reach the tube, where they meet the ovum usually in the ampulla. The sperm mature and become capable of releasing an enzyme called hyaluronidase, which allows penetration of the zona pellucida and the cell membrane surrounding the ovum. Many sperm are needed for this to take place, but only one will enter the ovum. After this, the membrane is sealed to prevent entry of any further sperm. The tail of the sperm is left behind. Nuclei of the two cells fuse resulting in the formation of a zygote. The sperm and ovum are known as the male and female gametes.

Neither the sperm nor the ovum can survive for longer than 2–3 days and hence fertilization is most likely to occur when intercourse takes place around the time of ovulation, within 48 hours prior to 24 hours following ovulation.

Development of Fertilized Ovum (Fig. 8.1)

The fertilized ovum (zygote) continues its passage through the fallopian tube and reaches the uterus in 3–4 days. During this time it undergoes segmentation or cell division to form *blastomeres*. The ovum divides into 2 cells, then 4, 8 and 16, and so on until a mulberry-like ball of cells is formed, known as the *morula*. The divisions occur quite slowly, about once in every 12 hours. Gradual accumulation of fluid in the morula results in the formation of the blastocyst. At one pole of the blastocyst there is a compact mass of cells, called the inner cell mass. Around the outside of it there is a single layer of cells, known as the trophoblast. The trophoblast will form the placenta and chorion, while the inner mass will become the fetus and the amnion. On its journey, the zygote is nourished by glycogen from the goblet cells of the uterine tubes and later the secretory glands of the uterus.

IMPLANTATION

When the blastocyst falls into the uterus, it lies free for 2–3 days. The part of the trophoblast that lies over the inner cell mass, then becomes quite sticky and adheres to the endometrium. It then begins to secrete enzymes that cause erosion of the epithelium (endometrial cells) allowing the blastocyst to sink into the endometrium. This is called embedding or nidation (nesting) and it normally is complete by the 11th day after ovulation. The endometrium closes over it completely and the only evidence of the presence of the blastocyst will be a small bulge on the surface **(Fig. 8.2)**. Implantation usually occurs on the posterior uterine wall, though it may sometimes occur on the anterior wall of the fundus.

Postimplantation Changes in the Uterus

Decidua is the name given to the uterine endometrium during pregnancy. It differs from the non-pregnant

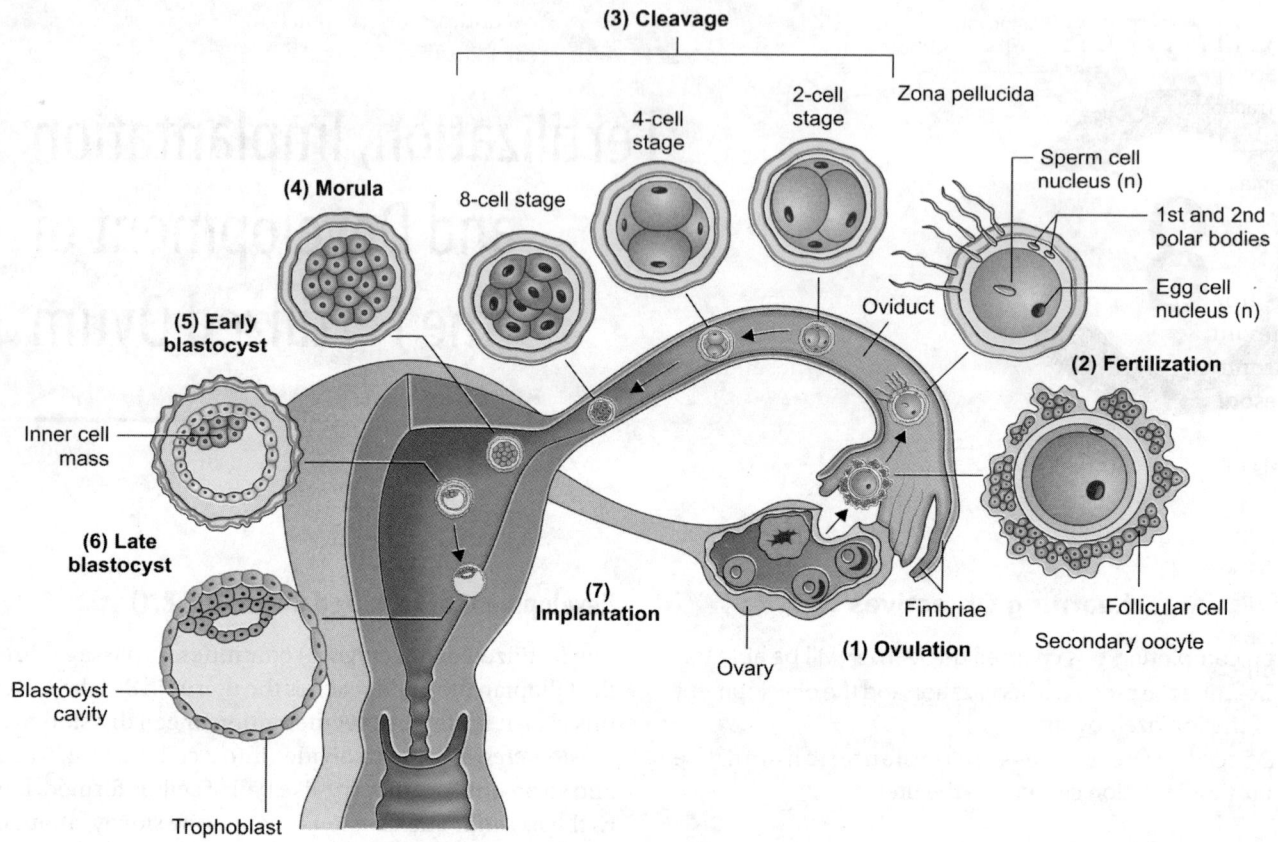

Figure 8.1: Development of fertilized ovum.

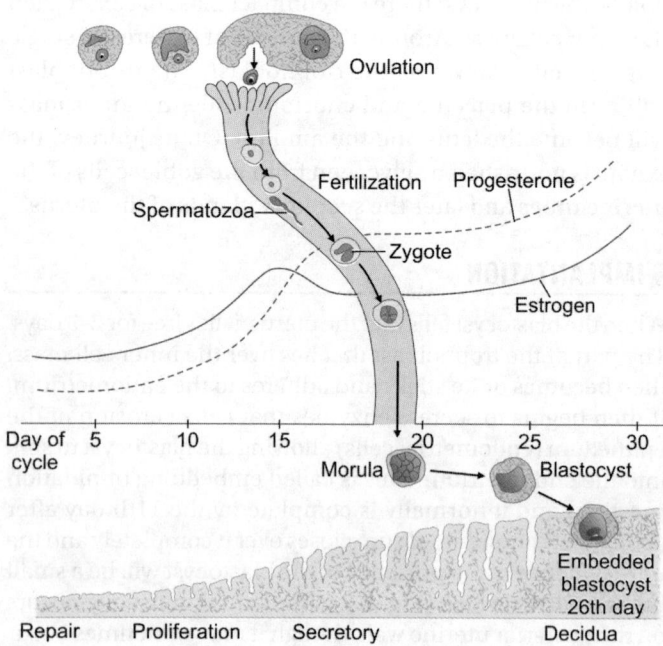

Figure 8.2: Fertilization and nidation.

endometrium because of the changes that undergoes in pregnancy. Increased secretion of estrogens causes the endometrium to grow four times of its original thickness. Progesterone from the corpus luteum stimulates the endometrial glands and increases the size of the blood vessels. It becomes a soft, vascular and spongy bed in which the fertilized ovum implants. With the exception of the zona basalis, the decidua is shed after birth giving meaning to the Latin origin of the word *deciduous* meaning 'a falling off'. There are three areas of decidua:

1. *Decidua basalis*: This is the decidua beneath the site of implantation of the embryo. It lies immediately above the myometrium and remains unchanged. This part of the decidua is the maternal contribution to the placenta. It regenerates to form the new endometrium during the puerperium.
2. *Decidua capsularis*: The decidua surrounding the remainder of the embryo that serves as a covering between the embryo and the uterine cavity. With fetal growth, the decidua capsularis bulges into the uterine cavity and fuses with the decidua parietalis. The uterine cavity is thus obliterated by the end of the 4th month.
3. *Decidua parietalis or decidua vera*: This is the decidua lining the rest of the uterine cavity.

DEVELOPMENT OF THE FERTILIZED OVUM (FIG. 8.3)

Trophoblast

Small projections begin to appear all over the surface of the trophoblast becoming most abundant at the area of contact.

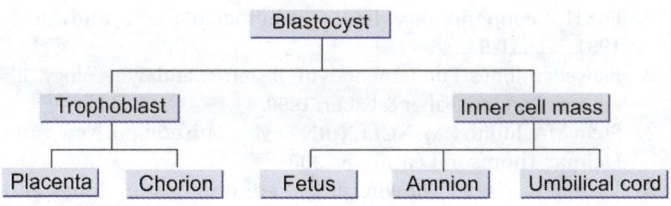

Figure 8.3: Development of the fertilized ovum.

These trophoblastic cells differentiate into three layers such as the outer syncytiotrophoblast (syncytium), the inner cytotrophoblast and below that the primitive mesenchyme or mesoderm.

The *syncytiotrophoblast* erodes the walls of the blood vessels of the decidua, to make the nutrients in the maternal blood accessible to the developing embryo.

The *cytotrophoblast*, which is a well-defined single layer of cells, produces a hormone known as human chorionic gonadotropin (hCG). This hormone is responsible for informing the corpus luteum that pregnancy has begun. As a result, corpus luteum continues to produce estrogen and progesterone. Progesterone maintains the integrity of the decidua so that menstruation does not occur. The high level of estrogen suppresses the production of follicle-stimulating hormone (FSH) stopping further follicle development in the ovary.

The *mesenchyme* develops to chorionic vesicle with its membrane called chorion. It condenses about the embryo to form the body stalk that connects the embryo to the nutrient chorion and forms the umbilical cord later on.

Inner Cell Mass

While the trophoblast develops to form the placenta, which will nourish the fetus, the inner cell mass develops to form the fetus itself. The cells differentiate into three layers, i.e. ectoderm, endoderm and mesoderm; each of which will form particular parts of the fetus (**Fig. 8.4**).

The *ectoderm* develops into the central and peripheral nervous systems and the epidermis with its appendages.

The *endoderm* forms the dermis, the skeleton, the connective tissue, vascular and the urogenital systems, and most skeletal and smooth muscles.

The *mesoderm* forms certain internal organs such as the heart and blood vessels, liver, pancreas, and also the bones and the muscles. The three layers together are termed as the embryonic plate. As the development continues, two cavities appear in the inner cell mass, one on either side of the embryonic plate. These are termed the *amniotic* cavity and the yolk sac.

The amniotic cavity is lies on the side of the ectoderm. It is filled with fluid and gradually enlarges to envelop the embryo. The amnion forms from its lining.

The yolk sac is lies on the side of the ectoderm and provides nourishment for the embryo until the trophoblast is sufficiently developed to take over. Part of it forms the primitive gut and remainder atrophies under the amnion on the surface of the placenta.

Embryo

The developing offspring is termed as embryo until 8 weeks after implantation. During this period all the organs and systems of the body are laid down in rudimentary form, which in further months grow and mature. After 8 weeks until term, the conceptus is known as fetus.

▎STUDY QUESTIONS

Short Notes

1. Fertilization.
2. Implantation.

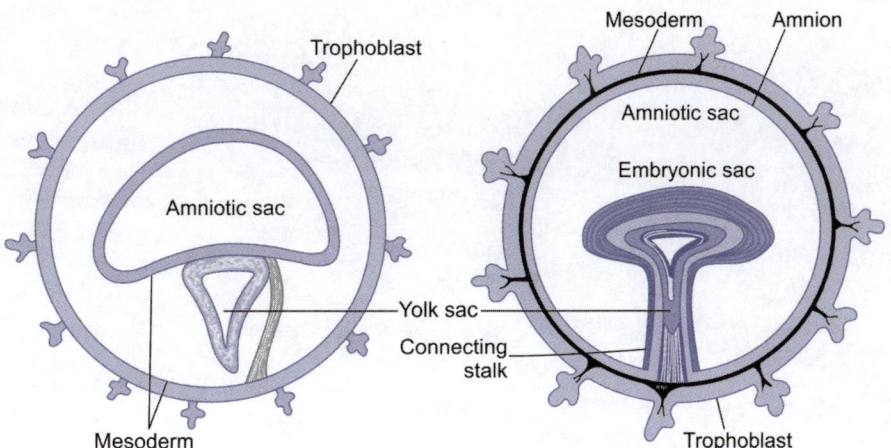

Figure 8.4: Development of the embryo.

Short Answer Questions

1. The trophoblast.
2. Postimplantation changes in the uterus.

Essay Question

1. Describe the development of the fertilized ovum.

BIBLIOGRAPHY

1. Bennett VR, Brown LK. Myles Textbook for Midwives, 13th edition. Edinburgh: Churchill Livingstone; 1999. pp. 963-80.
2. Fox H. A contemporary view of the human placenta. Midwifery; 1991:7(1):31-9.
3. Llewellyn-Jones. Fundamentals of Obstetrics and Gynecology, 5th edition. London: Faber & Faber; 1990.
4. Stein MA, Judith CM. NCLEX-RN Review, 4th edition. New York: Delmar Thomson Learning; 2000.
5. Varney H. Nurse Midwifery, 2nd edition. Boston: Jones and Bartlett Publishers; 1999.pp. 93-111.

CHAPTER 9

Development of the Placenta and Fetus

Learning Objectives

Upon completing this chapter, the learner will be able to:
- Enumerate the developmental stages of the fertilized ovum
- Describe the development of the placenta and circulation through the placenta
- List the functions, variations, anomalies and abnormalities of placenta.

The placenta is partly fetal and partly maternal in origin. It connects closely with the mother's circulation to carry out functions, which the fetus is unable to perform for itself during intrauterine life. The survival of the fetus depends on the integrity and efficiency of the placenta.

DEVELOPMENT OF THE PLACENTA (FIG. 9.1)

The small projections that appear on the trophoblastic layer of the blastocyst proliferate (grow by multiplication) and branch from about 3 weeks after fertilization, forming the chorionic villi. The villi become most profuse in the area where the blood supply is richest, i.e. in the basal decidua. This part of the trophoblast is known as the chorion frondosum. It will eventually develop into the placenta.

The villi under the capsular decidua get less nourishment and gradually atrophy and form the chorion laeve or bald chorion, which is the origin of the chorionic membrane.

The villi erode the walls of maternal blood vessels as they penetrate decidua, opening them up to form a lake of maternal blood in which they float. The opened blood vessels are known as sinuses and the area surrounding the villi as blood spaces. Maternal blood circulates slowly in these vessels, enabling the villi to absorb food and oxygen, and to excrete waste. A few villi are attached more deeply to the decidua and are called the anchoring villi. Placental circulation is established by the 17th day.

Each chorionic villus is a branching structure. Its center consists of mesoderm and branches of umbilical vein and artery. Four layers of tissue separate the maternal blood from the fetal blood making it impossible for the two circulations (maternal and fetal) to mix unless the villi are damaged **(Fig. 9.2)**.

The placenta is completely developed and functioning from the 10th week after gestation. In its early stages, it is a relatively loose structure, but becomes more compact as it matures. Between 12 and 20 weeks of gestation, the placenta weighs more than the fetus. At this stage the fetal organs are insufficiently developed to cope with the metabolic processes of nutrition. Later in pregnancy as the fetus matures some of the fetal organs, such as liver begin to function resulting in easier exchange of oxygen and carbon dioxide.

Each main stem villus and its branches form a cotyledon. The total number of cotyledons remains constant, but the individual cotyledons continue to grow until term.

CIRCULATION THROUGH THE PLACENTA (FIG. 9.3)

Fetal blood that is low in oxygen is pumped by the fetal heart towards the placenta along their branches to the capillaries of the villi. The blood returns to the fetus via umbilical vein after giving up carbon dioxide and absorbing oxygen.

Maternal blood is delivered to the placental bed in the decidua by the spiral arteries that flow into the blood spaces

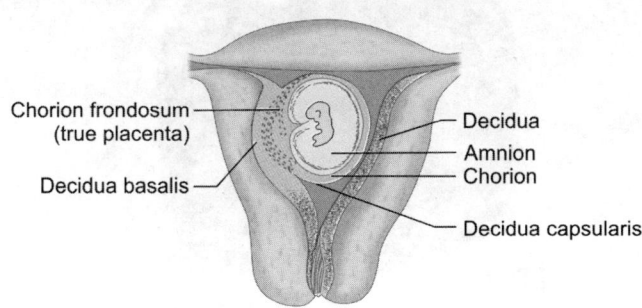

Figure 9.1: Development of placenta.

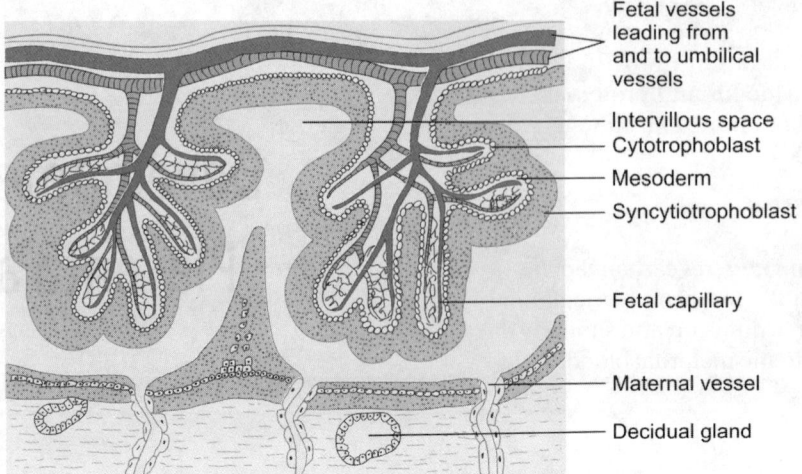

Figure 9.2: Diagrammatic representation of the chorionic villi.

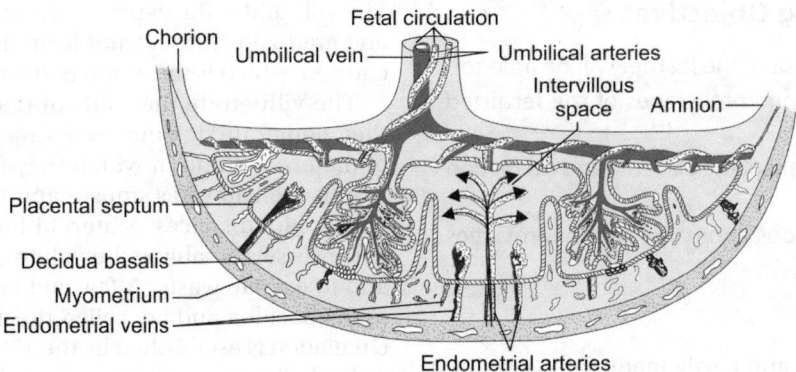

Figure 9.3: Placental circulation.

surrounding the villi. The blood enters the sinuses in a funnel-shaped stream similar to a fountain and as it passes upwards, bathes the villus and drains back into a branch of uterine vein.

MATURE PLACENTA

The normal term placenta is a flattened disk-like mass with a circular or oval outline. Its average volume is 500 mL and ranges from 200 to 900 mL. Average weight of the placenta is 500 g and the range is 200–800 g. It often weighs approximately one-sixth of the baby's weight at term. Average diameter is 20 cm and thickness is 2.5 cm.

The fetal surface of the placenta is smooth, shiny and transparent. The underlying chorion can be seen through it. The umbilical cord is attached to the fetal surface near the center and branches of the umbilical vessels radiate out under the amnion at this point, the veins being larger and deeper than the arteries. The amnion can be peeled off the surface leaving the chorionic plate **(Fig. 9.4A)**.

The maternal surface is finely granular and divided into 15–30 lobes (average 20) that are called cotyledons by a series of fissures or furrows termed as sulci. The lobes are made up of lobules, each of which contains a single villus with its branches **(Fig. 9.4B)**.

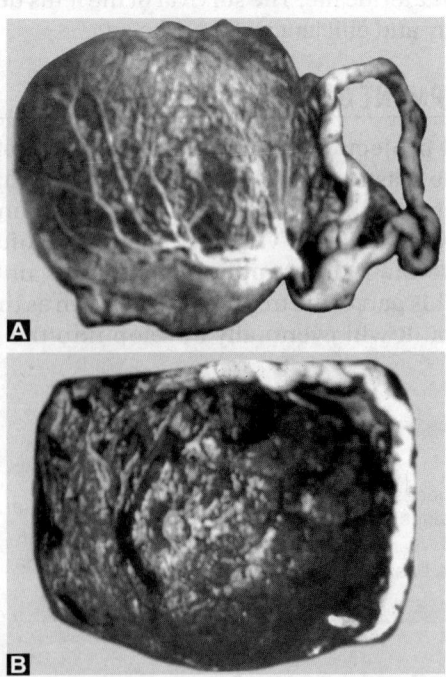

Figures 9.4A and B: Placenta at term. (A) Fetal surface of the placenta; (B) Maternal surface of the placenta (*For color version, see Plate 1*).

FUNCTIONS OF THE PLACENTA

The placenta truly is an organ of life with a number of functions designed to provide for and protect the fetus. Its functions include respiration, nutrition, storage, protection and endocrine.

Respiration

The fetus obtains oxygen and excretes carbon dioxide through the placenta. Oxygen from the mother's hemoglobin passes into the fetal blood by simple diffusion and similarly the fetus gives off carbon dioxide into the maternal blood.

Nutrition

The fetus requires all the nutrients like anyone. Amino acids, glucose, vitamins, minerals, lipids, water and electrolytes are transferred across the placental membrane. Food from the maternal diet gets broken down into simpler forms by the time it reaches the placental site. The placenta selects those substances required by the fetus. It can breakdown complex nutrients into compounds that can be used by the fetus. Protein gets transferred as amino acids; carbohydrates as glucose and fats as fatty acids.

Storage

The placenta stores glucose, iron and vitamins. Glucose stored in the form of glycogen gets reconverted to glucose when required.

Excretion

Carbon dioxide is the major substance excreted from the fetus. Other substances include bilirubin from the breakdown of red blood cells and small amounts of urea and uric acid.

Protection

The placental membrane has a limited barrier function. Certain antibodies which the mother possesses gets passed on to the fetus to provide immunity for the baby for 3 months after birth. Certain viruses such as the rubella virus and bacteria such as *Treponema Pallidum* of syphilis and *Mycobacterium* of tuberculosis also cross the barrier. Most drugs given to mother also cross the barrier and reach the baby. However, most bacteria and certain drugs do not cross the barrier. It is important for the midwife to know which substances cross or does not cross the placental membrane.

Endocrine

The cytotrophoblastic layer of the chorionic villi produces human chorionic gonadotropin (hCG). It is present in large quantities between the 7th and 10th week when the production is at its peak and then gradually decreases as the pregnancy advances. In many pregnancy tests, hCG forms the basis as it is excreted in the mother's urine. Estrogens are produced by placenta in the large amount throughout pregnancy. The amount of estrogen produced is an index of fetoplacental well-being.

Progesterone is produced in the syncytial layer of the placenta in increasing quantities until immediately before the onset of labor, when its level falls.

Human placental lactogen (HPL) is another hormone produced by the placenta. It is involved in lactogenic and metabolic processes in pregnancy. The production of HPL increases as the level of hCG falls and continues throughout pregnancy.

Mechanisms for Transfer of Materials

As an organ of transfer, the placenta has several mechanisms by which to transfer materials between the maternal and fetal circulations in the intervillous space across the placental membrane. These include the following:

- *Diffusion:* The transfer of substances across a membrane from an area of higher concentration to an area of lower concentration. Low-molecular-weight substances diffuse readily across the placental membrane. Substances concerned with biochemical homeostasis are transferred by diffusion, e.g. water, oxygen, carbon dioxide, urea and certain simple amines.
- *Active transport:* This transfer is against usual physiological principles. It includes the transfer of substances, which are in low concentration in the maternal blood and in high concentration in the fetal blood. It is a metabolic process requiring energy and enzymatic transfer systems. The transport of iron and ascorbic acid from the mother to the fetus are examples.
- *Pinocytosis or phagocytosis:* A substance is taken and moved across the cells of the fetal membrane to the fetal bloodstream by invaginations (infoldings) of the chorionic villi simply engulfing the material. Large protein molecules with a higher molecular weight, such as immune gamma globulin G, are thought to be taking place by this mechanism. The direction of cellular transfer may depend on such factors as whether the mother is erect or supine.
- *Breaks between cells:* A break in the chorionic villi allows for the direct transfer of cells. An example of this is the sensitization of an rhesus negative (Rh negative) woman from the receipt of erythrocytes from her Rh-positive fetus.
- *Placental infection:* Conditions in which the placenta is infected and the lesions in the placenta caused by the infectious organisms serve as a means of access into the fetal bloodstream. Protozoal and bacterial infections are transferred this way. Viral infections may pass through the placental membrane and infect the fetus without infecting the placenta.

AMNIOTIC FLUID

Amniotic fluid, also termed as liquor amnii, is the fluid, which distends the amniotic sac and allows for the growth and free movement of the fetus. It equalizes pressure and protects the fetus from jarring (sudden vibrations) and injury. The fluid maintains a constant temperature for the fetus and provides small amounts of nutrients. In labor, it aids effacement of cervix and dilation of the os. As long as the membranes remain intact, the amniotic fluid protects the placenta and umbilical cord from pressure of uterine contractions.

Constituents

Amniotic fluid is a clear, pale straw-colored fluid, consisting of 99% water. The remaining 1% is dissolved in solid matter including food substances and waste products. It contains fetal urine, respiratory tract secretions and skin cells shed by the fetus, vernix caseosa and lanugo.

Source

Amniotic fluid comes from both maternal and fetal sources. Some fluid is exuded from maternal vessels in the decidua and some from fetal vessels in the placenta. It is also secreted by the amnion and umbilical cord. Fetal urine also contributes to the volume from the 10th week of gestation.

Volume

The volume of amniotic fluid increases throughout pregnancy. At 38 weeks, it is about 1 liter (1,000 mL). Then it diminishes slightly and at term the amount is about 800 mL. If the total amount exceeds 1,500 mL, the condition is termed as polyhydramnios (often referred to as hydramnios) and if less than 300 mL, the term oligohydramnios is used. Such abnormalities are often associated with congenital malformation of the fetus. As the normal fetus swallows amniotic fluid, conditions which interfere with swallowing increases the amount of fluid. Similarly, the normal fetus passes urine and when urine production is affected due to congenital problems, amount of liquor tends to be less.

UMBILICAL CORD (FIG. 9.5)

The umbilical cord or funis extends from the fetus to the placenta. It transmits the umbilical blood vessels, which are two arteries and one vein.

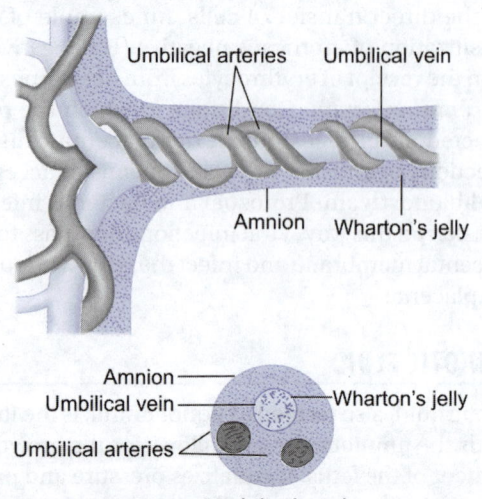

Figure 9.5: Umbilical cord.

These are enclosed and protected by a gelatinous substance known as Wharton's jelly. The whole cord is covered in a layer of amnion continuous with that covering the placenta.

The length of the average cord is 50 cm. A cord is considered to be short when its length is less than 40 cm. Certain cords are longer and with longer cords, problems can arise. It may become wrapped round the neck or body of the fetus or become knotted. A true knot occurs when the fetus has passed through a loop in the cord and a real knot has been created. False knotting of the cord occurs when the cord appears to be knotted, but instead has kinking of the blood vessels within the cord or accumulation of lumps of Wharton's jelly on the side of the cord. True knotting is most likely to occur in one of two situations:

1. *Small fetus, long cord and large amount of amniotic fluid:* The higher ratio of amniotic fluid to fetal size in early pregnancy makes this the time of greatest incidence. These knots are usually benign because they are kept from tightening by pulsations in the blood vessels. However, with true knots there is possibility of occlusion of blood vessels during labor.
2. *Multiple gestation within a single amnion:* All sorts of cord entanglements and knots are possible because the fetuses have greater freedom of movement within the fetal sac, thereby increasing the chance of knot forming and its tightening.

VARIATIONS, ANOMALIES AND ABNORMALITIES OF PLACENTA

1. Larger and heavier than normal placentas are seen with excessively large fetuses, fetal syphilis and erythroblastosis.
2. Smaller and lighter than normal placentas may occur with general systemic diseases or local uterine conditions, which cause undernourishment of the placenta and resultant intrauterine growth retardation.
3. The color of placental tissue is markedly lighter. This condition may be caused by fetal anemia, such as those found in erythroblastosis.
4. *Excessive infarct formation:* Infarction of cotyledons happen due to disease processes, such as severe maternal hypertension, severe preeclampsia or eclampsia. Extensive infracting reduces effective placental functioning, which may result in intrauterine growth retardation or if a substantial portion of the placenta is infarcted, may result in fetal death.
5. *Edema of the placenta:* Edematous placenta is mushy, thick and pale, and fluid can be squeezed from it. This may be caused by severe maternal heart disease, diabetes or nephritis and by severe erythroblastosis. The fetus usually dies in utero either as a stillbirth or earlier as an abortion.
6. Tumors are found in association with prematurity and polyhydramnios. Perinatal mortality and maternal hemorrhage are both increased.
7. *Syphilitic placenta:* It is abnormally large, pale and yellow-gray placenta.

8. *Succenturiate placenta or placenta succenturiata (Fig. 9.6):* One or more separate accessory lobes in the membranes, a variable distance away from the main placental mass. These accessory lobes are usually connected to the main placental mass.

    The primary significance of this anomaly lies in the possibility that the succenturiate lobe(s) will be retained in the uterus after expulsion of the main placental mass. Retained succenturiate lobes may cause severe postpartum hemorrhage. The retention of succenturiate lobes can be detected during inspection of the placenta and membranes by noting:
    a. Torn blood vessels at the margin of the placenta or extension of blood vessels into the membranes.
    b. Rough or torn roundish defects, or holes in the membranes at a short distance from the placenta. The midwife must examine every placenta for evidence of a retained lobe. Manual exploration of the uterus and removal of the succenturiate lobe(s) is indicated if retention has occurred.
9. *Extrachorial placenta:* A placental anomaly observed on the fetal surface as a thick white ring, which gives the impression that the central portion is somewhat depressed.

    There are two varieties of extrachorial placenta, which are determined by the location of the ring. Both may be complete or incomplete as dictated by whether or not the ring circumscribes a full circle:
    a. *Placenta circumvallata or circumvallate placenta:* The ring situated at a variable distance between the margin and center of the placenta. A double fold of both chorion and amnion, with fibrin and degenerated decidua forms the ring giving it a raised appearance **(Fig. 9.7)**.
    b. *Placenta marginata or circummarginate placenta:* The ring is located at the edge or margin of the placenta and is raised by the presence of degenerated decidua and fibrin.
10. *Lobulated placenta:* There appears to be multiple placentas for a single baby. In fact, it is one placenta divided into two or more parts either completely separated or joined in part. Either way, the lobes are held together by the one set of membranes and blood vessels. The number of lobes determines the name as bipartite placenta [placenta duplex **(Fig. 9.8)**] or tripartite placenta (placenta triplex). This anomaly is thought to be due to abnormalities in the blood supply to the decidua. Its main significance is that the midwife must be alert to make sure that all lobes have been expelled from the uterus.

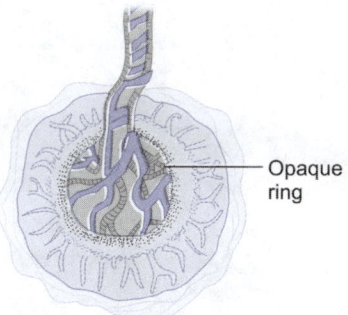

Figure 9.7: Circumvallate placenta.

VARIATIONS, ANOMALIES AND ABNORMALITIES OF THE UMBILICAL CORD AND ITS INSERTION

1. *Battledore placenta:* A variation in which the umbilical cord is inserted at the edge or margin of the placenta **(Fig. 9.9)**. Marginal insertion of the cord occurs in less than 10% of placentas and it is considered a normal insertion.
2. *Velamentous insertion:* The cord is inserted into the membranes at some distance from the edge of the placenta **(Fig. 9.10)**. The umbilical vessels from the cord run through the membranes for a variable distance before each enters the placenta. Velamentous insertion occurs approximately 1% of the time with an increased incidence in the event of multiple gestations.

    A velamentous insertion can be dangerous for the fetus. Rupture of the membranes may also rupture a fetal blood vessel because their portion is flimsy since they are covered only with amnion. A ruptured vessel may cause hemorrhage and exsanguination (without blood) of the fetus.

    A velamentous insertion when noticed upon inspection of the placenta after its delivery, a disaster might have already happened. In such cases, noting the anomaly would be of diagnostic value.

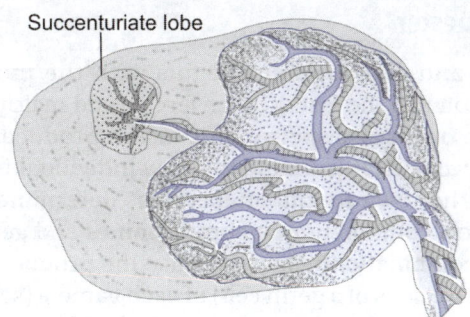

Figure 9.6: Succenturiate lobe of placenta.

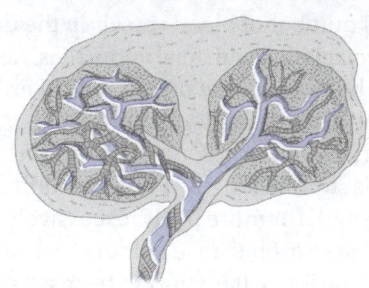

Figure 9.8: Bipartite placenta.

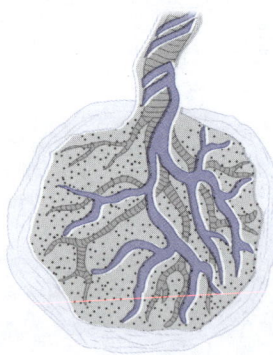

Figure 9.9: Battledore insertion of the cord.

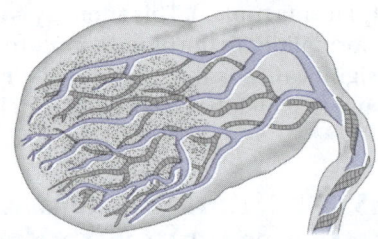

Figure 9.10: Velamentous insertion of the cord.

3. *Vasa previa:* It is a dangerous anomaly with a high perinatal mortality, if rupture occurs. Vasa previa refers to blood vessels, covered only with amnion and running between the chorion and amnion, which present first at the cervical os by crossing it ahead of the fetal presenting part. With fetal descent and rupture of the membranes, the vessels are subject to compression and rupture with resulting exsanguinations and anoxia of fetus.

   Vasa previa occurs in conjunction with a velamentous insertion of the cord. Vasa previa may also occur when there is a succenturiate placenta, since the vascular connections to the succenturiate lobe are also unprotected vessels coursing between the chorion and amnion.

   Vasa previa is extremely rare. However, it should be thought of as a possibility when the midwife is not sure of what is felt at the cervical os on vaginal examination. Examination should include feeling for pulsations synchronous (coinciding) with the fetal heart, in questionable presenting part.

4. Abnormal number of blood vessels in the umbilical cord has high correlation with fetal anomalies. About one third of babies born with only one umbilical artery will have multiple and severe malformations.

5. *Short cord (relative or absolute):* An absolute short cord is one, that is short in length. A relative short cord is one of average length (or more likely, excessively long), which has become short because of looping around the body or neck of the fetus. It is short in terms of reaching from its placental insertion to the umbilicus of the newborn, outside the maternal vulva as is necessary for normal delivery. A short cord may be a causative factor in failure of the fetus to descend. In such an event it might additionally cause abruptio placentae, umbilical hernia, fetal distress, rupture of the cord, shoulder dystocia or a combination of these. Recognition of a short cord usually does not take place until there is evidence of a problem. Therefore, it should be considered as a possibility whenever descent does not take place in the presence of an adequate pelvis and good contractions. Fetal distress in such situations compounds the urgency for action.

6. *Excessively long cord:* Long cords are more common than short cords. Generally it has no significance. However, a long cord becomes looped around the fetal body or neck causing a relative short cord. It can also become knotted or prolapsed in front of the presenting part.

7. *Cord looping:* The average length of a cord is 50–55 cm. Cords longer than 100 cm will become looped. Single or multiple looping may cause a short cord with all its complications. Looping of the cord around the neck may cause fetal distress due to tightening of the cord around the neck during descend, especially if the distance is short between the loop and the placental insertion. Therefore, it is important to check for a cord around the neck as soon as the baby's head is born.

8. *Cord knotting:* False knotting occurs when the cord appears to be knotted, but instead has kinking of the blood vessel within the cord or accumulation of Wharton's jelly on the cord.

   A true knot occurs when the fetus has passed through a loop in the cord and a real knot has been created. True knots are liable to occur with small fetus, long cord, large amount of amniotic fluid and multiple gestations within a single amnion.

9. Markedly decreased amount of Wharton's jelly may be seen in malnourished and postmature newborns.

10. *Rarities:* Other conditions that may occur in the umbilical cord are hematomas, tumors, cysts and edema. Hematomas usually are the result of rupturing of the umbilical vein. Edema is common with an edematous or macerated fetus.

DEVELOPMENT OF THE FETUS (FIG. 9.11)

First Trimester

Growth and development begins with the moment of fertilization and the fusing of the female and male pronuclei from the ovum and sperm. This fusion produces what is called zygote. At this moment a new individual is created with his/her own unique makeup, as determined by the totally new combination of chromosomes and genes. This unique combination results because the pronucleus (fully matured nucleus of a germ cell) of each gamete (sex cell, i.e. ovum and sperm) contains only half (23) of the total number (46) of chromosomes in human beings. The halving of the

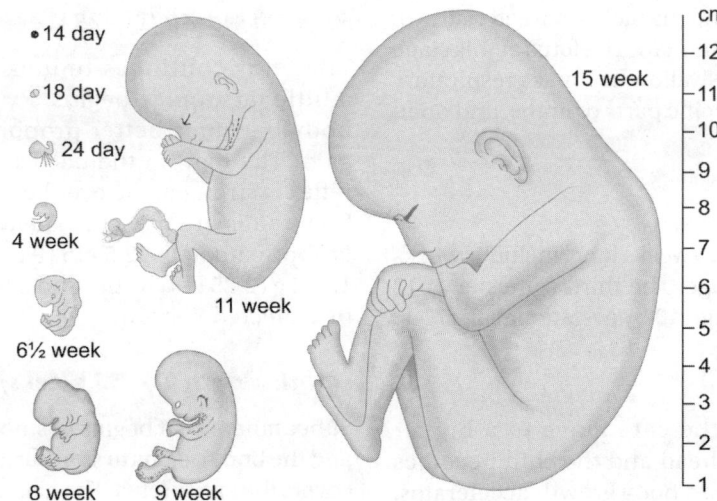

Figure 9.11: Changes in the body size of the embryo and fetus during development in the uterus.

chromosome number is a result of gametogenesis, the process by which mature ova and spermatozoa are developed. At the moment of fertilization, the fusion of the pronucleus of the two gametes restores the diploid (doubled) number of chromosomes. As a result of this fusion and restoration of the diploid number, the sex of the new individual is determined at the moment of fertilization. The males determine the sex as they carry two dissimilar sex chromosomes XY. Females carry two similar sex chromosomes XX. Each spermatozoa will carry either X or Y chromosome, whereas the ovum always carries X chromosome. Upon fusion, a XX combination normally develops into a female, while XY combination normally develops into a male. Immediately following fertilization, the resulting zygote begins to undergo mitotic cellular division called cleavage. Going through sequential stages, the dividing cellular mass is called morula. With cellular reorganization and the entry of fluid, the morula becomes a blastocyst. It is the blastocyst, which implants in the uterine lining. The process of implantation is completed on the 10th or 11th day after fertilization after which the embryonic period begins.

Embryonic period is roughly the period of life from the 2nd through 7th week after fertilization. At the time of implantation (6th week), the embryo known as a bilaminar embryo because the embryonic disk arising from the inner cell mass has two layers of cells:
1. The embryonic ectoderm.
2. The embryonic endoderm.

The embryonic endoderm is the first of the three germ layers from which all tissues (e.g. bone, muscle, connective and skin), organs, and structures derive. Structures such as the fetal membranes, the umbilical cord and part of the placenta also develop from these layers.

From the beginning of the 3rd week, the primitive stalk, arising from the embryonic disk, is the growth center for the embryo for about 2 weeks after which it disintegrates. During the 3rd week, the neural tube (rudiment of the brain and spinal cord), notochord (rudiment of the vertebrae), coelomic spaces (rudiment of body cavities) and primitive blood cells develop.

The heart starts to beat at the beginning of the 4th week. During the 4th week, a longitudinal and transverse folding of the embryonic disk takes place. The longitudinal folding, involving a head fold and a tail fold, converts the embryo from a straight form to a curved form. The transverse folding involving right and left transverse folds, folding towards the midline converts the embryo from a flat form to a cylindrical form. By the end of the 4th week, the embryo has assumed its often called salamander look and has the rudiments of ears (otic pit), arms (arm buds), legs (leg buds) and facial and neck structures.

During the 5th week rapid development of the brain results in extensive growth of the head and makes it much larger in relation to the rest of the body. Development takes place from cephalic to caudal, with development of the legs almost a week behind development of the arms. The eyes begin development with lens, vesicles, optic cups and retinal pigment.

During the 6th week, nose, mouth and palate begin to take form and the eyelids become visible. Arms and legs undergo extensive development and by the end of 7th week, arms and legs are formed with clearly defined fingers and toes.

During the 7th week, the neck region is established, the abdomen is less protuberant and urogenital development begins. The external ears are evident, although they are not fully developed. The embryo by the end of 7th week has distinctive human characteristics. The end of the 7th week also marks the end of the embryonic period. All essential internal and external structures are formed. They undergo further elaboration and growth, including the replacement of cartilage with bone cells. The embryonic period is a critical period during which any teratogen (e.g. drugs, X-rays, viruses) may either be lethal (deadly) or cause major congenital malformations.

By the end of the first trimester or the 12th gestational week calculated from the last menstrual period (LMP), the intestines are fully into the abdomen, the external genitalia have male or female characteristics, but neither are fully formed, the anus has formed and the facial characteristics of the fetus now look undeniably human. The fetus at this stage weighs about 0.5–1 ounce, can swallow and make respiratory movements, urinate, move specific parts of limbs, and open and shut his/her mouth.

Second and Third Trimester

The second trimester, which is 15 weeks long, includes weeks 13 through 27 by gestational age. The third trimester of 13 weeks includes weeks 28 through 40 by gestational age.

Fourth Month (13–16 Weeks)

Head growth slows, while the ears move to a higher elevation on the sides of the head and the chin becomes evident. Eyes remain closed and body growth accelerates. Reflex responses and muscular activity begin. Sex is clearly distinguishable by 14th week. Bone development takes place by 16th week and they could be seen with roentgenography. The average crown-rump (top of head to buttocks) length is 11.5 cm (4.5 inch), and the fetus weights between 99 g and 113 g (3.5–4 ounce) by the end of 16th week.

Fifth Month (17–20 Weeks)

Rapid body growth continues; legs reach their full length and toe nails develop. The eyelids remain fused. The fetus moves freely inside the uterus. Stronger fetal movements and thinner uterine wall result in the mother's experiencing quickening around the 18th week. The fetus hiccups and the mother may feel it as a series of slight rhythmic jerks or jolts. By the end of the 5th month the vernix caseosa covers the entire body. Vernix caseosa, a mixture of sebum (secretion from the sebaceous glands) and surface epithelial cells, a thick cheesy substance that is protective to the delicate skin of the fetus. The fetal heart may be heard with a fetoscope by the end of the month. By the end of the 20th week the average crown-rump length of the fetus is about 16.5 cm (6.5 inch) and the average weight is almost 341 g (0.75 lbs).

Sixth Month (21–24 Weeks)

Hair growth is prominent. The fetus is completely covered with lanugo, a fine downy (soft) hair. Eyebrows, eyelashes and head hair are present. The head remains large compared to the rest of the body. The skin is wrinkled, translucent (imperfectly transparent) and red, giving an aged appearance to the fetus. Buds for the permanent teeth are present. The fetus being small has room in the uterus to somersault (turn heels overhead) and can make motions of crying and sucking. The hands make fists. Brown fat, which is a source of energy, heat production and heat regulation in the newborn forms. The average crown-rump length of the fetus reaches just over 20 cm (8 inch) and the weight is approximately 568 g (1.25 lbs).

Seventh Month (25–28 Weeks)

The fetus continues to look old and wrinkled though a little fat storage begins. By the end of the month, the body becomes better proportioned because of weight gain. The hair on the baby's head is longer, the sucking reflex is stronger, the eyes begin to open and shut, and the fingernails are present. The average crown-rump length is approximately 22.5 cm (9 inch) and the weight is about 1,023 g (2.25 lbs) by the end of the 28th week. Survival may be expected, if born.

Eighth Month (29–32 Weeks)

Subcutaneous fat begins to smooth out some of the wrinkles and the body begins to store fat and iron. Thick vernix caseosa covers the entire fetus. The hair on the head continues to grow and the lanugo is plentiful except on the face from where it has now disappeared. Fingernails reach the ends of the fingers; toenails are present, but do not reach the ends of the toes. The fetus has control of rhythmic breathing and body temperature. The eyes are open. The average crown-rump length is about 27.5 cm (11 inch) and weight is approximately 1.7 kg (3.75 lbs).

Ninth Month (33–36 Weeks)

By the end of 9th month the skin is smooth and without wrinkles as the subcutaneous fat becomes thicker from additional deposits. The baby is rounder, the hair is larger, the toenails have reached the ends of the toes, and the left testicle has usually descended into the scrotum and plantar creases are visible. The average crown-rump length is a little over 31 cm (12.5 inch) and the weight is approximately 2.5 kg (5.5 lbs) in the 36 weeks.

37 to 40 Weeks

The fetus receives the finishing touches during this period. Full growth and development are attained. The fetus is now well rounded with a prominent chest and protuberant mammary glands in both sexes. Both testes are in the scrotum. The lanugo has disappeared from most of the body. The nails project beyond the tips of both fingers and toes. The skull is firm. The skin varies in color from white to pink to bluish pink regardless of race because the melanin that colors the skin is produced only after exposure to light. The crown-rump length now averages 31 cm (14 inch). The weight depends on a number of variables, but has a general average of 3.2 kg (7 lbs). Term is reached and birth is due.

An understanding of fetal development is essential for the midwife in order to estimate the approximate age of a baby born before term. It is also helpful to know the outline of organogenesis in order to appreciate the ways in which developmental abnormalities arise. When making reference to the age at which various events happen, it is important for the midwife to distinguish between the gestational age (the time since the first day of last menstrual period) and the conceptional age (the interval since fertilization). In obstetric practice, gestational age is commonly used.

STUDY QUESTIONS

Short Notes

1. Chorionic villi.
2. Succenturiate placenta.
3. Battledore placenta.
4. Velamentous insertion of cord.
5. Vasa previa.

Short Answer Questions

1. Blood circulation through the placenta.
2. The mature placenta.
3. The amniotic fluid.
4. Enumerate the constituents, source and volume of amniotic fluid.

Essay Questions

1. Describe the functions of placenta.
2. Describe fetal development from fertilization to term.

BIBLIOGRAPHY

1. Bennett RV, Linda KB. Myles Textbook for Midwives, 13th edition. Edinburgh: Churchill Livingstone; 1999. pp. 973-94.
2. Dutta DC. Textbook of Obstetrics, 5th edition. Kolkata: New Central Book Agency; 2001. pp. 28-45.
3. Johnson M, Evereitt B. Essential Reproduction, 4th edition. Oxford: Blackwell Science; 1995.
4. Moore KL. Before We are Born, 5th edition. London: Saunders; 1998.
5. Varney H. Nurse-Midwifery, 2nd edition. Boston: Jones and Bartlett Publishers; 1999. pp. 93-110.

CHAPTER 10

Fetal Organs and Circulation

> **Learning Objectives**
>
> Upon completing this chapter, the learner will be able to:
> - Describe the fetal development and fetal circulation.
> - Describe the features of fetal skull, its regions, diameters and mechanism of molding.

FETAL ANATOMY

Blood

The origin of fetal blood is from the inner cell mass. The fetus will inherit the genes, which determine its blood group from both its parents. The ABO group and Rhesus factor may therefore be the same or different from those of its mother.

The fetal hemoglobin termed as HbF is of a different type from adult hemoglobin. It has a much greater affinity for oxygen and is found in greater concentration (18–20 g/dL) at term. Towards the end of pregnancy the fetus begins to make adult-type hemoglobin (HbA). In utero red blood cells (RBCs) have a shorter life span. This is about 90 days by the time the baby is born.

Urinary Tract

The kidneys begin to function and fetus begins to pass urine from 10th week. The superior vesical arteries arise from the hypogastric arteries, which lead to the umbilical arteries. If a single umbilical artery is found instead of the normal two, abnormalities of the renal tract are suspected.

Liver

The fetal liver is comparatively large in size occupying much of the abdominal cavity especially in the early months. From the 3rd to 6th month, the liver is responsible for the formation of RBCs after which they are produced in the red bone marrow and spleen.

Alimentary Tract

The digestive tract is nonfunctional before birth. It forms from the yolk sac as a straight tube first, later growing out into the base of the umbilical cord and finally rotating back into the abdomen. Sucking and swallowing of amniotic fluid begins about 12 weeks after conception. Most digestive juices are present before birth and they act on the swallowed substances (shed skin cells and other debris), and discarded intestinal cells to form meconium. This is normally retained in the gut until after birth when it is passed as the first stool of the newborn.

Lungs

The lungs originate from a bud growing out of the pharynx, which divides and subdivides repeatedly to form the bronchial tree. The process continues until about 8 years of age when the full number of bronchioles and alveoli will have developed. The chances of survival are reduced for babies born before 24th week of gestation because of the immaturity of lungs. At this stage the alveolar surface is limited, the capillary system is immature and surfactant is insufficient. Surfactant is a lipoprotein which reduces the surface tension in the alveoli and assists gaseous exchange. At term the lungs contain about 100 mL of lung fluid. About one-third of this is expelled during delivery and the rest is absorbed, and carried away by the lymphatics and blood vessels as air takes its place.

There is some movement of the thorax from the 3rd month of fetal life and more definite diaphragmatic movements from the 6th month.

Central Nervous System

Central nervous system is derived from the ectoderm. It folds inwards to form the neural tube which is then covered over by skin. This process is occasionally incomplete leading to open neural tube defects.

The fetus is able to perceive strong light and to hear external sounds. Periods of wakefulness and sleep occur.

Skin

The fetus is covered with a white, creamy substance called *vernix caseosa* from 18th week onwards. At 20th week the fetus will be covered with a fine downy hair called *lanugo* and at the same time the head hair and eyebrows begin to form.

Fingernails develop from about 10th week and toenails from about 18th week.

FETAL CIRCULATION (FIG. 10.1)

Fetal circulation differs from adult circulation in several ways and is designed to ensure a high oxygen blood supply to the brain and myocardium.

Characteristics

- Placenta is the source of oxygen for the fetus.
- Fetal lungs receive less than 1% of the blood volume; lungs do not exchange gas.
- Right atrium of fetal heart is the chamber with the highest oxygen concentration.

Structures

Fetal circulation contains five unique structures:

1. *Umbilical vein*: Carries oxygen and nutrients to the fetus.
2. *Two umbilical arteries*: Carry deoxygenated blood and waste products from the fetus.
3. *Ductus venosus (from a vein to a vein)*: Shunts blood from the umbilical vein to the inferior vena cava, bypassing the liver and organs of digestion.
4. *Foramen ovale (oval opening)*: Shunts blood from the right atrium to the left atrium, bypassing the lungs.
5. *Ductus arteriosus (from an artery to an artery)*: Shunts blood from the pulmonary artery to the aorta, bypassing the lungs.
6. *Hypogastric arteries*: Blood from descending aorta returns to the placenta through the two hypogastric arteries which become umbilical arteries when they enter the umbilical cord.

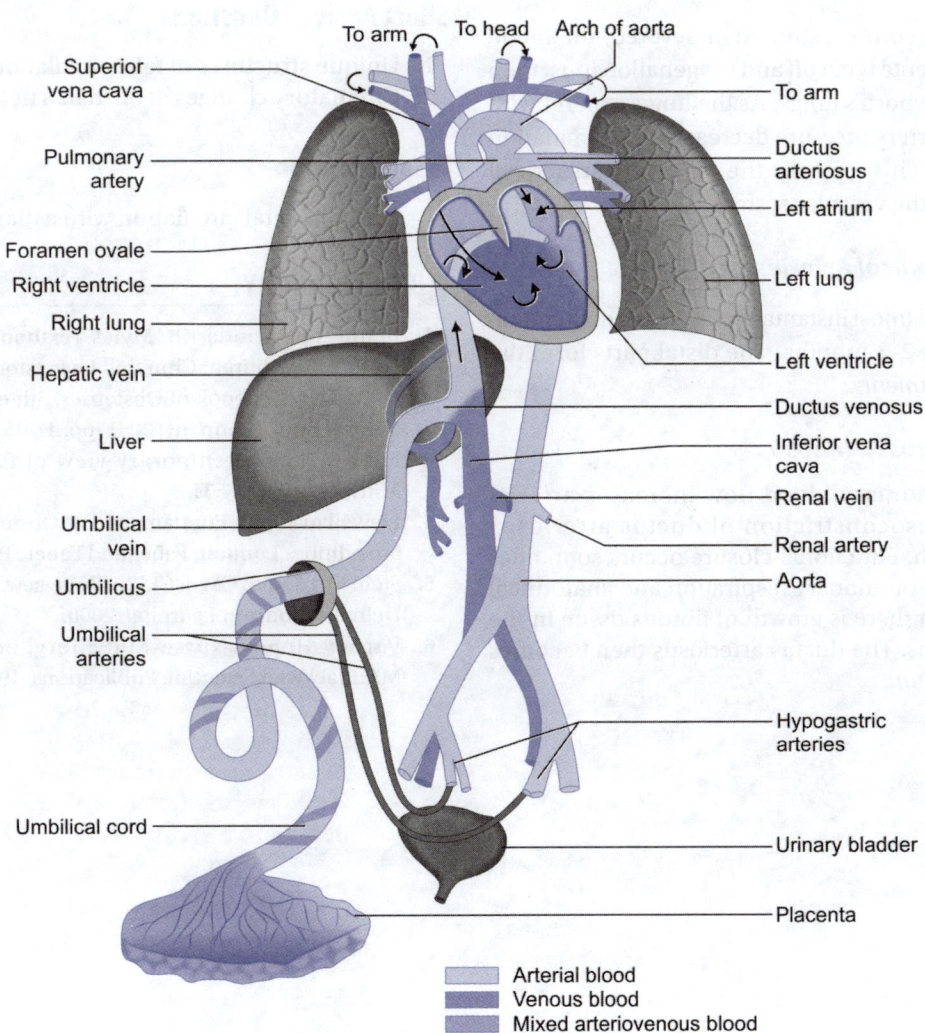

Figure 10.1: Fetal circulation (*For color version, see Plate 2*).

Pattern of Altered Blood Flow

Blood is carried from the placenta through the umbilical vein and enters the inferior vena cava through the ductus venosus. This permits most of the highly oxygenated blood to go directly into the right atrium, bypassing the liver. This right atrial blood flows directly into the left atrium through the foramen ovale, an opening between the right and left atria. From the left atrium, blood flows into the left ventricle and aorta and through the subclavian arteries, to the cerebral and coronary arteries resulting in the brain and heart receiving the most highly oxygenated blood. Deoxygenated blood returns from the head and arms through the superior vena cava, enters the right atrium and passes into the right ventricle.

Blood from the right ventricle flows into the pulmonary artery, because the fetal lungs are collapsed, the pressure in the pulmonary artery is very high. Because pulmonary resistance is high, most of the blood passes into the distal aorta through the ductus arteriosus, which connects the pulmonary artery and the aorta distal to the origin of the subclavian arteries. From the aorta, blood flows to the rest of the body.

Normal Circulatory Changes at Birth

When the umbilical cord is clamped or severed, the blood supply from the placenta is cut off and oxygenation must then take place in the newborn's lungs. As the lungs expand with air, the pulmonary artery pressure decreases and circulation to lungs increases. This leads to the following structural changes to occur in the vascular system.

Closure of the Umbilical Arteries

Functional closure is almost instantaneous. Actual obliteration takes place in about 2–3 months. The distal parts form the *lateral umbilical ligaments*.

Closure of the Ductus Arteriosus

The increased pulmonary blood flow increases arterial oxygen, causing vasoconstriction of ductus arteriosus within hours of birth. Functional closure occurs soon after the establishment of pulmonary respiration and anatomical closure occurs when there is growth of fibrous tissue in the lumen by 1–3 months. The ductus arteriosus then becomes *ligamentum arteriosum*.

Closure of the Umbilical Vein

Obliteration of the umbilical vein occurs a little later than the arteries, allowing a little extra volume of blood (80–100 mL) to be received by the baby from the placenta. After obliteration, the umbilical vein forms the *ligamentum teres*.

Closure of the Ductus Venosus

When the umbilical cord is severed, blood flow through the ductus venosus decreases and eventually ceases. It constricts in 3–7 days and eventually becomes *ligamentum venosum*.

Closure of Foramen Ovale

Expansion of pulmonary artery and increased pulmonary blood flow increases the left ventricular and left atrial pressure. Functional close of this valve-like opening occurs when the pressure in the left atrium exceeds pressure in the right. The anatomical obliteration occurs in about 12 months with deposits of fibrin and becomes *fossa ovalis*.

STUDY QUESTIONS

Short Answer Questions

1. Unique structures of fetal circulation.
2. Circulatory changes at birth in a neonate.

Essay Question

1. Describe fetal circulation with a diagram.

BIBLIOGRAPHY

1. Bennett RV, Linda KB. Myles Textbook for Midwives, 13th edition. Edinburgh: Churchill Livingstone; 1999. pp. 981-94.
2. Dutta DC. Textbook of Obstetrics, 5th edition. Calcutta: New Central Book Company; 2001. pp. 41-45.
3. Fox HA. A contemporary view of the human placenta. Midwifery. 1991;7:31-9.
4. Llewellyn-Jones. Fundamental of Obstetrics and Gynecology, 5th edition. London: Faber and Faber; 1990. p. 1.
5. Stein MA, Judith CM. NCLEX-RN Review, 4th edition. New York: Delmar Thomson Learning; 2000.
6. Varney Helen. Nurse-Midwifery, 2nd edition. Boston: MA:Blackwell Scientific Publications, 1987.

CHAPTER 11

Fetal Skull

Learning Objectives

Upon completing this chapter, the learner will be able to:
- Identify the bones of the vault of the fetal skull.
- List and explain the sutures of the fetal skull.
- Identify and describe the regions and diameters of the fetal skull in the mechanism of molding.
- Explain the mechanism of molding.

The fetal skull is oval shaped. At term, it is larger in proportion to the fetal body and in comparison with the true pelvis. The baby's head is wider than its shoulders and one quarter of its length.

The bones of the fetal head originate in two different ways. The face is laid down in cartilage and is almost completely ossified at birth, the bones being fused together and firm. The bones of the vault are laid down in membrane and are much flatter, and pliable. They ossify from the center onwards and this process is incomplete at birth leaving small gaps, which form the sutures and fontanels. The ossification center on each bone appears as a protuberance.

BONES OF THE VAULT

The vault of the skull consist of five main bones. It includes:
1. Two frontal bones.
2. Two parietal bones.
3. Occipital bone.

Two Frontal Bones

The two frontal bones form the forehead or sinciput. At the center of each is a frontal eminence. The frontal bones fuse into a single bone by 8 years of age.

Two Parietal Bones

The two parietal bones lie on either side of the skull. The ossification center of each is called parietal eminence.

Occipital Bone

The occipital bone lies at the back of the head and forms the region of the occiput. Part of it contributes to the base of the skull as it contains foramen magnum which protects the spinal cord as it leaves the skull. At the center is the occipital protuberance.

SUTURES

Sutures are cranial joints and are formed where two bones adjoin. They are composed of fibrous tissue and allow mobility between the cranial bones. There are four sutures in the vault which are of obstetrical significance (**Fig. 11.1**):
1. *Frontal suture:* It is between the two frontal bones.
2. *Sagittal suture:* It is between the two parietal bones.
3. *Coronal suture:* There are two coronal sutures, each between the frontal and parietal bones on either side of the head.
4. *Lambdoidal suture:* There are two lambdoidal sutures, each between the parietal bones and the upper margin of the occipital bone on either side of the head. It is shaped like the Greek letter lambda (λ).

FONTANELS

Fontanels are areas of fibrous tissue membrane found at the angles of the parietal bones where ossification is incomplete at birth (**Fig. 11.1**).

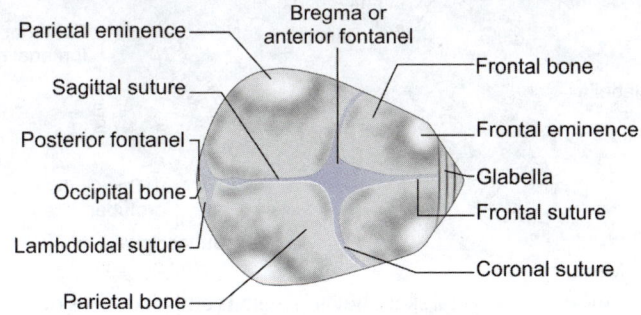

Figure 11.1: Fetal head at term showing fontanels and sutures.

Anterior Fontanel or Bregma

The anterior fontanel or bregma is formed by the meeting of the frontal, sagittal and two coronal sutures. This is roughly in the shape of a diamond (◊) and four sutures can be felt leading from the anterior fontanel in four different directions as indicated by the points on the diamond. It measures 3–4 cm long and 1.5–2 cm wide and normally closes by the time the child is 18 months old. Pulsations of cerebral vessels can be felt through it.

Posterior Fontanel

The posterior fontanel is formed by the meeting of the sagittal and the two lambdoidal sutures. This is roughly in the shape of a triangle (Δ) and three sutures can be felt leading from the posterior fontanel in three different directions as indicated by the points of the triangle. It is small and normally closes by 6 weeks of age.

REGIONS OF THE FETAL SKULL (FIG. 11.2)

1. **Vertex:** It is bounded by the anterior fontanel, the two parietal eminences and the posterior fontanel. Of the 96% of babies born head first, 95% present by the vertex.
2. **Sinciput** or brow extends from the anterior fontanel and the coronal suture to the orbital ridges.
3. **Face:** It extends from the orbital ridges and the roof of the nose to the junction of the chin, and neck. The point between the eyebrows is known as the *glabella*. The chin is termed as mentum and is an important landmark.
4. **Occiput:** It lies between the foramen magnum and posterior fontanel. The part below the occipital protuberance is known as the suboccipital region.

LANDMARKS OF THE SKULL (FIG. 11.2)

The skull is considered as divided into three parts such as vault, face and base. The vault is the large, dome-shaped part above the imaginary line, drawn between the orbital ridges

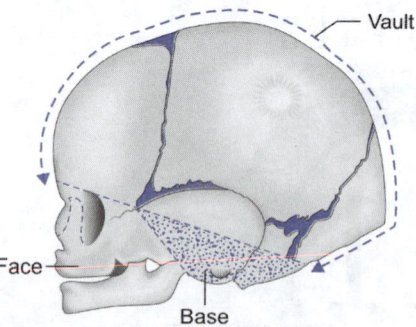

Figure 11.3: Regions of the skull showing the vault, face and base.

and nape of the neck. In the vault, the bones are relatively thin and pliable which allows the skull to alter slightly in shape during birth. The face is composed of 14 small bones which are also firmly united and noncompressible. The facial part forms one-third of the cranium compared to half in an adult. The base is comprised of bones, which are firmly united to protect the vital centers in the medulla **(Fig. 11.3)**.

The fetal head is large in comparison with the true pelvis; therefore some adaptation between the skull and pelvis must take place during labor. The head is the most difficult part to deliver whether it comes first or last. The knowledge of the landmarks and measurements of the skull enables the midwife to recognize normal presentations and positions, and to facilitate delivery with the least possible trauma to mother and baby. Where malpresentation or disproportion exists, she will be able to identify it and alert the physician.

DIAMETERS OF THE FETAL SKULL (FIG. 11.4)

* *Biparietal diameter (9.5 cm)*: It lies between the two parietal eminences.
* *Bitemporal diameter (8.5 cm)*: It lies between the furthest points of the coronal suture.
* *Suboccipitobregmatic (9.5 cm)*: From below the occipital protuberance to the center of the anterior fontanel or bregma.
* *Suboccipitofrontal (10 cm)*: From below the occipital protuberance to the center of the frontal suture.
* *Occipitofrontal (11.5 cm)*: From the occipital protuberance to the glabella.
* *Mentovertical (13.5 cm)*: From the point of the chin to the highest point on the vertex.
* *Submentovertical (11.5 cm)*: From the point where the chin joins the neck to the highest point on the vertex.
* *Submentobregmatic (9.5 cm)*: From the point where the chin joins the neck to the center of the bregma.

Knowledge of the measurements of the skull is important for the midwife because some diameters are more favorable for easy passage through the pelvic canal.

Attitude of the Fetal Head

The term attitude used to describe the degree of flexion or extension of the head on the neck. The attitude of the head determines which diameters will present in labor.

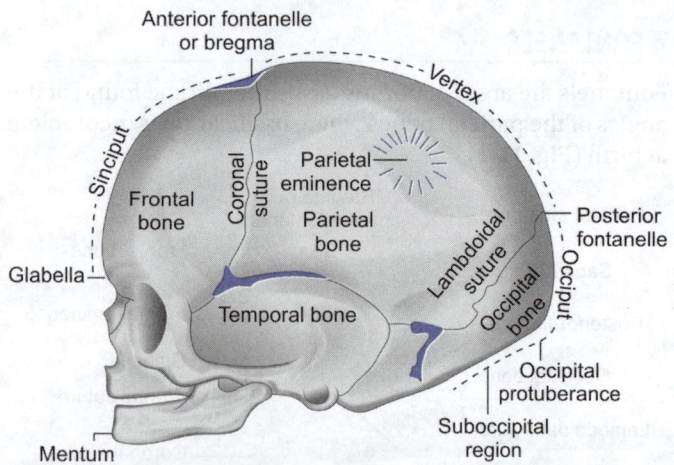

Figure 11.2: Fetal skull showing regions and landmarks of obstetrical importance.

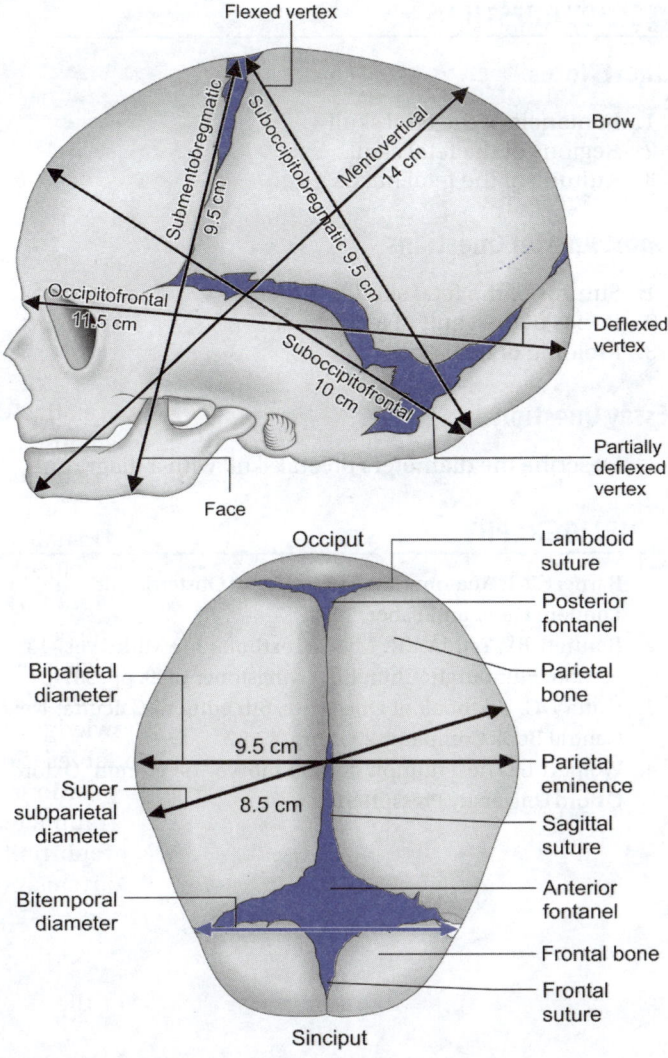

Figure 11.4: Diameters of the fetal skull.

Presenting Diameters

The presenting diameters are those which are at right angles to the curve of Carus. Presenting diameters are always two, a longitudinal diameter and transverse diameter. The diameters presenting in cephalic or head presentations **(Figs. 11.5A to E)**.

Vertex Presentation

When the head is well-flexed, the suboccipitobregmatic diameter and the biparietal diameter are present. As those two diameters are more or less the same length (9.5 cm), the presenting area is round and most favorable for dilating the cervix. The diameter distending the vaginal orifice will be suboccipitofrontal (10 cm). When the head is erect and not flexed, the presenting diameters are the occipitofrontal (11.5 cm) and biparietal (9.5 cm). This situation often arises when the occiput is in a posterior position. The diameter distending the vaginal orifice will be occipitofrontal (11.5 cm).

Brow Presentation

When the head is partially extended, the mentovertical diameter (13.5 cm) and the bitemporal diameter (8.5 cm) are present. With these diameters, vaginal delivery is unlikely.

Face Presentation

When the head is completely extended, the presenting diameters are submentobregmatic (9.5 cm) and bitemporal (8.5 cm). The submentovertical diameter (11.5 cm) will distend the vaginal orifice.

Presenting diameters of the fetal trunk are as follows:

1. *Bisacromial diameter (12 cm):* This is the distance between the acromion processes on the two shoulder blades and is the dimension that needs to pass through the pelvis for the shoulders to be born.
2. *Bitrochanteric diameter (10 cm):* This is the distance between the greater trochanters of the femurs and is the presenting diameter in breech presentation.

MOLDING

Molding is the term applied to the change in shape of the fetal head that takes place during its passage through the birth canal. Alteration in shape is possible because the bones of the vault allow a slight degree of bending and the skull bones are able to override at the sutures **(Fig. 11.6)**.

In a normal vertex presentation with the fetal head in a fully flexed attitude, the suboccipitobregmatic and biparietal diameters will be reduced as much as 1.25 cm and the mentovertical will be lengthened **(Fig. 11.7)**. The skull of the preterm infant, being softer and having wider sutures, may mold excessively. The skull of the postmature infant does not mold well and its greater hardness tends to make labor more difficult. Molding is a protective mechanism and prevents the fetal brain from being compressed as long as it is not too excessive or too rapid.

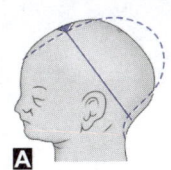 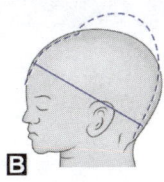 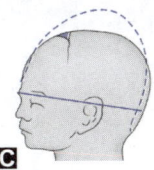 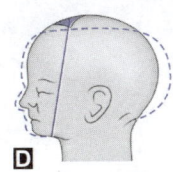 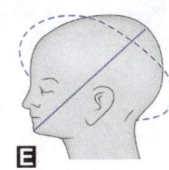

Figures 11.5A to E: Molding of the head presents in varying degrees of flexion: (A) Vertex presentation, head is well-flexed; (B) Vertex presentation, head partially flexed; (C) Vertex presentation, head deflexed; (D) Face presentation; (E) Brow presentation.

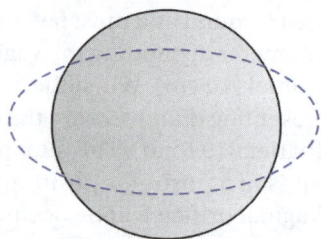

Figure 11.6: The principle of molding of fetal skull.

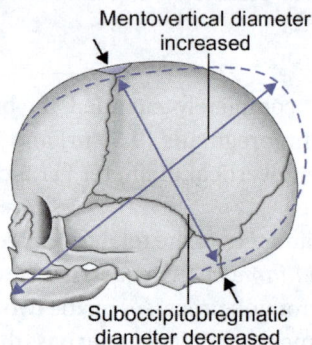

Figure 11.7: Molding in a normal vertex presentation.

STUDY QUESTIONS

Short Notes

1. Fontanels of the fetal skull.
2. Regions of the fetal skull.
3. Attitude of the fetal head.

Short Answer Questions

1. Sutures of the fetal skull.
2. Bones of the vault of fetal skull.
3. Molding of fetal skull.

Essay Question

1. Describe the diameters of fetal skull with a diagram.

BIBLIOGRAPHY

1. Barnet CWF. Anatomy and Physiology of Obstetrics, 6th edition. London: Faber and Faber; 1979.
2. Bennett RV, Linda KB. Myles Textbook for Midwives, 13th edition. Edinburgh: Churchill Livingstone; 1999. pp. 987-94.
3. Dutta DC. Textbook of Obstetrics, 5th edition. Calcutta: New Central Book Company; 2001. pp. 87-92.
4. Wolpert L. The Triumph of the Embryo, 1st edition. Oxford: Oxford University Press; 1991.

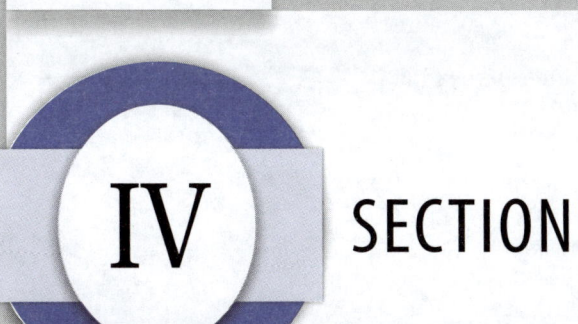

SECTION IV

NORMAL PREGNANCY

Section Outline

12. Physiological Changes due to Pregnancy
13. Diagnosis of Pregnancy
14. Minor Disorders in Pregnancy
15. Antenatal Care
16. Specialized Investigations and Fetal Evaluation in the Antenatal Period

CHAPTER 12

Physiological Changes due to Pregnancy

Learning Objectives

Upon completing this chapter, the learner will be able to:
* Explain the changes occurring in different body systems during pregnancy.
* Identify those physiological changes that cause discomfort or inconvenience to the mother.
* Define the terms that describe the specific changes in the pregnant woman due to hormonal influence.

Physiological changes that take place in a mother's body during pregnancy are associated with and caused by the effects of specific hormones. These changes enable her to nurture the fetus, prepare her body for labor and develop her breasts for the production of milk during the puerperium.

CHANGES IN THE REPRODUCTIVE SYSTEM

The changes in pregnancy that take place in the reproductive system are the temporary adaptation to meet the needs and demands of the fetus.

Body of Uterus

After conception the uterus develops to provide a nutritive and protective environment in which the fetus will develop and grow.

Changes in Uterine Shape

The uterus changes to a globular shape to accommodate the growing fetus, increasing amounts of liquor and placentaltissue **(Fig. 12.1)**.

The lower part of the uterus consisting of the isthmus softens and elongates to three times its original length during the first trimester giving the appearance of a stalk below the

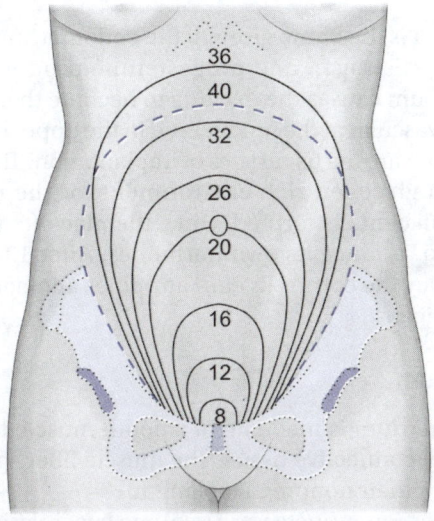

Figure 12.1: Changes in uterine shape during pregnancy

globular upper segment. This is the beginning of the upper and lower segments of the uterus.

By 12th week of pregnancy, the uterus rises out of pelvis and becomes upright. It is no longer anteverted and utflexed. It is about the size of a grapefruit and may be palpated abdominally above the symphysis pubis.

By 16th week, the conceptus has grown enough to put pressure on the isthmus causing it to open out, so that the uterus becomes more globular in shape.

By 20th week of pregnancy, the uterus becomes spherical in shape and has a thicker, more rounded fundus. As the uterus continues to rise in the abdomen, the uterine tubes, being restricted by attachments to the broad ligaments, become progressively more vertical. At 20th week, the fundus of the uterus may be palpated at or just below the umbilicus.

By 30th week, the lower uterine segment can be identified. It is the portion of the uterus above the internal os of the cervix. The fundus can be palpated midway between the umbilicus and xiphisternum.

The uterus reaches the level of the xiphisternum by 38th week. A reduction in fundal height known as lightening may occur at the end of pregnancy when the fetus sinks into the lower pole of the uterus. This is due to softening of the tissues of the pelvic floor and further formation of the lower uterine segment. In the primigravida, this also encourages the beginning of a gradual descend of the fetus into the pelvis and the head becomes engaged. In the multiparous women, descend often does not occur until the labor begins.

When the formation of the lower uterine segment is complete in labor it measures approximately one-third of the body of the uterus.

Decidua

The decidua is the name given to the endometrium during pregnancy. Estrogen and progesterone produced by the corpus luteum causes the decidua to become thicker, richer and more vascular at the fundus, and in the upper body of the uterus which are the usual sites of implantation. The decidua provides a glycogen rich environment for the blastocyst until the placenta is formed. Once the placenta is formed, it is able to produce its own hormones. After 13-17 weeks of pregnancy the corpus luteum atrophies and becomes the corpus albicans.

Myometrium

The myometrium is made up of smooth muscle fibers held together by connective tissue. The muscle fibers grow up to 15-20 times their nonpregnant length.

The hypertrophy (increase in size) and hyperplasia (increase in number) of the uterine muscle is due to the effects of estrogen and progesterone. The uterus continues to grow in this way for the first 3 months, after which the growth is related to distention by the growing fetus.

At term, the uterus measures 30 × 23 × 20 cm and weights 750-1,000 g. Individual muscle cell grows 17-40 times. The walls of the myometrium becomes thicker in the first few months of pregnancy and as gestation advances, the walls become thinner owing to the gross enlargement of the uterus, being only 1.5 cm thick or less at term.

Throughout most of the pregnancy, the uterus generates small waves of irregular and usually painless contractility known as Braxton Hicks contractions. These are infrequent and nonrhythmic, and facilitate the formation of the lower uterine segment. They usually increase in frequency and intensity from about 36th week of pregnancy causing some discomfort. These prelabor contractions are associated with 'ripening' of the cervix and eventually become the contractions of labor as the effects of estrogen supersede those of progesterone (progesterone normally suppresses myometrial activity). During pregnancy, the muscle layers

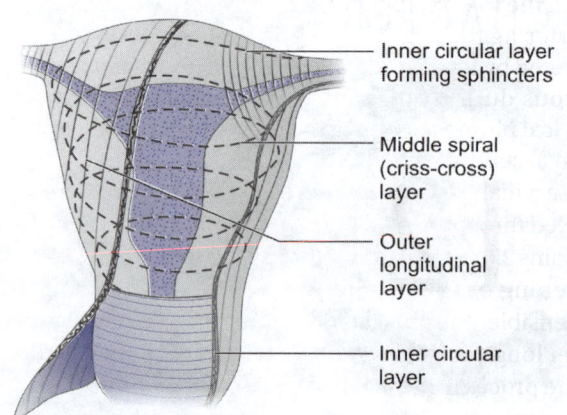

Figure 12.2: Muscle layers of the uterus in pregnancy.

become more differentiated and organized for their part in expelling the fetus.

Muscle Layers (Fig. 12.2)

The outer longitudinal layer of muscle fibers is thin. The middle layer of spiral myometrial fibers is thick. During labor, the synchronous contraction and retraction of these fibers cause them to become heaped up in the upper uterine segment making it thicker and shorter in length, while the lower uterine segment becomes thinner and more stretched.

The thickness of the upper uterine segment acts as a piston to force the fetus into the receptive passive lower uterine segment. Contraction of these muscle fibers is necessary to entrap and enmesh bleeding vessels and ligate them after the placenta is delivered.

The inner circular layer is thin and forms sphincters around the openings of the uterine tubes at the cornua, and around the lower uterine segment and cervix. During labor, the stretching and pulling up of the circular layer of muscles around the cervix into the lower uterine segment causes the cervix to become effaced and dilated.

Blood Supply

The uterine blood vessels increase in diameter and new vessels develop under the influence of estrogen. The blood supply to the uterus through the uterine and ovarian arteries increases to about 750 mL/min at term to keep pace with its growth and also to meet the needs of the functioning placenta.

Fallopian Tubes

The fallopian tubes on either side are more stretched out in pregnancy and are much more vascular. The uterine end of the tube is usually closed and the fimbriated end remains open.

Cervix

The cervix remains tightly closed during pregnancy providing protection to the fetus and resistance to pressure from above when the woman is in standing position. It acts as an effective barrier against infection during pregnancy. The mucus secreted by the endocervical cells becomes thicker and more viscous during pregnancy. The thickened mucus forms a cervical plug called the *operculum* which provides protection from ascending infection.

Cervical vascularity increases during pregnancy and if viewed through a speculum, it looks bluish in color. The cervix remains 2.5 cm long throughout pregnancy. In late pregnancy, softening or ripening of the cervix occurs making it more distensible. The muscles of the fundus enhance tension in the outer longitudinal layer of muscles of the cervix contributing to the process of effacement. Effacement or tinning up of the cervix normally occurs in the primigravida during the last 2 weeks of pregnancy, but does not usually take place in the multigravida until labor begins.

Vagina

Estrogen causes changes in the muscle layer and epithelium of the vagina. The muscle layer hypertrophies and the capacity of the vagina increases. Changes in the surrounding connective tissue make it more elastic.

These changes enable the vagina to dilate during the second stage of labor. The epithelium becomes thicker with marked desquamation (peeling off) of the superficial cells which increases the amount of normal vaginal white discharge known as *leukorrhea*.

The epithelial cells have high glycogen content. These cells interact with Doderlein's bacillus which is normally found in vagina and produce more acid environment. The acid environment provides an extra degree of protection against some organisms and an increasing susceptibility to others, such as *Candida albicans*.

The vagina becomes more vascular and appears violet in color probably due to increased blood supply.

CHANGES IN THE CARDIOVASCULAR SYSTEM

In the cardiovascular system, profound changes take place during pregnancy. For the care of women with normal pregnancies as well as for the management of women with pre-existing cardiovascular diseases, an understanding of these changes is important.

Heart

The heart muscle particularly the left ventricle, hypertrophies leading to enlargement of the heart. The growing uterus pushes the heart upwards and to the left. During pregnancy, the heart rate and stroke volume (the amount of blood pumped by the heart with each beat) increases. This is due to the increased blood volume and increased oxygen requirements of the maternal tissues and the growing fetus.

The cardiac output (the rate at which blood is pumped by the heart expressed as liters per minute) increases markedly by the end of the first trimester. In the third trimester, a rise, fall or no change at all has been shown to occur depending on individual variations.

Although the cardiac output is increased in pregnancy, the blood pressure does not rise because of the reduction in peripheral resistance. The capacity of veins and venules increases. Arterial walls relax and dilate due to the effect of progesterone. The increased production of vasodilator prostaglandin also contributes to this.

During the midtrimester, changes in blood pressure may occur causing fainting. In later pregnancy, hypotension may occur in 10% of women in unsupported supine position.

This is termed as the supine hypotensive syndrome. The pressure of the gravid uterus compresses the vena cava reducing the venous return. Cardiac output is reduced by 25–30% and the blood pressure may fall by 10–15%, which produces the feelings of dizziness, nausea and even fainting.

Poor venous return in late pregnancy along with increased distensibility and pressure in the veins of the legs, vulva, rectum, and pelvis can lead to edema in the lower leg, varicose veins and hemorrhoids.

Blood flow increases to the uterus, kidneys, breasts and skin during pregnancy. Much of the increased cardiac output goes to the uteroplacental circulation which is about 750 mL/min at term.

Regulation of uterine blood flow is of critical importance to the welfare of the fetus. Hemorrhage, uterine contractions and lying in the supine position in late pregnancy all can reduce uterine blood flow. Chronic impairment can lead to intrauterine growth retardation and ultimately fetal death. Renal blood flow increases during pregnancy. Blood flow to the capillaries of the skin and mucous membranes, and in particular to hands and feet increases. The associated peripheral vasodilatation causes the women to sweat profusely at times. Some may suffer nasal congestion.

There is increased blood flow to the breasts throughout pregnancy and dilated veins may be seen on the surface of the breasts along with enlargement and tingling from early pregnancy.

Blood Volume

The increase in blood volume in pregnancy varies according to the size of the woman, the number of pregnancies she has had, her parity and whether the pregnancy is singleton or multiple. The increase begins at about 10th week gestation and progresses up to 30–34 weeks of gestation. The increase may be as much as 100% in some women. A higher circulating volume is required for the following functions:

- ❖ To provide extra blood flow for placental circulation
- ❖ To supply the extra metabolic needs of the fetus
- ❖ To provide extra perfusion of kidneys and other organs
- ❖ To counterbalance the effects of increased arterial and venous capacity
- ❖ To compensate for blood loss at delivery.

There is an increase in plasma volume, which reduces the viscosity of the blood and improves capillary blood flow.

The total volume of red blood cells in the circulation (red cell mass) increases as a result of increased production in response to the extra oxygen requirements of maternal and placental tissue. There is constant increase throughout the pregnancy from about 10th week resulting in a total increase of 18–25%.

As the increase in plasma volume is much greater than that of the red blood cell mass, hemodilution occurs. It is characterized by a lowered red blood cell count and hemoglobin level (in spite of the rise in total circulating hemoglobin). The hematocrit concentration or packed cell volume falls from an average non-pregnant figure of 35–29% at around 30th week. The effect is referred to as *physiological anemia*.

Plasma Protein

During the first 20 weeks of pregnancy, the plasma protein concentration reduces as a result of the increased plasma volume. This leads to lowered osmotic pressure, contributing to edema of the lower limbs seen in late pregnancy. In the absence of disease, moderate edema is seen as physiological.

Iron Metabolism

Iron requirement increases significantly in the last trimester, during this time iron absorption from the gut is enhanced. The purpose of iron supplementation in pregnancy is to prevent iron deficiency in the mother, not to raise the hemoglobin.

Clotting Factors

The clotting and fibrinolytic systems undergo major changes during pregnancy. Plasma fibrinogen (factor I) increases from the 3rd month of pregnancy progressively until term. Prothrombin (factor II) increases only slightly. Factors VII, VIII, IX and X increases leading to change in coagulation time from 12 to 8 minutes.

The capacity for clotting is thus, increased in preparation for the prevention of hemorrhage at placental separation. However, there is a higher risk of thrombosis and embolism.

White Blood Cells

The neutrophils increase in pregnancy, which enhances the blood phagocytic and bactericidal properties. In the second and third trimester the action of the polymorphonuclear leukocytes (PMNLs) may be depressed, perhaps accounting for the increased susceptibility of pregnant women to infection. The lymphocyte and monocyte numbers remain the same throughout pregnancy.

Immunity

Immune response is reduced in pregnancy. Levels of immunoglobulins IgA, IgG and IgM decrease steadily from the 10th week to the 30th week and then remain at these levels until term resulting in reduced immune response. Antibody titers against viruses, such as measles, influenza A virus and herpes simplex are reduced in proportion to the hemodilution effect therefore, viral resistance is unchanged.

CHANGES IN THE RESPIRATORY SYSTEM

The shape of the chest changes and the circumference increases in pregnancy by 6 cm. As the uterus enlarges the diaphragm is elevated as much as 4 cm and the rib cage is displaced upwards. The lower ribs flare out and may not always fully recover their original position after pregnancy.

There is a progressive increase in oxygen consumption which is caused by the increased metabolic needs of the mother and fetus.

The mucosa of the respiratory tract becomes hyperemic and edematous with hypersecretion of mucus, which can lead to stuffiness and epistaxis. As a result women may suffer chronic cold during pregnancy. Long-term use of nasal decongestant sprays should be avoided because of their effect on the mucosa.

Progesterone causes an increase in the sensitivity of the respiratory center to stimulation by carbon dioxide (CO_2). This causes a little hyperventilation and lowering of blood pCO_2. The alveolar CO_2 concentrations are lower than that in the nonpregnant woman that causes the maternal CO_2 tension to be lower leading to a respiratory alkalosis. The mild alkalemia (arterial pH 7.44) facilitates oxygen release to the fetus. The maternal pCO_2 is lower (5–4 kPa) than that in the fetus (6 kPa). This facilitates transfer of CO_2 from the fetus to the mother.

Hyperventilation (overbreathing) can lead to discomfort, dyspnea and dizziness. Women may complain of shortness of breath, when their need to breathe becomes a conscious one.

The stress on respiratory system imposed by pregnancy is very little in comparison with the cardiovascular system. The changes however, can cause some discomfort or inconvenience to the pregnant woman and diseases of the respiratory tract may be more serious during pregnancy.

CHANGES IN THE URINARY SYSTEM

Renal blood flow increases by as much as 70–80% by the second trimester. After 30 weeks it decreases slowly, although it is still above nonpregnant levels at term. The kidneys enlarge and glomerular filtration increases. The increase is maintained throughout the second trimester, but decreases significantly during the last weeks of pregnancy.

Plasma levels of urea, uric acid and creatinine fall in pregnancy, although uric acid level returns to nonpregnant level in late pregnancy.

Protein and amino acids are less efficiently reabsorbed and as a result found in much greater amounts in the urine of pregnant women. Proteinuria does not usually occur in normal pregnancy.

Glucose excretion increases as a result of increased glomerular filtration rate of glucose. Glycosuria is therefore, quite common in pregnancy and is not usually related to a high blood glucose level. Glycosuria can be a cause of urinary tract infection. It should, however, be monitored to exclude diabetes mellitus.

Urinary output is diminished because of an enhanced tubular reabsorption of water. An accompanying increase in the reabsorption of sodium is seen which is possibly due to hormonal effect.

The urine of pregnant women is more alkaline due to the alkalemia of pregnancy. In early pregnancy, increased production of urine causes frequency of micturition. In later pregnancy, frequency is caused by the pressure of the growing uterus on the bladder.

The ureters become relaxed and are dilated, elongated and curved above the brim of the pelvis due to the influence of progesterone. This along with compression of the ureters against the pelvic brim can result in stasis of urine in the ureters leading to bacteriuria and infection of the urinary tract. Hydroureter and hydronephrosis may be associated with stasis of urine.

The muscle of the bladder is relaxed owing to raised levels of progesterone. Bladder vascularity increases and bladder capacity is reduced. Toward the end of pregnancy, as the head engages, the entire bladder may be displaced upward.

CHANGES IN THE GASTROINTESTINAL SYSTEM

In the mouth, the gums become edematous, soft and spongy which can bleed when mildly traumatized as with a toothbrush. Increased salivation (ptyalism) is a common complaint in pregnancy. This problem seems to be associated with nausea which prevents women from swallowing their saliva.

Around 4–8 weeks, most women (about 70%) start complaining of nausea and vomiting, this may continue until about 14–16 weeks. Relaxation of the smooth muscles of the stomach and hypomotility may also contribute to this problem. It can be quite distressing and sometimes causing weight loss in early pregnancy. It occasionally causes nutritional or electrolyte imbalance.

Occasionally vomiting may become excessive. Excessive vomiting is common in multiple pregnancies or hydatidiform mole and hence excessive hormone levels are thought to be the cause for it.

In earlier period of pregnancy, a change in the sense of taste can occur. It can be metallic taste in the mouth, distaste for something usually enjoyed or craving for a food usually not eaten. Craving for bizarre substances such as coal, wall plaster, mothball, mud, etc. may be seen occasionally. This is termed as pica.

Many women notice an increase in thirst during pregnancy. This may be due to the fall in plasma osmolarity and rising levels of prolactin. An increase in appetite is also experienced by most of women which may be due to the fall in plasma glucose and amino acids in early pregnancy.

The enlarging uterus misplaces the stomach and intestines. Raised intragastric pressure without accompanying increase in tone of the cardiac sphincter causes reflux of acid mouthfuls with epigastric pain. The resulting symptom of heartburn is quite common in pregnancy.

The tendency to constipation is more in pregnancy, as the passage of food through the intestines is so much slower that there is increased absorption of water from the colon. This probably is due to raised levels of aldosterone and angiotensin. A high residue diet which helps to hold water in its passage through the colon will help to relieve this problem. Constipation may also be caused by mechanical obstruction by the uterus and by the relaxing effect of progesterone on smooth muscle. Oral iron may also contribute to the problem. Constipation may worsen hemorrhoids, which are caused by the increased pressure in the veins below the level of the enlarged uterus.

The gallbladder increase in size and empties more slowly during pregnancy. Stagnation of bile which is almost physiological in pregnancy is probably a hormonal effect and can lead to pruritus or gallstone formation. There are many changes in liver functions that mimic liver disease; therefore liver function tests in pregnancy should be interpreted with caution. Following are the common alterations:

- Serum albumin levels fall progressively throughout pregnancy and at term are 30% lower than the nonpregnant level.
- Serum alkaline phosphatase levels rise progressively and at term are at two to four times the nonpregnant values.
- Serum cholesterol levels are raised two-fold by the end of pregnancy.
- Many liver proteins are raised.
- Fibrinogen levels are increased 50% by the end of the second trimester.

CHANGES IN METABOLISM

There is increased food intake during pregnancy. this along with the gastrointestinal changes, lead to characteristic alteration in the metabolism of carbohydrate, protein and fat. These changes which are brought about by human placental lactogen ensure that glucose is readily available for body and brain growth in the developing fetus, and protects against nutritional deficiencies.

Fasting plasma glucose concentration falls during the first trimester, rises between 16 and 32 weeks and then falls again toward term.

Insulin secretion correspondingly rises in the second trimester and then falls to nonpregnant levels toward term. As human placental lactogen levels rise with advancing pregnancy, insulin resistance increases leading the diabetogenic effect of pregnancy. As a result a glucose load takes longer time to reach maximal plasma concentration. When the maximum concentration is reached, it is higher than normal and remains elevated for longer allowing more time for placental exchange.

A continuous supply of glucose must be available to transfer to the fetus. Pregnant women should not fast or skip meals for the following reasons:

1. Maternal blood glucose levels are critically important for the fetal well-being.
2. Fasting in pregnancy produces more intense ketosis known as accelerated starvation that may be dangerous to fetal health.

As the nutritional demands of the fetus increases in the second half of pregnancy and insulin resistance increases, mobilization of fat stores laid down in the first half of pregnancy occurs providing the mother with extra energy. However, because of the increased concentration of fatty acids resulting from this process, the mother is more prone to ketosis. Even an overnight fast of 12 hours will result in hypoglycemia and increased production of ketone bodies.

Restriction of carbohydrate in any diet may be avoided and the mother may be encouraged to take bedtime snacks.

Plasma albumin concentration is reduced due to increased plasma volume. This causes reduction of colloid osmotic pressure resulting in limb edema in late pregnancy. Plasma amino acid concentrations also fall because amino acids are used to make glucose.

Plasma calcium concentrations fall as a result of both fetal needs and the normal hemodilation of pregnancy. If the intake of vitamin D is sufficient, calcium absorption from the intestines increases by the end of second trimester, which provides for fetal needs as well as protecting the mother's skeleton. Pregnant clients should therefore be advised to increase their calcium intake by about 70%.

MATERNAL WEIGHT CHANGES

A continuing weight increase in pregnancy is considered to be a favorable indicator for maternal adaptation and fetal growth. Analysis of studies on weight gain in pregnancy suggests the following as the expected increase in primigravida:
- 4 kg in first 20 weeks
- 8.5 kg in second 20 weeks (0.4 kg per week in the last trimester)
- 12.5 kg approximate total.

The average weight gain in a multigravida is approximately 1 kg less than in the primigravida.

There is a wide range of normality in weight gain and many factors influence it, which include maternal edema, maternal metabolic rate, dietary intake, vomiting or diarrhea, amount of amniotic fluid and size of the fetus.

Maternal age, prepregnancy body size, parity and diseases like diabetes and hypertension also seem to influence the pattern of weight gain. Distribution of average weight gain in pregnancy is illustrated in **Figure 12.3**.

SKELETAL CHANGES

Relaxation of pelvic ligaments and muscles occurs because of the influence of estrogen and relaxin. This reaches the maximum during the last weeks of pregnancy allowing the pelvis to increase its capacity in readiness to accommodate the fetal presenting part at the end of pregnancy and in labor.

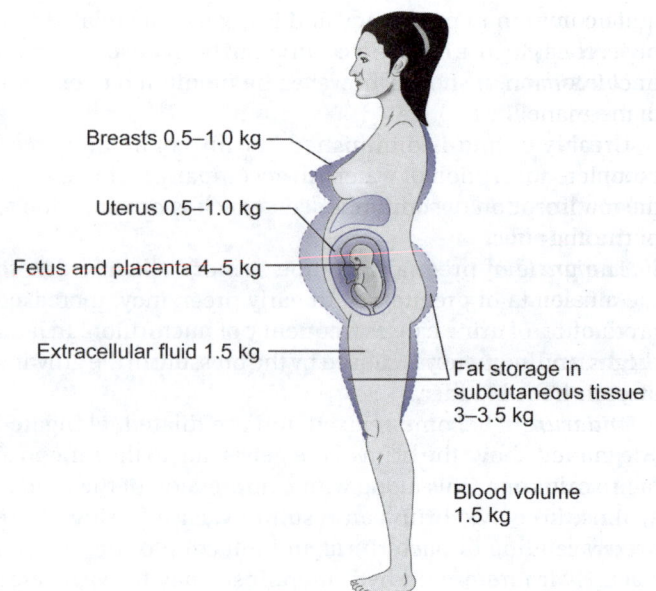

Figure 12.3: Distribution of average weight gain in pregnancy.

The ligaments of the symphysis pubis and the sacroiliac joints loosen. The symphysis pubis widens by about 4 mm by 32 weeks gestation and sacrococcygeal joint loosens allowing the coccyx to be displaced backwards. Increased mobility of the pelvic joints facilitates vaginal delivery. It also results in a rolling gait in late pregnancy which is the likely cause of backache and ligament pain.

Posture of the pregnant woman alters to compensate for the enlarging uterus anteriorly. The woman leans backwards exaggerating the normal lumbar curve and causing a progressive lordosis (an abnormal curvature of the spinal column with convexity toward the front), which shifts her center of gravity back over her legs. The side effect is low back pain and sometimes shoulder pain by which most women suffer during pregnancy. Relaxation of the joints and lordosis can also lead to unsteadiness of gait and the tendency to fall. The teeth are prone to decay during pregnancy, perhaps due to calcium deficiency resulting from increased demand for it by the growing fetus.

SKIN CHANGES

Increased activity of the melanocyte-stimulating hormone from the pituitary causes varying degrees of pigmentation in pregnant women from the end of 2nd month until term. The depth of pigmentation varies according to skin color and race.

The areas most commonly affected are areola of breasts abdominal midline, the perineum and axillae. On the breasts, darkening of the nipple primary areola (areola around the nipple) and secondary areola (mottling of the skin around and beyond the primary areola) are seen. The face is less frequently involved. It is speculated that these areas become more pigmented than others, either because of increased sensitivity of the melanocytes to the hormone or because of a greater number of melanocytes in these areas.

The irregular brownish discolorations of the forehead, nose, cheeks and neck are known as the 'mask of pregnancy' or *chloasma* (Fig. 12.4A) usually develops in the second half of pregnancy in about 50–70% of women. Chloasma is most noticeable in dark-haired, brown-eyed women. It regresses completely after delivery. In the most of pregnant women, a narrow line of dark skin pigmentation appears in the midline of the abdomen from the symphysis to the umbilicus called *linea nigra* (Fig. 12.4B).

As maternal size increase, stretching occurs in the collagen layer of the skin particularly over the breasts, abdomen, thighs and occasionally buttocks. The areas of maximum stretch become thin and stretch marks known as *striae gravidarum* (Fig. 12.4C) appear as red stripes during the pregnancy. Hair growth increases during pregnancy over face, scalp and body. The excess hair is shed after delivery.

A rise in body temperature of 0.5°C with an increased blood supply causing vasodilatation makes women feel hotter and sweaty. Many women develop angiomas during pregnancy, which are red elevations on the skin of the face, neck, arms and chest. Palmar erythema, which is reddening of the palms, is another frequent occurrence. Both are likely to be due to high levels of estrogen and disappear after delivery.

BREAST CHANGES

Marked changes take place in the breasts. The changes are more obvious in primigravida than in multipara. The breasts increase in size and sensitiveness, and bluish discoloration appears in the form of streaks. The nipple becomes more erectile with the areola more deeply pigmented. Prominent tubercles, Montgomery's follicles appear in the primary areola.

About the 5th month, a less pigmented area forms around the primary areola which is known as the secondary areola and on this also some Montgomery's tubercles may be seen. After the first trimester, a little clear, sticky fluid may be expressed from the nipples which later becomes yellowish in color. This is known as colostrum (Figs. 12.5A and B).

CHANGES IN THE ENDOCRINE SYSTEM

Placental Hormones

Placenta produces several hormones. These hormones cause a number of physiological changes that aid in the diagnosis of pregnancy. The high levels of estrogen and progesterone produced by the placenta are responsible for breast changes, skin pigmentations and uterine enlargement in the first trimester. Human chorionic gonadotropin (hCG) is the basis for the immunologic pregnancy tests. Human placental lactogen (HPL) stimulates the growth of the breasts has lactogenic properties and affects a number of metabolic changes. The secretion of HPL and hCG by the fetoplacental unit alters the function of the mother's endocrine organs either directly or indirectly. Raised estrogen levels increase the production of globulins that bind thyroxine and corticosteroids, and sex steroids. As a result, the total plasma

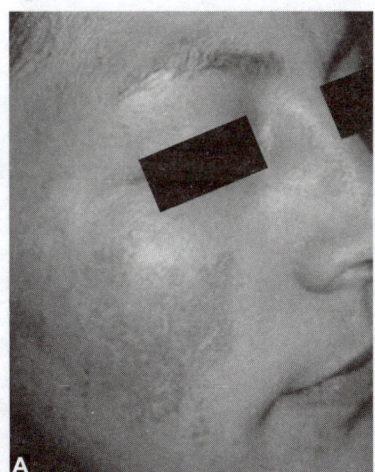
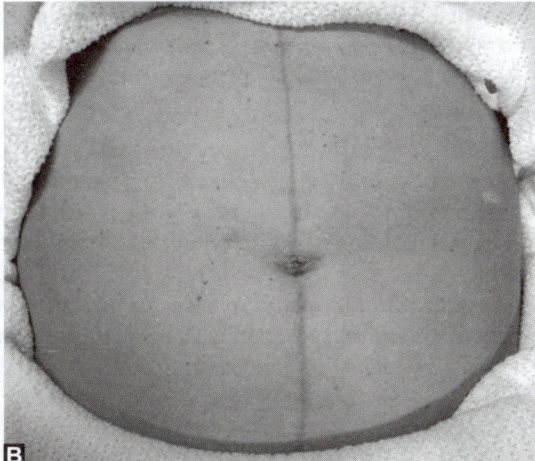
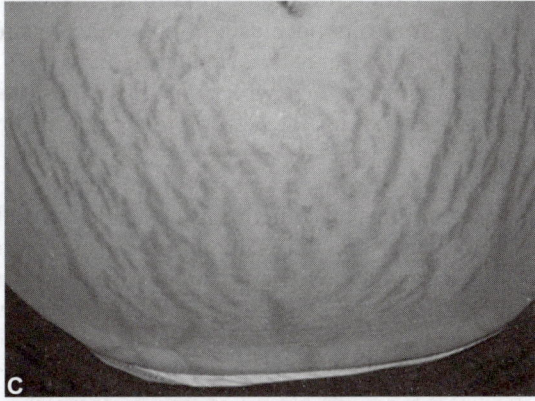

Figures 12.4A to C: (A) Chloasma gravidarum; (B) Linea nigra; and (C) Striae gravidarum *(For color version, see Plate 2).*

content of these hormones is increased, but the levels of free (physiologically active) hormones are not necessarily raised.

Pituitary Hormones

The secretion of prolactin, adrenocorticotropic hormone (ACTH), thyrotropic hormone and melanocyte-stimulating hormone (MSH) increases. Follicle-stimulating hormone (FSH) and luteinizing hormone secretion are the greatly inhibited by placental progesterone and estrogen.

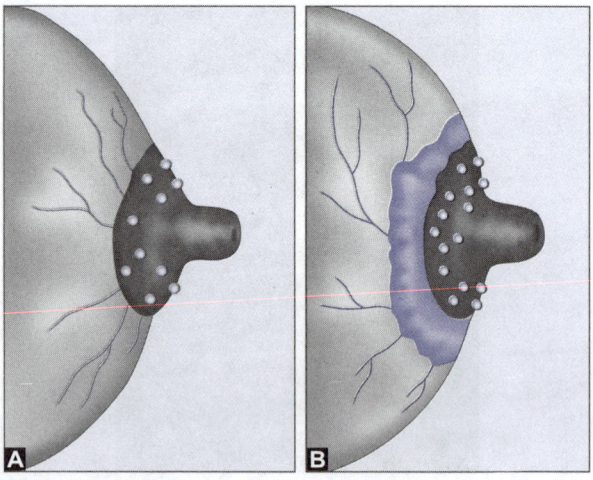

Figures 12.5A and B: (A) Pronounced pigmentation of the primary areola and nipple; (B) Appearance of secondary areola, development of Montgomery tubercles and increased vascularity.

The effects of prolactin secretion are suppressed during pregnancy. Following delivery of placenta, plasma concentrations of prolactin decrease, but is subsequently secreted in pulsatile bursts with sucking to stimulate milk production.

The posterior pituitary gland releases oxytocin in low frequency pulses throughout pregnancy. At term, the frequency of pulses increases which stimulates uterine contractions.

Thyroid Function

In normal pregnancy the thyroid gland increases in size by about 13% due to hyperplasia of glandular tissue and increased vascularity. There is normally an increased uptake of iodine during pregnancy, which may be to compensate for renal clearance of iodine leading to a reduced level of plasma iodine.

Although pregnancy can give the impression of hyperthyroidism, thyroid function is basically normal. The basal metabolic rate is increased mainly because of increased oxygen consumption by the fetus and the work of the maternal heart and lungs. Rising levels of T4 (thyroxin) and T3 (triiodothyronine) may also contribute to the increased metabolic rate.

Adrenal Glands

The adrenal glands are stimulated by estrogen to produce increasing levels of total and free plasma cortisol and other corticosteroids including ACTH from 12th week to term.

It is thought that the raised levels of free cortisol have an antagonistic action to insulin. More glucose is made available to the fetus by raising the levels of glucose in the blood, mobilizing maternal fatty acids and amino acids for the production of glycogen, and decreasing the uptake of glucose by muscle. Increase in free plasma cortisol may also be responsible for some of the Cushingoid features of normal pregnancy, such as fat deposition and striae gravidarum.

Because of the stimulus of progesterone and estrogen there is large increase in the concentration of renin by the adrenal cortex in the first 12 weeks of pregnancy. This activates the renin-angiotensin system, which is associated with maintaining blood pressure. It also balances the saltlosing effect of progesterone by enhancing aldosterone secretion from the adrenal cortex. Effects of aldosterone for promoting sodium absorption are most likely to be the key factor in maintaining the delicate balance of salt and water excretion.

Imbalance of these substances can cause pregnant women to reabsorb excess sodium from renal tubules and therefore to retain fluid which can cause hypertension. High levels of angiotensin II would also cause the blood pressure to rise.

CHANGES IN THE NERVOUS SYSTEM

The nervous system is in a more excitable condition in pregnant women. Temperamental changes are frequently noticed. Mood changes and symptoms of psychosis may develop in those with a family history.

Hemodynamic changes occur during pregnancy due to neurohormonal responses to pregnancy. Nitric oxide and prostaglandins are vasodilators that may be responsible for the observed drop in peripheral resistance and for changes in uterine and renal blood flow.

Activation of the sympathetic nervous system typically occurs in response to a decrease in peripheral vascular resistance and arterial pressure. Overactivity of the autonomic nervous and renin-angiotensin systems, and impairment in production or activity of vasodilators, such as nitric oxide and prostaglandins have all been implicated in the pathogenesis of preeclampsia.

The system wise physiological changes during pregnancy are summarized in **Figure 12.6**.

STUDY QUESTIONS

Short Notes

1. Breast changes in pregnancy.
2. Decidua.
3. Myometrium.

Short Answer Questions

1. Maternal weight gain in the normal pregnancy.
2. Hormones in pregnancy.
3. Skin changes in pregnancy.
4. Placental hormones.

Essay Question

1. Describe the cardiovascular changes that occur in women during pregnancy.

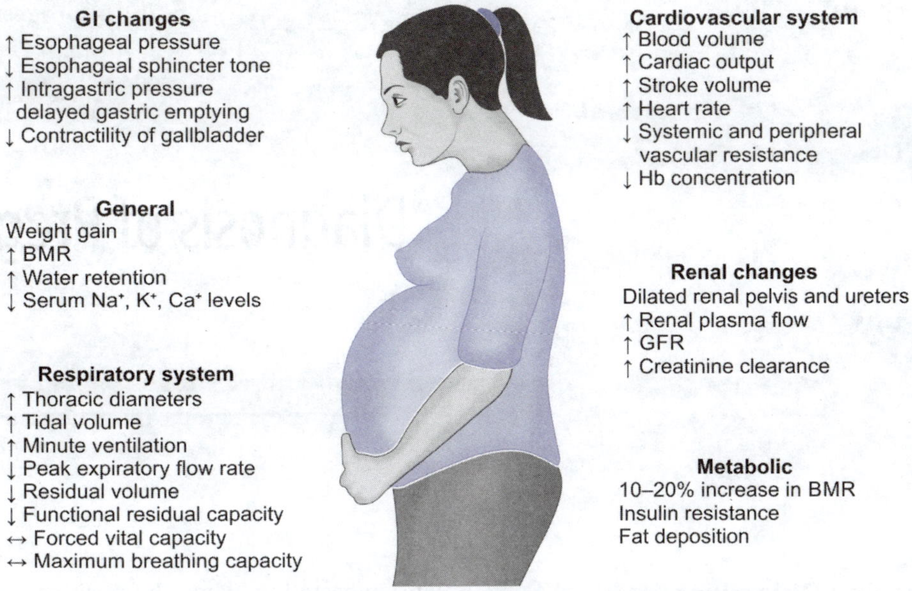

GI changes
↑ Esophageal pressure
↓ Esophageal sphincter tone
↑ Intragastric pressure
  delayed gastric emptying
↓ Contractility of gallbladder

General
Weight gain
↑ BMR
↑ Water retention
↓ Serum Na⁺, K⁺, Ca⁺ levels

Respiratory system
↑ Thoracic diameters
↑ Tidal volume
↑ Minute ventilation
↓ Peak expiratory flow rate
↓ Residual volume
↓ Functional residual capacity
↔ Forced vital capacity
↔ Maximum breathing capacity

Cardiovascular system
↑ Blood volume
↑ Cardiac output
↑ Stroke volume
↑ Heart rate
↓ Systemic and peripheral vascular resistance
↓ Hb concentration

Renal changes
Dilated renal pelvis and ureters
↑ Renal plasma flow
↑ GFR
↑ Creatinine clearance

Metabolic
10–20% increase in BMR
Insulin resistance
Fat deposition

Figure 12.6: Physiological changes during pregnancy.

BIBLIOGRAPHY

1. Beischer N, Mackay E, Colditz P. Obstetrics and the Newborn, 3rd edition. London: WB Saunders; 1997.
2. Bissonette J. Placental and fetal physiology. In: Gabbe S, Niebyl J, Simpson J (Eds). Obstetrics: Normal and Problem Pregnancies, 2nd edition. Edinburgh: Churchill Livingstone; 1991.
3. Case RM. Variations in Human Physiology, Manchester: Manchester University Press; 1985.
4. Case RM, Waterhouse J. Human Physiology, 2nd edition. Oxford: Oxford University Press; 1994.
5. Chamberlain G. The changing body in pregnancy. BMJ. 1991;302:719-2.
6. Cruikshank D, Hays P. Maternal Physiology in Pregnancy. In: Gabbe S, Niebyl J, Simpson J, Mark BL, Galan HL, Jauniaux, Driscoll (Eds). Obstetrics: Normal and Problem Pregnancies, 2nd edition. Edinburgh: Churchill Livingstone; 1991.
7. Cunningham FG, McDonald P, Gant N. William's Obstetrics, 18th edition. London: Prentice Hall; 1989.
8. Davison J, Dunlop W. Urinary Tract in Pregnancy. In: Chamberlain G (Ed). Turnbulls Obstetrics, 2nd edition. Edinburgh: Churchill Livingstone; 1995.
9. de Swiet M. The Cardiovascular System. In: Hytten F, Chamberlain G (Eds). Clinical Physiology in Obstetrics, 2nd edition. Oxford: Blackwell Scientific Publications; 1980.pp. 3-42.
10. Guyton A. Textbook of Medical Physiology, 8th edition. London: Saunders; 1991.
11. Hytten F. The alimentary system in pregnancies. Midwifery. 1990;6(4):201-4.
12. Llewellyn-Jones D. Fundamentals in Obstetrics and Gynecology, 6th edition. St Louis: Mosby; 1994.
13. McFadyen R. Maternal physiology in pregnancy. In: Chamberlain G (Ed). Turnbulls, Obstetrics, 2nd edition. Edinburgh: Churchill Livingstone; 1995.
14. Miller A, Hanretty K. Obstetrics Illustrated, 4th edition. Edinburgh: Churchill Livingstone; 1989.
15. Moore PJ. Maternal physiology during pregnancy. In: De Cherney AH, Pernoll ML (Eds). Current Obstetric and Gynecologic Diagnosis and Treatment, 8th edition. New York: McGraw-Hill.
16. Murray Irene. Change and adaptation in pregnancy. In: Bennett RV, Linda KB (Eds). Myles Textbook for Midwifes, 13th edition. Edinburgh: Churchill Livingstone; 1999.
17. Nilsson L. A Child is Born. London: Doubleday; 1990.
18. Silversider K, Coleman M. (1998). Physiological changes in Pregnancy. [online]. Available from http://www.metadogerar.com.br/wp
19. Symonds EM. Essential Obstetrics and Gynecology. Edinburgh: Churchill Livingstone; 1992.
20. Van Oppen AC, Stigler RH, Bruinse HW. Cardiac output in normal pregnancy: a critical review. Obstet and Gynecol. 1997;87:310-7.
21. Verralls S. Anatomy and Physiology Applied to Obstetrics, 3rd edition. Edinburgh: Churchill Livingstone; 1993.
22. Wade T. Skin disorders. In: Brudenell M, Wilds P (Eds). Medical and Surgical Problems in Obstetrics. Bristol: John Wright; 1984.

CHAPTER 13

Diagnosis of Pregnancy

Learning Objectives

Upon completing this chapter, the learner will be able to:
- List the signs of pregnancy and explain the changes evident in the mother's body.
- Diagnose pregnancies at different stages of gestation based on the findings of examination.
- Explain the different pregnancy tests.

The antepartum period covers the time of pregnancy from the first day of the last menstrual period (LMP) to the start of true labor, which marks the beginning of the intrapartum period.

The antepartal period is divided into three trimesters, each consisting of approximately 13 weeks or 3 calendar months. This derives from the calculation of pregnancy as being approximately 280 days or 40 weeks from the 1st day of LMP. In reality gestation is not that long. Fertilization takes place at the time of ovulation, i.e. approximately 14 days after the LMP. This makes actual gestation approximately of 266 days or 38 weeks. Adding 14 days gives a total of 280 days from the LMP.

A pregnancy period is divided into three semesters:
- The first semester is from week 1 to the end of week 12
- The second semester is from week 13 to the end of week 26
- The third semester is from week 27 to the end of the pregnancy.

DIAGNOSIS OF PREGNANCY

Pregnancy may be diagnosed by the woman herself even before she has missed a period because she feels different. Changes in the breasts can occur as early as 5-6 weeks after conception.

Diagnosis of pregnancy in the first trimester and early second trimester is based on a combination of presumptive and probable signs of pregnancy. Pregnancy is self-evident later in gestation, when the positive signs of pregnancy are readily observed:
- Presumptive signs of pregnancy are maternal physiological changes which the woman experiences and which in most cases indicate to her that she is pregnant.
- Probable signs of pregnancy are maternal physiological changes other than presumptive signs which are detected upon examination and documented by the examiner.
- Positive signs are those directly attributable to the fetus as detected and documented by the examiner.

Following is an outline of all the presumptive, probable and positive signs of pregnancy.

Presumptive Signs

- Abrupt cessation of menstruation (amenorrhea) at 4th week.
- Nausea and vomiting (morning sickness) from 4th to 14th week.
- Tingling, tenseness, nodularity and enlargement of the breasts, and enlargement of the nipples around 3-4 weeks.
- Increased frequency of micturition (bladder irritability) around 6-12 weeks.
- Fatigue.
- Color changes of breasts, i.e. darkening of the nipples, primary and secondary areolar change.
- Appearance of Montgomery's tubercles.
- Continued elevation of basal body temperature in the absence of an infection.
- Expression of colostrum from nipples.
- Excessive salivation.
- Quickening (the first movement felt by the mother around 18-20 weeks).
- Skin pigmentation and conditions, such as chloasma, breast and abdominal striae, linea nigra and palmar erythema.

Probable Signs

- Enlargement of the uterus.
- Change in shape of the uterus.
- Presence of human chorionic gonadotropin (hCG) in blood (4–12 weeks) and in urine (6–12 weeks)—positive pregnancy tests.
- *Hegar's sign:* Softening and compressibility of the isthmus (6–12 weeks) **(Fig. 13.1)**.
- *Jacquemier's sign/Chadwick's sign:* The violet-blue discoloration of the vulva and vaginal mucosa including vaginal portion of the cervix due to increased vascularity evident by about 6 weeks gestation.
- *Osiander's sign:* Pulsation in the lateral fornices (8th weeks).
- *Palmer's sign:* Regular, rhythmic and painless contraction resembling systole and diastole of the heart that can be elicited during bimanual examination in early pregnancy (as early as 8 weeks).
- *Goodell's sign:* Softening of the cervix from a nonpregnant state of firmness similar to the tip of a nose to the softness of lips in the pregnant state (from 6th week).
- Presence of Braxton Hicks contractions (16th week).
- Ballottement of fetus (16–28 weeks) **(Fig. 13.2)**.

Positive Signs

- Visualization of fetus by ultrasound (6th week and above).
- Visualization of fetal skeleton by X-ray (16th week).
- Fetal heart sounds by ultrasound (6th week).
- Fetal heart sounds with fetoscope (20th week).
- Palpable fetal movements (22th week).
- Visible fetal movements (late pregnancy).
- Palpation of fetal parts (24th week and above).

It is not always appropriate to seek findings regarding all of the signs of pregnancy outlined here when examining a woman

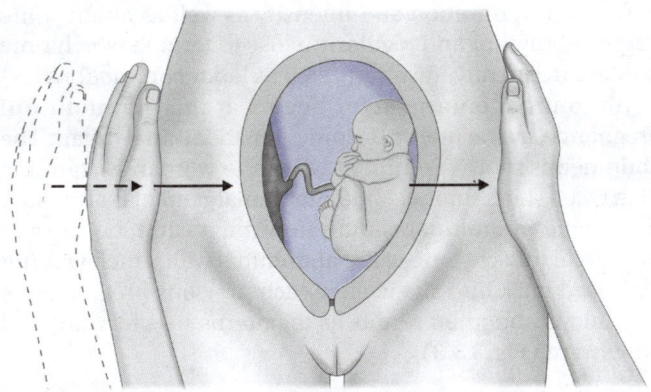

Figure 13.2: External ballotment.

who thinks she is pregnant. This is because of not all the signs are manifested at the same time. It is also important to know that the majority of these signs can be due to other conditions and a diagnosis of pregnancy can be made only in the presence of several of these changes.

Uterine Enlargement

Estrogen and progesterone are primarily responsible for the hypertrophy of the uterine wall during the early months of pregnancy. Uterine enlargement is the result of a considerable increase in the size and stretching of the muscle cells. The hypertrophy of the muscle cells is accompanied by a marked increase in the elastic and fibrous tissue, which strengthens the uterine wall.

After the 3rd month of pregnancy, the uterine enlargement is also due to the mechanical effect of inside pressure on the uterine wall by the growing products of conception. In the early months of pregnancy, there is a marked increase in the size of the uterine blood vessels and lymphatics. The resulting vascularity, congestion and edema most likely account for the overall softening of the uterus. These along with hypertrophy of the cervical glands give rise to Chadwick's/Jacquemier's sign and Hegar's sign.

The softness and compressibility of the uterine isthmus (Hegar's sign) has the effects of nonsupport to the enlarging body of the uterus with its increasing heaviness in the fundus. The result is an exaggerated uterine anteflexion during the first 3 months of pregnancy, while the uterus is still a pelvic organ. This causes the fundus to press on the bladder resulting in urinary frequency. Urinary frequency is relieved early in the 4th month of pregnancy as the uterus rises out of the pelvis.

As the uterus enlarges, it changes from its non-pregnant pear shape to globular and then to ovoid. Early uterine enlargement may not be symmetrical. The ovum implants in the upper uterine wall, more frequently on the posterior side.

Uterine enlargement contributes to two other maternal signs of pregnancy—the Braxton Hicks contractions and abdominal enlargement. Braxton Hicks contractions are nonrhythmic, sporadic, painless uterine contractions that start about the 6th week of pregnancy. These are detectable on bimanual examination in the second trimester and during abdominal examination in the third trimester. They increase

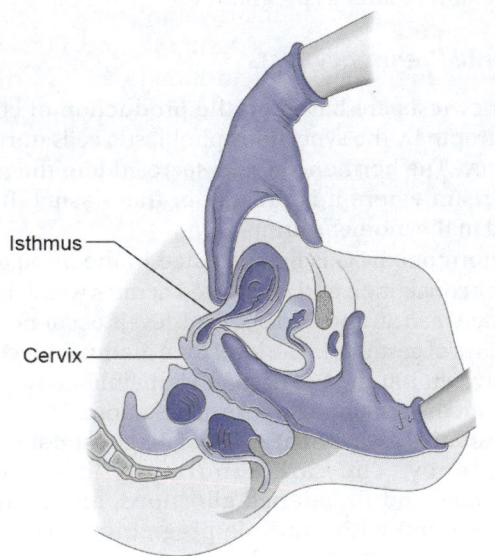

Figure 13.1: Hegar's sign.

in frequency, duration and intensity as well as attain some degree of rhythm and regularity close to term at which time they are frequently misinterpreted as labor contractions.

Abdominal enlargement begins at the 4th month of pregnancy, as the uterus becomes an abdominal organ. The abdomen is more prominent when the woman is standing than when she is supine. Abdominal enlargement is also more noticeable in multiparas than in primigravida, because of the loss of muscle tone of the abdominal wall which was not exercised back into shape after each previous pregnancy. A pendulous abdomen results as the uterus sags forward and downward **(Fig. 13.3)**.

Other Signs of Pregnancy

It is thought that the basal metabolic rate (BMR) initially falls during pregnancy and then progressively rises throughout the pregnancy as a direct result of the metabolic activity of the products of conception.

The initial fall in the BMR might account for the fatigue often encountered during the first trimester. Nausea and vomiting have been attributed to a number of possible causes, but their actual etiology is not yet known. Normal nausea and vomiting in pregnancy rarely extend beyond the first trimester. Excessive salivation (ptyalism) is an unusual occurrence, which may be caused either by increased acidity in the mouth or by the intake of starch stimulating the salivary glands in women who are susceptible to excessive secretion. Women who have ptyalism frequently, are nauseated also.

Fetal Contributions to the Diagnosis of Pregnancy

Anatomic

The combination of uterine enlargement, thinning of the uterine wall and the uterus becoming an abdominal organ enable the detection of a number of signs of pregnancy in the second trimester which was previously inaccessible. The precise time, when the fetal heart tones are heard and the quickening is felt vary with the thinness or obesity of the individual woman as well as with parity. In multiparous women, as the abdominal musculature has hypertrophied and stretched earlier, it may be thin enough to facilitate eliciting of the following signs of pregnancy a week or two earlier than in a primigravida.

The fetal heart starts beating at the 6th week (4th week postfertilization) and can be heard by 20th week with a fetoscope during abdominal examination of the mother. However, it can be heard between 12th and 20th week with ultrasonic instruments. Fetal heart tones must be differentiated from two other sound:

1. *Uterine souffle:* A soft blowing and systolic murmur heard low down at the sides of the uterus, best on the left side. The sound is due to increase in blood flow through the dilated uterine vessels and is synchronous with the maternal pulse.
2. *Funic souffle:* The sound of blood rushing through the umbilical arteries. It is a soft blowing murmur synchronous with the fetal heart sounds.

Weak fetal movements start in the 3rd month of pregnancy and by 20th week they are strong enough and the uterine wall is thin enough for them to be felt and properly diagnosed during abdominal examination. The mother may be aware of fetal movements around 18th week. These movements increase in intensity over the weeks from gentle flutterings to unmistakable fetal kicks. The time when she feels the first fetal movement is called **quickening,** meaning the perception of life.

After the 20th week, fetal outline can be palpated during abdominal examination. This is not a definitive diagnostic sign, because subserous myomas may feel like fetal parts. Ballottement can be elicited abdominally around the same time. In this sign, a sudden tap on the uterus causes the fetus to sink in the amniotic fluid and rebound to strike gently against the fingers of the examiner. Ballottement is possible at this time because there is a large volume of amniotic fluid in relation to the size of the still small fetus. This proportion grossly changes later in pregnancy.

Hormonal Pregnancy Tests

Pregnancy tests are based on the production of chorionic gonadotropin by the syncytiotrophoblastic cells during early pregnancy. The hormone hCG is secreted into the maternal bloodstream where it is present in the plasma. It is then excreted in the mother's urine.

The hormone hCG is first detected in the urine about 26 days after conception and is excreted at rates which increases rapidly between 30 and 60 days. Peak levels occur between 60 and 70 days of gestation. The level then gradually decreases to a low between 100 and 130 days and is maintained at this level throughout the remaining weeks of gestation.

Quantitative assays of hCG are of diagnostic significance in pregnancy. They are abnormally low in ectopic pregnancies and threatened abortions, and abnormally high in women with multiple pregnancy, hydatidiform mole or choriocarcinoma. The hormone hCG in the urine has been used for pregnancy tests since the late 1920s

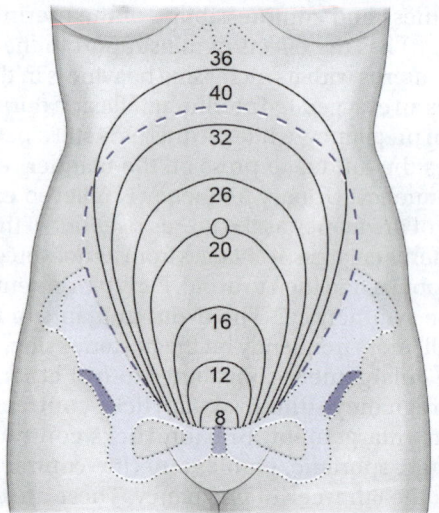

Figure 13.3: Fundal development in different weeks.

when Aschheim and Zondek originated **biologic assay** of its presence. These tests utilized small immature animals such as mice, rabbits, frogs and toads, and were based on the response of the animals' ovaries or testes after being injected with either serum or urine of the woman suspected of being pregnant.

These tests have been largely superseded by the immunologic assays of hCG. The immunologic assays of hCG test utilizes specific antisera, obtained from animals (rabbits) in which antibody response to hCG has been stimulated. It is based on the fact that hCG is a protein and therefore antigenic. The antisera are mixed with urine of the woman suspected of being pregnant. This mediates the response of the antisera when mixed with either latex particles coated with hCG or with erythrocytes, which have been sensitized to hCG. This will neutralize the antibodies in the antiserum and inhibit agglutination, which is a positive pregnancy test. If the woman is not pregnant, her urine does not contain hCG and agglutination will occur, which is a negative pregnancy test.

More recently, radioreceptor assay and radio-immunoassay (RIA) tests have become available. Both require expensive equipment and trained technicians. These are extremely sensitive tests, able to detect hCG at far lower levels than previous tests. The RIA blood test commonly known as beta-preg; can be used as early as 1 week after conception if laboratory facilities are available. Because the radioreceptor assay test cross-reacts with luteinizing hormone, it is more limited in its sensitivity than the RIA.

Pregnancy Test Kits for Home Use (Figs. 13.4A to D)

Several self-use pregnancy test kits are now available in India. These Food and Drug Administration (FDA) approved products are easy to use and give quick results. The strip tests are performed to discover the level of hCG hormone in urine. The kits contain instructions for use and give results in 1–5 minutes. The results (strip reading) indicate if the test is positive or negative for pregnancy, or needs to be repeated. Some of the pregnancy detection kits for home use that are presently available in India are —'i-can' one step pregnancy, test device,' 'First response pregnancy test kit,' 'Velocit eazy' pregnancy detection kit and 'Makesure pregnancy test kit' (**Figs. 13.4A to D**).

■ STUDY QUESTIONS

Short Notes

1. Ballottement.
2. Human chorionic gonadotropin.
3. Braxton Hicks contractions.

Short Answer Questions

1. Presumptive signs of pregnancy.
2. Probable signs of pregnancy.
3. Positive signs of pregnancy.

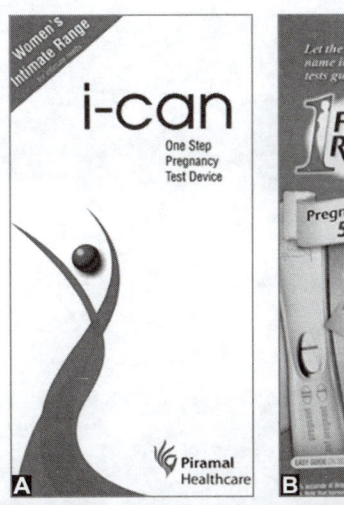
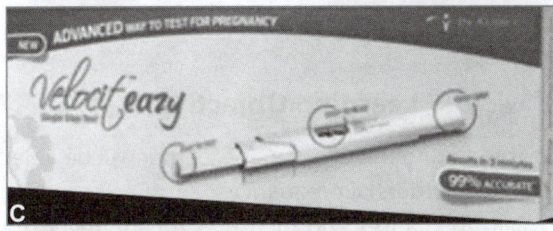
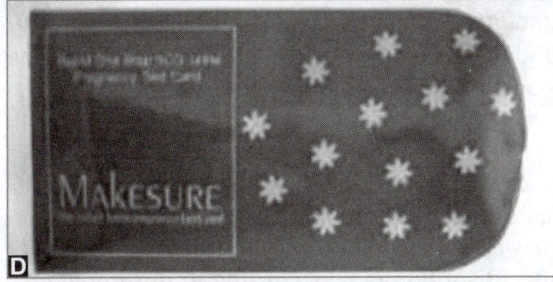

Figures 13.4A to D: Pregnancy test kits for home use. (A) 'i-can' test kit; (B) 'First response' pregnancy test; (C) 'Velocit eazy' test device; (D) 'Makesure' test kit.

Essay Question

1. Describe the signs of pregnancy and the tests used for diagnosing pregnancy.

■ BIBLIOGRAPHY

1. Dutta DC. Textbook of Obstetrics, 5th edition. Calcutta: New Central Book Company; 2001. pp. 66-77.
2. Ladewig PW, London ML, Olds SB. Essentials of Maternal-Newborn Nursing. New York: Addison-Wesley; 1990.
3. Murray Irene. Change and adaptation in pregnancy. In: Bennett RV, Linda KB (Eds). Myles Textbook for Midwives, 13th edition. Edinburgh: Churchill Livingstone; 1999. pp. 186-7.
4. Neeson JD. Clinical Manual of Maternity Nursing, 3rd edition. Philadelphia: JB Lippincot; 1989.
5. Varney Helen. Nurse-midwifery, 2nd edition. Boston: MA:Blackwell Scientific Publications, 1987.
6. Home check instant pregnancy test. [online]. Available from/ www. healthkart.com/SV
7. Pregnancy test kits. [online]. Available from/www.velocit.com

CHAPTER 14

Minor Disorders in Pregnancy

Learning Objectives

Upon completing this chapter, the learner will be able to:
- List the disorders of pregnancy.
- Explain the causes and measures for the relief of discomforts.
- Outline the disorders that can possibly escalate requiring immediate intervention.

Figure 14.1: Minor disorders during pregnancy.

Many women experience some minor disorders during pregnancy. These disorders should be treated adequately as they may escalate and become life-threatening.

Minor disorders may occur due to hormonal changes, accommodation changes, metabolic changes and postural changes. Every system of the body is affected by pregnancy. The mother needs knowledge to cope with the experience of pregnancy. She also needs knowledge when she presents with discomforting or worrying symptoms **(Fig. 14.1)**.

DIGESTIVE SYSTEM

Nausea and Vomiting

Nausea and vomiting is a common disorder seen in about 50% women between 4th and 16th week of gestation. Hormonal influences are thought to be the most likely cause. Human chorionic gonadotropin (hCG), which is present in large amounts in the first trimester, estrogen and progesterone are all contributors to this. The sickness is confined to 'early morning', but can occur at any time in the day. The smell of food cooking will often cause the mother to retch.

The midwife can explain the probable reasons and encourage the mother to look positively toward the resolution of the problem, which may happen between 12th and 16th week. Women have found the following as helpful practices:
- Salads and light snacks are more tolerable than full meals
- Carbohydrate snacks at bedtime can prevent hypoglycemia, which is often shown as a cause of nausea and vomiting
- Dry toast or biscuit on waking up and breakfast after half an hour.

If vomiting becomes severe, the mother may lose weight and become dehydrated and ketotic. This condition is called hyperemesis gravidarum and warrants specialized care, and appropriate referral **(Box 14.1)**.

Heartburn

Heartburn is a burning pain in the mediastinal region caused by reflux of stomach contents into the esophagus. It occurs because the cardiac sphincter relaxes during pregnancy due to the effect of progesterone. The condition tends to worsen as pregnancy advances, because the stomach is displaced upward by the enlarging uterus. Heartburn is most troublesome at about 30–40 weeks of gestation, because at this stage the stomach is under pressure from the growing uterus.

The advice varies according to the severity of the condition, which includes:

> **BOX 14.1:** Client education.
>
> **Nausea and vomiting in pregnancy**
> - Drink soups and liquids between meals, rather than with meals to avoid dehydration
> - Avoid fluids that contain caffeine or carbonation
> - Eat a diet that is high in protein and carbohydrates in 5–6 meals daily
> - Eat small, low fat meals and snacks every 2–3 hours
> - Avoid aromatic foods and cooking odors that may trigger nausea
> - Take a walk after meals, to help with digestion
> - Limit stressful events and get plenty of rest
> - Avoid being in a hurry, especially in the morning
> - Eat 2 or 3 crackers or dry toast in the morning before getting out of bed and avoid taking fluids with it
> - Do not take any medication for vomiting or any other condition without consulting your physician
> - Wear loose-fitting clothes

- If the heartburn is occasional, the reflux can be prevented by avoiding bending and kneeling, while doing household chores
- Small meals take less room in the reduced stomach space and are digested more easily
- Fried and fatty foods should be avoided
- Sleeping with more pillows than usual and lying on the right side semireclining can sometimes help
- For persistent heartburn antacids may be prescribed by the physician (**Box 14.2**).

Excessive Salivation

Excessive salivation (ptyalism) occurs from 8th week of gestation and it is thought that the hormones of pregnancy are the cause for it. It may accompany heartburn.

Pica

Pica is the term used when the mother craves certain foods or unnatural substances such as coal. The cause is unknown, but hormones and changes in metabolism are thought to contribute to this. If the substances craved are harmful to the unborn baby, the mother must be helped to seek medical advice.

> **BOX 14.2:** Client education.
>
> **Heartburn in pregnancy**
> - Monitor your diet for foods that cause upset. Keep a list
> - Avoid drinking large amounts of fluid with meals. Instead, spread fluid intake throughout the day
> - Remain sitting upright for at least 30 minutes after a meal and sleep with an extra pillow at night to keep the head elevated
> - Do not bend at the waist; always bend at the knees maintaining a more upright posture
> - Try lying on your right side and using relaxation techniques to calm your stomach and promote digestion

Constipation

Constipation is due to smooth muscle relaxant effect of progesterone causing decreased peristalsis of the gut. Pressure of the gravid uterus on the colon near term makes it worse as the colon gets displaced. It is usually overcome by adjusting the diet. The women may be advised to:
- Increase the intake of water
- Add green leafy vegetables, fruits and bran cereals to her diet
- Take a glass of warm water in the morning before tea or breakfast, which would activate the gut and help regular bowel movements
- Exercise by regular walking.

Constipation is sometimes associated with taking oral iron and it can aggravate hemorrhoids.

MUSCULOSKELETAL SYSTEM

Backache

The gradual weight gain and the change in the body's center of gravity combined with the stretching of weak abdominal muscles often lead to a hollowing of the lumbar spine. There is a tendency for back muscles to shorten as the abdominal muscles stretch and extra strain is put on the ligaments. This results in backache, usually of sacroiliac or lumbar origin. Women with this problem must be helped with:
- Postural re-education including correction of the 'pelvic tilt'
- Advise relating to comfortable positions in sitting, standing, lying, general mobility and how to lift correctly.

Lying on the side away from the discomfort, with the affected leg uppermost may relieve the problem. Pillows should be placed to support the whole limb.

Backache must never be dismissed lightly as it is associated with urinary tract infection and with the onset of labor, especially when the fetal occiput is posterior (**Box 14.3**).

> **BOX 14.3:** Client education.
>
> **Backache in pregnancy**
> - Be aware of your posture; be sure your neck, shoulders, and back are straight and your pelvis is tilted slightly forward
> - Bend the knees and never at the waist
> - Wear comfortable, low heeled shoes
> - Elevate one foot when standing for extended periods of time
> - Practice deep breathing and relaxation exercises that focus on the upper body
> - Get a massage to relax tired muscles

Cramps

Cramps are quite common, usually in the leg. They are worse at night. The cause of leg cramps in pregnancy is not known, but has been attributed to deficiency of vitamin B_1 and decreased levels of calcium. It may be due to ischemia or changes in pH or electrolyte status. It may be helpful to:

- Make gentle leg movements whilst in a warm bath prior to settling for the night
- Sleep with the foot end of the bed elevated by 20–25 cm
- Take vitamin B complex and calcium supplements.

An attack can be aborted by sharply stretching the involved muscle. Once a cramp has occurred, gentle kneading is effective.

GENITOURINARY SYSTEM

Frequency of Micturition

Micturition occurs in the first trimester when there is pressure of the gravid uterus on the urinary bladder. It is spontaneously relieved when the uterus rises up in the abdomen. It may recur late in pregnancy when the fetal head descends into the pelvis. Urinary tract infection should always be ruled out before attributing the frequency to pregnancy. Reassurance is sufficient.

Leukorrhea

Leukorrhea is the term used for the increased white, non-irritant vaginal discharge in pregnancy. If the mother finds the discharge disturbing, it is helpful to offer simple advice of personal hygiene.

Frequent washing of the vulva (3–4 time a day) with plain water would be sufficient. She should wear cotton underwear and avoid tights. The midwife should exclude the possibility of infection such as thrush and *Trichomonas*.

CIRCULATORY SYSTEM

Fainting

In early pregnancy, fainting may occur due to vasodilation under the influence of progesterone. It may subside following the compensatory increase in blood volume. Measures for relief include avoiding long periods of standing as well as sitting or lying down when she feels slightly faint.

Later in pregnancy, mother may feel faint, while lying flat on her back. This is because the weight of the uterine contents presses on the inferior vena cava and slows the return of blood to the heart. Turning the mother quickly on to her side will bring rapid recovery. She should be advised not to lie on her back except during abdominal examination.

Varicosities

Progesterone relaxes the smooth muscles of the veins and results in sluggish circulation (slow moving). The valves of the dilated veins become inefficient and varicosities result. Varicose veins occur in legs, anus (hemorrhoids) and vulva. The situation is often compounded by pelvic congestion.

Pregnant women with a family history of varicose veins and those doing work, which demands long periods of standing and sitting usually, develop varicose veins **(Box 14.4)**. Measures to reduce the discomfort of leg varicosities include:

BOX 14.4: Client education.

Varicose veins in pregnancy
- Maintain good circulation in your legs; avoid sitting, standing or crossing your legs for long periods
- Elevate your legs as often as you are able or flex your feet several times every few minutes while sitting
- Take breaks and short frequent walks while performing intense, stationary work
- Wear clothes that fit loosely and avoid wearing knee-high hose that may constrict the blood vessels in the legs

---

- Exercising the calf muscles by rising onto the toes or making circling movements with the ankles
- Resting with the legs vertical against the wall for a short time
- Wearing support tights before rising or after resting with legs elevated.

Those with hemorrhoids or tendency to develop them should be advised about:
- Avoidance of constipation by including fiber in the diet and adequate fluids
- Seeking medical advice for topical applications.

Vulvar varicosities are rare and very painful. A panty girdle or sanitary pad may give support. Vulval varicosities may rupture and bleed during delivery. Occasionally numerous spider varices develop on the skin. Most of those enlarged veins disappear after delivery.

Hemorrhoids

Hemorrhoids are varicosities of the rectum, which may occur outside the anal sphincter or inside the anal sphincter. Typically, hemorrhoids that are already present are exacerbated by the changes that occur in the body during pregnancy. Other factors that may exacerbate hemorrhoids are prolonged sitting or standing, straining at stool and pushing in the second stage of labor. Hemorrhoids may continue to be problematic in the postpartum period **(Box 14.5)**.

Edema

Edema is the result of venous and lymphatic stasis. Additional factors responsible are—changes in osmotic pressure of blood and tissue fluids, and altered capillary permeability. The blood pressure should be checked to see if the patient

---

BOX 14.5: Client education.

Hemorrhoids in pregnancy
- Maintain healthy and regular bowel habits.
- Try sitz bath: Sit for about 20 minutes in a tub filled with warm water.
- If hemorrhoids are protruding from the anus, gently push them back into the rectum: Using a glove and lubricant, gently press the hemorrhoid back through the anus and hold for a few seconds. This may be comfortably achieved after a sitz bath.

has pregnancy-induced hypertension. The treatment of gestational edema of feet is elevation of legs, sleeping in left lateral position and avoid sitting with the feet hanging down.

INTEGUMENTARY SYSTEM

Skin

Some pregnant women complain generalized itching, which often starts over the abdomen. This is thought to have some connection with the liver's response to the hormones in pregnancy and with raised bilirubin levels. It clears soon after the baby is born and comfort can be gained from local applications. An antihistamine is often prescribed. If a mother complains of vulvar irritation, infection such as thrush and glycosuria as a result of diabetes must be excluded. Washing with mild soap and cotton underwear might help to ease the irritation.

NERVOUS SYSTEM

Carpal Tunnel Syndrome

Pregnant women complains numbness and pins, and needles in their fingers and hands. This usually happens in the morning, but it can occur at any time of the day. It is caused by fluid retention, which creates edema and pressure on the median nerve. Wearing a splint at night, with the hands and resting on two or three pillows sometimes help. Restriction of salt intake and flexing the fingers, while the arm is held above the head can be recommended. Carpal tunnel syndrome usually resolves spontaneously following delivery.

Intercostal neuralgia may develop in late pregnancy due to muscle spasm. It may be unilateral or girdle type. Sitting in a straight-backed chair, using a cushion for lumbar support and lateral flexion exercises relieves it.

Bell's palsy may rarely develop in the last trimester due to edema compressing the facial nerve. It is relieved spontaneously in 3–4 weeks following delivery.

Insomnia

Insomnia is relatively common in late pregnancy owing to the discomfort caused by the fetal movements, frequency of micturition and difficulty in finding a comfortable position. It may also be due to some deep-seated anxiety or fear. Women with such problems can be advised to:
- Take rest in the afternoon
- Drink a glass of warm milk at bedtime
- Tuck a pillow under the abdomen when lying in a lateral position
- Talk about her fears and anxieties, so that she can have a sense of normality and lightness.

DISORDERS THAT REQUIRE IMMEDIATE ACTION

Most minor disorders can escalate into a more serious complication of pregnancy. Mothers should be encouraged to seek advice if at any time they feel unwell or the signs exceed what they have been led to expect. In addition there are incidents, which should always be reported to the physician. These are:
- Vaginal bleeding
- Reduced fetal movements
- Frontal or recurring headaches
- Sudden swelling/edema
- Rupture of the membranes
- Premature onset of contractions
- Sudden nausea or sickness
- Epigastric pain.

Mothers must be reassured about their pregnancy status. Knowledge that the pregnancy proceeds without complications, would add to their security and confidence. They should also know when to seek the help of a professional.

STUDY QUESTIONS

Short Notes

1. Ptyalism in pregnancy.
2. Pica in pregnancy.
3. Leukorrhea in pregnancy.

Short Answer Questions

1. Nausea and vomiting in pregnancy and helpful measures a nurse can teach the pregnant client.
2. Heartburn as a minor disorder of pregnancy and measures to deal with the problem.
3. Classification of minor disorders of pregnancy and measures to deal with them.
4. Cramps as a minor disorder of pregnancy and measures that can be advised to reduce and cope with them.

Essay Question

1. Describe the minor disorders commonly experienced by pregnant women and the measures that can be taught to deal with them.

BIBLIOGRAPHY

1. Jamieson L. Preparing for parenthood: Daily life in pregnancy. In: Bennett RV, Linda KB (Eds). Myles Textbook for Midwives, 13th edition. Edinburgh: Churchill Livingstone; 1999. pp. 203-7.
2. Karpen M, Conrad L, Chitwood L. Essentials of Maternal Child Nursing, 2nd edition. 1995. pp. 25-32.
3. Light HK, Fenster C. Maternal concerns during pregnancy. Am J Obstet Gynecol. 1974;118:46.
4. Moore P. Maternal physiology during pregnancy. In: De Chermey A, Pernoll M (Eds). Current Obstetric and Gynecologic Diagnosis and Treatment, 8th edition. London: Prentice Hall; 1994.
5. Parulekar SV. Textbook for Midwives, 2nd edition. Mumbai: Vora Medical Publications; 1998. pp. 134-6.
6. Helen V. Nurse-Midwifery, 2nd edition. Boston: Jones and Bartlett Publishers; 1996.

Antenatal Care

Learning Objectives

Upon completing this chapter, the learner will be able to:
- Explain the meaning and objectives of antenatal care.
- List the objectives and procedure of initial assessment, and review of body systems.
- Describe the physical examination of the mother during the initial and subsequent visits.
- Describe the steps of abdominal examination.
- Enumerate the steps of nursing process for an antenatal mother.

MEANING

Antenatal care refers to the care given to an expectant mother from the time conception is confirmed until the beginning of labor. It includes monitoring the progress of pregnancy, providing appropriate support to the woman and her family, and providing information, which will assist them to make sensible choices.

OBJECTIVES

The objectives of prenatal care are to:
- Promote, protect and maintain the health of the mother during pregnancy
- Detect 'high-risk' pregnancies, and give the mothers special attention
- Foresee complications and take preventive measures
- Remove anxiety and fear associated with pregnancy
- Reduce maternal-infant morbidity and mortality
- Teach the mother elements of nutrition, personal hygiene and newborn care
- Sensitize the mother to the need of family planning.

ANTENATAL VISITS

Ideally, the antenatal mother should visit the antenatal clinic once a month during the first 7 months; twice a month during the 8th month and thereafter once a week, if everything is normal. A large proportion of mothers in India are from lower socioeconomic group and many are working women. For women who find regular attendance at the clinic difficult due to economic reasons, if the pregnancy is uncomplicated, a minimum of three visits covering the entire period of pregnancy should be the target as outlined below (Park, 2000). First visit at 20th week or as soon as the pregnancy is known. Second visit at 32nd week and third visit at 36th week **(Box 15.1)**.

BOX 15.1: Client education.

Antenatal/prenatal visits
- Up to 28 weeks of gestation, every 4 weeks
- 29–32 weeks of gestation, every 2 weeks
- 33 weeks till delivery, every week

INITIAL EXAMINATION

The first visit, irrespective of when it occurs, should include the client's health history, obstetric history, physical and pelvic examinations and laboratory examinations.

Health History

1. Identifying information.
2. Chief complaints in her own words. Medical conditions that affect pregnancy may vary from common urinary tract infections (UTIs) to severe cardiac conditions. Some of the medical conditions that require special care are:

a. Urinary tract infection.
b. Essential hypertension that may lead to pregnancy-induced hypertension (PIH).
c. Asthma, epilepsy, psychiatric disorders.
d. Medical conditions such as diabetes and cardiac conditions.

Family History

History of conditions that are genetic in origin, familial or have racial characteristics such as:
- Diabetes in a first-degree relative
- Hypertension
- Multiple pregnancies
- Conditions like spina bifida, sickle cell anemia and thalassemia.

Menstrual History

- Age at menarche
- Frequency, duration and amount of menstrual flow
- Dysfunctional uterine bleeding, i.e. menorrhagia, metrorrhagia or intermenstrual spotting
- Premenstrual spotting.

Obstetric History

Obstetric history includes obtaining the date of her last menstrual period (LMP), calculation of her expected date of delivery (EDD), determination of the present number of weeks of gestation and calculation of her gravida and para status.

Gravida

Gravida refers to the number of times a woman has been pregnant. It does not take into account at what time during pregnancy it (the pregnancy) was terminated; nor does it matter how many babies were born from the pregnancy. It is the pregnancy that counts and not the number of babies. A woman who had one pregnancy from which she issued triplets would still be a gravida 1 until she becomes pregnant again at which time she would be gravida 2. A woman who is pregnant for the first time is called *primigravida* and a woman who is pregnant for the second time is called *secundigravida*. Thereafter, if she becomes pregnant again, she is called *multigravida*. A woman who has never been pregnant is called *nulligravida*.

Para

Para refers to the number of pregnancies that terminated in the birth of a fetus or fetuses that reached the point of viability (the ability of the fetus to survive, if born). This point is considered to be 28 weeks of gestation or 1,000 g (in India). It is the number of pregnancies carried to the point of the fetus or fetuses reaching the point of viability that determines parity and not the number of fetuses reaching the point of viability. Para is not affected whether the fetus or fetuses are born alive or are stillbirths.

A *primipara* is a woman who has given birth to a fetus or fetuses that has reached the point of viability. A *multipara* is a woman who had given birth to two or more babies, live or still excluding abortions.

A *grand multipara* is a woman who has given birth five times or more. A woman who has not carried a pregnancy to the point of viability is called *nullipara*. The items to be included in obstetric history are:
- Gravida, para
- Rhesus (Rh) and ABO blood type
- Previous pregnancy and delivery:
  - Weeks of gestation and dates of termination
  - Delivery in the hospital or at home
  - Length of labor
  - Type of delivery, i.e. spontaneous, instrumental or cesarean section
  - RhoGAM [Rho(D) immune globulin human] received
  - Any obstetric, medical problems during pregnancy, labor or delivery.
- Status of newborn at birth:
  - Cried immediately, problems and death
  - Sex and weight of the baby
  - Any congenital anomalies or neonatal problems.

Present Pregnancy

History of the present pregnancy is designed to detect complications, discomforts and any complaints about pregnancy; the woman may have experienced since her last menstrual period (LMP).

The date of the 1st day of the last normal menstrual period is used as the baseline for determining gestational age and estimated EDD. Hence, it is important to obtain the accurate date of this event. When the accuracy of pinpointing the LMP is impossible, other parameters may be used to arrive at the expected date of delivery. Ascertaining the approximate date on which the baby was conceived, is important to predict the date of giving birth and to calculate the gestational age at any point of pregnancy.

The EDD is calculated by *Naegele's* rule in which 7 days are added to the date of the first day of LMP and 3 months are subtracted from that date. It is also calculated by adding 9 calendar months and 7 days to the date of the 1st day of the woman's last menstrual period.

The actual period of gestation is from the time of fertilization. Since, ovulation is generally considered to occur approximately 14 days before the next menstrual period; the length of a woman's menstrual cycle will affect the accuracy of the EDD. A woman with a longer menstrual cycle (more than 28 days) will actually begin her pregnancy later in relation to her LMP and subsequently will deliver at a correspondingly later date. The reverse is true for women with shorter menstrual cycle. The majority of women will deliver within 10–14 days either earlier or later of their EDD and this is considered physiologically normal.

It is useless to calculate the EDD by Naegele's rule in the presence of the following situations:
- Irregular menstrual periods in which one or more months are amenorrheic

- Conception occurring, while the mother is breastfeeding and ovulating, but amenorrheic
- Conception occurring before regular menstruation is established after termination of pregnancy or discontinuation of oral contraceptive pills.

In such instances, an estimated date of delivery is arrived at based on clinical findings and if indicated an ultrasound scan is taken between 18th and 26th weeks of gestation. The woman may be seen for her initial antenatal examination at any time during the present pregnancy and therefore the present pregnancy history here covers the symptoms of possible problems in all three trimesters of pregnancy:

- Headache, dizziness, visual disturbances
- Syncope, fatigue
- Nausea, vomiting, heartburn
- Breast changes
- Shortness of breath
- Abdominal pain, back pain, dyspareunia
- Vaginal discharge, vaginal bleeding
- Dysuria, urinary frequency
- Constipation, hemorrhoids
- Leg cramps, varicosities
- Edema—ankles, pretibial, face, hands
- Feelings about pregnancy—body image, feeling about the baby.

Physical Examination

A complete screening physical examination is done during the initial antepartum examination in order to ascertain whether the woman has any medical disease or abnormalities. It includes a structured review of body systems through observation, inspection, examination and measurements. The physical examination should be carried out in an organized manner. As the midwife begins, the procedure she should be respectful to the client and gentle. The components of physical examination are:

1. Physical measurements, i.e. temperature, pulse, respirations and blood pressure.
2. General observations and client's own evaluation:
   a. Appropriateness of appearance.
   b. Apparent state of health.
   c. Mental and emotional state.
   d. Posture, gait and body movements.
   e. Striking obvious findings such as pallor, cyanosis or respiratory distress.
   f. Client's own evaluation of health, dietary patterns and ability to carry-out daily living activities.

Review of Systems

1. *Integumentary system:* Rashes, moles, lesions, pruritus, bruises, hirsutism, pigmentation, moisture, scars, tumors and turgor.
2. *Hair and scalp:* General character, scalp infections, lice, dandruff, alopecia and lumps.
3. *Head:* Headache, dizziness, fainting, sinusitis and involuntary movements.
4. *Eyes:* Blurring of vision, blind spots in vision, diplopia, photophobia, lacrimation discharge, redness, burning, glasses or contact lenses, injuries, infection, color of conjunctiva, pupillary size and reaction to light.
5. *Ears:* Hearing acuity, ear aches or discharges, tinnitus, vertigo, infection, mastoid, tenderness, lesions and placement on head.
6. *Nose:* Size, placement, patency of nostrils, epistaxis, discharge, sense of smell and septal deformity.
7. *Mouth and throat:* Condition of lips, gum, teeth, tongue and mucosa; sense of taste, voice, speech, odor of breath, any inflammation or surgery.
8. *Neck:* Movement, lymph node enlargement, vein distention, position of trachea.
9. *Breasts:* Nipples—normal flat or inverted, discharge, skin and glandular changes.
10. *Gastrointestinal system:* Appetite, nausea, vomiting, heartburn, belching, flatulence, bowel pattern, hemorrhoids food allergies and hernias.
11. *Cardiorespiratory system:* Breathing pattern, cough, wheezing, infection, respiration rate and rhythm, auscultation findings.
12. *Genitourinary system:* Urination difficulties and deviations, genital lesions and infections, history of hormone therapy.
13. *Muscular, skeletal and vascular systems:* Status of joints, muscles and extremities, appearance of nails and fingers.
14. *Central nervous system:* There are as follows:
    a. Speech and memory, complaints of vertigo and convulsions or loss of consciousness.
    b. Mental status.
    c. Motor symptoms.
    d. Sensory symptoms.
15. *Lymphatic and hematopoietic system:* Lymph nodes, bruising tendencies, blood dyscrasias.

Assessments and Laboratory Tests

General Assessments

1. *Height:* The woman height is checked at the time of first visit. Height over 160 cm is an indication of normal pelvis. A woman who is short in stature may belong to a small-sized race or family, or may be stunted because of poor nutrition in utero or childhood. In individual situations, the size of the fetus will determine the adequacy of the pelvis. At about 36th week, when the fetus is almost fully grown the pelvic size is reassessed. If the fetal head will engage in the pelvic brim, there is little cause for concern about cephalopelvic disproportion.
2. *Weight:* At every visit weight has to be checked and the rate of gain to be assessed. Obesity is associated with an increased risk of gestational diabetes and PIH.

3. *Blood pressure:* To provide a baseline reading for comparison throughout pregnancy, BP is checked. An adequate blood pressure is required to maintain placental perfusion. A blood pressure of 140/90 mm Hg at the first visit is indicative of hypertension.

Urinalysis

Urinalysis is done to exclude certain abnormalities. Pyelonephritis can readily develop because of changes in the renal tract during pregnancy. Possible findings in urinalysis include:
- Ketones due to increased maternal metabolism or vomiting
- Glucose caused by higher circulating blood levels, reduced renal threshold or disease
- Protein due to contamination by vaginal leukorrhea and diseases such as UTI or PIH.

Blood Tests (Box 15.2)

1. *ABO blood group and Rh factor:* Blood tests are done as part of the initial assessment to determine ABO blood group and Rh factor. Antibody screening is done followed by titration, if present. Follow-up of a woman, whose blood group is Rh negative will include further blood tests at 28th, 32nd, 36th and 40th week for Rh antibody titer to ensure that the pregnancy is not stimulating antibody activity. If the titration demonstrates a rising antibody response, more frequent assessment will be done in order to plan the management.
2. *Hemoglobin and hematocrit:* These are performed in order to assess the adequacy of iron stores. Hemoglobin estimation is repeated at 28th week, when the physiological effects of hemodilution become more apparent and at 36th week to ensure that any anemia is treated prior to delivery. The decision to use supplements is made on an individual basis. However, most women in the rural population are given iron and folic acid supplements. Health education about including iron-rich foods in diet should also be given.
3. *Venereal disease research laboratory (VDRL) test:* This test is done for all pregnant women. Early testing will allow the women to be treated adequately in order to prevent infection of the fetus. It is to remember that all positive results do not indicate active syphilis.
4. *Human immunodeficiency virus (HIV) test:* Routine screening to detect HIV infection is done in many centers. It is important to gain informed consent prior to the blood test and to offer appropriate counseling.
5. *Rubella immune status:* This is done by measuring the rubella antibody titer. Women who are not immune must be advised to avoid contact with anyone suffering from the disease. Other blood tests such as screening for blood disorders or hepatitis are done on individual cases based on the history.

Abdominal Examination

Abdominal examination of the pregnant woman should be done in addition to the physical examination and assessment. The examination includes:
- Observation of the size of the uterus, the shape of the uterus, the contour of the abdominal wall, any scar or injury marks, linea nigra and striae gravidarum
- Determination of the lie, presentation, position and variety of the fetus
- Measurement of fundal height, abdominal girth, palpation of fetal position and auscultation of fetal heart tones.

Each of these items provides informative data useful in diagnosis of pregnancy, evaluation of fetal well-being and growth and serves as indicators of possible problems.

INSPECTION

The examiner's eyes assess the size of the uterus roughly. A distended colon or obesity may give a false impression. Multiple pregnancy or polyhydramnios will enlarge both the length and breadth of the uterus, whereas a large baby increases only the length.

The shape of the uterus is longer than it is broad when the lie of the fetus is longitudinal. If the lie of the fetus is transverse, the uterus is low and broad, which occurs only in small percentage (0.5%). The multiparous uterus lacks the sung avoid shape of the primigravid uterus. Occasionally, it is possible to see the shape of the fetal back or limbs. In posterior positions of the occiput, a saucer-like depression is seen at or below the umbilicus.

A full bladder may be visible and may be more obvious in the later weeks of pregnancy. The umbilicus becomes less dimpled as pregnancy advances and may protrude lightly in later weeks. Lightening may be evident when the woman is erect. The uterus may sag forwards in multiparous women with lax abdominal wall. This is known as pendulous abdomen or anterior obliquity. In the primigravida, it is a sign of pelvic contraction.

Observation of *linea nigra* and *abdominal striae* are presumptive signs of pregnancy. Observation or palpation of fetal movement and hearing fetal heart sounds (FHSs) are positive signs of pregnancy. The normal range of fetal heart tones is 120–160 beats per minute (bpm).

BOX 15.2: Nursing tips.

Laboratory tests at the initial visit
- Blood work: Complete blood count, hemoglobin, hematocrit, Rh status, ABO blood group. Serology for rubella titer, syphilis, human immunodeficiency virus (HIV), hepatitis screening, glucose screening
- Urinalysis (with culture, if indicated); glucose, protein, erythrocytes, leukocytes, and bacteria
- Pelvic laboratory tests; Pap smear, culture for gonorrhea and *Chlamydia*. Presence of group B *Streptococcus* if the first visit is after 24 weeks of gestation

Determination of the lie, presentation, position and variety of the fetus varies in importance with the length of pregnancy. Prior to the 20th week of gestation, it is not possible to ascertain these informations because of the smallness of the fetus, the thickness of the uterus and the high ratio of amniotic fluid to baby in the amniotic sac. The baby will continue to turn and somersault in the amniotic sac until the bulk of the baby's body is far greater than the amount of fluid and there is no longer room for the fetus to turn easily. By the 36th week, most babies have settled into what will be their lie and presentation for the intrapartal period. This is not absolute, however, as some babies will turn again. Malpresentation prior to 36 weeks is not a cause for concern because the baby is still turning. Malpresentation after this time, however, may be cause for possible concern and intervention. Lie, presentation, position and variety (anterior or posterior) are informations obtained by doing Leopold's maneuvers of abdominal examination by palpation.

Measurements of the Fundal Height (Table 15.1 and Fig. 15.1)

Fundal height provides information regarding the progressive growth of the fetus as a gross screening tool for detection of problems related to fundal height, which is too large or too small for the presumed gestational age by dates.

This method of assessment does not always produce an accurate result because the size and number of fetuses, and the amount of amniotic fluid vary. A fundal height that is not increasing, but remains the same over a period of time is ominous. Signs and symptoms of possible intrauterine fetal growth retardation or fetal death must be looked for and these possibilities ruled out.

The fundal height can be measured in one of three methods. All have an inherent degree of inaccuracy because each depends on the examiner's identifying the top of the fundus correctly.

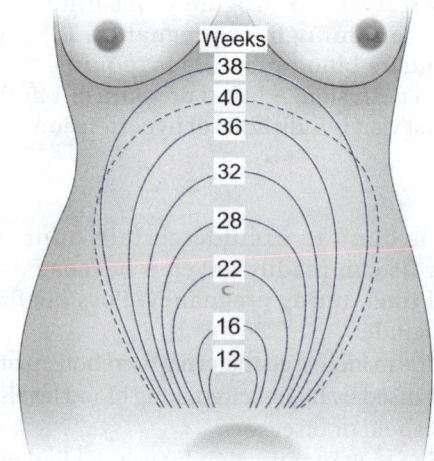

Figure 15.1: Approximate height of the fundus as the uterus enlarges.

TABLE 15.1: Approximate expected locations of the fundal height at various weeks of gestation.

Week of gestation	Approximate expected location of fundal height
12	Level of the symphysis pubis
16	Halfway between symphysis pubis and umbilicus
20	1–2 fingerbreadth below the umbilicus
22–24	1–2 fingerbreadth above the umbilicus
28–30	1/3 of the way between umbilicus and xiphoid process (3 fingerbreadth above the umbilicus)
32	2/3 of the way between umbilicus and xiphoid process (3–4 fingerbreadth below the xiphoid process)
38	Level of the xiphoid process
40	2–3 fingerbreadth below the xiphoid process, if lightening occurs

First Method

The first method combines knowledge of where to expect the fundal height to be at various weeks of gestation in relation to the woman's symphysis pubis, umbilicus and the tip of the xiphoid process, and the use of the examiner's fingerbreadths as the measuring tool.

In order to determine the height of the fundus, the midwife places her hand just below the xiphisternum pressing gently. She moves her hand gently down the abdomen until she feels the curved upper border of the fundus. She notes the number of fingerbreadths, which can be comfortably accommodated between the two.

This method of measuring the fundal height combines knowledge of where to expect the fundal height to be at various weeks of gestation in relation to the woman's symphysis pubis, umbilicus and tip of the xiphoid process and the use of the examiner's fingerbreadths as the measuring tool. Though it is a time-honored method, it has inherent inaccuracies. First, there is considerable variation between women in the distance from their symphysis pubis to their xiphoid process and in the location of the umbilicus between these two points. Second, there is a considerable variation between examiners in the width of their fingers. For example, two fingerbreadth of a thick-fingered person can be the same as three fingerbreadths of a thin-fingered person.

Second Method

The caliper method of measuring fundal weight is probably the most accurate method of measuring the fundal height after the 22–24 weeks of gestation. In order to use a caliper or external pelvimeter **(Fig. 15.2)**, place one tip on the superior border of the symphysis pubis and the other tip at the top of the fundus. Both placements are in the abdominal midline. The measurement is then read on a centimeter scale located on an arc close to where the two ends of the calipers come together. The number of centimeters should be equal approximately to the weeks of gestation after about 22–24 weeks of gestation.

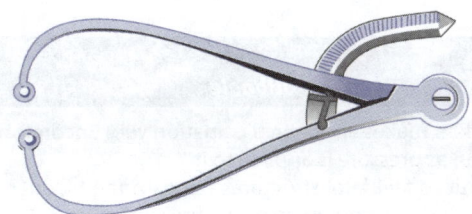

Figure 15.2: External pelvimeter.

ABDOMINAL PALPATION AND LEOPOLD'S MANEUVERS

The term abdominal palpation is often used to mean doing Leopold's maneuvers for determining fetal lie, presentation, position and engagement. While doing Leopold's maneuvers, other information is also obtained and further palpation may be involved than that strictly needed for doing Leopold's maneuvers. The following information is obtained from abdominal palpation:

- Evaluation of uterine irritability, tone, tenderness, consistency and any contractility present
- Evaluation of abdominal muscle tone
- Detection of fundal movement
- Estimation of fetal weight
- Determination of fetal lie, presentation, position and variety
- Determine whether the head is engaged.

Before performing abdominal palpation and Leopold's maneuvers, several preparatory steps are done **(Table 15.2)**.

Inspection of the Abdomen

Before actual palpation, the abdomen should be inspected for what its contours can tell you about the fetal lie, presentation and position. Palpation then gives you further information with which to confirm or rule out this initial impression **(Table 15.3)**.

Leopold's Maneuvers (Figs. 15.4A to D and Table 15.4)

There are four maneuvers starting at the fundus and ending at the pelvic brim. It is suggested that learners go through the steps sequentially due to the fact that, in this pattern they form a thought process and create a mental image for determining fetal position that will most quickly aid in developing skill and accuracy. Consistently following an orderly sequence will also aid in remembering to include all the maneuvers and gathering all necessary information. In doing the Leopold's maneuvers, stand on the side of the bed most convenient and comfortable for you. Right-handed people usually stand on the right side of the women.

The findings from the first and third maneuvers must be compared and final determination made of the lie and presentation before proceeding to the fourth maneuver. For a final determination of the fetal lie and presentation, a combined Pawlik's grip may be performed. In this case, Pawlik's grip is done with one hand and the fundus is grasped in the same way with the other hand at the same time. This combination enables you to compare simultaneously what are in the two poles for final determination of the fetal lie and presentation.

AUSCULTATION (FIG. 15.5)

Auscultation usually forms part of each abdominal examination and follows any procedure in order to assess fetal well-being. Abdominal palpation determining the lie,

Third Method (Fig. 15.3)

Measuring fundal height with a tape is the most frequently used method for obtaining an exact measurement. It is probably the second most accurate method of measuring fundal height after 22–24 weeks of gestation. The zero line of the tape measure is placed on the superior border of the symphysis pubis and the tape measure stretched across the contour of the abdomen to the top of the fundus. The abdominal midline is used as the line of measurement. In order to avoid error in locating the superior border, you must palpate for the symphysis pubis. The number of centimeters measured should be approximately equal to about 22–24 weeks of gestation.

All of the three methods described above have an inherent degree of inaccuracy because each depends on the examiner's identifying the top of the fundus correctly. Some unidentifiable point on the anterior slope of the fundus is often mistaken for the top of the fundus. This error can be avoided by doing the following.

Facing the woman's head, as she lies supine, place your hands on each lateral side of the uterus approximately midway between the symphysis pubis and the fundus. Ballotte the uterus between your hands with gentle pressure and being sure to stay on the lateral portion of the uterus, palpate up to the fundus. As you near the top, your hands will begin to come together and they will meet at the top of the fundus. Staying on the lateral portion of the uterus assures reaching the actual top of the fundus and keeping off its anterior slope.

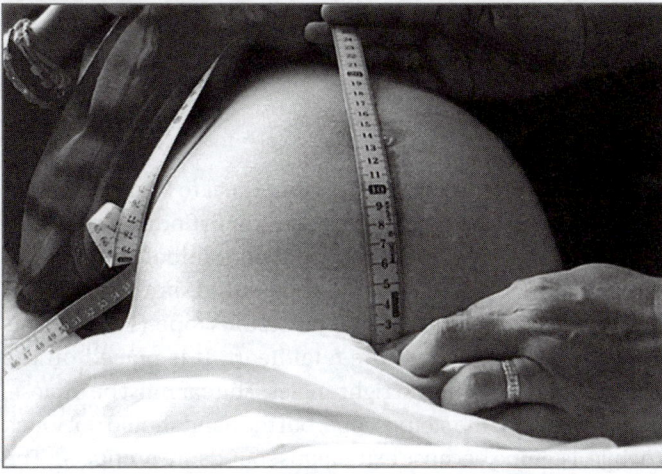

Figure 15.3: Measuring fundal height with tape measure *(For color version, see Plate 3).*

TABLE 15.2: Preparation for abdominal palpation.

Sl. No.	Preparatory steps of the procedure	Rationale
1.	The woman's bladder should be empty	• A full bladder makes abdominal palpation very uncomfortable for the woman as pressure is applied to it • It is difficult to feel fetal structures beneath the bladder, thereby obscuring findings pertaining to the presenting part
2.	The woman's abdomen is completely exposed from just below the breasts to the symphysis pubis	• Complete exposure of the abdomen at one time is essential for visual observation of the contours of the abdomen • Expose no more than that necessary for examination
3.	The women's abdominal muscles should be relaxed. This is achieved by the following: a. Placing a pillow under her head and upper shoulders b. Having her arms by her sides c. Explaining what you will be doing d. Helping her with relaxation breathing e. Having her knees bend slightly	Palpation is difficult for both the woman and the examiner if the abdominal muscles are contracted. It is difficult for the examiner to feel the fetus and therefore leads to longer and more forcible palpation. This causes the woman discomfort and she tenses her muscles more. This is avoided by starting with relaxed abdominal muscles, with warm hands and with smooth and gentle, but firm palpation
4.	Be sure your hands are warm. If not, rub them together or dip in warm water	Cold hands are uncomfortable to the woman. They may cause muscle contraction
5.	Before palpating, lightly rest your hands on the woman's abdomen. A good time for this is while you are explaining what you are going to do	This action gives the woman an opportunity adjust and become acquainted to your touching her. Since, this is not uncomfortable to her; the initial muscle tightening reaction gets dissipated
6.	The technique of palpation is as follows: a. Use the flat palmar surface of your fingers for palpating, not your fingertips b. Keep the fingers of your hands together c. Apply smooth, deep pressure as firm as necessary to obtain accurate findings d. Avoid any sudden movement, jabbing, poking or prodding	This technique is designed for the least possible discomfort for the woman and the gathering of the greatest amount of information for the examiner

TABLE 15.3: Inspection of abdomen.

Sl. No.	Observations	Significance
1.	A longitudinal ovoid, fundal height as expected for gestational age	Indicative of a longitudinal lie
2.	A transverse ovoid, fundal height lower than expected for gestational age	Indicative of a transverse lie
3.	Long-smooth curve prominent on one side of the abdomen	Indicative that the fetal back is on the side of abdomen
4.	A saucer-like depression just below the umbilicus and bulge like a full bladder above the symphysis pubis	Indicative of a posterior position
5.	Movement of fetal small parts all over the abdomen	Indicative of a posterior position

presentation and position of the fetus enable you to locate the fetal heart tones. This is because; the sound of the fetal heart is transmitted through the convex portion of the fetus closest to the anterior uterine wall. Therefore, the fetal heart tones are best heard through the fetal back in vertex and breech presentations, and through the chest in face presentations. Thus, if you know the position you can readily locate the fetal heart tones allowing for some variation depending on the amount of descend of the fetus into the pelvis.

Conversely, location of the fetal heart tones is an additional piece of data that serves to confirm or question your diagnosis of the fetal position. If you find the fetal heart tones loudest in a location different from where you expect to find them, then the question is raised, if you were in error in findings or in your interpretation of your findings from abdominal palpation.

Like all heartbeats, it is double sound, but more rapid than the adult heart. Pinard fetal stethoscope (**Fig. 15.6**) is commonly used to hear the fetal heart. It is placed on the mother's abdomen and at right angles. The ear must be in close, firm contact with the stethoscope, but the hand should not touch it, while listening because extraneous sounds are produced. The fetal stethoscope (fetoscope) should be moved about until the point of maximum intensity is located where the fetal heart is

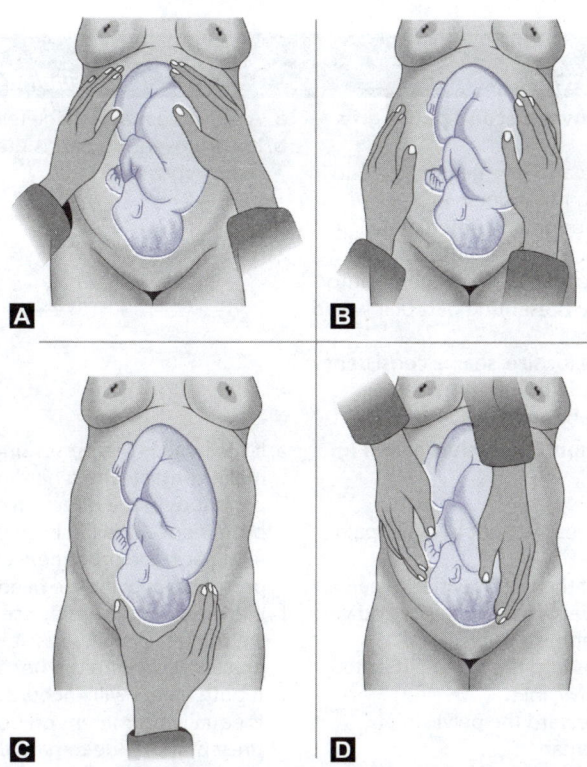

Figures 15.4A to D: Abdominal palpation (Leopold's maneuvers). (A) First maneuver (fundal palpation); (B) Second maneuver (lateral palpation); (C) Third maneuver (Pawlik's grip/second pelvic grip); (D) Fourth maneuver (pelvic palpation/first pelvic grip).

TABLE 15.4: Abdominal palpation (Leopold's maneuvers).

Sl. No.	Procedure steps	Findings and significance
1.	**First maneuver/Fundal palpation (Fig. 15.4A):** a. Face the woman's head. Place both hands on the woman's fundus and curve the fingers around the top of the fundusee b. Palpate for shape, size, consistency and mobility of the fetal part in the fundus.	a. Fetal parts that feel round and hard, which are readily movable and ballotable between fingers of two hands are indicative of fetal head. The mobility is due to the head being able to move independently of the trunk. The lie is longitudinal b. Fetal part that feels irregular, large or bulkier and less firm than a head, which cannot be readily moved or balloted is indicative of fetal breech. The breech cannot move independently of the trunk. The lie is longitudinal c. If neither of the above is felt in the fundus, it is indicative of transverse lie
2.	**Second maneuver/Lateral palpation (Fig. 15.4B):** a. Continue to face the woman's head. Place your hands on both sides of the uterus about midway between the symphysis pubis and the fundus b. Apply firm gentle pressure with one hand against the side of the uterus, thereby pushing the fetus to the other side of the abdomen and with your examining hand, stabilizing it there. Maintaining pressure on one side, palpate the other side of the uterus c. With the examining hand, palpate the entire area from the abdominal midline to the lateral side and from the symphysis to the fundus. Use firm, smooth pressure and rotary movement. d. Reverse the procedure for examination of the other side of the uterus	a. A firm, convex, continuously smooth and resistant mass extending from the breech to the neck is indicative of the fetal back. The location of the back in the left or right side of the woman's abdomen determines the position in longitudinal lie b. Small knobby, irregular masses, which move when pressed or may kick, or hit your examining hand is indicative of the small parts—hands, feet, knees and elbow c. These should be felt in the opposite side of the abdomen than the side where the fetal back is in d. Small parts all over the abdomen and the fetal back difficult to feel as it may seem just out of reach in the posterior portion of the abdomen is indicative of a posterior position

Contd...

Contd...

Sl. No.	Procedure steps	Findings and significance
3.	**Third maneuver/Pawlik's maneuver/Second pelvic grip (Fig. 15.4C):** a. Continue to face the woman's head. Have her knees bend in order to avoid discomfort during this maneuver b. Grasp the portion of the lower abdomen immediately above the symphysis pubis between the thumb and middle finger of one of your outstretched hands. Press gently into the abdomen in order to feel the presenting part below and between your thumb and finger c. As in the first maneuver, palpate for size, shape, consistency and mobility in order to differentiate if it is the head or breech in the lower pole of the abdomen	a. A movable mass will be felt, if the presenting part is not engaged b. If the presenting part is the head that is engaged, it may not be readily movable
4.	**Fourth maneuver/Pelvic palpation/First pelvic grip (Fig. 15.4D):** a. Turn and face the woman's feet b. Make sure that the woman's knees are bent to avoid pain during the maneuver c. Place your hands on the sides of the uterus with the palms of your hands just below the level of the umbilicus and your fingers directed toward the symphysis pubis d. Press deeply with your fingertips into the lower abdomen and move them towards the pelvic inlet e. Continue to move your hands toward the pelvic inlet f. Share your findings with the woman g. Offer to help her feel and identify various fetal parts if she would like to	a. If the head is the presenting part, one of your hands will make contact with a hard round mass, while your other hand continues in the direction of the pelvis. This is the cephalic prominence and if it is on the same side of the woman as the fetal back, the prominence is occiput and indicates a face presentation with the head extended b. If the cephalic prominence is on the same side of the woman as are the fetal small parts, it is the sinciput and indicates a vertex presentation with the head well-flexed c. If both hands will encounter simultaneously a hard mass, which is equally prominent on both sides, it is indicative of brow presentation due to partial flexion of the head. The occiput and sinciput are felt at the same time: • At the brim of the pelvis, your hands will converge around the presenting part with the fingertips of your two hands touching in the midline indicating the presenting part is not engaged. It is above the pelvic brim or floating d. If the presenting part is the breech, it will be readily movable: • The hands will diverge away from the presenting part and the midline indicating the presenting part is either engaged or dipping e. If the presenting part is the breech, it will have a feeling of give along with the trunk of the fetus: • If you are unable to feel the cephalic prominence because it is out of reach in the pelvis, the head is engaged

Note: *Leopold's maneuvers third and fourth:
1. Performing the third maneuver/Pawlik's grip/Second pelvic grip following lateral palpation (second maneuver) enables the midwife to complete this stage without taking her hands off the woman's abdomen and still facing her head.
2. Performing the fourth maneuver/Pelvic palpation/First pelvic grip following the third maneuver enables the midwife to change her position to face the woman's feet and place her hands with fingers directed toward the woman's symphysis pubis in order to palpate and feel the degree of flexion and descend of fetal presenting part. The maneuver that might give more discomfort to the client is then performed last.

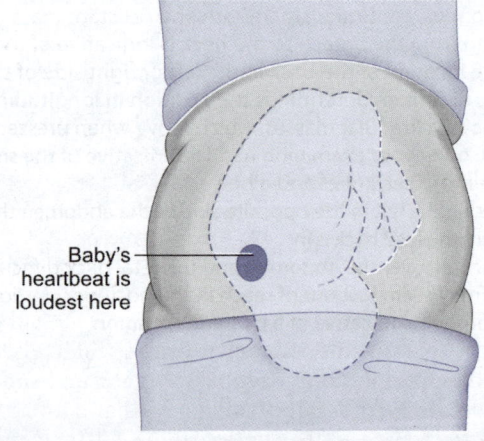

Figure 15.5: Auscultation of the fetal heart sounds.

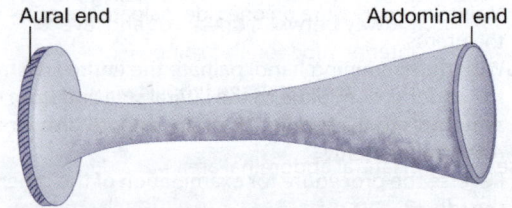

Figure 15.6: Pinard fetal stethoscope.

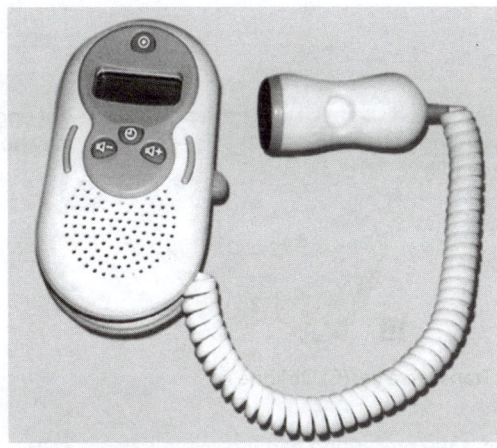

Figure 15.7: Ultrasonic Doppler device
(For color version, see Plate 3).

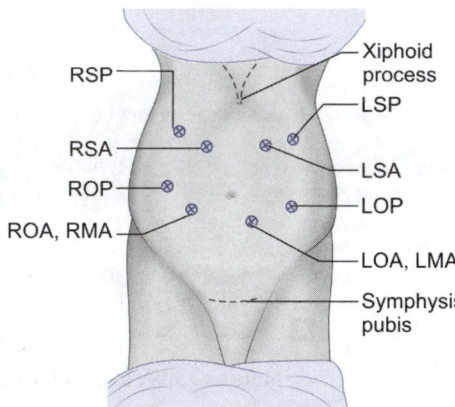

Figure 15.8: Location of the point of maximum intensity of the fetal heart tones for specific fetal positions.
(LMA: left mentoanterior; LOA: left occipitoanterior; LOP: left occipitoposterior; LSA: left sacroanterior; LSP: left sacroposterior; RMA: right mentoanterior; ROA: right occipitoanterior; ROP: right occipitoposterior; RSA: right sacroanterior; RSP: right sacroposterior).

heard more clearly. In recent times, increasingly ultrasound equipment such as ultrasonic Doppler device **(Fig. 15.7)** and fetal monitor are used for this purpose. When the monitor is used, the woman may also hear the fetal heartbeat.

In a full-term infant with an unengaged presenting part, the fetal heart tones are best heard in the following locations in relation to presentations and positions **(Table 15.5 and Fig. 15.8)**.

The nurse-midwife in making her diagnosis must assess all the information she had gathered from inspection, palpation and auscultation, and draw the conclusion, which accounts for all the factors. If one factor does not fit in with the rest she must think again **(Box 15.3)**.

OTHER FINDINGS

Gestational Age

During pregnancy, uterine size will usually equate with the gestation estimated by dates (*refer* **Table 15.1**). Later in pregnancy, increasing uterine size gives evidence of continuing fetal growth, but is less reliable as an indicator of gestational age.

Multiple pregnancies increase the overall uterine size and should be diagnosed by 24th week of gestation. In a singleton

TABLE 15.5: Location of fetal heart tones in various fetal presentations and positional varieties.

Presentations and positional varieties	Locations
Cephalic	Midway between umbilicus and level of anterior superior iliac spine
Breech	At the level or above umbilicus
Anterior	Close to abdominal midline
Transverse	In lateral abdominal area
Posterior	In flank area or close to abdominal midline on other side of abdomen

> **BOX 15.3:** Nursing tips.
>
> **Accurate detection of the fetal heart rate**
> To ensure an accurate diagnosis of the fetal heart rate, it must be distinguished from the maternal pulse. To do this, the fetal heartbeat should be auscultated while simultaneously assessing the maternal radial pulse

pregnancy, the fundus reaches the umbilicus at 22–24 weeks and the xiphisternum at 36th week. In the last month of pregnancy, lightening occurs and the fetus sinks down into the lower pole of the uterus. The uterus becomes broader and the fundus lower.

Lie

Lie is the relationship of the long axis of the fetus to the long axis of the uterus. There are three possible lies—longitudinal, transverse and oblique **(Figs. 15.9A to C)**.

In 95% of cases, the lie is longitudinal owing to the ovoid shape of the uterus; the remainder is oblique or transverse. Oblique lie that results when the fetus is diagonally across the uterus must be distinguished from obliquity of the uterus, when the whole uterus is tilted to one side (usually right) and the fetus lies longitudinally within it. When the lie is transverse, the fetus lies at right angle across.

Presentation

Presentation refers to the part of the fetus, which lies at the pelvic brim or in the lower pole of the uterus. This is the first portion of the fetus to enter the pelvic brim or inlet. There are three possible presentations—cephalic, breech and shoulder. The first two are further subdivided—cephalic into vertex, sinciput, brow and face and breech into frank, full (or complete) and footling, which can be single or double **(Figs. 15.10A to F)**.

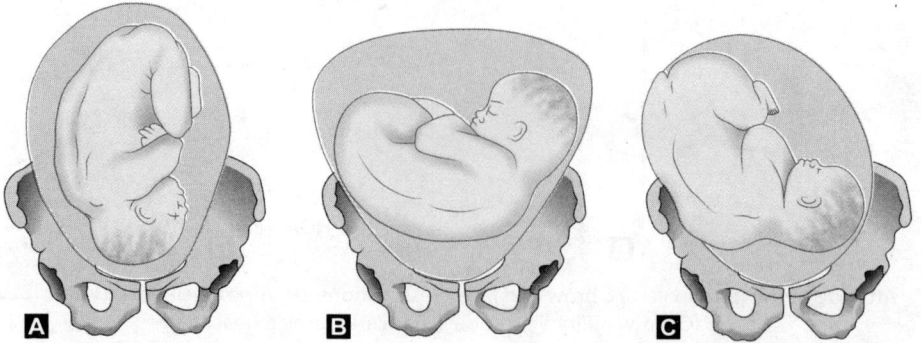

Figures 15.9A to C: Fetal lie. (A) Longitudinal lie; (B) Transverse lie; (C) Oblique lie.

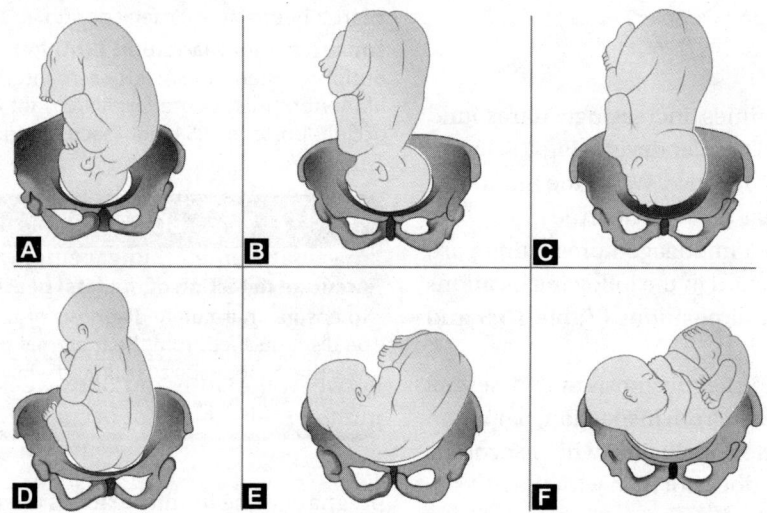

Figures 15.10A to F: Fetal presentations. (A) Vertex; (B) Brow; (C) Face; (D) Breech; (E) Shoulder—dorsoanterior; (F) Shoulder—dorsoposterior.

When the head is well-flexed, the vertex presents; when it is fully extended the face presents and when partially extended the brow presents. It is common for the head to present because the bulky breech finds more space in the fundus, which is the widest diameter of the uterus and the head lies in the narrower lower pole.

Attitude

Attitude is the relationship of the fetal head and limbs to its trunk. The attitude of the fetus varies according to its presentation. For example, a fetus in a vertex presentation has a well-flexed head, flexion of the extremities over the thorax and abdomen and a convexcurved back; while a fetus with a face presentation has a head, which is acutely extended, flexion of the extremities on the thorax and abdomen and a vertebral column, which not only is straightened but also has some degree of arching. Flexion of the fetal head enables the smallest diameters to present to the pelvis and results in an easier delivery **(Figs. 15.11A to D)**.

Denominator

The denominator is the name of the part of the presentation that is used when referring to fetal position. Each presentation has a different denominator, which are as follows:
- *Occiput* in vertex presentation
- *Sacrum* in breech presentation
- *Mentum* in face presentation
- *Acromion process* in shoulder presentation.
   In brow presentation, no denominator is used.

Position

Position is the arbitrarily chosen point on the fetus for each presentation in relation to the left or right side of the mother's pelvis. It is also expressed as the relationship between the denominator and six points on the pelvic brim **(Figs. 15.12A to F)**.

Anterior positions are more favorable than posterior positions because when the fetal back is in front, it conforms to the concavity of the mother's abdominal wall and can

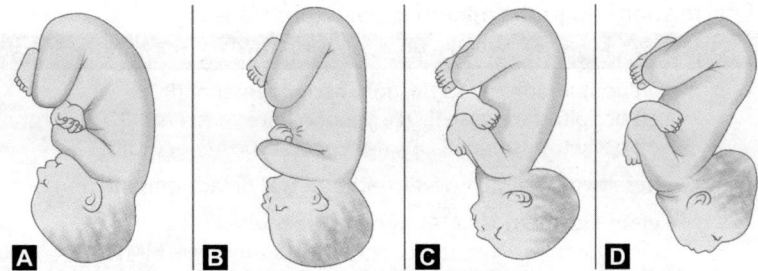

Figures 15.11A to D: Attitude of the fetus in vertex, brow and face presentations. (A) Vertex well-flexed head; (B) Vertex-deflexed head; (C) Brow military attitude; (D) Face-extended head.

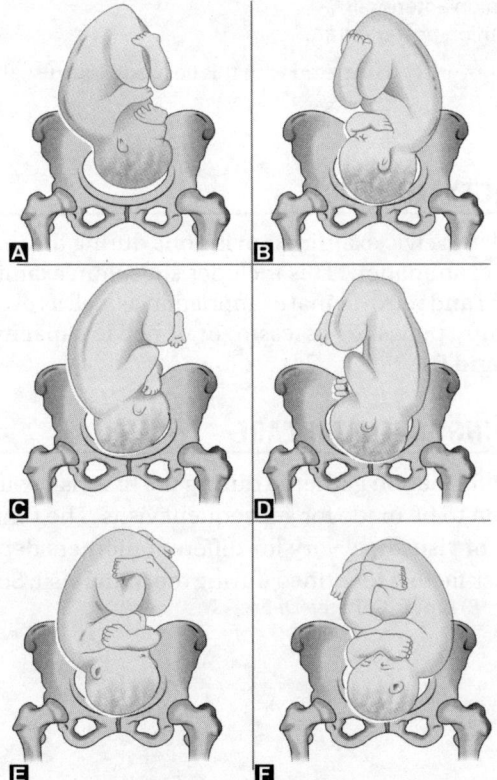

Figures 15.12A to F: Diagrammatic presentation of six positions of the vertex. (A) Right occipitotransverse (ROT); (B) Left occipitotransverse (LOT); (C) Right occipitoanterior (ROA); (D) Left occipitoanterior (LOA); (E) Right occipitoposterior (ROP); (F) Left occipitoposterior (LOP).

therefore flex better. When the back is flexed, the head also tends to flex and a smaller diameter presents to the pelvic brim. There is more room in the anterior part of the brim for the broad biparietal diameter of the head.

Engagement

Engagement may occur when the widest presenting transverse diameter of the fetal part has passed through the brim of the pelvis **(Fig. 15.13)**. In head presentations, this is biparietal diameter. Engagement is an important sign that the maternal pelvis is adequate for the particular fetus and that vaginal delivery may be expected **(Table 15.6)**.

In a primigravid woman, the head normally engages between the 36th and 38th week of pregnancy, but in a multipara this may not occur until after the onset of labor.

When the vertex presents and the head is engaged, the following will be evident on clinical examination:
- The head is not mobile
- Less than half the head is palpable above the brim
- The anterior shoulder is little more than 5 cm above the brim.

If the head is not engaged, the findings are as follows:
- More than half the head is palpable above the brim
- The head may be high and freely movable
- The sinciput may be 7.5 cm above the brim.

If the head remains unengaged in a primigravid woman at 38th week, the possibility of cephalopelvic disproportion should be ruled out.

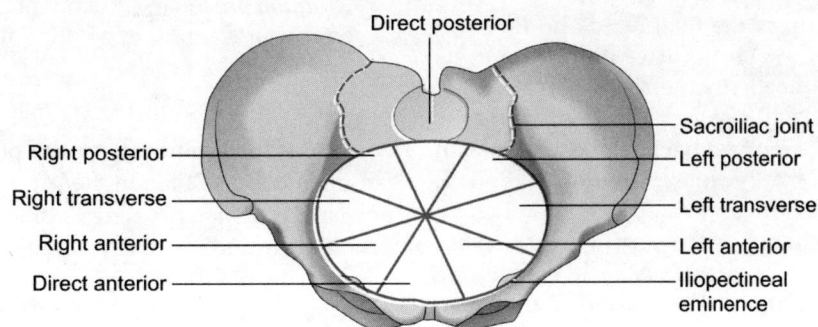

Figure 15.13: Segments of pelvis showing positions of fetus.

TABLE 15.6: Possibilities of fetal relationship to the maternal pelvis (positions).

Lie	Presentation	Position and variety
Longitudinal	Cephalic, vertex	Left occipitoanterior (LOA), right occipitoanterior (ROA) Left occipitotransverse (LOT), right occipitotransverse (ROT) Left occipitoposterior (LOP), right occipitoposterior (ROP)
	Sinciput, brow	These two usually convert to either vertex or face presentation
	Face	Left mentoanterior (LMA), right mentoanterior (RMA) Left mentotransverse (LMT), right mentotransverse (RMT) Left mentoposterior (LMP), right mentoposterior (RMP)
	Breech—frank, full and footling	Left sacroanterior (LSA), right sacroanterior (RSA) Left sacrotransverse (LST), right sacrotransverse (RST) Left sacroposterior (LSP), right sacroposterior (RSP)
Transverse	Shoulder	Left acromion anterior (LAA), right acromion anterior (RAA) Left acromion posterior (LAP), right acromion posterior (RAP)
Oblique		Nothing is felt at the inlet and there is no presentation, position or variety associated with this lie; an oblique usually is a transitory condition

Transverse and oblique lies in labor are abnormal conditions and they require cesarean section. Approximately 0.5–3.5% of women will enter labor with a breech presentation and 0.5% with a face presentation.

Although the breech of the fetus (podalic pole) is smaller than the fetal head (cephalic pole), the combination of the breech and the flexed lower extremities is bulkier because the flexed lower extremities are kept close to the breech **(Figs. 15.14A and B)**.

PELVIC EXAMINATION

A complete pelvic examination is done during the initial antepartal examination. This includes speculum examination, bimanual and retrovaginal examination as well as evaluation of the bony pelvis for assessment of pelvic capacity **(Figs. 15.15A and B)**.

ONGOING ANTENATAL CARE

All the information gathered during the first visit will enable a decision to be made for subsequent visits. The timing and number of visits may vary for different mothers depending on the risk factors identified during the initial visit. Someone

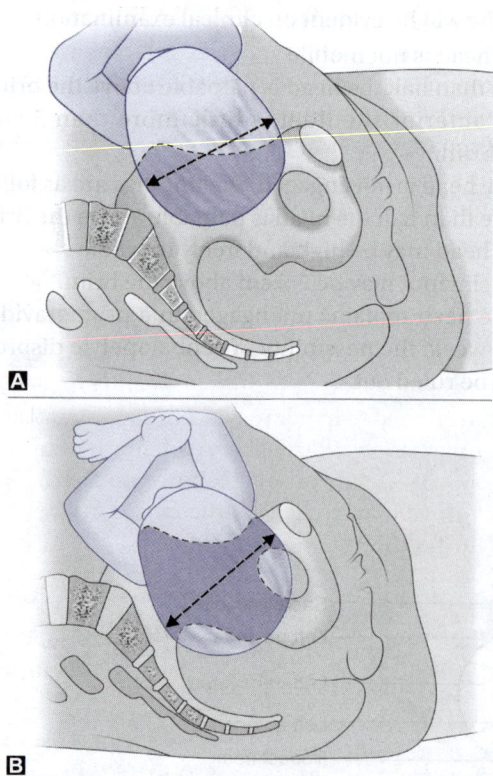

Figures 15.14A and B: Diagrammatic presentation of engagement of fetal head. (A) Head fixed, not engaged; (B) Head engaged.

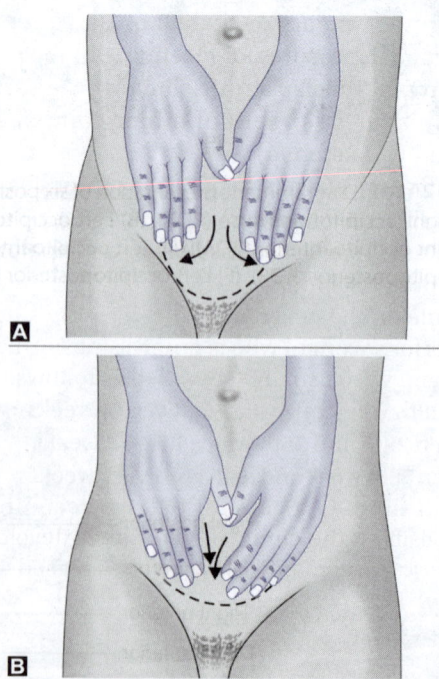

Figures 15.15A and B: Pelvic palpation. (A) Fingers diverge when head is engaged; (B) Fingers converge when head is not engaged.

who develops complications during pregnancy will have more frequent visits. Each revisit consists of:
- A chart review
- A history and physical examination geared toward evaluation of the well-being of mother and fetus
- A speculum and/or pelvic examination when indicated
- Laboratory and adjunctive studies when indicated
- Explanations and teaching appropriate to the patient's needs and her baby's gestational age.

Nursing Process for the Antenatal Mother

Step 1: Collection of the Database

Data may be collected from the following:
- Chart review for evaluation of preceding concerns and their management
- History of any symptoms of complications or discomforts, use of medicines and any medical care
- Physical examination
- Pelvic examination
- Laboratory studies.

Step 2: Interpretation of Database

Interpretation of database to identify the client's problems and needs to:
- Determine normality
- Identify the discomforts and possible complications
- Identify the signs and symptoms of complications.

Step 3: Development of a Comprehensive Plan of Care

Development of a comprehensive plan of care includes the following components:
- Measures for dietary re-evaluation and intervention
- Instructional measures for meeting learning needs
- Measures for relief of any discomfort
- Measures for treatment of minor complications (e.g. vaginitis, UTI, anemia)
- Measures for referrals to other health professionals (e.g. nutritionist, social worker)
- Measures for special counseling or anticipatory guidance by the physician
- Schedule for the next revisit.

Revisits for a woman who is progressing normally through her pregnancy are usually scheduled as follows:
- Up to 28th week of gestation: Every 4 weeks
- Between 28th and 36th week: Every 2 weeks
- Between 36th week and delivery: Every week.

Though there is a general pattern recommended for prenatal visits to the clinic, if the mother develops any risk factors during pregnancy, she must be advised to visit more frequently.

Risk Factors

Following risk factors can arise during the course of pregnancy:
- Change in fetal movement pattern
- Weight loss or poor weight gain
- Proteinuria, glycosuria
- Hypertension
- Uterus large or small for dates
- Excess or decreased liquor
- Malpresentation
- Head not engaged by 38 weeks in primigravid women
- Vaginal bleeding
- Vaginal or urinary infection
- Premature labor.

Record Keeping

In order to evaluate the effectiveness of advice and treatment during prenatal period, good record keeping is essential. Legibly written and signed entries are important for different health workers to know the well-being of mother and baby.

Indicators of Fetal Well-being

- Increasing maternal weight in association with increasing uterine size compatible with the gestational age of the fetus
- Fetal movements, which follow a regular pattern throughout pregnancy
- Fetal heart rate between 110 and 150 bpm.

Evidence of at least 10 movements a day is considered normal. The movements are usually observed for 12 hours starting at 9:00 AM. The same time period should be used each day to allow for comparison. If the fetus takes longer time to achieve these 10 movements, this indicates that the fetus is becoming compromised in utero. It is important that the woman is asked to seek help if the fetus has not moved 10 times in the 12 hours labor period or if its pattern of activity changes greatly (fetal activity is often greatest during late afternoons). She should not wait for the next clinic appointment.

Preparation for Labor

During the last weeks of pregnancy, labor should be discussed with the mother. A woman who has decided to give birth at home must be visited by the public health nurse or the female health worker to help her make the final arrangements. Most women choose hospital delivery and they should be explained how to recognize the onset of labor, emphasizing the normal pattern of events with clear instructions as to when they should reach the hospital.

■ STUDY QUESTIONS

Short Notes

1. Fetal lie.
2. Fetal presentation.
3. Fetal attitude.
4. Denominator in different fetal positions.
5. Engagement of fetal head.

Short Answer Questions

1. Approximate levels of fundal height as uterus enlarge in pregnancy.
2. Laboratory tests and assessments in prenatal period.
3. Indicators of fetal well-being in pregnancy.

Essay Questions

1. Explain the examination of a pregnant woman at the time of first visit to the hospital or health center.
2. Explain the abdominal palpation and Leopold's maneuvers on a mother of 34 weeks of gestation.

BIBLIOGRAPHY

1. Das S. Antenatal Care. In: Bennett RV, Linda KB (Eds). Myles Textbook for Midwives, 13th edition. Edinburgh: Churchill Livingstone; 1999. pp. 209-234.
2. Dutta DC. Textbook of Obstetrics, 5th edition. Calcutta: New Central Book Company; 2001. pp. 100-9.
3. Park K. Park's Textbook of Preventive and Social Medicine, 16th edition. Jabalpur: M/s Banarsidas Bhanot Publishers; 2000. pp. 352-8.
4. Helen V. Nurse-Midwifery, 2nd edition. Boston: Jones and Bartlett Publishers; 1996. pp. 63-112.

CHAPTER 16

Specialized Investigations and Fetal Evaluation in the Antenatal Period

Learning Objectives

Upon completing this chapter, the learner will be able to:
- Describe the screening methods for congenital abnormalities.
- Discuss the technologies used to screen and diagnose anomalies of the fetus.
- Describe the procedures for fetal evaluation in the antenatal period.

The fetal evaluation measures are used when the fetus is suspected of being at risk. Because many of them are expensive or carry with them an element of risk in the procedure involved, or both, the value of their use must be weighed against any possible risk and the expense in each given situation.

ULTRASONOGRAPHY

Ultrasound (US) is the production of high-frequency sound waves, which are reflected or echoed when beamed into the body and an interface is encountered between different types of tissues or structures with different densities. These echoes can be translated into visible images of the tissues or structures encountered. When the transducer, which transforms electrical energy to sound, is placed on the body, a sound wave passes into the body and encounters a structure; a fraction of that sound is reflected back. The amount of sound from each organ varies according to the type of tissue encountered (**Fig. 16.1**):
- Strong echoes give bright white dots, e.g. bone
- Weaker echoes give various shades of gray according to their strength
- Fluid-filled areas cause no reflection and give rise to a black image.

The procedure is simple and painless. Prior to 20th week of gestation, it is necessary to have a full bladder for the procedure.

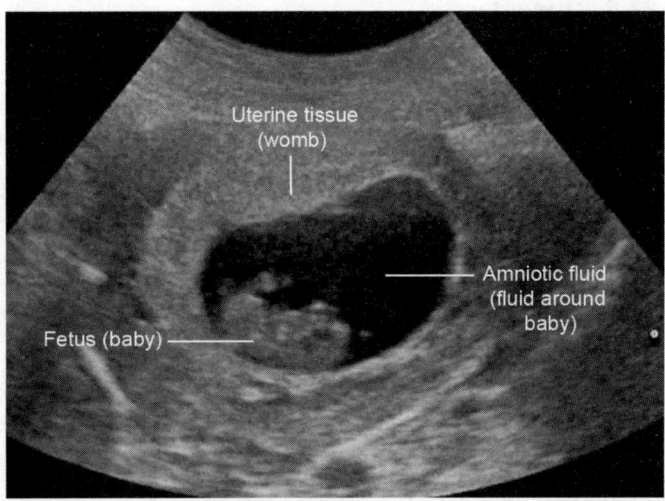

Figure 16.1: Ultrasound in pregnancy.

Diagnostic Uses in Obstetrics

1. *Early pregnancy:* Pregnancy can be diagnosed by ultrasound by 5th week of gestation.
2. Ectopic pregnancy.
3. *Hydatidiform mole:* Produces a characteristic image of scattered echoes. Diagnosis is reliable to the exclusion of other tests.
4. *Gestational age and fetal maturity:* An approximated fetal age is determined by using specific measurements at different stages:
   - At 5–10 weeks, by measuring the gestational sac
   - At 8–14 weeks, by measuring the crown-rump length—this is the length of the embryo from the top of the head to the rump or base of the sacrum
   - At 14–20 weeks, by measuring the length of the femur
   - At 18–26 weeks, by measuring the biparietal diameter
   - The fetal head is demonstrable by US by the 12th week of gestation.

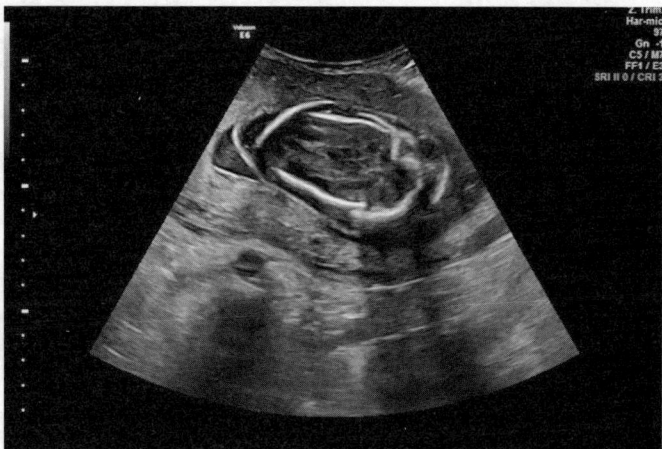

Figure 16.2: Spalding sign.

5. *Multiple gestations:* These may be diagnosed as early as first trimester.
6. Localization of placenta:
   - Aids in diagnosis of third trimester bleeding
   - Useful to locate the placenta prior to amniocentesis.
7. *Fetal anomalies:* A number of fetal anomalies can be identified including, abnormalities of the head and spine, the genitourinary tract, gastrointestinal defects, cardiac, thoracopulmonary and musculoskeletal anomalies.
8. *Fetal death:* Separation and overlapping of skull bones will be evident (Spalding's sign) **(Fig. 16.2)**.
9. Estimated fetal weight.
10. Fetal lie and presentation.
11. Intrauterine growth retardation.
12. *Polyhydramnios:* Indicated by a large intrauterine space that projects no echoes.
13. Oligohydramnios.
14. *Placental grading:* It is used for estimating fetal maturity and fetal pulmonary maturity.
15. *Biophysical profile:* This is used to evaluate the fetal well-being, e.g. in postdated pregnancy:
    - Biparietal diameter
    - Fetal movement
    - Respiratory movements
    - Amniotic fluid volume
    - Height-weight ratio (Ponder's index)
    - Heart rate pattern.
16. Localization of intrauterine contraceptive devices.

Ultrasonography (USG) is reliably replacing former diagnostic methods, especially roentgenography as a far safer methodology. The US does not carry the known risks that accompany irradiation. The USG is still in its developmental period and data are inconclusive about any adverse or long-term effects, which would develop or evidence themselves years later.

AMNIOCENTESIS AND AMNIOTIC FLUID STUDIES

Amniocentesis is the aspiration of amniotic fluid by way of a needle passed transabdominally into the gestational (amniotic) sac. The technique of amniocentesis can also be used for the injection of solutions into the amniotic sac. It is generally not possible to perform an amniocentesis until the second trimester, when the uterus has enlarged to become readily accessible to abdominal organ and the entire uterine cavity is filled with the amniotic sac. This change occurs when the chorion laeve fuses with the decidua parietalis around the uterine cavity other than the site of implantation, at approximately the 3rd or 4th month of gestation.

The ratio of amniotic fluid to fetus is high in the first trimester, about 3:2 by 20th week of gestation and decreases thereafter as the fetus grows. The average fluid volume during the third trimester is 800 mL; this quantity decreases to around 450 mL by term and further decreases post-term.

Amniocentesis is performed by physicians and usually is indicated when the fetus is in jeopardy or suspected of being at high risk. The physician weighs the reason for performing amniocentesis against the risks involved in the technique. These include the following:
1. Perforation of the placenta or fetal placental vessels, which may result in:
   a. Hemorrhage.
   b. Transfer of fetal cells, which could cause or aggravate isoimmunization and hemolytic disease in the newborn.
   c. Fetal death.
2. Infection, which may result in:
   a. Maternal morbidity or mortality.
   b. Fetal or neonatal morbidity, or mortality.
3. Abortion.
4. Premature labor or premature rupture of membranes.
5. Fetal trauma resulting from needle puncture.
6. Trauma to the umbilical cord or umbilical vessels.
7. Amniotic fluid leakage.
8. Hematoma.

The risk of amniocentesis is reduced when performed after the 20th week of gestation. Rho(D) Immune Globulin (Human), i.e. RhoGAM is given to Rh-negative women when the amniotic fluid is bloody and there is the possibility of an Rh-positive fetus.

Early in pregnancy, amniotic fluid is light yellow or straw-colored with slight turbidity. It then becomes essentially colorless and clear, reflecting light and containing white particulate matter (*vernix caseosa*). The color of the amniotic fluid thus may indicate conditions or diseases even before definite testing is done. The following are examples:
1. *Opaque with green-brown discoloration:* May be thick depending on the amount of meconium in the amniotic fluid. May indicate fetal distress.
2. *Yellow with slight turbidity:* Colored by products of hemolysis especially bilirubin may indicate hemolytic disease of the newborn.
3. *Opaque with some degree of dark red:* Indicates the presence of blood in the amniotic fluid. May indicate perforation of a placental vessel.
4. *Opaque, yellow-brown fluid:* Referred to as tobacco juice characteristic of fetal intrauterine death.

Reasons for Amniocentesis (Fig. 16.3)

1. *Diagnosis of genetic disorders or abnormalities:* Early amniocentesis is done when US scan suggests a fetus having Down syndrome. Fetal cells can be extracted from very small amounts of fluid and used to determine the karyotype. If a fetal abnormality is detected and the mother wishes to terminate the pregnancy, it can be undertaken at an early stage.
2. Maternal illness, which may affect the fetus, e.g. rubella infection.
3. Parents being carriers of genetic disease, e.g. cystic fibrosis.
4. Suspected infection of the fetus, e.g. toxoplasmosis.
5. Assessment of lecithin-sphingomyelin ratio to determine fetal maturity.
6. Determination of the severity of the fetal hemolytic disease (erythroblastosis fetalis).
7. Determination of fetal maturity by measurement of the creatinine level in the amniotic fluid.

Technique of Amniocentesis

An US examination is performed, the placenta localized and a pool of liquor is found. The woman's bladder should be empty and strict asepsis to be observed throughout the procedure. The skin is cleaned and dried, and the physician inserts a needle and a stilette through the abdominal wall into the uterus under direct US guidance. The needle is inserted under direct US visualization into the pool of liquor identified, so that the tip is seen to be in the center of the pool. The needles most commonly used are 20- or 22-gauge spinal needles. A local anesthetic may be used, but is not always considered necessary. About 10–20 mL of amniotic fluid is withdrawn for analysis or a smaller amount if the amniocentesis is performed in the first trimester.

Following the procedure, the fetal heart must be auscultated, if necessary with a Sonicaid or demonstrated on scan.

Diagnostic Studies Possible with Amniotic Fluid

1. *Diagnosis of genetic disorders and abnormalities:* Amniocentesis for this purpose is done sometime between 14th and 18th week of gestation, when there is sufficient number of shed fetal cells in the fluid. For diagnosis of chromosomal abnormality, the amniotic fluid is centrifuged, the cells cultured and karyotyping done. For abnormalities caused by biochemical disorders, amniocentesis is done around the 20th week of gestation.
2. *Measurement of the lecithin-sphingomyelin (L/S) ratio:* The L/S ratio is used to determine fetal maturity. It is used to predict the potential development of respiratory distress syndrome (RDS), since lecithin is essential to preventing collapse of the alveoli during respiratory expiration after birth. Prior to the 34th week of gestation, lecithin and sphingomyelin are present in the amniotic fluid in approximately equal amounts. Thereafter, lecithin increases in relation to sphingomyelin when the proportion becomes 2:1 or 2:0, the chance of RDS is slight unless the mother is diabetic. An L/S ratio of two or above is considered indicative of a mature fetus.
3. *Determination of fetal maturity by the 'rapid surfactant test':* It is also called the 'shake test', or the 'foam test'. This test is used to determine the amount of surfactant properties of lecithin present as an indicator of fetal maturity. This is determined by, whether or not there is a complete circle of foam or bubbles around the circumference of a test tube in which amniotic fluid has been shaken with ethanol and isotonic saline for 15 seconds and then allowed to sit for 15 minutes. A complete ring of bubbles is interpreted as fetal maturity.

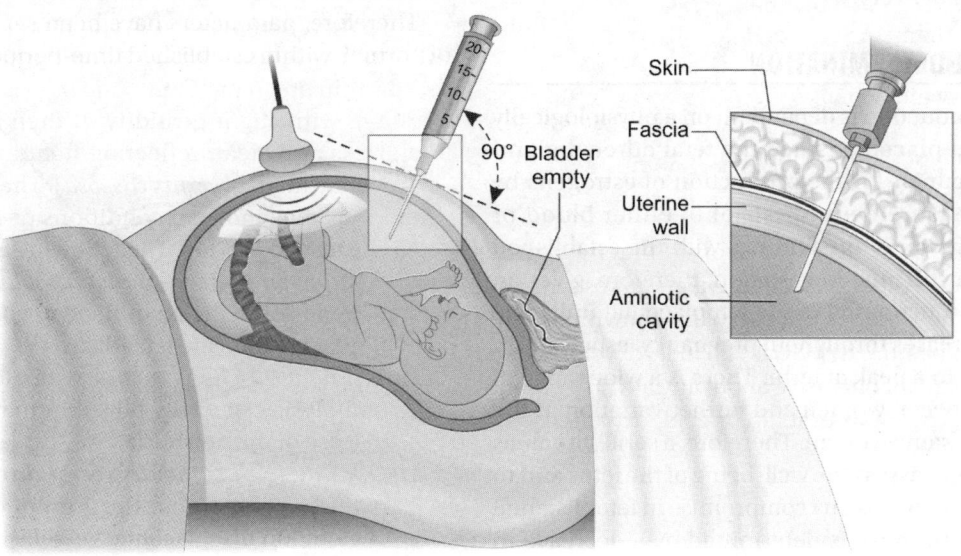

Figure 16.3: Amniocentesis.

4. *Determination of the severity of fetal hemolytic disease (erythroblastosis fetalis):* It is done when the result of maternal indirect Coombs' test is positive and an antibody titer indicates the possibility of severe hemolytic disease in the fetus.

ALPHA-FETOPROTEIN TESTING

Alpha-fetoprotein (AFP) testing is done to identify women at risk for having a baby with a neural tube defect (e.g. spina bifida, anencephaly) or a number of other congenital defects.

This is a normally occurring fetal protein. It is found in abnormally concentrated amounts in the amniotic fluid of a fetus with a neural tube defect and in the mother's blood. AFP testing is most accurate between 15th and 18th week of gestation. AFP testing is a sequence of tests. The first two are of maternal serum and the final test is of amniotic fluid. An elevated AFP level is indicative of significant fetal pathology. A low level of AFP may be associated with Down syndrome. The normal AFP concentration in liquor amnii at the 16th week is about 20 mg/L.

AMNIOSCOPY AND FETOSCOPY

Amnioscopy and fetoscopy both involve direct visualization through the fetal membranes. In amnioscopy, the amniotic fluid is viewed through the fetal membranes at the cervical os. In fetoscopy, the fetus and placenta are visualized through the fetal membranes with an endoscope inserted through a small abdominal incision.

Amnioscopy can be done only when the cervix is fully dilated. It is possible that the membranes will be ruptured inadvertently during the procedure. It may also be uncomfortable for the woman. Amnioscopy may be done during late pregnancy in multiparas with patulous cervices or during labor. Detection of meconium-stained amniotic fluid indicates a probable episode of fetal hypoxia and need for a closely monitored delivery.

ESTRIOL LEVEL DETERMINATION

Normal estriol production is dependent on a physiologically normal fetus and placenta, since the fetal adrenal gland provides the precursor for the production of estrogens by the placenta. Measurement of estriol in either blood or urine and comparison of the findings with the established normal values for the time in gestation, therefore, gives an indication of the functioning of the fetoplacental unit. The level of estriol increases throughout pregnancy, especially in the last trimester, to a peak at term. There is a wide range of normal values between women and further variation in the daily values of the same woman. Therefore, a series of values is needed in order to assess the well-being of the fetus and to determine whether there is any compromise in fetoplacental functioning. Compromise is determined by a decrease in estriol as reflected in a curve of descending values from a series of measurements.

A value above 12 mg indicates fetal well-being. Values between 4 and 12 mg may indicate fetal jeopardy if late in pregnancy, with the probability of jeopardy being higher the closer the value is to 4 mg. Values below 4 mg indicate severe fetal jeopardy or even impending death of fetus.

Estriol series may be ordered when there is a potential concern such as in the following conditions:
- Postmaturity by dates
- Unsure dates and possibility of postmaturity
- Elderly primigravida
- Toxemia/hypertensive disorders of pregnancy
- Diabetes
- Intrauterine growth retardation
- Suspected fetal death
- Suspected fetal abnormality such as anencephaly.

FETAL BLOOD SAMPLING (CORDOCENTESIS)

Cordocentesis technique is used to take a sample of fetal blood during pregnancy in order to screen for chromosomal abnormalities, hemoglobinopathies and other disorders affecting blood or cells. Under US guidance, a needle is passed into the base of the umbilical cord and samples are drawn. These samples are then sent for fetal karyotyping (Fig. 16.4).

FETAL EVALUATION PROCEDURES

Fetal Movement

Fetal movement is generally thought to be an indication of fetal well-being. The obvious and ideal person to count fetal movement is the mother; but two difficulties have been encountered. One is the variation in maternal sensitivity to fetal movements and the other is the wide range of factors, which affect fetal movement, sound, touch and external stimulation.

Therefore, parameters have been set for the lower limits of normal, within established time-periods during which the

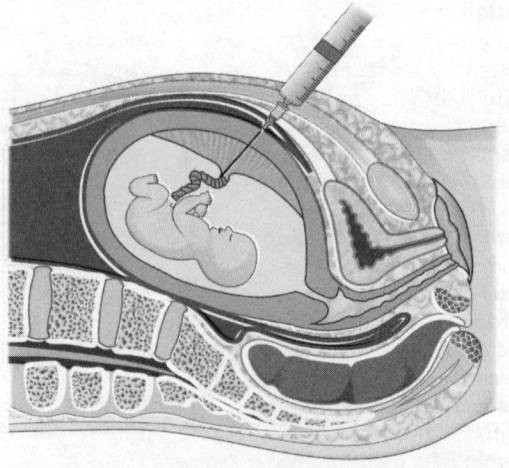

Figure 16.4: Cordocentesis.

mother counts and records daily fetal movements. The lower limit of normal is generally agreed to be 10 movements in 12 hours. Fewer than this constitutes a movement alarm signal (MAS). If the mother's count results in MAS, she immediately reports this and a non-stress test (NST) and/or a contraction stress test (CST) is arranged. The absence of MAS correlates well with good outcomes in over 90% of mothers. When there is a MAS, special note must be made of any progressive decrease in fetal movement; progressive decrease is ominous. A sudden or progressive fall in the movement count, even if it stays within normal range, may not be normal for a particular fetus and may be an indicator of fetal distress and impending death.

Non-stress Test

The non-stress test monitors the fetal heart rate in response to fetal movement in order to assess fetal well-being. It has the advantage of involving no external stimulation (e.g. oxytocin stimulation) in the conduct of the test. Because of this, it can be done for women for whom the CST might be contraindicated. Such women include those with previous cesarean section, placenta previa or threatened premature labor. Otherwise, the indications for an NST are the same as those for CST. The other advantage is that its simplicity and absence of risk factors allow it to be done in an outpatient setting **(Box 16.1)**.

The preparation and positioning of the woman are the same as for the CST. The fetal heart rate is then monitored for approximately 20–30 minutes. It is important that the fetus not be in a fetal sleep state for the entirety of the test as sleep may cause decreased fetal heart rate variability. If necessary, an abdominal palpation can be used to rouse the fetus. During the test, the woman presses a button whenever she feels fetal movements, which produce marks on the monitor strip so that fetal movements and fetal heart rate can be correlated.

> **BOX 16.1:** Nursing tips.
>
> **Indications for NST**
> - Suspected postmaturity.
> - Maternal diabetes mellitus.
> - Maternal hypertension; chronic and pregnancy-related disorders.
> - Suspected or documented intrauterine growth restriction (IUGR).
> - Sickle cell disease.
> - History of previous stillbirth.
> - Isoimmunization.
> - Older gravida.
> - Chronic renal disease.
> - Decreasing fetal movement.
> - Severe maternal anemia.
> - Multiple gestation.
> - High risk antenatal conditions; premature rupture of fetal membranes, preterm labor, bleeding.

Interpretation of the non-stress test is based on patterns of fetal heart rate reactivity to fetal movement. Normally, the fetal heart rate decreases (within the normal range of 120–160 beats per minute) and variability increases with gestational age, probably in relation to the development of the central nervous system. The fetus normally has a transient accelerated heart rate with average baseline variability when moving or to external stimuli such as abdominal palpation. An abnormal fetal heart rate reactivity response to fetal movement is evidenced by a persistent reduction in baseline variability with an absence of fetal heart rate acceleration. This pattern may indicate a distressed fetus and occurs when the fetal central nervous system is depressed by drugs, hypoxia or acidosis.

A *reactive test* is one in which a normal fetal reactivity pattern is demonstrated. This is evidenced by fetal heart rate acceleration of 15 beats per minute above the baseline lasting for 15–30 seconds in association with fetal movement. Two or more occurrences of this acceleration pattern within a 10-minute period or five or more accelerations within a 20-minute period are considered normal. A normal fetus near term will also evidence a baseline fetal heart rate between 120 and 160 beats per minute, variability between 10 and 25 beats per minute and no deceleration of any type.

A *non-reactive test* is one in which there is a persistent decreased variability with an absence of accelerations in fetal heart rate in response to fetal movement. This is evidenced by fetal heart rate accelerations of less than 15 beats per minute above the baseline or lasting less than 15 seconds in association with fetal movement.

A *suspicious (equivocal) non-stress test* is one in which there are definite fetal heart rate accelerations associated with fetal movements, but the number of accelerations, the increase in beats per minute above the baseline or the length of their duration does not meet the criteria for being either reactive or non-reactive.

A reactive test indicates fetal well-being and predicts a good outcome if birth were to occur within 1 week. If the test is non-reactive, further assessment of fetal status should be initiated to aid in determining fetal well-being. If the test is suspicious, it should be repeated in 24–48 hours. The non-stress test can be repeated or continued at any desired frequency without concern for adverse effects to the fetus.

Contraction Stress Test

Contraction stress test assesses fetal placental functioning and the fetus's projected ability to cope with the continuation of a high-risk pregnancy and the stress of labor. It aids the physician in selecting the optimal time for delivery of a high-risk fetus. The underlying physiological and technological bases for the CST are as follows:
1. Contractions decrease the blood flow through the intervillous space.
2. If the uteroplacental reserve is normal, this intermittent decrease in blood flow by contractions will not negatively affect the fetus.

3. If the uteroplacental reserve is diminished or suboptimal, the intermittent decrease in blood flow by contractions will affect the fetus.
4. This negative effect on the fetus is reflected as a fetal heart pattern of late deceleration.
5. A fetal heart pattern of late deceleration is thought to be due to uteroplacental insufficiency.

This is a test that ascertains the fetus's response to contractions—naturally occurring, or induced by nipple stimulation or oxytocin—by using external fetal monitoring to record simultaneously the fetal heart rate and the uterine contractions.

Some of the conditions in which a CST might be helpful in selection of an optimal time for delivery include the following:
- Postmaturity—suspected or actual
- Intrauterine growth retardation as suspected by a small for gestational age (SGA) fetus
- History of previous stillbirth
- Meconium-stained amniotic fluid obtained at amniocentesis
- Falling or abnormal estriol values
- Diabetes
- Toxemia/hypertensive disorders of pregnancy
- Chronic hypertension
- Chronic lung disease
- Cyanotic heart disease
- Chronic renal disease
- Hyperthyroidism
- Collagen disease
- Severe isoimmunization
- Sickle cell disease or other hemoglobinopathies

Procedure

The woman's bladder should be empty (to promote comfort and avoid disruption) and she should be in either a semi-Fowler's or left lateral position (to avoid supine hypotensive syndrome). Her blood pressure should be checked to obtain a baseline recording. There are two methods of inducing the contractions needed for a CST—nipple stimulation and intravenous oxytocin administration.

Nipple stimulation test

Nipple stimulation causes the neurohypophysis to release endogenous oxytocin. This method of producing naturally occurring oxytocin avoids the risks, discomfort and expenses associated with the intravenous infusion of oxytocin. At the beginning of the test, warm washcloths are applied to the breasts. A+D ointment or K-Y lubricating jelly is applied to the nipples to prevent soreness. The woman then stimulates her nipples by either rolling them or gently pulling them. Stimulation is initially unilateral. If contractions are inadequate (fewer than three contractions in the first 10 minute), the woman then simultaneously stimulates both nipples for another 10 minutes. If contractions are still inadequate, intravenous oxytocin is used. Nipple stimulation provides adequate contractions approximately in 75% of women using this method.

Oxytocin challenge test

The administration of oxytocin to induce contractions is called oxytocin challenge test or oxytocin contraction test (OCT). A venipuncture is done, an intravenous line is established and a very dilute solution of oxytocin, controlled by an infusion pump, is administered via a piggyback setup to another bag of intravenous solution. The rate of infusion is increased at intervals until the contractions are occurring at a frequency of at least three in a 10-minute period and lasting at least 30 seconds (preferably 40–60 second). The recording is then interpreted and the infusion stopped. Both the monitoring and the intravenous solution, without oxytocin in it, are continued until the contractions have diminished to their baseline activity. This is to assure that the OCT has not put the woman into labor without your knowing about it.

A negative CST is one in which no late decelerations occur with contractions as frequent as three in a 10-minute period. A negative CST indicates fetal well-being and predicts that the fetus will continue to be alright for another week without needing the intervention of delivery, if the woman's clinical status does not change. Negative CSTs are repeated weekly or sooner depending on the continuing clinical status.

A positive CST is one in which there have been repeated late decelerations of fetal heart rate patterns during the test. A positive CST indicates that the fetus may not withstand continuation of the pregnancy. Serious consideration needs to be given to immediate termination of the pregnancy by delivery. A positive CST is a valuable piece of information in decision-making, but urge caution and encourages use of a total picture of assessment methods and clinical judgment, as there can be a 25% rate false-positive results.

Other categories of interpretation of CST

1. *Hyperstimulation* in which the contractions are more frequent than 2 minutes or have duration of more than 90 seconds. This is more apt to occur with the use of oxytocin than with nipple stimulation. Hyperstimulation renders the test invalid. The late decelerations in the presence of hyperstimulation may not be due to uteroplacental insufficiency. The test should be repeated within 24–48 hours with an even more dilute solution of oxytocin.
2. *Suspicious (equivocal)* in which there has been an occasional late deceleration, but this is not repetitive and does not occur with continued contractions. The CST should be repeated within 24–48 hours.
3. *Unsatisfactory* in which the recording (tracing) is not of good enough quality to be interpreted. This may be due to the problems inherent with external fetal monitoring.

STUDY QUESTIONS

Short Notes

1. Alpha-fetoprotein testing.
2. Amnioscopy and fetoscopy testing.
3. Fetal blood sampling.
4. Nipple stimulation testing.
5. Indications for non-stress testing.

Short Answer Questions

1. Diagnostic uses of ultrasonography in pregnancy.
2. Amniocentesis and its uses in pregnancy.
3. Contraction stress test.

Essay Questions

1. Discuss the preparation of a patient and assisting with amniocentesis procedure and nursing care following the procedure.
2. Discuss the significance, indications and method of performing non-stress test (NST).
3. Explain the indications, use and procedure of performing a contraction stress test (CST).

BIBLIOGRAPHY

1. Das S. Antenatal care. In: Bennett RV, Linda KB (Eds). Myles Textbook for Midwives, 13th edition. Edinburgh: Churchill Livingstone; 1999. pp. 371-88.
2. Dutta DC. Textbook of Obstetrics, 5th edition. Kolkata: New Central Book Company; 2001. pp. 683-93.
3. Park K. Park's Textbook of Preventive and Social Medicine, 16th edition. Jabalpur: M/s Banarsidas Bhanot Publishers; 2000. pp. 352-9.
4. Helen V. Nurse-Midwifery, 2nd edition. Boston: Jones and Bartlett Publishers; 1996. pp. 63-74.

SECTION V

NORMAL LABOR

Section Outline

17. Physiology of the First Stage of Labor
18. Management of the First Stage of Labor
19. Physiology of the Second Stage of Labor
20. Management of the Second Stage of Labor
21. Physiology and Management of the Third Stage of Labor
22. Management of the Fourth Stage of Labor

CHAPTER 17

Physiology of the First Stage of Labor

Learning Objectives

Upon completion of this chapter, the learner will be able to:
- Define the term labor and describe the onset and stages of labor.
- Describe the signs and symptoms of impending labor.
- Enumerate the physiological changes in the uterus as labor progresses.
- Explain the mechanical factors that contribute to the progress of labor.
- Describe the assessment of a pregnant client for evaluation of maternal and fetal conditions.
- Explain the procedure of vaginal examination and enumerate the probable findings.

The first stage of labor usually starts with the onset of regular uterine contractions and culminates in the complete dilatation of the cervix. There are number of premonitory signs and symptoms that may alert a midwife to a woman's approaching labor. A woman may exhibit any, all or none of these, but it is useful to keep them in mind when seeing a woman late in pregnancy so that appropriate counseling, guidance and care can be given.

DEFINITION OF LABOR

Labor may be defined as rhythmic contraction and relaxation of the uterine muscles with progressive effacement (thinning) and dilatation (opening) of the cervix, leading to expulsion of the products of conception.

Labor is described as the process by which the fetus, placenta and membranes are expelled through the birth canal.

Labor can and does occur at any time during pregnancy, but takes place most frequently at term or about 40 weeks after the normal menstrual period.

Normal Labor

Normal labor occurs at term and is spontaneous in onset with the fetus presenting by the vertex. The process is completed within 18 hours and no complications arise.

Three P's of Normal Labor

The labor process involves a relationship between the three P's such as the *powers* or uterine contractions; the *pelvis* including the size and shape; and the *passenger*, which includes the size, position and presentation of the fetus as well as the bag of waters or amniotic sac. Normal labor assumes that the powers are sufficient, the pelvis is adequate and passenger is of average size and is in a normal position. Complications of labor occur when there are problems with one or more of the P's.

STAGES OF LABOR

Labor is divided into four stages (Table 17.1):
1. The *first stage* is that of dilatation of cervix. It begins with regular rhythmic contractions (true labor) and is complete when the cervix is fully dilated and effaced.
2. The *second stage* is the stage of expulsion of the fetus. It begins with complete dilation of the cervix through complete birth of the baby.
3. The *third stage* of labor is that of separation and expulsion of the placenta and membranes. It lasts from the birth of the baby through the delivery of the placenta and membranes with contraction and retraction of uterus.
4. The *fourth stage* is the first 4 hours after delivery of the placenta. This is an arbitrary time during which, the vital signs must stabilize and any tendency for immediate hemorrhage must be controlled. This is a critical period for every mother.

TABLE 17.1: Average length of labor stages.

Characteristics	First stage			Second stage	Third stage	Fourth stage	Total duration
	Latent phase	Active phase	Transition phase				
Duration of labor	Primigravida 8–10 h	5–6 h	2 h	1–1½ h	10–15 min	1 h	16–24 h
	Multigravida 4–5 h	3–4 h	1–1½ h	25–30 min	10–15 min	1 h	8–10 h
Cervical dilatation	0–4 cm	4–8 cm	8–10 cm	–	–	–	–
Contractions frequency	15–20 min progressing to 5–7 min	3–5 min	2–3 min	1½–2 min	–	–	–
Duration of contractions	10–20 s progressing to 30–40 s	40–60 s	60–90 s	60–90 s	–	–	–
Intensity of contractions	Mild progressing to moderate	Moderate progressing to strong	Strong	Strong	–	–	–

First Stage (Fig. 17.1)

The first stage of labor begins with the onset of regular contractions and ends when the cervix is fully dilated. The stage is divided into three phases such as latent, active and transition phases.

Latent Phase

The latent phase of labor begins with the onset of true labor contractions, which are usually mild. During this phase, contractions may be 15–20 minutes apart, lasting 20–30 seconds. As this phase progresses, however, the contractions

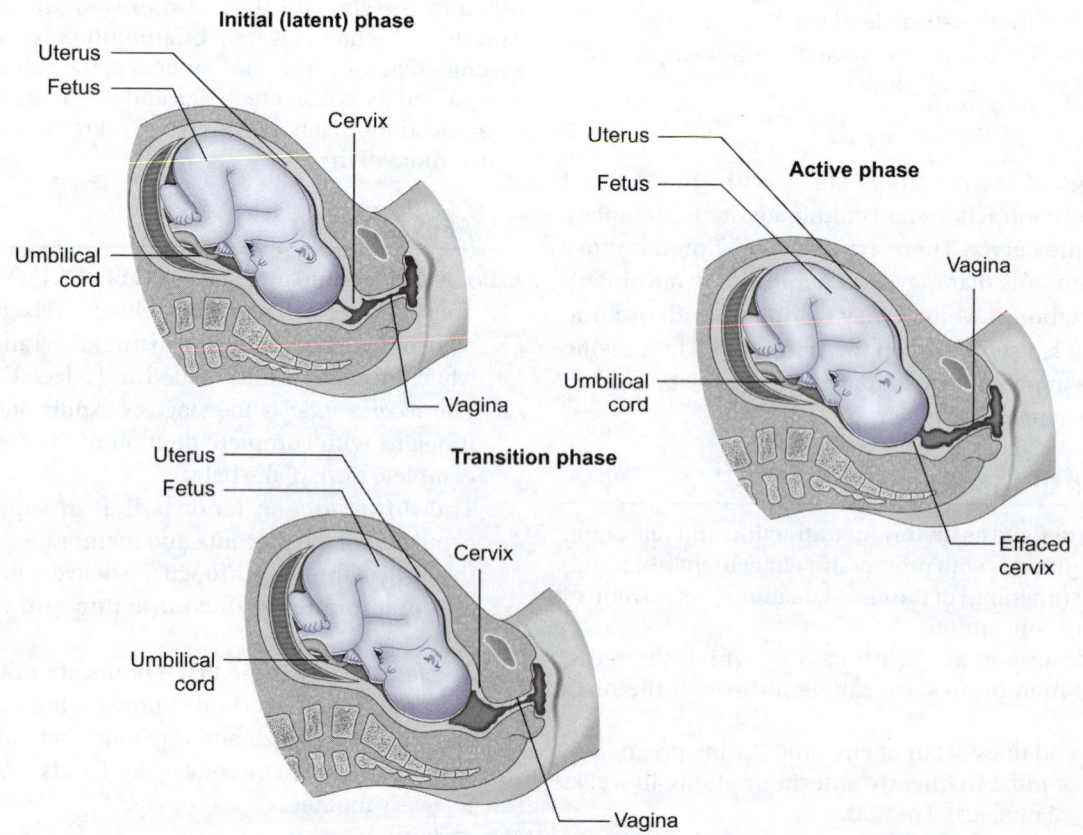

Figure 17.1: First stage of labor.

will occur every 5–7 minutes and the duration will lengthen to 30–40 seconds. This phase usually begins with little or no cervical dilation and ends when the cervix is 3–4 cm dilated. For the primigravida, the latent phase lasts an average of 9 hours; whereas in the multigravida, the latent phase generally lasts an average of 5 hours. Although, the woman may exhibit some anxiety during this phase, she often is comfortable enough to verbalize her concerns.

Active Phase

The active phase of labor begins when the woman is 3–4 cm dilated and ends when she is 8 cm dilated. During this phase, contractions occur every 3–5 minutes and last up to 60 seconds. The intensity of each contraction begins as moderate and continues to increase as the woman gets closer to transition phase. The average length of the active phase in the primigravida is 6 hours and in the multigravida 4 hours. Dilation rate should be at least 1.2–1.5 cm/h.

Transition Phase

The last and shortest part of the first phase of labor is transition, which typically is the most intense phase for the laboring woman. In transition, contractions occur every 2–3 minutes lasting 60–90 seconds. The intensity of contractions is very strong in the transition phase. The woman often becomes restless and agitated, may have difficulty focusing during contractions. They hyperventilate, complain of nausea and vomiting, tremble and experience rectal pressure. During this time the nurse will need to prepare the women for the second stage of labor. The average length of transition phase is 2 hours in primigravida and 1 hour in multigravida **(Box 17.1)**.

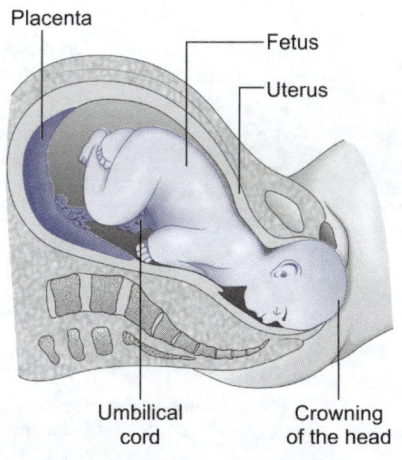

Figure 17.2: Second stage of labor.

Second Stage (Fig. 17.2)

The second stage of labor with the cervix completely dilated and effaced and ends when the fetus is expelled; it is also known as the expulsion stage. The average length of the second stage of labor in primigravida is 1 hour and in the multigravida 25 minutes. Many factors influence the length of the second stage of labor, including maternal parity, fetal size, uterine contractile force, presentation, position, pelvic size, method of anesthesia (if used) and magnitude of maternal expulsive effort. During contractions, the woman will bear down, causing the abdominal muscles to contract and helping the fetal head to descend through the birth canal. As the fetal head continues into the birth canal, the perineum begins to bulge. Crowning is defined as the point at which the fetal head is visible at the vulval opening. When crowning occurs, birth is imminent. At this time, women develop an urge to push. Some women describe intense pain and burning of the perineum as the pressure increases on the vulva. Nurses need to be aware of prolonged second stage of labor, because intervention may be required.

Third Stage (Fig. 17.3)

The third stage of labor or placental stage begins as soon as the fetus is delivered and lasts until the placenta is delivered. The mechanism of placental separation is a combination of uterine contractions and involution. After expulsion of the fetus, the uterus continues to contract every 3–4 minutes. As the uterus contracts and begins the process of involution (reduction in size) shrinkage of the site of implantation of the placenta occurs. Within 10–15 minutes after delivery of the infant, most of the placenta gets detached from the uterine wall. At this point, vaginal bleeding from the uncovered implantation site increases and delivery of the placenta generally follows.

The classic signs of placental separation are founding up of the uterus, upward movement of the fundus, lengthening of the umbilical cord and a rush of blood from the vagina. Once the placenta is delivered, the uterus continues to contract, closing the spiral arterioles. As the uterus continues to shrink, the bleeding decreases.

BOX 17.1: Nursing alert.		
True versus false labor		
	True labor	**False labor**
Contraction	• Regular, uterus hardens	• Irregular, no hardening occurs
	• Intervals shorten	• Intervals do not shorten
	• Intensity increases	• Intensity remains unchanged
	• Intensify with walking	• Do not intensify with walking
	• Lying down has no effect	• Lying down lengthens interval
Cervix	Dilates and becomes effaced	Does not dilate or efface
Sedation	Does not stop true labor	Tends to stop false labor
Show	Often is present	Usually is absent

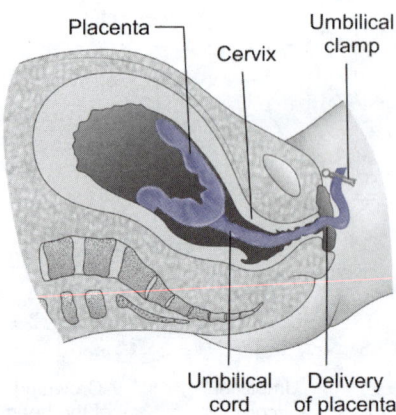

Figure 17.3: Third stage of labor.

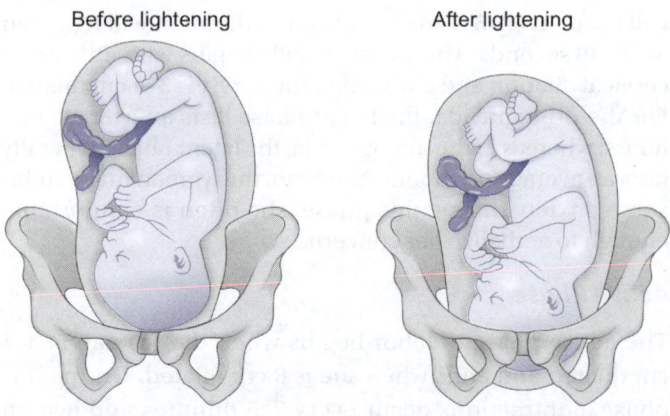

Figure 17.4: Before lightening and after lightening.

Fourth Stage

The *fourth stage of labor* or recovery stage is defined as the first 1 hour after delivery of the placenta. During this time, many internal physiologic readjustments occur. The average blood loss from a vaginal delivery is 250–300 mL. Because of the blood loss and the return of a more normal abdominal anatomy as the uterus returns to a more normal size (involution), there is a decreas in blood pressure and pulse rate. The fundus is in midline and at the level of the umbilicus. The fundus should remain firm, contracted and midline. Most of the discomforts of labor, such as nausea and vomiting should be subsiding.

SIGNS AND SYMPTOMS OF IMPENDING LABOR

The signs and symptoms of impending labor are lightening, cervical changes, false labor, premature rupture of membranes, bloody show, energy-spurt and gastrointestinal upsets. The last weeks of pregnancy during which these changes occur is termed as *prelabor*.

Lightening (Fig. 17.4)

About 2–3 weeks before the onset of labor, the lower uterine segment expands and allows the fetal head to sink lower. The baby's head, if there is a cephalic presentation, usually is fixed or engaged afterwards. The symphysis pubis widens and the pelvic floor becomes more relaxed and softened, allowing the uterus to descend further into the pelvis.

In a primigravid woman, when the abdominal muscles are in good tone, the uterus will be braced into an upright position, which helps the fetal head to engage. The increasing intensity of the Braxton Hicks contractions in late pregnancy may also contribute to lightening. In the multigravida, the abdominal muscles tend to be more lax and as a result, the abdomen becomes somewhat pendulous so that the fetal head may not engage.

The woman will experience a decrease in the minor discomfort of shortness of breath she has had during the third trimester, because lightening will give her more room in the upper abdomen for lung expansion. However, lightening will cause other discomforts due to the pressure of the presenting part on structures in the area of the true pelvis. Specifically, she will have:

- Frequency of urination, because the bladder feels pressure and has less room for expansion
- An uncomfortable feeling of generalized pelvic pressure, which may make her feel awkward and produces the constant sensation that something needs to come out or that a bowel movement is needed
- Leg cramps, which may be caused by the pressure of the presenting part on the nerves that course through the foramen obturator and lead to the legs
- Increased venous stasis producing dependent edema, because the pressure of the presenting part inhibits blood return from the lower extremities
- Vaginal secretion becomes more profuse at this time.

Lightening lowers the height of the fundus to a position similar to that of the 8th month of pregnancy and the ballottement of fetal head is no longer possible.

The nurse's knowledge of lightening is of value in being able to reassure the woman of the normality of the bodily changes she is experiencing and explain why they are occurring. This also provides a good opportunity to review with the woman her plans for labor. It provides an indication of the adequacy of the pelvic inlet. Lightening tends to encourage the woman that the long-awaited end of pregnancy is within sight.

Cervical Changes (Fig. 17.5)

As labor approaches, the cervix becomes 'ripe'. The cervix becomes softer, like the consistency of pudding and evidences some degree of effacement and perhaps slight dilatation. Evaluation of ripeness is relative to the individual woman. For example, a grand multipara's cervix may normally be 2 cm dilated as opposed to a primigravida's normally closed cervix.

Ripeness indicates a readiness of the cervix for labor. It is of value in assuring the patient that she will go into labor with the onset of labor contractions and that the time of labor is relatively close.

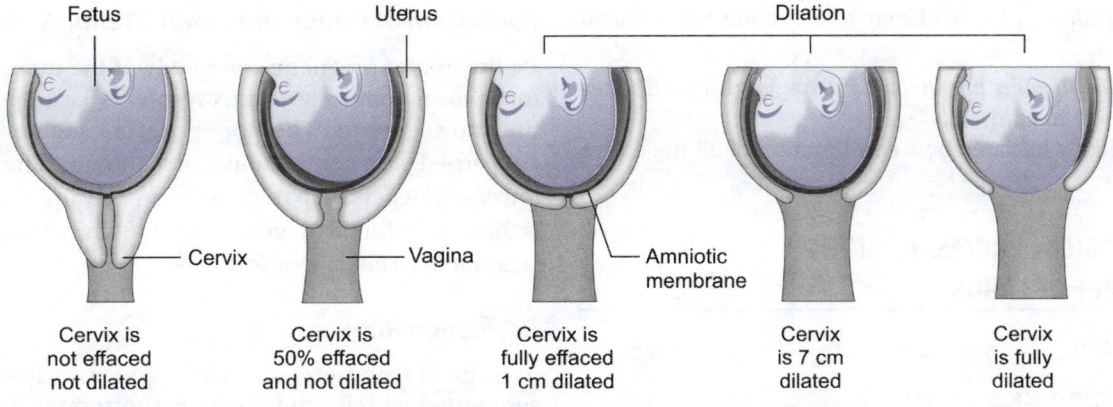

Figure 17.5: Cervical changes during labor.

False Labor

False labor consists of painful uterine contractions that have no measurable progressive effect on the cervix and are in actuality an exaggeration of the usually painless Braxton Hicks contractions, which have been occurring since about 6 weeks of gestation.

False labor may occur for days or intermittently even 3–4 weeks before the onset of true labor. False labor is genuinely painful and a woman may lose sleep and energy coping with it. She has no way of knowing for sure whether she is in true labor, since this can be determined only by vaginal examination. Such women need a great degree of understanding, patience, support, reassurance and explanation from the midwife, as they may get frustrated of making trips to the hospital. False labor, however, does indicate the approach of labor.

The midwife can confirm the presence of false labor pains when the following features are present:
- Pain remains stationary in lower abdomen
- Pain is continuous without any rhythm
- No associated hardening of the uterus
- No dilation of cervix and no 'show'
- Pain diminishes after enema.

Premature Rupture of Membranes

Normally, the membranes rupture at the end of the first stage of labor. When rupture occurs before the onset of labor, it is termed as premature rupture of membranes and occurs in about 12% of women. Approximately, 80% of women with premature rupture of membranes begin labor spontaneously within 24 hours.

Bloody Show

A mucus plug, created by cervical secretions from proliferation of the glands of the cervical mucosa early in pregnancy, serves the function of a protective barrier and closes the cervical canal throughout pregnancy. Bloody show is the expulsion of this mucus plug. Bloody show is most often seen as a tenacious, blood-tinged mucus discharge, which must be carefully differentiated from frank bleeding. Bloody show is a sign of imminent labor, which usually takes place within 24–48 hours.

ENERGY SPURT

Many women experience an energy spurt approximately 24–48 hours before the onset of labor. After days or weeks of feeling tired (physically tired and tired of being pregnant), they get up 1 day to find themselves full of energy and vigor. Typically these women do lot of household tasks, which they either have not had the energy to do or now feel need doing before the baby's arrival.

There is no known explanation for this energy spurt, other than it is a nature's way of giving the woman the energy she needs for the work of labor. Women should be informed of the possibility of their having this energy spurt and advised to deliberately refrain from expending it and instead to conserve it for use during labor.

Gastrointestinal Upsets

In the absence of any causative factors for the occurrence of diarrhea, indigestion, nausea and vomiting, it is thought that they might be indicative of impending labor. No explanation for this is known, but some women do experience one to all of these signs.

CAUSES FOR THE ONSET OF LABOR

Theories regarding initiation of labor include the following:

Oxytocin stimulation theory: Although the mechanism is unknown, the uterus becomes increasingly sensitive to oxytocin as the pregnancy progresses.

Progesterone withdrawal theory: A decrease in progesterone production may stimulate prostaglandin (PG) synthesis and enhance the effect of estrogen, which has a stimulating effect on uterine muscles.

Estrogen stimulation theory: Estrogen stimulates irritability of uterine muscles and enhances uterine contractions.

Fetal cortisol theory: Cortisol may affect maternal estrogen levels.

Prostaglandin stimulation theory: Prostaglandin stimulates smooth muscle to contract.

Labor is likely initiated by a combination of all the above mechanisms.

PHYSIOLOGICAL PROCESSES IN THE FIRST STAGE OF LABOR

Uterine Action

Fundal Dominance

Each uterine contraction starts in the fundus near one of the cornua and spreads across and downwards. Each contraction is longest and intense in the fundus, but the peak is reached simultaneously over the whole uterus and fades from all parts together. This pattern permits the cervix to dilate and the fundus to expel the fetus.

Polarity

A neuromuscular harmony prevails between the two poles or segments of uterus throughout labor, which is termed as polarity. During each contraction, these two poles act harmoniously. The upper pole contracts stronger and retracts to expel the fetus; the lower pole contracts slightly and dilates to allow expulsion to occur. If polarity is disorganized, the progress of labor is inhibited.

Contraction and Retraction (Fig. 17.6)

During labor the contraction does not pass off entirely, the muscle fibers retain some of the shortening of contraction instead of becoming completely relaxed. This is termed retraction, which is a unique property of the uterine muscle. Because of this, the upper segment of the uterus becomes gradually shorter and thicker and its cavity diminishes assisting in the progressive expulsion of the fetus.

When labor begins, uterine contractions occur every 15–20 minutes and may last for 30 seconds. They are weak to begin with and occur with rhythmic regularly and intervals between them gradually lessen, while the length and strength of the contractions gradually increase. By the end of first stage, they occur at 2–4 minutes interval, last for 50–60 seconds and are very powerful.

Formation of Upper and Lower Uterine Segments

By the end of pregnancy, the body of the uterus is divided into two anatomically distinct segments, i.e. upper and lower uterine segments. The upper uterine segment is mainly concerned with contraction and is thick and muscular. The lower segment is prepared for distension and dilatation, and is thinner. The lower segment develops from the isthmus and is about 8–10 cm in length.

Retraction Ring

A ridge forms between the upper and lower uterine segments, which are known as the retraction ring (**Fig. 17.7**). The physiological retraction ring gradually rises as the upper uterine segment contracts and retracts, and the lower uterine segment thins out to accommodate the descending fetus. Once the cervix is fully dilated and the fetus can leave the uterus, the retraction ring rises no further.

The retraction ring is normally not visible over the abdomen. When the phenomenon is exaggerated in an obstructed labor, the retraction ring becomes visible above the symphysis pubis; it is termed as *Bandl's ring*.

Cervical Action

Cervical Effacement

Cervical effacement is defined as the thinning of the cervix and shortening of the cervical canal from its usual length of 2–3 cm to one in which the cervical canal is obliterated leaving only the external os as a circular orifice with thin edges.

This shortening results from the lengthening of the muscular fibers around the internal os, as they are taken up into the lower uterine segment. Effacement is facilitated by the cleft-like arrangement of the endocervix, which in effect unfolds like an accordion, as it is stretched and taken up to become part of the lower uterine segment. The process of effacement is also facilitated by the expulsion of the mucus plug. Effacement is clinically evaluated in terms of percentages, e.g. 50% effaced, 80% effaced or completely effaced, which is often paper thin. The degree of effacement depends upon the examiner's evaluation and judgment, and the estimation varies among examiners. In the primigravida, this usually occurs prior to the onset of labor, while in the multigravida, this occurs simultaneously with cervical dilatation (**Fig. 17.8**).

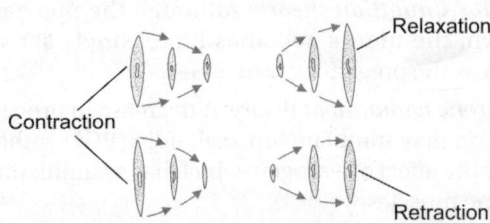

Figure 17.6: Contraction and retraction of uterine muscle fibers during labor.

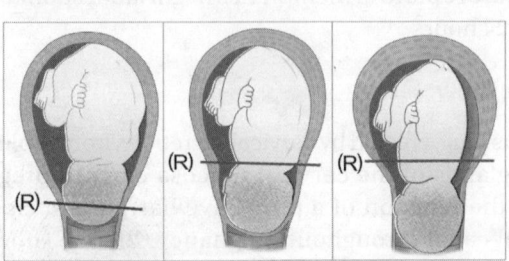

Figure 17.7: Formation of retraction ring.

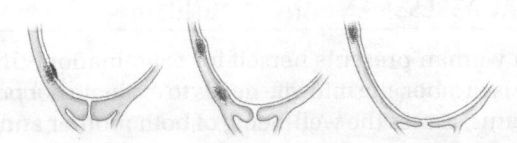

Figure 17.8: Dilatation and effacement of the cervix.

Cervical Dilatation

Dilatation of the cervix is the process of enlargement of the external cervical os from an orifice of a few millimeters to an opening large enough for the baby to pass through. Dilatation is effected primarily by the action of contractions and facilitated by the hydrostatic action of the amniotic fluid under the influence of contractions, causing the membranes to serve as a dilating wedge in the area of least resistance in the uterus. If the membranes have ruptured, the pressure of the presenting part on the cervix and the lower uterine segment has a dilating effect.

Dilatation is clinically evaluated by measuring the diameter of the cervical opening in centimeters, with 0 cm being a closed external cervical os and 10 cm being complete dilatation **(Fig. 17.9)**.

Because of the dilatation of the cervix, the operculum, which formed the cervical plug during pregnancy, is lost. This blood-stained mucoid discharge is termed as the *show*. The blood comes from the ruptured capillaries in the parietal decidua where the chorion has become detached from the dilating cervix.

Ripening of the Cervix

The term 'ripe' cervix is often used. It is believed that the Braxton Hicks contractions help to prepare the cervix or ripen it for the job ahead. The cervix moves from its posterior position during pregnancy to an anterior position and the normally firm tissue softens considerably. The cervix may be described as 'pudding soft', 'butter soft' or 'very pliable'.

A certain number of contractions and time are required to first ripen the cervix, and then to efface and dilate it.

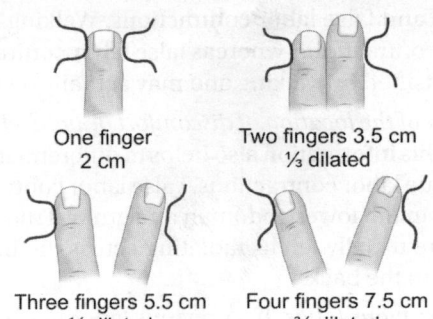

Figure 17.9: Clinical estimation of dilatation of cervix.

Mechanical Factors that Contribute to the Progress of Labor in the First Stage

Formation of the Forewaters (Fig. 17.10)

As the lower uterine segment stretches, the chorion becomes detached from it and the increased intrauterine pressure causes this loosened part of the sac of fluid, to bulge downwards into the dilating internal os, to the depth of 6–12 mm. The well-flexed head fits snugly into the cervix and cuts off the fluid in front of the head from that, which surrounds the body. The fluid in front of the head is termed *forewaters* and that which surrounds the body as *hindwaters*.

The effect of separation of forewaters is to keep the membranes intact during the first stage by preventing the pressure applied to the hindwaters during uterine contractions from being applied to the forewaters.

General Fluid Pressure

While the membranes remain intact, the pressure of the uterine contractions is exerted on the fluid and, as fluid is not compressible, the pressure is equalized throughout the uterus and over the fetal body, which is known as general fluid pressure. This equalization of pressure is lost when the membranes rupture and a quantity of fluid escapes causing compression of the placenta between the uterine wall and fetus during contractions lending to diminution of oxygen supply to the fetus. Preserving the integrity of the membranes, therefore, optimizes the supply of oxygen to the fetus and helps to prevent intrauterine infection.

Rupture of the Membranes

The physiological moment for the membranes to rupture is at the end of the first stage of labor when the cervix becomes fully dilated and no longer supports the bag of waters.

Spontaneous rupture of membranes may sometimes occur days or hours before labor begins or during the first stage. With a badly fitting presenting part, the forewaters are not cut off effectively and the membranes rupture early. In some cases, it happens without any apparent reason. It may sometimes rupture during the second stage just before the delivery of the head. Occasionally the membranes do not rupture even in the second stage and appear at the vulva as a bulging sac covering the fetal head as it is born; this is known as the *caul*.

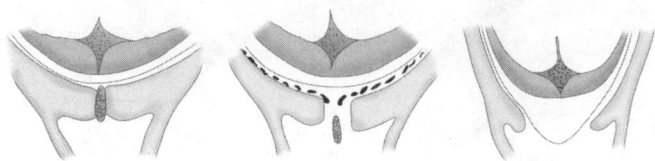

Figure 17.10: Formation of bag of membranes and forewaters.

Fetal Axis Pressure

During each contraction the uterus rears forward (becomes upright) and the force of the fundal contraction is transmitted to the upper pole of the uterus, down the long axis of the fetus and is applied by the presenting part to the cervix. This is known as fetal axis pressure. It becomes more significant after rupture of the membranes and during the second stage of labor.

Descent of the Presenting Part

Descent of the presenting part refers to the downward and outward movement of this part through the pelvis. The normal well-flexed head (vertex) twists and turns, flexes and extends to maneuver through the pelvis, just as one might twist and turn a hand, and flex and extend the fingers to get the hand into a jar. There are three planes or obstacles involved in the process of descent, i.e. the pelvic inlet, the pelvic brim and the pelvic outlet. When the examiner can feel the presenting part at the level if the ischial spines, a midplane (pelvic brim) mark, it indicates the largest part of the head has come through the inlet. The head is thus engaged. The presenting part is now at zero (0) station. When the vertex has descended to the perineum, the largest part has passed the ischial spines, another obstacle. The head is now at +2 station. Delivery of the head brings it past the third obstacle, i.e. the outlet, which is under the pubic arch, between the ischial tuberosities and over the coccyx. Station is the relationship of the lowermost part of the presenting part to an imaginary line drawn between the ischial spines of the woman's pelvis. The lowermost part at the level of the ischial spines is called '0' station. Station is measured in terms of centimeters above or below the level of ischial spines with above being designated as –1, –2, –3, – 4 and –5 station, and below being designated as +1, +2, +3, +4 and +5 station. The –5 station is equivalent to a floating head and the +5 is equivalent to a head at the perineum **(Fig. 17.11)**.

Station is at times difficult to ascertain if there has been considerable molding of the fetal skull and development of caput succedaneum. In cephalic presentation, the skull bones may be a centimeter or so higher than the caput, which is what an examiner's fingers may feel.

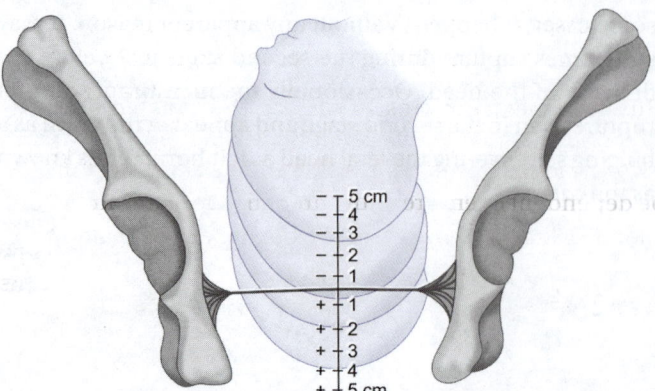

Figure 17.11: Diagrammatic representation of the stations of presenting part.

INITIAL ASSESSMENT AND DIAGNOSIS

When a woman presents herself for examination, thinking that she is in labor, the midwife needs to evaluate her possible labor status, assess the well-being of both mother and baby, and screen for immediate complications. On the basis of these findings and other related factors, a decision of whether or not the woman is in labor or needs any medical help or intervention is made.

Evaluation of labor status refers to that information needed to determine whether a woman is in the progress of her labor and to anticipate her continued progress. Requirements for this are history, physical examination (general and abdominal) and pelvic (vaginal) examination. Steps of the evaluation process with the significance of each are explained below.

History

Age

An age under 16 or over 35 predisposes the woman to a number of complications.

Gravida and Para

Parity has an effect on both duration of labor and on the incidence of complications. A cervix, which has been completely dilated in a previous labor offers less resistance to being dilated again, thereby shortening the length of labor. In addition multiparas have more relaxed pelvic floors, which offer less resistance to the passage of the baby and decrease the length of labor. However, in grand multiparas the duration of labor may be longer, i.e. exhaustion of uterine muscle due to changes in the uterine musculature. Increased parity increases the incidence of complications.

Time of onset of contractions and the frequency and duration of the contractions: This information is necessary in order to establish the start of labor, usually timed from when the contractions became regular and to differentiate between false and true labor. False labor contractions do not increase in frequency, duration and intensity; are irregular and are of short duration. True labor contractions may start as irregular and of short duration, but then become regular with increased frequency, duration and intensity.

Intensity of contractions when lying down contrasted to when walking around: This information helps to differentiate between true and false labor contractions. Walking intensifies true labor contractions, whereas false labor contractions are rarely intensified by walking and may actually be relieved.

Description of the location of discomfort or pain felt with contractions: This information also helps to differentiate between false and true labor contractions. False labor contractions are usually felt in the lower abdomen and groin. True labor contractions are usually felt as radiating across the uterus from the fundus to the back.

Length of previous labor: If a previous labor has been within the past few years, the length of that labor is a good indication of the potential length of this labor.

Number of years since the last baby: If there are a number of years between babies, a woman may have a length of labor more similar to her first one. If 10 or more years have passed since her last baby, she is predisposed to prolonged labor and to the complications of antepartum hemorrhage and perinatal mortality.

Delivery method of previous deliveries: This is to rule out previous cesarean section and instrumental deliveries.

Size of the largest and smallest previous babies: The size of the largest baby delivered vaginally assures the adequacy of the woman's pelvis for up to that size baby. It also provides baseline information for anticipating possible complications when compared with the estimated fetal weight of this baby. History of a baby over 4 kg and/or abortions and preterm babies are an indication to screen the woman for diabetes.

Expected date of delivery and present weeks of gestation: This is baseline data for evaluating gestational size and if labor is at term or premature.

Absence, presence or increase in bloody show: Bloody show is a premonitory sign of labor. An increase in bloody show is indicative of impending second stage of labor.

Absence or presence of vaginal bleeding: Bleeding is abnormal. Any frank bleeding requires immediate consultation and attention.

Membranes ruptured or not: Rupture of membranes is a premonitory sign of labor. Because ruptured membranes predispose both mother and baby to high risk factors due to the increased risk of intrauterine infection. A history of ruptured membranes demands determining by examination whether or not they have indeed ruptured. Women are not always clear as to whether their membranes have ruptured or not because a slow leak can always be confused with incontinence of urine. A history of sudden gush of water, which ran down her legs wetting her clothes, is a good history that the membranes have ruptured. A definitive test may be done to confirm the history. A strongly alkaline reaction or deep blue color on nitrazine test paper indicates a positive result. A fern test may also be done, which is a microscopic examination of a fern-like crystallization of the sodium chloride in amniotic fluid on a slide on which it is allowed to dry.

Any prenatal problems: It is essential to screen the woman quickly for antepartal complications, which may affect the intrapartal period, e.g. preeclampsia and anemia.

Physical Examination

Vital Signs

Temperature, pulse, respiration and blood pressure: An elevated temperature is indicative of an infectious process. An elevated pulse may indicate infection, shock or anxiety. An elevated respiratory rate may indicate shock and anxiety. An elevated or lowered blood pressure is indicative of hypertensive disorders of pregnancy or shock respectively. An elevated systolic, but normal diastolic blood pressure may indicate anxiety.

Physical Measurements

Height and weight.

Fetal Heart Tones

To assess the status of the baby; normal fetal heart rate is 120–160 beats per minute. A fetal heart rate below 120 or above 160 may be indicative of fetal distress and warrants immediate evaluation.

Contraction Pattern

The frequency, duration and intensity of the contractions must be accurately assessed to determine labor status.

Engagement

Engagement is determined by abdominal palpation. An unengaged or unfixed head in a primigravida in labor is indicative of possible cephalopelvic disproportion. Such finding requires repeating clinical pelvimetry during vaginal examination.

Estimated Fetal Weight and Fundal Height

A smaller than expected estimated fetal weight (EFW) and fundal height indicates either that the woman's dates are incorrect or that she has a small for date baby.

A larger than expected EFW and fundal height indicates that the woman's dates are in error or a large baby indicative of diabetes, or multiple gestation or polyhydramnios. A large baby also forewarns of the possibility of postpartum uterine atony producing hemorrhage or possible shoulder dystocia.

Lie, Presentation, Position and Variety

To ascertain an abnormal lie (i.e. transverse), presentation (i.e. breech) or position (i.e. mentum or brow), also to determine variety, as a posterior variety may lengthen or increase the discomfort of the first stage of labor. A woman in even early labor must be admitted, if she has a transverse lie. A primigravida with a breech presentation is also at risk and should be admitted.

Edema of Extremities

Edema of extremities is one of the classic signs of preeclampsia. Ankle, pretibial, finger and facial edema is checked for and evaluated. Ankle edema alone may simply be dependent edema resulting from the decrease in venous blood flow caused by pressure from the enlarged uterus.

Pelvic Examination/Vaginal Examination

Effacement and Dilatation

To determine, if progressive cervical changes have occurred and to diagnose labor. Also, to determine what stage and phase of labor the woman is in, if in labor.

To confirm abdominal findings: Sometimes, it is easier to obtain these findings upon vaginal examination, e.g. suture lines, fontanels and skull bones in cephalic presentation, a hand or foot in podalic presentation.

Position of the Cervix

The cervix is usually directed posteriorly prior to labor. Movement of the cervix anteriorly so that it is in the midline indicates readiness for or entry into labor.

Station

To determine descent of the fetal head. Descend of the fetal head is one of the mechanisms of labor and is indicative of progress and pelvic adequacy.

Whether or not the Membranes have Ruptured

To confirm or rule out a history of ruptured membranes, or to detect a rupture of membranes not reported.

If the membranes are not easily felt over the presenting part or as bulging, it is helpful to have the woman bear down or to apply fundal pressure, which may cause the membranes to bulge if they are there. Membranes in close contact with a head feel smooth and slick to the touch.

Diagnosis is definitive for ruptured membranes when the amniotic fluid is seen escaping from the cervical os and pooled in the vaginal vault or when the membranes are not felt over the presenting part at the cervical os.

When you feel the membranes bulging against your examining fingers during vaginal examination of the cervix, other possibilities must also be considered. They are:
1. Unruptured membranes.
2. A high leak that is occluded by pressure from the presenting part or escape of fluid trapped between the membranes with rupture of the chorion only and not amnion.

VAGINAL EXAMINATION FOR THE WOMAN IN LABOR

A vaginal examination must follow an abdominal examination so that the midwife can combine the external and internal findings to arrive at a clearer picture of the progress of labor.

Purposes

A vaginal examination for the client in labor will help to:
- Make a positive diagnosis of labor
- Make a positive identification of the presentation
- Determine if the presenting part is engaged
- Ascertain if the forewaters have ruptured or rupture them artificially
- Exclude cord prolapsed after rupture of the forewaters
- Assess progress or delay in labor
- Apply fetal scalp electrode.

Under no circumstances should a midwife make a vaginal examination if there is any frank bleeding.

Procedure

Prepare the client for the procedure by giving adequate explanation. This would enable her to relax and cooperate during the examination:
1. The bladder must be empty so that discomfort during the procedure will be minimized.
2. Assemble sterile articles such as a vaginal examination pack containing sterile swabs and bowls along with sterile disposable gloves. This is important to avoid introducing microorganisms into the vagina.
3. Position the woman on her back with thighs separated and knees bent, taking care to avoid unnecessary exposure.
4. Be sure that the woman's arms are down by her sides or across her abdomen to aid relaxation of her abdominal muscles.
5. Wash hands thoroughly and put on sterile gloves.
6. Swab the client's vagina.
7. Dip the first two fingers of the dominant hand in the antiseptic cream to get them lubricated.
8. Holding the labia apart with the thumb and index fingers of the other hand, insert the lubricated fingers into the vagina palm side down, pressing downwards. Direct the fingers along the anterior vaginal wall and should not be withdrawn until the required information has been obtained. With the fingers inside, explore the vagina for required data, taking care not to touch the clitoris where it may cause great discomfort or the anus where it may be contaminated.

Findings

External genitalia: Before cleansing the vulva, observe and note the following:
1. Any signs of varicosities, edema, vulval warts or sores.
2. Scar from previous episiotomy or tear.
3. Any discharge or bleeding from the vaginal orifice.
4. Color and odor of amniotic fluid if the membranes have ruptured. Offensive liquor suggests infection and green fluid indicates the presence of meconium, which may be a sign of fetal distress.

Condition of the Vagina

1. The vagina should feel warm and moist, and the walls soft and distensible. A hot dry vagina is a sign of obstructed labor. If the woman has raised temperature, the vagina will feel hot, but not dry.
2. Firm and rigid wall may suggest a longer labor.
3. Presence of scars from previous perineal wound may cause delay in the second stage.
4. In a multiparous woman, a cystocele may be found through the anterior wall.
5. A loaded rectum may be felt through the posterior wall.

Cervix

As the examining fingers reach the end of the vagina, they are turned so that the sensitive pads face upwards and come in contact with the cervix:

1. Palpate around the fornices and sense the proximity of the presenting part of the fetus to the examining finger. A spongy feeling between the fingers and presenting part may indicate the possibility of a placenta previa.
2. The cervical os is located by sweeping the fingers from side to side. It will normally be situated centrally, but sometimes in early labor, it will be posterior.
3. Length of the cervical canal must be assessed.
4. A long tightly closed cervix indicates that labor has not yet started. The cervical canal may be obliterated (without margins), partially or completely depending on the degree of effacement. In a primigravida, the cervix may be completely effaced, but still closed. As it will be closely applied to the presenting part, the os may be felt as a small depression in the center.
5. The consistency of the cervix is then noted. It should be soft, elastic and applied closely to the presenting part. If it is tight, rigid or unyielding, labor may be prolonged or it may be poor application associated with an ill-fitting presenting part.

Uterine os: Dilatation of the cervix that is the distance across the opening is estimated in centimeters. About 10 cm dilatation equates to full dilatation. At the point where the maximum diameters of the fetal head have passed through the os, the cervix can no longer be felt. It is important that the midwife feel for the cervix in every direction as a lip of cervix frequently remains in one quarter only, usually anteriorly.

Forewaters: Intact membranes can be felt through the dilating os. Between contractions, they feel slack, but will become tense when the uterus contracts. The consistency of the membranes will be similar to thin plastic film. When forewaters are very shallow, it may be difficult to feel the membranes.

If the presenting part does not fit well, some of the fluid from the hindwaters escape into the forewaters, causing the membranes to protrude through the cervix. This will be more exaggerated in obstructed labor. Bulging membranes are more likely to rupture early and in such case they will not be felt at all. Following rupture of membranes, there is possibility that the cord may prolapse and the midwife must feel for any cord. Following leakage of amniotic fluid, if forewaters are felt, it may be supposed that the hindwaters have ruptured.

Level or Station of the Presenting Part

In order to assess descend of the fetus in labor, the level of the presenting part is estimated in relation to the maternal ischial spines. The distance of the presenting part above or below the ischial spines is expressed in centimeters.

As a caput succedaneum may form over the presenting part, care must be taken to relate the bony part of the spines and not the edematous swelling. Molding of the fetal skull can also result in the presenting part becoming lower without any appreciable advance of the head as a whole. It is not possible to make an accurate judgment of the station vaginally. The purpose of making this estimate is to assess progress and it is therefore valuable for the same person to make all the vaginal examinations on any particular mother.

Identity of the Presentation

In 96% of cases, the vertex presents and is recognized by feeling the hard bones of the vault of the skull, fontanels and sutures. For details of finding in other presentations.

Position

By feeling the features of the presenting part, the position of the presentation can be derived. In vertex presentations the first feature to be felt even in early labor, is the sagittal suture. It may be felt in the right or left oblique diameter of the pelvis or it may be transverse. Later, as further descent occurs, it rotates to the anteroposterior diameter of the pelvis.

The sagittal suture is to be followed with the finger until a fontanel is reached. If the head is well-flexed, the posterior fontanel will be felt. The location of the fontanel(s) in relation to the pelvis, give information as to the whereabouts of the occiput.

Molding

Molding can be judged by feeling the amount of overlapping of the skull bones and can give additional information as to position. The parietal bones override the occipital bone.

Completion of the Examination

As the midwife withdraws her fingers from the vagina, she should note any blood or amniotic fluid and compare this with the observations made earlier. Finally, she should remove her gloves and auscultate the fetal heart prior to assisting the mother to find a comfortable position.

The woman must be kept informed of her progress in labor. Findings of examination must be recorded accurately after each examination.

STUDY QUESTIONS

Short Notes

1. Cervical changes in labor.
2. False labor.
3. Cervical effacement.
4. Lightening.
5. Define the term labor and the three 'P's of labor.

Short Answer Questions

1. Stages of labor.
2. Signs and symptoms of impending labor.
3. Explain cervical effacement and dilatation.

Essay Questions

1. Explain the physiological processes that occur in the first stage of labor.
2. Describe the initial assessment and diagnosis of a client admitted in labor.

BIBLIOGRAPHY

1. AJN/Mosby. Nursing Board's Review for NCLEX-RN Examination, 10th edition. St. Louis, Baltimore: Mosby; 1997.
2. Cassidy P. Management of the first stage of labor. In: Bennett RV, Linda KB (Eds). Myles Textbook for Midwives, 13th edition. Edinburgh: Churchill Livingstone; 1999. pp. 411-28.
3. Dick-Read G. Childbirth without Fear, 2nd edition. Harper & Row; 1957.
4. Friedman EA. Labor: Clinical Evaluation and Management, 2nd edition. New York: Meredith; 1978.
5. Pritchard JA, McDonald PC, Gant N. Williams Obstetrics, 17th edition. Connecticut: Appleton Century Crafts; 1885.
6. Helen V. Nurse-Midwifery, 2nd edition. Boston: Jones and Bartlett Publishers; 1996. pp. 229-76.

CHAPTER 18

Management of the First Stage of Labor

Learning Objectives

Upon completion of this chapter, the learner will be able to:
- List the responsibilities of midwives in the care of women during first stage of labor.
- Describe the physiological changes that occur during labor and their significance.
- Describe the measures for continuing evaluation of the progress of labor.
- Describe the measures for continuing evaluation of the maternal and fetal well-being.
- Describe the bodily care of the laboring client.
- Enumerate the supportive care of the woman and her significant others/family.

Management of the first stage of labor includes the diagnosis of labor; management of false labor; management of early labor and initial evaluation; and care of mother and fetus.

ADMISSION TO LABOR AND DELIVERY UNIT

When the woman is admitted, she undergoes an admission procedure. This procedure may not be same in all the hospitals or healthcare centers, but generally includes the following:
- Changing from street clothing to a hospital gown
- Safeguarding the woman's personal belongings or returning them to family
- Applying identification band for the woman
- Filling out the chart forms
- Carrying out the admission orders
- Carrying out an evaluation of the woman and fetus including history, physical and pelvic examinations, and laboratory tests.

Admission orders and procedures for a woman in labor include enema, perineal shave, oral or intravenous (IV) fluids, ambulation, medication and monitoring of maternal and fetal well-being.

Enema

The purposes of an enema are:
- To stimulate uterine contractions
- To assure a clean field without fecal contamination at the time of delivery
- To eliminate a possible deterrent to accurate and comfortable examination.

Though most women require an enema for the above reasons, it is to be avoided in the following situations:
1. A woman in the late first stage of labor or in rapidly progressive labor, especially a multipara. Expulsion of the enema may be accompanied by expulsion of the baby.
2. The membranes are ruptured; if the membranes are ruptured, there is an increased risk of possible intrauterine infection.
3. Unengaged presenting part.
4. The presence of complications, such as vaginal bleeding with suspected placenta previa or abruptio placentae (danger of severe bleeding), premature labor (to avoid stimulating labor) and severe preeclampsia (need for the woman to be as quiet and undisturbed as possible).

Perineal Shave

The purpose of a perineal shave is to prevent infection. Preparation of the perineum involving the shaving of the mons pubis, vulva and anal region, provides for cleanliness and easy viewing of the perineum. The decision about shaving may be made according to the practice established in the particular institution or setting. There are practitioners today, who believe in no preparation at all, especially if delivery over an intact perineum is expected. There are others, who believe that long hairs, which extend to the vulval area, can be clipped.

Food and Fluid by Mouth

A woman in labor, even in early labor, should not eat solid food. If she does, it will most likely remain in her stomach throughout labor or be vomited during transition. This is because of the severe decrease in secretion of gastric juice, gastric motility and absorption during labor. These decreases do not affect liquids, which leave the stomach in the usual amount of time. Liquids therefore may be ingested during labor.

The best liquids for women to have are clear liquids to which sugar (for energy) has been added, such as tea or coffee and water to provide fluid. Excessive fluids are not desirable as they may produce nausea. Most women want to only moisten their dry mouths and parched throats, and should be given the means for continuing relief.

If general inhalation anesthesia is anticipated, restrict even fluids.

Intravenous Infusion

Intravenous infusion serves as a means to maintain maternal nutrition and as a lifeline for medications, fluid or blood in the event of an obstetric disaster. An IV infusion is mandatory if one of the following conditions is present:

- Gravida 5 or greater
- An over distended uterus for any reason including multiple gestation, polyhydramnios and excessively large baby
- A Pitocin induction or augmentation
- Maternal dehydration or exhaustion
- Any obstetric or medical condition, which is life-threatening, such as abruptio placentae, placenta previa, preeclampsia or eclampsia
- History or presence of any other condition that predisposes an immediate postpartum hemorrhage.

Some obstetricians want all their clients to have an IV and some want none of their clients to have an IV unless there is an indication for it.

The usual IV solution for a woman in labor consists of 5% dextrose in water (D5W) or 5% dextrose in Ringer's lactate (D5RL). An IV intracatheter is used to permit the woman more free movement of her arm without trauma to the involved blood vessel and has the best chance of staying in the vein if she becomes physically active during labor.

Position and Ambulation

A woman in labor should assume a position, that is comfortable for her, provided there are no contraindications to it. Positions may include supine or flat, lateral recumbent, sitting, standing or walking. If the membranes have ruptured and the fetus presents problems such as transverse lie, breech presentation or small size (less than 2,000 g), it poses a risk of prolapsed cord. Then the positions are to be supine or lateral recumbent.

The lateral recumbent position has several beneficial effects, which are as follows:

- Better coordination and greater efficiency of uterine contractions
- Facilitation of kidney function (urine flow is increased in lateral position)
- Facilitation of fetal rotation in posterior positions
- Relief of uterine pressure on and compression of the major maternal blood vessels (the inferior vena cava and the aorta).

In order to avail these benefits, women with the following conditions should be instructed to assume lateral recumbent position during first stage of labor:

- Maternal supine hypotensive syndrome
- Fetal distress (to reduce uterine activity and pressure on the umbilical cord)
- Severe preeclampsia (for best urine flow)
- Mild hypertonicity or ineffectual uterine contractions.

A woman in labor should be allowed to ambulate for as long as she desires, if provided there are no complications. Walking in early labor may stimulate labor. Many women cope with their labor better when they can walk. The woman's freedom to walk, sit in a chair and use the toilet is certainly more conducive to normal process than the sickness orientation of being confined to bed.

Times when the woman should not be out of bed or ambulating are the following:

1. When the membranes are ruptured and the fetus is either small, in a footling or ill-fitting breech presentation, or transverse lie. In such events, there is a risk of cord prolapse, which is increased when the woman is upright.
2. When the woman has been medicated with any drug, which might make her lightheaded, dizzy or unsteady on her feet.
3. During rapidly progressive labor or late first stage labor in multiparas.
4. Any obstetric or medical complication requiring that the woman remains in bed (e.g. abruptio placentae, placenta previa and severe preeclampsia).

Medication

Medications used during labor are for the following purposes:
- Pain relief
- Decrease of anxiety and apprehension
- Sedation
- Control of vomiting.

The commonly used drugs are Demerol (meperidine), Phenergan (promethazine), Vistaril (hydroxyzine) and Seconal (secobarbital). The midwife may have to administer these drugs combined (adding them together) in divided doses and repeat doses. It is to be remembered that tranquilizers (ataractics) potentiate the action of analgesics.

In making decisions regarding medication administration, the midwife must consider the following factors.

Woman's Desire for Medication

Some women want as much medication as they can get. Usually such women do not understand why you cannot give them enough to take the pain away even after explanation. On the other hand, there are women who want to experience or tolerate as much as they can without medication. There may be women, who have had some preparation for labor.

The art of administering medication during labor comprises achieving a balance on the woman's desire, need and facilitation of her coping abilities within the parameters of safety.

Timing of Medication

Timing of medication is important in the care of women in labor. The following principles should be observed:
1. The progress of labor evaluated carefully and the giving of medication timed, so that it will not be at its peak action at the time of baby's birth. Otherwise, the baby might be sleepy and have some respiratory depression. This principle does not apply if a single small dose (e.g. 25 mg of Demerol) given early in labor.
2. A narcotic analgesic should not be given until the woman is in active labor. Given before the contractions are well established, as in the latent phase of labor the drug will most likely render the contractions ineffectual by diminishing their frequency, duration and intensity. The total labor may be lengthened. After the woman is in well-established active labor, a narcotic analgesic will not affect the contraction pattern.
3. Tranquilizers do not affect uterine contractions and will not slow down or delay the progress of labor. Because of their calming effect on the woman, progress of labor is often facilitated.
4. The sedatives are for use:
   – When the woman is in false labor
   – When the woman is in early labor, exhausted and needs a rest
   – As part of the treatment for hypertonic uterine dysfunction and to stop the present labor with its abnormal contraction pattern.

Fetal Size

Because of developmental immaturity and a high risk of respiratory distress in a preterm (premature) or small for gestational age fetus, all medications are withheld from the woman during labor in order not to distress the baby. Unlike full-term babies, small or premature babies cannot handle any amount of drugs crossing the placental barrier.

Fetal Condition

If there is any fetal distress, regardless of fetal age and size, all medications are withheld from the woman in order not to further stress the fetus, which no longer is able to handle drugs crossing the placental barrier.

For any fetus at risk, such as those of diabetic mothers, preeclamptic mothers or those who are post-term, judicious very small dosages must be tried and fetus carefully monitored for the drugs effect. In such cases, internal fetal monitoring will be used for comprehensive monitoring of the fetal response.

Maternal Size

The amount of medication is limited by the fact that the fetus cannot tolerate the levels it would take to totally alleviate the woman's pain. Thus, if a woman is large, additional medication cannot be given in accordance with her increased body size. On the other hand, you need to consider the body size of the small, petite woman in determining the amount of medication within the limits imposed by the fetus.

Woman's Response to Support in Labor

Women who have undergone preparation for childbirth and have practiced relaxation and breathing exercises often require less medication. The presence and help of a significant other (spouse or coach) during labor, where it is permitted or possible, makes coping easier and such women require less medication generally.

Need for Medication

In addition to and underlying all the factors discussed is the amount of real pain or discomfort the woman is feeling. This varies in each woman depending on her pain threshold and on the amount of anxiety and tension she has and their effect on intensifying the amount of pain. For some women, supportive care alone or in conjunction with a small dose of tranquilizer would be sufficient to cope with labor. In medicating a woman in labor, the midwife should always be anticipating when she is going to really need it most, which is during transition and plan to give it accordingly. A woman's pain in labor, as she is experiencing it, should never be scoffed at regardless of your findings, she is feeling it and needs to have it respected.

Monitoring Maternal Physiological Changes

In order to plan the care during the first stage, the midwife needs to know the normal physiologic changes that take place during labor and their significance. This knowledge is important to accurately interpret certain signs, symptoms and laboratory findings as normal or abnormal during the first stage of labor. They may also be significant factors to consider in the management of care of the woman.

Vital Signs

Blood pressure (BP) rises during contractions with the systolic rising an average of 15-20 mm Hg and the diastolic rising an average of 5-10 mm Hg. Between contractions the BP returns to its prelabor level. A shift of the woman's position from supine to lateral eliminates the change in BP during contractions. Pain, fear and apprehension may also raise the blood pressure. In order to ascertain the true BP, it is to be checked between contractions.

An increase in pulse rate during the increment of contractions, a decrease during the acme and an increase during the decrement are usual. A slightly elevated pulse may be normal.

A slight increase in respirations may be due to the increased metabolism. Prolonged hyperventilation may result in alkalosis.

Renal System

Bladder distention commonly occurs due to increased glomerular filtration. The bladder must be evaluated and emptied every 2 hours to prevent obstruction of labor and trauma to the bladder. Slight proteinuria (trace to +1) is common in a third to half of women in labor. This is seen more frequently in women, who have anemia or are in prolonged labor.

Gastrointestinal Changes

Gastric motility and absorption of solid foods taken are severely reduced. Secretion of gastric juice is reduced. Digestion is stopped and gastric emptying is prolonged. Oral intake should be limited to liquids. Nausea and vomiting are not uncommon during the transition stage. Pain, medications, fear and apprehension may be the contributing factors.

Hematological Changes

Blood coagulation time decreases and plasma fibrinogen level increases. These changes decrease the risk of postpartum hemorrhage. The white cell count increases during the first stage.

Blood glucose decreases during labor dropping markedly in prolonged and difficult labors probably as a result of the increased uterine and skeletal muscle activity.

Monitoring of Fetal Well-being

Assessment of fetal well-being includes continuing evaluation of the following:
- Normality of the fetal lie, presentation, attitude, position and variety
- Fetal adaptation to pelvis
- The fetal heart rate and pattern.

Evaluation of the fetal lie, presentation, attitude, position and variety is done first by abdominal palpation and confirmed by vaginal examination. Information needed to evaluate fetal adaptation to the pelvis includes synclitism/asynclitism, molding of the fetal skull, the formation of caput succedaneum and the parameters of normal for each.

All the information in these two categories of evaluating fetal well-being is obtained when the client is evaluated upon admission to the labor and delivery suite and at any other time a vaginal examination is done during labor.

The fetal heart rate and pattern are checked by any one of the following methods:
- Intermittent auscultation of the fetal heart
- Intermittent external fetal monitoring
- Continuous external fetal monitoring
- Continuous internal fetal monitoring.

The decision should be based on the indicated need and the established policy of the institution (**Table 18.1**).

The frequency of evaluation of the fetal heart rate and the pattern, using auscultation with a fetoscope or ultrasonic method (e.g. Doptone/Doppler) is every 30 minutes during active labor. In addition, the fetal heart rate is checked at other times during the course of a normal labor including the following:
- When the membranes rupture
- After expulsion of an enema
- Whenever there is sudden change in the contraction or labor pattern
- After giving medication, at its peak action time
- Whenever there is any indication that an obstetric or medical complication is developing.

In using a fetoscope, it helps to be able to hear the fetal heart if you remember that the fetoscope is constructed to take advantage of bone conduction of sound. For this reason, keep your fingers off the fetoscope while listening. Fingers on the fetoscope disrupt the conduction of sound.

External and internal fetal monitoring is discussed under Evaluation of Fetal Well-being in this Chapter.

CONTINUING CARE AND EVALUATION

As the mother continues in labor, the midwife is responsible for carrying out all of the following, which may be going on simultaneously:
- Evaluation of the maternal well-being
- Evaluation of the fetal well-being
- Evaluation of the progress of labor
- Screening for maternal or fetal complications
- Bodily care of the woman
- Supportive care of the woman and her significant others/family.

Evaluation of Maternal Well-being

Evaluation of maternal well-being includes continuing evaluation of the following:
- Vital signs:
  - Blood pressure
  - Temperature
  - Pulse
  - Respiration.
- Bladder care
- Urine testing:
  - Protein
  - Ketones.
- Hydration:
  - Fluids
  - Nausea/Vomiting.
- General condition:
  - Fatigue
  - Behavior and response to labor
  - Pain and coping ability.

TABLE 18.1: Fetal heart rate pattern, significance and nursing interventions.

Sl. No.	Pattern	Features and causes	Significance	Nursing interventions
1.	Normal pattern	• Baseline rate 120–160 bpm • Average variability • Absence of late or variable decelerations	• Fetus can respond to environment • A reassuring pattern	None needed
2.	Acceleration	• Increased FHR during contractions • Fetal movement can also cause acceleration	• Response to stress • Lowered oxygen or fetal movement	None needed
3.	Variability of FHR	• Beat to beat variation (short-term) • 3–5 fluctuations per minute (long-term)	• Indicates fetus can respond to environment	None needed
4.	Early deceleration	• Uniform • Inversely mirrors uterine contractions • Starts and ends with uterine contractions • Caused due to compression of fetal head associated with contractions	• Caused by head compression	None needed
5.	Late deceleration	• Inversely mirrors contractions • Occurs after the peak of contraction • Does not end until after contraction ends • Cause may be uteroplacental insufficiency	• May indicate fetal distress	• Turn mother to left side (to maximize uteroplacental perfusion) • Administer oxygen at 7–10 L/min by face mask • Increase IV fluids (to treat hypotension and to decrease intensity of contractions) • Discontinue IV oxytocin (if it is being used) • Maintain continuous monitoring
6.	Variable deceleration	• Varies in onset, occurrence and waveform • Cause may be umbilical cord compression	• Indicates compression of umbilical cord • May be associated with fetal distress	• Chan e maternal position • Administer oxygen at 7–10 L/min via face mask • Look for prolapsed cord
7.	Decreased variability	• Minimal variations • Causes may be anoxia, fetal sleep and CNS depression due to medications taken by mother	• Short term if associated with fetal sleep or medications • If pattern persists more than 30 minutes or variability continues to decrease, it is ominous	• Carefully evaluate pattern • Maintain continuous FHR monitoring • Notify physician

(FHR: fetal heart rate; IV: intravenous; CNS: central nervous system).

Vital Signs

All of the vital signs are checked upon admission to the labor and delivery suite. Thereafter, the frequency of checking vital signs may vary with the hospital since each may have a policy regarding this to assure a minimum standard. A generally accepted norm of frequency for a normal laboring woman during the active phase of first stage is as follows:

1. Blood pressure—every hour.
2. Temperature, pulse and respirations:
   a. Every 2 hours (or every 4 hour) when the temperature is normal and the membranes are intact.
   b. Every hour (or every 2 hour) after, the membranes have ruptured.

Bladder Care

During the active phase of first stage of labor, the woman's bladder should be evaluated for distention, at least every 2 hours. With the descent of the fetal presenting part into the true pelvis, the bladder is compressed, so that distention occurs even with 100 mL of urine in the bladder. This distention is visible above the symphysis pubis.

If the bladder is not carefully attended to and emptied, the following may result:

1. *Obstructed labor:* An overdistended bladder can impede the progress of labor by preventing fetal descend.
2. *Difficulty in management of an immediate postpartal hemorrhage resulting from uterine atony:* An

overdistended bladder displaces the postpartal uterus, thereby inhibiting its ability to contract and effect uterine hemostasis.
3. *Difficulty in delivering the shoulders:* An overdistended bladder interferes with descend of the shoulders and decreases the amount of room in the true pelvis (shoulder dystocia).
4. *Discomfort to the woman:* A distended bladder increases the discomfort or pain in the lower abdomen that women frequently experience during labor.
5. Bladder hypotonicity, urine stasis and infection during postpartal period resulting from trauma due to pressure exerted on the distended bladder during labor.

Every time the woman's abdomen is uncovered for abdominal examination or taking fetal heart tones, the contour of her abdomen should be noted for bladder distention. A distended bladder appears as a bulge above the symphysis pubis and in severe cases, may extend as high as the umbilicus. When the fetus is in a posterior position, the contour of the woman's abdomen may look as though she has a full bladder; distention must then be excluded.

If bladder distention occurs, all measures must be taken to facilitate the woman's efforts to void. The best method is to make her walk to the toilet if there are no contraindications to her ambulating. If she is unable to be out of bed, following measures can be tried:
- Having her listen to the sound of running water
- Dabbling her fingers in water
- Running warm water over her perineum
- Applying light suprapubic pressure.

If these measures do not result in her voiding, then the midwife must decide for catheterization. The decision for catheterization is to be taken on the basis of the severity of the distention, her labor status and her progress in labor.

Urine Testing

Subsequent to the initial specimen collected at the time of admission for a routine microscopic examination, when a woman voids during labor, the urine should be examined for protein and ketones. Dipstick may be used if available for this test. If there is protein in the specimen it is vital to know whether this is proteinuria or not. Urine, contaminated with bloody show, may have positive result due to the contamination of blood protein. The results from carefully collected clean-catch specimens may be considered valid.

Examination of the urine for ketones is for the purpose of screening the patient for maternal exhaustion and distress due to dehydration, electrolyte imbalance and nutritional deficiency during labor. It is most important to use dipstick testing of the urine for ketones to evaluate the well-being of a laboring woman, who does not have an IV infusion in order to evaluate the adequacy of her oral intake of liquids for maintenance of hydration. Ketonuria would indicate the need for an IV infusion.

Hydration

The maintenance of hydration throughout labor is essential for the well-being of the woman. Signs of dehydration, such as dry or cracked lips, a dry mouth or a parched throat may not always be due to dehydration at all in a woman in labor, but may instead be due to the type of breathing she is doing with her contractions. Evaluation thus, is based on the screening for ketonuria and knowledge of the woman's intake (by whatever route) and loss (output). Concentration of the urine should also be noted.

Excessive nausea or vomiting in a woman with or without IV fluids must be counterbalanced with IV fluids. Maintain strict intake and output record, note fluid intake, urinary output and the amount of emesis if any.

For details, refer Monitoring of Fetal Well-being in this Chapter.

Evaluation of Fetal Well-being

Cardiotocograph (OTG)

A technical means of recording (-graphy) the fetal heart beat (-cardio) and uterine contractions (-toco) in pregnancy, typically in the third trimester and during labor. The machine (electronic device) used to perform the monitoring is called a cardiotocography, more commonly known as an electronic fetal monitor (EFM).

Schematic explanation of cardiotocography

- Fetal heart rate is calculated from motion determined by ultrasound using a fetal heart sensor strapped to the abdomen (in external monitoring) and a fetal scalp electrode (FSE) in internal monitoring.
- Uterine contractions are measured by a pressure transducer strapped to the abdomen (in external monitoring) and an intrauterine pressure catheter (IUPC), a sensing device introduced directly into the uterus.

External Monitoring (Fig. 18.1)

In external monitoring, electronic monitoring is the use of electronic devices for monitoring frequency, intensity and duration of contractions and for continuous recording of fetal heart rate patterns. It should be obvious that continuous monitoring of the fetus is more accurate, in terms of detecting fetal distress, than is periodic evaluation with fetoscope. Intermittent stethoscopic monitoring during labor and delivery, when the fetus is at the highest risk of the entire pregnancy, allows detection of only gross changes in the fetal heart rate and therefore provides little useful information. Only ominous changes are likely to be detected by fetoscopic or stethoscopic monitoring as usually practiced. It has been established that simultaneous graphic recording of the fetal heart rate and

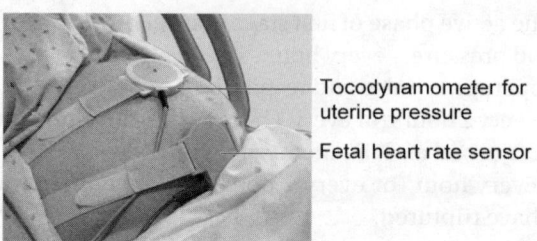

Figure 18.1: External monitoring.

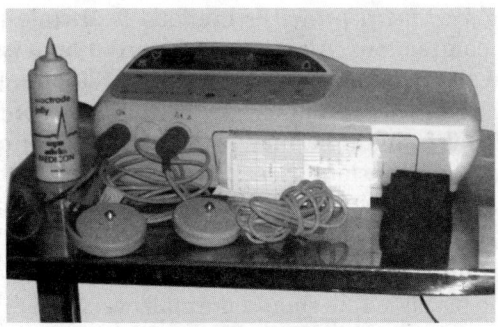

Figure 18.2: Electronic fetal monitor |
(For color version, see Plate 3).

uterine activity can give an accurate picture of the status of the fetus **(Fig. 18.2)**.

Continuous recording of the uterine activity and response of the fetal heart are done using an electronic apparatus in the form of a fetal heart monitor. The recording combines a fetal cardiograph and a maternal tocograph.

The ultrasound transducers are strapped on the abdomen, one over the uterine fundus and the other at the point where the fetal heart is heard at a maximum intensity. This method is noninvasive and does not require rupture of membranes. One drawback to external monitoring is that women doing abdominal breathing to help them cope with their contractions find it difficult to breathe deeply. If the straps are too loose, however, the transducer will not pick up the contraction or monitor the fetus. Correct placement of the transducers for comfort and accuracy is a legitimate nursing function. The quality of the recording on the graph paper may be affected by the thickness of the abdominal wall, fetal position and maternal or fetal movement.

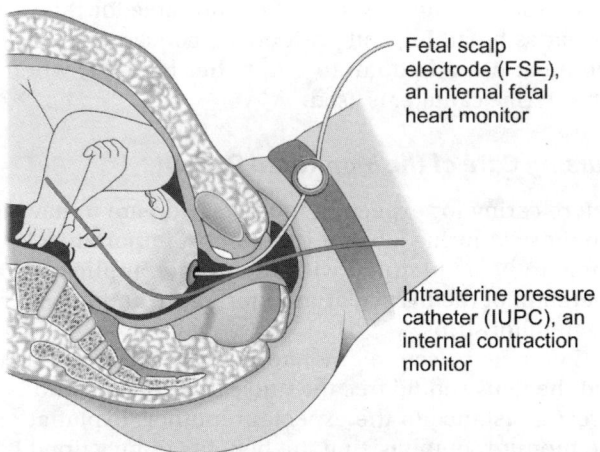

Figure 18.3: Internal monitoring.

Internal Monitoring (Fig. 18.3)

Internal monitoring means the sensing devices are introduced directly into the uterus. The contraction transducer is a special fluid-filled catheter, which transmits exact pressure in terms of 'centimeters of water' (cm H_2O) to the monitor. The fetal monitoring device is a pronged scalp electrode, which is applied to the fetal scalp over a bone by the physician and transmits the electrocardiogram of the fetus to the graphic display **(Figs. 18.4 and 18.5)**.

In order to achieve this, the membranes must be ruptured and the cervix is at least 2–3 cm dilated. A small scalp wound is inevitable, but this rarely causes problems.

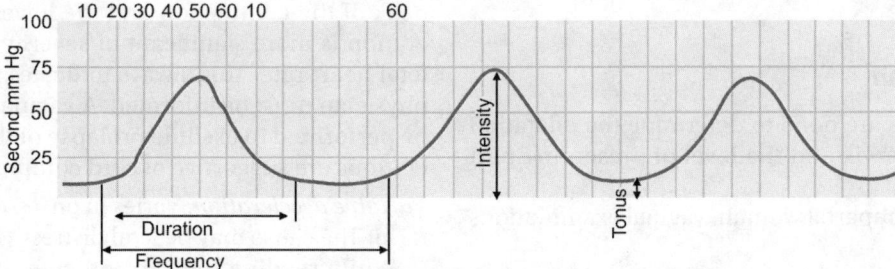

Figure 18.4: Terms used in describing uterine contractions.

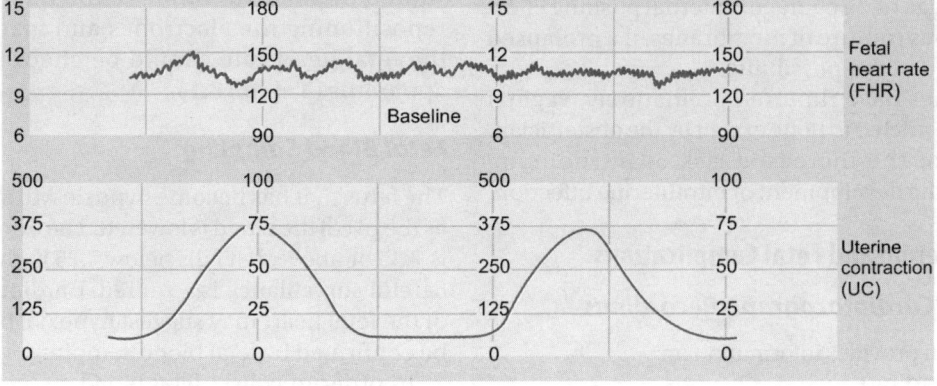

Figure 18.5: Tracing of normal fetal heart rate and uterine contractions.

Internal monitoring is more comfortable for the patient insofar as breathing and position are concerned. However, she must use a bedpan to empty her bladder, when the intrauterine catheter is used.

Nursing Care of the Monitored Patient

Before caring for expectant mothers, who are to have fetal monitoring during labor, it is of utmost importance for the nurse to be acquainted with the proper application and operation of the particular monitor in use and how to read the monitor strips.

Continuous electronic monitoring of the labor contractions and the fetus should free the nurse to give more and better direct assistance to the expectant mother. Explanation of the monitor, emphasizing the benefits to be gained by its use, is essential to the psychological well-being of the client. Although readjustments of the transducers is a common necessity with external monitoring, when the woman moves the monitoring should not be affected. Nurses should readjust the abdominal transducers and note on the graph paper any changes in position.

Evaluation of the Progress of Labor

In the continuing evaluation of the progress of labor, the following informations are used:
- Contraction pattern, frequency, duration, intensity
- Maternal behavior changes
- Signs and symptoms of transition and impending second stage
- Position of low back pain
- Position of location of maximum intensity of fetal heart tones.

Vaginal Examination

Vaginal examinations are done to determine the dilatation and effacement of cervix and the level of presenting part (fetal station).

For the normal intrapartal woman, vaginal examinations are indicated:
- Upon admission, to establish an informational baseline
- Before administering medication
- As labor progresses, to verify complete dilatation in order to either encourage or discourage maternal pushing effort
- After spontaneous rupture of membranes, if a prolapsed cord is suspected or is a possibility.

If the membranes have ruptured prematurely, vaginal examinations are restricted to none except by the obstetrician. This is because of the increased risk of introducing contaminants and the development of intrauterine infection.

Screening for Maternal and Fetal Complications

Interpretation of Cardiotocograph Recordings

The cardiotocograph provides information on:
- Baseline fetal heart rate
- Baseline variability
- Response of the fetal heart to uterine contradictions.

Baseline fetal heart rate: It is the fetal heart rate between uterine contractions. A rate more than 160 bpm is termed *baseline tachycardia*. A rate slower than 120 bpm is called *baseline bradycardia*. Either may be indicative of fetal hypoxia. Fetal tachycardia may be associated with maternal ketosis also. A constant baseline rate between 110 and 120 bpm may indicate cord compression as in cord prolapse.

Baseline variability: The tracing on the graph paper appears uneven due to the minute variations in the length of each beat. The baseline rate should normally vary by at least five beats over a period of 1 minute. Loss of this variability may indicate fetal hypoxia. It may also be seen for a short period after the administration of pethidine to mothers, which depresses the cardiac reflex center in the fetal brain. Periods of 'fetal sleep' also cause reduction in variability, which usually last for 20–30 minutes during labor.

Response of the fetal heart to uterine contractions: The fetal heart rate will normally remain steady or accelerate during contractions (**Fig. 18.6**). Decelerations (slow down) of fetal heart rate, if recorded must be assessed for their relationship to uterine contractions.

Early deceleration: Begins at or after the onset of a contraction and returns to the baseline rate by the time the contraction has finished. An early deceleration is commonly associated with compression of the fetal head. For example, as it engages, but may also indicate early fetal hypoxia (**Fig. 18.7A**).

Late deceleration: Begins during or after a contraction, reaches its lowest point after the peak of the contraction and has not recovered by the time that contraction has ended. Sometimes the deceleration has barely recovered by the onset of the next contraction. The time lag between the peak of the contraction and the lowest point of the deceleration is more significant of severity than the drop in the fetal heart rate. This always indicates fetal hypoxia and the physician must be informed. A vaginal examination should be performed to exclude prolapse of the cord, as late decelerations are suggestive of cord compression (**Fig. 18.7B**).

Variable deceleration: Varies in onset, occurrence and waveform. The cause may be fetal distress (**Fig. 18.7C**).

While reading the cardiotocograph the midwife must be careful not to be confused with the artifacts, which may appear on the tracing if the contact is lost. An attempt should be made to improve the quality of recording by repositioning the electrodes and maternal position and the fetal heart rate should be checked using a Doppler apparatus (**Table 18.1**).

Fetal Blood Sampling

The fetus that has become hypoxic will also become acidotic as the pH of the blood is lowered. The normal pH of fetal blood is 7.35 or above. If it falls below 7.25 in the first stage of labor, careful surveillance is required. Cardiotocograph recording of the fetal heart may suggest hypoxia, but acidosis can only be confirmed by fetal blood sampling.

In order to collect fetal blood, an amnioscope is passed through the cervix to obtain access to the fetal scalp. A small puncture is made on the fetal scalp and 0.5 mL of blood is

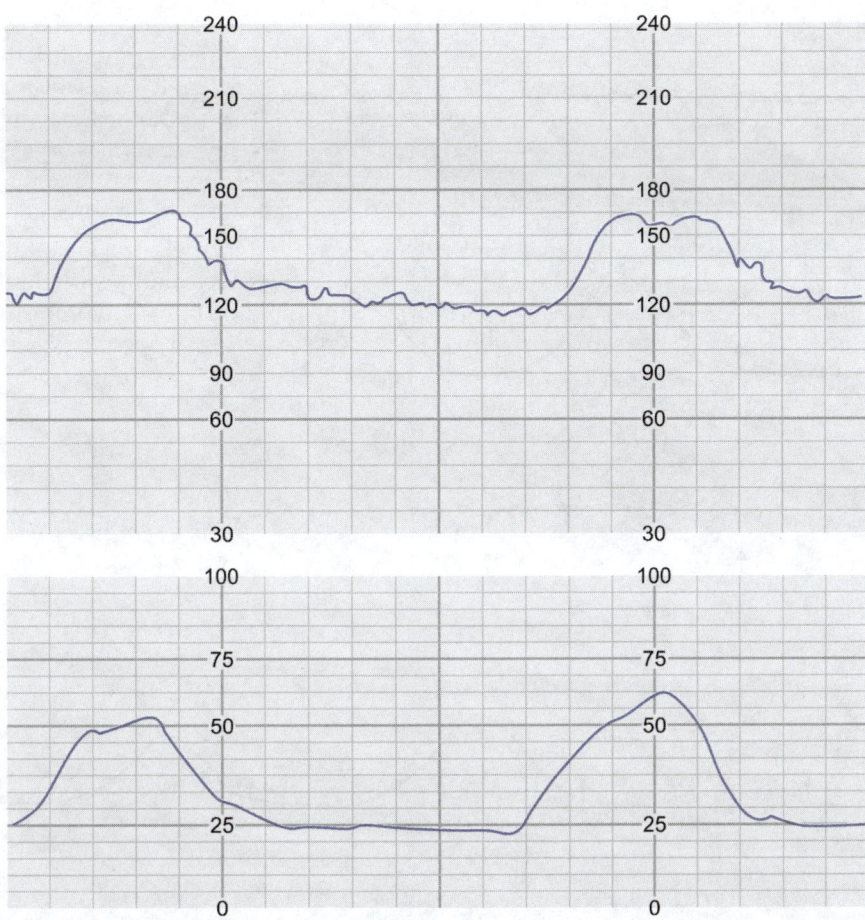

Figure 18.6: Acceleration of the fetal heart rate in response to uterine activity.

collected in a heparinized capillary tube. The specimen must be analyzed immediately for accurate result. Care must be taken to prevent clotting of blood while transporting the sample to the laboratory.

Observation of Amniotic Fluid

Following rupture of membranes amniotic fluid escapes from the uterus continuously and may provide information about the condition of the fetus. The fluid should normally remain clear. If the fetus becomes hypoxic, meconium may be passed as hypoxia causes relaxation of the anal sphincter. As a result of meconium staining, the amniotic fluid becomes green. Amniotic fluid, which is a muddy yellow color or which is only slightly green, may signify previous distress from which the fetus has recovered.

If the fetus presents by breech and is compacted in the pelvis, the fetus may pass meconium because of the compression of abdomen. Thus, green amniotic fluid with the fetus in the breech presentation is considered normal. However, a fetus presenting by the breech is also prone to fetal distress and may pass meconium as a result of hypoxia.

If a fetus is severely affected by rhesus (Rh) isoimmunization the amniotic fluid may be golden yellow due to an excess bilirubin.

In case of a vasa previa, at the time of rupture of membranes the blood vessel may also become torn causing bleeding. Blood in the amniotic fluid is an acute emergency.

Fetal Distress

Fetal distress occurs when the fetus suffers oxygen deprivation and becomes hypoxic. In severe hypoxia the baby may be asphyxiated at birth and suffer brain damage or result in stillbirth **(Box 18.1)**.

> **BOX 18.1:** Nursing alert.
>
> **Management of fetal intolerance of labor**
> - Reposition client to a side-lying position
> - Turn off the oxytocin infusion if present
> - Increase the main line IV fluid
> - Administer oxygen per face mask at 8 – 10 L/minute
> - Perform a vaginal examination to check for umbilical cord prolapse
> - Notify physician
> - Prepare to administer terbutaline(Brethine) 0.25 mg SQ if prescribed; to decrease uterine activity
> - Continuously monitor contractions and FHR

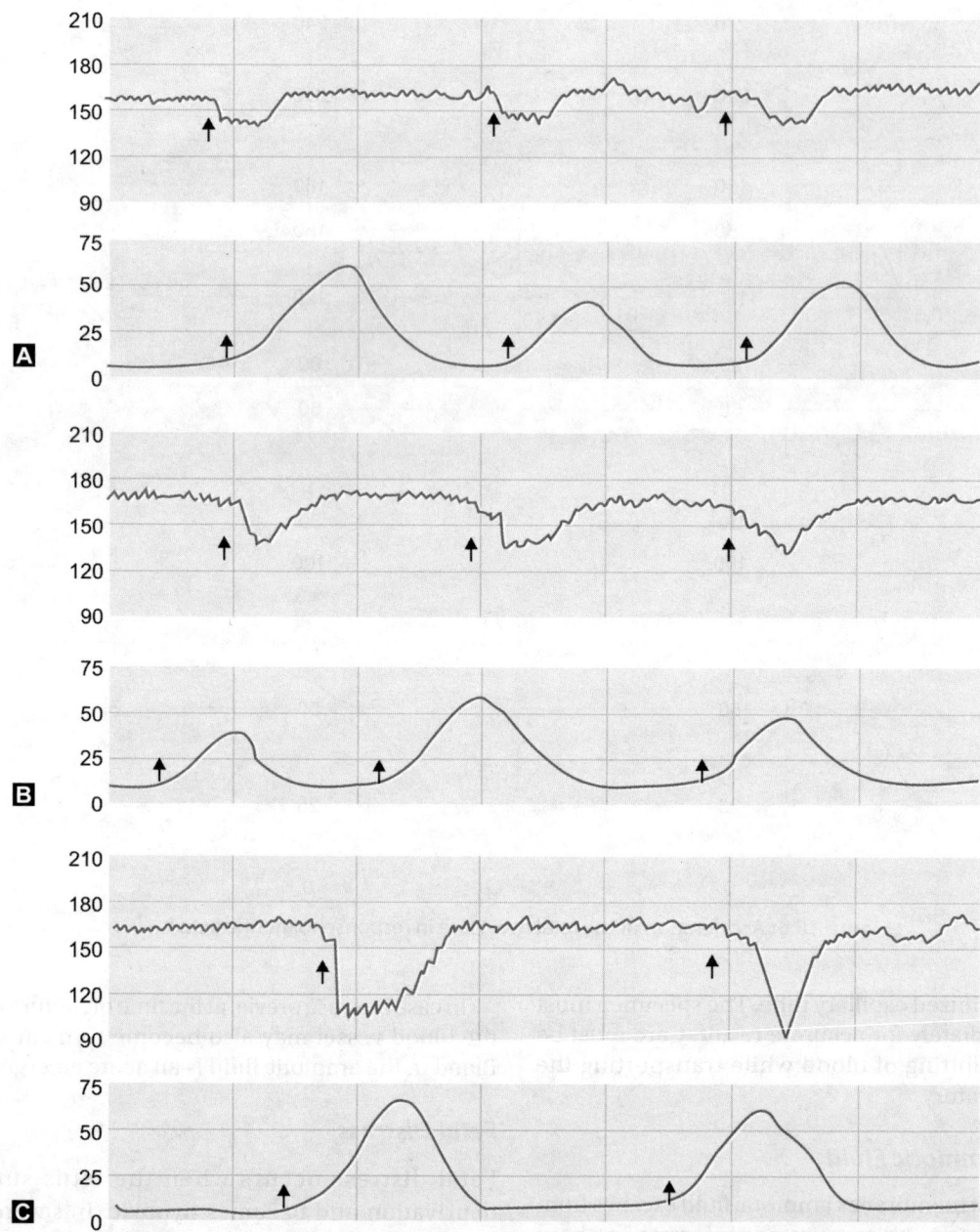

Figures 18.7A to C: Types of decelerations in fetal heart rate. (A) Early deceleration; (B) Late deceleration; (C) Variable deceleration.

Signs of fetal distress
- Fetal tachycardia, which is an early sign of oxygen deprivation
- Fetal bradycardia, which may be shown as fetal heart rate deceleration in the monitor tracing
- Passage of meconium-stained amniotic fluid.

Management of fetal distress
When signs of fetal distress are noticed, the midwife must call the physician. If Pitocin is being administered, it must be stopped and the woman placed on her left side. The mother may be given oxygen via a facemask especially in cases of maternal oxygen lack such as eclampsia or antepartum hemorrhage. Fetal blood sample may need to be taken.

If the fetal distress does not get corrected, delivery will be expedited. In the first stage of labor, this will necessitate cesarean section. In the second stage of labor a quicker vaginal delivery may be affected with an episiotomy, a forceps delivery or a ventouse extraction. In all cases of delivery following fetal distress, the baby will require resuscitation and the midwife must be prepared for it. Presence of a pediatrician is necessary whenever possible to resuscitate the newborn.

Bodily Care of the Woman

A woman in labor needs constant care throughout labor. This care refers to an active and participative presence in the room to manage the care of the woman obstetrically and to provide or facilitate the provision of indicated supportive care.

Keeping Clean and Dry

Cleanliness and dryness promote comfort and relaxation and decrease the risk of infection. A possible combination of bloody show, perspiration, amniotic fluid, solutions for vaginal examinations and feces creates a feeling of messiness, discomfort and general misery for the woman.

A shower can change a woman's entire outlook and feeling to one of well-being, if there are no contraindications to ambulation and there are available facilities. If a shower is not possible, a sponge bath is also refreshing.

Subsequent attention to perineal care and keeping dry continues the feeling of well-being. This is done by changing the gown if one becomes damp with perspiration, changing sheets if they become wet from solutions, discharges, or perspiration; giving perineal care to remove any solutions or discharges and frequently changing the absorbent pad beneath her buttocks. Emphasis on cleanliness of the perineum and anything that comes close to the perineum, as well as scrupulous attention to handwashing by both the woman and all in contact with her decreases the chance for intrauterine infection developing from contamination at the vaginal introitus.

Mouth Care

A woman in labor will develop bad breath, a dry mouth, dry or cracked lips, a parched throat and coated teeth, especially if in labor for a number of hours without oral fluids and without mouth care. If all these develop the woman is uncomfortable and it is unpleasant to those attending her. Some of this can be avoided if the woman is able to ingest liquids during her labor. Some of it develops because of mouth breathing, slight dehydration and lack of moisture in the mouth or passage of time without mouth care. Mouth care consists of the following:
1. Brushing teeth: Women should be encouraged to bring their toothbrush and toothpaste with them to the hospital.
2. Mouthwash: Diluted or undiluted according to the client's preference.
3. Glycerin swabs or Vaseline for lips.
4. Sips of water or clear liquids with sugar for hydration and moistening of the mouth and throat.

A washcloth can save several useful purposes for a woman in labor:
- To refresh by cleaning/washing
- To wipe away facial perspiration
- To serve as a moist pack or as a cold compress
- To moisten dry lips.

Back Rub

Two types of back rubs are useful in providing support and comfort to a woman in labor. One is the usual generalized, overall back rub, which is used to promote relaxation. The second is called the OB back rub. This is done just during contractions, when the woman experiences the greatest discomfort or pain in her lower back. Some women experience localized pain caused by the pressure of the fetal head against her spine. This pain is exaggerated if the fetus is in an occipital posterior position. The obstetrical (OB) back rub is application of external pressure on the spine to counteract the internal pressure on the spine by the fetal head and thus reduces the pain. You will need to recheck with the woman frequently about the proper location of the pressure you are applying as the pain will move downwards as descent of fetal head occurs.

The OB back rub is offered by placing the palm of your hand against the spot identified by the woman and applying pressure. You can massage the spot and adjacent area at the same time by circularly moving your palm on that spot without lifting your palm or moving it off the identified spot. The woman can also guide you as to the proper amount of pressure. Too much pressure is painful and too little pressure is ineffective. In order to give the rub effectively and without strain for the midwife, the client needs to be in lateral position. Lotion or powder should be used to reduce friction and prevent skin irritation.

Both types of back rubs have the effect of expressing care for the woman and assuring a sustaining human presence for as long as the back rub is given. At times, some degree of relief can be obtained by folding a small towel and placing it at the specific spot, where the woman feels pain, so she lies on it. It will provide counter pressure.

Abdominal Rub

The abdominal rub is a light rubbing (massage) of the entire abdomen usually done in a circular fashion. The midwife/attendant or significant other can do it while using one hand for feeling a contraction or holding the woman's hand. This is very comforting to the woman and it expresses caring in a strange environment. It also increases circulation to the area, thereby dilating blood vessels, which have become constricted from contractions and caused tissue anoxia. The increased blood flow combats the tissue hypoxia and provides a physiological basis for a decrease in pain.

Effleurage

Effleurage is a technique used in the Lamaze and other psychoprophylactic methods of childbirth preparation. By definition effleurage means 'feather touch', which describes the amount of pressure to be used in doing it. It is usually done by the laboring woman, using both hands and following definite pattern over primarily her lower abdomen (symphysis pubis to just above her umbilicus) as illustrated in **Figure 18.8**. Using all her fingers of both hands, with the fingers loosely separated, the woman covers the entire lower abdominal area with the two circular patterns—up and outwards from her umbilicus, down and around or in a reverse pattern. Its effectiveness is both psychological and physiological.

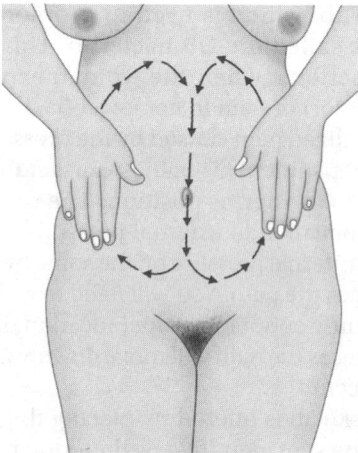

Figure 18.8: Effleurage pattern.

Psychological in that it is one more thing to concentrate on along with her breathing other than discomfort and physiologic in that the action also increases circulation to the area, combating tissue hypoxia and thus decreasing pain.

Alleviation of Leg Cramps

Leg cramps during labor are usually so acute that they capture the woman's total attention and demand immediate relief. Cramps probably are caused by pressure of the presenting part on the nerves of the extremities as they cross through the obturator foramen in the pelvis.

The woman's legs must never be massaged because of the risk of unwittingly dislodging unknown thrombi developed during months of trouble with venous return and possible varicosities. In order to obtain immediate relief straighten the woman's leg and dorsiflex her foot. Alternating relaxation with dorsiflexion of her foot increases the rapidity of the effectiveness. The dorsiflexion should be forcibly exaggerated to effect relief.

Supportive Care of the Woman and her Significant Others

Use of Physical Touch

Physical touch means the touching of the woman by the midwife (e.g. on her leg, head or arm) for no other reason. Most people who touch mean to convey caring, comfort and understanding in an effort to soothe, calm, dispel loneliness and so forth. However, touching is effective only if the one touching is comfortable with touching others and if the woman is comfortable with being touched. Touching can be extremely effective when both the toucher and the touched are comfortable with it. Some clients who are extremely frightened, especially young women may throw their arms around your neck and forcibly hang on to you during a contraction. It is important that you do not reject such a client because her touch is more like a cry for help. Between contractions, ascertain the problems and location of pain and either find a significant other for her to hang on to (if it is possible) or tell her you have to be free bodily to do other things to help her, but she can hang on to one of your hands.

Significant Others

In places where a significant other is allowed to stay with the laboring woman, it is found as the most important of all support and comfort measures. The first step is to identify the woman's significant other who she wants with her during the childbirth process—spouse, parent, sibling, friend or relative. In hospitals where it is practiced, the woman has to identify one person, who is so designated and accepted as the person and who will be with her in the labor room.

The family member should be made to feel welcome and wanted in the labor room by the staff and viewed as important participants in the ongoing events. They should be given territorial space at the side of the woman. Unprepared significant others usually are glad to do anything you suggest and show them how to do. Prepared significant others have probably planned beforehand with the woman what they will do. Find out their plans, so that you will facilitate rather than frustrate them.

They will do anything within their capacity that is agreeable to the laboring women, themselves and the midwife. The woman will respond to the prepared significant other with whom she has practiced and on whom she relies for coaching. Unprepared attendants usually learn quickly and do well in coaching breathing. The significant other can be involved in such activities as the use of a wet washcloth, hand holding, fanning and abdominal rubbing. Men usually make the best back rubbers.

The most important thing in working with women and their significant others is to facilitate their relationship as it involves a continuing commitment in their daily life.

RECORDS

Throughout the first stage of labor, the midwife must keep meticulous records of all the events of the woman's physical and psychological condition and the condition of the fetus. While observing the progress of labor, she should be alert for signs of second stage of labor. A comprehensive record of the progress of the labor must be evident. Vital parameters, treatments and nursing care must be clearly documented.

PARTOGRAPH (FIG. 18.9)

Description

The partograph is a graphical presentation of the progress of labor and of fetal and maternal condition during labor. It is the best tool to detect whether labor is progressing normally or abnormally and to warn if there are signs of fetal distress or if the mother's vital signs deviate from the normal range.

Purposes

1. To record the clinical observations accurately during the period of labor.

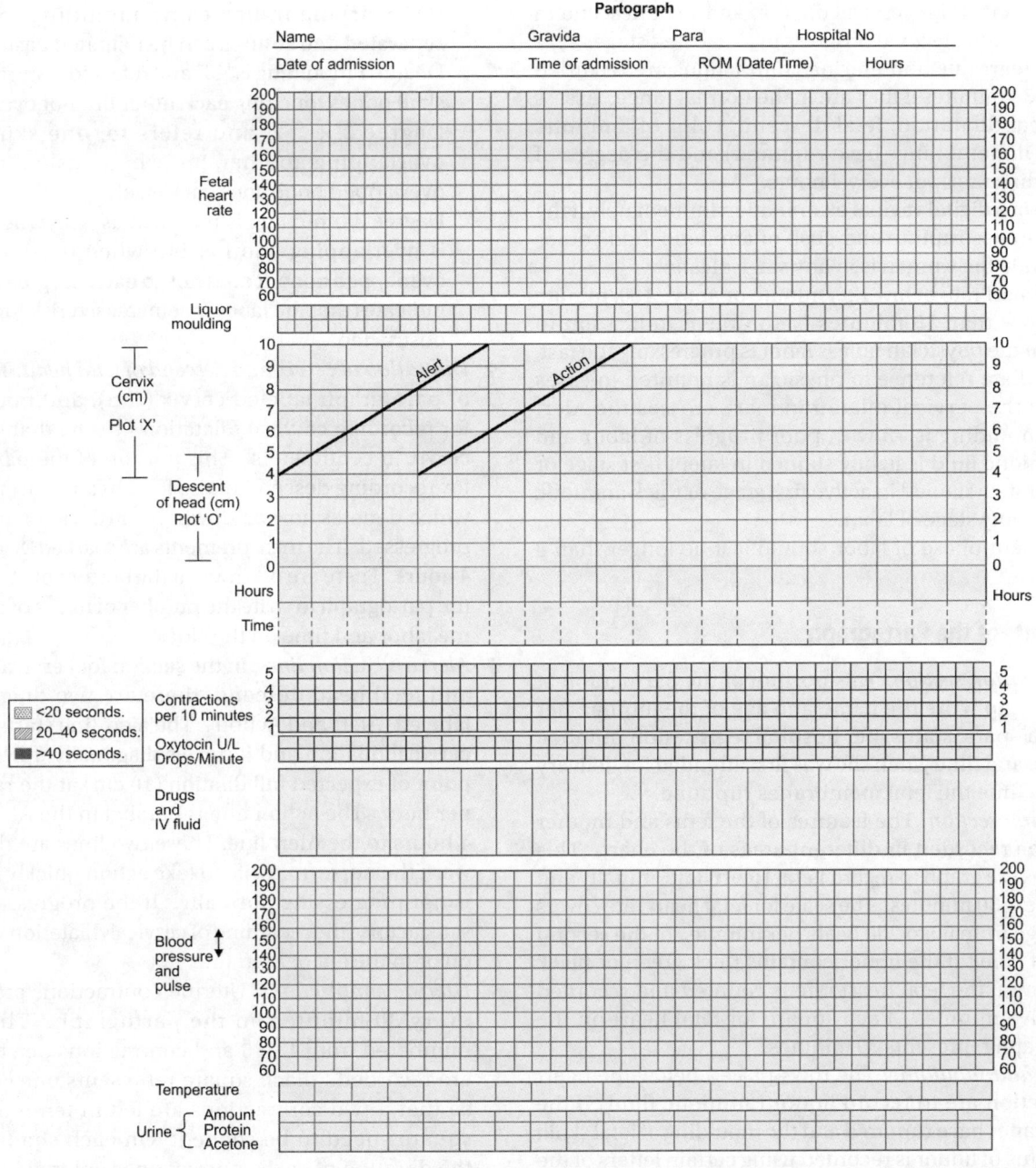

Figure 18.9: Partograph.
(EDD: expected date of delivery; IV: intravenous)

2. To monitor the progress of labor and to organize the need for action at the appropriate time for timely referral.
3. To interpret the recorded partograph and to identify any deviation from normal.
4. To monitor the wellbeing of mother as she goes through labor.
5. To clearly identify the different stages of labor for providing appropriate attention and care.

Principal Features

1. The partograph is a valuable tool to assess the progress of labor.
2. Partograph is useful to detect deviations from normal such as abnormal progress, fetal distress, or maternal exhaustion.
3. The partograph is designed for recording maternal identification data, fetal heart rate, color of amniotic fluid, moulding of the fetal skull, cervical dilatation, fetal descend, uterine contractions, whether oxygen was administered or intravenous fluids were given, maternal vital signs and urine output.
4. Partograph reading to be started when labor is in active stage (4 cm cervical dilation or above).
5. Cervical dilatation, descend of the fetal head and uterine contractions are used in assessing the progress of labor.

About 1 cm/hour cervical dilation and 1 cm descend in 4 hours indicate good progress in active first stage.
6. Fetal heart rate and uterine contractions are recorded every 30 minutes if they are in the normal range. Assess cervical dilatation, fetal descent, color of amniotic fluid (if membranes have ruptured) and the degree of moulding or caput every 4 hours.
7. Perform a digital vaginal examination immediately if the membranes rupture and gush of amniotic fluid comes out while the woman is in any stage of labor.
8. Fetal heart rate below 120/minute or above 160/minute for more than 10 minutes is an urgent indication to inform the physician unless labor is progressing too fast.
9. Immediate reference to physician is required in cases where the cervical dilatation mark crosses the Alert line, moulding is +3 with poor progress of labor and if amniotic fluid is lightly stained in latent first stage or moderately stained in active first stage or thick amniotic fluid in any stage of labor.
10. The latent phase of labor should last no longer than 8 hours.

Components of the Partograph

* *Identification section:* This portion of the partograph at the top is to write the name and age of the mother, her 'gravida', 'para' status, her hospital registration number, the date and time when she was first attended for delivery and the time the fetal membranes ruptured.
* *The graph section:* The features of the fetus and mother are to be recorded in different areas of the chart. This includes the graph to record Fetal Heart Rate, initially and then every 30 minutes. The scale for fetal heart rate covers the range from 60 to 200 beats per minute. In the second stage of labor, if the liquor contains thick green or black meconium, the fetal heart rate is counted and recorded every five minutes. Each square for fetal heart on the partograph represents 30 minutes.
* *Liquor and moulding:* The rows placed below the heart rate section are to record liquor (amniotic fluid) if the membranes have ruptured and the moulding of fetal skull. The status of liquor is recorded using certain letters of the alphabet.
    I: Intact membranes
    A: Membranes have ruptured and liquor is absent
    C: Clear liquor
    B: Blood stained liquor
    M1: Lightly meconium stained
    M2: Little bit thick meconium stained
    M3: Very thick liquor with meconium which has soup-like appearance
  The color of liquor should be recorded every four hours.
* *Moulding:* Moulding denotes the extent to which the bones of the fetal skull are overlapping each other as the head is forced down the birth canal. The degree of moulding to be recorded every 4 hours. Moulding is recorded in the partograph as degrees 1 to 3.

"O" marking indicates no moulding. Bones are separated and sutures can be palpated easily.
Degree 1 moulding is '+1' and refers to; sutures apposed, skull bones touching each other but not overlapping
Degree 2 is '+2' and refers to; one skull bone is overlapping another, but when pushed gently, the overlapped bone goes back easily.
Degree 3 moulding is recorded as '+3'. One skull bone is overlapping another but when tried to push the overlapped bone, it does not go back. Degree 3 moulding indicates that the labor is at increased risk for becoming obstructed.

* *Dilatation of cervix and descend of fetal head:* The portion of partograph labeled cervix (Cm), and marked 'X' is for recording cervical dilatation i.e., the diameter of the cervix in centimeters. This portion of the partograph is for recording descend of the fetal head (Cm) marked 'O' which denotes how far down the birth canal the baby has progressed. The measurements are marked 'X' or 'O' every 4 hours. There are two rows at the bottom of this section of the partograph to write the number of hours of monitoring the labor and time on the clock.
* *Alert and action lines:* In the section for cervical dilatation and fetal head descend, there are two diagonal lines labeled "Alert and Action". The alert line starts at 4 cm of cervical dilation and it travels diagonally upwards to the point of expected full dilation (10 cm) at the rate of 1 cm per hour. The action line is parallel to the Alert line and 4 hours to the Alert line. These two lines are designed to warn the nurse/midwife to take action quickly if the labor is not progressing normally. If the progress of labor is satisfactory, the recording of cervical dilatation will remain on or to the left of Alert line.
* *Uterine contractions:* Uterine contractions are recorded every 30 minutes on the partograph. The scale is numbered from 1 to 5 and contractions per 10 minutes are recorded. Each square represents one contraction so that if two contractions are felt in ten minutes, two squares need to be shaded. On each shaded square, the duration of each contraction is entered by using the symbols shown below:
  – Dots represent mild contractions of less than 20 seconds duration.
  – Diagonal lines indicate moderate contractions of 20 – 40 seconds duration
  – Solid shading represents strong contractions of longer than 40 seconds duration.
* *Oxytocin:* There are two rows for recording administration of oxytocin during labor and the amount given
* *Drugs and IV fluids:* Medications and intravenous fluids given to the mother are recorded in these columns
* *Maternal well-being:* Maternal well-being is assessed by measuring the mother's vital signs; blood pressure, pulse, temperature and urine output. Pulse is recorded every 30

minutes and temperature every 2 hours. Urine output is recorded every time urine is passed. Any deviation from normal needs to be informed the physician.

NURSING PROCESS DURING THE FIRST STAGE OF LABOR

Assessment

Nursing History (On Admission)

1. Name and age.
2. Personal data such as blood type, Rh, current weight and amount of weight gain, allergies to medications, and other substances.
3. Data regarding this pregnancy such as gravida, para.
4. Status of labor: Characteristics of contractions and whether membranes have ruptured.

Physical Assessment

1. Assess maternal vital signs.
2. Assess uterine contractions, determine frequency, duration and intensity.
3. Assess contractions either by palpation or by an electronic monitor.
4. Assess fetal station, presentation and position by Leopold's maneuvers and/or vaginal examination.
5. Assess cervical dilatation and effacement.
6. Assess FHR.
7. Evaluate FHR pattern—variability, acceleration, deceleration.
8. Assess coping skills, level of anxiety and response to labor.

Analysis/Nursing Diagnosis

- Discomfort related to uterine contractions
- Fatigue related to labor process
- Anxiety related to labor and delivery process
- Powerlessness related labor process
- Risk for infection related to labor progress and interventions
- Ineffective individual coping.

Planning

1. Orient the client and significant other to surroundings.
2. Promote physical comfort and safety.
3. Promote maternal and fetal well-being during the birth process.
4. Provide support and counseling to client and spouse/significant other during labor.
5. Encourage self-care activities and support measures during labor and delivery.
6. Monitor woman and fetus.

Implementation

1. Complete maternal and fetal physical assessment:
   a. Maternal vital signs.
   b. Determine if membranes are ruptured.
   c. Assess FHR.
2. Evaluate uterine contractions.
3. Evaluate progression of cervical dilatation, effacement and fetal descend.
4. Provide support measures for mother:
   a. Quiet environment.
   b. Reassurance and encouragement.
   c. Rest between contractions.
5. Maintain comfort measures.
6. Support breathing methods.
7. Provide teaching and associated nursing care.
8. Identify the signs of any developing complications:
   a. Decreased fetal movement.
   b. Abnormalities in FHR.
   c. Meconium-stained liquor.
   d. Abnormal presentation and position.
   e. Maternal fever, pregnancy-induced hypertension (PIH), diabetes.
   f. Bleeding.
9. Encourage woman to empty bladder every 2 hours.
10. Provide clear fluids and/or IV fluids.
11. Monitor labor for signs of fetal distress:
    a. Meconium-stained amniotic fluid.
    b. Fetal hyperactivity or lack of activity.
    c. Fetal tachycardia or bradycardia.
    d. Loss of baseline variability.
    e. Presence of late or variable decelerations.

Note: Entries d and e for clients on continuous fetal monitoring.

Evaluation

Ensure that:

1. The woman and significant other have knowledge regarding the surroundings and labor process.
2. The woman understands and practices safety measures.
3. The woman and her fetus experience a safe labor and birth.
4. The woman acknowledges that support was received during labor and birth.

STUDY QUESTIONS

Short Notes

1. Variability of fetal heart rate.
2. Features of early deceleration and nursing interventions.
3. Features of decreased variability and nursing interventions.

Short Answer Questions

1. Assessment of fetal well-being in first stage of labor.
2. External method of fetal monitoring.
3. Use and significance of partograph.

Essay Questions

1. Explain the nursing care of a mother in labor undergoing electronic fetal monitoring.
2. Describe the observations and physical care of a mother in first stage of labor.

BIBLIOGRAPHY

1. AJN/Mosby. Nursing Boards Review for NCLEX-RN Examination, 10th edition. St Louis, Baltimore: Mosby; 1997.
2. Cassidy P. Management of the first stage of labor. In: Bennett RV, Linda KB (Eds). Myles Textbook for Midwives, 13th edition. Edinburgh: Churchill Livingstone; 1999. pp. 391-410.
3. Dick-Read G. Childbirth Without Fear, 2nd edition. Harper and Row; 1957.
4. Friedman EA. Labor: Clinical Evaluation and Management, 2nd edition. New York: Meredith; 1978.
5. Pritchard JA, McDonald PC, Gant N. Williams Obstetrics, 17th edition. Connecticut: Appleton-Century-Crofts; 1885.
6. Helen V. Nurse-Midwifery, 2nd edition. Boston: Jones and Bartlett Publishers; 1996. pp. 225-76.

CHAPTER 19

Physiology of the Second Stage of Labor

Learning Objectives

Upon completing this chapter, the learner will be able to:
* Explain the second stage of labor.
* Describe the physiological processes during the second stage of labor.
* Enumerate the presumptive signs and differential diagnosis of second stage.
* Describe the mechanisms of labor.
* Describe the maternal physiological changes and the limits of normality for each.

The second stage of labor begins with complete dilatation of the cervix and ends with the birth of the baby. It is known as the stage of expulsion. It is the period when the baby descends from the uterus through the birth canal and is expelled.

PHYSIOLOGICAL PROCESSES

The physiological changes result from a continuation of the same forces, which have been at work during the first stage of labor.

Descend

Descend of the fetal presenting part, which began during the first stage of labor and reached its maximum speed toward the end of the first stage of labor, continues its rapid pace through the second stage of labor until reaching the pelvic floor. The average maximum rate of descend is 1.6 cm per hour in nulliparas and 5.4 cm per hour in multiparas.

Uterine Action

Contractions during the second stage are frequent, strong and slightly longer that is approximately every 2 minutes, lasting 60–90 seconds. They are of strong intensity and become expulsive in nature. After the painful contractions, she experienced during the transition, the woman usually feels relief to be in second stage and be able to push if she so desires.

In the natural course of labor, there is often a lull or quiet period between first and second stage. The hard contractions of transition are now past and the cervix is fully dilated. The woman's body seems to 'take a breath' before starting expulsive efforts. The contractions space out and are not so intense. The woman rests and may even nap. This quiet period may last as long as an hour and is longer in primigravida than in multigravida. Gradually, momentum builds as the fetal head descends through the pelvis, the contractions become more forceful and the woman begins to voluntarily bear down with expiratory, grunty, short pushes.

Rupture of Membranes

The membranes often rupture spontaneously at the onset of the second stage. The consequent drainage of liquor allows the hard, round fetal head to be directly applied to the vaginal tissues and aid distention. Fetal axis pressure increases flexion of the head, which results in smaller presenting diameters, more rapid progress and less trauma to both mother and fetus. As the fetus further descends into the vagina, pressure from the presenting part stimulates nerve receptors in the pelvic floor and the woman experiences the need to push.

Soft Tissue Displacement

As the hard fetal head descends, the soft tissues of the pelvis become displaced. Anteriorly, the bladder is pushed upwards into the abdomen where it is at less risk of injury during fetal descent. Posteriorly, the rectum becomes flattened into the sacral curve and the pressure of the advancing head expels any residual fecal matter. The levator ani muscles dilate, thin out and become displaced laterally; the perineal body is flattened, stretched, and thinned. The fetal head becomes visible at the vulva, advancing with each contraction and receding during the resting phase until crowning takes place and the head is born.

PRESUMPTIVE SIGNS OF SECOND STAGE AND DIFFERENTIAL DIAGNOSIS

Expulsive Contractions

The woman's verbal expression—"my baby is coming" often signals an imminent delivery. It is possible for a woman to feel strong desire to push before the cervix is fully dilated if the fetus is in an occipitoposterior position, the rectum is full or the woman is highly parous.

Rupture of Membranes

Membranes normally rupture at the onset of second stage. However, this may occur at any time during labor.

Dilatation, Gaping of Anus and Perineal Bulging

Deep engagement of the presenting part and premature maternal effort may produce this sign during the latter part of the first stage.

Progressive Visibility of the Fetal Head at the Introitus

Excessive molding may result in the formation of a large caput succedaneum, which can protrude through the cervix prior to full dilatation. Similarly, a breech presentation may be visible when the cervix is only 7–8 cm dilated.

Congestion of the Vulva

Enthusiastic premature pushing may also cause this. The average length of the second stage is 1 hour for primigravida and 15 minutes for multipara. Generally, a second stage that lasts longer than 2 hours for primigravida or 1 hour for multipara is considered abnormal.

MATERNAL PHYSIOLOGICAL CHANGES IN THE SECOND STAGE

The normal physiological changes that occur in the first stage of labor continue through the second stage of labor.

Blood Pressure

Blood pressure may rise another 15–20 mm of mercury with contractions during the second stage. Maternal pushing effort affects the blood pressure, causing variation from an increase to a decrease and ending at a level slightly above normal. It is important, therefore, to evaluate the blood pressure well between contractions. A rise of 10 mm of mercury between contractions, when a woman has been pushing, is normal.

Metabolism

The steady rise in metabolism continues through the second stage. The maternal pushing effort adds further skeletal muscle activity that contributes to the increase in metabolism.

Pulse Rate

Pulse rate increases during each pushing effort. It is elevated throughout the second stage with a definite tachycardia reaching a peak at the time of delivery.

Temperature

The highest elevation of temperature is at the time of delivery and immediately thereafter. An increase of 0.5–1°C is considered normal.

Gastrointestinal Changes

The reduction in gastric motility and absorption continues through the second stage. Usually, the nausea and vomiting of transition subside during the second stage, but they may persist for some women.

Renal and Hematological Changes

The changes are same as discussed for the first stage of labor.

MECHANISM OF NORMAL LABOR

The mechanisms of labor are the positional movements that the fetus undergoes to accommodate itself to the maternal pelvis. This is necessary in as much as the larger diameters of the fetus must be in alignment with the larger diameters of the maternal pelvis in order for the full-term fetus to negotiate its way through the pelvis to be born.

At the onset of labor, the most common presentation is the vertex and the most common position is either left or right occipitoanterior; therefore, this mechanism that will be described below. When the fetus presents in left or right occipitoanterior position, the way the fetus is normally situated can be described as follows:

- The lie is longitudinal
- The presentation is cephalic
- The position is right or left occipitoanterior
- The attitude is one of flexion
- The denominator is the occiput
- The presenting part is the posterior part of the anterior parietal bone.

Positional Movements (Figs. 19.1A to G)

There are several basic positional movements, which take place when the fetus is in a cephalic vertex presentation. These are as follows:

- Engagement
- Descend throughout
- Flexion
- Internal rotation of the head
- Crowning
- Birth of the head by extension
- Restitution

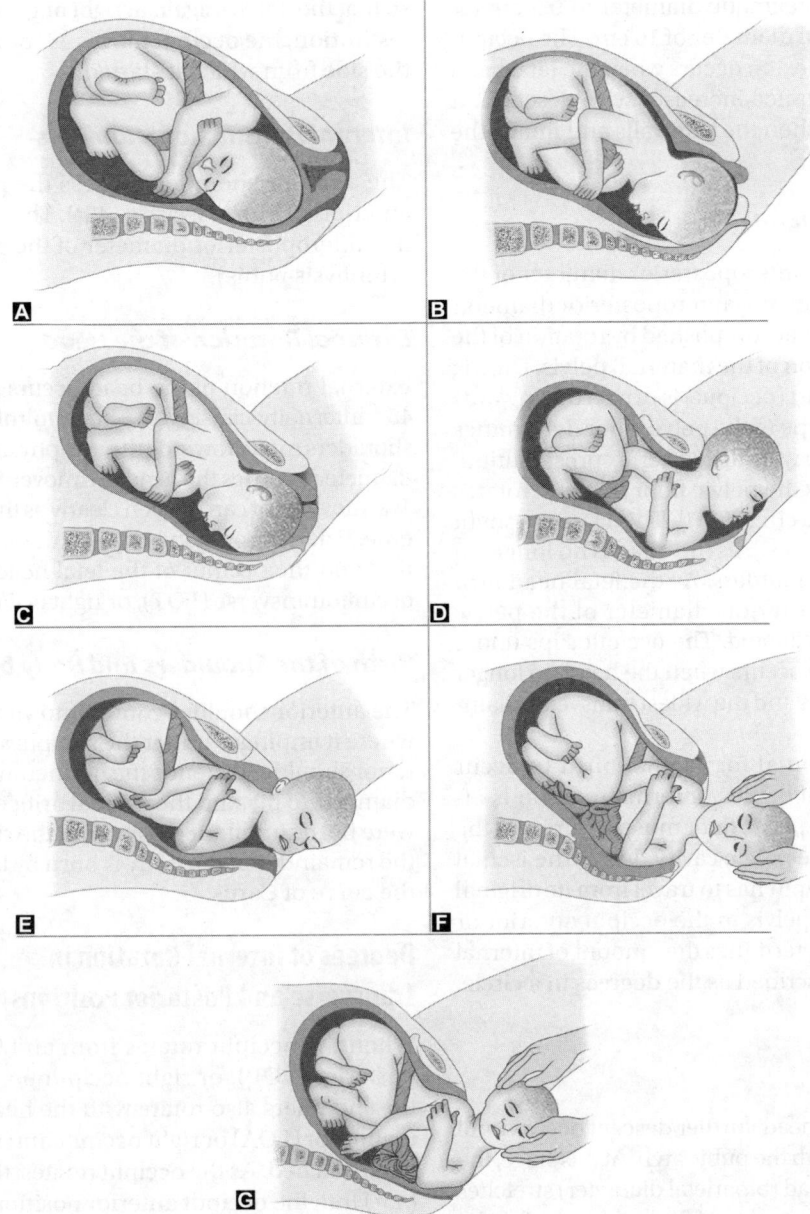

Figures 19.1A to G: Mechanisms of labor. (A) Engagement descent, flexion; (B) Internal rotation; (C) Extension beginning; (D) Extension complete; (E) Restitution; (F) External rotation; (G) Lateral flexion (expulsion).

- Internal rotation of the shoulders
- External rotation of the head
- Birth of the shoulders and body by lateral flexion.

Although the mechanisms of labor are listed separately, some of these overlap or occur simultaneously (internal rotation of shoulders and external rotation of the head).

Engagement

Engagement takes place when the biparietal diameter of the fetal head has passed through the pelvic inlet. In primigravida, it usually occurs during the latter weeks of pregnancy. In multigravida, as the muscle tone is lax engagement may not occur until labor actually begins.

Descend

Descend occurs throughout the mechanisms of labor and is therefore both requisite to and simultaneous with the other mechanisms. Descend is the result of a number of forces including contractions (which straighten the fetal spine, bring the fundus into direct contact with the breech and exert pressure of the fundus on the breech) and maternal pushing effort with contraction of her abdominal muscles.

Flexion

Flexion is essential to further descend. The pressure exerted down the fetal axis will be transmitted to the occiput. The effect is to increase flexion, which results in the substitution of the smaller suboccipitobregmatic diameter of 9.5 cm for the larger suboccipitofrontal diameter of 10 cm. The occiput becomes the leading part. Flexion occurs when the fetal head meets resistance; this resistance increases with descend. It is first met from the cervix, then the sidewalls and finally the pelvic floor.

Internal Rotation of the Head

Internal rotation brings the anteroposterior diameter of the fetal head into alignment with the anteroposterior diameter of the maternal pelvis. This is accomplished by rotation of the occiput to the anterior portion of the maternal pelvis. During a contraction, the leading part (occiput) is driven downwards onto the pelvic floor. The slope of the pelvic floor determines the direction of rotation. In a well-flexed vertex presentation, the occiput leads and meets the pelvic floor first and rotates anteriorly through 1/8th of a circle (45°). This causes a slight twist in the neck of the fetus (45°), as the head is no longer in direct alignment with the shoulders. As the fetal head now lies in the widest (anteroposterior) diameter of the pelvic outlet, an easy escape is facilitated. The occiput slips under the pubic arch and *crowning* occurs when the head no longer recedes between contractions and the widest transverse diameter (biparietal) is born.

Internal rotation is essential for vaginal birth to occur except for abnormally small babies. Internal rotation is effected by the 'V' shape of the pelvic floor musculature and the decreased dimensions of the pelvic cavity due to the ischial spines. The distance the occiput has to travel from its original position upon entering the pelvis to the occiput anterior or occiput posterior position determines the amount of internal rotation. The distance is described as the degrees in a circle, which is being traversed.

Crowning

After internal rotation of the head, further descent occurs until the subocciput lies underneath the pubic arch. At this stage, the maximum diameter of the head (biparietal diameter) stretches the vulval outlet without any recession of the head even after the contraction is over. This is called 'crowning of the head'.

Birth of the Head by Extension

Once crowning has occurred, the fetal head can extend. The suboccipital region or nucha impinges under the symphysis pubis and acts as a pivotal point. The fetal head is now positioned so that further pressure from the contracting uterus and maternal pushing serves to further extend the head as the vaginal orifice opens. Thus, the head is born by extension as the sinciput face and chin sequentially sweep over the perineum.

Restitution

Restitution is the rotation of the head either to the left or right depending on the direction from which it rotated into the occipitoanterior position. In effect, restitution untwists the neck so that the head is again at right angle with the shoulders. With restitution, the occiput moves 45° or 1/8th of a circle towards the side from which it started.

Internal Rotation of Shoulders

The anterior shoulder reaches the pelvic floor and rotates anteriorly 1/8th of a circle (45°). The shoulders come to lie in the anteroposterior diameter of the pelvic outlet (under the symphysis pubis).

External Rotation of the Head

External rotation of the head occurs as the shoulders rotate 45°, internally causing the head to rotate another 45° (as the shoulders rotate towards the symphysis pubis from the oblique diameter it carries the head in a movement of external rotation). The movement can be seen clearly as the head turns at the same time. External rotation occurs in the same direction as restitution and the occiput of the fetal head now lies laterally [left occipitotransverse (LOT), or right occipitotransverse (ROT)].

Birth of the Shoulders and Body by Lateral Flexion

The anterior shoulder comes into view at the vaginal orifice, where it impinges under the symphysis pubis, while the posterior shoulder distends the perineum. This enables a smaller diameter to distend the vaginal orifice than if both shoulders were born simultaneously. After the shoulders are delivered, the remainder of the body is born by lateral flexion following the curve of Carus.

Degrees of Internal Rotation in Transverse and Posterior Positions

When the occiput rotates from an LOT, ROT, left occipitoposterior (LOP), or right occipitoposterior (ROP) position, the shoulders also rotate with the head until the left occipitoanterior (LOA) or right occipitoanterior (ROA) position has been reached. As the occiput rotates, the final 1/8th of a circle (45°) into the occiput anterior position, the shoulders do not continue their rotation with the head, but instead enter the pelvic inlet in one of the oblique diameters (the left oblique diameter for an LOA and the right oblique diameter for an ROA). The entire mechanism therefore has the effect of twisting the neck 1/8th of a circle (45°).

Internal rotation in transverse positions (LOT and ROT) is 90° and in posterior positions (LOP and ROP) 135°. When the rotation is 135°, it is termed as *long arc rotation*.

Curve of Carus

The curve of Carus is the pelvic curve at its lower end as determined by the pelvic structure. The products of conception must follow this curve for birth. The pelvic cavity actually resembles a curved cylinder, so that the direction of either the baby or the placenta coming through it is first downward from the axis of the inlet to just above the tip of the sacrum and then forward, upward and outward to the vaginal orifice.

Summary of Mechanisms in Left Occipitoanterior Position (Figs. 19.2A to H)

1. Lie is longitudinal.
2. Presentation is cephalic.
3. Position is left occipitoanterior.
4. Attitude is one of flexion.
5. Denominator is the occiput.
6. Presenting part is the posterior part of the anterior parietal bone.
7. Engagement takes place with sagittal suture of the fetal head in the right oblique diameter of the pelvic inlet and the biparietal diameter of the fetal head in the left oblique (opposite) diameter of the pelvis. The occiput points to the left iliopectineal eminence and the sinciput to the right sacroiliac joint.
8. Descend occurs throughout.
9. Flexion substitutes the suboccipitobregmatic diameter for the diameter, which entered the pelvic inlet (suboccipitofrontal).
10. Internal rotation takes place and the occiput turns 1/8th of a circle (45°) to the right. The sagittal suture comes to the anteroposterior diameter of the mother's pelvis.
11. The occiput escapes under the symphysis pubis and crowning occurs when the head no longer recedes between contractions.
12. The head is born by extension, pivoting on the suboccipital region around the pubic arch.
13. Restitution—the occiput turns 1/8th of a circle (45°) to the left to undo the twist on the neck.
14. Internal rotation of the shoulders—the anterior shoulder reaches the pelvic floor and rotates anteriorly to lie under the symphysis pubis. This movement can be seen as the head turns at the same time (external rotation of the head).
15. External rotation of the head—the head turns another 1/8th of a circle (45°) to the mother's left. The bisacromial diameter of the shoulders comes into the anteroposterior diameter of the maternal pelvis. This occurs in the same direction as restitution and at the same time as internal rotation of the shoulders.
16. The anterior shoulder escapes under the symphysis pubis and the body is born by lateral flexion.

For every presentation and position that is delivered vaginally, there is a mechanism. These are the series of passive movements taken by the fetus to negotiate the birth canal. Knowledge of these movements enables the midwife to recognize the level of descend and anticipate the next step in the process. Monitoring of the movements, aids in assessment of the progress, safe completion of delivery and intervention for any delay.

Principles

Principles are common to all mechanisms:
- Descend occurs throughout
- The part that leads and first meets the resistance of the pelvic floor will rotate forwards until it comes under the symphysis pubis
- The part that escapes under the symphysis pubis will pivot around the pubic bone
- During the mechanism, the fetus turns slightly to take advantage of the widest available space in each plane of the pelvis, i.e. transverse at the brim and anteroposterior at the outlet.

FETAL NORMALITY DURING THE SECOND STAGE

Evaluation of the fetus during the second stage of labor includes evaluation of the amount of caput succedaneum and molding as well as the normalcy of progress being made in the mechanisms of labor and the fetal heart tones.

Periodic fetal heart rate—changes of the early deceleration type may occur as delivery nears. Early deceleration caused by compression of the head, is a uniform-shaped pattern reflecting the uniform shape of the contractions. Head compression occurs at this time because of the pressure exerted on the fetal head by the pelvic floor and perineum during contractions, and further exaggerated by the woman's pushing effort. Usually, the fetal heart rate does not fall below 100 beats per minute (bpm) during the deceleration period and the baseline fetal heart rate is usually within normal range in an early deceleration pattern. Early deceleration is not considered an indication of acute fetal distress, but needs to be differentiated carefully from

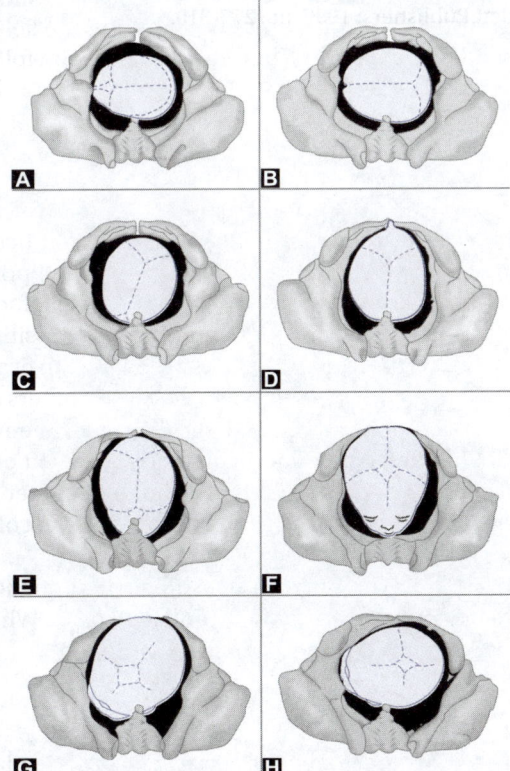

Figures 19.2A to H: Diagrammatic representation of the positions of fetal skull in left occipitotransverse (LOT) to left occipitoanterior (LOA) mechanism. (A) At onset of labor; (B) Descend and flexion; (C) Internal rotation: LOT to LOA; (D) Internal rotation: LOT to occipitoanterior (OA); (E) Extension beginning; (F) Extension complete; (G) Restitution: OA to LOA; (H) External rotation: LOA to LOT.

a late deceleration pattern, which is due to uteroplacental insufficiency. A baseline bradycardia may occur when the fetal head descends rapidly into the pelvis and needs to be carefully evaluated.

DURATION OF THE SECOND STAGE

The duration of the second stage is difficult to predict with any degree of certainty. In multigravida, it may last as little as 5 minutes; in primigravida, the process may take 2 hours (average length for multigravida is 15 minute and for primigravida 1 hour). More important than the time factor is the evidence of progressive descent and the condition of mother and fetus. Once the onset of second stage has been confirmed, a woman should not be left without a midwife in attendance.

STUDY QUESTIONS

Short Notes

1. Signs of second stage of labor.
2. Maternal physiological changes in second stage of labor.
3. Spontaneous rupture of membranes.

Short Answer Questions

1. List the positional movements of the fetus in a normal delivery.
2. List the principles of labor common to all mechanisms.

Essay Question

1. Describe the mechanisms of labor in the left occiput anterior position (LOA).

BIBLIOGRAPHY

1. Caldero Barcia P. Effects of position changes on the intensity and frequency of uterine contractions during labor. American Journal of Obstetrics and Gynecology. 1971;109:274.
2. Dutta DC. Textbook of Obstetrics, 5th edition. Kolkata: New Central Book Company; 2001. pp. 118-28.
3. Friedman EA. The functional divisions of labor. American Journal of Obstetrics and Gynecology. 1971;109:274-80.
4. Hillan EM. Physiology and management of the second stage of labor. In: Bennett RV, Brown KB (Eds). Myles Textbook for Nurses, 13th edition. Edinburgh: Churchill Livingstone; 1999. pp. 447-64.
5. Hon EH. An Introduction to Fetal Monitoring, 2nd edition. North Haven Corometrics. Connecticut: Medical Systems; 1971.
6. Peterson G. Birthing Normally: A Personal Growth Approach to Childbirth, 2nd edition. Berkeley, California: Mind-Body Press; 1984.
7. Singh R. Modified WHO Partograph in Labor Room, https://careus.com; 2022.
8. Schrag K. Maintenance of pelvic floor integrity during childbirth. Journal of Nurse Midwifery. 1979;24(6):26-31.
9. Varney Helen. Nurse-Midwifery, 2nd edition. Boston: Jones and Bartlett Publishers; 1996. pp. 277-310.

CHAPTER 20

Management of the Second Stage of Labor

Learning Objectives

Upon completing this chapter, the learner will be able to:
- Enumerate the nursing care activities for a woman in the second stage of labor.
- Describe the sequence of events during the second stage in a normal labor.
- Describe the process and conduct of delivery.
- Discuss the rationale for an episiotomy and explain its risks and benefits.
- Describe the midwife's role in the immediate care of the newborn.

Management of the second stage of labor is a continuation of the responsibilities included in the management of the first stage of labor and additional responsibilities for preparation for delivery and management of delivery.

EVALUATION OF MATERNAL WELL-BEING

Continuing evaluation of maternal well-being during the second stage of labor includes the following items:
- Vital signs
- Bladder care
- Hydration and general condition
- Maternal pushing effort
- Analgesia and anesthesia
- Perineal integrity.

Vital Signs

The frequency with which vital signs are checked, is increased during the second stage of labor. This frequency may vary somewhat from hospital to hospital or from obstetrician to obstetrician, but the following schedule reflects generally accepted standards for a normal woman during the second stage of labor. Temperature, pulse and respirations are to be evaluated every hour and blood pressure every 15 minutes.

It is important to remember that the blood pressure should be taken between contractions and it is normally increased by an average of 10 mm Hg, if the woman has been pushing.

Bladder Care

Management of the woman's bladder during the second stage of labor and the rationale for this management is same as discussed for the first stage of labor.

In addition, a decision may have to be made about catheterizing the woman immediately prior to delivery, which is toward the end of the second stage of labor. If catheterization is to be done, it is usually done after the woman is scrubbed and draped, and before any other procedure such as pudendal block or cutting of an episiotomy. This timing is important so that the catheter can be inserted before the fetal head gets any lower in the pelvis, since further descend makes the catheterization more difficult.

In making a decision whether or not to catheterize a woman at this time, the following factors are considered:
1. Whether the bladder needs emptying or not:
   a. Is it distended?
   b. Has the woman voided within the last 2 hours?
   c. What has been her fluid intake since her last voiding?
2. There is increased risk of bladder infection with catheterization.
3. Whether or not a possible potential complication is being anticipated:
   a. Immediate postpartum hemorrhage.
   b. Shoulder dystocia.
      Management of both of these complications includes having an empty bladder. Precious time can be gained if an empty bladder is already assured.

Careful monitoring of the bladder during the first and second stage of labor and use of all measures to get the woman void naturally, often avoids the need for catheterization. However, if the bladder is obviously distended, a decision must be made to catheterize the woman in order to avoid further trauma to the bladder, decrease the discomfort in her lower abdomen and circumvent a problem with the bladder in the event of aforementioned complications. A high probability for complications warrants catheterization even if a distended bladder is not obvious, as the woman should end this phase of labor with an empty bladder.

Catheterization for a client in the second stage of labor with the fetal head in the true pelvis is different from usual as regards the direction of the catheter is concerned. The urethra is displaced to conform to the contour of the fetal head, which is displacing it.

Therefore, immediately upon entry of the catheter into the urethra, it is necessary to direct the catheter upward and over the fetal head, while going inward. Otherwise, by going straight in as usual, the catheter simply will not go in and the urethra will be traumatized. Going up and over the fetal head also means that more than usual length of the catheter will be inserted before reaching the bladder.

Hydration and General Condition

Management of these three areas during the second stage of labor and the rationale for their management is the same as for the first stage of labor.

Hydration, however, is further affected during the second stage of labor by fluid loss through the skin in the form of perspiration. The woman may perspire profusely from the effort of pushing.

The general condition of the woman in the second stage of labor depends on the manner in which it was maintained in the first stage of labor. If she enters the second stage of labor exhausted, she is going to have difficulty in mustering the energy required for pushing, especially if she is a primigravida. This is because the average length of a primigravida second stage is longer than that of a multipara.

Maternal Pushing Effort

The maternal pushing effort occurs in response to a reflex mechanism, which is initiated when the head is pressing against and distending the pelvic floor. The reflex mechanism is thereafter triggered with each contraction; the maternal response of pushing is activated shortly after the onset of the contractions, after it has started to build toward its acme.

The maternal pushing effort must be evaluated for effectiveness. Proof of effectiveness is the progressive descend and sequence of mechanisms of labor by the fetus. The sequential bulging of the rectum, then the perineum and finally visualization of an ever-increasing amount of the fetal presenting part at the enlarging vulval orifice generally evidence this. In the absence of progress, it is essential to re-evaluate pelvic adequacy and rule out arrest in the mechanisms of labor by careful vaginal examination. If neither of these difficulties exists, the problem is probably either ineffectual pushing or a psychological obstacle (e.g. a frightened woman).

There are those who believe that the word pushing should never be used and the woman should bear down only as she feels like it. There are others, who believe in vigorously encouraging the maternal pushing effort as soon as the cervix is completely dilated. Management by most obstetricians and midwives lies somewhere between these two extremes.

The breathing used in the natural pushing effort is that of a series of short pushes often during the expiratory phase of respiration. This reduces the possibility of fetal hypoxia and acidosis, which may result from repeated breath holding after inspiration and prolonged bearing down. Natural bearing down and slow distension of the perineal musculature serves the following advantages:
1. Reduced possibility of lacerations or the need for an episiotomy.
2. Lessened incidence of uterine prolapse and cystocele because of less strain on the cardinal ligaments.
3. Lessened trauma to the fetal head because of gradual even pressure against the head.

Taking all these into consideration, it seems reasonable to use an approach that combines the best of the two methods. In this approach, the 'natural' method is used unless or until there is evidence of a need for the woman to push deliberately as in the case of spinal anesthesia.

Women, who have not had preparation for childbirth in the prenatal period, must be taught the techniques of breathing and bearing down, before she reaches the second stage of labor. If the natural efforts of pushing are ineffectual, such women should be taught how to push effectively.

Analgesia and Anesthesia

Analgesia during the second stage of labor usually is the continuation of analgesia given during the first stage of labor.

Anesthesia is achieved by one of the following methods.

Local Infiltration (Fig. 20.1)

Local infiltration of the perineal body is carried out to provide anesthesia when an episiotomy is planned.

Pudendal Block

Pudendal block is used when a larger area of the perineum is to be anesthetized. It anesthetizes the perineum and vulva

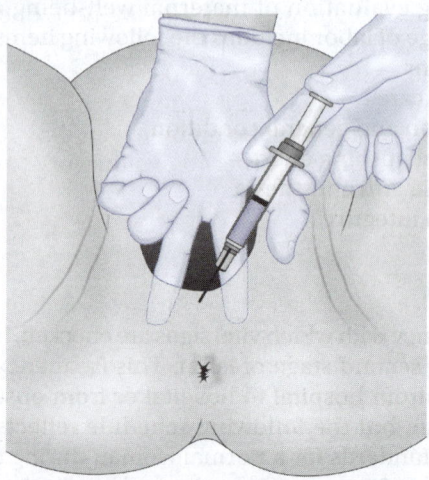

Figure 20.1: Local infiltration.

including the clitoris, labia majora, perineal body and rectal area without tissue distortion.

Lumbar Epidural Block

For lumbar epidural block, the anesthetic is introduced between lumbar vertebrae two and three or three and four as a single shot, intermittent technique or continuous technique.

Perineal Integrity

Evaluation of perineal integrity is for determining if delivery can possibly occur over an intact perineum or if episiotomies are needed. This decision is continually re-evaluated until the baby is born. There are several techniques, which facilitate delivery over an intact perineum. The commonly used techniques include:
1. 'Ironing out' the perineum by sweeping the midwife's fingers back and forth from side to side in the vagina just ahead of the fetal head. The pressure applied to iron out or stretch the muscles also stimulate the pushing reflex.
2. Perineal support at the time of birth: Some midwives do this by directly bracing the perineal body with their hand. Other midwives place their thumb and middle finger across from each other in the left and right groin and press inward to provide a little extra support across the perineal body.
3. Fetal head control by asserting pressure against the fetal head to keep it well-flexed and then allowing gradual extension as the perineum stretches. This is essential in lithotomy and dorsal positions in order to prevent tears.

Some midwives believe that if fetal head control is done properly, there is no need to touch the perineum. Others combine fetal head control and perineal support.

Maternal self-control is the key to whatever method of delivering over an intact perineum is used. A woman who is out of control, is more likely to tear or need an episiotomy.

EPISIOTOMY (FIG. 20.2)

An episiotomy is a surgical incision of the perineal body. The perineum is evaluated prior to the time of delivery to determine whether or not an episiotomy is indicated and if so, what kind of episiotomy. The perineum is evaluated for its length, thickness and distensibility. A short perineum may indicate performing a mediolateral episiotomy rather than a median episiotomy in order to avoid injury to the rectal sphincter and wall.

Indications

Any condition that places the woman at risk for perineal tearing:
1. Large size baby: A baby estimated to be 4,000 g or more may cause need for an episiotomy either to prevent laceration or in anticipation of a possible shoulder dystocia.
2. Preterm or small for gestational age (SGA) baby in order to minimize the risk of intracranial hemorrhage.

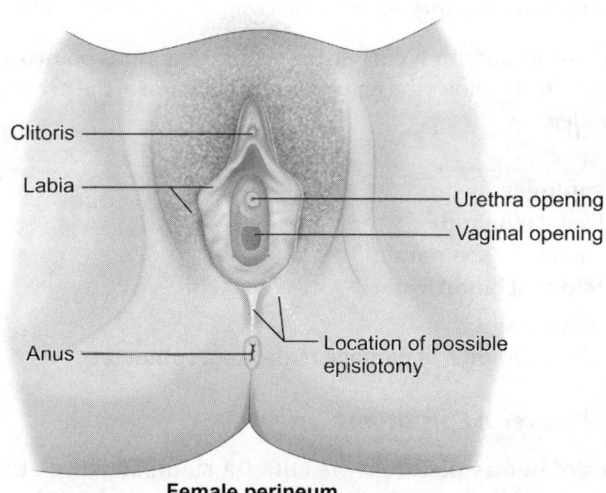

Figure 20.2: Episiotomy.

3. An uncontrolled woman who is unable to respond for the instructions given to push and to breathe in order to slowly ease the head out.
4. Anticipation of shoulder dystocia.
5. Fetal malpresentations and malpositions: In these situations, the widest diameter of the fetal head coming through the pelvic outlet and vaginal orifice is larger than usual.
6. A thick perineum, which is rigid and resistant to distention.
7. An inevitable laceration evidenced by narrow white lines resembling stretch marks and visible just beneath the skin. These appear just prior to laceration and probably represent beginning of tearing of the underlying tissues. A quick episiotomy prior to the moment of crowning is indicated to avoid an inevitable tear.
8. Prior to an assisted delivery such as forceps or vacuum extraction.
9. To speed up delivery, if there is fetal distress.

Types of Episiotomies (Fig. 20.3)

There are two main types of episiotomies:
1. Midline or median.
2. Mediolateral, which may be to the right or left.

Lateral and J-shaped episiotomies are mentioned in the literature. Both are not done currently due to several drawbacks.

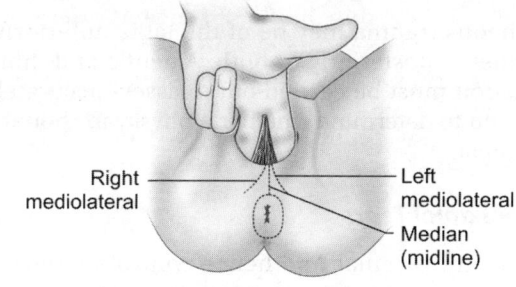

Figure 20.3: Types of episiotomies.

Midline or Median

Midline episiotomy is cut into the central tendinous point of the perineum. It follows the natural line of insertion of the pectineal muscles.

Advantages
- Easily repaired
- Generally less painful
- Minimal blood loss.

Disadvantage
Higher incidence of damage to the anal sphincter.

Mediolateral Episiotomy

Mediolateral episiotomy is cut at a slant, starting at the midpoint of the posterior fourchette and is directed at 45° angle towards a point midway between the ischial tuberosity and the anus. The cut may be to either the left or right and about 2.5 cm.

Advantages
- Extension into the rectum is less likely
- Avoids danger of damage to anal sphincter and Bartholin's gland.

Disadvantages
- Blood loss is greater
- Repair is more difficult
- During healing, the area is more painful
- Possible damage to pubococcygeal muscle.

Principles

The following principles should be observed regardless of which type of episiotomy is cut:
1. The presenting part of the fetus is protected from injury.
2. A single cut in any direction is far preferable to repeated snipping because the latter will leave jagged ends.
3. The episiotomy should be large enough to meet the purpose for deciding to cut it.
4. The timing of the cut should be such that lacerations are prevented (too late) and unnecessary blood loss avoided (too early). The perineum should be bulging, the vaginal orifice distended by approximately 3 cm diameter of presenting part between contractions and delivery of the presenting part should be expected to occur within the next two to four contractions.

Perineal Tears (Fig. 20.4)

Spontaneous trauma may be of the labia anteriorly and the perineum posteriorly or both. A gentle and thorough examination must be carried out to assess accurately the trauma and to determine whether a physician should carry out the repair.

Anterior Labial Tears

The labia are vascular and hence control of bleeding is important. A suture may be necessary to secure hemostasis.

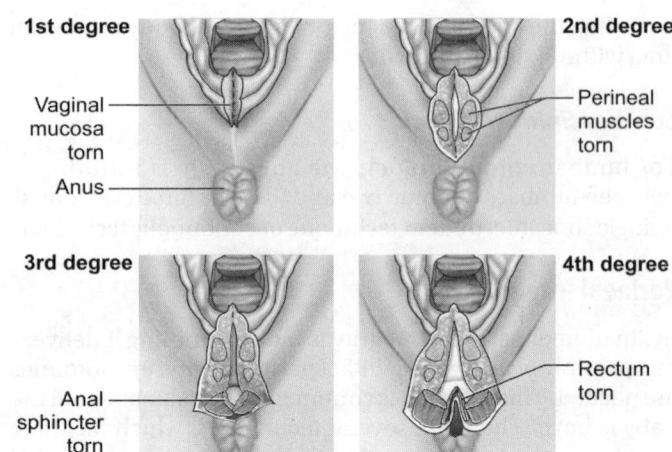

Figure 20.4: Perineal tear.

Posterior Perineal Trauma

Spontaneous tears of the perineum are usually classified in degrees, which are related to the anatomical structure, which have been traumatized. This classification only serves as a guideline because it is difficult to identify the structures precisely:
1. First degree tear involves the fourchette, perineal skin and mucous membrane.
2. Second degree tear involves the fourchette and the superficial perineal muscles. Namely, the bulbocavernosus and the transverse perineal muscles and in some cases the pubococcygeus.
3. Third degree tear involves damage to the anal sphincter in addition to the above structures.
4. Fourth degree tear is one, which extends into the rectal mucosa.

Note: Third and fourth degree tears should be repaired by an experienced obstetrician under a general anesthetic or effective epidural or spinal anesthetic.

EVALUATION OF THE FETAL WELL-BEING

Continuing evaluation of the fetal well-being during the second stage of labor is a continuation of the evaluation of the well-being of the fetus during the first stage of labor. It consists of evaluating the following:
1. Normalcy of the fetal lie, presentation, attitude and position.
2. Fetal adaptation to the pelvis (synclitism or asynclitism, molding, formation of caput succedaneum).
3. Fetal heart rate (FHR) pattern.
4. The normalcy of progress being made in the mechanisms of labor.

Progress in the mechanisms of labor is determined during vaginal examinations done prior to delivery. The frequency for checking fetal heart rate is increased to every 15 minutes during the second stage. Some obstetricians believe that it should be checked at the end of and after each contraction during which the woman pushes.

In interpreting the FHR and pattern, it must be remembered that toward the end of second stage when the resistance on the fetal head from pelvic floor and perineum increases, there may be a resultant early deceleration pattern. This is not considered an indication of acute fetal distress. Increased pressure on the head occurs as the delivery nears.

EVALUATION OF THE PROGRESS OF LABOR

Continuing evaluation of the progress of the second stage of labor is based on the following:
1. Contraction pain.
2. Length of second stage.
3. Descend and station.
4. Progress through the mechanisms of labor.

The decisions regarding moving the woman to the delivery room (timing) and consulting with the physician be made, based on evaluation of progress.

Evaluation of the progress through the mechanisms of labor is essential to detecting deep transverse arrest and concomitant second stage hypotonic uterine dysfunction. The fetus is in danger in the situation in which there are strong expulsive contractions and maternal pushing effort, but failure to progress because of some fetopelvic disproportion including deep transverse arrest.

Detection of progressive descends includes the following:
1. Progressively lower location (on the woman's spine) of back pain due to pressure from the fetal head.
2. Progressively lower location in the woman's abdomen of the maximum point of intensity of the fetal heart tones.
3. Increasing desire of the woman to push, which indicates descend of the fetal head to the pelvic floor and subsequent initiation of the reflex mechanism for pushing.
4. Change in station of the presenting part noted during vaginal examination.
5. Rectal and perineal bulging.
6. Appearance of the presenting part at the vaginal orifice.
7. The woman's assertion that the 'baby is coming', confirmed by either observation or examination.

Engagement should have occurred during the active phase of the first stage of labor in the primigravida and by the onset of the second stage of labor in the multipara. Failure of engagement if noted in the second stage is a signal of a potential problem.

BODILY AND SUPPORTIVE CARE OF THE WOMAN

Bodily and supportive care during the second stage of labor are continuations of the care begun during the first stage of labor, modified to meet the woman's changing needs as she progresses through labor. Additional measures specific to the second stage of labor are breathing and pushing. The woman's significant other may be permitted if the policy of the institution permits it.

Breathing

The usual instruction for the woman is to take one or two cleansing breaths (a deep breathe in and out) when she feels the start of the contraction and while the contraction is building. A controlled form of breathing should be used through the contractions if the woman does not yet feel like pushing. A woman needs help with her breathing and in making effective use of either her natural pushing desire or a deliberate pushing effort.

The woman needs to be instructed to pant if she feels like pushing and you do not want her to push. Panting may be a quick inhalation followed by a forcible exhalation and repeated immediately. It may also be rapid, shallow throat breathing. The woman's ability to pant and not push can be critical in the second stage and should be taught when she enters this stage of labor as a form of anticipatory instruction if it has not been taught before.

Pushing

A woman who feels like or needs to push can be helped in a number of ways in order to make her effort as effective as possible. Her significant other (if present) can also be involved in helping her push in a way that will make the person feel important, contributing and participating in the experience.

The urge to push may come before the vertex is visible. In order to conserve maternal energy and to allow vaginal tissues to stretch passively, the mother should be helped to avoid pushing at this stage. She should be instructed to lie in left lateral position and take breathing exercise at this time.

When the head becomes visible, the woman should be encouraged to follow her own inclinations in relation to expulsive effort. The usual instruction for the woman is to take one or two deep breaths when she feels the start of the contraction and while the contraction is building to hold the breath and give 4-5, 6 seconds pushes. Pushing for longer than 6 seconds at one breath holding, may produce fetal hypoxia and acidosis because the breath holding closes the glottis, while bearing down and increases the intrathoracic pressure. This combination results in a drop in arterial pressure caused by decreased cardiac output leading to decreased blood flow to the placenta and decreased oxygen content in the placental circulation causing fetal hypoxia.

In cases where there is delay in the delivery of the fetus, the woman may be given a different instruction, which is to push after expiration as forced exhalations, for short periods of time (5–6 second). This often will be accompanied by a grunt. In such an effort, the glottis is at least partially open and the intrathoracic pressure does not increase to interfere with venous return to the heart that produce its resulting effect on cardiac output and arterial pressure **(Box 20.1)**.

> **BOX 20.1:** Nursing alert.
>
> **Pushing technique**
> - Encourage spontaneous bearing down
> - Allow the mother to rest until the fetal head has descended low enough in the pelvis to stimulate Ferguson's reflex (a reflex stimulated by stretch receptors in the pelvic floor, which usually occurs at the +1 station that stimulates in the mother an involuntary urge to push)
> - Consider fetal situation and position in addition to dilation of cervix for determining a woman's readiness for pushing
> - Discourage prolonged maternal breath-holding (more than 6 seconds) during pushing
> - Encourage four or more pushes per contraction
> - Support the woman's involuntary pushing efforts whether they include grunting, groaning, exhaling or breath holding for less than 6 seconds
> - Validate the normalcy of sensations and maternal sounds
> - The woman who has received epidural anesthesia may require more directed support for expulsive efforts during the second stage

PREPARATION FOR DELIVERY

Location of the Delivery

Once the onset of second stage has been confirmed, it is the midwife's responsibility to assure that all is in readiness for the delivery when managing the labor and delivery of the woman. The alternatives for delivery within a hospital are the delivery room, the labor room or a birthing room. Newer hospitals often are designed for combination of labor and delivery rooms or birthing rooms for normal women. The planned location of the delivery may change due to unforeseen circumstances such as development of fetal distress and need for forceps delivery, and availability of immediate newborn resuscitation equipment.

Positions for the Delivery

The usual positions in a hospital delivery room are lithotomy or dorsal. Other positions used for delivery are left lateral, supported sitting, squatting, kneeling, standing and knee-chest. When the dorsal position is the choice, the woman can be encouraged to be in a semisitting or back up and legs down modification.

In deciding, which of the two positions to utilize for the delivery of a woman in the hospital, the following should be considered:
1. A woman with varicosities should be delivered in dorsal rather than lithotomy position. This position avoids pressure on the legs in the popliteal space, which is exerted by stirrups and cause circulatory interference. The risk of thrombophlebitis would be quite high with the woman in stirrups.
2. A dorsal delivery is more effective when the woman is cooperative and in control.
3. The lithotomy position gives the midwife better control in the event when the woman is out of control.
4. In the event of any existing complications (e.g. malpresentations, multiple gestation) or anticipated complications (e.g. shoulder dystocia), the woman should be in lithotomy position because the obstetrician needs all possible visualization and room in which to function with ready, direct access to the woman.

General Preparation

1. The room in which the delivery is to take place should be warm with a spotlight available so that the perineum can be easily observed.
2. A clean area should be prepared to receive the baby and waterproof covers provided to protect the bed and floor.
3. A sterile delivery pack, which includes articles for cutting and suturing an episiotomy, two cord clamps, a pairs of scissors for cutting the cord and a bulb syringe for oropharyngeal and nasal suctioning of the baby are placed at hand.
4. An oxytocic agent (methergine, ergometrine or syntometrine) is prepared in readiness for the active management of third stage or for use during an emergency. It must be kept separate from any neonatal drugs to avoid risk of error.
5. A warm cot and blankets should be prepared for the baby. In hospital a warmed mattress, a radiant warmer or an incubator may be used. At home, a warm (not hot) water bottle can be placed in the cot.
6. Neonatal resuscitation equipment must be thoroughly checked and readily available.
7. A cap and a mask must be worn in the delivery room (if available) prior to opening the sterile packs.
8. A surgical hand scrub is done as soon as the head becomes visible for a multigravid woman. In primigravida, the head usually takes a little longer to advance over the perineum.
9. Once she has put on her sterile gown and gloves (after hand scrub), the midwife must prepare her sterile articles on the instrument table. This includes antiseptic solution, cotton wool and pads.

During delivery, both mother and baby are particularly vulnerable to infection. Care must be taken to observe meticulous aseptic technique when preparing sterile equipment. Sterile surgical gloves must be worn during the delivery for the protection of both mother and the midwife.

CONDUCTING THE DELIVERY

Management of the delivery includes the hand maneuvers used to assist the baby's birth, the immediate care of the newborn, and the following management decisions (**Figs. 20.5A to J**).

Delivery of the Baby's Head

In preparation for the delivery of the baby, the mother's perineum needs to be swabbed, the delivery area draped with sterile linen and a pad used to cover the anus.

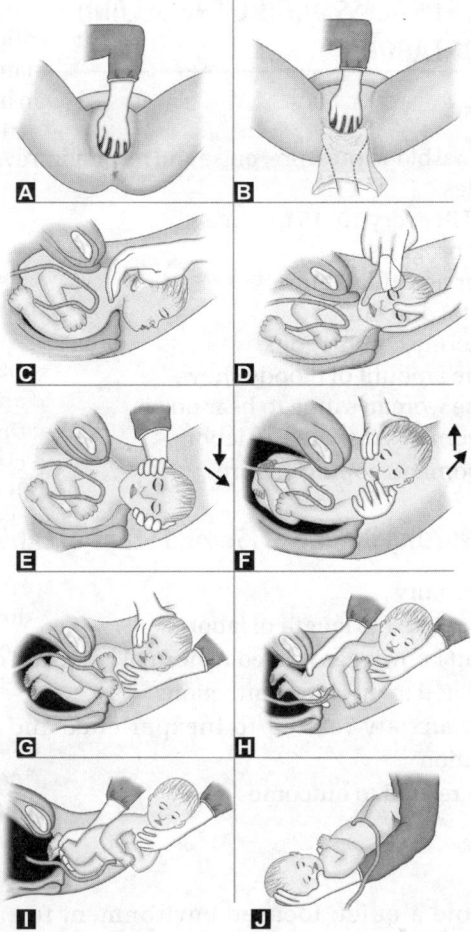

Figures 20.5A to J: Hand maneuvers for delivery of the baby in occiput anterior position. (A and B) Controlling the head; (C) Feeling for nuchal cord; (D) Wiping the baby's face and head; (E) Delivery of the anterior shoulder; (F and G) Delivering of the posterior shoulder; (H and I) Delivery of the trunk; (J) Safety hold.

Delivery of the Head Between Contractions

The idea behind delivering the baby's head between contractions is that the combination of the contractions and the maternal pushing effort actually constitutes exertion of a double force at the moment of birth. This makes the birth of the head more rapid and the release of restraining pressure more abrupt both of which increase the risk of intracranial damage to the baby and laceration to the woman. If the woman is in control of herself, it is possible for her to follow the midwife's instructions and then gently push in between contractions, an action that will ease the baby's head out with the least amount of trauma to the baby and woman.

Ritgen's Maneuver

The midwife or obstetrician controls the delivery of the head by this technique. It is performed as follows:
1. Place the pads of your fingertips on the portion of the vertex showing at the vaginal introitus. As more of the head is accessible at the vaginal introitus, spread your fingers over the vertex of the baby's head with the fingertips pointing toward the yet unseen face and your elbow pointing upward towards the mother.
2. Allow the head to gradually extend beneath your hand by exerting control, but not prohibitive, pressure with your hand. Use the length of your fingers in doing this and not just the fingertips. Proper control of the head in this manner will prevent explosive crowning and preserve the perineum.
3. An additional maneuver of supporting the perineum may also be used. For this, cover the hand not being used on the baby's head with a towel. Place the thumb in the crease of the groin midway on one side of the perineum. Place the middle finger in the crease of the groin midway on the other side of the perineum. Apply pressure with the thumb and finger downward and then inward toward each other across the perineal body.
4. While doing this, combination of head control and perineal support observe the perineum in the space between the thumb and middle finger. As the perineum distends, the decision is made as to whether an episiotomy is required.
5. Infiltrate the perineum, cut a mediolateral episiotomy and secure hemostasis, if required.
6. Watch the perineum, while the head born by extension.
7. As soon as the head is born (during the resting phase before the next contraction), place the fingertips of one hand on the occiput and then slide them down the curve of the baby's head at the level of the top of the shoulders and sweep them in both directions, feeling for the umbilical cord (nuchal cord). Most midwives use their dominant hand for this maneuver as it is the hand most accustomed to and sensitive for touching.

Management of a Nuchal Cord

1. If the cord is loose, slip it over the baby's head.
2. If the cord is too tight to slip over the baby's head, but not tight around the neck, slip it back over the shoulders as the baby's body is born.
3. If the cord is tight, immediately clamp (about 3 cm apart) and cut the cord at the neck before the baby's body is born. Tell the mother to pant, while you are clamping, cutting and unwinding the cord.
4. Wipe the baby's face and head, and wipe off fluid from the nose and mouth with a soft absorbent cloth.
5. Suction the nasal and oral passages of the baby with a soft, rubber bulb syringe or mucus sucker.

Delivery of the Shoulders

Wait for a contraction and watch the head return to anatomical alignment with the body (restitution) and external rotation. External rotation shows that the shoulders are rotating into the anteroposterior diameter of the pelvic outlet, which is the largest space. The midwife proceeds to deliver one shoulder at a time to avoid overstretching of the perineum.

A hand is placed on each side of the baby's head, over the ears and downward traction is applied. This allows the anterior shoulder to slip beneath the symphysis pubis, while the posterior shoulder remains in the vagina.

When the axillary crease is seen, the head and trunk are guided in an upward curve to allow the posterior shoulder to escape over the perineum. The baby is then grasped around the chest to aid the birth of the trunk and lift the baby towards the mother's abdomen. This allows the mother immediate sighting of the baby and provides close skin contact. The time of birth is noted.

Clamping and Cutting the Umbilical Cord

Clamping the umbilical cord is done by placing two instrument clamps on the cord about 8–10 cm from the umbilicus with enough room between them to allow for easy cutting of the cord. Application of a gauze swab over the cord, while cutting it will prevent blood spraying the delivery field. The timing of clamping the cord is not crucial unless asphyxia, prematurity or Rhesus (Rh) incompatibility is present. Some centers advocate delay until respiration are established and cord pulsation has ceased, thus ensuring that the infant receives a placental transfusion of some 70 mL of blood. This view is countered by those who maintain that the placental transfusion so acquired may predispose to neonatal jaundice.

Immediate Care of the Newborn

After the cord is severed at whatever time is considered appropriate, the baby is dried and warmly wrapped to prevent cooling. Subsequent actions vary, but may include the use of:
- Bodily contact with the mother
- Radiant warmer
- Warmed blankets.

The baby is then shown to the mother and her significant other. A 1 minute Apgar score must also be done by the midwife. If the baby is taken to a warmed crib or radiant warmer, the bulb syringe is also taken as well as the cord clamp and scissors for the final clamping and cutting of the cord. During this minute of life, while doing the above, the baby must be grossly examined for any visible deformities or congenital defects. When the cord will be shortened, care must be taken to apply the clamp nearer the baby, some authors recommend clamping the cord 3–4 cm clear of the abdominal wall to avoid pinching the skin. A greater length of the cord is left when the umbilical vessels are expected for needed transfusion as in cases of preterm and Rh hemolytic disease.

RECORDS

It is the responsibility of the midwife conducting the delivery to complete the labor record. This should include details of any drugs administered, the duration and progress of labor, and if an episiotomy was performed and repaired. The information is entered in the mother's records as well as in the birth register. Details of the baby's condition including Apgar score are also recorded.

NURSING PROCESS DURING THE SECOND STAGE OF LABOR

Assessment

1. Maternal blood pressure, pulse and respiration every 5–15 minutes.
2. The FHR every 10–15 minutes.
3. Labor progress:
   a. Cervical dilatation.
   b. Fetal descent.
   c. Uterine contractions.
   d. The amount of bloody show.
   e. The woman's urge to bear down.
4. The woman's response to labor.
5. The woman's coping pattern.

Analysis/Nursing Diagnosis (Second Stage of Labor)

- Risk for injury
- Fatigue related to length of labor
- Deficient knowledge related to normal labor and delivery
- Pain related to uterine contractions
- Fear or anxiety related to inexperience and lack of preparation
- Anxiety related to outcome

Planning

1. Promote a quiet, focused environment to enhance pushing efforts.
2. Monitor maternal and fetal status.
3. Provide encouragement for pushing efforts.
4. Support ongoing comfort measures and pushing efforts.

Implementation

1. Continue assessment of maternal blood pressure, FHR and uterine contractions.
2. Assist laboring woman into position of comfort and pushing efforts.
3. Observe for approaching birth such as:
   a. Perineal bulging.
   b. Appearance of the fetal head.
4. Provide comfort measures such as:
   a. Wiping face with wet washcloth.
   b. Moistening the lips.
   c. Supporting the woman's body and/or extremities during pushing efforts.
5. Prepare for the delivery.
6. Complete perineal cleansing.

Evaluation

Ensure that:
1. The laboring woman is able to remain focused on pushing.

2. The woman and the fetus maintain physical parameters within normal limits.
3. The woman feels encouragement.
4. The woman feels comfortable.

STUDY QUESTIONS

Short Notes

1. Clamping and cutting of the umbilical cord.
2. Breathing pattern recommended for mothers in first and second stages of labor.

Short Answer Questions

1. Episiotomy: Indications, types and principles.
2. Analgesia and anesthesia during second stage of normal labor.
3. Perineal lacerations.
4. Immediate care of the newborn.

Essay Questions

1. Evaluation and nursing care of a mother in second stage of labor.
2. Explain 'the conduct of' delivery using different hand maneuvers (Ritgen's maneuver).

BIBLIOGRAPHY

1. Caldero Barcia P. Effects of position changes on the intensity and frequency of uterine contractions during labor. American Journal of Obstetrics and Gynecology. 1971;109:274.
2. Dutta DC. Textbook of Obstetrics, 5th edition. Kolkata: New Central Book Company; 2001. pp. 130-52.
3. Friedman EA. The functional divisions of labor. American Journal of Obstetrics and Gynecology. 1971;109(2):274-80.
4. Hillan EM. Physiology and management of the second stage of labor. In: Bennett RV, Brown KB (Eds). Myles Textbook for Nurses, 13th edition. Edinburgh: Churchill Livingstone; 1999. pp. 430-47.
5. Hon EH. An Introduction to Fetal Monitoring, 2nd edition. North Haven Corometrics: Connecticut: Medical Systems; 1971.
6. Peterson G. Birthing Normally: A Personal Growth Approach to Childbirth, 2nd edition. Berkeley, California: Mind-Body Press; 1984.
7. Schrag K. Maintenance of pelvic floor integrity during childbirth. Journal of Nurse Midwifery. 1979;24(6):26-31.
8. Helen V. Nurse-Midwifery, 2nd edition. Boston: Jones and Bartlett Publishers; 1996. pp. 277-310.

CHAPTER 21

Physiology and Management of the Third Stage of Labor

Learning Objectives

Upon completing this chapter, the learner will be able to:
- Describe the mechanism of placental separation, descend and the physiological factors that ensure hemostasis.
- Enumerate the use of oxytocic drugs in third-stage management.
- Outline the nursing management of the mother immediately after delivery of the placenta and membranes.
- Describe the causes and management of postpartum hemorrhage.

The third stage of labor begins upon completion of the birth of the baby and ends with the birth of the placenta. It is known as the placental stage of labor. The third stage of labor averages between 5 and 15 minutes, but any period up to 1 hour may be considered within normal limits.

PHYSIOLOGICAL PROCESSES OF PLACENTAL SEPARATION AND EXPULSION

These are a continuation of the processes and forces at work during the earlier stages of labor. The processes of the third stage of labor and parameters of normal for this period must be known by the midwife for effective practice.

The third stage of labor consists of two phases. The first phase is the placental separation and the second phase is that of placental expulsion. Both separation and expulsion are brought about by contractions, which begin again after a brief pause at birth. The contractions must have been approximately every 2–2½ minutes apart during the second stage of labor. After the birth of the baby, the next contraction may not occur for 3–5 minutes. Contractions then follow every 4–5 minutes until there has been separation and expulsion of the placenta and membranes. After that, the emptied uterus contracts down on it and remain contracted if the muscle tone is good. Otherwise, recurrent contraction and relaxation constitute after birth pains if the muscle tone is not as good.

Placental Separation

Placental separation **(Figs. 21.1A and B)** is the result of the abrupt decrease in size of the uterine cavity during and following delivery of the baby. As the uterine cavity empties progressively, the retraction process accelerates (the unique characteristic of the uterine muscle). This decrease in uterine size necessarily means a concomitant decrease in the area of placental attachment. The placenta, however, remains the same size and at the site of attachment, it is unable to withstand the stress and buckles. The result is a separation of the placenta from the uterine wall, which takes place in the spongiosa layer of the decidua.

Separation usually begins at the center, so that a retroplacental clot is formed. This may further aid separation by exerting pressure at the midpoint of placental attachment, so that the increased weight helps to strip the adherent lateral borders. This increased weight also helps to peel the membranes off the uterine wall.

While the formation of the retroplacental clot is the result rather than the cause of placental separation, it does facilitate the completion of placental separation.

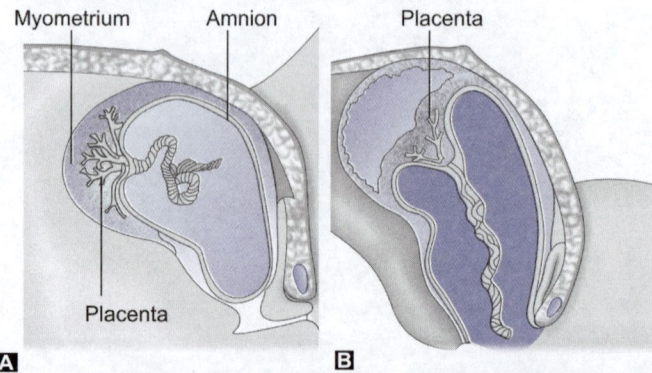

Figures 21.1A and B: Mechanism of placental separation. (A) Placenta attached to the uterine wall; (B) Placenta separated from the uterine wall.

Descend of the Placenta

After the placenta has separated, it descends into the lower uterine segment or into the upper vaginal vault, causing the clinical signs of placental separation to become evident. These are as follows:
1. Sudden trickle or gush of blood.
2. Lengthening of the amount of umbilical cord visible at the vaginal introitus.
3. Change in the shape of the uterus from a discoid (circular) to globular, as the uterus now contracts upon itself.
4. Change in the position of the uterus as it rises in the abdomen, because the bulk of the placenta is in the lower uterine segment or upper vaginal vault.

Expulsion of the Placenta

Placental expulsion begins with descend of the placenta into the lower uterine segment **(Fig. 21.2)**. It then passes through the cervix into the upper vaginal vault from where it is expelled. Expulsion of the placenta is by one of two mechanisms:
1. The Schultz mechanism of placental expulsion is delivery of the placenta with the fetal side presenting **(Fig. 21.3A)**. This is thought to occur when separation begins centrally with corresponding formation of a central retroplacental clot, which weights the placenta, so the central portion descends first. This in effect inverts the placenta and amniotic sac, and causes the membranes to peel off the decidua and trail behind the placenta. The majority of bleeding occurring with this mechanism of separation is not visualized until the placenta and membranes are delivered, since the inverted membranes catch and hold the blood. This method is more common of the two.
2. The Duncan mechanism of placental expulsion is delivery of the placenta with the maternal side presenting **(Fig. 21.3B)**. This is thought to occur when separation first takes place at the margin or periphery of the placenta. Blood escapes between the membranes and uterine wall, and is visualized externally. The placenta descends sideways and the amniotic sac, therefore, is not inverted, but trails behind the placenta for delivery.

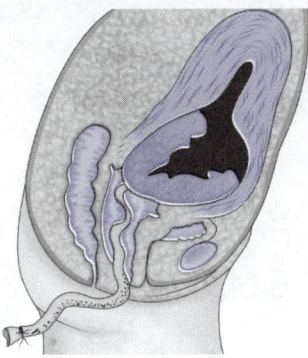

Figure 21.2: Placenta in the lower uterine segment.

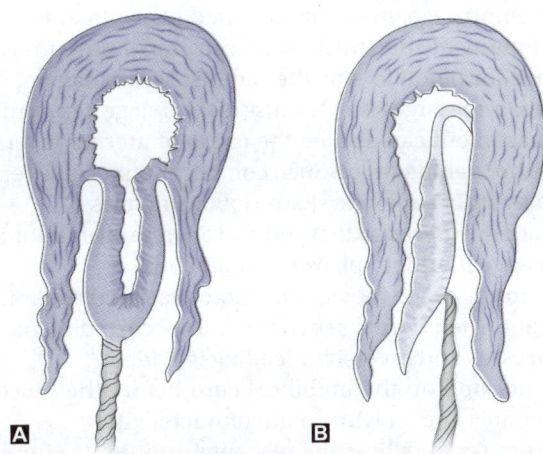

Figures 21.3A and B: Methods of placental expulsion. (A) Schultz method; (B) Matthew Duncan method.

The memory aid for correctly identifying the mechanisms of placental expulsion is based on the appearance of two different sides of the placenta. The fetal side is shiny and glistening, because it is covering the fetal membranes, while the maternal side is rough and red looking. Hence, the sayings 'shiny Schultz' and 'dirty Duncan'.

Hemostasis

The normal volume of blood flow through the placental site is 500–800 mL/min. At placental separation, this has to be arrested within seconds to prevent serious hemorrhage. The interplay of three factors within the normal physiological processes control the bleeding. They are:
1. Retraction of the oblique uterine muscle fibers in the upper uterine segment through which tortuous blood vessels intertwine. The resultant thickening of the muscles exerts pressure on the torn vessels, acting as clamps, thus securing a ligature action. Oblique fibers are absent in the lower uterine segment that explains the greatly increased blood loss in placenta previa, when placental separation occurs.
2. The presence of vigorous uterine contraction following placental separation brings the walls into apposition, so that further pressure is exerted on the placental site.
3. The achievement of hemostasis: There is a transitory activation of the coagulation and fibrinolytic systems during and immediately following, placental separation (Bonner et al. 1970). This protective response is especially active at the placental site, so that clot formation in the torn vessels is intensified. Following separation, the placental site is rapidly covered by a fibrin mesh utilizing circulating fibrinogen.

MANAGEMENT OF THE THIRD STAGE OF LABOR

Care of the mother in the third stage of labor should be based on an understanding of the normal physiological processes at work. Prompt nursing actions can reduce the risk of hemorrhage, infection, retained placenta and shock. Management of the third stage can make considerable difference for blood loss by the mother. Mismanagement of third stage is the largest single cause of third stage hemorrhage. Mismanagement can also be the cause of uterine inversion and life-threatening shock. Such complications can be readily avoided by strict adherence to the following rules:

1. Guard the uterus so that you and anyone else should not massage it prior to placental separation.
2. Do not massage the uterus before placental separation, except when partial separation has occurred by natural processes and excessive bleeding is evident.
3. Do not pull on the umbilical cord before the placenta separates or ever with an uncontracted uterus.
4. Do not try to deliver the placenta prior to its complete separation unless in the emergency of third stage hemorrhage.
5. Wait for the natural process to occur and do not interfere.

During the third stage of labor, the nurse is also responsible for initial management of the baby (i.e. drying the baby, providing for warmth, assuring a clear airway), and for the initial mother-baby bonding unless there is another nurse to receive and attend the baby soon after birth. During the initial care of the baby, the nurse midwife must keep one eye on the mother's perineum in order to watch for signs of placental separation and for excessive bleeding (by the same token, when she returns to the mother's perineum to manage third stage, she must keep one eye on the baby to continually evaluate the baby's well-being). Upon return to the mother to evaluate the progress of labor and the mother's condition, she places one hand on the mother's abdomen to feel, without massaging, the shape and position of the uterus, and whether or not it is contracted.

If cord blood is to be collected, she can guide the cut end of the umbilical cord into the open end of the blood tube and hold it in position with the fingers of the same hand, which is holding the blood tube. The other hand may release the clamp on the cord. The cord can be reclamped as soon as the tube is filled. This procedure is repeated for more blood tubes, if required. Care must be taken to hold the umbilical cord in position in the upper end of the blood tube to avoid sudden spray of blood, when the clamp is released due to the sudden pressure of blood flowing through the depleted cord. The sample may also be collected using a syringe and needle from the fetal surface of the placenta, where the blood vessels are congested and easily visible. This must be done before the blood clots.

The cord is wound around the clamp until the clamp is at the vaginal introitus, so that traction can be effectively exerted on the cord when needed. This clamp is held with one hand, while the other hand continues to guard the uterus. Guarding the uterus from massaging is essential to avoid partial separation of the placenta and resulting hemorrhage. Normal placental separation from the uterine wall is accomplished by the effect of uterine contractions.

If you are unsure whether the placenta has separated, it can be checked by using a modification of the Brandt-Andrews maneuver. For this, hold the cord taut at the vaginal introitus with one hand, using the clamp for leverage. With the fingers of the abdominal hand held together press down into the lower abdomen above the symphysis pubis. If the cord recedes into the vagina, the placenta is not separated **(Fig. 21.4)**.

If the cord has a feeling of give (lack of resistance) and lengthens beyond its position at the vaginal introitus, the placenta is separated and you may proceed with facilitating placental expulsion.

Delivery of the Placenta and Membranes

At the beginning of the third stage, the fundus is palpable below the umbilicus. It feels broad as the placenta is still in the upper segment. As the placenta separates and falls into the lower segment the following signs are evident:

1. A small fresh blood loss.
2. Lengthening of the cord.
3. Fundus becoming rounder, smaller and more mobile in the abdomen.

It is important not to manipulate the uterus until a strong contraction is palpable. In the management of third stage, strict vigilance and correct practice are important to prevent disastrous consequences. The methods are generally followed:

1. Expectant management.
2. Assisted expulsion:
   a. Controlled cord traction (modified Brandt-Andrews method).
   b. Expression by fundal pressure.

Expectant Management

In expectant management, the placental separation and its descent into the vagina are allowed to occur spontaneously. Mother's efforts are used to aid the expulsion. Minimal assistance is given if the mother's efforts fail to expedite the expulsion. This method can be practiced, when the mother has not received any anesthesia or an oxytocic drug has not been administered at the delivery of the anterior shoulder.

Steps of the method

1. A hand is placed over the fundus to feel the signs of placental separation, the state of uterine activity—

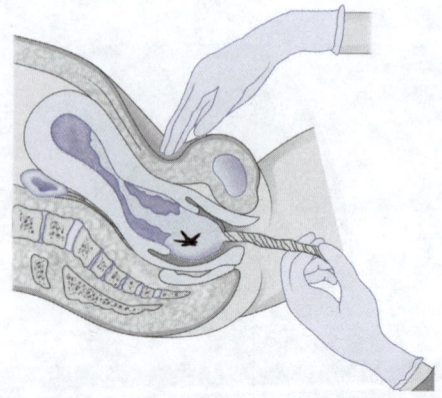

Figure 21.4: Checking for placental separation.

contraction and relaxation, and any collection of blood in the uterine cavity. The placenta generally separates within few minutes and 15–20 minutes may be allowed for the separation to occur.

2. When the features of placental separation and its descend into the lower segment are confirmed, the client is asked to bear down simultaneously with the hardening of the uterus. With a good uterine contraction, mother's bearing down effort will usually bring about expulsion of the placenta. The tendency to massage the uterus must be avoided. If the placenta fails to expel, one can wait for up to 10 minutes, if there is no bleeding. With another contraction and bearing down by the mother, it is likely to be expelled.

3. As soon as the placenta passes through the introitus, it is grasped by both hands and twisted round and round or slightly up and down with gentle traction applied as the membranes are stripped off intact. If the membranes threaten to tear, they are to be held by an artery forceps and gentle traction applied to deliver the rest of the membranes. Gentleness and patience are important in delivering the membranes completely.

Assisted Expulsion

Controlled cord traction (modified Brandt-Andrews method)

Controlled cord traction **(Figs. 21.5A and B)** method is used after an oxytocic drug has been administered and given time to act. The uterus must be well-contracted and signs of placental separation must be evident.

The left hand is placed above the level of the symphysis pubis with the palmar surface facing toward the umbilicus to exert pressure in an upward direction. The body of the uterus is displaced upwards and toward the umbilicus, while with the right hand, steady tension is given in a downward and backward direction following the line of birth canal (curve of Carus), by holding on the clamp placed on the cord at the vulva. It is important to apply steady traction by pulling the cord firmly and maintaining the pressure. Force and jerky movements must be avoided.

If the maneuver is not immediately successful, there should be a pause before another contraction is palpated and further attempt is made. Great care should be taken to avoid tearing the membranes. Tension on the umbilical cord without uterine contraction can cause inversion of the uterus, partial separation of placenta and hemorrhage or detachment of cord from the placenta, thereby requiring manual removal.

This method when used properly achieves reduced blood loss, shorter third stage of labor and as a result less risk of postpartum hemorrhage.

Expression by fundal pressure

Expression by fundal pressure is done by placing four fingers of the hand behind the fundus and the thumb in front of the uterus to use as a piston. The uterus is made to contract by gentle rubbing. When the uterus becomes hard, it is pushed downwards and backwards. The pressure is to be withdrawn as soon as the placenta passes through the introitus. This method is preferred in cases where the baby is premature or macerated, as the cord in such cases tends to have reduced tensile strength.

A sterile receiver should be placed against the woman's buttocks to catch blood and to hold the placenta, when it is born. If the woman is in a lithotomy position, the basin is braced between the woman's buttocks and the midwife's body, because the midwife needs both her hands free to manage the third stage of labor. Use of placenta basin to catch the blood makes it possible to measure the majority of the blood loss and minimize mess.

As the placenta is born it is allowed to slide gently down the side of the placenta basin, which is positioned more on its side at the vaginal introitus for this purpose or is delivered into the midwife's hands at the vaginal introitus. Either way, the purpose is not to let the placenta drop any distance from the level of the introitus, since this might cause the after coming membranes, which may still be peeling off the uterine wall as the placenta is delivered, to tear and break off and retained.

Third stage has ended if the membranes follow the placenta immediately, and are delivered with the placenta. However, sometimes the membranes trail behind and threaten to break off, if tension is applied to them. In such an instance, they may be teased out in one of the following two ways:

1. One way is to take a clamp (large Kelly clamp or large ring forceps) and place it on the membranes at the vaginal introitus. One hand continues to support the placenta or the basin with the placenta in it, in order to prevent tension on the membranes. The other hand manipulates the clamped membranes by gently rocking them up and down, and side to side, while exerting the slightest bit of traction on them. The appropriate amount of traction can be judged by the feeling of steady 'give' of the membranes being teased out. As the membranes are gradually teased out, the clamp moves away from the vaginal introitus. Therefore, it needs to be periodically reclamped on the membranes at the introitus whenever it gets an inch or two away, because you have better control of manipulating the membranes the closer the clamp is to the vaginal introitus. The process is continued until the membranes are delivered.

2. The other way to tease out the membranes is to hold the placenta in your hands and turn it repeatedly. This causes the membranes to twist, thereby having the effect of

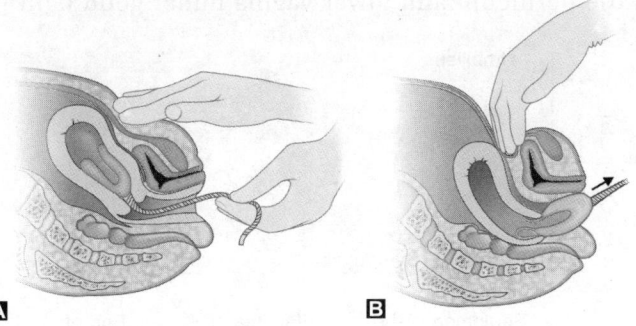

Figures 21.5A and B: Brandt-Andrews method of delivering placenta (controlled cord traction). (A) Traction on cord; (B) Traction on cord in the line of birth canal.

gradually teasing them out until they are delivered. This method may be more difficult for inexperienced hands because the placenta is slippery and it is not as easy to control the amount of tension on the membranes as it is in the first method.

If the membranes do break off, while trying to tease them out, third stage is considered ended. Sometimes the torn end of the membranes may be visualized during the cervical inspection and more teased out. The generally accepted management, if a portion of the membranes is retained, is that it does not warrant uterine exploration to remove them. Retention of a portion of the membranes is not a cause of hemorrhage as is true for retained placental fragments. The retained portion of the membranes will eventually be expelled with lochia. They need to be expelled as soon as possible as their retention increases the risk of endometritis. To achieve this more rapid expulsion, a full series of Methergine or ergometrine is usually ordered (methergine or ergometrine 0.2 mg q4h for 6 doses or tid for 3 days). If the estimated amount of membranes retained was a large amount, some obstetricians also give an immediate dose of Methergine 0.2 mg or ergometrine 0.5 mg intramuscularly unless the mother is hypertensive in which case it would be contraindicated. A uterine exploration is not done to remove the fragments of membranes as it is traumatic to the woman and increases the risk of intrauterine infection.

Use of Oxytocic Agents

Oxytocic drugs stimulate the uterus to contract. They may be administered at crowning of the baby's head, at delivery of the anterior shoulder of the baby, at the end of second stage of labor or following the delivery of the placenta.

Prophylactic use
Routine administration of an oxytocic at the time of birth of the baby, given as a precautionary measure for the prevention of postpartum hemorrhage regardless of the assessed risk status of the woman. This is a part of active management, a policy of labor management practiced in developed countries. It usually comprises the administration of an oxytocic drug at the time of delivery of the anterior shoulder, clamping to the umbilical cord immediately following birth of the baby and delivery of the placenta by controlled traction.

Therapeutic administration
Therapeutic administration implies the use of an oxytocic either to stop the bleeding once it has occurred or to maintain the uterus in a contracted state, when there are indications that excessive bleeding is likely to occur. This oxytocic administration practice is more consistent with a physiological or expectant philosophy of care. In this event, routine administration of an oxytocic drug is withheld, the umbilical cord is left unclamped until cord pulsation has ceased and the placenta is expelled by use of gravity and maternal effort. A procedure generally practiced in midwife, managed deliveries is the administration of ergometrine 0.5 mg or Methergine 0.2 mg intramuscularly soon after the expulsion of the placenta (**Box 21.1**).

BOX 21.1: Nursing alert.

Oxytocin administration after delivery of placenta

Oxytocin (Pitocin)	A polypeptide hormone
Action	Increases myometrial contraction by increasing the availability of intracellular calcium. Binds to oxytocin receptors in the decidua and myometrium
Indication	Delivery of placenta
Dosage and route	Oxytocin for control of postpartum bleeding may be diluted and administered by IV or 10-20 μ as IM. Oxytocin 20μ (range 10μ–40μ) in one liter lactated ringers (LR) or dextrose 5% (D5W) solution. Administer the first liter at a rapid rate. When second liter of solution is ordered, administer at 125 mL/h
Adverse reaction	With too rapid infusion, tachycardia may occur. Hypotension or hypertension may also occur. The antidiuretic effect may cause oliguria, fluid overload, arrhythmia, water intoxication, nausea, vomiting or headache
Nursing consideration	Assess the fundus for contraction. Assess the amount of lochia. Monitor vital signs. Record intake and output and assess the bladder

---

Fundal Height during Third Stage

At the beginning of the third stage, the fundus is palpable below the umbilicus. It feels broad as the placenta is still in the upper segment. As the placenta separates and falls into the lower uterine segment, there is a small fresh blood loss, the cord lengthens, and the fundus becomes rounder, smaller and more mobile as it rises in the abdomen to the level of the umbilicus or just above the umbilicus. At the end of third stage following the expulsion of the placenta, the fundus is about 4 cm below the umbilicus (**Fig. 21.6**).

Completion of the Third Stage

Continuing evaluation is essential at the completion of third stage. The midwife must ensure that the uterus is well-contracted and fresh blood loss is minimal. Careful inspection of the perineum and lower vagina under good light is

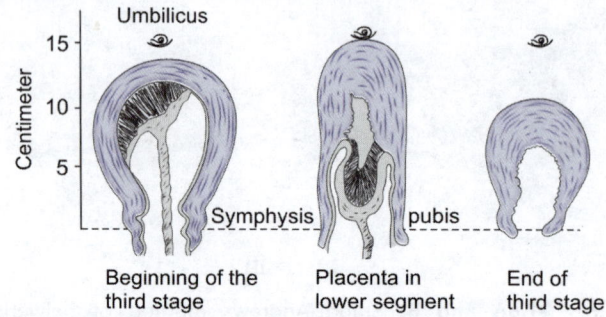

Figure 21.6: Fundal height relative to the umbilicus and symphysis pubis.

important. Slight lacerations are usually repaired immediately. If repair of a more extensive wound, such as an episiotomy or a second degree tear, is necessary, the mother should be made comfortable by changing soiled bed linen, while preparations are made for suturing.

The vulva and perineum are gently cleansed using antiseptic solution, softly dried and a clean pad placed in position. The mother's blood pressure, pulse and temperature should be taken and recorded at least once. Once the mother is comfortable, examination of the placenta and membranes is the next priority.

Examination of Placenta and Membranes

Examination of placenta and membranes should be performed as soon as after delivery as possible, so that if there is doubt about their completeness, further action could be taken before the mother leaves the labor room or the midwife leaves the home in case of home delivery. A thorough inspection must be carried out in order to make sure that no part of the placenta or membranes has been retained. The membranes often become torn during delivery and may be ragged and hence, care must be taken to piece them together to have an overall picture of their completeness. This is easier to see if the placenta is held by the cord, allowing the membranes to hang. The hole through which the baby was delivered can usually be identified and a hand spread out inside the membranes to aid inspection. The placenta should then be laid out on a flat surface and both placental surfaces examined carefully **(Fig. 21.7)**. The amnion should be peeled from the chorion right up to the umbilical cord, which allows the chorion to be fully viewed.

Assessment of the Placenta

Any clots from the maternal surface must be removed and kept for measuring. Broken fragments of cotyledons must be carefully replaced before an accurate assessment is made:

1. *Infarctions that are recent or old:* These areas on the placental surface indicate deprivation of blood supply. Recent infarctions appear bright red and old infarctions as gray patches.
2. *Localized calcifications:* These are seen as flattened white plaques that feel gritty (as small hard particles of sand) to touch.
3. *Lobes:* There are of a complete placenta fit neatly together without any gaps, the edges forming a uniform circle.
4. *Blood vessels:* They should not radiate beyond the placental edge. If they do, this denotes a succenturiate lobe. If the lobe has been retained, the vessels will end abruptly at a hole in the membrane.
5. *Insertion of the cord (on the fetal surface):* Normal insertion is central. Lateral insertion is abnormal.
6. *Umbilical vessels:* Two umbilical arteries and one vein should be present. The absence of one artery may be associated with congenital abnormality, particularly renal agenesis.
7. *Cord length:* Average length is 50 cm.
8. *Weight of placenta:* Approximately one-sixth of the baby's weight.

Immediate Care to Mother and Baby

The mother and baby should remain in the midwife's care for at least an hour after delivery. In some hospitals, the baby may be in a nursery unit and cared for by another nurse. Both need careful observation and specific care during this period.

The mother should receive cleansing body wash, mouthwash and perineal care. She should be encouraged to empty her bladder and a bedpan offered. Blood pressure, pulse, uterine contraction and bleeding should be checked every 15 minutes.

The baby's general well-being and security of the cord clamp needs to be checked. As the baby will quickly chill after birth, it is important to thoroughly dry and wrap the baby in a clean, dry towel or blanket. A full neonatal examination is done at an early stage and the baby is kept in a warm crib or cradle close to the mother.

Mothers intending to breastfeed may be encouraged to put their babies to the breast during early contact. Babies are usually alert and their sucking reflex strong at this time. For the mother, early breastfeeding causes a reflex release of oxytocin from the posterior lobe of the pituitary gland that stimulates the uterus to contract. The mother may experience a sudden fresh blood loss as the uterus empties and she should be reassured.

Records

The midwife is responsible for documentation of all the events of labor and observations. Her recording should include the following details—all the drugs administered, examination of the placenta, membranes and cord with attention drawn to any abnormalities and the amount of blood loss.

After the specified period of observation, the mother and baby are transferred to the postnatal ward.

COMPLICATIONS OF THE THIRD STAGE

Postpartum Hemorrhage

Postpartum hemorrhage is defined as excessive bleeding from the genital tract at any time following the baby's birth to 6 weeks after delivery. If it occurs during the third stage of labor or within 24 hours of delivery, it is termed *primary postpartum hemorrhage.*

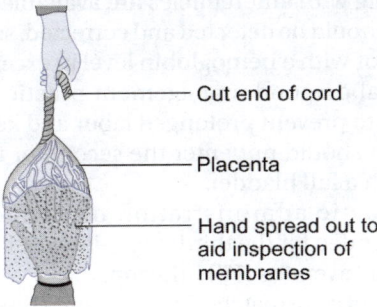

Figure 21.7: Examination of membranes.

If bleeding occurs subsequent to the first 24 hours following birth until the 6th week postpartum, it is termed *secondary postpartum hemorrhage*.

Primary Postpartum Hemorrhage

During the 1st or 2nd hour after birth, when blood loss is excessive, it is difficult to measure it accurately, especially when the fluid has soaked into dressings and linen. The measurable solidified clots only represent about half the fluid loss. If measured blood loss reaches 500 mL, it is treated as postpartum hemorrhage. Another yardstick is maternal condition and states that any blood loss, however, small which adversely affects the mother's condition, constitutes a postpartum hemorrhage.

Causes of primary postpartum hemorrhage are atonic uterus, retained placenta, trauma and coagulation disorders.

Atonic uterus: This is a failure of the myometrium at the placental site to contract and retract to compress torn blood vessels and control blood loss by a living ligature action. The volume of blood flow at the placental site, when the placenta is attached, is approximately 500–800 mL/min. Upon separation, the efficient contraction and retraction of the uterine muscle stops the flow of blood and prevents hemorrhage.

Factors that interfere with this phenomenon and cause bleeding are listed below:

1. *Incomplete placental separation:* If placental tissue remains partially embedded in the spongy decidua, efficient contraction and retraction are interrupted. If the placenta remains fully adhere to the uterine wall, it is unlikely to cause bleeding. However, once separation has begun, maternal vessels are torn open.
2. *Retained cotyledon, placental fragment or membranes:* These will similarly impede efficient uterine action.
3. *Precipitate labor:* When the uterus has contracted vigorously resulting in a short duration of labor that is less than 1 hour, the muscle may have insufficient opportunity to retract.
4. *Uterine inertia due to prolonged labor:* In a labor where the active phase lasts more than 12 hours, uterine inertia may result owing to muscle exhaustion.
5. *Uterine over distension due to polyhydramnios, multiple pregnancy or large baby:* The myometrium becomes excessively stretched and therefore less efficient.
6. *Placenta previa:* The placental site is partially or wholly in the lower uterine segment where the muscle layer contains few oblique fibers. This results in poor control of bleeding.
7. *Uterine relaxant anesthetic agents:* Volatile inhalational agents, such as halothane, cause uterine relaxation.
8. *Mismanagement of the third stage of labor:* Manipulation of the uterus or 'fundus fiddling' may precipitate arrhythmic contractions, so that the placenta separates only partially and retraction is lost.
9. *A full bladder may interfere with uterine action:* This is also considered as mismanagement.
10. *Grand multiparity:* With each successive pregnancy fibrous tissue replaces muscle fibers in the uterus, reducing its contractility and the blood vessels become more difficult to compress. Women who have had five or more deliveries are at increased risk.
11. *Uterine fibroids:* These may impede efficient uterine action.
12. *Anemia:* Women who enter labor with reduced hemoglobin concentration (below 10 g/dL) are more prone to bleed more.

Retention of the placenta or a part of the placenta due to:
- Cornual implantation
- Constriction ring below the placenta
- Placenta membranacea
- Placenta accreta, increta or percreta
- Placenta in one horn of the uterus, with the fetus in the other horn
- Firm adhesion of extraplacental chorion to the decidua
- Abruptio placentae.

Traumatic conditions: These include perineal tears, vaginal tears, cervical tears, lower segment tears and uterine rupture.

Previous history of postpartum hemorrhage or retained placenta: In such clients, there is a risk for recurrence in subsequent pregnancies.

Coagulopathy: Conditions such as disseminated intravascular coagulation, excessive fibrinolysis, inherited coagulation disorders and idiopathic thrombocytopenic purpura.

Clinical features

1. Visible bleeding per vaginam, which may be in the form of copious, continuous ooze or intermittent gushes.
2. *Enlarged uterus:* Sometimes there may be little or no visible loss of blood. Blood accumulates within the uterus and the fundal height increases. Uterus feels 'boggy' on palpation, i.e. soft and distended lacking tone.
3. Pallor.
4. Rising pulse rate.
5. Falling blood pressure (severe hypotension).
6. *Altered level of consciousness:* May become restless or drowsy.
7. Metabolic acidosis and shock.

Prophylaxis

1. Women, who are identified as having risk factors, should be instructed to have delivery in a unit, where facilities for dealing with emergencies are available.
2. Anemia should be detected and corrected, so that women enter labor with a hemoglobin level in excess of 10 g/dL.
3. During labor, good management practices should be followed to prevent prolonged labor and ketoacidosis.
4. A woman should not enter the second or third stage of labor with a full bladder.
5. Prophylactic administration of oxytocic agent is recommended for the third stage either by intramuscular (IM) or intravenous (IV) infusion.
6. Two units of crossmatched blood should be kept available for any woman known to have a placenta previa.

Management
Primary postpartum hemorrhage is an emergency, which requires prompt and efficient management. As soon as the midwife recognizes the occurrence, she must call the physician, if one is not already present in the delivery room. This initial step is important because the mother's condition can deteriorate very rapidly:

1. *Stop the bleeding:* Feel the fundus with the fingertips. If it is soft and relaxed (atonic), massage the fundus with a smooth, circular motion to make it contract. When a contraction occurs, the hand is to be held still.
2. *Give an oxytocic to sustain the contraction:* In many cases, Syntocinon 10 units must have already been administered and this may be repeated. Alternatively, ergometrine 0.25–0.5 mg may be given intravenously, which will be effective in 45 seconds.
3. *Resuscitate the mother:* An IV line should be commenced, while peripheral veins are easily negotiated. Fluid replacement and administration of oxytocics are done. Ringer's lactate and blood may be administered. As an emergency measure, the mother's legs may be lifted up in order to allow blood to drain from them into the central circulation. The foot of the bed should not be raised as this encourages pooling of blood in the uterus, which prevents uterus from contracting.
4. *Empty the uterus:* Once the midwife is satisfied that the uterus is well-contracted, she should ensure that it is emptied. With firm gentle pressure on the fundus expel residual clots. If the placenta is still in the uterus, it should be delivered by applying suprapubic pressure and controlled cord traction. If this fails, the placenta is removed manually.
5. *Bimanual compression:* If bleeding continues, bimanual compression of the uterus may be necessary in order to apply pressure to the placental site. In order to do this, the fingers of the right hand are inserted into the vagina like a cone, the hand is formed into a fist and placed into the anterior vaginal fornix, the elbow resting on the bed. The left hand is placed behind the uterus abdominally, the fingers pointing toward the cervix. The uterus is brought forward and compressed between the palm of the left hand and the fist in the vagina.
6. *Removal of the retained placenta:* If the placenta is retained by a constriction ring, it is removed manually after relaxing the ring with general anesthesia. Placenta accreta, increta and percreta require total abdominal hysterectomy. Very rarely, a totally adherent placenta that does not cause bleeding is left in situ to be absorbed during puerperium.
7. *Genital tract injuries or trauma:* If bleeding continues despite a well-contracted uterus, it may be due to trauma. In order to identify the source of bleeding, the mother must be placed in lithotomy position under good directional light. Any torn vessels identified must be clamped and ligated. Internal trauma to vagina, cervix or uterus, which may have occurred following instrumental or manipulative delivery, must be visualized through a speculum and suturing done under general anesthesia. If bleeding persists when the uterus is well-contracted and no evidence of trauma can be found, uterine rupture must be suspected. This needs repair following laparotomy or hysterectomy.
8. *Blood coagulation disorders:* Postpartum hemorrhage may be the result of coagulation failure. It can occur following severe preeclampsia, antepartum hemorrhage, amniotic fluid embolism, intrauterine death or sepsis. Transfusion of fresh blood is usually the best treatment, as this will contain platelets and coagulation factors. Fresh frozen plasma and fibrinogen are also transfused.

Observations of the mother following postpartum hemorrhage the woman will usually remain in the labor ward until her condition is stable. This allows her progress to be monitored closely.

Once bleeding is controlled, the total volume lost must be estimated as accurately as possible. Pulse and blood pressure are recorded every 15–30 minutes and temperature every 4 hours. The uterus must be palpated frequently to ensure that it remains well-contracted. IV fluid replacement must be carefully monitored. Monitoring of central venous pressure, fluid intake and output are done hourly and recorded. All records should be meticulously completed. Continued vigilance will be required for 24–48 hours.

Secondary postpartum hemorrhage
Secondary postpartum hemorrhage is bleeding from the genital tract more than 24 hours after delivery of the placenta and may occur up to 6 week later. It is most likely to occur between 10 and 14 days after delivery. Bleeding is usually due to retention of a fragment of the placenta or membranes, or the presence of blood clots. Subinvolution, infection and estrogen withdrawal following its use for suppression of lactation have also been identified as causes.

Clinical manifestations
1. The lochia are heavier than normal and recurrence of bright red flow.
2. Offensive lochia, if infection is a contributory factor.
3. Subinvolution of uterus.
4. Pyrexia and tachycardia.

Management
1. Massage the uterus if it is still palpable to bring about a contraction.
2. Express any clots.
3. Encourage the mother to empty her bladder.
4. Give an oxytocic drug such as ergometrine by IV or IM route.
5. Save all pads and linen to assess the volume of blood loss.
6. If retained products of conception are not seen on an ultrasound scan, the mother may be treated conservatively with antibiotic therapy and oral ergometrine.
7. If bleeding persists an exploration of the uterine cavity under general anesthesia and a blunt curettage is done. The material obtained by curettage is to be subjected to histopathological examination, if a choriocarcinoma is suspected.
8. Anemia is treated with iron supplement and in severe cases, blood is transfused.

Hematoma Formation

Postpartum hemorrhage may also be concealed because of hematoma formation. These form at sites such as the perineum, lower vagina, the broad ligament or vault of the vagina. A large volume of blood (up to 1 L) may collect insidiously. Involution of the uterus and lochia are usually normal. The main symptom is increasingly severe pain. The hematoma has to be drained in the operating room under general anesthetic. Secondary infection is a high possibility and broad-spectrum antibiotics are generally administered.

NURSING PROCESS DURING THE THIRD STAGE

Assessment

1. Determine that normal third stage progress is occurring:
   a. Rhythmic contractions until the placenta is born.
   b. Birth of placenta occurs 5–30 minutes after birth of the baby.
   c. Signs of placental separation are seen:
      - Fundus rises slightly in abdomen
      - Uterus changes in shape
      - Umbilical cord lengthens
      - Slight gush of blood noted.
   d. Placental expulsion occurs:
      - Schultz mechanism
      - Duncan mechanism.
   e. Following birth of placenta, the uterine fundus remains firm and is located two fingerbreadths below the umbilicus.
   f. The mother may experience chills or shivering.
2. Assess maternal blood pressure following birth of the baby.
3. Assess status of the uterus: Contractions will continue until birth of the placenta.
4. Assess the newborn Apgar score and complete newborn assessment.
5. Examine placenta to document that all cotyledons and membranes are present.

Analysis/Nursing Diagnosis

- Anxiety related to knowledge deficit regarding postpartum changes
- Pain related to altered perineal skin/tissue integrity
- Fatigue related to labor and delivery process
- Risk for ineffective individual coping related to delivery process
- Self-care deficit related to fatigue.

Planning

1. Complete initial assessment of the newborn.
2. Monitor maternal and newborn status.
3. Provide support in parental newborn interactions.
4. Provide support and comfort measures during the third stage.

Implementation

1. Observe and record birth of placenta.
2. Monitor maternal blood pressure.
3. Dry the baby completely.
4. Complete initial newborn assessments.
5. Provide initial newborn care:
   a. Provide warmth
   b. Prevent infection
   c. Promote mother-baby attachment.
6. Administer oxytocic drugs as per physician's order.

Evaluation

1. See that the newborn establishes and maintains adequate respiratory pattern.
2. Be sure that mother and newborn maintain normal physical parameters.
3. Monitor mother-baby attachment/bonding.
4. Make sure that mother feels comfortable and supported during the third stage.

STUDY QUESTIONS

Short Notes

1. Signs of placental separation.
2. Steps of expectant management for delivering the placenta.

Short Answer Questions

1. Mechanism of hemostasis following placental separation.
2. Examination of placenta and membranes.
3. Factors that can lead to primary postpartum hemorrhage.

Essay Questions

1. Explain the physiological processes of placental separation and expulsion.
2. Describe the care of the mother and management in the third stage of labor.
3. Describe the management of a mother who has developed primary postpartum hemorrhage.

BIBLIOGRAPHY

1. Helen V. Nurse midwifery, 2nd edition. Boston: Jones and Bartlett Publishers; 1996. pp. 277-310.
2. Klaus M, Kennell JH. Maternal-Infant Bonding. St Louis: Mosby; 1976.
3. Ladipo OA. Management of third stage of labour, with particular reference to reduction of feto-maternal transfusion. British Medical Journal. 1972;1(5802):721-3.
4. Levy V, Moore J. The midwife's management of the third stage of labour. Nursing Times. 1985;81(39):47-50.
5. McDonald S. Physiology and management of the third stage of labor. In: Bennett RV, Linda KB (Eds). Myles Textbook for Midwives, 13th edition. Edinburgh: Churchill Livingston; 1999. pp. 465-88.
6. Oliver CM, Oliver GM. Gentle birth: its safety and its effect on neonatal behavior. Journal of Obstetrics, Gynecology & Neonatal Nursing. 1978;7(5):35-40.
7. Phillips CR. The essence of birth without violence. MCN American Journal of Maternal Child Nursing. 1976;1(3):162-3.

CHAPTER 22

Management of the Fourth Stage of Labor

Learning Objectives

Upon completing this chapter, the learner will be able to:
- Explain the physiological changes during the fourth stage of labor.
- Describe the nursing actions required in the fourth stage of labor.
- Describe the observations and checks to be done on the mother.

The fourth stage of labor begins with the birth of the placenta and ends 1 hour later. This stage marks the completion of the tasks associated with the first three stages of labor. The mother may have expressions of relief and accomplishment, intermingled with excitement.

EVALUATION AND INSPECTION

The first postpartal hour is a critical time of initial recovery from the stress of labor and delivery, and requires close observations of the mother. A portion of this hour will be spent in activities directly related to the intrapartal period. These activities may include the following:
1. Evaluation of the uterus.
2. Inspection and evaluation of the perineum, vagina and cervix.
3. Inspection and evaluation of the placenta, membranes and umbilical cord.
4. Repair of episiotomy and laceration, if any.

In addition to these, vital signs and other physiologic manifestations are checked and evaluated as indicators of recovery from the stress of labor. This period is the beginning of family relationships and mother-baby bonding. The mother, and perhaps father, may want to see, hold and fondle the baby. Facilitation of this phase and encouraging the mother's participation in it are vital to the bonding process. Continuing evaluation of the baby's vital signs and physiologic manifestations are important, and should be ongoing during the fourth stage of labor. Evaluation of the baby is discussed in Chapter 39: Baby at Birth.

Evaluation of the Uterus

After delivery of the placenta, the uterus is normally found in the midline of the abdomen approximately two-thirds to three-fourths of the way up between the symphysis pubis and umbilicus. A uterus found above the umbilicus is indicative of blood clots inside, which need to be expressed and expelled. A uterus found above the umbilicus and to one side, usually the right side indicates a full bladder. In such an instance, the bladder must be emptied. A full bladder displaces the uterus from its position and prevents its contracting as it should, thereby allow a greater amount of bleeding.

The uterus should be firm to touch. A soft, boggy uterus is a hypotonic uterus that is not contracting as it should and therefore, more bleeding is occurring than should be. Uterine atony is the major cause of immediate postpartum hemorrhage. A firm uterus is indicative of effective uterine hemostasis.

Hemostasis

Uterine hemostasis occurs as a result of the interplay of certain physiological processes:
1. Retraction of the oblique uterine muscle fibers in the upper uterine segment through which the tortuous blood vessels intertwine. When contracted the entwining muscle fibers in the myometrium serve as ligatures to the open blood vessels at the placental site and bleeding is controlled (**Figs. 22.1A and B**). It is the absence of oblique fibers in the lower uterine segment that contributes to increased blood loss following placental separation in placenta previa.
2. The vigorous uterine contraction that occurs following separation of placenta brings the walls into apposition exerting further pressure on the placental site.
3. The third mechanism that contributes to the achievement of hemostasis is the transitory activation of the coagulation and fibrinolytic system during and immediately following

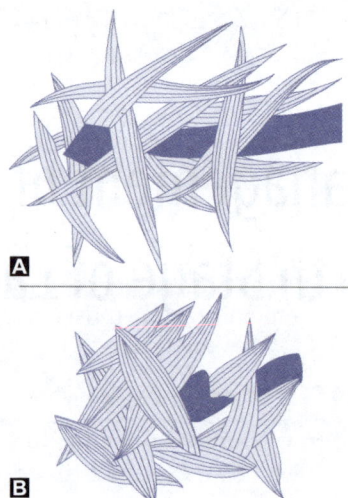

Figures 22.1A and B: Diagrammatic representation of clamping of blood vessels by the contracting muscle fibers.

placental separation. This protective response is especially active at the placental site, so that clot formation in torn vessels is intensified.

Inspection of the Cervix and Upper Vaginal Vault

The cervix and upper vaginal vault must be inspected in the presence of any (or a combination) of the following indications:
1. The uterus is well-contracted, but there continues to be a steady trickle or flow of blood from the vagina.
2. The mother was pushing prior to complete dilatation of the cervix.
3. The labor and delivery were rapid and precipitous.
4. There was manipulation of the cervix during labor such as manually pushing back an edematous anterior lip of cervix.
5. Traumatic procedures were necessary such as forceps application.
6. Traumatic second stage of delivery such as prolonged shoulder dystocia or large baby.

Following normal, spontaneous, vaginal deliveries, if none of these indications is present, it is not necessary to do a cervical and upper vaginal vault inspection. However, some obstetricians advocate routine inspection of these structures in order to rule out the possibility of a cervical laceration as the cause, if the woman bleeds excessively after an hour or two after the delivery.

Inspection and Evaluation of the Placenta, Membranes and Umbilical Cord

Inspection and evaluation of the placenta, membranes and umbilical cord are done before repairing any laceration or an episiotomy. This is because, if during the examination of the placenta, the midwife determines that the uterus needs to be explored manually because of a retained placental fragment, it needs to be done as soon as possible since it has the potential for causing hemorrhage.

Repairs

The repair of any laceration or an episiotomy is done after the examination of the placenta and membranes. If a uterine exploration for retained placental fragments is necessary, it is done prior to the repair. The uterus is checked again for consistency and repair is begun.

Perineal Cleansing and Positioning of Legs

When all the inspections and repairs if necessary, are completed the midwife must recheck the uterus for consistency, watch the effect of uterine massage on the amount of vaginal blood flow and express any blood clots. The next nursing action is to wash off the mother's entire perineal area including the perineum, vulva, inner thighs, buttocks and the rectal area.

A perineal pad is then placed against the perineum and the mother assisted to put her legs together. If the woman was in lithotomy position it is important to remove both legs from the stirrups at the same time in order to avoid undue back strain and discomfort, which may occur if one leg is down and the other is still up in a stirrup. It is also helpful to have put her legs together, while they still are in the air with the midwife supporting them and bicycle them down with help to a resting position. This stimulates circulation to the legs, and makes the transition of position less abrupt and more comfortable.

■ CONTINUING CARE AND MONITORING

Throughout the remainder of the fourth stage of labor the mother's vital signs, uterus, bladder, lochia and perineum are monitored and evaluated. This monitoring is maintained until all are stabilized within normal range. The technique of monitoring should be organized and include the following:
1. Vital signs check
2. Palpation of the fundus of the uterus for contractility
3. Massage of the fundus, and expression of clots and free blood from the uterus
4. Measurement of the fundus in relation to the umbilicus
5. Inspection of the perineum for discoloration and swelling
6. Inspection of the bladder
7. Inspection of the perineal pad and change, if necessary
8. Offering food and fluids if allowed and comfort and safety measures.

Vital Signs

The mother's blood pressure, pulse and respirations are evaluated every 15 minutes until stable at prelabor levels. The temperature is taken at least once during the fourth stage of labor. The temperature continues to be elevated with normal being less than 2°F increase or below 100.4°F (38°C).

In assessing the blood pressure and pulse rate, it must be remembered that the excitement after delivery may cause an elevation in some mothers. Injection of oxytocic drugs may also cause some women to experience elevated blood pressure and pulse rate. The optimum postpartum blood pressure and pulse rate is that, which most closely approximates the mother's blood pressure and pulse rate prenatally, provided these were within normal limits at that time.

A common complaint of mothers after delivery of the baby and placenta is a feeling of chill (the postpartum chill). It often occurs, while the mother is being prepared for transfer from the recovery room, while she is being transferred or immediately after transfer. The mother actually shakes as a manifestation of chill. The chill and the overt shaking usually do not last over 15 minutes. Some of the hypotheses regarding the cause of the chill are the following:

1. The mother's nervous reaction and exhaustion related to childbearing.
2. An aftermath of and due to release of nervous tension and energy output during labor and delivery.
3. The muscular exertion during labor and delivery cause disequilibrium between the external and internal body temperature.
4. The sudden release of intra-abdominal pressure after the uterus is emptied.
5. Previous maternal sensitization to elements of fetal blood, as well as maternal fetal transfusions at the time of delivery causing a reaction in the mother manifested as chills.

Whether this reaction is emotional, physiological or an interaction of the two, the midwife can be helpful by reassuring the mother that chills are not uncommon after delivery and that it will quickly pass. Comfort measures should be provided and include warm blankets, gown and warm fluids by mouth if not contraindicated.

Palpation of the Fundus of Uterus for Contractility

During the fourth stage of labor, the uterus continues to contract and relax. The uterus controls postpartum hemorrhage by contracting and compressing the patent blood vessels at the site, where the placenta was implanted. Therefore, the immediate precaution to postpartum hemorrhage is sustained contraction of the uterus.

Medications such as ergometrine, Methergine, Pitocin or Syntocinon may have been given to the mother intramuscularly or intravenously during the delivery of the anterior shoulder or immediately after the placenta is delivered. These medications stimulate uterine contractions, the effect of which may last several hours. Oxytocics work well in the prevention of uterine atony—the most common cause of postpartum hemorrhage. However, the tone of the uterus is dependent on many factors other than whether the mother has had oxytocics. Contractions of the uterus occur when the mother hears her newborn baby's cry or when she can see or hold the baby. These contractions are brought about by the sympathetic nervous system, which is activated by the mothers' emotions. In some hospitals, the baby is put to breast on the delivery table. This action tends to cause the uterus to contract and is prophylactic to postpartum hemorrhage.

The fundus of the uterus is palpated by placing the side of one hand on top of, and slightly cupped above the fundus, while the other hand is placed suprapubically with the exertion of slight pressure. Ideally, the fundus should lie on the midplane of the pelvis at or below the umbilicus (**Fig. 22.2**).

Massage of the Uterus and Expression of Clots

If the fundus is found boggy on palpation, it is massaged until it contracts and becomes firm. Care must be taken not to over massage or overstimulate the fundus. Overstimulation can result in undue muscle fatigue with subsequent relaxation of the organ and possible hemorrhage.

Expression of the fundus is done by utilizing the same maneuvers as shown in **Figure 22.2**. In addition, during expression, pressure is applied to the fundus with one hand, while equal pressure is applied suprapubically with the other hand. Expression is done in sequential 3–5 seconds, with several seconds rest between, until the nurse is sure that clots and free blood held in the uterus is expressed sufficiently. After palpation, massage and expression have been completed, the uterus usually stays firm for a period. However, there is always possibility that it may not remain contracted. If there is any doubt in the midwife's mind regarding the tone of the uterus or if during the check it is believed that bleeding and clotting is heavier than what it should be, the nurse should repeat the maneuvers more frequently than the suggested every 15 minutes and notify the physician.

Measurement of the Fundus

A measurement of the height of the fundus is taken after the fundus is expressed, measuring from the top of the fundus to the umbilicus using fingerbreadths. The fundus of the uterus tends to lie closer to the umbilicus in mother's who are multiparous than in those who are primiparous. Some factors, which affect the size, placement and muscular tone of the uterus include presence of antepartum hydramnios, multiple births, uterine inertia during labor, effects of oxytocic and the amount of urine in the bladder.

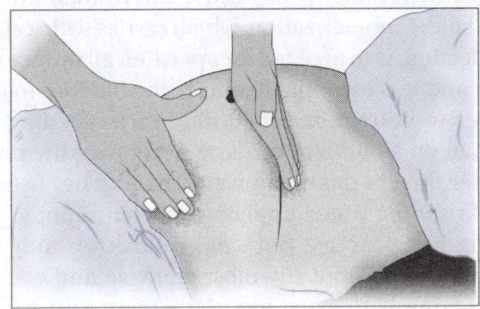

Figure 22.2: Hand maneuver involved in palpation of the fundus of uterus.

Inspection of the Perineum

Perineal discomfort is a common complaint of mothers during the 1st hour postpartum, particularly after the period of time during which the anesthetic used for perineal repair loses its effect. Some physicians order an ice bag placed to the perineum for several hours postpartum. The cold lessens the edema in the episiotomy area and tends to numb the area, so that the mother's discomfort is not as pronounced. This is especially useful if there has been extensive repair, such as third or fourth degree perineal repair or repair of an exceptionally sensitive area such as the clitoris. If chemical perineal 'ice' packs are not available, adequate ice packs can be created by putting crushed ice in a rubber glove or a sandwich bag. All ice packs should be covered with some form of clean cloth before being placed on the perineum.

While inspecting the perineal area, during the postpartum check, the nurse may observe swelling or ecchymosis. This is indicative of the formation of a perineal or perineal-vaginal hematoma. The midwife can make a positive nursing diagnosis of a hematoma by touching the area *very lightly* with sterile gauze or with the patient's perineal pad. If the swelling is more than edema and is in fact the beginning of a hematoma, the mother will complain of extraordinary tenderness when touched. The physician should be notified immediately. A hematoma should not be left unattended for it may continue to enlarge, causing the mother increasing pain. Continued extravasations can lead to circulatory shock.

Inspection of the Bladder (Fig. 22.3)

The bladder must be evaluated and emptied if it is full and displacing the uterus. In the event that the bladder is filling or full, a bladder bulge will be evident. It feels and appears as a spongy, fluid-filled mass below the uterus and above the symphysis pubis. A hypotonic bladder with urinary retention and bladder enlargement is common. This is due to trauma caused by pressure and compression placed on the bladder and urethra during labor and delivery. It is important for the bladder to be emptied, because a full bladder displaces the uterus and decreases its ability to contract properly. A poorly contracted uterus increases the amount of bleeding and the severity of after pains. On examination, the uterus can be seen elevated in the pelvis and displaced from the midline.

Bladder hypotonicity may cause the woman not to feel a desire to void. Catheterization, which carries with it significant risk of infection, is to avoided except when all inducements to void fail, and it is essential to empty the bladder in order for the uterus to better contract and reduce bleeding. Putting the woman on a bedpan, running water over the perineum, having her fingers dabble in water, having her listen to the sound of running water, applying light suprapubic pressure or having her practice perineal relaxation may work in getting her to void, but the most effective and comfortable method is simply to assist her to the bathroom. There is no contraindication to walking with assistance at this time, if she is not heavily medicated, did not have spinal anesthesia or has not had an excessive blood loss.

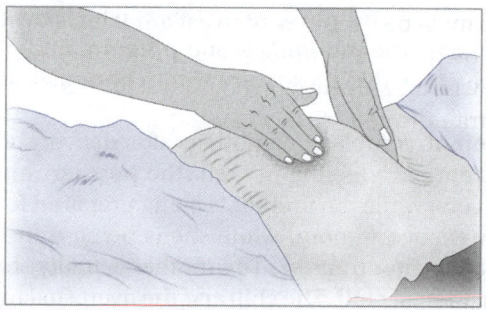

Figure 22.3: Palpation of a full bladder on a postpartum client.

Inspection and Change of Perineal Pad

It is not necessary to perform any particular type of perineal care during the 1st hour postpartum except to keep the area as clean and dry as possible. Regular change of perineal pad and linens under her buttocks is required in order to keep the lochia from becoming dry and adhering to mother's body. It is necessary to wash the perineal area and buttocks with mild soap and water to remove lochia not absorbed by the perineal pad.

When checking the perineal pads for lochia, the mother is rolled on her side, so that the midwife can better determine the amount of bleeding. The lochia is prone to collect under the buttocks and is obscured from sight if the patient is not turned on her side during the check.

The lochia during the fourth stage of labor is rubra, neither dark red nor bright red. Normally it has a fleshy odor, similar to that of fresh blood. The lochia consist of blood from the placental site, shreds of membranes, vernix, lanugo, decidua and meconium. Size and consistency of lochial clots are to be observed and noted in the chart. If the midwife has any doubt as to whether the clots contain placental tissue, they should be saved for inspection by the physician.

A constant bright red trickle of lochia from the vagina in the presence of a contracted uterus is an indication of fresh bleeding. This is the result of cervical or vaginal laceration or both. The physician is to be notified immediately, so that the laceration can be repaired as soon as possible.

If the bleeding is more than normal, the midwife must keep a perineal pad count, so that the estimation of blood loss is more accurate. Notations must be made in the mother's chart of how many pads were used, the degree of saturation of each pad, the size and character of clots and the color of lochia.

Fluids and Food

Any previous nausea and vomiting should have subsided and the mother most likely will be thirsty, and if all is progressing normally, she should be encouraged to take water, juices and tea or coffee with sugar. After her condition has stabilized within the limits of normal, which will usually be by the end of the 1st hour postpartum, she may also eat solid foods.

Mothers must be encouraged to eat a small amount first and to eat slowly. Comfort measures should be supplied and include warm blankets, gown and warm fluids by mouth if not contraindicated.

USE OF OXYTOCIC DRUGS

Oxytocic drugs stimulate uterine contractions. A number of factors should be considered in using oxytocics during the immediate postpartum period. They include determination of the need, action and effect, and dosage and route.

Determination of the Need

Determination of whether or not there is a need for an oxytocic drug is based on the following:
1. Uterine consistency: The uterus should be well-contracted, feeling firm and hard to touch in the immediate postpartum period.
2. Potential for the uterus to relax even if it is presently firm. A uterus is more likely to relax if:
   a. It has been overdistended due to multiple gestation, polyhydramnios or large baby.
   b. The patient had a Pitocin induction or augmentation.
   c. Labor and delivery have been rapid and precipitous.
   d. The patient is a grand multipara.
   e. There is a history of uterine atony during previous childbearing experience.
   f. The first and second stages of labor were prolonged.
3. Whether or not the membranes were delivered completely.
4. Whether or not the mother initiates breastfeeding immediately.

Action and Effect

The action and effect of different oxytocic drugs must be considered. The synthetic forms of oxytocin such as Pitocin and Syntocinon stimulate intermittent contractions. They have little or no effect on the blood pressure if given intramuscularly or added to intravenous (IV) fluids. These are the drugs of choice in most situations.

The natural and synthetic ergot preparations—Ergotrate and Methergine respectively—stimulate a sustained, tetanic contraction. Both of these drugs potentiate a hypertensive condition and may cause blood pressure increase in normotensive women because of their vasoconstrictive effect. However, of the two drugs, Methergine causes lesser elevation. Therefore, if the woman is bleeding excessively due to atony of uterus (which indicates a need for a drug that will stimulate a sustained contraction), but there is concern for a possible hypertensive effect, Methergine would be the drug of choice.

Drugs with the action of stimulating intermittent contractions may be used to supplement those effecting a sustained contraction by adding them to an IV infusion, which will last overtime or may be used by themselves when the bleeding is not excessive, but the uterus has a tendency to relax.

Dosage and Route

The standard single dose for each oxytocic drug is as follows:
1. Ergotrate (ergometrine):
   a. Injection: 0.2 mg (1 cc)
   b. Tablets: 0.2 mg per tablet.
2. Methergine (methylergonovine):
   a. Injection: 0.2 mg (1 cc)
   b. Tablets: 0.2 mg per tablet.
3. Pitocin injection: 10 USP units (1 cc).
4. Syntocinon injection: 10 USP units (1 cc).

The use of oxytocic drugs is invaluable in controlling postpartal uterine bleeding. The desired action, however, can be obtained rapidly by way of intramuscular route for the ergot preparations or by way of intramuscular or diluted IV infusion routes for the synthetic oxytocic drugs. *At no time should any of these drugs be given IV push (direct IV administration) because of the danger of cardiovascular complications.*

SUMMARY OF POSTPARTUM MANAGEMENT

The 1st hour postpartum is of critical importance to the well-being of the newly delivered mother. The uterus continues to relax and contract just as it did during the first three stages of labor. The newly delivered mother is a biopsychosocial being. Consequently, nursing care appropriate to the integration of these components must be rendered.

NURSING PROCESS DURING THE FOURTH STAGE OF LABOR

Assessment

1. *Physical assessment:* Determine that fourth stage is progressing within normal limits:
   a. Blood pressure returns to prelabor state.
   b. Pulse is slightly lower than in labor.
   c. Fundus remains contracted in the midline and is located 1-2 fingerbreadths below the umbilicus.
   d. Lochia is scant to moderate.
   e. Bladder is nonpalpable.
   f. Perineum is intact.
2. *Psychosocial assessment:*
   a. Assess the mother's emotional state. May vary from exhaustion to euphoria.
   b. Some mothers may want to interact with their baby, and others may wish to rest at this time.

Nursing Diagnosis

- Pain related to perineal injury
- Fatigue related to deprivation of rest and sleep
- Altered nutrition related to prolonged labor and delivery process

- Anxiety related to care of baby and self
- Risk for altered homeostasis related to blood loss and fluid intake.

Planning

1. Frequent assessments to monitor maternal recovery from delivery.
2. Enhance maternal-newborn attachment.
3. Teach self-care measures to prevent bleeding and enhance comfort.

Implementation

1. Complete maternal assessment every 15 minutes for the 1st hour, every 30 minutes for the 2nd hour and then hourly for the next 2 hours.
2. Provide comfort measures:
   a. Provide warm blankets and/or hot drinks for shivering or chilling.
   b. Place ice packs on perineum to decrease swelling and increase comfort.
   c. Carry out perineal cleansing.
   d. Offer sponge bath.
   e. Provide clean linen.
3. Massage and express fundus.

Evaluation

Ensure that the mother:
1. Has physical parameters monitored at frequent intervals.
2. Had uneventful recovery period and does not develop complications.
3. Has opportunity to interact with newborn as desired.
4. Can demonstrate fundal massage and practice comfort measures.

STUDY QUESTION

Essay Question

1. Describe the continuing assessment and nursing care of a mother in the fourth stage of labor.

BIBLIOGRAPHY

1. Helen V. Nurse Midwifery, 2nd edition. Boston: Jones and Bartlett Publishers; 1996. pp. 377-86.
2. Klaus M, Kennell JH. Maternal-Infant Bonding. St Louis: Mosby; 1976.
3. Ladipo OA. Management of third stage of labour, with particular reference to reduction of feto-maternal transfusion. British Medical Journal. 1972;1:721-3.
4. Levy V, Moore J. The midwife's management of the third stage of labour. Nursing Times. 1985;81(39):47-50.
5. McDonald S. Physiology and management of the third stage of labor. In: Bennett BV, Linda KB (Eds). Myles Textbook for Midwives, 13th edition. Edinburgh: Churchill Livingstone; 1999. pp. 475-8.
6. Oliver CM, Oliver GM. Gentle birth: its safety and its effect on neonatal behavior. Journal of Obstetrics, Gynecology & Neonatal Nursing. 1978;7(5):35-40.
7. Phillips CR. The essence of birth without violence. MCN American Journal of Maternal Child Nursing. 1976;1(3):162-3.

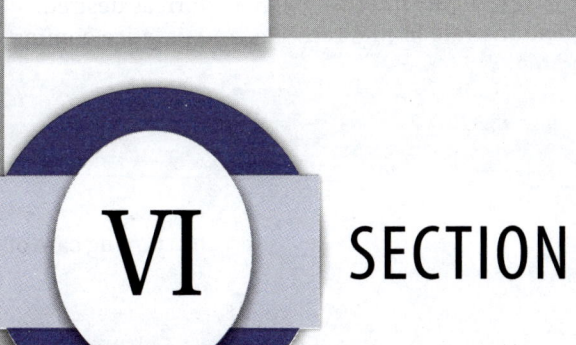

SECTION VI

NORMAL PUERPERIUM

Section Outline

23. Physiology and Management of the Normal Puerperium
24. Family Planning

CHAPTER 23

Physiology and Management of the Normal Puerperium

Learning Objectives

Upon completing this chapter, the learner will be able to:
- Discuss the anatomical and physiological changes of the puerperium.
- Describe the physical signs, symptoms and discomforts in the puerperal period.
- Describe the postnatal assessment as a basis for exploring normal physiology and potential complications.
- Enumerate the responsibilities of the midwife in care management of postnatal clients.

DEFINITION

Puerperium is the period following childbirth during which the body tissues, especially the pelvic organs, revert approximately to the prepregnant state both anatomically and physiologically. The retrogressive changes are mostly confined to the reproductive organs with the exception of the mammary glands, which show features of activity.

DURATION

The puerperium (postpartal period) is the time from the delivery of the placenta and membranes to the return of the woman's *reproductive tract to its nonpregnant condition and lasts for approximately 6 weeks*. The woman progressing through the puerperium is called puerpera. The postpartum period is arbitrarily divided into:
1. *Immediate—the first 24 hours.*
2. *Early—up to 7 days.*
3. *Remote—up to 6 weeks.*

ANATOMICAL AND PHYSIOLOGICAL CHANGES OF THE PUERPERIUM

The term *involution* is used to refer to the *retrogressive changes taking place* in all of the organs and structures of the reproductive tract.

Uterus

Immediately following delivery, the uterus becomes firm and retracted with alternate hardening and softening. It weighs approximately *1,000 g and measures 15 × 12 × '8 to 10' cm* in length, width and thickness, respectively. This is roughly about two to three times the size of the nonpregnant, multiparous uterus. Subsequently, the uterus weights approximately 500 g by the end of the first postpartal week, 300–350 g by the end of the second week, *100 g by the 6th postpartal week* and its usual non-pregnant weight of 60 g by the 8th week postpartum. This rapid decrease in size is reflected in the changing location of the uterus as it descends out of the abdomen and *returns to being a pelvic organ. Immediately after delivery, the top of the fundus is approximately two-thirds to three fourths of the way up between the symphysis pubis and the umbilicus*. It then rises to the level of the umbilicus *within a few hours*. It remains at approximately the level of or *one fingerbreadth below the umbilicus for a day then involutes at the rate of 1–2 cm/day (one fingerbreadth per day) and then* gradually descends into the pelvis, being abdominally nonpalpable above the symphysis pubis after *the 10th day*. The uterine descend is illustrated in **Figure 23.1**.

If at any postpartal time, the top of the fundus is above the umbilicus, the following should be considered—filling of the uterus with blood or blood clots in the early postpartal hours or displacement of the uterus by a distended bladder especially if also displaced to the right upper quadrant.

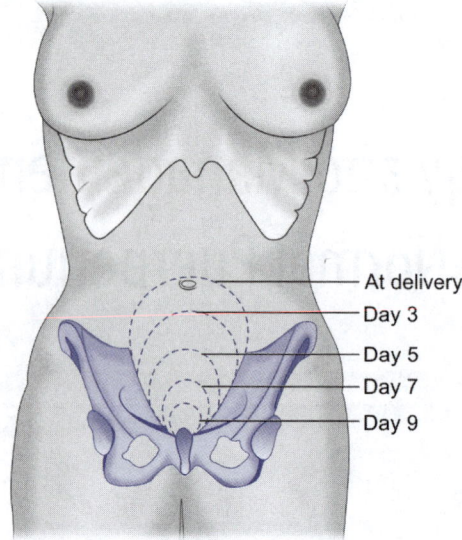

Figure 23.1: Fundal height and uterine involution.

Involution of the uterus involves the reorganization and shedding of the decidua/endometrium and the exfoliation of the placental site as evidenced by the decrease in size and weight and change in location of the uterus and by the color and amount of the lochia. Involution is hastened if the mother is breastfeeding.

The placental site contracts rapidly presenting a raised surface, which measures about 7.5 cm. It remains elevated even at 6 weeks, when it measures about 1.5 cm. By this time, complete regeneration of the endometrium at the placental site takes place.

The blood vessels degenerate and become obliterated followed by thrombosis. New blood vessels grow inside the thrombi.

Cervix

Immediately after delivery, the cervix is extremely soft, flabby and floppy. It may be bruised and edematous, especially anteriorly if there was an anterior lip during labor. It looks congested and readily admits two to three fingers. The cervix contracts slowly, the external os admits two fingers for a few days and by the end of 1st week, narrows down to admit the tip of a finger only. The contour of the cervix takes longer time to regain (6 weeks) and the external os never reverts to the nulliparous state.

The broad and round ligaments, which accompanied the uterus during its increase in size, are now lax because of the extreme stretching. This accounts for the easy displacement of the uterus by the bladder. By the end of the puerperium, the ligaments regain their nonpregnant length and tension.

Lochia

Lochia is the name given to the uterine discharge that escapes vaginally during the puerperium. As it changes color, it changes its descriptive name, i.e. rubra, serosa and alba.

Lochia rubra is red, as it contains blood. It is the first lochia that starts immediately after delivery and continues for the first 3–4 days postpartum. Lochia rubra contains primarily blood and decidual tissue.

Lochia serosa is the next lochia. It is paler than lochia rubra and is serous and pink, as it contains fewer red blood cells (RBCs) but more leukocytes, wound exudates, decidual tissue and mucus from the cervix. Lochia serosa lasts for 5–9 days.

Lochia alba is the last lochia. It starts about the 10th postpartum day and dwindles to nothing in about a week or so (10–15 day). It is pale, creamy white and consists primarily of leukocytes, decidual cells and mucus.

Lochia has a characteristic odor, which is heavy but not offensive. The odor is strongest in the lochia serosa. It is still stronger if mixed with perspiration and must be carefully differentiated from a foul odor indicative of infection.

Lochia begins as a heavy discharge in the early postpartum hours. Subsequently, it decreases to a moderate amount as lochia rubra, a small amount as lochia serosa and a scant amount as lochia alba. It is common for a woman to have small amount of lochia, while lying down and to flood when she gets out of bed. This occurs because the discharge pools in the upper vaginal vault in the recumbent position and then drains out of the vagina with the positional change of standing up. Pooling may cause some clotting, particularly on the day of delivery. A slight increase in the amount or in the blood content may be seen, when the mother becomes more active and during breastfeeding. The average lochial discharge for the first 5–6 days is estimated to be approximately 250 mL.

The normal duration of lochial discharge may extend up to 3 weeks. The discharge may be scanty following premature labor or may be excessive in twin delivery or hydramnios.

Vagina and Perineum

The immediate postdelivery vagina remains quite stretched may have some degree of edema and bruising, and gapes open at the introitus. In a day or so it regains enough tone that the gaping reduces and the edema subsides. It is now smooth-walled, larger than usual and lax. Its size decreases with the return of the vaginal rugae by about the 3rd postpartal week. It will always be a little larger than it was prior to the first childbirth. Perineal muscle tightening exercises will restore its tone. This can be accomplished by the end of the puerperium with daily practice. The torn hymen heals by scar formation, leaving several tissue tags called myrtiform caruncles (carunculae myrtiformes). Abrasions and lacerations of the vulva and perineum heal readily including those requiring repair.

Breasts

For the first 2 days following delivery, no further anatomic changes occur in the breasts. The secretion from the breasts called colostrum, which starts during pregnancy and becomes more abundant during this period.

Colostrum is a deep yellow, serous fluid that is alkaline in reaction. It has higher specific gravity, protein, sodium, chloride and vitamin A content than breast milk. Carbohydrates, fat and potassium content are lower than in the breast milk. It contains antibodies (immunoglobulins like IgA, IgG and IgM) and humoral factors (lactoferrin) that provide immunological defense to the newborn. Colostrum has a laxative action on the baby because of the large fat molecules in it and facilitates passage of meconium.

Physiology of Lactation

Lactation is initiated in all puerperal women normally and naturally unless effectively prohibited by a lactation suppressant. Though some secretary activity is present (colostrum) during pregnancy, it is accelerated following delivery and milk secretion actually starts on 3rd or 4th postpartum day. Around this time, the breasts become engorged, tense and tender and feel warm. In spite of a high prolactin level during pregnancy, milk secretion is kept in abeyance. The steroids estrogen and progesterone circulating during pregnancy are thought to make the breast tissues unresponsive to prolactin. When estrogen and progesterone are withdrawn following delivery of the placenta, prolactin begins its milk secretary activity in previously fully developed mammary glands. The secretary activity (lactogenesis) is enhanced by growth hormone, thyroxine, glucocorticoids and insulin.

Discharge of milk from the mammary glands (galactokinesis) depends on the suction exerted by the baby during suckling and the contractile mechanism, which expresses the milk from the alveoli into the ducts.

After initiation of lactation, its subsequent continuation is dependent on the suckling stimulus of the baby to the breast. During suckling, a conditioned reflex is set-up. The ascending impulses from the nipples cause the posterior pituitary to liberate oxytocin, which enters the circulating blood in the breasts and causes contraction of the myoepithelial cells surrounding the alveoli and ducts. The contraction of these cells expels the milk out of the alveoli, through the ductile to the lactiferous (storage) sinuses, where it is readily accessible to the baby by compression of the sinuses as the baby sucks.

The milk ejection reflex is inhibited by factors such as pain, breast engorgement or adverse psychic condition. The ejection reflex may be deficient for several days following initiation of milk secretion in some women and results in breast engorgement.

Maintenance of lactation (galactopoiesis) is achieved by the continued release of prolactin from the anterior pituitary. For maintenance of effective and continuous lactation, sucking is essential. It is not only essential for the removal of milk from the glands but also causes the release of prolactin. Secretion of milk is a continuous process unless suppressed by congestion, emotional disturbances or medication. Milk pressure reduces the rate of production and hence periodic breastfeeding is necessary to relieve the pressure, which in turn maintains the secretion.

The sucking propels the milk to final distance through the lactiferous ducts into the baby's mouth. The movement of milk from the lactiferous sinuses is called 'let-down' or 'milk ejection' and is felt by the woman as a specific event. Eventually the let-down can be triggered without the actual sucking of the baby, by the mother's simply hearing the baby cry or thinking about the baby. This is due to the influence of emotions on this mechanism. In such an event, the milk may stream from the breasts and leak on to the mother's clothing. As the demand and supply of milk stabilizes and lactation is well-established, this profuse ejection of milk from the breasts is less apt to happen.

Milk production

In the 1st postpartum week, the total amount of milk yield in 24 hours is calculated to be 60 multiplied by the number of postpartum days and is expressed in terms of milliliters. Thus, the milk yield on the 4th day is about $60 \times 4 = 240$ mL. Milk yield of 120–180 mL per feeding is usual by the end of 2nd week.

Stimulation of lactation

The methods that can be adopted during pregnancy include:

- Improving the maternal desire to breastfeed the baby through education regarding breastfeeding.

Care and Preparation of the Nipple

After delivery the mother should be encouraged to:

- Put the baby to breast as soon as possible after delivery
- Nurse the baby every 2–3 hours without missing any feeding
- Take plenty of oral fluids.

Suppression of lactation

Suppression becomes necessary if the baby is born dead, dies in the neonatal period, when the woman does not want to breastfeed her baby or if breastfeeding is contraindicated. Either hormones or mechanical means may be used to achieve suppression.

Drugs

1. Bromocriptine (Parlodel) 2.5 mg orally twice daily for 2 weeks. This inhibits prolactin secretion.
2. Ethinyl estradiol 0.05 mg twice daily for 5 days.
3. Combination of estrogen and testosterone preparation (Mixogen), intramuscularly soon after delivery.

Use of Parlodel may be associated with early return of ovulation and hormonal preparations carry the risk of thromboembolic complication.

Mechanical methods can be used effectively when lactation is to be suppressed after the establishment of milk secretion. For this the woman should:

- Stop breastfeeding
- Not express or pump out milk from breasts
- Apply a tight compression bandage or binder for 2–3 days. Analgesic tablets may be given to relieve pain.

GENERAL PHYSIOLOGICAL CHANGES (FIG. 23.2)

Vital Signs

The blood pressure should be stabilized within the realm of normal. The pulse rate is likely to be raised for a few hours after normal delivery, which settles down to normal during the 2nd day. In some mothers it may be slowed down for 1–2 days, may be due to rest, diminished fluid intake and excessive fluid excretion. The pulse rate is often unstable and often rises with afterpains or excitement. Any pulse rate above 100 during the puerperium is abnormal and may be indicative of infection or delayed postpartal hemorrhage.

Respirations should be within the realm of normal. The temperature should return to normal from its slight elevation during the intrapartal period and stabilized within the first 24 hours postpartum. There may be slight reactionary rise following delivery by 0.5°F, but comes down to normal within 12 hours. The temperature should not be above 37.2°C (99°F) within the first 24 hours. However, on the 3rd day, there may be slight rise of temperature due to breast engorgement, which should not last for more than a day.

Renal System Changes

The renal pelvis and ureters, which were stretched and dilated during pregnancy, return to normal by the end of the 4th postpartum week.

Immediately postpartum, the bladder is edematous, congested and hypotonic, which may result in overdistension, incomplete emptying and excessive urine residual, unless care is taken to encourage periodic voiding even when the woman does not feel like it. The urethra is insensitive because of trauma during labor. Unless urinary tract infection develops, the effects of trauma during labor on the bladder and urethra diminish within the first 24 hours.

Approximately 40% of postpartal women have non-pathologic proteinuria from immediately after delivery up to the 2nd day postpartum. To avoid contamination with protein-laden lochia, only 'clean catch' sample of urine should be collected for examination. A nonpathological condition of proteinuria can be assumed only in the absence of signs and symptoms of a urinary tract infection or preeclampsia. Stagnation of urine along with a devitalized bladder wall contributes to the urinary tract infection in puerperium.

There is considerable diuresis starting shortly after delivery and lasting up to 5th day postpartum. The urine output may be more than 3,000 mL/day. This is thought to be one of the means the body uses in ridding itself of the increased extracellular water (interstitial fluid) that is a normal part of pregnancy. Other routes are also used for this purpose and this is the explanation for a rather profuse perspiration that may occur during the early postpartum days.

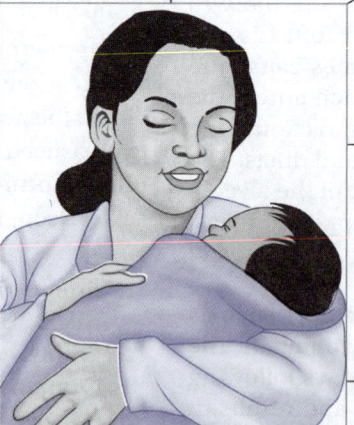

Vital signs
- Temperature may be elevated to 38° C for up to 24 hours
- BP rises early and then returns to normal
- Bradycardia occurs for first 6–10 days

Endocrine system
- ↓estrogen and progesterone levels
- ↑prolactin in lactating mothers and vice versa

Breast
Initiation of lactation

Blood and fluid changes
- Blood volume returns to its normal pre-pregnancy level by first or second week after birth
- Relative lymphopenia and an absolute eosinopenia
- Cardiac output ↑ for 24 to 48 hours postpartum and ↓ to non-pregnant values by 10 days

Digestive system
- Digestion and absorption begin to be active again soon after birth
- Bowel evacuation may be difficult because of the pain of episiotomy sutures or hemorrhoids
- Weight loss

Integumentary system
- Stretch marks in women's abdomen still appear reddened and may be even more prominent than pregnancy
- Excessive pigment on face and neck (chloasma) and on abdomen (linea nigra) barely detectable in 6 weeks' time
- Abdominal wall and ligaments require 6 weeks' time to return to their former state

Urinary system
- Renal pelvis and ureters return to normal
- The bladder wall becomes edematous and hyperemic and often shows evidence of submucous extravasation of blood
- Considerable diuresis starting shortly after delivery and lasts up to 5th day

Reproductive system
- Uterine involution
- Presence of lochia
- Cervical involution
- Resumption of normal function by the ovaries
- Menstruation returns by 6th week following delivery
- Ovulation in non-lactating mothers, ovulation occurs as early as 4 weeks and in lactating mothers about 10 weeks after delivery

Figure 23.2: Physiological changes during puerperium.

Gastrointestinal Changes

In early puerperium there is increased thirst, due to loss of fluid during labor, in the lochia, diuresis and perspiration. Women are usually hungry and ready for a regular meal an hour or two after delivery.

Constipation may be a problem in the early puerperium due to lack of solid foods during labor and self-restraint, because her perineum is sore. Lack of tone of the perineal and abdominal muscles and reflex pain in the perineal region are contributing factors for constipation.

Weight Loss

In addition to the weight loss because of the expulsion of the uterine contents, a further loss of about 2 kg (5 lb) occurs during the 1st postpartal week because of fluid loss through diuresis. Most women return to their prepregnant weight by the end of the puerperium.

Fluid Loss

There is a net fluid loss of about 2 liters during the 1st week and an additional 1.5 liters during the next 5 weeks. The amount of loss depends on the amount retained during pregnancy, dehydration during labor and blood loss during delivery.

Abdominal Wall

The abdominal striae are never eradicated completely but they do change to fine, silvery white lines. The abdominal walls are flabby after delivery because of their stretching during pregnancy. All puerperal women have some degree of diastasis recti, which is the separation of the rectus muscles of the abdomen. Women who take exercises regain their abdominal muscle tone and close the diastasis to some extent, however regaining complete muscle tone becomes difficult with increasing parity. If the abdominal wall muscle tone is not regained, the space between the rectus muscles fills in with peritoneum, fascia and fat. Subsequent pregnancies do not have the necessary muscle support, which accounts for the pendulous abdomen often seen in multiparas. The rapidity of pregnancies, where there is no time to regain the muscle tone before being into another pregnancy and over distention in conditions such as multiple gestation, also contribute to pendulous abdomen. This condition may lead to extreme back pain for the woman and difficulties with fetal engagement at the time of labor and delivery.

Hematologic Changes

Immediately following delivery, there is slight decrease of blood volume due to dehydration and blood loss. The blood volume returns to the nonpregnant level by the 2nd week. Cardiac output rises soon after delivery to about 60% above the prelabor value, but gradually returns to normal within 1 week.

Red blood cell volume and hematocrit values return to normal by the end of 1st week after the hydremia disappears. Leukocytosis to the extent of 30,000/mm^3 occurs following delivery probably in response to the stress of labor. However, the various types of possible infections should be ruled out in the presence of such finding. Platelet count decreases soon after separation of the placenta, but secondary elevation occurs with increase in platelet adhesiveness between 4 and 10 days. Fibrinogen level remains high up to the 2nd week puerperium, resulting in persistent high level of erythrocyte sedimentation rate (ESR) in puerperium as during pregnancy. A hypercoagulable state persists and fibrinolytic activity is enhanced.

Normal nonpregnant levels for all the constituents of the blood are reached by the end of the puerperium.

Menstruation and Ovulation

The onset of the first menstrual period following delivery is very variable and depends more than anything on lactation. If the woman does not breastfeed her baby, the menstruation returns by 6th week following delivery in about 40% and by 12th week in 60% of cases. If the woman breastfeeds her baby, the menstruation may be suspended in about 70% until the baby stops breastfeeding. However, menstruation may start even before cessation of breastfeeding in the remaining 30%.

In non-lactating mothers, ovulation may occur as early as 4 weeks and in lactating mothers about 10 weeks after delivery. Thus, lactation provides a natural method of contraception and contributes to spacing of pregnancies. However, ovulation may precede the first menstrual period in about one-third and it is possible for the woman to become pregnant before she menstruates following her delivery.

MANAGEMENT OF EARLY PUERPERIUM

The principles in management of postpartal clients are:
- To restore the health of the mother
- To prevent infection
- To take care of the breasts
- To motivate the mother for contraceptive acceptance.

Immediate Attention

Immediately following delivery, the mother should be closely observed as outlined in the management of the fourth stage of labor. She may be given a drink or something to eat, if she is in hungry. Measures to promote sleep must be instituted.

Rest and Ambulation

Physician's order for rest and ambulation may vary by virtue of the intrapartal course, the mother's condition, type of analgesia and anesthesia used and so on. For example, a woman who had a long, difficult labor and is exhausted, who hemorrhaged or who is still groggy from medication may be ordered bed rest for a specified period. A woman who has had spinal or epidural anesthesia may be ordered 6–8 hours flat in bed to prevent spinal headache. For a woman who entered labor rested, progressed normally and is alert, the order may be ambulate pro re nata (PRN) with assistance at first.

Each woman should be assisted and accompanied the first time she gets up and thereafter as indicated until she feels no dizziness, weak knees, light headedness or any other indication that she might faint or fall. For most women 8–10 hours of rest is sufficient after which they become fresh and can breastfeed the baby or move about. The practice of early ambulation decreases the incidence of postpartal thrombophlebitis, bladder complications and constipation. It facilitates uterine drainage and hastens involution of the uterus.

Diet

The woman may be given regular diet (normal diet) after delivery. For a woman who hemorrhaged, high-protein diet may be given to promote tissue healing. Women, who breastfeed, require high calories, adequate protein, plenty of fluids, minerals and vitamins.

Perineal Care

Routine perineal care varies from setting to setting. An elaborate washing of the perineum using sterile equipment two to three times is practiced in some settings.

At its minimum, the woman should be instructed clearly about how to cleanse herself after urination, defecation and provision of supplies and equipment made available. Basics related instructions to patients should include:

- Washing hands before and after, perineal care
- Not touching her stitch area with her fingers; if uncomfortable or concerned, she should call for help
- Wipe with wet cotton or disposable wipe from front to back across the stitches, rinse and pat dry from front to back
- Application of perineal pads snugly enough, so it would not move back and forth with movements
- Application and removal of perineal pad from front to back
- Not to touch the side of the perineal pad that will be worn next to her perineum.

Care of the Bladder

The anatomical changes described earlier necessitate extra attention to the urinary bladder, especially in the early puerperium. The woman is encouraged to pass urine 6–8 hours following delivery and thereafter at 4–6 hours interval. At times, the woman fails to pass urine due to unaccustomed position or reflex from perineal injuries. Allowing the woman to use the toilet if not contraindicated, usually serves the purpose. If measures such as running water, pouring water on her perineum and perineal relaxation fail, catheterization should be done. Catheterization is also indicated in case of incomplete emptying of the bladder evidenced by the presence of residual urine of more than 60 mL. The principle of bladder care is to ensure adequate drainage of urine, so that infection may not occur.

Care of the Bowel

The problem of constipation is much less because of early ambulation and liberalization of dietary intake. A diet containing sufficient roughage and fluids is enough to move the bowel. If necessary, mild laxatives such as milk of magnesia may be given at bedtime.

Sleep

The postpartal woman is in need of rest both physical and mental. She should be protected against undue fatigue and worries, as she is in a hypersensitive state of the nervous system. Sleep may be ensured by administering diazepam 5 mg or phenobarbitone 30–60 mg orally at bedtime. If she has discomfort due to afterpains, painful piles or engorged breasts, they should be dealt with adequate analgesics such as Aspirin with codeine orally (30–60 mg) 4–6 hours as necessary.

Care of the Breasts

The breasts should be examined daily, regardless of the chosen feeding method. Following enquiry as to any discomfort or concerns, the midwife should inspect the breasts for areas of redness. Then proceed to gently palpate the breasts to exclude areas of heat, redness or pain. The mother should be instructed to give scrupulous attention to handwashing and hygiene to prevent infection, which is a serious and painful complication of the puerperium. The nipples should be washed before each feeding, cleansed and dried after the feeding is over. A nursing brassiere provides comfortable support.

Uterus and Involution

The uterine fundus should be carefully palpated each postnatal day to ensure adequate involution. It is helpful if the woman has emptied her bladder prior to the palpation as a full bladder may make the uterine fundus appear high and deviated to one side. On palpation, the uterus should feel evenly contracted, smooth and firm and it should not be painful. Specific daily measurement of fundal descends, either by tape measure or manual palpation is done in some settings though it is of questionable value. Subinvolution is identified if the uterus remains the same size for several days. Uterine fibroids could also lead to delayed involution. Tenderness of the uterus is suggestive of infection.

Rooming-in or Bedding-in

Following a normal delivery, the baby should be kept with the mother in a cot (basinet) beside her bed or when the mother is awake in her bed. This not only establishes mother-child relationship, but the mother is conversant with the art of baby care, so that she can take full care of the baby, while at home.

Immunization

Unimmunized Rh-negative mothers, who delivered Rh-positive babies are given anti-D-gammaglobulin. Women who are susceptible to rubella infection must be vaccinated and instructed about postponement of pregnancy for at least 2 months. The booster dose of tetanus toxoid should be given at the time of discharge, if it is not given during pregnancy.

Monitoring and Charting of Postpartum Events

During the postpartum period, assessment of maternal condition must be done on a regular basis and a progress record to be maintained noting the following:
1. Blood pressure, pulse, respiration and temperature recording every 4–6 hours.
2. Measurement of the height of the uterine fundus above the symphysis pubis once a day at a fixed time with prior evacuation of the bladder and preferably the bowel too.
3. Character, color and amount of lochia.
4. Voiding and bowel movement.
5. Perineal status such as healing, edema, inflammation, hematomas and bruising.
6. Extremities for varicosities, calf tenderness and heat, edema and reflexes.

Postpartum Exercises

The objectives of postpartum exercise are:
1. To improve the tone of abdominal and perineal muscles, which were stretched during pregnancy and labor.
2. To educate the mother about correct posture in different working positions, while lifting during day-to-day activities.

Practicing the exercises would help the mother:
1. To minimize the risk of puerperal venous thrombosis by preventing venous stasis.
2. To prevent backache.
3. To prevent uterine prolapse and stress incontinence of urine.

The nursing interventions are:
1. Initially, the mother is taught *deep abdominal breathing* to strengthen the diaphragm. This may be begun on the 1st postpartum day. She is taught to take a deep breath raising her abdominal wall and exhale slowly. To ensure exercise is being done correctly, place one hand on the chest and one on the abdomen. When inhaling, the hand on the abdomen should be raised and the hand on the chest should remain stationary. Repeat the exercise five times.
2. To tone up the abdominal muscles, she may be taught head and shoulder raising exercise, leg raising exercise, pelvic tilt exercise and sit-ups:
   a. *Head and shoulder raising*: On the 2nd postpartum day, lie flat without pillow and raise head until the chin is touching the chest. On the 3rd postpartum day raise both head and shoulders off the bed and lower them slowly. Increase gradually until able to do 10 times.
   b. *Leg raising*: This exercise may be begun on the 7th postpartum day. Lying down on the floor with no pillow under the head, point toe and slowly raise one leg keeping the knee straight. Lower the leg slowly. Gradually increase to 10 times each leg. On the 9th postpartum day, slowly raise both legs together.
   c. *Pelvic tilt*: Lie flat on the floor with knees bent, inhale and while exhaling, flatten the back against the floor, so that there is no space between the back and the floor. While doing this, tighten abdominal muscles and the muscles of the buttocks.
   d. *Sit-ups*: In 2 weeks, the mother may begin sit-ups, slowly increasing the number until she is able to do at least 10 times. Lie flat on the back with hands on hips. Slowly raise head, shoulder and trunk until attaining a sitting position.
3. *Kegel exercise:* This exercise is used to strengthen and tone the muscles of the pelvic floor. The mother should be instructed to do this daily for the rest of her life. Exercise can be done lying on the floor with ankles crossed or sitting in a chair with knees apart and feet flat on the floor. Tighten the muscles around the anus as if to control a bowel movement and then tighten the muscles around the vagina and urethra as if to stop urine in midstream. Now hold these muscles tightly to the count of 6 and then relax. This exercise can be done on the 1st postpartum day. It also increases the circulation to the perineal region, hence promoting faster healing of the episiotomies.

After 2 weeks, the mother may do almost any exercise she chooses. She must be reminded that if she notices that the lochia turns bright red after she has been exercising, she should stop for a few days until the bleeding is no longer bright red. If the mother does these six exercises faithfully and follows a sensible diet, she will most likely be able to regain her figure quickly.

CONTINUING PHYSICAL ASSESSMENT AND DAILY CARE

The nurse should follow an organized method when examining the postpartum client, which provides a consistent, quality approach to nursing care. The acronym, BUBBLE-HE can serve a helpful reminder of the elements in a postpartum assessment.

BUBBLE-HE stands for:
- **Breasts**
- **Uterus**
- **Bladder**
- **Bowel**
- **Lochia**
- **Episiotomy**
- **Homans' sign**
- **Emotional status**.

The nurse should assess these elements every 8 hours along with vital signs.

Breasts

On palpation after delivery, breasts usually are enlarged, soft and warm and contain only small amount of colostrum. The nipples should be intact without redness, tenderness, cracks or blisters. Colostrum may be expressed. If the mother is not breastfeeding, the breast changes that occurred as a result of pregnancy regress in 1-2 weeks postpartum.

The mother may experience breast engorgement (enlargement and filling of the breasts with milk), which may begin as a tingling sensation in her breasts, 2-4 days after delivery. The breasts feel very full, tender and uncomfortable until the milk is released through infant sucking, manual expression or pumping. The discomfort from engorgement normally subsides once stimulation to produce milk is decreased. The nursing mother's breasts should be inspected for the presence of inverted nipples, cracks, blisters, fissures and palpated for fullness and tenderness.

For non-breastfeeding mothers, suppression can be achieved through a variety of methods that decrease simulation to the breasts such as securely binding the breasts with a snug support bra or a binder, avoiding warmth (e.g. hot shower water) on breasts and applying ice packs to the breasts. The mother may be prescribed analgesics for breast discomfort and manual expression of milk and simulation of nipples to be avoided. These methods can be used until milk production stops.

Uterus

Immediately after delivery, the uterus begins the process of involution or reduction in size. It generally takes 6 weeks for complete physiologic involution and for the reproductive system to be restored to its nonpregnant state, except for the nursing mother's breasts. Subinvolution or the failure of the uterus to return to a nonpregnant state occurs, when the process of involution is prolonged or stopped as a result of hemorrhage, infection or retained placental parts.

Uterine involution involves diminishing in size and weight, and anatomic location back into the pelvis. The endometrial decidua is shed as the lochial vaginal bleeding. By the end of 3 weeks postpartum, the endometrial lining and site of placental attachment return to a nonpregnant state. The placental site usually is completely healed without scarring by 6 weeks postpartum.

Immediately after delivery, the uterus weighs about 100 g, measuring 8-10 cm, which is two to three times of the non-pregnant size. At the end of 6 weeks postpartum, the uterus weighs 50-100 g. Breastfeeding assists in hastening the speed of uterine involution. There generally is no difference between primiparas and multiparas regarding healing time. Multiparas may have less abdominal muscle tone and their cervix does not completely return to its closed, nonpregnant appearance. The parous cervix is easily distensible and appears as a slit.

Assessment of Fundus

For assessing the location and firmness of the uterine fundus (the top portion of the uterus), the nurse should place the client in a supine position with the bed flat. Immediately after delivery, the fundus usually can be located midline at the level of or one to two fingerbreadths below the umbilicus. The fundus is approximately 1 cm below the umbilicus at 12 hours after delivery. After the 1st postpartum day, the fundus descends or involutes 1-2 cm (1 fingerbreadth) each day. The fundus becomes nonpalpable on or about 9 days postpartum, as it gradually descends into the true pelvis.

Immediately after delivery of the placenta, the fundus should be firm upon palpation. If the fundus is not firm or palpable, it may feel soft or boggy. A boggy uterus may be related to an over distended uterus or structural anomalies (e.g. fibroid uterus). A fundus that remains boggy is a warning sign of uterine atony and potential postpartal hemorrhage. Assessment will also include monitoring for risk factors for hemorrhage such as tocolytics, high parity and prolonged labor.

The position of the fundus should also be noted. An overfilled bladder easily displaces the uterus. It is palpated above the umbilicus and deviated to the right. This displacement interferes with the ability of the uterus to contract after delivery, resulting in uterine atony and hemorrhage.

Management of Bleeding

After delivery of the placenta 20-40 units of oxytocin (Pitocin) often is added to the intravenous (IV) solution if an IV line is in place, oxytocin is prescribed to hasten uterine contractility and control bleeding. When IV access is not present, other options such as administering oxytocin (10 unit) intramuscularly (IM), initiating early breastfeeding or performing nipple stimulation is employed.

When the uterus remains boggy despite massage and oxytocin administration, other reasons for bleeding must be determined. When bleeding continues, a second pharmacological agent such as methylergonovine (Methergine) 0.12 mg IM may be given to clients, who do not have a current history of high blood pressure. Another medication used for controlling bleeding is a prostaglandin called carboprost tromethamine (Hemabate), which can be given when Methergine does not stop bleeding or is contraindicated. If the fundus is firm and lochia is heavy, the nurse should suspect cervical laceration. Common causes of postpartum hemorrhage are:
- Uterine atony
- Retained placenta
- Cervical or perineal laceration
- Subinvolution and bleeding disorders.

Assessment of Uterine Pain

Abdominal cramping or afterpains are caused by uterine tonic contractions, which are the efforts of the uterus to expel blood clots and placental fragments. The contractions are enhanced with oxytocin and breastfeeding. Afterpains usually will seem more intense and occur at regular intervals in multiparous women. The cramping becomes milder after 3 days. When the pain becomes significantly more intense or the uterus tender to palpation, the nurse should assess for problems such as endometritis (an infection of the uterine lining).

Bladder

In the immediate postpartum period, the bladder is congested, edematous and hypotonic from the effects of labor. Unless a urinary tract infection is present these effects should resolve within 24 hours of delivery. Diuresis up to 3,000 mL/day occurs in the first 2-3 days postpartum due to decreasing production of aldosterone causing removal of excess fluid. In the immediate postpartum period, bladder distension, incomplete emptying and residual urine may occur due to edematous perineum, pain, reflex spasms and bladder desensitization.

Nursing responsibilities include teaching the newly delivered mother to empty the bladder often after birth to assist in controlling pain and bleeding. After delivery, the client should be assisted to the toilet the first two to three times to protect against falls due to orthostatic hypotension and dizziness. Early ambulation and comfort facilitate urination. After delivery, the client should be able to urinate within 4 hours, at least 300 mL, with complete emptying of the bladder. Complaints of urinary frequency, dysuria, retention and inability to void for 6-8 hours after delivery should be noted and informed to the physician.

After urination the fundus should be palpated for location and bladder for appropriate emptying. The bladder normally should be nonpalpable. Presence of residual urine (palpable bladder) can result in urinary infection. For clients who cannot urinate, a straight catheterization may be done after considering individual circumstances such as the degree of bladder distension, location of the displaced uterus, amount of bleeding, amount of fluid or IV intake since the last voiding and the techniques used to encourage voiding.

An indwelling catheter inserted before cesarean delivery generally is kept in place for 24 hours. For the client who cannot empty her bladder completely, an indwelling catheter may be inserted and retained for the minimum required period as it carries the risk of bacteriuria.

Bowels and Gastrointestinal System

The client's appetite typically will return to normal in 1-2 hours after delivery. If there are no complications from anesthesia, regular food may be resumed. The client who had vomited during labor may not have an appetite. She should be encouraged to increase her fluid intake. The new mother after a long and difficult labor will need food and fluids to regain her strength. Diet rich in protein and iron is needed to promote tissue healing and to restore iron levels due to blood loss.

Following vaginal delivery, bowel movement normally occurs 2-3 days later. When gastric motility does not return by 2-3 days, constipation occurs. Causes of constipation include increase in progesterone levels in late pregnancy, decreased bowel motility and fluid intake during labor, side effects of medications, and hesitancy to defecate owing to perineal discomfort. In order to avoid this problem, the client should be encouraged to drink 6-8 glasses of fluids daily and eat a high-fiber diet (e.g. whole grains, legumes, vegetables and fruits). Sitz baths, topical medications and stopping medications that cause constipation are helpful.

When constipation is severe administering an analgesic and a stool softener before ambulation may facilitate bowel movement by 2-3 days postpartum. Mineral oil, bisacodyl (Dulcolax) suppository or fleet enema (evacuant enema) may be given to stimulate intestinal activity.

Examination of the bowels includes assessment for the presence of hemorrhoids. Hemorrhoids present during pregnancy may enlarge during labor. If the hemorrhoids are large, they may cause pain if they become thrombosed and may subsequently cause constipation. Treatment with topical ointment or spray may relieve discomfort.

Lochia

The usual uterine discharge of blood, mucus and tissue after childbirth is called lochia. Lochia contains the sloughing of decidual tissues, including erythrocytes, epithelial cells and bacteria. Lochia is assessed according to its amount, color and change with activity and time.

The descriptive name of lochia changes with the change in color. Lochia rubra is the term given for the discharge in the first 3 days after delivery. Lochia rubra has bright red color and consists mainly of decidual tissue and blood.

Lochia serosa, which occurs 4-10 days after delivery, is watery, pink or brown-tinged and lesser in amount than lochia rubra. Lochia serosa primarily contains serous fluid, leukocytes, erythrocytes and decidual tissue. The lochia changes into lochia alba, a whitish-yellow creamy discharge in 10-15 days. Many women may have minimal discharge by day 14; however, it is not uncommon for lochia alba to last until 6 weeks postpartum. Lochia alba consists of a mixture of leukocytes, decidual tissue and decreasing fluid content.

When the client is bleeding heavily, the nurse needs to ensure that the bleeding is not coming from another source such as cervical or vaginal laceration. Lacerations are highly suspected when heavy bleeding continues despite a firm uterus. Saturation of a perineal pad within 15-30 minutes may indicate hemorrhage. A complete blood count (CBC) may indicate a 1.0-1.5 g/dL decrease in hemoglobin and a 3-4% decrease in hematocrit, which is consistent with a loss of 500 mL of blood.

The amount of lochia varies with position changes, but should continually decrease throughout the first 4-6 weeks postpartum. Blood pools in the vaginal vault, when the client is recumbent and drains standing up. Clot formation occurs as a result of the pooling in the uterus or vagina. An increase in bright red bleeding and the passage of clots may also occur during physical activity or breastfeeding. Lochia with a reddish color that persists after 2 weeks of delivery may indicate subinvolution of the placental site or retained placental parts.

The client should be instructed to report to the physician if blood clots larger than 1 cm are passed. Nursing actions include assessing the fundus for firmness and amount of lochia. Further examination may be required to evaluate for other sources of continued bleeding.

Lochia has a characteristic menstrual like musky or fleshy smell. A foul-smelling discharge, along with other indicators, such as fever or uterine tenderness, may suggest an infection such as endometritis. Because lochia is an excellent medium for bacterial growth, clients should be taught to change the perineal pad after each voiding.

The first menstrual period usually begins within an average of 8 weeks after delivery for most non-lactating women. The timing may be delayed from 2 to 18 months in breastfeeding mothers and ovulation may occur without the onset of first menstrual period. Thus, it is possible for a woman to become pregnant before the return of menses. Consistent, continuous breastfeeding increases prolactin levels, thus postponing the resumption of ovulation. Once breast stimulation decreases, prolactin levels decrease, and follicle-stimulating hormone (FSH) and luteinizing hormone (LH) hormone levels increase, inducing ovulation.

Episiotomy

An episiotomy is the surgical incision made to enlarge the vaginal opening for delivery of the baby's head. The episiotomy may be incised midline down the center of the perineum or mediolaterally, which extends in a diagonal angle to either the left or right side. With or without episiotomy, the perineum may suffer from lacerations during childbirth. Lacerations are classified as first, second, third or fourth degree. First degree involves only the skin and superficial structures above the muscle. Second degree extends to the perineal muscles. Third degree reaches into the anal sphincter muscles. Fourth degree continues into the anterior rectal wall.

To assess an episiotomy and condition of the perineum, it is best to have the client lie on her side, flexing her upper leg toward her hip. The nurse can then lift her buttocks examine the perineum. Using a good light source facilitates visualization of incision and for inspection. The REEDA (i.e. redness, edema, ecchymosis, discharge and approximation) scoring scale can be used when assessing the episiotomy.

Care of the vulva includes applying ice packs to the perineum, for the first 24 hours, to help decrease edema and pain. Ice packs also assist in constricting blood vessels, minimize the risk of hematoma formation and decrease muscle irritability and spasm. Ice packs should not be applied directly to the skin; they should be wrapped with an absorbent disposable type of covering.

After the first 24 hours following delivery, a sitz bath with warm water may be used to reduce the local discomfort, increase circulation and healing. Use of heat lamp or infrared lamp two to three times a day also will assist in the healing process. The client should be taught perineal hygiene, including daily washing with warm water and mild soap. The perineum should be cleansed after each voiding and bowel movement. The perineum should be wiped from front to back (anterior to posterior) to avoid contamination from the anal region. Practices such as changing the perineal pad frequently after each voiding and bowel movement or at least four times a day, removing pad from front to back and handwashing will help decrease the risk of infection. Soiled pads should be placed in appropriate disposal container. Pain should be assessed and medication provided as needed.

Immediately after delivery, the vagina appears edematous, bruised and stretchable, and may gape at the introitus. By 4th week, the vaginal rugae return. The vagina returns to its prepregnant state (except for a slightly larger size than in pregnant state) by 6–8 weeks postpartum. The nurse should reach the client how to perform perineal exercises, such as Kegel exercises to assist in restoring vaginal perineal tone and elasticity, and to help reduce urinary incontinence.

Extremities

Assessment of the extremities should include examination of varicosities, deep tendon reflexes (DTRs), tenderness and presence of edema or nodular areas on the legs. DTRs should be no greater than +1 to +2. Brisk DTRs (+3 to +4) or hyperactive reflexes are suggestive of pregnancy-induced hypertension (PIH). Pretibial or pedal edema may be present, especially in the client with PIH.

Risk factors for developing deep vein thrombosis (DVT) are severe anemia, traumatic delivery and obesity. Pain, erythema or local swelling on the legs, especially the calves may signify thrombophlebitis.

The client's legs should be assessed for sensation and mobility, when epidural anesthesia has been administered. With appropriate return of mobility, the client should be able to move her toes and lift her buttocks off the bed within 2–4 hours after discontinuation of anesthesia.

Homans' Sign (Fig. 23.3)

Assessment of Homans' sign must be done for all postpartum clients, to check for presence of thrombophlebitis. In order to perform the test, have the client straighten her legs flat on the bed. Place one hand under the knee in the popliteal region for support. Place the other hand on the foot and dorsiflex (flexing the foot toward the body) it. Presence of calf pain during sharp dorsiflexion in either foot is a sign of DVT.

Prevention of Thrombophlebitis

Clients who remain in bed up to 8 hours should perform leg exercises to prevent formation of clots (thrombus) in the legs, which can develop into thrombophlebitis or thromboembolism. A clot formed in the deep leg vein may fragment from the original clotted site and lodge in the lungs

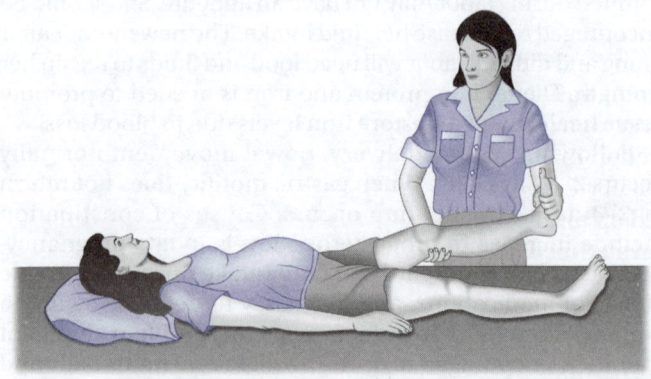

Figure 23.3: Homans' sign—check to identify thrombosis in the calf.

as pulmonary embolus, which is a serious complication. Superficial thrombophlebitis is noted as hard, painful, warm and red vein. Unlike DVT, there is little potential for pulmonary embolism with superficial thrombophlebitis.

It is important to teach clients to flex and extend both feet and legs alternatively while in bed. In a rhythmic motion, press and then relax the backs of the knees into the mattress. Clients should also be taught other ways to prevent thrombus formation, such as:

- Keeping the legs uncrossed while seated
- Not flexing the legs at the groin
- Resting the legs without putting pressure on the back of the knees
- Wearing support shoes or antiembolism stockings when varicosities are present
- Padding pressure points during lithotomy position.

Examine the calves for redness, hardness or nodules along leg veins. In addition, check the ankles and pretibial areas for edema. Assess the client for signs of pulmonary embolism such as dyspnea, cough and chest pain.

Emotional Status

The immediate postpartum period is an emotional roller coaster and almost any emotion may be observed. The nurse should be continually assessing the mother for appropriate responses to her infant. Clients often experience a sense of elation immediately after the birth of their babies. They are excited and relieved that labor is finally over. They may want to relive the experience by talking about the process of labor and delivery. However, they may also be exhausted; need sleep and rest to restore their bodies to health.

In this 'taking in phase', mother's wish to meet their own rest and nutritional needs before focusing their energy on newborns. The attainment of parental roles, infant care and family adaptations should also be assessed.

OTHER ASSESSMENTS

In addition to the basic postpartum assessments addressed in the approach using the acronym BUBBLE-HE, other important body systems need to be assessed.

Hemodynamic Status

Blood values return to normal within the first 6 weeks after delivery. A CBC may show marked leukocytosis, predominantly neutrophils, both during and after labor. The leukocyte count may increase during labor up to 25,000/mm^3 and up to 30,000/mm^3 during a prolonged labor and remain elevated for the first 2 days postpartum. The average leukocyte count is 14,000–16,000/mm^3. A possible infectious process must be ruled out in the presence of such increased counts, especially during the first 6 hours after delivery.

Hemoglobin, hematocrit and erythrocyte levels may fluctuate during the 1st postpartum days. When considerable blood loss occurs, the levels may decrease below those measured before labor. Immediately after delivery, the hematocrit level begins to rise owing to hemodilution, increase in plasma volume and dehydration. By 4–5 weeks, the hematocrit returns to normal values.

Blood coagulation normalizes a few days after delivery. Depending on the amount of blood lost during delivery, it takes 3–4 weeks for the blood volume to return to prepregnant levels. Cardiac output remains increased for at least 48 hours after delivery.

Integumentary System

The striae on breasts, thighs and abdomen eventually fade to a pale color, but may never completely disappear. Skin discolorations that appeared during pregnancy such as chloasma usually disappear toward the end of pregnancy. However, hyperpigmentation of the areolae and linea nigra may be permanent.

After giving birth, the mother may complain of profuse perspiration, especially at night, which is normal during the 1st week as the body rids itself of excess fluid from pregnancy. Some women may have a mild eruption of acne from hormonal changes. Other changes include hair loss for the first 2 months after delivery. The nurse should reassure her that this is normal owing to hormonal changes. The rapid decrease in estrogen also induces the regression of vascular abnormalities such as palmar erythema and spider angiomas.

Musculoskeletal System

Because the abdomen stretches during pregnancy, the mother's abdominal wall relaxes or becomes flaccid after delivery. When visually assessing and palpating the abdomen and fundus, the nurse may notice some degree of muscle separation, called diastasis recti, along the center of the abdomen. This separation occurs due to pressure from an enlarging uterus and may increase with each subsequent pregnancy. The severity depends on the client's general physical condition, muscle tone, timing between pregnancies, parity and other circumstances that distend the uterus and abdomen. Conditions such as multiple gestation, macrosomia and hydramnios also distend the uterus to a larger than average size, making it difficult for the client to regain her prepregnant muscle tone.

Activity

After childbirth many mothers complain of fatigue and require time to recuperate and recover from the effects of labor and delivery. Once the mother is stable, the nurse should encourage her to ambulate often. Women who deliver vaginally often are able to ambulate to the toilet within few hours of delivery.

Before rising from the bed, the client should be assessed for dizziness and motor weakness from weak knees or legs. When assisting the client in getting up from bed for the first time, the nurse should accompany her because she may experience orthostatic hypotension and be at risk of falling. When the mother is very tired or has received an epidural or analgesic that may cause drowsiness, she may not have the ability to stand and walk independently.

The client should be encouraged to return to normal activities of daily living as soon as possible. She should be able to provide independent self-care before going home. After going home she may perform light household chores depending on physician's instructions.

The client would feel better and stronger, if she ambulates early after delivery. Specific medical advantages of early ambulation are:
- Fewer bladder infections
- Less frequent constipation
- Decreased incidence of DVT
- Decreased incidence of the pulmonary embolism.

Exercise

A woman who has had an uncomplicated vaginal delivery can begin moderate exercise soon afterward. Vigorous exercise should be delayed until 6-8 weeks because joints do not stabilize earlier. She may be instructed to perform mild stretching and flexing of muscles especially abdominal muscles, which may relieve tension and muscle strain. These include deep breathing, head raising, arm raising, knee flexes and leg raising. Other safe exercises include Kegel exercises and pelvic tilts. Exercising too much and too soon may result in bright-red vaginal flow. The client must not lift anything heavier than her baby for the first 2 weeks after childbirth. She should avoid climbing stairs for 2-3 weeks.

Pain Management

After delivery, the mother is at risk for various types of discomfort. She may complain of perineal discomfort, uterine cramping, sore nipples or a headache, if she received incorrectly administered spinal anesthesia. The most common discomfort is from the *afterpains* related to uterine contractions.

Analgesics may be administered orally every 4-6 hours as needed. Emptying the bladder every 1-2 hours or so is an effective measure to relieve afterpains. Another useful method is for the client to lie on her abdomen with a pillow against her lower abdomen because this creates pressure that keeps the uterus contracted.

Topical anesthetics provide temporary relief from episiotomy pain. Ice packs and sitz baths also provide relief for the mother. When medications do not relieve complaints of perineal pain, the site should be assessed more carefully. Pain not relieved by the usual means may indicate a possible hematoma. Episiotomy pain normally is relieved by 3 weeks.

Sexuality

Mothers must be instructed to avoid sexual activity until their episiotomy has healed, which may take 6 weeks or more, or until they are comfortable and desire to have sex. Because of perineal discomfort or swelling, most mothers wait to resume sexual intercourse until after the 6 weeks checkup.

Contraception

The decision about contraception depends on many things; the client's and her spouse's motivation, the number of children desired, the state of the child's health, whether she is breastfeeding and the couple's religious beliefs.

If an intrauterine device is the method of choice, it usually is inserted after the 6 weeks postpartum checkup. Some physicians may decide to insert it in the immediate postpartum period; however, the risk of expulsion is higher with rates from 10% to 20%.

For clients who prefer to go on oral contraceptives it may be prescribed to start after breastfeeding has been firmly established. The mother who is not breastfeeding can begin to take oral contraceptives as early as 2-3 weeks after delivery.

If the couple is sure about permanent sterilization, this can often be accomplished during a cesarean delivery or 24-48 hours following vaginal delivery.

Immune System

Unsensitized mothers who are Rh (D) negative and have given birth to an infant who is Rh positive should receive 300 µg of Rh (D) immune globulin (RhoGAM) within 72 hours of delivery. RhoGAM is administered even if the mother received RhoGAM in the antepartum period. Depending on the extent of hemorrhage and exchange of maternofetal blood, a larger dose may be necessary in some instances.

Before discharge, the client's rubella status needs to be checked. If the mother is rubella nonimmune with a titer below 1:8, she should be vaccinated before leaving the hospital. It is important to counsel the woman against becoming pregnant again, for next 4 weeks, after receiving the vaccine. The client should also be informed that she might experience a brief period of rubella-like symptoms such as a rash, lymphadenopathy, joint symptoms and low-grade fever for 5-21 days after vaccination. The vaccine is safe to be given to breastfeeding mothers. If the client declines to receive the vaccine in the hospital, she should be counseled about the devastating teratogenic effects on the fetus if she conceives before receiving the vaccine.

Documentation

Careful documentation is the closing step of each assessment encounter. Daily care of the woman after delivery includes the parameters such as episiotomy, lochia and breastfeeding. If written in narrative format, the nurse may use the acronym BUBBLE-HE to assist her in ensuring that all pertinent assessment are charted completely at least every shift or more frequently depending on the client's acuity. Nursing documentation should follow the nursing process and the facility's policy on documentation.

Discharge Preparation

Client education comprises much of the nurse's responsibilities throughout the postpartum stay with shortened hospital stays. The nurse must streamline her teaching methods, assessing the new mother's and her family's personal teaching needs. Focused client interactions should be directed toward desired client outcomes, empowering the woman and her family. The nurse should assess the mother's current knowledge regarding self-care and infant care because the mother's prior experiences with pregnancy and infant care may change the direction of the nurse's teaching plans. New mothers must learn how to care for herself and her infant. Self-care topics include those activities that help her to manage, anticipate and recognize health problems and danger signs. Infant care encompasses activities such as feeding, dressing and recognition of health problems.

General instructions in addition to self and infant care activities include the following:
- Do not lift anything heavier than the baby for the first 2–3 weeks
- Do not move furniture or vacuum cleaner for the 1st few weeks
- Get lots of rest and sleep when the baby sleeps
- Get help from family for household chores for 1st few weeks and enjoy the baby
- If an episiotomy is present, avoid having sexual intercourse until it heals or the bottom feels better
- Take medications as prescribed
- Keep track of postpartum follow-up appointment
- Seek medical help if any warning sign of sickness occurs.

A postpartum follow-up examination usually is scheduled for 6 weeks after delivery or earlier depending on the agency policy.

DISCOMFORTS OF THE PUERPERIUM AND RELIEF MEASURES

There are number of discomforts of the puerperium. While they are considered normal, there is no reason for a woman to have to suffer with them.

Afterbirth Pains

Afterbirth pains, sometimes called afterpains, can be quite painful. They are continuing sequential contraction and relaxation of the uterus. They are much more common with increasing parity and in women who breastfeed. With increased parity, there is decrease in uterine muscle tone, which causes the uterus to relax thereby subject it to recontraction. In the instance of breastfeeding women, the suckling of the baby stimulates the production of oxytocin by the posterior pituitary. The release of oxytocin not only triggers the let-down reflex in the breasts but also causes the uterus to contract; even the well-contracted uterus of a primipara will contract even more.

The key to effective relief from afterbirth pains is an empty bladder. The reason for this is the fact that a full bladder displaces the uterus from its normal and proper position. When the uterus is so displaced, it is unable to contract as it should and tends to relax, thus prohibiting relief from afterpains. Sometimes afterbirth pains are totally relieved just by the act of emptying the bladder.

Once the bladder is empty, the woman may lie prone with a pillow under her lower abdomen. The prone position places constant pressure against her uterus (the pillow creates even greater pressure), which keeps it contracted and thus eliminates afterbirth pains, since there is no uterine relaxation. The woman needs to be forewarned that when she first lies on stomach, she will have severe cramps or pain for about 5 minutes before she experiences complete and total relief.

Analgesia can be effective for afterbirth pains, but not for very long if the woman's bladder is not emptied. For nonbreastfeeders, generally analgesia is not needed because the prone position usually alleviates the discomfort even in multipara. It is important to remember that the let-down essential to breastfeeding is inhibited by pain. The amount of analgesic that gets into the milk will not hurt the baby.

Excessive Perspiration

Excessive perspiration is due to the body's using this route as well as diuresis to rid itself of the excess interstitial fluid that resulted from the hormonal effect during pregnancy. Keeping the mother clean and dry will provide comfort. The woman may want to change her gown frequently. Bed sheets should be changed as necessary. Care must be taken to assure that the woman is hydrated. Drinking a glass of water or any fluid of her liking during each hour she is awake, will assure this.

Breast Engorgement

It is thought that engorgement of the breasts is due to a combination of milk accumulation and stasis, and increased vascularity and congestion. It occurs on approximately the 3rd postpartal day in both breastfeeding and non-breastfeeding mothers and lasts approximately 24–48 hours. Signs and symptoms of engorgement include the following, which are experienced to a greater or lesser degree by individual woman:
- Sense of increasing breast heaviness or filling on the day prior to engorgement
- Enlargement of breasts from distention
- Skin becomes tight, shining and reddened
- Breasts are warm to touch
- Veins become visible
- Breasts are tender, throbbing and painful
- Breasts feel firm, full and hard.

Because this is not an inflammatory process, there is no temperature elevation caused by breast engorgement.

Relief measures for a woman, who is not breastfeeding is geared toward relief of discomfort and cessation of lactation. Relief for a breastfeeding woman aims for relief of discomfort and continuation of lactation. Treatment of breast engorgement is important to the breastfeeding mother as unrelieved breast engorgement suppresses the milk supply. With the current short hospital stay, many women will be home before breast engorgement occurs and need to be instructed about what to do when it happens.

Relief Measures for Non-breastfeeding Mothers

1. Give the breasts good support. A breast binder should be used to provide upward and inward thrust and support. If a binder is not available, one may be prepared using a pillowcase or towel, which will go around the woman and two shorter strips to be used as shoulder straps. The binder has to be secured with safety pins to fit each woman. A tuck is to be given beneath each breast to provide support and the ends are overlapped and fitted in front. Applied this way a breast binder is extremely comfortable for the woman, because it imparts support and prevents painful movement.
2. Apply ice bags or packs to the breasts. Ice relieves discomfort, has a certain numbing effect and does not encourage milk flow.
3. Take analgesics such as aspirin or paracetamol to relieve pain.
4. *Avoid massaging* the breasts in an effort to get the milk out. Such actions will only extend the length of time of breast engorgement. Any emptying of the breasts by any means stimulates the breasts to further lactation.
5. *Do not apply heat* to breasts, as heat dilates the blood vessels and ductile system causing the milk to flow. This causes partial emptying and stimulates the breasts to further lactation.

Relief Measures for Breastfeeding Mothers

Relief measures for the breastfeeding woman are designed to get the milk flow and empty the breasts. This also alleviates the mother's discomforts. The following are the relief measures:
1. Carry out breast massage, manual expression and nipple rolling.
2. Nurse the baby every 2–3 hours without missing any feeding or using any of the supplements.
3. Use both breasts at each feeding. Start on the breast, which is used last during the previous feeding. The baby should be on each breast for 5–10 minutes to start with and then build-up to complete emptying of one breast, which may take about 20 minutes before switching to the other to finish the feeding. Sucking for shorter period initially helps to accustom the nipples to the baby's sucking and minimizes soreness.

Many breastfeeding mothers, who had antenatal breast preparation, begin breast-feeding within an hour of delivery, feed frequently thereafter and use both breasts to avoid undue breast engorgement:
1. Apply warmth to the breasts, prior to each breastfeeding to promote milk flow. This can be accomplished with warm washcloth on breasts or warm shower.
2. Manually express the milk if there is engorging of the areola, to soften the area prior to nursing the baby. This will help the baby latch on to the nipple properly and easily.
3. Use manual expression of milk to empty the breasts after the baby has nursed if they are still uncomfortably full and engorged.
4. Maintain good support to the breasts without any pressure points. A nursing brassiere may be worn for this purpose.
5. Ice bags may be used between feedings to deduce swelling and pain.
6. Analgesics may be used if needed.

Perineal (Stitch) Pain

Before any measures are instituted, it is essential to examine the perineum to ascertain, if the woman is experiencing normal pain or if a complication, such as hematoma or infection, is developing. Perineal comfort measures are as following:
1. Ice pack, ice bags or rubber gloves filled with crushed ice or ice chips can be applied. Ice bags or packs should be wrapped in sterile towel or any clean disposable soft material. These are most useful in reducing the swelling and numbing the area in the immediate postpartum period especially if the woman had a third or fourth degree laceration.
2. Topical anesthetic spray or ointment may be used as ordered. If an ointment is to be used the woman should be instructed to wash her hands before applying it.
3. Sitz bath two to three times a day.

Many women consider the sitz bath most soothing of all the measures. A modification of the same idea is to pour warm water over the perineum. This can be a part of routine perineal care after voiding and defecation. The warmth of the water increases circulation and promotes healing. The warmth and motion of the water are soothing.

Constipation

Stool softeners or mild laxatives are usually ordered for women with third or fourth degree repair of perineum. Multiparas with lax abdominal wall may also require measures to avoid constipation.

Hemorrhoids

If the woman has hemorrhoids, they may be quite painful for a few days. Relief measures include the following:
- Ice bags or packs
- Medicated compresses
- Analgesic or anesthetic spray or ointment
- Heat lamp
- Warm water compresses
- Stool softeners
- Rectal suppositories
- Replacement of external hemorrhoids inside the rectum.

BREASTFEEDING DIFFICULTIES AND MANAGEMENT

A mother who is breastfeeding for the first time is in a vulnerable position and requires support, encouragement and knowledgeable assistance. She has to make the transition from being insecure, anxious and self-doubt to being self-assured and confident in herself and her abilities.

Preparation for Mother

The mother should be prepared for each breastfeeding and helped with the following measures:
1. Assume a comfortable position, which also allows proper positioning of the baby. Side lying, reclining or sitting position with generous use of pillows for support and comfort.
2. Her bladder should be empty and should have received comfort measures for any afterpains or perineal discomfort prior to breastfeeding time.
3. Assure of available help as necessary.
4. Rested and relaxed.
5. Hands should be washed and nipples cleansed by gently wiping them off with plain water.

Preparation for Baby

1. The baby's immediate preparation includes having a clean diaper and if absolutely necessary to be swaddle wrapped.
2. Position the baby so that he or she will not be doubled up or have a twisted neck when sucking and the head and body are supported.

Positioning

In bringing the baby and breast together, the following steps are helpful:
1. Let the baby find the breast and grasp the nipple. Do not thrust the breast in the baby's face.
2. Help the mother to hold the breast beyond the areolar area, so her fingers will not interfere with proper positioning of the baby's mouth and gums on the nipple.
3. Touch the baby's cheek with the nipple, so the baby will turn toward the breast (use the rooting reflex).
4. Express few drops of colostrum, so they are on the surface of the nipple. This provides the baby with instant gratification and reinforces learning.
5. As the baby grasps the nipple, the mother must make sure that the baby has enough of it for proper positioning in the mouth. The baby must grasp more than just the end of the mother's nipple to compress the lactiferous sinuses located beneath the areolae in order to obtain colostrum or milk.
6. Once the baby's mouth is properly positioned well on to the areola; the mother releases her grasp of her breast. As the baby starts sucking and swallowing, she must provide breathing space for the baby, if needed, by pressing with a finger on her breast where the baby's nose is. This is needed only during the learning period and when the breast is engorged. Babies usually suck a bit, rest a bit (maintaining their hold on the nipple while they rest) and then suck some more. The mother must be prepared for this.
7. Suction must be broken before trying to remove the baby from the breast by slipping a finger into the corner of the baby's mouth and between the baby's gums. Once the suction is broken, the baby is removed from the breast without injury to the nipple. The baby is then burped and put to the other breast.

Establishing Lactation

Lactation is established by a combination of the following:
1. Starting breastfeeding as soon as possible after delivery.
2. Frequent feedings during the first few days, using both breasts.
3. No missed feedings.
4. No supplementary feedings. Rotation of breasts as the starting and ending to provide for complete emptying of both breasts.
5. Tension free, painless, rested and relaxed mother during feeding times.
6. Baby properly positioned on the breast.
7. Supportive spouse.

After first few days, the baby will settle into his/her own pattern of feeding frequency. A self-demand scheduling (i.e. feeding the baby when he/she is hungry) can be adopted rather than a rigid scheduling.

Breast Care

The final factor in successful breastfeeding is effective breast care. Breast care and preparation for breastfeeding begin in the antenatal period. Breast care while breastfeeding, is as follows:
1. Wash the nipples only with water. Soap, alcohol or any other drying agent can lead to cracking of the nipples.
2. Expose the nipples to air for 15–30 minutes after a feeding.
3. While exposing the nipples to air, expose them also to sunlight and/or use dry heat from a 25-watt electric bulb or sunshine.
4. Following exposure, rub a nipple cream, vitamin 'A and D ointment' or other prescribed ointment.
5. Provide good support to the breasts.
6. If breasts become engorged, care for them, as discussed earlier in this chapter.
7. If the nipple becomes tender:
    a. Enhance the let-down before feeding with warmth, as discussed for care of the breast during engorgement.
    b. Nurse on the less sore nipple first until there is let-down, then switch the baby to the sorest nipple to empty that breast, then switch back to the less sore nipple to finish the feeding.
    c. Use a pacifier to meet the baby's sucking needs rather than the end of feedings on the nipple.
    d. Breastfeed more frequently for shorter periods of time.
    e. Be sure to use a combination of exposure to air and heat after each breastfeeding, followed by thorough application of nipple cream.
8. Be sure to break the suction, before removing the baby from the breast.

GUIDANCE AND INSTRUCTIONS IN PREPARATION FOR HOME CARE

Following normal delivery, mothers are discharged on the second or third postpartum day. Prior to discharge from the hospital, the midwife must appraise the mother's need for instructions and guidance for the care of self, baby and self in relation to others.

Self

1. Measures to improve her general health.
2. Perineal care.
3. Breast care.
4. Caring of the breasts during breast engorgement.
5. Postnatal exercises (abdominal and perineal muscle tightening).
6. Gradual return to day-to-day activities.
7. Avoid lifting anything heavier than the body.
8. Return for 6 weeks postpartum check-up.

Self in Relation to Others

1. Sibling and husband rivalry.
2. Family planning.
3. Resumption of sexual intercourse after 6 weeks.

Baby

1. Breastfeeding (as discussed earlier in this Chapter).
2. If being bottle fed:
   a. Care and preparation of formula.
   b. Care and preparation of bottles, nipples or container and spoon or feeding dish.
   c. How to hold the baby during feeding?
   d. How to hold the feeding bottle to prevent the baby sucking air (the nipple to be full)?
3. Burping.
4. Baby bathing and dressing including care of genital area.
5. Cord care.
6. Prevention and treatment of diaper rash.
7. Checking baby's temperature.
8. Recognizing baby's needs.
9. Checkup and immunization for the baby.

NURSING PROCESS DURING THE PUERPERIUM

Assessment

Assess for the following manifestations:
1. *Vital signs:* Blood pressure (BP), pulse, temperature, respirations.
2. *Breasts:* Soft or engorged.
3. *Abdomen:* Soft and loose.
4. *Gastrointestinal system:*
   a. Appetite (increased normally).
   b. Thirst (more thirst).
   c. Bowel movements (sluggish).
5. *Uterus:*
   a. Location on different days.
   b. Consistency (firm normally).
   c. Rate of involution.
   d. Afterpains especially for multiparas and breastfeeding mothers.
6. *Lochia:*
   a. Color: Rubra to serosa to alba.
   b. Smell: Any foul smell indicates infection.
7. Small clots.
8. *Urinary output:*
   a. Large amounts normal.
   b. Difficulty in emptying.

Analysis/Nursing Diagnosis

- Ineffective individual management related to fatigue and baby care needs
- Impaired home maintenance related to lack of availability of assistance
- Potential for altered nutrition related knowledge deficit
- Alteration of comfort related to reduced rest and sleep
- Potential for anxiety related family process and sexuality pattern

Planning

- Create an environment to parent-newborn interaction/bonding
- Promote maternal-neonatal well-being
- Provide support and counseling to new mothers
- Provide teaching regarding postpartal self-care measures and newborn care.

Implementation

1. Complete postpartum assessment every 4-6 hours. Include the following areas:
   a. Take and record vital signs.
   b. Palpate breasts, note firmness and complaints of breast tenderness. Assess nipples for tenderness/soreness, blisters and cracking in breastfeeding mothers.
   c. Palpate the abdomen and note any tenderness.
   d. Palpate fundus, note height, position (midline or to the side) and firmness.
   e. Inspect perineum for bruising, edema and hematoma. Note presence of hemorrhoids.
   f. Inspect legs for reddened, tender areas and inquire about areas of tenderness. Check Homans' sign.
   g. Inquire about urinary and bowel elimination.
   h. Assess comfort level and need for pain medication.
2. After initial recovery period, assess vital signs every 8 hours according to the protocol.
3. Promote urinary and bowel function:
   a. Urine elimination:
      - Encourage voiding within 6-8 hours; catheterization to relieve bladder distention
      - Measure urinary output for the first three voidings
      - Note frequent voidings of small amounts (less than 100 mL), which may indicate retention with overflow

- Teach woman regarding:
  - Adequate fluid intake
  - Emptying bladder on regular basis
  - Wiping from front to back.
b. Feces elimination:
  - Encourage adequate fluid intake
  - Administer stool softeners as needed and desired
  - Teach client regarding:
    - Daily exercise
    - Adequate fluids
    - Including fiber and roughage in diet.
4. Promote perineal healing and teach self-care measures:
   a. Apply ice packs for 6–12 hours.
   b. Cleanse perineum by applying warm water and rinse.
   c. Offer sitz baths two to four times a day.
   d. Use local anesthetics.
   e. Apply perineal pads from front to back and change after each voiding.
   f. Teach client to report:
      - Blood clots
      - Foul-smelling lochia
      - Change from lochia alba to serosa and back to lochia rubra.
5. Provide breast care and teach self-care measures:
   a. Breastfeeding mothers should:
      - Cleanse breast with warm water (no soap)
      - Wear a supportive bra
      - Apply cream (as prescribed) for nipple soreness
      - Be taught breast massage
      - Be assisted with breastfeeding technique.
   b. Non-breastfeeding mothers should:
      - Wear a supportive bra
      - Use a breast binder if desired
      - Avoid breast stimulation
      - Be offered cold/ice packs to decrease swelling and inflammation from engorgement.
6. Teach abdominal and pelvic strengthening exercises:
   a. Modified sit-ups.
   b. Woman should be advised that increase in vaginal flow or return to lochia rubra may occur, if activity becomes excessive.
7. Provide the information regarding sexual activity:
   a. Sexual activity may be resumed in about 6 weeks postdelivery.
   b. Ovulation may occur, so contraceptive measures are needed to prevent pregnancy.
8. Provide infant-care teaching:
   a. Common variations in infants.
   b. Cord care.
   c. Elimination.
   d. Diapers.
   e. Feeding.
   f. Temperature.
   g. Signs of illness should be reported to the physician/pediatrician.
   h. Newborn bath.
   i. Formula preparation and feeding.
   j. Breastfeeding.

Evaluation

1. Ensure that parents have opportunities for interaction with their baby.
2. Ensure that mother and baby remain within normal physiological parameters.
3. Provide parents with the support and counseling.
4. Confirm that mother is able to demonstrate self-care measures and infant care.

STUDY QUESTIONS

Short Notes

1. Lochia.
2. Homans' sign.
3. Perineal discomfort due to stitches and hemorrhoids.

Short Answer Questions

1. Physiology of lactation.
2. Postpartum exercises.
3. Afterbirth pain and management.
4. Breastfeeding difficulties and instructions to mother for management.

Essay Questions

1. Describe the physical assessment and nursing care of a client on the second postpartum day.
2. Explain breast engorgement and relief measures to be provided for breastfeeding and non-breastfeeding mothers.

BIBLIOGRAPHY

1. Helen V. Nurse-Midwifery, 2nd edition. Boston: Jones and Bartlett Publishers; 1996. pp. 363-73.
2. Hynes L. Physiology, complications and management of the puerperium. In: Bennett RV, Linda KB (Eds). Myles Textbook for Midwives, 13th edition. Edinburgh: Churchill Livingstone; 1999. pp. 589-614.
3. Kitzinger S. The Complete Book of Pregnancy and Childbirth, New York: Knopf; 1980.
4. Llewellyn Jones D. Fundamentals of Obstetrics and Gynecology, 6th edition. London: Mosby; 1994.
5. Montgomery E, Alexander J. Assessing postnatal uterine involution: a review and a challenge. Midwifery. 1994;10:73-6.
6. Royal College of Midwives. Successful breast-feeding, 2nd edition. Edinburgh: Churchill Livingstone; 1991. pp. 45-6.

CHAPTER 24

Family Planning

Learning Objectives

Upon completing this chapter, the learner will be able to:
- Describe the magnitude of population increase and the urgency for measures to reduce the rate of growth.
- Describe the concept and objectives of family planning.
- Describe the contraceptive methods.
- Explain the role of the midwife regarding family planning and related issues.
- Explain the provision of family planning services.

People throughout the world are becoming increasingly aware of and concerned about the steadily rising population and the inherent effect this will have on the quality of life and the delicate balance of nature. Man continues to seek for answers to the question of how a level of population can be maintained through reproduction that will not exploit the environment.

The disparity between the death rate and the birth rate results in the rapid rise of population. This is specially pronounced in the developing countries comprising about 70% of the total world population.

MAGNITUDE OF THE PROBLEM

In the beginning of the 20th century, the rate of population increase was about 10 million per year. It is now increasing at a much faster rate of 100 million per year. As the population growth continues unabated, India's population has reached 1,027 million in 2001 from 944.5 million in 1996.

India with 2.5% of the world's land surface area has to accommodate about 16% of the world population. India is the second most populous country in the world, next to China. The density of the population is 267/km^2. The death rate was 9 per 1,000 in 1997. Thus, there is a wide gap between births and deaths resulting in rapid rise of population.

Impact of Population Increase

The rapid increase of population has an adverse effect on the national economy. The benefits of improvement in the different sectors are being eroded by the growing population. At the level of families, the increasing number of births has a deleterious effect on the health of the mother and the child, and hinders social and economic upliftment of the family. High parity is associated with increased maternal and infant mortality, various other obstetric and gynecological complications and nutritional problems. For these reasons, population control by appropriate family welfare program is considered a branch of preventive and social medicine. Many developing countries, India in particular, have taken family planning as a national program of vital importance.

FAMILY PLANNING

Definition

An expert committee of World Health Organization (WHO) (1971) defined family planning as "a way of thinking and living that is adopted voluntarily, upon the basis of knowledge, attitudes and responsible decisions by individuals and couples, in order to promote the health and welfare of the family group and thus contribute effectively to the social development of the country".

Another expert committee defined and described family planning as "Family planning refers to practices that help individuals or couples to attain certain objectives". These are as follows:
1. To avoid unwanted births.
2. To bring about wanted births.
3. To regulate the interval between pregnancies.
4. To control the time at which births occur in relation to the ages of the parent.
5. To determine the number of children in the family.

Basic Human Rights

The United Nations Conference on human rights in 1968 recognized family planning as a basic human right. The 1974 conference on world population endorsed the same view and stated in its 'plan of action' that all couples and individuals have the basic human right to decide freely and responsibly the number and spacing of their children and to have the information, education and means to do so. The world conference of the International Women's Year in 1975 also declared the right of women to decide freely and responsibly on the number and spacing of their children and to have access to the information and means to enable them to exercise that right. Thus, family planning has become the focus of international concern as a basic human right and a component of family health and social welfare.

Modern Concept of Family Planning

Family planning is not synonymous with birth control. A WHO expert committee in 1970 has stated that family planning in its purview includes all the following:
- The proper spacing and limitation of births
- Advice on sterility
- Education for parenthood
- Sex education
- Screening for pathological conditions related to the reproductive system (e.g. cervical cancer)
- Genetic counseling
- Premarital consultation and examination
- Carrying out pregnancy tests
- Marriage counseling
- The preparation of couples for the arrival of their first baby
- Providing services for unmarried mothers
- Teaching home economics and nutrition
- Providing adoption services.

These activities vary from country to country according to national objectives and policies with regard to family planning.

Health Aspects of Family Planning

The principal health outcomes of family planning, as listed by a WHO scientific group on health aspects of family planning, include women's health, fetal health and child health.

Women's Health

Pregnancy can mean serious problems for women. It may damage the mother's health or even endanger her life. The risk increases as the mother grows older and after she has had three or four children. Family planning by intervening in the reproductive cycle of women helps them to control the number, interval, timing of pregnancies and births, and thereby reduces maternal mortality and morbidity, and improves health.

The health impact of family planning occurs through the avoidance of unwanted pregnancies, limiting the number of births and proper spacing, and timing the births, particularly the first and last in relation to the age of the mother.

Fetal Health

A number of congenital anomalies are associated with advancing maternal age (e.g. Down syndrome). Such congenital anomalies can be avoided by timing the births in relation to the mother's age. Further, the 'quality' of population can be improved only by avoiding unwanted pregnancies.

Child Health

Mortality among children is high, when pregnancies occur in rapid succession. A birth interval of 2–3 years is considered desirable to reduce child mortality. Family planning is therefore an important means for birth spacing and limiting family size thereby insuring the survival of all children in the family.

Small Family Norm

The objective of family welfare program in India is that people should adopt the 'small family norm' to stabilize the country's population at the level of some 1,533 million by the year 2050. In the 1970s and 1980s, the models adopted in India for family size were three children and two children respectively. The current emphasis is on three themes, i.e. 'sons or daughters—two will do' 'second child after 3 years' and 'universal immunization'.

The national target is to achieve a net reproduction rate of one, by the year 2006, which is equivalent to attaining approximately the two-child norm.

Objectives of Family Planning Program in India

Conception Control

1. To bring down the birth rate to a realistic minimum during a given period. There were about 168 million eligible couples in India in 1999. These are couples with wives in the reproductive age group of 15-45 years and who require the use of some sort of family planning method. According to the latest available report, about 44% of the eligible couples in the country are practicing effective methods of contraception.
2. To bring about certain special changes such as:
   a. To educate and motivate the sexually active and fertile couples to accept the small family norm.
   b. To increase the literacy rate especially among women in rural areas.
   c. To raise the marriageable age of both boys and girls. Low age of marriage not only contribute to the increased birth rate but also adversely affects the

health of the woman. In 1948, the Indian parliament approved the bill fixing the minimum age of marriage at 21 years for men and 18 years for women.
d. To maximize the access of good quality family planning services.

Maternity and Child Health Services

1. To extend maternity services through antenatal, intranatal and postnatal care with immunization against tetanus, and prevention and correction of anemia.
2. To offer protection to children through immunization schedule and vitamins supplement program.

Other Services

1. To provide sex education and marriage guidance.
2. To promote research on normal reproduction, investigation and treatment of infertility and recurrent abortion. It also includes evaluation of pregnancy termination as a method of family limitation.

Birth Control, Contraception and Family Planning

The words birth control, contraception and family planning are often used interchangeably, although they are not identical in meaning. The term birth control refers to regulation of the number of children that are conceived or born. Contraception refers to the prevention of pregnancy, which is accomplished by specific contraceptive or birth control methods. Family planning has the broadest connotation. It encompasses the additional considerations of the physical, social, psychological, economic and theological factors that govern the family's attitudes and influence decisions pertaining to the size of the family, the spacing of children and the selection and utilization of a contraceptive method.

Contraception plays an important role in the lives of many women. It should be viewed in the wider context of sexual and reproductive health. The capacity to enjoy and control sexual and reproductive behavior is a key element of sexual health.

Role of the Midwife in Family Planning

The role of the midwife in family planning has been acknowledged by the WHO and the International Confederation of midwives. She must be able to facilitate client knowledge and choice by providing valid, current information in a way, which is easily understood by the woman and possibly by her partner or spouse. Her counseling skills, attributes such as being nonjudgmental and positive listening skills are of supreme importance.

Discussion regarding family planning may well be appropriate at all stages of reproductive period. Preconceptionally, contraception is advocated for 2 months after rubella vaccination. Antenatally, the woman and her partner may wish to have information on which to base future choices and following delivery they may require further information.

A mother who has chosen not to breastfeed will need to commence contraception, so that it is effective before postpartum ovulation that occurs on an average between 40 and 50 days after delivery. The midwife needs to be aware that general factors governing individual contraceptive choices vary greatly and can include religion and culture, relationship, age, motivation to avoid pregnancy, lifestyle and socioeconomic considerations. After childbirth, these may be compounded by issues such as breastfeeding, because their chosen method of contraception must not affect lactation, health of their baby, body image and adjustment to motherhood.

The midwife will also need to be aware of the family planning services available in the area where she practices. Guillebaud (1993) suggested that the ideal contraceptive would be 100% effective, perfectly safe, reversible, inexpensive, free of side effects, simple to obtain and use, and not related to the time of coitus. Although, some of these ideal standards have been achieved, no single method meets all the criteria.

METHODS OF CONTRACEPTION

1. Temporary methods:
   a. Barrier methods.
   b. Natural contraception.
   c. Intrauterine contraceptive devices (IUCDs).
   d. Steroidal/hormonal contraception.
2. Permanent methods:
   a. Female: Tubal occlusion/tubal ligation.
   b. Male: Vasectomy.

TEMPORARY METHODS OF CONTRACEPTION

Temporary methods of contraception are commonly used to postpone or to space births. However, these are also used frequently by couples, who desire to have no more children.

Barrier Methods

Barrier methods prevent sperm deposition in the vagina or sperm penetration through cervical canal. The objective is achieved by mechanical devices or by chemical means, which produce sperm immobilization or by combined means. The following are included:

❖ Mechanical:
  – Male: Condom
  – Female: Condom, diaphragm, cervical cap.
❖ Chemical (vaginal contraceptives):
  – Creams: Delfen, velpar
  – Foam tablet: Durofoan tablet
  – Aerosol foam: Nonoxynol-9
  – Contraceptive sponge: Today sponge.
❖ Combination: Combined use of mechanical and chemical methods.

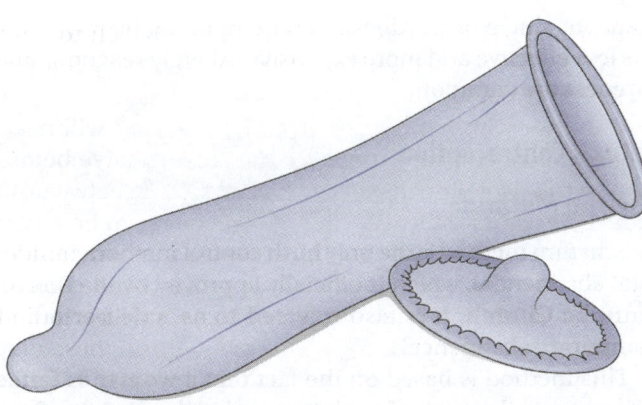

Figure 24.1: Male condom.

Male Condom (Fig. 24.1)

Condoms are made of polyurethane or latex. Polyurethane condoms are thinner and suitable to those who are sensitive to latex rubber. It is the most widely practiced method used by the male. A widely marketed brand in India is 'Nirodh'. The efficacy of condoms can be augmented by adding spermicidal agents during its use. Protection against sexually transmitted disease is an additional advantage. The method is suitable for couples who want to space their pregnancies and who have contraindications for the use of oral contraceptive or IUCD. These are also suitable to those who have infrequent sexual intercourse.

Instructions for use

The condom is unrolled over the erect penis before any genital contact. The rim of the condom should be held against the base of the penis during withdrawal making sure the condom does not become dislodged from the penis. The condoms are tested for holes electronically by the manufacturer and need not be tested before use. The condom should be grasped at its open end and held in place during withdrawal of penis. However, after use it should be checked for tears before throwing it away. If it is found torn, a spermicidal jelly should be put into the vagina immediately. The condom should be thrown away after single use.

Use of condom
1. As an elective contraceptive method.
2. As an interim form of contraception during pill use, following vasectomy operation and if an IUCD is thought lost, until a new IUCD can be fitted.
3. During the course of treatment of the wife for *Trichomonas vaginalis*.

Advantages
1. Easily available and inexpensive.
2. No contraindications or side effects.
3. Easy to carry, simple to use and disposable.
4. Protection against sexually transmitted diseases like chlamydia, gonorrhea and human immunodeficiency virus (HIV).
5. Protection against pelvic inflammatory diseases.
6. Suitable for use during lactation, for teenagers and in cases where pills and IUCDs are contraindicated.
7. Useful where sexual intercourse is infrequent and irregular.

Disadvantages
1. It reduces sexual pleasure to a small extent due to reduced sensitivity for the male and interruption of sexual act.
2. May accidentally break or slip off during coitus.

Female Condom (Femshield) (Fig. 24.2)

Female condom is a pouch made of polyurethane, which lines the vagina and external genitalia. It is about 15 cm in length with one flexible polyurethane ring at each end. The condom is inserted into the vagina in such a manner that the closed inner end is anchored in place by the polyurethane ring, while the open outer edge lies flat against the vulva. The inner ring at the closed end is smaller compared to the outer ring. It gives protection against sexually transmitted disease and pelvic inflammatory disease.

Female condoms were not accepted well though they were not expensive or required no prescription from physician.

Diaphragm (Figs. 24.3A and B)

Diaphragm is an intravaginal device made of rubber with flexible metal or spring ring at the margin. Its diameter varies

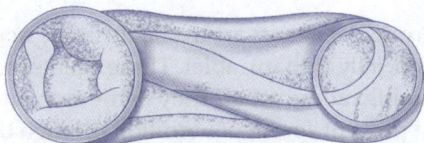

Figure 24.2: Female condom—Femidom.

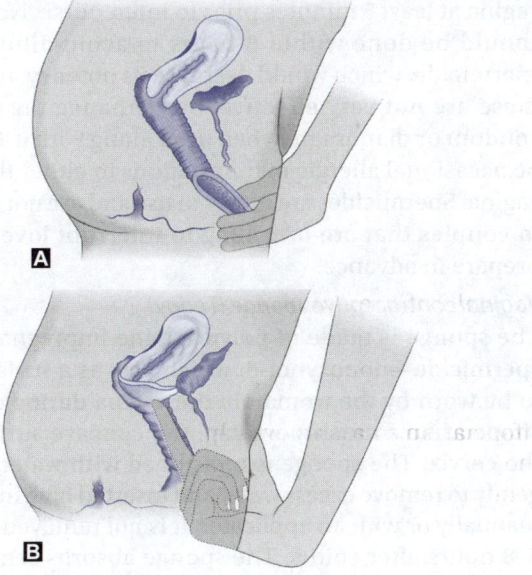

Figures 24.3A and B: Diaphragm—insertion and checking. (A) Insertion of a diaphragm; (B) Checking the position of diaphragm using finger.

from 5 to 10 cm. It is not a popular method. It requires a medical person to measure the size required.

Instructions for use

The diaphragm of the right size is selected that is of the same length as the distance between the top of the posterior fornix and the undersurface of the symphysis pubis. It is inserted dome pointing down with some spermicidal jelly within the cup and along the rim. The diaphragm is pinched between the thumb and index finger and released only after insertion into the vagina. The device should be introduced up to 3 hours before intercourse and kept for at least 6 hours after the last coital act. Ill-fitting and accidental displacement during intercourse increases the failure rate.

Advantages
1. Inexpensive.
2. Can be used repeatedly for long time.
3. Highly effective if used properly.
4. No interruption in love making as with condom.

Disadvantages
1. Requires help of a physician to measure the size required.
2. Risk of vaginal irritation and urinary tract infection.
3. More difficult to use than condom and requires high degree of motivation for the user.
4. Not suitable for women with uterine prolapse.

Vaginal Contraceptives

Chemicals

Several spermicidal agents are available in the market in the form of cream, jelly or foam tablet. These agents mostly cause sperm immobilization, when they come in contact and to some extent prevent sperm penetration through the cervical canal. The cream or jelly is introduced high in the vagina with plastic applicators at least 15 minutes before sexual intercourse. Foam tablets are to be introduced high in the vagina at least 5 minutes prior to intercourse. No douching should be done within 8 hours to avoid dilution of the spermicide, which would decrease its potency. In isolation, these are not very effective, but enhance the efficacy of condom or diaphragm when used along with it. There may be occasional allergic manifestations in either the vulva or vagina. Spermicides are messy to use and are not acceptable to couples that are unwilling to interrupt lovemaking or prepare in advance.

Vaginal contraceptive sponge (Today)

The sponge is made of polyurethane impregnated with a spermicide—nonoxynol-9, which acts as a surfactant. It is to be worn by the woman in the vagina during coitus. It is shaped like a mushroom cap, the concave surface facing the cervix. The sponge is moistened with water, squeezed gently to remove excess water and inserted high in the vagina manually or with an applicator. It is not removed for at least 6–8 hours after coitus. The sponge absorbs semen as it is deposited in the vagina, prevents its entry into the cervix and releases nonoxynol-9 during coital thrust, which inactivates sperm. The sponge measures about 2 cm in diameter and is made for single use. It does not require fitting by physician. It is less effective and more expensive. Allergic reactions and soreness are common.

Natural Contraception

Rhythm Method

The rhythm method is the only birth control method (besides total abstinence), which is officially approved by the Roman Catholic Church. It is also referred to as 'safe period' or 'temporary abstinence'.

This method is based on the fact that a woman is fertile only around the time of ovulation and if she abstains from intercourse during that time, she is unlikely to conceive. Usually a woman ovulates once during each menstrual cycle. The ovum has an active life of 12–24 hours during which it can be fertilized. Sperm cells, once within the birth canal are viable for 72 hours during which they can fertilize the ovum. Thus, there is a minimum total of 96 hours (4 days) during each cycle when conception is possible. To these 4 days, an additional margin of several days is added to allow for variation in the exact day of ovulation.

The method to determine the approximate time of ovulation and the fertile period include:
1. Recording of the previous menstrual cycles (calendar rhythm).
2. Recording the basal body temperature (temperature rhythm).
3. Taking note of the excessive mucoid vaginal discharge (mucus rhythm).

The users of the calendar method obtain the period of abstinence from calculations based on the previous 12 menstrual cycle records. From this record the number of days in each cycle is listed. From this list the longest cycle and the shortest cycle are noted. The number 20 is subtracted from the number of days in the shortest cycle to get the 1st day of the fertile or unsafe period and the number 10 is subtracted from the number of days in the longest cycle to get the last day of the fertile or unsafe period. Thus, if a woman had cycles ranging from 25 to 31 days, she would abstain from intercourse from the 5th day of her current menstrual cycle (25 − 20 = 5) until the 21st day of her current cycle (31 − 10 = 21).

Users of the temperature rhythm require abstinence until the 3rd day of the rise of temperature. This is because the basal temperature (taken immediately on awakening and before any activity) of a woman is more or less constant during the first part of menstrual cycle until the day of ovulation. At that time, it drops slightly and then rises to a level somewhat higher (usually five tenth to seven tenth of a degree) than it has been and remains at that higher level for the rest of the cycle. If there is no cold or infection to account for this elevation, the woman can consider beyond the fertile period, when the elevation has persisted for 3 days.

Users of mucus rhythm require abstinence on all days of noticeable mucus and for 3 days thereafter.

The effectiveness of rhythm method can be considered satisfactory for highly motivated, carefully selected women with fairly regular cycles, who have the intelligence and self-discipline as well as cooperative marital partner to understand and practice it correctly. However, many couples find it difficult to have sex by the calendar instead of by inclination.

Advantages
1. No cost.
2. No side effects.

Disadvantages
1. Difficult to calculate the safe period.
2. Compulsory abstinence from sexual act during certain periods.
3. Not applicable during lactational amenorrhea or when periods are irregular.
4. Higher rate of ectopic or congenital abnormality of the fetus because of chances of the union of aging sperm and ovum.

Coitus Interruptus

Coitus is the oldest and probably the most widely accepted contraceptive method used by man. It necessitates withdrawal of penis shortly before ejaculation. It requires sufficient self-control by the man, so that withdrawal of penis precedes ejaculation.

Disadvantages
1. Requires sufficient self-control by the men.
2. The woman may suffer anxiety, vaginismus or pelvic congestion.
3. Chance of pregnancy is more:
   – Precoital secretion may contain sperm
   – Accidental chance of sperm deposition in the vagina.

Breastfeeding (Lactational Amenorrhea)

Prolonged and sustained breastfeeding offers a natural protection of pregnancy. This is more effective in women, who are amenorrheic than those who are menstruating. The risk of pregnancy to a woman who is fully breastfeeding and amenorrheic is less than 2% in the first 6 months.

Contraceptive Effectiveness of Conventional Methods of Contraception

Conventional methods of contraception are:
1. Condoms.
2. Vaginal diaphragms.
3. Spermicides.
4. Rhythm method.

The failure rate of any contraceptive is calculated in terms of pregnancy rate per hundred women years (HWY) of use. It is calculated according to the following formula (Pearl Index).

Pregnancy failure rate

$$= \frac{\text{Number of accidental pregnancies} \times 1{,}200}{\text{Number of patients observed} \times \text{Months of use}}$$

Where,
1,200 = Number of months in 100 years.

For example, if 100 couples have used a method for a period of 2 years (24 months) and have resulted in 20 pregnancies, the pregnancy rate is calculated to be:

$$\frac{20 \times 1{,}200}{100 \times 24} = 10$$

When the pregnancy rate is below 10, the effectiveness of the particular method is considered to be high. If it is more than 20, it is said to be low. The failure rates of the commonly used contraceptive methods is given in **Table 24.1**.

TABLE 24.1: Failure rates of contraceptive methods.

Method of contraception	Failure rate (HWY)
Condom	14
Diaphragm	12
Vaginal contraceptives (spermicides)	9–27
Rhythm method	20–30
Coitus interruptus	18

(HWY: hundred women years)

Intrauterine Contraceptive Devices

Intrauterine devices (IUD), often referred to as IUCDs, are small plastic or metal forms to which a 'tail' of nylon threads is usually attached. These are worn by women in their uterine cavity. During the last couple of decades, there has been a significant improvement in its design and content.

Types of IUD

There are two basic types of IUD, non-medicated and medicated. Both are usually made of polyethylene or other polymers; in addition, the medicated or bioactive IUD, release either metal ions (copper) or hormones (progestogens).

The non-medicated IUDs are often referred to as *first generation* IUDs. The copper IUDs comprise the *second* and the hormone-releasing IUDs—the *third generation* IUDs. The medicated IUDs were developed to reduce the incidence of side effects and to increase the contraceptive effectiveness.

First generation IUDs: Include Lippes loop, Margulies spiral, Saf-T-coil and Dana super **(Figs. 24.4A to D)**. Of these, the Lippes loop was widely used in India since 1965, when it was introduced in the national family planning program.

Second generation IUDs: Were introduced in the 1970s. It was found that metallic copper had a strong antifertility effect. The addition of copper has made it possible to develop smaller devices, which are easier to fit, even in nulliparous

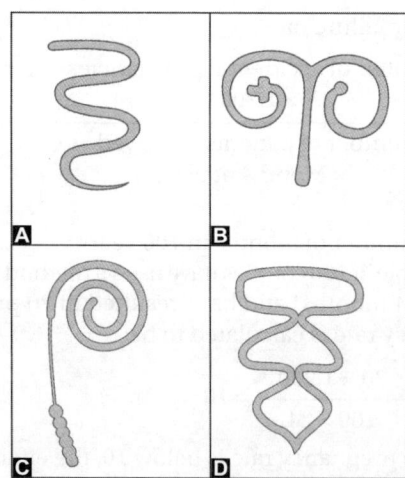

Figures 24.4A to D: First generation intrauterine devices (IUDs). (A) Lippes loop; (B) Saf-T-coil; (C) Margulies spiral; (D) Dana super.

women. A number of copper bearing devices are now available **(Figs. 24.5A to C):**
1. Earlier devices:
   a. Copper-7.
   b. Copper T-200.
2. Newer devices:
   a. Variants of the T device:
      » Copper T-220C (Cu T-220C)
      » Cu T-380A or Ag.
   b. Nova T.
   c. Multiload devices:
      » Multiload copper-250 (ML Cu-250)
      » ML Cu-375.

The numbers included in the names of the devices refer to the surface area (in mm^2) of the copper on the device. Nova T and Cu T-380Ag are distinguished by a silver core over which is wrapped the copper wire.

According to recent reports, copper devices have become very popular in India, accounting for 99.7% of the total IUD insertions in 1990–1991. Lippes Loop, which was widely used in the 1970s and 1980s is being phased out.

Advantages of copper devices are:
❖ Lower expulsion rate
❖ Lower incidence of side effects, e.g. pain and bleeding
❖ Easier to fit even in nulliparous women

❖ Better tolerated by nullipara
❖ Increased contraceptive effectiveness.

Third generation IUDs: These are based on still another principle, i.e. release of a hormone **(Figs. 24.6A to C)**. The most widely used hormonal device is *Progestasert*. It has a direct local effect on the uterine lining, on the cervical mucus and possibly on the sperms. Because the hormone supply is gradually depleted, regular replacement of the device is necessary.

Another hormonal device that has been tested is a T-shaped IUD, the *levonorgestrel* intrauterine system (LNG-IUS) releasing 20 µg of the potent synthetic steroid.

Long-term clinical experience with levonorgestrel-releasing IUD has shown to be associated with lower menstrual blood loss and fewer days of bleeding than the copper devices.

Description of Devices

Copper T-200: This is the widely used medicated device. It carries 215 mm^2 surface area of fine copper wire wounded around the vertical stem of the device. The stem of the T-shaped device is made of a polyethylene frame. It has a polyethylene monofilament tied at the end of the vertical stem. These two threads are used for detection and removal. The device contains 120 mg of copper. The device is to be removed after 3 years **(Fig. 24.5A)**.

Multiload Cu-375: It has 375 mm^2 surface area of copper wire wound around its vertical stem. The device is to be replaced in every 5 years **(Fig. 24.5B)**.

Copper T-380A: Carries 380 mm^2 surface area of copper wire wound around the stem (175 mg) and sleeves on the horizontal arms (66.5 mg). Replacement is after 10 years (copper is lost at the rate of 50 µg per 24 hours during a period of 1 year) **(Fig. 24.5C)**.

Multiload Cu-250: The device is available in a sterilized, sealed packet with an applicator. The device emits 60–100 µg of copper per day during a period of 1 year. The device is to be replaced in every 3 years **(Fig. 24.6A)**.

Progestasert: Bioactive core-containing microcrystals of progesterone (38 mg) enclosed within the plastic wall, which releases about 65 µg of progesterone daily into the uterine cavity. It should be replaced after 1 year **(Fig. 24.6B)**.

Levonorgestrel intrauterine system: It is a T-shaped device, with a polydimethylsiloxane membrane around the stem, which contains levonorgestrel (a potent synthetic steroid). It releases the hormone at the rate of 20 µg/day. The device is to be replaced in every 5 years. The third generation devices are more expensive, to be used on a wider scale **(Fig. 24.6C)**.

Mode of Action of IUDs

The precise mode of action of IUDs by which they prevent pregnancy, is not clear even after three decades of use and study. At present, the most widely accepted views are the following:

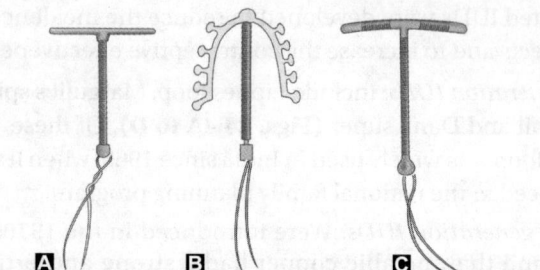

Figures 24.5A to C: Second generation IUCDs. (A) Copper T-200 (B) Multiload Cu-375; (C) Copper T-380A.

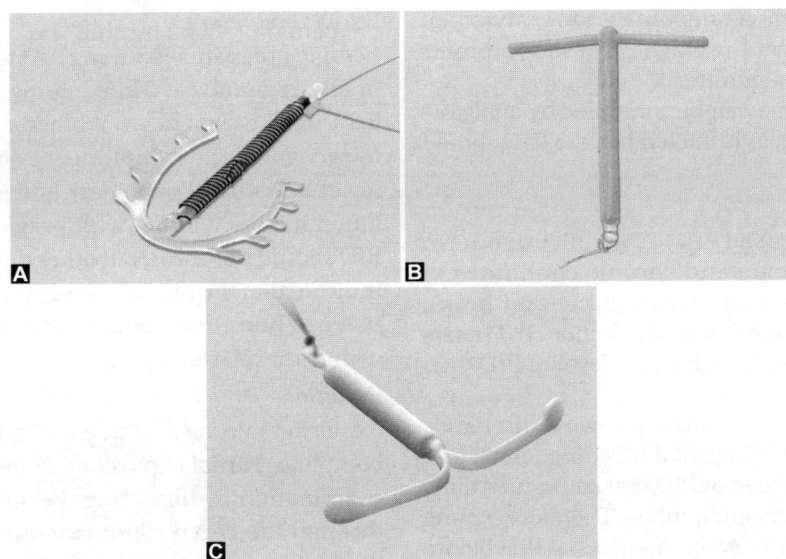

Figures 24.6A to C: (A) Multiload Cu-250; (B) Progestasert; (C) Levonorgestrel intrauterine system (lNG-IUS).

1. The IUD causes a foreign body reaction in the uterus causing cellular and biochemical changes in the endometrium and uterine fluids, and it is believed that these changes impair the viability of the gamete and thus reduce its chance of fertilization rather than its implantation.
2. Medicated IUDs produce other local effects that may contribute to their contraceptive action. Copper seems to enhance the cellular response in the endometrium. It also affects the enzymes in the uterus. By altering the biochemical composition of cervical mucus, copper ions may affect sperm motility, capacitation and survival.
3. Hormone-releasing devices increase the viscosity of the cervical mucus and thereby prevent sperm from entering the cervix. They also maintain high levels of progesterone and low levels of estrogen in the endometrium, thereby sustaining it unfavorable to implantation.

Time of Insertion

1. During menstruation or within 10 days of the beginning of a menstrual period. During this period, insertion is technically easy because the diameter of the cervical canal is greater at this time than during the secretary phase. The uterus is relaxed and myometrial contractions, which might tend to cause expulsion, are at a minimum. In addition, the risk that a woman is pregnant is remote at this time.
2. Postpartum insertion is done 6–8 weeks after delivery. Postpuerperal insertion has several advantages. It can be combined with the follow-up examination of the woman and her child.
3. Postabortion insertion can be taken up immediately after a legally induced first trimester abortion.
4. Immediate postpartum insertion of IUD can also be done during the 1st week after delivery before the woman leaves the hospital. Special care is required with insertions during the 1st week after delivery because of the greater risk of perforation during this time. Furthermore, immediate insertion is associated with a high expulsion rate.

Follow-up and Client Instructions

The objectives of follow-up examination are:
1. To provide motivation and emotional support.
2. To confirm the presence of IUD.
3. To diagnose and treat any side effects or complication.

The IUD wearer should be examined after her first menstrual period, for chances of expulsion of the device are high during this period; and again after the third menstrual period to evaluate the problems of pain and bleeding, and thereafter annually. The IUD wearer should be given the following instructions:
1. She should regularly check the threads or 'tail' to be sure that the IUD is in the uterus. If she fails to locate the thread, she must consult the physician.
2. She should visit the clinic whenever she experiences any side effects such as fever, pelvic pain or bleeding.
3. If she misses a period, she must consult the physician.

Side Effects and Complications

Bleeding

The most common complaint of women, fitted with IUD (inert or medicated), is increased vaginal bleeding. It may be greater volume of blood loss during menstruation, longer menstrual periods or mid-cycle bleeding. Copper devices and hormone-releasing devices cause less average blood loss.

If the bleeding is heavy or persistent, or if the woman develops anemia despite the iron supplement, the IUD should be removed. In most women, removal of the device is rapidly followed by a return to the normal menstrual pattern.

Pain

Pain is the second major side effect leading to IUD removal. Pain may be experienced during IUD insertion and for a few days thereafter, as well as during menstruation. It may manifest itself as low backache, cramps in the lower abdomen and occasionally pain down the thighs. These symptoms usually disappear by the 3rd month.

Slight pain during insertion can be controlled by analgesic or antispasmodic drugs. If pain is intolerable, the IUD should be removed.

Pelvic infection

Pelvic inflammatory disease (PID) is a collective term that includes acute, subacute and chronic conditions of the ovaries, tubes, uterus, connective tissue and pelvic peritoneum, and is usually the result of infection. IUD users are about two to eight times more likely to develop PID than non-contraceptive users.

The clinical manifestations of PID are vaginal discharge, pelvic pain and tenderness, abnormal bleeding, chills and fever. Even one or two episodes of PID can cause infertility, permanently blocking the fallopian tubes. Therefore, young women should be fully counseled on the risks of PID before choosing an IUD.

When PID is diagnosed, it should be treated promptly with broad-spectrum antibiotics. Most clinicians recommend removing IUD if infection does not respond to antibiotics within 24–48 hours.

Uterine perforation

The reported incidence ranges from 1:150 to 1:9,000 insertions depending upon the time of insertions, design of IUD, technique of insertion and operator's experience. In the hands of experienced physicians, it should not be higher than 0.3%. Perforations occur more frequently, when insertions are performed between 48 hours and 6 weeks postpartum.

The device may migrate into the peritoneal cavity causing serious complications such as intestinal obstruction. The perforation may be completely asymptomatic and discovered only when searching for a missing IUD. The conclusive diagnosis of perforation is usually made by a pelvic X-ray. Any IUD that has perforated the uterus should be removed because the risks of intra-abdominal inflammatory response, leading to adhesions or perforation of organs within the abdominal cavity outweigh the risks associated with removal.

Pregnancy

Pregnancy may occur in 3–5 per hundred users per year. About 50% of uterine pregnancies occurring with the device in situ end in a spontaneous abortion. Removal of the IUD in early pregnancy has been found to reduce this abortion rate by half. In women who continue the pregnancy with the device in situ, a four-fold increase in the occurrence of premature births has been reported.

Lowest pregnancy rates are observed with Cu T-380A and LNG-IUS. Should pregnancy occur with a device in situ, there is risk of ectopic pregnancy (1–2%).

If the thread is visible through the cervix, it is best to remove the device. However, if the thread is not visible it is better to leave it alone after counseling the woman about the risks involved in continuing the pregnancy. The device may be expelled spontaneously with the delivery of the placenta.

Ectopic pregnancy

Ectopic pregnancies among IUD users are estimated at 3–4% of all pregnancies, while among nonusers, the estimate is 0.8% of all pregnancies. Women using IUDs must be taught to recognize the symptoms of ectopic pregnancy such as lower abdominal pain, dark and scanty vaginal bleeding or amenorrhea. Women with previous ectopic pregnancy or PID should not use IUD if other methods are feasible. Studies indicate that the rate of ectopic pregnancies is higher among users of hormone-containing devices than among women using other IUDs.

Expulsion

Expulsion rate vary between 4% and 30%. It can be partial or complete. Partial expulsion can be diagnosed on speculum examination by observing the stem of the IUD protruding through the cervix. Spontaneous expulsion occurs during the 1st few weeks or during menstruation. Expulsion is more common among young women, nulliparous women and women who have postpartum insertion. Expulsion rates are somewhat lower for copper than for inert devices. In general, expulsion in itself is not a serious problem, but if expulsion is unnoticed, pregnancy may occur.

Fertility after removal

Fertility does not seem to be impaired after removal of a device provided there has been no episode of PID, whilst the device was in situ. Over 70% of IUD users conceive within 1 year of removal. It is now established that PID is a threat to woman's fertility.

Mortality

Mortality with IUD use is extremely rare and has been estimated to be one death per 100,000 woman years of use. The deaths usually occur following complications such as septic spontaneous abortion or ectopic pregnancy. In this regard, IUD is safer than oral contraceptive, particularly in older or high-risk women.

Cancer or teratogenesis

There is no evidence to date that IUD use increases cancer risks. Nor there is any evidence of developmental abnormality or congenital malformations among the offspring of either former IUD users or those who conceive with an IUD in situ.

Indications for Removal of IUD

The indications for removal are:
1. Persistent excessive regular or irregular bleeding and/or severe cramp-like pain in the lower abdomen.
2. Flaring up of salpingitis.
3. Perforation of the uterus with the device in the peritoneal cavity.
4. Downward displacement of the device into the cervical canal or partly protruding outside into the vagina.
5. Patient desirous of a baby.
6. Missing thread.

Missing thread

The thread may not be visible through the cervical os due to:
1. Thread coiled inside.
2. Thread torn through.
3. Device expelled outside unnoticed by the woman.
4. Device perforated the uterine wall and lying in the peritoneal cavity.
5. Device pulled up by the growing uterus in pregnancy.

Identification of the missing IUD is done by straight X-ray or ultrasonography.

Removal may be done with a specially designed hook, an artery forceps or by uterine curette. Removal under hysteroscopic visualization is the best procedure.

Advantages of Third Generation IUDs over the Others (Cu T-380A, ML Cu 375, LNG-IUS)

1. Higher efficiency with lower pregnancy rate (< 1% women per year).
2. Significant reduction in menorrhagia, dysmenorrhea and premenstrual tension syndrome is observed with LNG-IUS.
3. Risk of ectopic pregnancy is significantly reduced (0.02/HWY).
4. Risk of PID is reduced.
5. Longer duration of action (5–10 year).
6. Low expulsion rate and fewer indications for medical removal.

Disadvantages of Third Generation IUDs

1. Expensive.
2. Not available through government channel in India currently.
3. Deposition of calcium salts over the device on prolonged use may prevent the diffusion of copper.

Copper T (Cu T) is distributed free of cost through government channel in India. Because of the prolonged contraceptive protection, it is suitable for the rural population of developing countries. With Cu T, there are no systemic side effects and reversibility to fertility is prompt soon after removal. Local reactions include menstrual abnormalities, pelvic pain, heavy period and pelvic inflammatory disease. Ectopic pregnancy is a risk and failure rate is 0.1–2.0 HWY.

Steroidal/Hormonal Contraceptives

Hormonal contraceptives when properly used are the most effective spacing methods of contraception. Oral contraceptives of the combined type are almost 100% effective in preventing pregnancy. More than 65 million people in the world are estimated to be taking the 'pill' of which about 10 million are estimated to be in India.

Gonadal Steroids

Estrogens and progestogens are the gonadal steroids used for contraception:
1. *Synthetic estrogens*: Two synthetic estrogens are used in oral contraceptives. These are ethinyl estradiol and mestranol. Both are effective.
2. *Synthetic progestogens*: These are classified into three groups—pregnanes, estranes and gonanes.

Estranes, which are also known as 14-nortestosterones and gonanes, are used in oral contraceptives.

Classification of Hormonal Contraceptives

Hormonal contraceptives currently in use and/or under study are classified as follows:
1. Oral pills:
   - Combined pill
   - Progestogen-only pill (POP)—minipill
   - Postcoital pill
   - Once a month (long-acting) pill.
2. Depot (slow-releasing) formulations:
   - Injectables
   - Subdermal implants
   - Vaginal rings.

Combined pill

The combination pill is one of the major spacing methods of contraception. Most formulations of the combined pill of the present time contain 30–35 μg of synthetic estrogen and 0.5–1.0 mg of progestogen.

The pill is given orally for 21 consecutive days beginning on the 5th day of the menstrual cycle, followed by a break of 7 days of no hormonal intake (7 pills contain no hormones and are inert) during which menstruation occurs. When bleeding occurs, this is considered the 1st day of the next cycle. The bleeding is not like normal menstruation, but is an episode of uterine bleeding from an incompletely formed endometrium caused by the withdrawal of exogenous hormones. Therefore, it is called 'withdrawal bleeding' rather than menstruation. The loss of blood, which occurs, is about half that occurring in a woman having ovulatory cycle. If bleeding does not occur, the woman is instructed to start the second cycle 1 week after the preceding one. Ordinarily, the woman menstruates after the second course of pill intake.

The pill should be taken every day at a fixed time, preferably before going to bed at night. The first course should be started strictly on the 5th day of the menstrual period, as any deviation in this respect may not prevent pregnancy. If the user forgets to take a pill, she should take it as soon as she remembers and that she should take the next day's pill at the usual time. If she forgets her pill for 2 days in a row, she should be advised to continue the daily schedule, but to use an additional contraceptive, such as condom for the remainder of the cycle. Cessation of pill taking at any point prior to completion of the full cycle of pills will result in withdrawal bleeding.

Biphasic and triphasic preparations are two different formulations of the combined pills. In these pills, there are two and three different levels of progestogens respectively during a 21-day cycle of pills followed by 7 days of no hormonal pills. These are prepared to mimic the natural hormonal fluctuations during the menstrual cycle.

Types of pills
The department of family welfare, in the Ministry of Health and Family Welfare, Government of India has made available two types of low dose oral pills under the brand names of Mala N and Mala D:
1. *Mala N* **(Fig. 24.7A)**: Norgestrel 0.3 mg and ethinyl estradiol 0.03 mg.
2. *Mala D* **(Fig. 24.7B)**: Norgestrel 0.3 mg and ethinyl estradiol 0.03 mg.

Mala D is available in a package of 28 pills (21 of oral contraceptive pills and 7 brown, ferrous fumarate coated tablets at a price of ₹ 2/packet). Mala N is supplied free of coast through all Primary Health Centers and Urban Family Welfare Centers.

Mode of action
The probable mechanisms of contraception are:
1. *Inhibition of ovulation:* Both the hormones act synergistically on the hypothalamic-pituitary axis. The release of gonadotropic-releasing hormones from the hypothalamus is prevented through a negative feedback mechanism. There is thus no peak release of follicle-stimulating hormone (FSH) and luteinizing hormone (LH) from the anterior pituitary, so the follicular growth is not initiated.
2. *Production of static endometrial hypoplasia:* There is stromal edema, residual reaction and regression of glands.
3. *Alteration of the character of the cervical mucus:* Thick, viscid and scanty to prevent sperm penetration.

Contraindications
The contraindications are either absolute or relative:
1. Absolute:
   a. Circulatory diseases (past or present):
      » Arterial or venous thrombosis
      » Severe hypertension
      » Valvular disease, ischemic heart disease, angina
      » Hyperlipidemia
      » Focal migraine.
   b. Diseases of the liver:
      » Active liver disease
      » History of cholestatic jaundice in pregnancy
      » Liver adenoma, carcinoma.
   c. Others:
      » Pregnancy
      » Genital tract bleeding
      » Breast cancer.
2. Relative:
   a. Obesity.
   b. Varicosities.
   c. Epilepsy.
   d. Bronchial asthma.
   e. Depression, mood fluctuation.
   f. Age over 35.
   g. Smoking.
   h. Nursing mothers who are in the first 6 months.

Follow-up
The woman should be examined after 3 months, 6 months and then once a year. Women above 35 years should be checked more frequently. Any adverse symptoms are to be noted at each visit. Examinations of breasts, weight, blood pressure and pelvic examination including cytology are to be done and compared with the previous records.

Length of pill use
For spacing of births, use of 3–5 years is considered adequate and safe. However, with careful monitoring, pill use may continue until the age of 40. Beyond 40 years, pills may not be continued because of the risk of cardiovascular complications.

Beneficial effects
The most important benefit is prevention of unwanted pregnancy (failure rate is 0.1 per HWY).
The non-contraceptive benefits are:
1. Relief of:
   – Menorrhagia (less by 50%)
   – Dysmenorrhea (less by 40%)
   – Premenstrual tension syndrome
   – Mittelschmerz syndrome.
2. Improvement of:
   – Iron deficiency anemia
   – Endometriosis

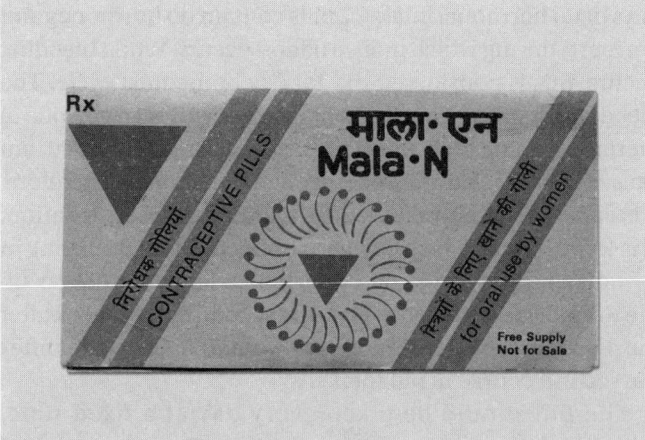
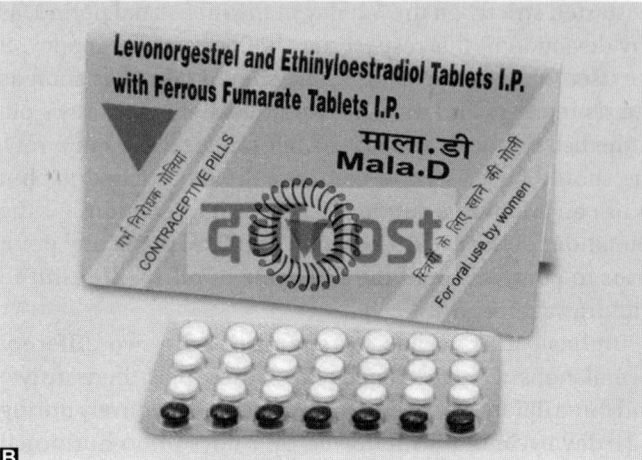

Figures 24.7A and B: (A) Mala N; (B) Mala D.

- Hirsutism
- Rheumatoid arthritis.
3. Reduction in risk of:
    - Pelvic inflammatory disease
    - Benign breast disease
    - Fibroid uterus
    - Functional ovarian cysts
    - Carcinoma of endometrium and ovary
    - Osteoporosis.

Adverse effects
1. Nausea, vomiting and headache—these are transient and often subside following continuous use.
2. Mastalgia—heaviness and tenderness of breasts are transient.
3. Weight gain and edema of legs.
4. Chloasma and acne.
5. Menstrual abnormalities—breakthrough bleeding, hypomenorrhea, menorrhagia and amenorrhea.
6. Reduced libido.
7. Leukorrhea.

Major complications
1. Depression, change of mood and sleep disturbances.
2. Hypertension (less than 1% of cases).
3. Vascular complications—venous thromboembolism, arterial thrombosis.
4. Cholestatic jaundice (due to stasis of bile).

Effects on reproduction
1. Ovulation returns within 3 months of withdrawal of the drug in 90% of cases.
2. Lactation may be affected by a reduction in the milk production.

Progestogen-only pill
Progestogen-only pill is commonly referred to as the minipill or micropill. It contains only progestogen, which is given in small doses throughout the cycle. The commonly used progestogens are norethisterone (350 µg) and levonorgestrel (30 µg).

Mechanism of action
Progestogen-only pills works mainly by making cervical mucus thick and viscous, thereby prevents sperm penetration. Endometrium becomes atrophic. In about 2% of cases, ovulation is inhibited.

Advantages
1. No adverse effects on lactation and hence, can be suitably given to lactating women and as such is known as lactation pill.
2. It can be given to women having hypertension, fibroid, diabetes or epilepsy.

Drawbacks
1. There may be breakthrough bleeding or at times amenorrhea in about 20–30% of cases.
2. Simple cysts in ovary may be seen.
3. Failure rate is about 0.5–2 per HWY.

Postcoital pill
Postcoital (or 'morning after') contraception is recommended within 48 hours of unprotected intercourse. Two methods are available:

1. IUD, especially a copper device.
2. Hormonal: More often, a hormonal method may be preferable.

The combined oral pill has been generally accepted as the preparation of choice for postcoital contraception, as it is less likely to cause adverse side effects. The method is to give a double dose of the standard combined pill. The recommended regimen is to take two pills immediately, followed by another two pills 12 hours later, if pills containing 50 µg, are used. If pills containing 30–35 µg estrogen are available, four of these must be taken at one time rather than two in each dose.

Postcoital contraception is advocated as an emergency method, e.g. after unprotected intercourse, rape or contraceptive failure. Although, the failure rate of postcoital contraception is less than 1%, some experts think, a woman should not use this method unless she intends to have an abortion, if the method fails. Though there is no evidence of fetal abnormalities, some doubts remain regarding this.

Once a month (long-acting) pill
Experiments with once a month pill in which quinestrol, a long-acting estrogen is given in combination with a short-acting progestrogen, have been disappointing. The pregnancy rate was too high to be acceptable.

Depot (slow-releasing) formulations
The need for depot formulations, which are highly effective, reversible, long-acting and estrogen free for spacing pregnancies in which a single administration suffices for several months or years led to the development of injectable contraceptives and subdermal implants.

Injectable contraceptives
There are two types of injectable contraceptives:
1. Depot medroxyprogesterone acetate (DMPA) or Depo-Provera.
2. Norethisterone enanthate (NET-EN).

Both are administered intramuscularly. DMPA is given in a dose of 150 mg every 3 months or 300 mg every 6 months. NET-EN is given in a dose of 200 mg at 2-monthly intervals.

Mechanism of action
1. Inhibition of ovulation by suppressing the midcycle LH peak.
2. Cervical mucus becomes thick and viscid thereby prevents sperm penetration.
3. Endometrium becomes atrophic preventing blastocyst implantation, if fertilization occurs, which is extremely unlikely.

Advantages
1. It eliminates regular medication as imposed by oral pill.
2. It can be used safely during lactation.
3. No estrogen related side effects.
4. Menstrual symptoms such as menorrhagia and dysmenorrhea are reduced.
5. Protective against endometrial cancer.
6. Can be used as an interim contraception before vasectomy becomes effective.

Drawbacks
1. Failure rate for DMPA is 0–1 per HWY.
2. There are chances of irregular bleeding and an occasional phase of amenorrhea.
3. Return of fertility after their discontinuation is usually delayed for several months (4–8 months).
4. The preparations are available only in selected centers in India. The potential long-term effects of DMPA and NET-EN are not yet known.

Subdermal implants (Fig. 24.8)
The population council, New York has developed a subdermal implant known as *Norplant* for long-term contraception. It consists of six silastic (silicone rubber) capsules containing 35 mg (each) of levonorgestrel. More recent devices comprise fabrication of levonorgestrel into two small rods, *Norplant (R)-2*, which are comparatively easier to insert and remove. It initially releases 80 µg and later on reduced to 30 µg levonorgestrel per day over 5 years.

Norplant capsules measure 34 mm × 24 mm and provide effective contraception for 5 years.

Insertion
The capsules are inserted subdermally, in the inner aspect of the non-dominant arm, 6–8 cm above the elbow fold. It is done under local anesthetic. It is ideally inserted on day 1 of menstrual cycle, immediately after abortion and 3 weeks after delivery.

Removal
Norplant should be removed within 5 years of insertion. Loss of contraceptive action is immediate.

Advantages
Advantages are same as with DMPA and additional ones are:
1. Improvement of anemia due to control of menorrhagia.
2. Suitable for women who have completed their family and do not desire permanent sterilization.

Efficacy is comparable to the combined pills. Failure rate is 0.7 per HWY.

Disadvantages
1. Frequent irregular, menstrual bleeding, spotting, especially in the 1st year.
2. Surgical procedure necessary to insert and remove implants.

Implanon
Single implant rod of 4 cm long, containing 60 mg of ketodesogestrel is used. It releases the hormone about 60 µg per day over 3 years. Use of single rod makes Implanon easier for insertion and removal. Efficacy and side effects are the same as that of Norplant.

Vaginal ring (Nova ring)
A ring-shaped device that contains the hormone estradiol and etonogestrel (a progestin) can be placed in the vagina. It remains in place for 3 weeks continuously and releases low levels of hormone into the bloodstream. Then it is removed for a week to allow for menstrual period.

PERMANENT METHODS (STERILIZATION)

Voluntary sterilization is a well-established contraceptive procedure for couples desiring no more children. Currently female sterilizations account for 85% and male sterilizations for 10–15% of all sterilizations in India. Voluntary sterilization is a surgical method whereby the reproductive function of an individual male or female is destroyed purposefully and permanently. The operation done on male is vasectomy and that on female is tubal ligation or tubal occlusion.

Sterilization offers many advantages over other contraceptive methods:
- It is a one-time method
- It does not require sustained motivation of the user for its effectiveness
- It provides the most effective protection against pregnancy
- The risk of complications is small if the procedure is performed according to accepted medical standards
- It is most cost-effective.

Guidelines for Sterilization

Sterilization services are provided free of charge in government institutions. Guidelines issued by the Government of India covers various aspects of sterilization. These are:
1. The age of husband should not ordinarily be less than 25 years or more than 45 years.
2. The age of wife should not be less than 20 years or more than 45 years.
3. The motivated couple must have two living children at the time of operation.
4. If the couple has three or more living children, the lower limit of age of the husband or wife may be relaxed at the discretion of the operating surgeon.
5. The couple knows that for all practical purposes, the operation is reversible.

Vasectomy or Male Sterilization

Vasectomy is a permanent sterilization operation done in the male, where a segment of vas deferens of both the sides is resected (1 cm) and the cut ends are ligated. The ligated ends are then folded back on them and sutured into position, so that the cut ends face away from each other. This will reduce the risk of recanalization later.

Following vasectomy, sperm production and hormone output are not affected. The sperm produced are destroyed intraluminally by phagocytosis. This is a normal process in the male genital tract, but the rate is increased after vasectomy.

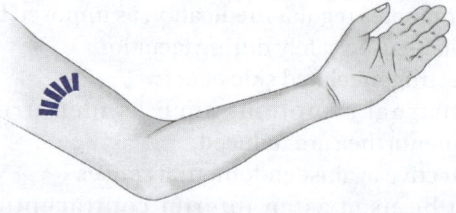

Figure 24.8: Subdermal implant—norplant.

The vasectomized person is not immediately sterile after operation, usually until approximately thirty ejaculations have taken place, as the semen is stored in the distal part of the vas deferens for about 2–3 months. During this period, another contraceptive must be used.

Advantages

1. The vasectomy operation is simple and can be performed as an outpatient or outdoor procedure.
2. Complications—immediate or late, are few.
3. Failure rate is about 0.15% and there is a fair chance of success of reversal anastomosis (recanalization) operation (50%).
4. The overall expenditure is minimal in terms of the equipment, hospital stay and doctor's training. Cost wise the ratio is about five vasectomies to one tubal ligation.

Drawbacks

1. Additional contraception is needed for about 2–3 months following operation, i.e. until the semen becomes free of sperm.
2. Frigidity or impotency when occurs is mostly psychological.

Selection of Candidates

Sexually active and psychologically adjusted husband having the desired number of children is an ideal candidate. Any misconception about the fear of castration, loss of hormones and impotency are to be removed by sympathetic explanation. Eczema or scabies in the scrotal area is a temporary contraindication. In the presence of hydrocele or inguinal hernia, vasectomy can be done only along with the operative correction of these conditions.

Postoperative Advices

1. Antibiotic injection (Penidure) is administered as a routine and an analgesic is prescribed.
2. Weight lifting, heavy work and cycling are restricted for about 2 weeks while usual activities can be performed forthwith.
3. To wear a scrotal support (T-bandage) for 15 days.
4. The patient should report for checkup after 1 week or earlier, if any complication arises.
5. To have the stitches removed on the 5th day.
6. Additional contraceptive should be used for 3 months.
7. Semen should be examined once a month and if two consecutive semen analyzes show an absence of spermatozoa, the man is declared sterile. Until then additional contraceptive (condom or DMPA) should be advised.

Complications

1. Immediate:
    a. Wound sepsis, which may lead to scrotal cellulitis or abscess.
    b. Scrotal hematoma.
2. Remote:
    a. Frigidity or impotency: It is mostly psychological in origin. They may complain of diminution of sexual vigor, impotence, headache or fatigue.
    b. Sperm granuloma or sperm granules caused by accumulation of sperm. They appear in 10–14 days after the operation. The most frequent symptoms are pain and swelling. The mass is hard and approximate size is 7 mm. The sperm granules eventually subside. This can be prevented by cauterization or fulguration of the cut ends.
    c. Autoimmune response: Vasectomy is said to cause an autoimmune response to sperm. Blocking of the vas causes reabsorption of spermatozoa and subsequent development of antibodies against sperm in blood. Normally 2% of men have circulating antibodies against their sperm. In vasectomized men, the figure can be as high as 54%. Such antibodies are harmless to physical health. It is likely that they can cause a reduction in subsequent fertility despite successful reanastomosis of the vas.
    d. Spontaneous recanalization: The incidence of recanalization is variously placed between 0% and 6%. Its occurrence is serious. Therefore, the surgeon should explain the possibility of this complication to every acceptor prior to the operation and have written consent acknowledging this fact. Regular follow-up for up to 3 years is recommended to avoid this possibility.

No-scalpel Vasectomy (Figs. 24.9 and 24.10)

No-scalpel vasectomy is a new technique, i.e. safe, convenient and acceptable to males. This new method is now being canvassed for men as a special project, on a voluntary basis under the family welfare program. This method, which is popular in China, is performed under local anesthetic. Stretched skin over the vas is punctured with one blade of sharp-pointed dissecting scissors, instead of using a scalpel. Then the hole is increased and the vas is dissected out by using the tip of the scissors. The testicular end is dropped back into the scrotum and the upper end is cauterized. The procedure is repeated for the second vas through the same incision. The rest of the steps are same as for the regular vasectomy procedure.

Open-ended Vasectomy

The abdominal end of the resected vas is coagulated. The testicular end is left open. This will prevent congestive epididymitis.

Female Sterilization

Occlusion of the fallopian tubes in some form is the underlying principle to achieve female sterilization. It is the most popular method of terminal contraception, specially adopted in the developing countries, where high parity births prevail in a comparatively younger age group. It is also widely accepted in the affluent countries.

Female sterilization also known as *tubal ligation* or *tubectomy* is a surgical procedure in which the fallopian

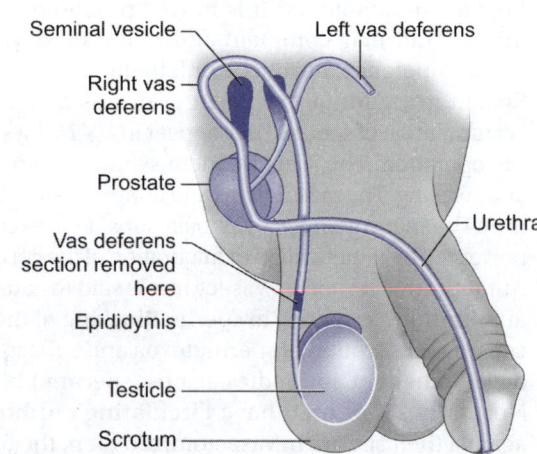

Figure 24.9: Vasectomy operation showing the site of vasectomy.

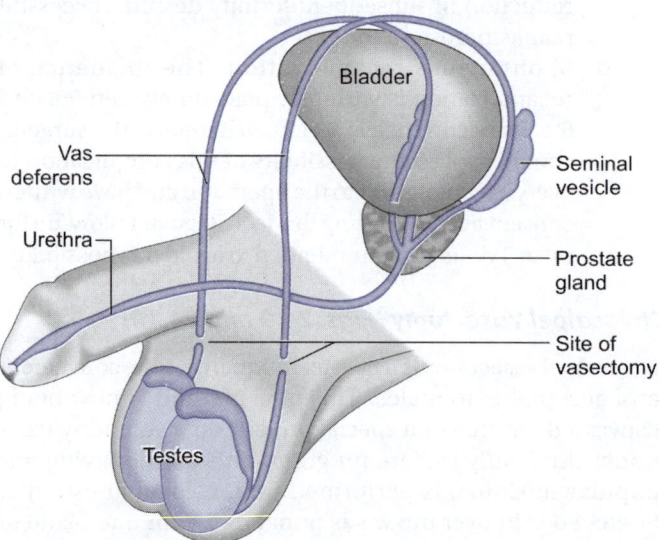

Figure 24.10: Vasectomy site on the scrotum.

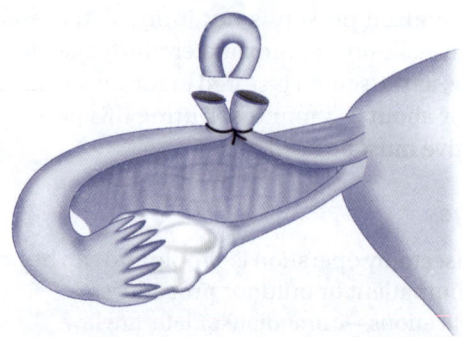

Figure 24.11: Partial salpingectomy (Pomeroy method).

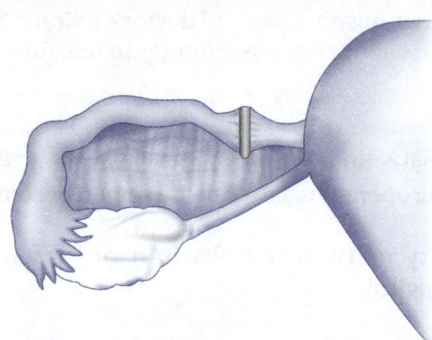

Figure 24.12: Hulka clip on fallopian tube.

tubes are severed and sealed or 'pinched shut' in order to prevent fertilization. It is a highly effective, safe and simple procedure that involves cutting, tying or removing a part of the fallopian tubes. Consequently the passage of eggs from the ovaries to the uterus is blocked and sperm will not be able to reach the eggs. The eggs released from the ovaries after tubal ligation break and get absorbed harmlessly by the body. Tubal ligation is performed in a hospital as inpatient or outpatient procedure under general or regional anesthesia, using various techniques.

Methods of Tubal Ligation

1. *Occlusion method:* It is for tubal ligation are typically carried out on the isthmic position of the fallopian tube that is the thin portion of the tube closest to the uterus:
   a. Partial salpingectomy: The Pomeroy technique is widely used for achieving partial salpingectomy. This method involves tying a small loop of the tube by suture and cutting off the top segment of the loop. This can be done via laparoscopy or laparotomy **(Fig. 24.11)**.
   b. Clips: It clamps the tube and inhibit blood flow to that portion causing a small amount of scarring or fibrosis, in turn preventing fertilization. The most commonly used clips are *Filshie clip* made of titanium and the *Hulka clip* or *Wolf clip* made of stainless steel and spring loaded. Clips are simple to insert, but require a special instrument to put it in place **(Fig. 24.12)**.
   c. The clip is introduced into the abdominal cavity via laparoscopic clip applicator. It is placed across the fallopian tube and when closed, a small spring holds it firmly. The Hulka clip has the advantage of damaging only a very small portion of the fallopian tube—approximately 7 mm. The squeezed portion is deprived of its blood supply and eventually undergoes a vascular necrosis.
   d. Falope rings: Tubal rings are similar to clips and they are used to block the tube mechanically. When placed, it encircles a small loop of the fallopian tube, blocking the blood supply to that small loop, resulting in scarring that blocks passage of sperm or egg. A commonly used type of ring is the *Yoon ring* made of silicone. The procedure is performed by inserting a laparoscope just under the umbilicus. After identifying the fallopian tube, the device with the ring is slid over 2–3 cm 'knuckle' of tube that is kinked off by the ring. This is done once for each side **(Fig. 24.13)**.

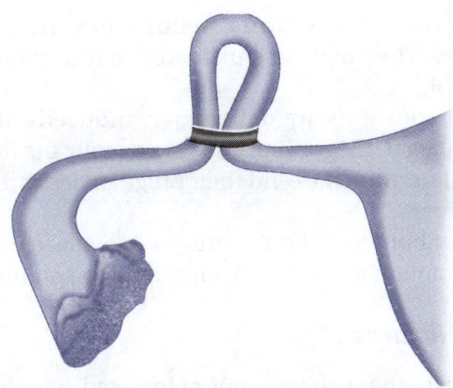

Figure 24.13: Falope ring on fallopian tube.

e. Electrocoagulation or cauterization: Electric current is used to coagulate or burn a small portion of each fallopian tube. It mostly uses bipolar coagulation, where electric current enters and leaves through two ends of a forceps applied to the tubes. The procedure is usually done via laparoscopy.

2. *Method of tubal ligation by entry sites or routes:*
   a. Laparotomy method:
      i. Pomeroy method: An occlusion type procedure in which a part of the fallopian tube on each side is elevated to create a loop or knuckle. An absorbable suture is tied around the base of the elevated segment and the segment is severed (**Fig. 24.12**).
      In modified Pomeroy method, a silk stitch is applied medial to the tubal stump after the conventional steps. Pomeroy method is usually performed after delivery by cesarean section.
      ii. Irving tubal ligation: In this procedure two ligatures are placed around the tube in its proximal to midsegment and a tubal segment between the two ligatures is removed. The tied end of the tube attached to the uterus is then sutured into the back side of uterus and the other end is buried in the connective tissue underlying the fallopian tube. This method keeps the two cut ends of the tubes healthy, should reversal microsurgery become a need.
      iii. Uchida method: The fallopian tube is dissected at the midpoint and the proximal end is ligated and allowed to drop back into a sac that has been created in the serosa. The distal end is tied and left to project into the abdominal cavity. This method has been abandoned, as it was associated with higher failure rates. Earlier techniques that used fimbriectomy were also abandoned.
   b. Laparoscopic tubal ligation: The procedure is done under general or regional anesthesia. The surgeon makes an incision of about 1½ inches just inside the naval. The laparoscope (a fine tube that conducts light connected to a telescope) is inserted through the opening. The instrument for blocking the tube is then introduced through another opening on the side. Application of clips, rings or cauterization is then performed.
   c. Minilaparotomy: This procedure is done under general anesthesia and involves making a small incision just above the pubic hairline. The surgeon lifts the fallopian tubes through the incision and blocks them using electrocoagulation, clips or rings. This method differs from laparoscopy that no visualizing instrument is inserted.
   This method is recommended for women for whom laparoscopy is contraindicated, such as those who had previous abdominal surgery for other reasons, recent or chronic tubal infections, or serious heart or respiratory illness.
   d. Vaginal tubal ligation (colpotomy): This procedure is done for women, who cannot have a laparoscopy or laparotomy. This involved making a small incision in the vaginal wall through which the surgeon can draw the tubes and ligate them using suture material.
   The procedure can be performed under local anesthesia and there will be no visible scar. However, the woman is more susceptible to infection because of high bacterial count in vagina. Some women find sexual intercourse painful for several months after surgery.

Timing for Tubal Ligation

1. *Postpartum or puerperal tubal ligation:* This procedure is basically a minilaparotomy done following childbirth. It is done through a small incision just below the umbilicus. This operation may be performed any time within the first 3 days of childbirth.
2. *Cesarean ligation:* The procedure is done, following cesarean childbirth for women who have completed their families.
3. *Interval tubal ligation:* The operation is done beyond 3 months following delivery or abortion. The ideal time of procedure is following the menstrual period in the proliferative phase.
4. *Concurrent with metatarsophalangeal (MTP):* Sterilization is done along with termination of pregnancy.

Advantages of Female Sterilization

- Very effective as a method of contraception
- Gives permanent or lifelong protection
- Nothing to remember, no supplies needed and no repeated clinic visits required
- No interference with sex
- No known long-term side effects or health risks

Disadvantages or Possible Problems

- Pain for few days after surgery
- Infection or bleeding at the incision site
- Injury to internal organs
- Anesthetic risks:

- Allergic reaction or overdose of local anesthesia or sedation
- Delayed recovery and side effects of general anesthesia.
❖ Reversal surgery is difficult and expensive.

Failure Rate

The overall failure rate for tubal ligation is about 0.7%, the Pomeroy technique being the lowest 0.1–0.3%.

Mortality rate following tubal ligation is estimated to be 72 per 100,000 for all methods. Laparoscopic procedures carried a mortality rate of 5–10 per 100,000 compared to 7 per 100,000 for puerperal ligations [Indian Council of Medical Research (ICMR), 1982].

POSTCONCEPTION METHODS OF BIRTH CONTROL (TERMINATION OF PREGNANCY)

Menstrual Regulation

Menstrual regulation is a relatively simple method of birth control. It consists of aspiration of the uterine contents 6–14 days of a missed period, but before most pregnancy tests can accurately determine whether a woman is pregnant. Cervical dilatation is indicated only in nullipara or in apprehensive subjects. No aftercare is necessary as a rule.

The immediate complications are uterine trauma and perforation. Late complications (after 6 week) include a tendency to abortion or premature labor (if the aspiration was not successful), infertility, menstrual disorders and an increase in ectopic pregnancies. Menstrual regulation differs from abortion in three respects:
1. The lack of certainty, if a pregnancy is being terminated.
2. The lack of legal restrictions.
3. Increased safety as the procedure is done early in pregnancy.

Menstrual Induction

Menstrual induction is based on disturbing the normal progesterone prostaglandin balance by intrauterine application of 1–5 mg solution (or 2.5–5 mg pellet) of prostaglandin F_2. Within a few minutes of the prostaglandin impact, performed under sedation, the uterus responds with a sustained contraction lasting about 7 minutes, followed by cyclic contractions continuing for 3–4 hours. The bleeding starts and continues for 7–8 days.

Abortion

Abortion is defined as termination of pregnancy before the fetus becomes viable (capable of living independently). This has been fixed administratively at 28 weeks, when the fetus weighs approximately 1,000 g. Abortion is sought by women for a variety of reasons including birth control.

Abortions usually are categorized as *spontaneous and induced*.

Spontaneous abortions occur once in every 15 pregnancies. They may be considered 'nature's method of birth control'.

Induced abortions are deliberately induced—they may be legal or illegal. Illegal abortions are usually the last resort of women determined to end their pregnancies at the risk of their own lives.

In India, about 6 million abortions take place every year of which 4 million are induced and 2 million spontaneous.

Abortion Hazards

Abortions, whether spontaneous or induced, whether in the hands of skilled or unskilled persons are usually fraught with hazards, resulting in maternal morbidity and mortality. The mortality ratio ranges from 1 to 3.5 per 100,000 in developed countries (WHO technical report, 1978). In India, mortality is reported to be 7.8 per 1,000 'random abortions'. This is because most of the random abortions are illegally induced.

The early complications of abortion include hemorrhage, shock, sepsis, uterine perforation, cervical injury, thromboembolism and anesthetic and psychiatric complications.

The late complications include infertility, ectopic gestation, increased risk of spontaneous abortion and reduced birth weight of newborns. The optimum time for termination of pregnancy is the 7th and 8th weeks of gestation. Studies indicate that the risk of death is seven times higher for women, who wait until the second trimester to terminate pregnancy. The Indian law [The Medical Termination of Pregnancy (MTP) Act, 1971] allows abortion only up to 20 weeks of pregnancy.

The MTP Act is a healthcare measure, which helps to reduce maternal morbidity and mortality resulting from illegal abortions. It also affords an opportunity for motivating such women to adopt some form of contraception.

Although, abortion has been greatly liberalized, the annual number of legal abortions are about 0.6 million, which contribute hardly 10% of the abortions done in the country. The numerous abortion hazards, which are inherent, should serve as a warning that abortions even under the best of circumstances can never be as safe as efficient contraception.

STUDY QUESTIONS

Short Notes

1. Natural contraception.
2. Postcoital contraception.
3. Menstrual induction.

Short Answer Questions

1. Oral contraceptives.
2. Subdermal implants.
3. Hazards of induced abortion.

Essay Questions

1. Explain the types of intrauterine contraceptive devices, their mode of actions and client instructions.
2. Explain the puerperal tubal ligation, advantages, disadvantages and patient instructions.

BIBLIOGRAPHY

1. Bounds W. Contraceptive efficacy if the diaphragm and cervical caps are used in conjunction with spermicides—A fresh look at the evidence". British Journal of Family Planning. 1994;20:84-7.
2. Calderone MS. Manual of Contraceptive Practice. Baltimore: Williams and Wilkins; 1964.
3. Dutta DC. Textbook of Obstetrics, 5th edition. Kolkata: New Central Book Company; 2001. pp. 368-98.
4. Ford N, Mathie E. The acceptability and experience of the female condom. British Journal of Family Planning. 1993;19:187-92.
5. Franey J. Family Planning. In: Bennett RV, Linda KB (Eds). Myles Textbook for Midwives, 13th edition. Edinburgh: Churchill Livingstone; 1999. pp. 629-50.
6. Government of India, Yearbook-Family Welfare Program in India. New Delhi: Ministry of Health; 1983. p. 4.
7. Guillebaud J. Combined hormonal contraception. In: Loudon N, Glasier A, Gebbie A (Eds). Handbook of Family Planning and Reproductive Health Care, 3rd edition. Edinburgh: Churchill Livingstone; 1995.
8. Hawkins DF, Elder MC. Human Fertility Control: Theory and Practice. London: Butterworth; 1979.
9. Huchings JE. International Family Planning Perspectives. 1985;11(3):77-85.
10. ICMR Bulletin; 1983.
11. Liskin L. Intrauterine Devices. The John Hopkins University, Population Report Series B:4, 1980.
12. Park K. Park's Textbook of Preventive and Social Medicine, 16th edition. Jabalpur: Banarsidas Bhanot Publishers; 2000. pp. 319-50.
13. Vlugt T, et al. Pregnancy Termination. The George Washington University Population Report Series F; 1973.
14. WHO. Global Health Situations and Projections; 1992.

SECTION VII

ABNORMALITIES OF PREGNANCY, LABOR AND PUERPERIUM

Section Outline

25. Abnormalities of Early Pregnancy
26. Sexually Transmissible and Reproductive Tract Infections
27. Disorders of Pregnancy
28. Hypertensive Disorders of Pregnancy
29. Medical Disorders, Gynecological Disorders and Psychiatric Disorders Associated with Pregnancy
30. Multiple Pregnancy
31. Preterm Labor, Premature Rupture of Membranes and Intrauterine Fetal Death
32. Post-term Pregnancy, Induction of Labor, Prolonged Labor and Disorders of Uterine Action
33. Malpositions and Malpresentations
34. Obstetric Operations
35. Obstetric Emergencies
36. Complications of Third Stage of Labor
37. Injuries to the Birth Canal
38. Complications of Puerperium

CHAPTER 25

Abnormalities of Early Pregnancy

Learning Objectives

Upon completing this chapter, the learner will be able to:
- Discuss the types of spontaneous and induced abortions, and the medical and nursing management of patients.
- Describe the varieties of ectopic gestation, their presentation, outcome and management.
- Enumerate the pathology, clinical presentation and treatment of hydatidiform mole in pregnancy.
- Discuss the clinical presentation and management of clients who suffer hyperemesis in pregnancy.
- Describe ABO and Rhesus (Rh) disease and retroversion.

ABORTION

Any bleeding in pregnancy is abnormal. Vaginal blood loss in early pregnancy should be thought of as a threatened miscarriage until shown otherwise. The term miscarriage and spontaneous abortion are synonymous.

Classification

The classification of abortion is shown in **Figure 25.1**.

Definition

Abortion is the process of partial or complete separation of the products of conception from the uterine wall with or without partial or complete expulsion from the uterine cavity before the age of viability.

The age of viability is 28 weeks in India. Abortions are usually categorized as spontaneous and induced.

SPONTANEOUS ABORTION

Spontaneous abortion is defined as the involuntary loss of the products of conception prior to 28 weeks of gestation, when the fetus weighs approximately 1,000 g or less.

Spontaneous abortions occur once in every 15 pregnancies. In India it has been computed that about 6 million abortions take place, every year of which 2 million are spontaneous and the 4 million are induced.

Causes

The causes of spontaneous abortion in most cases are not known. Where a cause is determined, 50% of miscarriages are due to chromosomal abnormalities of the conceptus. Genetic and structural causes are also attributed to pregnancy loss. Maternal causes are:
- Structural abnormalities of the genital organs such as retroversion of uterus, bicornuate uterus and fibroids
- Infections such as rubella and chlamydia
- Medical conditions such as diabetes, renal disease and thyroid dysfunction, when not well controlled.

Types

Threatened Abortion (Fig. 25.2)

Threatened an abortion is characterized by vaginal bleeding with or without recognizable uterine contractions. The blood loss may be scanty with or without accompanying backache and cramp-like pain. The pain may resemble dysmenorrhea or period pains. The cervix remains closed and the uterus soft with no tenderness when palpated.

The outcome of a threatened abortion could be either stoppage of bleeding and continuance of pregnancy to term

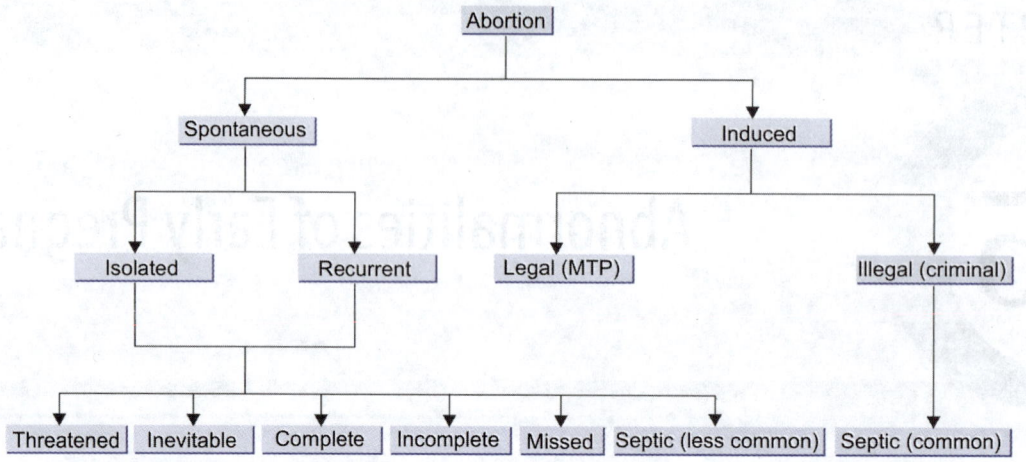

Figure 25.1: Classification of abortion. (MTP: medical termination of pregnancy)

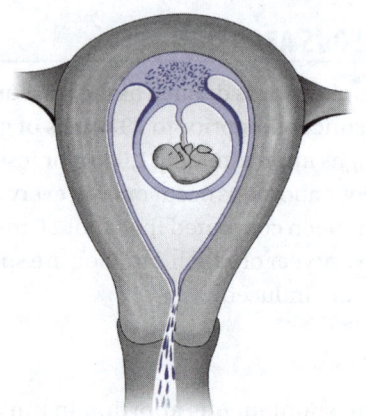

Figure 25.2: Threatened abortion.

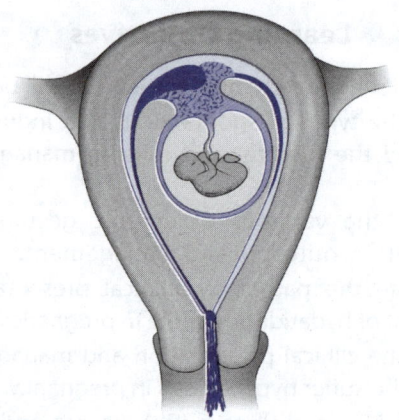

Figure 25.3: Inevitable abortion.

or continuance of bleeding and uterine contractions to expel the products of conception.

Management: General and systemic examination may reveal the cause of threatened abortion. Investigations include hemoglobin, ABO grouping and Rh, venereal disease research laboratory (VDRL), urine routine and blood glucose. Thyroid function tests are done if thyroid dysfunction is suspected. Plasma progesterone estimation is done if corpus luteum insufficiency is suspected. The patient is admitted and given complete rest in bed. If any specific cause is found, it is treated accordingly. If pregnancy continues, the possibility of intrauterine growth retardation, due to poor placental function must be considered. There is also an increased risk of preterm labor.

Inevitable Abortion (Fig. 25.3)

The woman presents with bleeding, often heavy, with clots or products of conception. Blood loss may be heavy and the mother in a shocked state. The cervix is dilated and on examination, products may be seen in the vagina or protruding through the os. The uterus if palpable may be smaller than expected.

Management: Blood loss may be controlled by administering injection syntocinon or ergometrine. The pain may be intense and appropriate analgesics are prescribed. The woman and her family must be given information and reassurance.

Incomplete Abortion (Fig. 25.4)

In this type of abortion, remnants of placenta remain within the uterine cavity, contributing to heavy and profuse bleeding. Intravenous or intramuscular ergometrine is given to control bleeding. Evacuation of the uterus to remove any retained tissue should be done under general anesthesia, when the mother is in a stable condition. Incomplete miscarriage is a cause of maternal mortality.

Complete Abortion (Fig. 25.5)

The conceptus, placenta and membranes are expelled completely from the uterus. The pain stops. Signs of pregnancy will regress. The uterus on palpation is contracted. No further medical intervention is required.

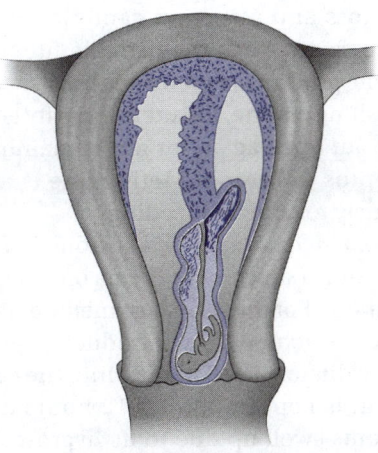

Figure 25.4: Incomplete abortion.

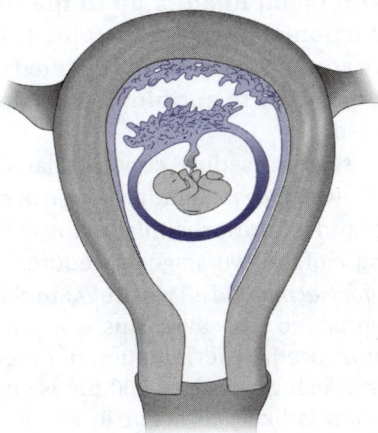

Figure 25.5: Complete abortion.

Missed Abortion

In missed abortion, the embryo dies despite the presence of a viable placenta and the sac is retained. Death of the embryo occurs before 8 weeks of gestation, but the mother's body fails to recognize the demise.

A brown discharge from the degeneration of placental tissue may present and threatened miscarriage is suspected. There may be a regression of signs and symptoms of pregnancy. Often there is failure to gain weight. The uterus is smaller than expected for the period of amenorrhea, firm rather than soft in consistency.

Thromboplastin may be liberated from the placental bed into the maternal circulation causing disseminated intravascular coagulation (DIC) usually about 5 weeks after fetal death.

Ultrasonography will show smaller than expected uterus with distorted or broken sac and an absence of fetal heart movements.

A coagulation profile is done because of the risk of hypofibrinogenemia. Treatment of a missed abortion of first trimester is evacuation of the uterus by dilation and curettage. In the second trimester, it is achieved by administration of prostaglandins intramuscularly.

Habitual Abortion

In this type, of spontaneous abortions in three or more successive pregnancies may occur. Usually abortions occur at the same gestational age. Cervical incompetence occurs when painless dilatation of the cervix occurs as pregnancy progresses allowing the membranes to bulge through the cervical os into the vagina. As the intrauterine pressure increases, the membranes may rupture, resulting in miscarriage. Abortions due to incompetent os, usually occurs after 16 weeks.

Causes of incompetence are uncertain. Genetic causes, endocrine factors and immunological factors are thought as possible causes.

Treatment: As follows:
- The patient is given complete bed rest from before the time of occurrence of the earliest abortion to after the time of occurrence of the latest abortion.
- Specific treatment is given for any cause identified.
- Cervical cerclage at 14 weeks gestation by Shirodkar's or McDonald's method; nonabsorbable suture is inserted at the level of the cervical os. This remains in situ until 38 weeks or the onset of labor, when it is removed.

INDUCED ABORTION

Induced abortion is deliberate interruption of an intact pregnancy. Induced abortions are performed legally in India since the Medical Termination Pregnancy (MTP) Act of 1971 (revised in 1975).

Medical Termination of Pregnancy (Legal Abortion)

Legal abortion is the deliberate induction of abortion prior to 20 weeks gestation by a registered medical practitioner in the interest of mother's health and life.

Provisions for MTP Under the MTP Act

1. The continuation of pregnancy would involve serious risk of life or grave injury to the physical and mental health of the pregnant woman.
2. There is substantial risk of the child being born with serious physical and mental abnormalities so as to be handicapped in life.
3. The pregnancy is the result of rape.
4. The pregnancy is caused as a result of failure of contraceptive.
5. Where there are actual or reasonably foreseeable environments (social or economic), which could lead to risk or injury to the health of the mother.

Indications for MTP

Therapeutic
- Deteriorating health due to pulmonary tuberculosis
- Cardiac diseases grade III and IV with history of decompensation

- Chronic glomerulonephritis
- Malignant hypertension
- Intractable hyperemesis gravidarum
- Cervical or breast malignancy
- Diabetes mellitus with retinopathy
- Psychiatric illness.

Social
- Parous women having unplanned pregnancy with low socioeconomic status
- Pregnancy caused by rape
- Pregnancy due to failure of contraceptive.

Eugenic
Risk of baby being born with various physical and mental abnormalities and include:
- Inherited chromosomal and gene disorders
- Exposure to teratogenic drugs or radiation
- Rubella infection in first trimester
- One or both parents being mentally defective
- Congenital malformations for siblings.

Consultation with geneticists will be required prior to deciding on MTP.

Conditions to be Met Prior to the Procedure

1. The act provides safeguards to the mother by authorizing only a registered medical practitioner having experience in gynecology and obstetrics to perform abortion where the length of pregnancy does not exceed 12 weeks. In order to terminate pregnancies, which exceed 12 weeks and are not more than 20 weeks, the opinion of two registered medical practitioners is necessary.
2. The procedure can only be performed in hospitals established or maintained by the government or places approved by the government for this purpose.
3. A pregnancy can be terminated only with the written consent of the woman.
4. Pregnancy in a minor (below the age of 18 years) or lunatic can only be terminated with the written consent of parents or legal guardians.
5. The procedure has to be reported to the Directorate of Health Services of the state.

Methods of Termination in the First Trimester

- *Menstrual regulation:* This is aspiration of uterine cavity and extraction of endometrium within 14 days of the missed period, when the presence of an early pregnancy is suspected. The procedure is performed by introducing a 4–5 mm flexible plastic cannula into the uterine cavity and sucking out the endometrium with a 50 mL plastic syringe attached to it. Menstrual regulation is done as an outpatient procedure.
- *Suction evacuation and curettage:* This is a procedure in which the products of conception are sucked out from the uterus with the help of a cannula attached to a suction apparatus. The cervix is dilated with small metal dilators and a suction cannula introduced into the uterine cavity. With the cannula fitted to a suction machine, the products of conception are sucked out. With a small flushing curette, the uterine cavity is curetted and suctioned out once again for any remaining portion of the conceptus. A dose of Methergine is administered intravenously to control bleeding.
- *Dilation and evacuation:* This is done either as a two-stage procedure (slow method) or a one-stage procedure (rapid method). For the two-stage method, slow dilatation of the cervix is achieved by introducing laminaria tents or synthetic dilators like Dilapan into the cervical canal. The woman is kept in bed for 12 hours during which time the tents swell up due to its hygroscopic property dilating the cervix. In the second stage of the procedure (after 12 hours), the tents are removed and cervix further dilated with metal dilators up to the desired extent for introduction of an ovum forceps. The products of conception are then removed and curetted with a flushing curette. Prophylactic antibiotic and Methergine are administered.
- For the one-stage procedure, cervical dilatation with metal dilators followed by evacuation is done at one stage. The steps of the procedure are similar to those followed in the second phase of the two-stage procedure.
- *Pharmacological methods:* Two drugs are commonly used.
    1. Mifepristone (RU 486): This is a progesterone antagonist used for termination of pregnancy up to 9 weeks. A single dose of 600 mg is given orally and abortion is likely to occur in about 36 hours. If it fails, prostaglandin E_1 methyl ester pessary (1 mg) is introduced vaginally to complete the abortion process. Abortion occurs within 4 hours.
    2. Methotrexate: Termination with methotrexate has been used effectively up to 8 weeks of pregnancy. A single dose of methotrexate is given intramuscularly followed by application of prostaglandin E_1 analog (misoprostol) vaginally. The products of conception are usually expelled in 3–4 hours.

Second Trimester Terminations (up to 20 weeks)

- *Intrauterine instillation* of hypertonic saline may be of intra-amniotic or extra-amniotic type.
- *Intra-amniotic instillation:* Hypertonic saline (20%) is instilled through a polythene tube connected to a drip set into the amniotic cavity. An amount of 10 mL multiplied by the number of weeks gestation is infused at a rate of 10 mL per minute. Uterine contraction and expulsion of the products of conception occurs in about 32 hours. Hypertonic urea (40%) with Syntocinon or prostaglandin is also used for intra-amniotic instillation.
- *Extrauterine instillation:* This is done by instillation of ethacridine lactate 0.1% solution vaginally about 10 cm above the internal os. Presence of the solution between

the membranes; and myometrium results in stripping of the membranes and dilatation of the cervix by the catheter (No. 16 Foley's) in about 4 hours. Expulsion of the products of conception follows.

- *Prostaglandins:* These are used in women for whom hypertonic saline is contraindicated. Vaginal, intramuscular, extra-amniotic and intra-amniotic methods are used for termination of pregnancy in the second trimester.
- *Oxytocin:* It is administered intravenously in conjunction with chemical agents used intra-amniotically or extra-amniotically, to augment the abortion process.
- *Hysterotomy:* It is used as a method of termination of midtrimester pregnancy where other methods of termination have failed or are contraindicated. The products of conception are extracted out of the uterus by cutting through the anterior wall of the uterus.

SEPTIC ABORTION

It is an abortion characterized by infection of the products of conception and the uterus. This condition is most commonly a complication of induced or incomplete abortion. Illegal abortions carried out in non-sterile conditions often lead to septic abortion.

Causes

- Criminal abortion, which is inexpert attempts at termination of pregnancy by passing sticks, catheters, pastes or soap solution into the uterine cavity
- Inevitable abortion with infection
- Medical termination of pregnancy with infection.

Clinical Manifestations

The patient may present with pyrexia (fever with chills), headache, nausea and foul smelling discharge per vagina. There is tenderness in the lower abdomen.

Examination may reveal localized infection in the uterine cavity and tubes, adnexal masses and pelvic abscess or generalized septicemia with peritonitis. They may even present with signs of septic shock and gas gangrene of the uterus. Blood culture and vaginal swabs should be taken to identify the cause of infection. Ultrasonography may be done for evaluation of adnexal masses.

Treatment

Intravenous antibiotics commencing with a broad-spectrum antibiotic and one effective against anaerobic infection are given. Pelvic abscess if present will be drained. When adequate blood levels of antibiotics have been reached, uterine evacuation by gentle curettage is done. Heparinization is done to prevent intravascular coagulation and in certain cases, an exchange transfusion is given to remove damaged red blood cells (RBCs).

NURSES' ROLE WITH PATIENTS UNDERGOING ABORTION

All women have an emotional response to learning or having confirmed that they are pregnant. For some it is very happy news, perhaps a much desired and planned for event; for some others the news has all the events of a catastrophe; for still others the response is that of not caring one way or the other. For all women, it requires a number of adjustments. The first trimester is the period of adjustment.

For a woman in the first category who desired having a baby, symptoms of miscarriage or termination of pregnancy brings lot of anxiety and grief. She may express feelings of inadequacies and failure, and even blame herself for the loss of her baby. She is incapable of bearing children. Some parents may want to see and hold the baby.

Midwives need to support the mother and her family at the time when they are grieving for their lost baby. Parents must be helped to meet their wishes. Depending on the type of abortion, they need advice regarding follow-up and future pregnancies.

The legalization of abortion means that every woman, upon being diagnosed as pregnant, now has a choice as to whether or not to carry the pregnancy to its natural conclusion. The woman's decision to have an abortion or to terminate her pregnancy is not lightly made. In many cases, she may approach the nurse for counsel, information and advice prior to the procedure. A calm and relaxed atmosphere and psychological support are import to the client during the procedure.

Women who undergo MTP as an inpatient procedure require close monitoring, support and care during therapy and as they develop uterine contractions and expel the products of conception.

It is important that all women going home after an abortion be aware of possible complications. Vaginal bleeding will continue for 1–3 weeks, but if it becomes heavier than a menstrual period, or if the patient passes large clots with bleeding, she should consult the physician, she should also seek medical advice if she develops fever, persistent pain or burning on micturition. The first menses usually occurs 2–8 weeks after the abortion. The menses may be heavier or less in quantity and may be either of a longer or shorter duration.

If lactation begins, it is usually mild and lasts less than 48 hours if the breasts are not stimulated. Using a tight brassiere or binding the breasts and using an ice bag will ease the discomfort until the engorgement decreases.

Normal physical activity can be resumed as early as desired. Increased fatigue is often noted for a few days. Tub baths or immersion baths should be avoided for at least 1 week.

Follow-up visits must be made in 2–4 weeks after abortion. It is important for the patient to have this examination to ensure that the reproductive organs have returned to the prepregnancy state.

At some time during the abortion experience, the nurse should introduce the subject of family planning if she has not already requested for information. Counseling on contraception is of importance to those women who are or have been faced with the reality of an unwanted pregnancy.

Nursing Process for Clients with Abortion

Assessment

Assess for the following manifestations:
- Vaginal bleeding, spotting and clots
- Low abdominal cramping
- Passing of tissue through the vagina
- Shock decreased blood pressure, increased pulse rate
- Woman may verbalize fear, disappointment or feelings of guilt.

Analysis/Nursing Diagnosis

- Risk for fetal injury
- Risk for infection
- Ineffective airway clearance
- Actual risk for aspiration
- Anxiety
- Anticipatory grieving
- Altered family processes
- Actual risk for altered parenting
- Health-seeking behavior.

Planning

- Provide information regarding treatment plan
- Provide support and reassurance regarding nursing care
- Promote maternal physical well-being
- Provide opportunities for counseling and support
- Provide teaching related to self-care.

Implementation

- Observe for vaginal bleeding and cramping
- Save expelled tissues and clots used for examination
- Monitor vital signs every 5 minutes to 4 hours depending on maternal status
- Maintain woman on bed rest
- Observe for signs of shock and institute treatment measures
- Prepare for dilation and curettage if appropriate
- Provide support, but avoid offering false assurance.

Evaluation

Ensure that the woman:
- Is free from anemia and/or infection?
- Is free from vaginal bleeding?
- Returns to normal physiological status following the abortion
- Verbalize feelings regarding the event and the outcome as does her significant other/spouse
- Understands self-care measures.

ECTOPIC PREGNANCY/ ECTOPIC GESTATION

An ectopic pregnancy is one where implantation occurs at a site other than the uterine cavity. Sites can be in the uterine tube, ovary, cervix and the abdomen **(Fig. 25.6)**.

About 1% of all pregnancies are ectopic and the life-threatening outcome of this condition calls for appropriate treatment for the mother.

Tubal Pregnancy

Tubal pregnancy develops when the transport of the fertilized ovum into the uterine cavity is interfered with. Implantation can occur at any point along the tube, although the ampulla is the common site. The isthmus is next in frequency and the interstitial portion least common.

Causes

Any alteration of the normal function of the uterine tube in transporting the gametes contributes to the risk of tubal pregnancy:
- Congenital abnormalities of the tube such as hypoplasia, undue tortuosity and tubal diverticula
- Previous infection such as postabortal sepsis, puerperal sepsis, gonorrhea and tuberculosis.
  This may alter the ciliated lining, or the peristaltic action of the tube. Infection can also leave adhesions both inside and surrounding the tube restricting normal function.
- Surgery on the uterine tube—reconstructive surgery for infertility or reversal of tubal ligation

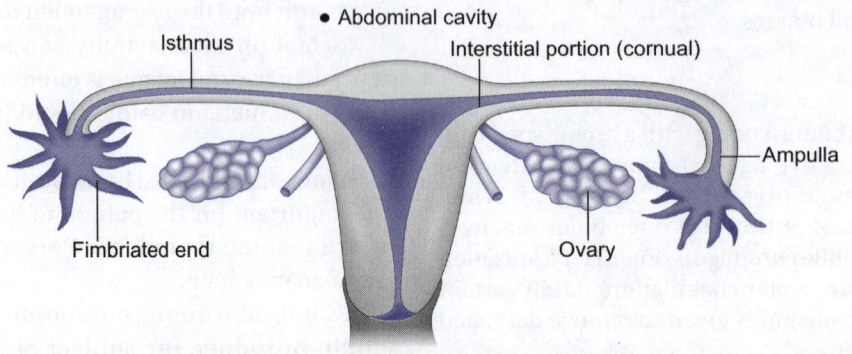

Figure 25.6: Sites of implantation in ectopic pregnancy.

- Use of intrauterine contraceptive devices—these devices protect from intrauterine pregnancy, but not from tubal pregnancy
- Assisted reproductive techniques like in vitro fertilization and embryo transfer—the transferred embryo may get injected into the tube
- Induction of ovulation with gonadotropic hormones
- Endometriosis.

Physiology

In tubal pregnancy, the blastocyst erodes the epithelium and attaches itself to the muscle layer. It grows and expands within the wall, distending the tube. Maternal vessels are exposed and the pressure caused by the resultant blood flow can destroy the embryo. The uterus enlarges in size and in the body, changes associated pregnancy occur under the influence of hormones.

Outcomes (Figs. 25.7A to C)

The result of a tubal ectopic gestation may be any of the following:

1. *Tubal abortion:* A pregnancy in the infundibulum or ampulla of the tube may be aborted into the pelvic peritoneal cavity through the fimbriated end of the tube.
2. *Tubal mole:* Bleeding around the embryo from the site of implantation causes death of the embryo and formation of layers of organized blood clots distending the tube. The mole may need to be removed.
3. *Tubal rupture:* The tubal wall is distended by the pregnancy and penetrated by the trophoblast to such an extent that it ruptures.
4. *Pelvic hematocele:* A considerable collection of blood forms in the pouch of Douglas or the uterovesical pouch. Initially, it is fluid, later forms as a mass. Finally, it becomes firm as it gets absorbed.
5. *Secondary abdominal ectopic pregnancy:* If the embryo is implanted on the pelvic peritoneum after expulsion from the ruptured tube, a secondary abdominal ectopic pregnancy develops.

Clinical Presentation

Amenorrhea is present in 75–95% of pregnancies. In the remaining cases, ectopic pregnancy ruptures before the woman misses a period. The woman may give the history of some vaginal spotting.

Acute lower abdominal pain, often localized in nature is present. This may be sharp and stabbing type, the mother may have dizziness, nausea and shoulder pain indicative of bleeding into the peritoneal cavity.

The woman will have severe pallor, rapid and thready pulse, tachypnea and low blood pressure. Abdominal examination will show lower abdominal tenderness, rebound tenderness, guarding and shifting dullness due to hemoperitoneum. Pelvic examination will show tenderness on transverse cervical movements, lateral forniceal tenderness, adnexal mass and vascular pulsations on the side of the ectopic pregnancy. Ultrasound examination enables an accurate diagnosis.

Treatment

The patient is resuscitated if she presents with an acute rupture. An exploratory laparotomy is carried out under controlled general anesthesia. The ruptured tube is removed by salpingotomy or salpingostomy may be done. If the tubal pregnancy is in the process of tubal abortion, the process is completed by suction of the ectopic pregnancy through the fimbriated end. The mother should be offered follow-up support and information regarding subsequent pregnancies. As with any loss during pregnancy, the client will need to grieve and the midwife must offer needed psychological support.

Abdominal Pregnancy

Abdominal pregnancy is rare. A primary abdominal ectopic pregnancy is the result of implantation of the fertilized ovum on the peritoneal surface. A secondary abdominal pregnancy forms when an embryo extruded through rupture or abortion of a tubal pregnancy. The embryo does not die because of its chorionic attachments to the uterine tube and grows by forming attachments to the pelvic peritoneum, omentum, intestines, etc. The fetus grows in the peritoneal cavity, but the majority of these pregnancies do not survive. If the fetus

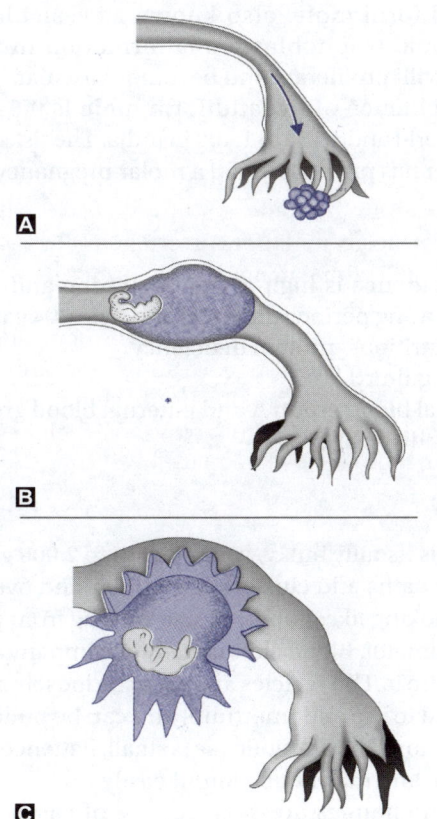

Figures 25.7A to C: Possible outcomes of tubal pregnancy. (A) Tubal abortion; (B) Tubal mole; (C) Tubal rupture.

dies early in pregnancy, it may be reabsorbed or calcification occurs.

If pregnancy continues, the woman complains of persistent lower abdominal pain, nausea, vomiting, constipation, diarrhea, distention and urinary frequency. There may be vaginal spotting or hemorrhage. Fetal movements are painful. On abdominal examination, there is tenderness and superficiality of fetal parts. Abnormal fetal lie and loud fetal heart sounds. Ultrasonography confirms the diagnosis.

Delivery is by laparotomy. Separation of placenta may be followed by major hemorrhage. If the placenta is attached to the intestines, it may be left in situ. When the placenta is left inside, the risk of infection is high, but is considered a safer option. Fetal mortality is very high. The fetus is growth retarded and deformed in 20%–40% of cases due to oligohydramnios. The fetus usually dies when the membranes rupture or in the immediate neonatal period from respiratory distress.

Cervical Pregnancy

Cervical pregnancy occurs due to implantation in the cervical canal. It may be due to rapid passage of the fertilized ovum or fertilization of the ovum after it reaches the cervical canal. It is rare and seldom lasts beyond the 20th week. Signs and symptoms include the following:
* Painless bleeding soon after the time of implantation
* Palpation of the cervical mass with distention and thinning of the cervical wall
* Partial dilatation of the external os and a slightly enlarged uterine fundus.

The treatment is removal of the products of conception by curettage and packing of the cervical canal or total abdominal hysterectomy.

Nursing Process for Clients with Ectopic Pregnancy

Assessment

Assess for the following clinical manifestations:
* Sharp localized pain in lower abdomen
* Syncope and referred shoulder pain
* Irregular vaginal bleeding
* Abdominal rigidity and distention
* Shock-decreased blood pressure, increased heart rate
* Palpable mass in the cul-de-sac or adnexa
* Lower than normal human chorionic gonadotropin (hCG) titers
* Disorientation and lack of cooperation due to severe pain
* Expression of fear if the woman was unaware of pregnancy
* Grief over loss of pregnancy.

Analysis/Nursing Diagnosis

* Risk for fetal injury
* Risk for infection
* Ineffective airway clearance
* Actual risk for aspiration
* Anxiety
* Anticipatory grieving
* Altered family processes
* Actual risk for altered parenting
* Health-seeking behavior.

Implementation

* Provide pain relief
* Manage shock:
  – Administer oxygen, IV fluids
  – Type and crossmatch blood.
* Prepare for surgery, laparotomy with removal of the ectopic pregnancy and perhaps the affected fallopian tube
* Provide postoperative care:
  – Give routine postoperative care
  – Assess vaginal bleeding
  – Offer emotional support.

Evaluation

Ensure that the woman:
* Has participated in decision-making
* Is free from pain?
* Is normotensive?
* Acknowledges support through the treatment process
* Demonstrates knowledge of self-care measures.

HYDATIDIFORM MOLE (FIG. 25.8)

A hydatidiform mole, also known as vesicular mole is a gestational trophoblastic malformation in which the chorionic villi proliferate and become avascular.

The incidence of hydatidiform mole is 0.5–2.5 in the western world and 1:160 to 1:400 in India. The risk rises where the mother has previously had a molar pregnancy.

Incidence

* The incidence is high at the beginning and the end of childbearing period (under 20 and over 40 years of age)
* Poor nutrition—protein deficiency
* Consanguinity
* Maternal blood group A and paternal blood group O
* Genetic disposition.

Pathology

The mole is usually bulky, weighing up to 2,000 g. There are bunched chains and clusters of globular and ovoid stalked vesicles looking like grapes, of size varying from pinhead to 3 cm in diameter. Blood clots usually accompany a mole and may obscure it. The vesicles appear to be loosely attached or unattached to the endometrium, and can be pulled away by gentle traction. The amniotic sac is small, flattened, displaced to one side and may not be found easily.

Ovarian changes are seen in 50% of cases. There are multiple cysts enlarging the ovaries. About 50% of molar pregnancies develop into choriocarcinoma, a malignant

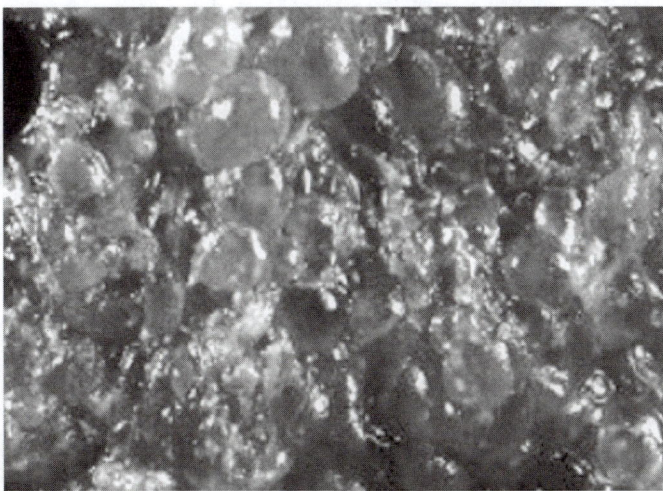

Figure 25.8: Hydatidiform mole.

trophoblastic tumor. It is a dull-red, liver like or spongy nodule in the myometrium, occasionally streaked with yellowish or greenish white areas. It may or may not reach the endometrium. It differs from hydatidiform mole in having no villi.

Two forms of moles have been identified, one of which carries an increased risk of the mother subsequently developing choriocarcinoma, the malignant gestational trophoblastic disease.

Complete Hydatidiform Mole

This type of mole contains no evidence of embryo, cord or membranes. Death of embryo occurs prior to the development of the placental circulation. The chorionic villi alter to form clear, hydropic, vesicles, which hang in clusters from small pedicles. The mass occupies the uterine cavity and can be large enough to mimic an advanced gestation. The developing mole penetrates the uterine wall beyond the site of implantation. Myometrium can be involved and more rarely the veins. Rupture of the uterus with massive hemorrhage is a possible outcome.

Complete moles usually have 46 chromosomes of paternal origin only. Choriocarcinoma can develop from complete mole.

Partial Mole

In this type, evidence of an embryo, fetus or amniotic sac may be found as death occurs at 8th or 9th week. Hyperplasia of the trophoblast is confined to a single syncytiotrophoblast layer and is less widespread than in complete moles. Chromosome analysis usually show this to be triploid with 69 chromosomes, i.e. three sets of chromosomes, one maternal and two paternal. The risk to the mother of developing choriocarcinoma from a partial mole is slight. Follow-up however, is still essential.

Clinical Features

- Apparently normal first trimester of pregnancy.
- Persistent nausea and vomiting.
- Uterine bleeding evident by 20th week of pregnancy—usually more brown than red, occurring intermittently or continuously overtime.
- Anemia: Often it is out of proportion to the amount of blood lost due to rapidly growing tumor.
- A large for dates uterus, which is clearly out of proportion to the presumed gestational age in about 50% of cases.
- On palpation, the uterus feels 'doughy' or elastic.
- Shortness of breath.
- Often enlarged, tender ovaries.
- No fetal heart tones (FHT).
- No fetal activity.
- Palpation of fetal parts is impossible.
- Hyperemesis gravidarum due to high levels of hCG.
- Pregnancy-induced hypertension (PIH), preeclampsia or eclampsia before 24 weeks of gestation.
- Vaginal discharge may rarely show vesicles of the mole.

Investigations

- Urinary pregnancy test, due to the large amounts of hCG produced by the tumor, the test is positive in a dilution 1:2,000 or more after 14 weeks of gestation
- Serum levels of hCG is high
- Ultrasound scan shows a characteristic pattern and a snowstorm appearance.

Possible Complications

- Hemorrhage and shock
- Pulmonary embolism and acute cor pulmonale
- Thyrotoxicosis due to production of thyrotrophic hormone by the mole
- Rupture of an invasive mole into the peritoneal cavity
- Disseminated intravascular coagulation
- Choriocarcinoma
- Recurrence in subsequent pregnancies.

Treatment

The aim of treatment is to remove all the trophoblastic tissues. If the patient presents with bleeding and shock, she is resuscitated. Then the mole is evacuated by vacuum aspiration or dilation and curettage. A slow dilatation of cervix may be achieved by using laminaria tents over 12–24 hours. Spontaneous expulsion of the mole carries less risk of malignant change.

The mole can be aborted by administration of prostaglandin intramuscularly. In about 10% of cases, the trophoblast tissue does not die off completely. For this reason and the possibility of developing malignancy, women confirmed as having complete mole require follow-up for over a 2 year period. Follow-up examinations are done every week for 8 weeks, monthly for 10 months and 3 monthly for 2 years. At each visit the patient is examined for vaginal metastasis, subinvolution of uterus and theca lutein cysts. Curettage is repeated if there is irregular vaginal bleeding, the uterus does not involute or hCG levels are still positive 6 weeks after evacuation. If serum hCG level is high (more than 20 IU/mL) or rising, chemotherapy is given. Usually actinomycin D or methotrexate is given for 5 days.

Pregnancy should be avoided during the follow-up period. Intrauterine contraceptive devices are contraindicated because of perforation and infection, and hormonal methods of contraception are not prescribed until levels of hCG have returned to normal.

The midwife has to provide support and explanations of the importance of the prolonged period of screening. The client should be helped to plan subsequent pregnancy and care during pregnancy.

CHORIOCARCINOMA

Choriocarcinoma is a malignant neoplasm, which can develop because of a molar pregnancy. The growth actively invades the myometrium, which can result in severe hemorrhage. The mother is also at risk for developing lung, hepatic and cerebral metastasis. It can also occur after a normal term gestation or a termination of pregnancy.

Nursing Process for Clients with Hydatidiform Mole

Assessment

Assess for:
- Vaginal bleeding by the 12th week that is intermittent, bright red or dark brown, slightly or profuse in amount
- Hyperemesis
- Fundal height in relation to estimated date of confinement (EDC)
- hCG levels
- 'Snowstorm' pattern in ultrasonography
- No FHT on auscultation
- Symptoms of PIH
- Fear of pregnancy and apprehension.

Analysis/Nursing Diagnosis

- Risk for fetal injury
- Risk for infection
- Ineffective airway clearance
- Actual risk for aspiration
- Anxiety
- Anticipatory grieving
- Altered family processes
- Actual risk for altered parenting
- Health-seeking behavior.

Planning

- Provide information regarding treatment plan
- Promote maternal physical well-being
- Provide opportunities for counseling and support
- Provide teaching related to self-care.

Implementation

- Coordinate diagnostic testing
- Prepare woman for uterine evacuation
- Observe for postprocedural hemorrhage and infection
- Instruct and facilitate follow-up care:
  – Monitor hCG level for 2 years
  – Instruct regarding birth control measures to prevent pregnancy for 2 years.
- Provide support during family's grieving period.

Evaluation

Ensure that the woman:
- Has rapidly decreasing hCG titers
- Recovers physically after evacuation of the molar pregnancy
- Verbalizes positive self-image
- Avoids conception during the follow-up period
- Voices understanding regarding need to avoid pregnancy as per the physician's recommendations.

HYPEREMESIS GRAVIDARUM

Hyperemesis gravidarum is excessive nausea and vomiting during pregnancy. This pernicious vomiting is differentiated from the more common and more normal morning sickness by the fact that it is of greater intensity and extends beyond the first trimester. Hyperemesis gravidarum may occur in any of the three trimesters. It is a condition affecting one in 1,000 pregnancies.

Causes

High levels of hCG or undue sensitivity to normal levels of hCG may cause vomiting. Psychological factors are thought to play an important role. Women with a previous history of hyperemesis are likely to experience it in subsequent pregnancies. It is known to be associated with first pregnancies. An allergic factor may also be operative, since large amounts of histamine are found in cases of hyperemesis. The sensitizing agents possibly are the woman's own corpus luteum, syncytial cells and gonadotropic hormones.

Clinical Presentation

- Pernicious vomiting (anything taken orally is rejected)
- Poor appetite and poor nutritional intake
- Loss of more than 25% of body weight

- Dehydration and electrolyte imbalance
- Acidosis due to starvation
- Alkalosis resulting from loss of hydrochloric acid in the vomitus
- Occasionally, jaundice develops in severe cases
- Low urine output
- Rapid pulse and low blood pressure
- Hemoconcentration with rising blood urea nitrogen and falling sodium, potassium and chloride.

The condition is said to be mild when there is loss of weight, but no dehydration. Moderate cases are those characterized by dehydration and circulatory changes. Severe cases have biochemical changes with complications.

Complications

- Circulatory failure
- Jaundice due to liver involvement
- Retinal hemorrhage
- Wernicke's encephalopathy and Korsakoff's syndrome (disorientation and loss of memory)
- Renal insufficiency
- Polyneuritis
- Delirium, coma, death.

Treatment

Women with hyperemesis gravidarum are admitted to the hospital. Initially nothing is given by mouth. Hypovolemia and electrolyte imbalance are corrected by intravenous infusion. Vitamin supplements are given parenterally. Fluids and diet are gradually introduced as the woman's condition improves.

The mother should be encouraged to rest and be cared for in a single room. Some women are prescribed a mild sedative if they are agitated. Supportive psychotherapy and counseling may help.

Small palatable meals, at regular intervals may help the mother to regain her appetite. Antihistamines may be prescribed for treatment of nausea and vomiting. Patient's weight is taken twice a week to monitor the recovery.

Termination of pregnancy is recommended in severe cases with jaundice, persistent albuminuria, and polyneuritis to reverse the condition and to prevent maternal mortality.

Nursing Process for Clients with Hyperemesis

Assessment

- Intractable vomiting
- Weight loss of 25% or more
- Ketosis, ketonuria (alkalosis)
- Dehydration—poor skin turgor, dry tongue
- Epigastric pain
- Drowsiness and confusion
- Uncoordinated movements, jerking
- Jaundice.

Analysis/Nursing Diagnosis

- Risk for fetal injury
- Risk for infection
- Ineffective airway clearance
- Actual risk for aspiration
- Anxiety
- Anticipatory grieving
- Altered family processes
- Actual risk for altered parenting
- Health-seeking behavior.

Planning

- Provide IV and/or oral fluids to re-establish fluid and electrolyte balance
- Create opportunities for the woman to explore feelings about pregnancy and coping abilities
- Provide teaching related to need for fluids.

Implementation

- Administer parenteral fluids, vitamins, and sedatives as prescribed
- Monitor intake, output and daily weight
- Assess state of hydration
- Begin oral feedings slowly with fluids; progress to six small feedings a day
- Obtain psychiatric consultation, if indicated.

Evaluation

Ensure that the woman:
- Is well hydrated
- Has normal electrolyte values
- Verbalizes feelings and ability to cope with the pregnancy
- Verbalizes knowledge of need for fluids.

Rh ISOIMMUNIZATION AND ABO INCOMPATIBILITY

Immunization is a process in which immune antibodies are produced in an individual in response to injection of antigens from another individual of the same species who possesses antigens that the first one lacks.

The Rh antibodies develop when Rh-positive cells enter the circulation of an Rh-negative person. This may occur due to a mismatched transfusion. In obstetrics, this happens due to fetomaternal hemorrhage during abortions, childbirth, rupture of ectopic pregnancy, antepartum hemorrhage, versions, amniocentesis, etc.

To the transfer of fetal (RBCs), the mother responds by producing antibodies against the Rh factor, which on the first exposure begin to show-up in her serum a few days after the event—usually delivery. Since the production of antibodies takes time, the first Rh-incompatible fetus usually escapes disease unless the mother has been sensitized earlier by an Rh-incompatible blood transfusion.

Incompatibility of the ABO groups occurs more frequently than that caused by the Rh factor. It usually occurs when the woman is type O and the fetus is A or B. Hemolytic disease due to ABO incompatibility can occur without prior sensitization since A, B antibodies are already present in the mothers blood, and thus the first-born can be affected. However, the disease is much less severe with ABO isoimmunization.

Screening for blood incompatibility between the mother and fetus is limited to Rh incompatibility because there is no generally accepted method for diagnosing ABO incompatibility during pregnancy. History taking, which may be relevant to ABO or Rh-incompatibility, includes the following:
- History of previous blood transfusion
- History of previous 'yellow baby' or baby needing blood transfusion or phototherapy
- History of stillbirth or neonatal death from causes not known to the mother
- History of taking RhoGAM after previous deliveries or abortions.

If a pregnant woman is found to be Rh- negative, her husband's Rh status should be determined. If it is Rh negative, the baby will also be Rh negative. The baby cannot be affected and nothing further needs to be done.

Investigations

Determination of Rh type is made during the initial prenatal visit. If the woman is Rh negative, an indirect Coombs test is ordered. This is a screening for Rh antibodies. If the test is positive, thereby indicating the presence of Rh antibodies, antibody titers are then ordered.

A woman who is Rh negative, with a negative indirect Coombs should have the test repeated every 4 weeks up to 28 weeks. Increasing titer indicates that the fetus is Rh positive.

If the Coombs test is negative at 28 weeks, a dose of Rh immunoglobulin (RhoGAM) is given to the mother to prevent the development of antibodies in the event of an antepartum hemorrhage or during intrapartum period. A dose of 300 µg offers protection against developing antibodies for approximately 12 weeks. If antibodies are found at any stage, the antibody titers are measured regularly and the fetus is monitored closely by ultrasound for any edema or hepatosplenomegaly. Rh-negative mothers are given 300 µg of RhoGAM after delivery, within 72 hours, if the baby is Rh positive. Rh-negative women who have ectopic pregnancies and evacuation of hydatidiform mole should also receive anti-D γ-globulin. The antibodies disappear from maternal blood within about 6 hours following an intramuscular administration of RhoGAM.

RETROVERSION OF THE GRAVID UTERUS

A gravid uterus is said to be retroverted when its long axis is directed backwards. In the first trimester, retroversion of the uterus occurs in 11% of all pregnancies. It is associated with a slightly increased risk of early pregnancy—bleeding and abortion. This is due to compression of the uterine vessels, decreasing blood flow to the decidua. As pregnancy progresses most cases correct spontaneously, the uterus rises out of the pelvis in to the abdomen, causing no further problems.

Incarceration of the Retroverted Gravid Uterus

If the retroverted gravid uterus fails to rise out of the pelvic cavity by 14th week it is considered as incarcerated. This occurs in 1–3,000 pregnancies. Congenital anomalies of the pelvis and uterus are identified as causes. Conditions such as pelvic adhesions, endometriosis, fibroids and ovarian tumors may contribute to incarceration.

The growing uterus is confined within the pelvis beneath sacral promontory. Pressure causes abdominal discomfort, feeling of pelvic fullness and low back pain. Frequency of micturition, dysuria and incontinence may be experienced because of the urethra being elongated. Compression of the bladder neck causes urinary retention and stasis resulting in urinary infection including pyelonephritis. The mother may complain of rectal pressure and constipation with impaction of feces.

The distended bladder will be palpable abdominally. Fetal heart sounds are difficult to auscultate. Management measures include:
- Catheterization to relieve the retention of urine
- Indwelling catheter to keep the bladder empty.

These measures may enable the uterus to rise out of the pelvis. In cases where correction does not occur, the uterus continues to expand and extend forming a pouch to accommodate the fetus. Uterine rupture can result. Rupture of the bladder can also happen due to over distension.

STUDY QUESTIONS

Short Notes

1. Complete abortion.
2. Threatened abortion.
3. Habitual abortion.
4. Missed abortion.
5. Choriocarcinoma.

Short Answer Questions

1. Septic abortion.
2. Medical termination of pregnancy.
3. Methods of termination of first trimester pregnancy.
4. Clinical features and management of clients with hydatidiform mole.

Essay Questions

1. Discuss the types of spontaneous abortions and management of each with relevant client instructions.
2. Discuss the management and nursing care of a client admitted with signs and symptoms of acute tubal rupture resulting from tubal pregnancy.

BIBLIOGRAPHY

1. Bracken MB. Incidence and aetiology of hydatidiform mole: an epidemiological review. Br J Obstet Gynaecol. 1987;94(12):1123-35.
2. Dutta DC. Textbook of Obstetrics, 5th edition. Kolkata: New Central Book Company; 2001. pp. 170-215.
3. Edmonds DK. Spontaneous and recurrent abortion. In: Shaw RW, Soutter PW (Eds). Gynecology. Edinburgh: Churchill Livingstone; 1972.
4. Fairweather DV. Nausea and vomiting in pregnancy. Am J Obstet Gynecol. 1968;102(1):135-75.
5. Gibbons JM Jr, Paley WB. The incarcerated gravid uterus. Obstet and Gynecol. 1969;33(6):842-5.
6. Shiers CV. Abnormalities early pregnancy. In: Bennett RV, Linda KB (Eds). Myles Textbook for Midwives, 13th edition. Edinburgh: Churchill Livingstone; 1999. pp. 235-52.
7. Szulman AE. The biology of trophoblastic disease: Complete and partial hydatidiform moles. In: Beard RW (Ed). Early Pregnancy Loss: Mechanisms and Treatment. London: Springer-Verlag; 1988.
8. Weekes AR, Atlay RD, Brown VA, et al. The retroverted gravid uterus and its effect on the outcome of pregnancy. Br Med J. 1976;1(6010):622-4.

CHAPTER 26

Sexually Transmissible and Reproductive Tract Infections

Learning Objectives

Upon completing this chapter, the learner will be able to:
- Outline the relevance of sexually transmissible infections for women of childbearing age.
- Describe the local infections of the vagina and vulva and their management.
- Describe the bacterial infections common in pregnancy and their impact on mother and baby.
- Discuss the commonly occurring viral infections and their impact on pregnant women and their newborn babies.

Sexually transmissible diseases (STDs) are a group of communicable diseases that are transmitted predominantly by sexual contact and caused by a wide range of bacterial, viral, protozoal and fungal agents. The true incidence of STDs is not known because of inadequate reporting and the secrecy that surrounds them. Minimal estimates of yearly incidence of four major bacterial STDs worldwide are (WHO, Health for All Series, 1981):
- *Gonorrhea:* 62 million
- *Genital chlamydial infection:* 89 million
- *Syphilis:* 12 million
- *Chancroid:* 2 million.

For viral STD, due to the importance of asymptomatic infection, incidence can only be very roughly estimated:
- *Genital herpes:* 20 million
- *Genital human papillomavirus (HPV) infection:* 30 million.

Trichomoniasis which is of much less public health importance than the bacterial and viral STD has an estimated annual incidence of 170 million cases (WHO, Health Situation in the Southeast Asia Region, 1994).

EXTENT OF THE PROBLEM IN INDIA

Sexually transmitted diseases are becoming a major public health problem in India.

Syphilis

Serological surveys continue to be the best source of information on the prevalence of syphilis. The extent of the problem can be gauged from the reports of surveys done in Aurangabad (Maharashtra) and Kerala which showed prevalence of 2.4 and 1.4, respectively (WHO, World Health Report, 1999), which are rather high figures.

Gonorrhea

Accurate information on the morbidity of gonorrhea is lacking, as most cases are not reported. However, the general impression is that gonorrhea is more prevalent than syphilis. About 80% of infected women are reported to be asymptomatic carriers.

Chancroid

Chancroid or soft sore is reported to be widely prevalent in India.

Chlamydia Infections

Chlamydia infections are more prevalent in the southern states of India than in the northern states.

Donovanosis

Donovanosis or granuloma inguinale is endemic in Tamil Nadu, Andhra Pradesh, Odisha, Karnataka and Maharashtra. A greater prevalence along the coastal areas has been reported (WHO, World Health Report, 1999). Information about this disease in other states is lacking.

Other STDs

Information about other STDs in India is not readily available, as there is no reporting system for these diseases.

HOST FACTORS

Age

For most notifiable STDs, the highest rates of incidence are observed in 20–24 years old followed by 25–29 and 15–19 years age groups. The most serious morbidity is observed during fetal development and in the neonate.

Sex

For most STDs, the overall morbidity rate is higher for men than for women, but the morbidity caused by infection is generally much more severe in women, e.g. pelvic inflammatory disease.

Marital Status

The frequency of STD infection is higher among single, divorced and separated persons than among married couples.

Socioeconomic Status

Individuals from the lowest socioeconomic groups have the highest morbidity rate.

Social Factors

Several social and behavioral factors are involved in the spread of STDs. These include the following:

Prostitution

Prostitution is a major factor in the spread, as prostitutes act as reservoir of infection. In Asia, most STDs are contracted from prostitutes. The male component of prostitution, the prostituant is also equally important in the spread, as prostitution supplies a demand.

Broken Homes

Social studies indicate that promiscuous women are usually drawn from broken homes, e.g. homes which are broken either due to death of one or both parents or their separation. Children reared in such unhappy atmosphere are likely to go astray in search of other avenues of happiness.

Sexual Disharmony

Married people with strained relation, divorced and separated persons are often victims of STDs.

Easy Money

In most of the developing world, prostitution is simply a reflection of poverty. It provides an occupation for earning easy money. It is fostered by lack of female employment and the prospect of a financial return impossible to achieve by other means.

Emotional Immaturity

Emotional immaturity has been often stressed as a social factor in acquiring STDs.

Urbanization and Industrialization

Urbanization and industrialization are conducive to the type of lifestyle that contributes to high level of infection.

Social Disruption

Social disruption caused by disasters, wars and civil unrest have always caused an increase in the spread of STDs.

International Travel

Travelers can import as well as export infection and their role in the transmission of STD is exampled by the rapid spread throughout the world of resistant strains of *Neisseria gonorrhoeae (N. gonorrhoeae)* and AIDS.

Changing Behavioral Patterns

In the modern society, there has been a relaxation of moral and cultural values. The tendency to break away from traditional ways of life is particularly marked among young people desiring more independence and freedom from supervision.

Social Stigma

The social stigma attached to STDs accounts for the nondetection of cases, not disclosing the sources of contact, dropping out before treatment is complete, going to quacks for treatment and self-treatment.

RELEVANCE FOR WOMEN

- A number of sexually transmitted organisms such as *N. gonorrhoeae* and *Chlamydia trachomatis* cause salpingitis which may lead to chronic pelvic inflammation and permanent damage to the uterine tubes resulting in reduced fertility and ectopic pregnancy.
- The presence of an organism within or around the genitalia or its presence in the blood and sexual secretions facilitate perinatal transmission of infection from the mother to her fetus or newborn baby.
- Some perinatally acquired infections have serious and prolonged consequences for the fetus or neonate, e.g. cardiac defects, hearing problems, cataracts and developmental delay.
- Pregnancy may have an impact on the presentation and course of infection giving rise to difficulties in diagnosis or management. Some infections such as HPV become more virulent; group B *Streptococcus* (GBS) are asymptomatic in the woman but may produce serious neonatal disease.
- The diagnosis of a sexually transmitted infection may have stressful consequences for the relationship between the woman and her husband.
- Women may experience high levels of anxiety and guilt about the implications for their babies of a perinatally transmissible infection.
- Some infections such as syphilis and cytomegalovirus (CMV) infection are important causes of stillbirths and neonatal deaths.

- Certain carcinomas occur as sequel of STDs which include hepatocellular carcinoma caused by hepatitis B, Kaposi's sarcoma, B-cell lymphomas and primary lymphoma of the central nervous system (CNS) in patients with AIDS.

CONTROL OF STDs

The aim of the control program for STDs is the prevention of ill health resulting from the conditions mentioned here through various interventions. These interventions have a primary prevention focus (prevention of infection), a secondary prevention focus (minimizing the adverse health effects of infection) or a combination of the two.

Case Detection

Case detection is an essential part of any control program. The methods of early detection in a STD control program are following:

Screening

Screening is the testing of apparently healthy volunteers from the general population for the early detection of disease. Priority is given to screening of special groups such as pregnant women, blood donors, industrial workers, army, police, refugees, prostitutes, convicts restaurant and hotel staff.

Contact Tracing

Contact tracing is the technique by which the sexual partners of diagnosed patients are identified, located, investigated and treated. This is one of the best methods of controlling the spread of infection.

Cluster Testing

The patients are asked to name other persons of either sex who move in the same sociosexual environment. These persons are then screened through blood testing.

Case Holding and Treatment

Adequate treatment of patients and their contacts is the mainstay of STD control. There is a tendency on the part of patients suffering from STDs to disappear or dropout before treatment is complete. Therefore, every effort should be made to ensure complete and adequate treatment.

Epidemiological Treatment

Treatment consists of the administration of full therapeutic dose of treatment to persons recently exposed to STD, while awaiting the results of laboratory tests. It is combined with a venereological examination and the tracing of contacts revealed by that examination.

Personal Prophylaxis

Contraceptives

Mechanical barriers such as condoms and diaphragms can be recommended for personal prophylaxis of STDs. These barrier methods especially when used with spermicides, will minimize the risk of acquiring STD infections. The exposed parts should be washed with soap and water as soon as possible after contact. Vaccine is now available for hepatitis B.

Health Education

Health education is an integral part of STD control programs. The principal aim of educational intervention is to help individuals alter their behavior in an effort to avoid STDs, i.e. to minimize disease acquisition and transmission.

LOCAL INFECTIONS OF THE VAGINA AND VULVA

The vagina is a host to a rich variety of microorganisms. These are subject to dynamic alteration in quantity and composition, reflecting at any given time, a woman's current physiological state, her immunological defense mechanisms and her past exposure. Transfer and sharing of microorganisms between partners occur during sexual intercourse, and may include the exchange of infective organisms.

Clinical disease may occur because of the introduction of organisms, which are new to the woman, or because of redistribution of existing microbiological flora due to the pathophysiological changes of pregnancy or the action of antibiotics. Changes may occur in a woman's susceptibility to or the pathogenicity of previously encountered organisms.

FUNGAL INFECTIONS

The most common of these is *Candida albicans* (thrush), which accounts for the vast majority of fungal vulvovaginal infections. A minority of infections is caused by organisms such as *Torulopsis glabrata* and *Candida tropicalis*.

Candida (**Fig. 26.1**) is a common inhabitant of the mouth, large intestine and vagina in 25–50% of healthy individuals and isolation of the organism does not correlate strongly the presence of clinical disease. Some women are more susceptible to candida infection. Predisposition to infection is associated with diabetes, pregnancy and the administration of antibiotics particularly those like penicillin which are effective against vaginal lactobacilli.

Resistance to fungal infection depends on cell-mediated immunity and therefore, compromise on this by disease such as HIV infection or immunosuppressive therapy increases infection risk. Some individuals develop *Candida*-specific reduced cell immunity. Tight clothes and mild skin abrasions may contribute to clinical presentation of infection.

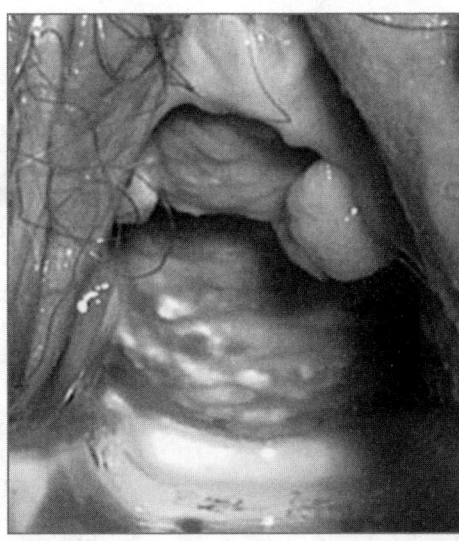

Figure 26.1: Candidia Infection *(For color version, see Plate 3)*.

Clinical Presentation and Diagnosis

The woman may complain of vulval pruritus (itchiness) and on examination, there may be evidence of vulvovaginitis and/or vulval, vaginal and cervical erythema. Dyspareunia (pain during intercourse) is a common complaint.

A vaginal discharge is common, but not universal and may be scant or thick and white with a curd-like consistency.

In less than 20% of cases, white thrush patches may be present on the vulva or walls of the vagina.

Half of the babies born to infected women will be infected by *Candida* generally involving oral or gastrointestinal infection. Treatment of the mother prior to delivery is desirable.

Treatment

Female

Vaginal infection is treated by insertion of vaginal suppositories at night with cream for application to the vulval and perineal area:

- Clotrimazole suppositories or pessaries for six nights:
  - Clotrimazole cream 1% for application to the vulva two to three times daily.
- Miconazole pessaries 150 mg for three nights.
- Nystatin pessaries × 2 of 100,000 IU for 14 nights with nystatin gel 100,000 IU/g for external use.

Male

Signs of clinical infection in a man usually small red spots or plaques on the glans penis should be treated with cream applied to the infected area.

Instructions

- Avoid sexual intercourse until the treatment is complete
- Avoid local irritation which might provoke reinfection
- Take daily bath to maintain cleanliness of the perineal area
- Avoid the use of harsh soaps and other irritants
- Wipe away from the vagina after defecation
- Use cotton underwear and avoid clothing which is tight or constricting in the crotch.

PROTOZOAL INFECTIONS

The protozoan, *Trichomonas vaginalis (T. vaginalis)* is an anaerobic organism which is highly pathogenic to the epithelium in the vagina. Its prevalence varies considerably in different populations.

The major mode of transmission is sexual intercourse. Around 80% of women whose partners are infected with *T. vaginalis* become infected, although the rate of female-male transfer is lower than this. Severe vaginitis is experienced by some women. Infection of the neonate seems to be uncommon **(Fig. 26.2)**.

Clinical Presentation and Diagnosis

About half to two-third of infected women will complain of symptoms. Pruritus, burning and increased vaginal discharge are commonly seen. Vaginal discharge may range from normal to copious, grayish in color and somewhat bubbly in character. The green, frothy discharge and friable erythematous cervix are the 'classic' presenting features of the infection. Urethritis may also be a feature.

Asymptomatic infection may sometimes be detected on the Papanicolaou smear. A wet swab examined immediately under a microscope will demonstrate the presence of the pear-shaped protozoan with three to five flagella and an undulating membrane. Swabs should be cultured to exclude the presence of gonococcal and chlamydial infection.

Treatment

A single oral dose of metronidazole 2 g or 5 days course of 400 mg twice daily is the treatment of choice. Clotrimazole

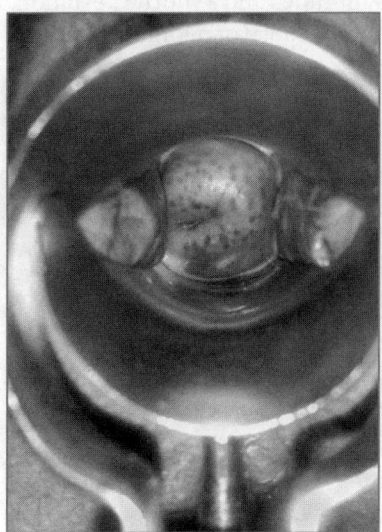

Figure 26.2: *Trichomonas vaginalis (For color version, see Plate 3)*.

may also be used as local treatment. The woman's partner should also be prescribed treatment with metronidazole.

Metronidazole potentiates the action of alcohol, anticonvulsant and warfarin. Alcohol should be avoided and use of other drugs monitored when the client is prescribed metronidazole. Because of its excretion in breast milk, it is contraindicated for breastfeeding mothers.

Clients must be advised to avoid sexual intercourse until treatment is complete.

BACTERIAL INFECTIONS

Bacterial Vaginosis

Bacterial vaginosis is a term applied to vaginal discharge associated with a variety of anaerobic organisms including *Gardnerella vaginalis* and *Bacteroides* species. It has been associated with postpartum pyrexia, amniotic fluid infection, preterm labor and pelvic inflammatory disease.

Presentation, Diagnosis and Treatment

The infection presents with a gray or white, fishy smelling discharge which may be adherent or of normal consistency and may be more profuse than normal.

The distinctive fishy odor of the discharge and a vaginal pH of greater than or equal to 4.5 are diagnostic clues.

Treatment is with metronidazole 400 mg twice daily for 5 days.

Chlamydial Infection (Fig. 26.3)

Chlamydia trachomatis (C. trachomatis) is one of a group of intracellular parasites, closely related to gram-negative bacteria. The organism is a major cause of salpingitis and pelvic inflammatory disease (PID) with their sequelae of ectopic pregnancy and infertility, and postpartum and postabortal infection. Chlamydial infection has been associated with increased risk of low birth weight, preterm rupture of membranes and a shorter gestation. It is currently the most common cause of neonatal conjunctivitis and it is

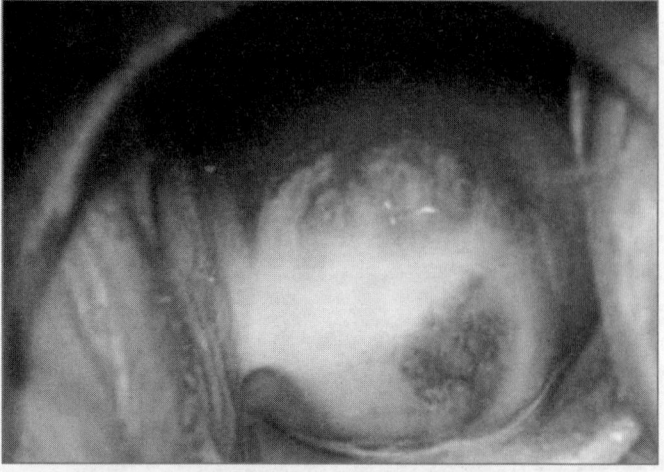

Figure 26.3: Chlamydia infection *(For color version, see Plate 3).*

estimated that from 3–18% of babies born to infected mothers will develop chlamydial pneumonia.

Presentation and Diagnosis

The condition is often asymptomatic in the woman, although a mucopurulent cervicitis may be detected clinically, or the woman may present with salpingitis or urethral syndrome.

In the light of its association with maternal and neonatal morbidity, detection of chlamydial infection during pregnancy could offer significant benefits. The Centers for Disease Control (CDC) in the US recommended that at least one prenatal culture for *C. trachomatis* be undertaken for pregnant women who fall into one of the following categories:
- Age less than 20 years
- Unmarried
- History of other STD
- Multiple sexual partners and a partner with multiple sexual partners.

Treatment

Erythromycin 500 mg four times a day for 7–10 days is the antibiotic of choice during pregnancy. Therapy should be instituted to the husband simultaneously. As a prophylaxis to ophthalmia neonatorum, tetracycline or erythromycin ointment 1% is to be applied to the neonate's eye, soon after birth. Neonatal infection is treated with erythromycin 50 mg/kg/day, four times a day for 14–20 days.

Group B *Streptococcus*

Group B *Streptococcus* (agalactiae) is part of the vaginal flora in 5–25% of women. One-third or more pregnant women may be vaginal carriers of GBS during pregnancy with intermittent and recurring colonization.

This asymptomatic maternal infection is significant in pregnancy, as the most frequent cause of overwhelming sepsis in neonates estimated to occur from 0.6 to 3.7 cases per 1,000 live births. The mortality rate of neonatal GBS in the US is 50%.

The GBS has been associated with early spontaneous rupture of membranes and with a three-fold increase in preterm delivery at or before 32 weeks' gestation.

Of the neonates of women with GBS colonization, 65–75% will be colonized with the organism, although only 1–2% of exposed neonates will develop invasive disease.

Treatment of GBS Colonization in Pregnancy

The recommended treatment is intravenous (IV) administration of ampicillin (or erythromycin if the woman is allergic to penicillin).

Gonococcal Infection

Gonorrhea **(Fig. 26.4)** is caused by *N. gonorrhoeae*, a gram-negative *Diplococcus* that has an affinity for columnar

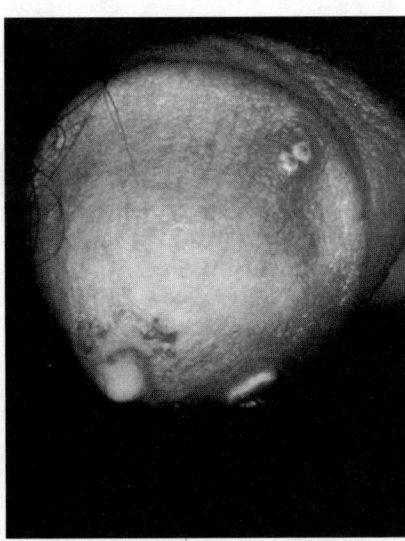

Figure 26.4: Gonorrhea infection *(For color version, see Plate 4).*

epithelial tissue. In women, infection occurs in the urethra or cervix.

Incidence of maternal infection varies greatly between populations ranging from 1 to 5%. The rate of asymptomatic infection is high; and as many as 50% of women diagnosed are usually asymptomatic.

Effects of Gonococcal Infection in Pregnancy

Gonorrhea in pregnancy may present as local infection (arthritis) or systemic disease.

Among nonpregnant women with endocervical infection, about 1%–20% show clinical evidence of pelvic inflammatory disease (PID). Acute PID is rare in pregnancy, although positive *N. gonorrhoeae* cultures are sometimes associated with fever and pain.

Manifestations of Gonococcal Infection in Pregnant Women

- Dysuria (urethral infection)
- Cervicitis (endocervical infection)
- Proctitis (rectal infection)
- Conjunctivitis (ophthalmic infection).

Less common manifestations noted include acute inflammation of the Bartholin's glands (bartholinitis), endometritis and salpingitis.

Arthritis is the most common manifestation of disseminated infection. Infection usually presents with fever and rigors, and there may be a characteristic purpuric petechial rash. Pregnancy complicated by gonococcal endocervicitis is associated with premature rupture of membranes, chorioamnionitis, early rupture of membranes and preterm delivery. Early infection is associated with septic abortion and chorioamnionitis.

Intrapartum infection is associated with postpartum endometritis and upper genital tract infection.

Neonatal infection most commonly presents as conjunctivitis, but infection at other body sites can occur and may be associated with a higher risk of disseminated infection.

Diagnosis

Swabs should be taken from the cervix and urethral meatus for culture. If culture is being done because of known contact with an infected partner, other sites of exposure such as throat and anus should be swabbed.

Screening

Screening of all women for gonococcal infection in pregnancy is recommended because of its serious effects on pregnancy and the risks of neonatal and puerperal infection and the fact that a high proportion of infection in women is asymptomatic. Repeat cultures in the last trimester are suggested for women with a previous history of gonorrhea or other sexually transmitted infection.

Treatment

Single dose of procaine penicillin 4.8 million units combined with probenecid 1 g orally or ampicillin 3 g in a single dose orally with probenecid 1 g orally. In cases of disseminated infection, penicillin is to be administered IV or intramuscularly (IM) for 10–14 days. If arthritis is a feature of infection, a longer therapy is indicated.

Syphilis (Fig. 26.5)

Syphilis is an infection caused by *Treponema pallidum (T. pallidum)*. In pregnancy, its particular significance is the devastating effect it has on fetal well-being. The natural course of adult infection is divided into stages which are also follows:

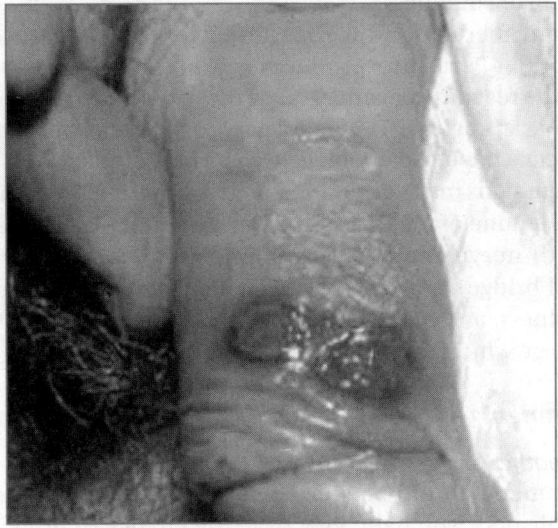

Figure 26.5: Syphilis *(For color version, see Plate 4).*

Early Infectious Stage

* *Primary stage:* 9–60 days after exposure.
* *Secondary stage:* 6 weeks to 6 months after exposure.
* *Early latent stage:* 2 years after exposure.

Late Noninfectious Stage

Late latent stage
More than 2 years after exposure. Examples are neurosyphilis, cardiovascular syphilis or gummatous syphilis.

Most pregnant women diagnosed are in the primary or secondary stages and untreated infection will affect almost all fetuses. Depending upon the intensity and time of occurrence of the infiltration, the fate of the fetus will be as follows:
* Abortion or intrauterine death—20%
* Preterm deliveries—20%
* Delivery of highly infected baby with neonatal death—20%
* Survival with congenital syphilis with resulting disability—40%.

Prenatal diagnosis and treatment through routine serological testing in early pregnancy is the key to prevention of congenital syphilis. This should be done as a routine in the first antenatal visit. Venereal disease research laboratory (VDRL) is commonly done. A positive VDRL test has to be confirmed by fluorescent treponemal antibody (FTA) test which is a specific test. Husband's blood should also be tested for VDRL. Detection of spirochetes from the cutaneous lesion, if any, is done by dark field examination. Fetal infection could be diagnosed by demonstration of *T. pallidum* in the amniotic fluid.

Congenital Syphilis

The syphilitic baby may appear normal at birth, but shows signs of infection within 1 or 2 weeks after birth. Purulent nasal discharge—often hemorrhagic, hoarse cry, maculopapular rash and pemphigus (highly contagious vesicles) on the soles and palms are common manifestations. Ulcers can occur on the lips and mouth, and if on the larynx, the baby's cry may be thin or soundless.

Poor feeding and weight loss may be the features of infection. Periostitis produces swelling of the long bones and the resulting pain may cause the baby to behave as if he/she has a fracture. The baby may also present with patchy alopecia, hepatosplenomegaly and mild jaundice.

Late signs may develop at any time from 2–30 years of life, even if none of the early signs was exhibited. These include eighth nerve deafness, saddle nose (depression on the nasal bridge), corneal scarring causing impaired vision or blindness, and mental disability. Prognosis depends on the damage which has occurred prior to treatment.

Treatment

For mother
Treatment should be started as soon as the diagnosis is established. The baby may have the chance of protection even if the treatment is begun late in pregnancy. For primary, secondary or latent syphilis (of less than 1 year duration), benzathine penicillin 2.4 million units IM as a single dose is administered. When the duration is more than 1 year, benzathine penicillin 2.4 million units weekly for 3 weeks is given. If the woman is allergic to penicillin, oral erythromycin 2 g daily for 15 days is given. If the treatment is given in early pregnancy, the treatment should be repeated in late pregnancy. Irrespective of the serological report, treatment should be repeated in subsequent pregnancies.

For baby
Infected baby with positive serological reaction requires:
* Isolation with the mother.
* Intramuscular administration of aqueous procaine penicillin G 50,000 units per kg body weight, each day in divided doses for 10 days.

In the presence of contagious lesions, the baby must be barrier nursed until antibiotics have been given for 48 hours.

Babies with positive serum reaction without clinical evidences of the disease may be treated with a single IM dose of penicillin G 50,000 units per kg body weight. The baby must be observed for 8 weeks and quantitative blood reactions are tested twice a week for 4 weeks and then at weekly intervals for another 4 weeks.

An apparently healthy baby of a syphilitic mother should be tested for serological reaction every week for the 1st month and then monthly for 6 months.

VIRAL INFECTIONS

Herpes Simplex Virus

Herpes simplex is one of a family of herpes viruses which includes varicella-zoster, CMV and Epstein-Barr virus. All within this family share the ability to establish lifelong, persistent infection in their host and to undergo periodic reactivation. Reactivated infection may have characteristics different from the primary episode.

Herpes simplex virus (HSV) type 1 is associated with infections of the lip and oropharynx, and type 2 associated with genital infection. Neonatal infection is most often associated with HSV type 2. However, postnatal infection of the newborn baby with HSV type 1 from maternal or non-maternal sources such as staff and visitors have also been documented.

For transmission to occur, the HSV virus must come into contact with mucosal surfaces or abraded skin. Viral replication occurs at the site of infection and then the virus or particles of it are transported along the neurons to the ganglia where they remain dormant until there is an alteration in the host environment that gives rise to occurrence of active infection.

Presentation of Infection with HSV

Primary infection of HSV type 1 is usually asymptomatic, though it may present with gingivostomatitis. In young adults, it is often associated with pharyngitis.

Primary infection with HSV type 2 usually presents with painful genital ulcers after an incubation period of less than 7 days. Skin lesions begin with erythema, progress to vesicles and then ulcers and finish with crusting. Local lesions with viral shedding may last about 12 days with complete healing taking another week. Both vulva and cervix are involved in most primary attacks, but single sites may be affected.

Recurrent infection involves reactivation of the same virus at the same site rather than reinfection. Clients may experience prodromal symptoms of local tingling and numbness at the site of the lesions about 24–48 hours prior to the onset of lesions. In recurrent attacks, there may be fewer lesions, milder symptoms and a shorter duration.

Both primary and recurrent infection may be asymptomatic in pregnancy, which is the situation in which the fetus is at greater risk. Primary infection is associated with an increased risk of spontaneous abortion, prematurity and the acquisition of serious infection by the neonate. Transmission of virus to the fetus or neonate is thought to occur at delivery and only very rarely transplacentally.

Management of HSV in Pregnancy

Because most genital herpes infection (**Fig. 26.6**) is unrecognized, it is important that a careful vulval inspection is done at the time of labor of all women, not just those with a history of genital herpes. When the infection occurs in the first or second trimester of pregnancy, the women are treated with oral or IV acyclovir.

When the first episode occurs in the third trimester, there is an increased risk of premature labor. If labor becomes established, the recommended management is IV administration of acyclovir and delivery by cesarean section, on the grounds of reducing maternal viremia and reducing exposure of the fetus to virus.

In the case of women who have recovered from the first episode without going into labor, because of the high-risk of continued viral shedding, an elective cesarean section at 38 weeks may be done; especially if symptoms began within 6 weeks of the expected date of delivery.

If following a first episode of infection in the third trimester, a vaginal delivery is unavoidable or if the membranes have been ruptured for more than 4 hours prior to cesarean section, the mother and baby must be treated with IV acyclovir to reduce the risk of neonatal infection.

Cytomegalovirus

Cytomegalovirus is another group of herpes viruses which can be found in saliva, urine, breast milk, semen and cervical secretions. Transmission between adults usually occurs by direct contact, e.g. by kissing and may be sexually. Primary infection may occasionally present similarly to glandular fever or influenza, with headache, sore throat and anorexia. There may be hepatitis with prolonged pyrexia. Subsequently the virus may remain dormant, but be subjected to reactivation and be excreted for many years.

Diagnosis is by culture of specimens of urine, blood or saliva, or of a swab taken from the cervix. Serology is performed for antibody levels.

Infection in Pregnancy

At any stage of pregnancy, both primary and reactivated CMV infection can result in transplacental transmission to the fetus. The results are probably more serious in primary infection. Abortion, stillbirth, growth retardation and premature labor may result.

The incidence is estimated to be about 4 per 1,000 live births. About 2% of these develop serious problems such as micro- or hydrocephaly, spastic quadriplegia, psychomotor retardation and deafness. About 8% develop minor problems like hepatosplenomegaly and thrombocytopenia. About 90% of babies are symptom-free at birth, but some will not attain their expected intellectual potential and/or will become deaf in later childhood. If transplacental infection is suspected, cord blood should be examined for specific immunoglobulin M (IgM), and a urine sample and nasopharyngeal swab sent for culture. Treatment is supportive only, and care should be taken to avoid infection of other babies and members of staff particularly pregnant staff. The virus may continue to be shed by the infected infant for a prolonged period.

Whilst it is estimated that 50% of women of childbearing age have been infected by CMV, but only about 1% of their infants will be infected.

Hepatitis B Infection

Hepatitis B virus is the most common cause of jaundice in pregnancy. It has an incubation period of 1–6 months. Perinatal transmission from an infected mother to her newborn is the major mode of transmission. It can also be transmitted sexually and by means of infected blood products or parenterally by use of unsterilized equipment contaminated by infected blood.

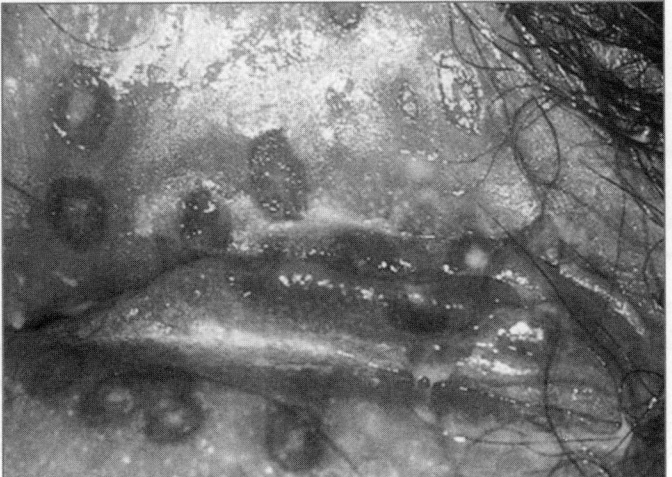

Figure 26.6: Genital herpes *(For color version, see Plate 4)*.

Transmission

The risk of transmission to fetus ranges from 10% in the first trimester to as high as 90% in the third trimester and it is specially high from those mothers who are seropositive to hepatitis surface antigen (HBsAg) and 'e' antigen (HBeAg). Approximately 10% of the infected individuals will go to the chronic state. They are at high-risk of developing chronic active hepatitis, cirrhosis and hepatocellular carcinoma. The presence of HBeAg indicates continued viral activity, although antibody to this indicates a lower level of infectivity.

Neonatal transmission: It mainly occurs at or around the time of birth through mixing of maternal blood and genital secretions. About 90% of infected babies become chronic carriers, who can infect others. About 25% of carrier neonates will die from cirrhosis or hepatic carcinoma between late childhood and early adulthood. HBV is not teratogenic.

Maternal infection: The acute infection is manifested by flu-like illness as malaise, anorexia, nausea, and vomiting and mild diarrhea. There may be arthralgia, skin rashes and pain over the liver. Majority may remain asymptomatic. Jaundice is rare and fever is uncommon. Spontaneous resolution occurs in 90% and 1% may die of fulminating hepatitis.

Diagnosis

Diagnosis is confirmed by serological detection of HBsAg, HBeAg (denote high infectivity) and antibody to hepatitis B core antigen. Chronic carriers are diagnosed by the presence of HBsAg or HBeAg and anti-HBe antibodies 6 months after initial infection. Liver enzymes are elevated during the initial phase.

Screening

All pregnant women should be screened for HBV infection at the first antenatal visit and it should be repeated during the third trimester for 'high-risk' groups (IV drug abusers, sexually promiscuous individuals, hemophiliacs or women having multiple sex partners).

Management

The babies of mothers who are chronic carriers or who have been infected with HBV during pregnancy should receive hepatitis B vaccine within 24 hours of birth which will be repeated at 1st and 6th months of age. In addition, the babies of mothers who had acute hepatitis B during pregnancy and those who do not have anti-HBe antibodies should receive 0.5 mL of hepatitis B immunoglobulin (HBIG) IM, administered in a different site from the vaccine, not later than 48 hours after birth to provide immediate passive immunity.

Infection control measures should be instituted where the mother is considered infectious. The woman should be given information about the disease and advice regarding sexual behavior. Household contacts and husband should be tested for HBsAg and offered immunization.

Rubella (German Measles)

The virus that causes rubella is particularly virulent during pregnancy. If the woman contracts rubella during the first trimester, there is approximately 20% chance that her baby will be born with congenital malformations. This figure is as high as 50% during the 1st month of pregnancy.

The most common malformations are cataracts, cardiac defects and deafness. There may also be glaucoma, microcephaly and other defects involving heart, brain and CNS. The most severely affected fetuses may abort spontaneously.

Diagnosis

Diagnosis of rubella is difficult because the disease may be subclinical, thereby infecting the fetus, but not exhibiting itself clinically in the mother.

Signs

Clinical signs of rubella when they are present include the following:
- Low-grade fever
- Drowsiness
- Sore throat
- Rash—pale or bright red on the 1st or 2nd day, spreading rapidly from the face over the entire body and fading rapidly
- Swollen neck glands
- Duration of 3–5 days.

Women who contract rubella in the first trimester are faced with the decision of whether or not to obtain a therapeutic abortion.

Genital Warts

Genital warts are caused by the HPV and nearly always transmitted by sexual contact. Rarely, a baby may acquire laryngeal papilloma because of exposure at the time of delivery.

The significance of warts in pregnancy is that they occasionally increase very dramatically in size which may be distressing to the woman and may occasionally jeopardize the possibility of vaginal delivery.

Women presenting with genital warts should be fully investigated to exclude other sexually transmitted infections. In addition, the cervix should be examined to exclude flat warts on the cervix, which may be associated with malignant changes. Because of the possible association between HPV and cervical intracellular neoplasia (CIN), cytological screening is recommended for women with vulval or vaginal warts or those whose husbands have penile warts.

The treatment suggested during pregnancy includes trichloroacetic acid cryotherapy or electrocautery. Treatment with podophyllin 10–25% is recommended for nonpregnant women. In pregnancy, it is contraindicated because of its toxicity. If the warts are smaller, they may be left untreated until delivery.

Acquired Immunodeficiency Syndrome in Pregnancy

Acquired immunodeficiency syndrome (AIDS) is caused by human immunodeficiency virus (HIV) which is a group of retrovirus, HIV-1 and HIV-2. The virus specifically reduces the CD4 receptor molecule of the T lymphocytes, monocytes, macrophages and other antigen-presenting cells leading to immunodeficiency. As a result, the individual is susceptible to infections by opportunistic microorganisms and specific tumors. The incubation period is from 2 months to 4 years. AIDS is the end stage of HIV infection.

Incidence in India

Estimate at the national level are that about 3.7 million people were suffering from HIV infection at the end of 1999. Serosurveillance findings from the states showed 98,451 persons positive for HIV by June 2000, a seropositivity rate of 26.88 per 1,000. The cumulative number of AIDS in the country has risen to 12,389 that include 2,632 females.

Mode of Transmission

The modes of transmission of HIV are:
- Sexual contact (homosexual or heterosexual)
- Transplacental
- Exposure to infected blood or tissue fluids
- Through breast milk.

HIV Infection in Pregnancy

The transmission from mother to fetus (vertical transmission) is about 30% in seropositive mothers. The fetus may be affected through uteroplacental transfer, during delivery by contaminated secretions and blood of the birth canal and through breast milk in the neonatal period.

Clinical Presentation

Initial presentation of an infected woman may be fever, malaise, headache, sore throat, lymphadenopathy and maculopapular rash. Primary illness may be followed by an asymptomatic period. Progression of the disease may lead to multiple opportunistic infections with candida, tuberculosis, pneumocystis and others. Patient may present with neoplasms such as cervical carcinoma, lymphomas (Hodgkin and non-Hodgkin) and Kaposi's sarcoma. There may be associated constitutional symptoms like weight loss, lymphadenopathy or protracted diarrhea.

Diagnosis of HIV Infection

The diagnosis of asymptomatic adult HIV infection is made on the basis of the presence in serum of antibodies to the virus. Most individuals will produce antibodies (seroconversion) within 3 months after the most recent exposure. During the so-called 'window of infectivity' (3 months), a negative result will require a repeat test in order to account for the late seroconversion.

Diagnostic HIV testing employs two tests. The enzyme-linked immunosorbent assay (ELISA) is highly sensitive to the presence of antibodies. Its sensitivity increases the possibility of false positive results and thus a 'Western blot' test which has a greater specificity for HIV is used to confirm the presence of the antibodies. A second specimen of blood may be tested to confirm the result **(Box 26.1)**.

Management

Prenatal care
- All clients should be offered voluntary serologic testing for HIV infection.
- In seropositive cases, additional investigations should be done to test for other STDs. Husbands should be offered serologic testing for HIV.
- Counseling about the risk of HIV transmission to the fetus and neonates should be made, and termination of pregnancy offered.
- Tuberculin test is to be done. If it is positive, a chest X-ray should be performed. Even if the chest X-ray is negative, chemoprophylaxis with isoniazid (INH) 300 mg orally daily should be administered.
- The woman should have T-lymphocyte count in each trimester. If the count falls to less than 200 cells/μL, the woman should be treated with zidovudine; she should receive prophylaxis against *Pneumocystis carinii* infection with trimethoprim 160 mg and sulfamethoxazole 800 mg orally thrice weekly. Nevirapine is found to reduce the viral transmission to breastfed infants.
- The progression of the disease is assessed by CD-4 lymphocyte count (gradual fall), presence of P24 core antigen and decrease of titer of P24 antibody.

Care during intrapartum period

Cesarean section does not protect the baby from vertical transmission. It should only be for obstetric indications:
- Procedures that might result in break in the skin or mucous membrane of the baby such as amniotomy, attachment of scalp electrode and fetal blood sampling (fetal scalp blood for pH) should be avoided.

BOX 26.1: Client education.

HIV positive results
- Offer immediate psychological support
- Help the client understand what the test results mean
- Review methods of transmission and assess the client's risk of transmitting HIV to others
- Explain that treatment is available
- Identify immediate healthcare resources
- Identify immediate psychiatric services as appropriate
- Offer counseling and education
- Offer contraception information
- Review safe sex practice and other risk-reduction strategies
- Advice client not to donate blood, plasma or organs

- Healthcare workers should be protected from contact with potentially infected body fluids.
- Caps, waterproof gowns, double gloves and goggles (protective eye wear) should be worn by physicians and midwives.
- Disposable needles and syringes should be used and the needles should be placed in puncture proof containers.
- Mechanical suctioning devices should be used to remove secretions from the neonates' air passages.
- Any blood contamination must be washed off the skin immediately.

Postpartum care
- Mothers must be counseled about the risks and benefits of breastfeeding and helped to make an informed choice.
- Zidovudine syrup 2 mg/kg is given to the neonate 4 times daily for first 6 weeks.
- Mother should be encouraged to manage the baby's care herself with the support of the midwife.
- Gloves must be worn for examining the perineum, lochia or cesarean wound.
- Disposal of sanitary napkins, disinfection and cleaning of any spilled blood must be done correctly (using recommended methods).

Contraception
Barrier methods of contraception are effective in preventing transmission of the virus. Simultaneous use of a spermicidal agent such as nonoxynol-9 is found to improve the efficacy.

Follow-up care of the baby
Babies born to HIV positive women will have passively acquired maternal antibodies to HIV and these may persist for as long as 18 months. Therefore, diagnosis of HIV cannot be achieved with antibody testing and confirmation of the infant's infection status may not occur for an extended period. Parents must be counseled with regard to this period of uncertainty and doubt.

Nursing Process for Pregnant Women with AIDS

Assessment
Assess for the following clinical manifestations:
- History of IV drug use, prostitution or infection for spouse
- Malaise
- Progressive weight loss
- Lymphadenopathy
- Diarrhea
- Evidence of opportunistic infection
- Fever
- Evidence of Kaposi's sarcoma (purplish, reddish brown lesions)
- Anxiety about future of self and baby.

Analysis/nursing diagnosis
- Discomfort related to disease process
- Risk for injury to self and/or fetus related to disease process
- Altered family process related to illness
- Anxiety related to pregnancy outcome
- Anticipatory grieving related to pregnancy outcome
- Altered nutrition related to lack of information and resources

Planning
- Protection from infection
- Isolation precautions
- Opportunities for counseling
- Education for self-care regarding isolation precautions and prevention of infection.

Implementation
- Observe blood and *body secretion precautions*
- Teach precautions to client
- Maintain isolation to prevent client from other organisms
- Follow blood and body fluid precautions during all contacts with expectant woman (antepartal, intrapartal, postpartal and for the newborn infant)
- Provide education regarding disease process and treatment.

Evaluation
Ensure that the expectant woman:
- Is protected from further infection?
- Participates in maintaining blood and body secretion isolation.
- Is able to verbalize feelings about her condition?
- Verbalizes knowledge of disease condition.

STUDY QUESTIONS

Short Answer Questions

1. Fungal infections of the vulva and vagina.
2. Protozoal infections of the vulva and vagina.
3. Group B streptococcal infection in pregnancy.
4. Herpes simplex virus infection in pregnancy.
5. Rubella infection in pregnancy.

BIBLIOGRAPHY

1. Abel E, von Unwerth L. Asymptomatic chlamydia during pregnancy. Res in Nurs Health. 1988;11(6):359-65.
2. Adler MW. The ABC of Sexually Transmitted Diseases, 5th edition. British Medical Journal Publishing Group Ltd: London; 1995.
3. Bell TA, Grayson JT. Centers for Disease Control guidelines for prevention and control of Chlamydia trachomatis infections. Summary and Commentary. Ann Intern Med. 1986;104(4):524-6.
4. Brunham RC, Holmes KK, Embree JE, et al. Sexually transmitted diseases in pregnancy. In: Holmes KK, Mardh PA (Eds). Sexually Transmitted Diseases, 2nd edition. New York: McGraw Hill; 1999.
5. Erikson SH, Oppenheim GL, Smith GH. Metronidazole in breast milk. Obstet Gynecol. 1981;57(1):48-50.
6. Hankins CA, Handley MA. HIV disease and AIDS in women: current knowledge and a research agenda. J Acquir Immune Defic Syndr. 1992;5(10):957-71.
7. Lossick JG. Sexually transmitted vaginitis. Semin Adolesc Med. 1986;2(2):131-42.

8. Park K. Park's Textbook of Preventive and Social Medicine, 16th edition. Jabalpur: M/s Banarsidas Bhanot Publishers; 2000. p. 310-8.
9. Roth C. Sexually transmissible and reproductive tract infections in pregnancy. In: Bennett RV, Linda KB (Eds). Myles Textbook for Midwives, 13th edition. Edinburgh: Churchill Livingstone; 1999. p. 329-50.
10. Sexually Transmitted Diseases. [online]. P3em.com Available from www.emedicinehealth.com
11. Wang E, Smaill F. Infection in pregnancy. In: Chalmers I, Murray E, Marc J, Keirse NC, et al. Effective Care in Pregnancy and Childbirth. Oxford: Oxford University Press; 1989.
12. WHO, Health for All Series, 1981.
13. WHO, World Health Report 1999; Report of the Director General, WHO.

CHAPTER 27

Disorders of Pregnancy

Learning Objectives

Upon completing this chapter, the learner will be able to:
- Define antepartum hemorrhage and explain its causes and effects on mother and fetus.
- Describe the role of midwife in relation to the identification, assessment and management of clients with placenta previa and abruptio placentae.
- Explain the disorders of amniotic fluid, their treatment and nursing care of patients admitted and management.

Medical disorders associated with pregnancy increase as women delay childbearing. They become more at risk with increasing age.

ANTEPARTUM HEMORRHAGE

DEFINITION

Antepartum hemorrhage is defined as bleeding from the genital tract after 28th week of pregnancy and before the birth of the baby.

TYPES

1. Placental bleeding:
   - Placenta previa
   - Abruptio placentae.
2. Extraplacental bleeding:
   - Due to local cervicovaginal lesions.

PLACENTA PREVIA

Definition

An implantation of the placenta in the lower uterine segment causing it to lie alongside or in front of the presenting part.

Incidence

Placenta previa occurs approximately 1 of every 250 births. It is 1 in 200 in India. One-third of all antepartum hemorrhage occurs due to placenta previa.

Causes

The exact cause of implantation of the placenta in the lower segment is not known. Following are the postulated theories.

Dropping Down Theory

The fertilized ovum drops down to the lower uterine segment. Poor decidual reaction in the upper segment may be the cause.

Multiple Pregnancies

The large placental bed of the twin placenta is prone to low implantation of at least a part of the placenta.

Defective Decidua

Defective decidua causes spreading of the chorionic villi over a wide area in the uterine wall encroaching on to the lower segment.

Degrees of Placenta Previa (Fig. 27.1)

Type 1: The lower margin of the placenta dips into the lower segment (lateral).

Type 2: The placenta reaches the internal os when closed, but does not cover it (marginal).

Type 3: The placenta covers the internal os when closed, but not when fully dilated (partial or incomplete).

Type 4: The placenta completely covers the internal os even when the cervix is fully dilated (central or complete).

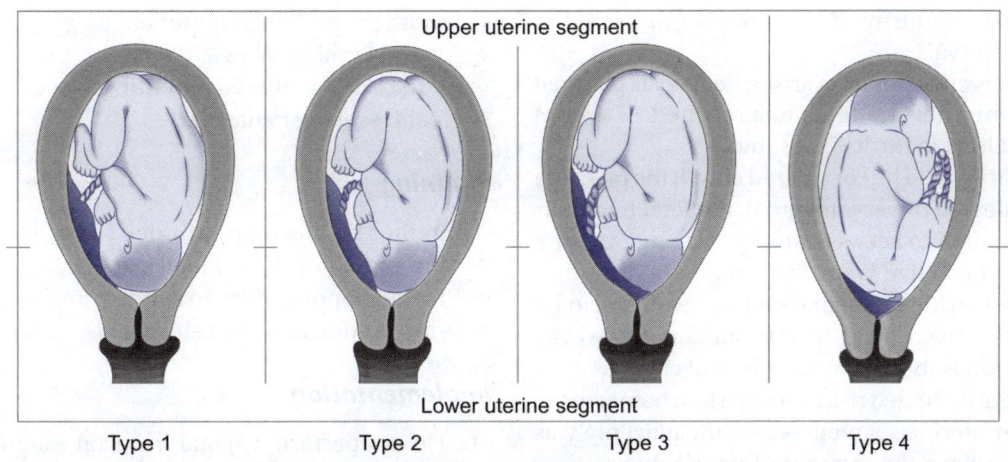

Figure 27.1: Types of placenta previa.

Predisposing Factors

1. Increased placental size, e.g. twin placenta
2. Previous uterine scar, e.g. previous cesarean or myomectomy scar
3. Multiparity
4. Advanced maternal age, over 35 years
5. Previous reproductive surgery, e.g. dilation and curettage
6. Placental abnormality, e.g. succenturiate lobe
7. Leiomyomas distorting the uterine cavity
8. Congenital malformations of the uterus.

Signs of Placenta Previa

1. Painless vaginal bleeding in the third trimester of pregnancy.
2. The bleeding is usually bright red and the amount varies with the proportion of separation of placenta. Bleeding occurs as the lower segment of the uterus begins to pull upward with cervical effacement and dilatation in late pregnancy, causing the placental villi to tear away from the uterine wall.
3. The bleeding may be scant at first and then become more profuse as more and more of the placenta separates.
4. There is no way that the bleeding from the placenta can be arrested other than delivering the fetus and complete removal of the placenta.

Risk to Mother and Fetus

The mother is at risk for severe hemorrhage, embolism and endometritis. The fetus is at risk for prematurity, asphyxia or hemorrhage.

Diagnosis

1. Clinical diagnosis is reached by an ultrasound examination in which the placenta is localized in relation to the cervix **(Fig. 27.2)**.

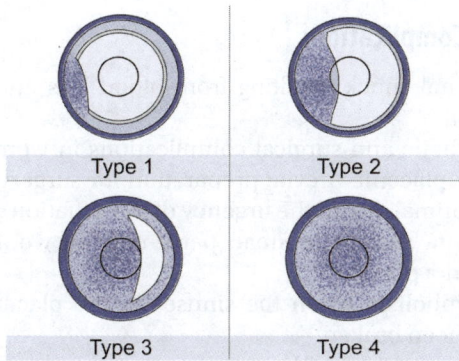

Figure 27.2: Relationship of placenta previa to cervical os.

2. The placenta may be visualized by means of an examination with a sterile speculum. This should be done only with a 'double setup' with personnel and equipment available for immediate cesarean delivery, when a sudden hemorrhage occurs.
3. The midwife should not attempt to do a vaginal examination as this could precipitate severe hemorrhage.

Management

After a diagnosis of placenta previa is established by ultrasonography, the gestational age is calculated. Management depends on the gestation of pregnancy:

1. If the gestational age is early, an attempt is made to prolong the pregnancy with the intention of optimizing the neonatal outcome. The woman is usually hospitalized to try and avoid preterm labor or hemorrhage.
2. Pregnant women mobility is usually restricted to bedrest at first.
3. Activity may be gradually increased as the pregnancy progresses to term.
4. The hemoglobin and hematocrit values are monitored.
5. Blood replacement therapy or iron therapy is instituted if anemia is present.

6. The pulmonary maturity of the fetus is monitored at appropriate intervals.
7. Unless an emergency situation arises, delivery is planned for some point after the fetus has reached 37 weeks gestation and lung maturity is assured.

A vaginal delivery would be considered only, if the placenta previa were first degree or very marginal, the fetal head has descended low enough to act as a tampon placing pressure against the placenta, active labor has begun and no other complications were evident. Vaginal delivery would also be considered if the fetus were dead. In most situations however, surgical intervention is the delivery method of choice.

The women are at increased risk of postpartum hemorrhage because the lower uterine segment where the placenta was attached, does not have the number of interlacing muscle fibers found in the upper portion of the uterus and thus, is not an efficient in contraction to control bleeding in the early postpartum period.

Possible Complications

1. Maternal shock resulting from blood loss and hypovolemia.
2. Anesthetic and surgical complications in women with major placenta previa; preparation for surgery may be suboptimal due to the urgency of the situation.
3. Placenta accreta in small percentage of women with placenta previa.
4. Air embolism when the sinuses in the placental bed have been broken.
5. Postpartum hemorrhage.
6. Puerperal sepsis.
7. Fetal hypoxia due to placental separation.
8. Fetomaternal hemorrhage and Rh isoimmunization if the mother is Rh negative and the fetus is Rh positive.
9. Fetal death depends on gestation and amount of blood loss.
10. Maternal death is a very rare outcome.

Summary of Nursing Process

Assessment

Assess for:
1. Painless unexplained vaginal bleeding after the 20th week (usually around week 27).
2. Intermittent gushes of blood.
3. Placental placement revealed by ultrasonography.
4. Maternal apprehension caused by the bleeding episode.

Analysis/Nursing Diagnosis

- Risk for fetal injury
- Risk for infection
- Ineffective airway clearance
- Actual/risk for aspiration
- Anxiety
- Anticipatory grieving
- Health promotion/maintenance
- Altered family process
- Actual/risk for altered parenting
- Health seeking behavior.

Planning

- Monitor for bleeding episodes
- Monitor maternal and fetal status
- Provide opportunities to support and counseling
- Provide education for self-care.

Implementation

1. Do not perform vaginal or rectal examinations, or give enemas.
2. Monitor fetal heart rate (FHR) and prepare client for ultrasound test.
3. Facilitate 'double setup', vaginal examination by the obstetrician:
   a. Prepare for cesarean section before vaginal examination.
   b. Vaginal examination is done in operating room.
   c. Type and crossmatch for possible blood transfusion.
4. Manage bleeding episodes:
   a. Keep woman nil per os (NPO).
   b. Monitor vital signs and FHR (by continuous electronic fetal monitor).
   c. Maintain woman on absolute bedrest.
   d. Start and/or maintain intravenous (IV).
   e. Maintain perineal pad count to estimate amount of bleeding (1 g of weight is approximately 1 mL).
   f. Prepare for cesarean delivery.
   g. Maintain meticulous sterile techniques.
5. Support mother, spouse and family, and encourage them to verbalize feelings.
6. Provide parents information about the nature of problem.
7. Prepare women for vaginal birth, if pregnancy is near term, the cervix is favorable and marginal placental placement is identified.

Evaluation

Ensure that the pregnant woman:
1. Maintains normal vital signs, hematocrit and hemoglobin.
2. Verbalizes her apprehension and feelings.
3. Demonstrates FHR between 120 and 160 beats per minute with average variability, and no late or variable decelerations.

ABRUPTIO PLACENTAE

Definition

Abruptio placentae are defined as premature separation of a normally situated placenta after 28 weeks gestation and before birth of the baby (**Figs. 27.3A to C**).

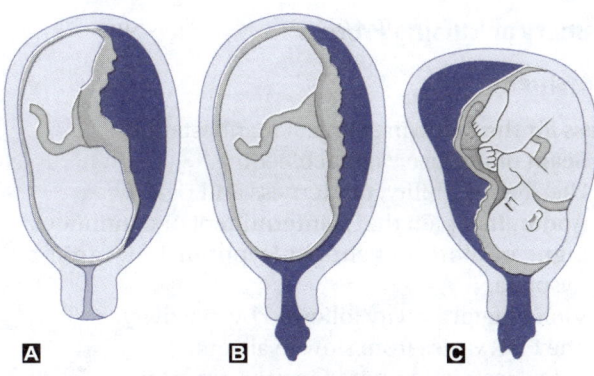

Figures 27.3 A to C: Abruptio placentae. (A) Concealed; (B) Revealed; (C) Mixed.

Types of Placental Abruption

Concealed (Fig. 27.3A)

The blood collects behind the separated placenta or between the membranes and decidua. The collected blood is prevented from coming out of the cervix by the presenting part, which presses on the lower segment. Sometimes, it is retained behind the placenta and forced into the myometrium where it infiltrates between the muscle fibers of the uterus, resulting in a condition known as couvelaire uterus.

Revealed (Fig. 27.3B)

Following separation of the placenta, the blood escapes from the placental site, separates the membranes from the uterine wall and drains through the vagina.

Mixed (Fig. 27.3C)

In this type, some portion of the blood collects inside (concealed) and a portion is expelled out (revealed). Usually one type predominates the other.

Causes

The exact cause is unknown, but several factors have been considered as causes:
- Spasm of the uterine vessels followed by flooding into the choriodecidual space
- Malnutrition
- Folic acid deficiency
- Traction of short cord
- Trauma from external cephalic version.

Abruptio placentae are seen associated with the following conditions:
- Multiparity, fifth pregnancy and over
- Major congenital malformations
- Abruption in previous pregnancy
- Pregnancy-induced hypertension.

Grading of Placental Abruption

Grade 1

1. Mild separation of the placenta.
2. Slight vaginal bleeding and some uterine irritability are present. Maternal blood pressure is unaffected. Fibrinogen level is unaffected. The FHR is normal.

Grade 2

1. Moderate separation of the placenta.
2. External bleeding is mild to moderate. The uterus is irritable. Tetanic contractions may be present. Maternal blood pressure may be normal. The fetal heart rate shows signs of distress. The maternal fibrinogen level is decreased.

Grade 3

1. Severe separation of the placenta.
2. The bleeding may be severe and may be concealed. Uterine contractions are titanic and painful. Maternal hypotension may be present. The fibrinogen level is greatly reduced with resultant coagulation problems.

Signs and Symptoms

1. Small to moderate amount of bright or dark red vaginal bleeding
2. Acute abdominal pain associated with vaginal bleeding
3. Uterine tenderness and high uterine tonicity often described as 'board-like abdomen'
4. Increase in the size of the uterus, particularly, if the bleeding is concealed
5. Failure of the uterus to relax between contractions
6. Fetal heart sounds absent with concealed or mixed type
7. Urine output usually diminished.

Diagnosis

1. Ultrasonography to visualize the location of the placenta and presence of clot or hematoma
2. Coagulation profile to rule out disseminated intravascular coagulation:
   - Clotting time
   - Bleeding time
   - Fibrinogen level
   - Platelet count
   - Prothrombin and partial prothrombin time
   - Fibrin degradation products.
3. Renal function tests.

Management

1. Fluid and blood replacement.
2. Vaginal delivery if bleeding is minimal, the mother's condition is stable, the labor is progressing and the presenting part is in the pelvis. Labor may have to be augmented (induced) if it is not progressing well.

3. Cesarean delivery if hemorrhage is severe, fetal heart tones are present, the presenting part is not in the pelvis, the cervix is closed or if it is anticipated that birth is not imminent.

If the fetus is dead, a cesarean section is performed only if the bleeding is life-threatening. A cesarean hysterectomy may be necessary if the bleeding cannot be controlled.

Possible Complications

1. Severe shock may cause renal failure with first hematuria, then oliguria or anuria due to necrosis of the nephrons.
2. Coagulation defect, if not treated successfully can lead to catastrophic bleeding due to disseminated intravascular coagulation (DIC).
3. Heavy blood loss and shock can cause pituitary necrosis leading to Sheehan's syndrome.
4. Postpartum hemorrhage may occur as a result of the couvelaire uterus and DIC.

Nursing Care

1. All maternal and fetal vital signs should be monitored frequently and recorded carefully.
2. The amount and nature of bleeding to be assessed, and recorded.
3. Contraction pattern and cervical status to be monitored if the woman is in active labor.
4. Urinary output and skin color should be observed, and recorded.
5. The woman should be grouped and cross-matched for packed red blood cells.
6. If the pain is extreme, an analgesic such as morphine is given, as pain can exacerbate shock, which must be avoided.
7. An IV line must be set up with a 16-gauge intracatheter to administer plasma expander and blood. Blood is collected for investigations.
8. A central venous line is usually inserted in order to monitor the central venous pressure 2 hourly or more frequently.
9. Physical comfort and emotional support must be provided. The woman must be assisted to rest in left lateral position, which relieves occlusion of vena cava and compression of aorta by the gravid uterus.
10. Fundal height and abdominal girth are to be measured hourly. An increase indicates continued bleeding behind the placenta.
11. If the fetus is alive, the FHR should be monitored continuously and oxygen to be administered to relieve hypoxia. Once the woman's condition is stabilized, cesarean section may be indicated.
12. Observation must be made for any developing complication such as hypotension, hypovolemia, shock and DIC.

Summary of Nursing Process

Assessment

Assess for the following clinical manifestations:
1. Scant or profuse vaginal bleeding.
2. Uterine irritability, tenderness and rigidity.
3. Abdominal pain that is intermittent or continuous.
4. Signs of maternal shock: Hypotension, rapid pulse, dyspnea.
5. Violent fetal activity followed by inactivity.
6. The FHR varies from slow to absent.
7. Late deceleration noted in monitor strip.
8. May have blood-stained amniotic fluid (port-wine stained).

Analysis/Nursing Diagnosis

1. Risk for fetal injury
2. Risk for infection
3. Ineffective airway clearance
4. Actual/risk for aspiration
5. Anxiety
6. Anticipatory grieving
7. Altered family processes
8. Actual/risk for altered parenting
9. Health seeking behavior.

Planning

1. Promote safe care environment
2. Monitor for presence of pre-existing conditions
3. Assess maternal-fetal status and initiate emergency care
4. Provide encouragement and support
5. Administer measures to treat shock and blood loss.

Implementation

1. Monitor maternal and fetal vital signs.
2. Treat shock symptoms:
   a. Assess vital signs every 5–15 minutes
   b. Administer oxygen by face mask at 7–10 L/min
   c. Increase IV flow rate
   d. Administer blood
   e. Monitor urinary output
   f. Monitor FHR continuously.
3. Observe for signs and systems of coagulation problems.
4. Measure abdominal girth.
5. Remain with woman.
6. Monitor labor pattern continuously, if allowed to progress or prepare for cesarean section.

Evaluation

Ensure that:
1. The woman and her spouse understand the treatment plan.
2. The physiological status of the woman and the fetus remains within normal limits.

3. The woman and her spouse verbalizes, decrease of anxiety and feelings of support.
4. The woman remains normotensive.
5. The hemoglobin and hematocrit levels are within normal limits.

DISSEMINATED INTRAVASCULAR COAGULATION

Disseminated intravascular coagulation is a condition of inappropriate coagulation within the blood vessels, which leads to the consumption of clotting factors. As a result clotting fails to occur at the bleeding site.

Etiology

Disseminated intravascular coagulation always occurs as a response to another disease process, it is never a primary disease. The response triggers widespread clotting with the formation of microthrombi throughout the circulation. Clotting factors get used up. The DIC triggers fibrinolysis and production of fibrin degradation products (FDPs). FDPs reduce the efficiency of normal clotting. A paradoxical feedback system is thus setup in which clotting is the primary problem, but hemorrhage is the predominant clinical finding.

When DIC occurs during or after delivery, the reduced level of clotting factors and the presence of FDPs prevent normal hemostasis at the placental site. FDPs inhibit myometrial action and prevent the uterine muscle from constricting the blood vessels in the normal way. Torrential bleeding may be the outcome. The lost blood may be observed to remain uncoagulated for several minutes and even when clotting does occur, the clot is unstable.

Microthrombi may cause circulatory obstruction in the small blood vessels. The effects of this vary from cyanosis of fingers and toes to cerebrovascular accidents, and failure of organs such as the liver and kidneys.

Obstetric Conditions, Which may Precipitate Disseminated Intravascular Coagulation

Placental Abruption

In placental abruption, due to the damage of tissue at the placental site large quantities of thromboplastins are released into the circulation, which may cause DIC. If the placenta is delivered, as soon as possible after the abruption, the risk of DIC is reduced.

Intrauterine Fetal Death

If a dead fetus is retained in uterus for more than 3–4 weeks, thromboplastins are released from the dead fetal tissue. These enter the maternal circulation and deplete clotting factors. If fetal death occurs and labor does not follow spontaneously, it should be induced. If fetal death is known to have occurred sometime previously, clotting studies should be performed prior to induction of labor and if DIC is diagnosed, appropriate management must be instituted.

Amniotic Fluid Embolism

Thromboplastin in the amniotic fluid is responsible for setting off the cascade of clotting. If death does not occur from maternal collapse, DIC may develop.

Intrauterine Infection

The causes of infection in obstetric patients include septic abortion, chorioamnionitis, placenta accreta and endometrial infection before or after delivery. In such conditions, DIC is caused by endotoxins entering the circulation and damaging the blood vessels. Therefore, while treating the DIC, the infection itself must be treated aggressively with antibiotics. If the woman develops hemolytic septicemia, the bacteria in the bloodstream may destroy any blood administered. In postpartum infection, any retained products must be evacuated from the uterus.

Preeclampsia and Eclampsia

The factors, which precipitate DIC in these patients is unclear, FDPs are seen increased in the serum and urine, which indicates fibrinolysis, is taking place.

Management

In patients suspected of having DIC, blood investigations such as blood grouping and crossmatching, clotting studies, platelets, fibrinogen and FDPs are done. Treatment involves the replacement of blood cells and clotting factors. Fresh frozen plasma and platelet concentrates are usually given. Whole blood may also be given.

Nursing Care

The midwife should be aware of the conditions in her patients, which may cause DIC. Her observation should include looking for signs of defective clotting and the nature of clot formation during the third stage of labor. Oozing from a venipuncture site or bleeding from the mucous membrane of the mother's mouth and nose during the third and fourth stage of labor must be noted and reported.

Disseminated intravascular coagulation is a frightening situation and an obstetric emergency. The nurse must be quick to recognize the signs and to take necessary action. She has to maintain her own calmness and clarity of thinking to deal with the situation. The patient, spouse and family need help to deal with the situation. Frequent and accurate observations must be made to monitor the mother's condition. This includes vital signs, fluid balance and other parameters to assess the patient's general condition. The death of the mother is a real possibility and if the midwife finds herself in such a situation, supporting the bereaved family will be an important responsibility.

DISORDERS OF AMNIOTIC FLUID

Amniotic fluid normally increases in amount throughout pregnancy from few milliliters to a liter at 38th week. The fluid is not static, the water and solutes in it are changing every few hours. There are two chief abnormalities of amniotic fluid—polyhydramnios and oligohydramnios.

POLYHYDRAMNIOS

Polyhydramnios is a state where the amount of amniotic fluid exceeds 1500 mL. Clinical definition states that the excessive accumulation of liquor amnii causing discomfort to the patient and/or when an imaging help is needed to substantiate the clinical diagnosis of the lie and presentation of the fetus.

Incidence

Polyhydramnios occurs in 1-2% of pregnancies. It is more common in multiparae than in primipare. Minor degrees of hydramnios are fairly common and occurs in 1 in 1,000 pregnancies.

Etiology

Exact cause for the excessive accumulation of amniotic fluid is still speculative. It may be the result of deficient absorption as well as the excessive production which may be temporary or permanent. While certain maternal and fetal factors are found to be associated with hydramnios in certain cases, the cause remains unknown in about 60%. The composition of liquor amni however remains normal.
1. *Fetal anomalies:* Congenital fetal malformations are associated with polyhydramnios in about 20% of cases. These include:
   - Anencephaly
   - Open spina bifida
   - Esophageal or duodenal atresia
   - Facial clefts and neck masses
   - Hydrops fetalis.
2. *Maternal causes:*
   - Diabetes mellitus
   - Cardiac or renal diseases
3. *Placental factors:* Choriocarcinoma of the placenta
4. *Multiple pregnancies:* Multiple pregnancies especially with monozygotic twins usually affecting the second sac.

Clinical Types

Depending on the mode of onset and progress, there are two types of polyhydramnios.
1. *Chronic polyhydramnios:* This is the most common type which is gradual in onset, usually from about 30th week of pregnancy.
2. *Acute polyhydramnios:* It is extremely rare and occurs at about 20th week and comes on suddenly. The uterus reaches the xiphisternum in 3-4 days. It is often associated with monozygotic and/or severe fetal abnormalities.

Signs and Symptoms

Signs and symptoms of polyhydramnios include the following:
1. *Uterine enlargement:* Abdominal girth and fundal height are far beyond the expected for gestational age.
2. Tenseness of the uterine wall, making it difficult or impossible to auscultate fetal heart tones and palpate fetal outline and fetal parts.
3. Elicitation of uterine fluid thrill (fluid thrill may be elicited by placing a hand on one side of the abdomen and tapping the other side with the fingers).
4. Mechanical problems such as:
   - Severe dyspnea
   - Lower extremity and vulvar edema
   - Pressure pains in the back, abdomen and thighs
   - Nausea and vomiting.
5. Frequent change of fetal lie (unstable lie).
6. Auscultation of the fetal heart is difficult because of the increased quality of fluid.

Acute Polyhydramnios

Acute polyhydramnios is extremely rare. The onset is acute and the fluid accumulates within a few days. It usually occurs before 20 weeks of pregnancy. It is often associated with uniovular twins or choriocarcinoma of the placenta.

Signs and Symptoms

Features of acute abdomen predominate and include:
1. Abdominal pain, nausea and vomiting
2. Edema of legs
3. Abdomen hugely enlarged in relation to the period of gestation with tense skin
4. Fetal parts cannot be felt nor is the fetal heart audible.
5. Fluid thrill is present
6. On internal examination, dilation of os, taking up of cervix and bulging of membranes may be felt.
7. Ultrasonography may reveal fetal or placental anomaly.

Management

Spontaneous abortion occurs most often. Decompression of the uterus has to be done. On rare occasion, where the baby is valuable, repeated amniocentesis is done to continue the pregnancy after excluding fetal congenital anomalies. Otherwise pregnancy is terminated by low rupture of membranes.

Severe degree hydramnios

In view of the risks involved and high perinatal morbidity rate, the patient should be managed in a hospital equipped to deal with high-risk patients. This is needed to avoid, and deal with fetal complications.

Supportive therapy
- Bed rest and treatment of associated conditions like preeclampsia
- Investigations to exclude congenital fetal malformation
- Further management depends on:
  - Response to treatment
  - Period of gestation
  - Presence of fetal malformation
  - Associated complicating factors
- In cases where response to treatment is good, pregnancy is continued.
- If unresponsive and pregnancy is less than 37 weeks amniocentesis and termination of pregnancy is done
- For unresponsive pregnancy above 37 weeks induction of labor is done
- During labor: Usual management measures are followed. If the uterine contractions become sluggish, oxytocin infusion may be started. To prevent postpartum hemorrhage, IV administration of Methergine is used.

Puerperium Maternal Complications

- Subinvolution of uterus
- Increased puerperal morbidity
- Increased blood loss.

Fetal Complications

There is increased perinatal mortality to the extent of 50%. The deaths are mostly due to prematurity, congenital abnormality and due to contributory factors such as cord prolapse, hydrops fetalis, accidental hemorrhage and increased operative delivery are possible.

Management

In recent times there has been a falling trend in the incidence of hydramnios of severe magnitude due to following reasons.
1. Early detection and control of disease
2. Prevention of Rhesus isoimmunization due to improved prenatal care
3. Genetic counseling in early months and detection of fetal congenital abnormalities with ultrasound and their termination.

Minor degree hydramnios
this is commonly detected in mid-trimester and usually requires no treatment except extra bed rest for few days. The excess liquor is expected to diminish as pregnancy advances. Presence of extra fluid allows the fetus to move away from the stethoscope, however its presence can be picked up by the Doppler ultrasound. Abdomen is markedly enlarged and appears globular with fullness at the flanks.

Diagnosis
- An ultrasound scanning (ultrasonography) to confirm the findings and identify any co-existing conditions
- Screening for diabetes
- Screening for ABO/Rh disease.

Complications
The complications of hydramnios are grouped into:
Maternal
- During pregnancy, there is increased incidence of:
  - Preeclampsia
  - Malpresentation
  - Prematuree rupture of membranes
  - Preterm labor
  - Antepartum hemorrhage due to placental abruption
  - Ureteral obstruction
- During labor:
  - Early rupture of membranes
  - Cord prolapse
  - Uterine inertia
  - Increased incidence of cesarean section due to malpresentation. Retained placenta, postpartum hemorrhage and shock.

OLIGOHYDRAMNIOS

Description

Oligohydramnios is a condition in pregnancy characterized by a deficiency of amniotic fluid. It is almost invariably associated with Potter's syndrome. It is an extremely rare condition, where the liquor amni is deficient in amount to the extent of less than 250 mL at term. Sonographically, it is diagnosed when the maximum vertical pool of liquor amnii is less than 2 cm and the amniotic fluid index (AFI) is less than 5 cm (<10 centile).

Characteristic Features

- Diminished amniotic fluid volume (AFV)
- Amount less than 500 mL at 32–36 weeks gestation.
- Single deepest pocket (SDP) of less than 2 cm
- Amniotic fluid index (AFI) is less than 5 cm or less than 5th percentile.

Etiology

The cause is unknown, but is often seen associated with:
- Fetal chromosomal abnormalities
- Intrauterine infection
- Drugs such as ACE inhibitors
- Renal agenesis or obstruction of the urinary tract in fetus
- Intrauterine growth retardation due to placental insufficiency
- Post maturity.

Pathophysiology

Oligohydramnios is secondary to either an excess loss of fluid or a decrease in fetal urine production. Oligohydramnios is associated with one or more of the following conditions.
1. Early rupture of fetal membranes (24–26 weeks)
2. Congenital anomalies such as:
   - Renal agenesis (absence of kidneys)

- Potter's syndrome (pulmonary hypoplasia)
- Cystic dysplasia
- Ureteral atresia
2. Post-mature pregnancy related to:
   - Decreased efficiency of placental function
   - Decreased fetal renal blood flow and decreased fetal urine production.

Frequency

Oligohydramnios is common in pregnancies beyond term because the amniotic fluid volume (AFV) normally decreases at term. It complicates as many as 12% of pregnancies that lasts 41 weeks or longer. In the US, Oligohydramnios is a complication in 0.5–5.5 % of all pregnancies and severe. Oligohydramnios is a complication in 0.7% of pregnancies.

Clinical Signs and Symptoms

These are because the amniotic fluid volume is below what is normally found for the particular gestational age.
- The uterus appears smaller than expected for the period of gestation.
- Reduced fetal movements compared to previous normal pregnancies.
- The uterus is small and compact, and fetal parts are easily felt.
- The fetus is not ballotable.
- Auscultation is normal.

Diagnosis

- Ultrasonography measurement of amniotic fluid volume. The criteria for diagnosis include:
  The absence of fluid pockets throughout the uterine cavity, crowding of the fetal limbs and the absence of packets surrounding the fetal legs, and overlapping of fetal ribs (in severe cases).
- Measurement of the single deepest pocket (SDP) and summation of SDPs in each quadrant or the amniotic fluid index (AFI). The test is done with the mother in supine or semi-Fowler's position. The ultrasound transducer is held along the maternal longitudinal axis and maintained perpendicular to the floor while the SDP of amniotic fluid is measured. Pockets should be free of fetal limbs and umbilical cord.

AFI as a Quantitative Measurement

The pregnant abdomen is divided into 4 quadrants by using the umbilicus as a reference point to divide the uterus into upper and lower halves and by using the linea nigra to divide the uterus into left and right halves. The 4 measurements are summed to obtain the AFI in centimeters. In gestations earlier than 20 weeks, measurements from the two halves are divided by the linea nigra to obtain the AFI. The Mean AFI for normal pregnancies is 11–16 cm. Oligohydramnios is diagnosed if AFI is less than 5 cm, although 8 cm has been occasionally considered.

Magnetic resonance imaging (MRI) and 3-dimensional ultrasonography are newer modalities for accurately diagnosing amniotic fluid volume.

Complications

Fetal

- Abortion
- Deformity due to intra-amniotic adhesions or due to compression.
- Fetal pulmonary hypoplasia (this condition includes alteration in skull bone, wry neck and even amputation of the limp).
- High fetal mortality
- Cord compression.

Maternal

- Prolonged labor due to inertia.
- Increased operative interference due to malpresentataion.
- Increased maternal morbidity.

Management

Premature rupture of membranes is common. Labor may be protracted and contractions may be stronger. Fetal distress occurs frequently. Because of frequent association of fetal malformation, vaginal delivery is favored.

1. *Before term:* Expectant management is often the most appropriate course of action, depending on maternal and fetal condition. Ongoing antepartum surveillance including assessment of fetal growth and follow-up monitoring of amniotic fluid volume are necessary.
2. *At term:* Delivery is often the most appropriate management. With reassuring fetal testing, delivery may be safely delayed on the basis of parity, the gestational age, the indelibility of mother's cervix and the severity of oligohydramnios.
3. *After term:* Oligohydramnios in the post-term patient is associated with more fetal decelerations, a higher incidence of meconium- stained fluid, and increased risk of cesarean delivery. Oligohydramnios is considered an indication for cesarean delivery in a post-term pregnancy.
   Amnioinfusion for increasing the amount of fluid within the amniotic cavity can be accomplished during delivery. Warm or room-temperature sodium chloride solution is transcervically infused through an intrauterine catheter. This procedure increases the amount of fluid to provide more padding around the umbilical cord, which has been shown to decrease the frequency and severity of variable decelerations secondary to decreased cord compression. Amnioinfusion lowers the rate of surgical delivery.
   Amnioinfusion via amniocentesis before labor to improve the intrauterine environment for the fetus is advocated by some. Duration of the effect of this therapy is not known.

Oligohydramnios is usually observed to return in one week. Amnioinfusion via amniocentesis has been used in the second trimester to better visualize the fetal anatomy and to confirm the diagnosis.
4. Vesicoamniotic shunts may be used to divert fetal urine to the amniotic cavity in patients in whom a fetal obstructive uropathy is determined to be the cause of oligohydramnios. Findings from human and animal studies suggest that the shunts can prevent or at least ameliorate pulmonary hypoplasia. Unfortunately such shunts are associated with rupture of membranes in about 12% of the cases at the time of shunt placement.

Summary of Nursing Process

Assessment

Assess for the following:
- Ballottement results in fluid waves
- Fundal height excessive for gestation
- Fetus difficult to outline with palpation
- Supine hypotension
- Fetal abnormalities of central nervous systems (CNS) or gastrointestinal (GI) tract
- Easy fatigability.

Analysis/Nursing Diagnosis

- Risk for fetal injury related to altered fluid amount in uterus.
- Impaired physical mobility related to abdominal size.
- Actual/risk for fluid volume deficit.
- Anxiety related to the health status.
- Altered family process.
- Health seeking behaviour related to change in physical condition.

Planning

- Promote maternal comfort
- Promote maternal-fetal well-being
- Provide opportunities for counseling and support
- Provide education for self-care measures in increasing comfort.

Implementation

1. Facilitate testing: Amniocentesis, sonogram.
2. Assess FHR.
3. Anticipate premature labor and postpartum hemorrhage caused by overdistention of the uterine muscle.
4. Instruct and explain the nature of problem:
   a. Need to obtain immediate medical attention for problems.
   b. Need to observe for preeclampsia.

Evaluation

Ensure that the expectant mother:
- Verbalizes increased comfort
- Progresses to uneventful birth, as does her baby
- Verbalizes support
- Verbalizes self-care measures.

STUDY QUESTIONS

Short Answer Questions

1. Definition and types of antepartum hemorrhage.
2. Types of placenta previa.
3. Disseminated intravascular coagulation as a complication of abruptio placentae.

Essay Questions

1. Describe the possible management and nursing care of a 24-year-old woman admitted in the inpatient unit, who is 38 weeks pregnant and diagnosed as having abruptio placentae.
2. Describe the types and clinical manifestations of placenta previa, and explain the management of a client admitted with type 2 placenta previa at 30th week.

BIBLIOGRAPHY

1. Beare PG. Davis's NCLEX-RN Review, 3rd edition. Philadelphia: FA Davis Company; 2001. pp. 186-221.
2. Crafter H. Problems of pregnancy. In: Bennet RV, Brown KS (Eds). Myles Textbook for Midwives, 13th edition. Edinburgh: Churchill Livingstone; 1999. pp. 255-76.
3. Dutta DC. Textbook of Obstetrics, 5th edition. Kolkata: New Central Book Company; 2001. pp. 256-76.
4. Helen V. Nurse-Midwifery, 2nd edition. Boston: Jones-Bartlett Publishers; 1996. pp. 188-92.
5. Knuppet RA, Drukker JE. High risk pregnancy: a team approach, 1st edition. Philadelphia: WB Saunders; 1993. pp. 98-116.
6. Nicholas FN, Zwelling E. Maternal newborn nursing: theory and practice. Philadelphia: WB Saunders Co; 1997. pp. 106-18.

CHAPTER 28

Hypertensive Disorders of Pregnancy

Learning Objectives

Upon completing this chapter, the learner will be able to:
- List the classifications of hypertensive disorders in pregnancy including the differentiating characteristics.
- Describe the signs, symptoms and potential complications of hypertensive disorders.
- Describe the management of different hypertensive disorders.
- Outline the nursing care and support for clients with hypertensive disorders.

Hypertension is one of the common disorders of pregnancy and contributes significantly to the maternal and perinatal morbidity and mortality. Hypertension may appear for the first time during pregnancy as a direct result of the gravid state or as a sign of underlying pathology, which may be pre-existing.

BOX 28.1: Classification of hypertension in pregnancy.

1. Pregnancy-induced hypertension (PIH):
   a. With proteinuria and/or edema:
      » Preeclampsia
      » Eclampsia.
   b. Without gross edema or proteinuria:
      » Gestational hypertension.
2. Chronic hypertension in pregnancy. Pregnancy is unrelated to the hypertensive state:
   a. Essential hypertension.
   b. Renovascular hypertension.
   c. Pheochromocytoma.
   d. Coarctation of aorta.
   e. Thyrotoxicosis.

PREGNANCY-INDUCED HYPERTENSION

The hypertension develops as a direct result of the gravid state. The woman does not have a history of previous hypertension or evidence of it. The clinical types of PIH are:
- Preeclampsia
- Eclampsia
- Gestational hypertension.

PREECLAMPSIA

Definition

Preeclampsia is a multisystem disorder of unknown etiology characterized by development of hypertension to the extent of 140/90 mm Hg or more with proteinuria induced by pregnancy after the 20th week in a previously normotensive and non-proteinuric woman (International Society for Study of Hypertension in Pregnancy, 1988).

Incidence

About 5–8% of all pregnancies are complicated by hypertension and of these preeclampsia accounts for 80%. It occurs more frequently in young primigravida and in mothers over 35 years of age. It is known to be associated with hydatidiform mole, multiple pregnancy and maternal diabetes.

Etiology

The exact nature of the primary event causing PIH is not known. The following are thought to be the possibilities:
1. There is a relative or absolute deficiency of vasodilator prostaglandin I2 (PGI2), synthesized in vascular endothelium and increased synthesis of thromboxane A2 (TxA2), a potent vasoconstrictor in platelets.

2. There is an increased vascular sensitivity to the pressor agent angiotensin II. The sensitizing substances are yet to be explored.
3. Nitric oxide, which normally relaxes vascular smooth muscle, inhibits platelet aggregation and prevents intervillous thrombosis, is found deficient in preeclamptic clients. Hence, preeclampsia is characterized by complex endothelial cell dysfunction.
4. In preeclampsia, trophoblastic invasion of the spiral arteries is thought to be inhibited by some immunological mechanism.

The cause of excessive accumulation of fluids in the extracellular spaces is not clear. Excessive retention of sodium in the edematous state is probably due to the increased aldosterone, out of activation of corticosterone by angiotensin II. Diminished renal blood flow, decreased glomerular filtration rate and increased tubular reabsorption are responsible for retention of sodium.

The probable events that contribute to proteinuria are spasm of the afferent glomerular arterioles, anoxic damage to the endothelium of the glomerular tuft, increased capillary permeability and increased leakage of proteins. Tubular reabsorption is simultaneously depressed.

Pathophysiology

The pathological changes that occur in the various organs in severe preeclampsia and eclampsia are well-documented:

1. *Uteroplacental bed:* There is an increased evidence of premature aging of the placenta. Areas of occasional acute infarcts are visible on the maternal surface of the placenta.
2. There is acute atherosis of spiral arteries with obliteration of the lumen. Intervillous circulation is impaired to the extent of about one-third, secondary to changes in the maternal blood vessels. This results in placental changes, which are responsible for fetal jeopardy.
3. In the kidneys, there is reduced blood flow and glomerular filtration rate, and impaired tubular reabsorption or secretary functions.
4. In the blood vessels, there is intense vasospasm. Circulation in the vasa vasorum is impaired leading to damage of the vascular walls including the endothelial integrity.
5. Hemorrhagic necrosis occurs in the liver due to thrombosis of the arterioles. Hepatic insufficiency seldom occurs because of the reserve capacity and regenerative ability of the liver.

Clinical Classification of Preeclampsia

The clinical classification of preeclampsia is principally dependent on the level of blood pressure for management purpose.

Mild preeclampsia is diagnosed when there is sustained rise of blood pressure of more than 140/90 mm Hg, but less than 160 systolic or 110 diastolic without significant proteinuria on two occasions of 6 hours apart.

Severe preeclampsia is diagnosed when the blood pressure exceeds 160/100 mm Hg, when there is an increase in the proteinuria (75 g/day) and where edema is marked. The woman may complain of frontal headaches, visual disturbances and upper abdominal pain with or without vomiting (imminent eclampsia). Reduced platelet count (less than 100,000/μL), elevated liver enzymes, retinal hemorrhages or papilledema, pulmonary edema and intrauterine growth retardation of the fetus are also seen.

Clinical Features

1. Preeclampsia frequently occurs in primigravida (70%).
2. It is often associated with obstetrical-medical complications such as multiple pregnancies, polyhydramnios, pre-existing hypertension, diabetes, etc.
3. The clinical manifestations usually appear after the 20th week.
4. The onset is usually insidious and the symptoms run a slow course. On rare occasions, however, the onset becomes acute and follows a rapid course.
5. Edema is seen in approximately 80% of women with preeclampsia. It may appear rather sudden and be associated with a rapid weight gain. Clinical edema may be mild or severe in nature and the severity is related to the worsening of the preeclampsia. The edema pits on pressure and may be found in the following anatomical areas such as face, hands, lower abdomen, vulva, sacral area, pretibial region, ankles and feet.
6. Elevated blood pressure: More than 140/90 mm Hg in mild cases and above 160/110 mm Hg in severe preeclampsia.

Alarming Symptoms and Signs

The following symptoms and signs may be evident either singly or in combination. These are usually associated with acute onset of the symptoms:

1. Headache over the occipital or frontal region.
2. Disturbed sleep.
3. Diminished urinary output (less than 500 mL in 24 hour).
4. Epigastric pain associated with vomiting, at times coffee colored due to hemorrhagic gastritis or subcapsular hemorrhage in the liver.
5. Blurring or dimness of vision or at times complete blindness (vision is usually regained 4–6 h following delivery).
6. A rapid gain in weight of more than 2.5 kg (5 lb) a month or more than 500 g (1 lb) a week in the later months of pregnancy.
7. Visible edema over the ankles on rising from the bed in the morning. Sudden and generalized edema may indicate imminent eclampsia.
8. Scanty liquor or growth retardation of the fetus.

Preeclampsia is principally a syndrome of signs and when symptoms appear it is usually late. Targeted assessments in clients with preeclampsia is depicted in **Box 28.2**.

> **BOX 28.2:** Nursing Alert
>
> **Targeted assessments in clients with preeclampsia**
> - Blood pressure measurements.
> - Intake and output measurements.
> - Physical assessment for:
>   – Presence and location of edema
>   – Deep tendon reflexes.
>   – Presence of headache and visual changes
>   – Presence of nausea, vomiting and epigastric, or right upper quadrant pain
> - Fetal evaluation appropriate for gestational age and fetal well-being
> - Proteinuria monitoring with 24-hours urine collection

Tests in Preeclampsia

Laboratory Tests

- Urine:
  - Urine quantity reduced.
  - Proteinuria of > 300 mg/24 h.
  - Urine dipstick > 1 +.
- Blood:
  - Protein/creatinine ratio > 0.3.
  - Serum creatinine >1.2 mg/dL.
  - Serum uric acid >5.6 mg/dL.
  - Platelet count < 100,000/mm^3.
  - Elevated PT or PTT.
  - Decreeased fibrinogen.
  - Peripheral smear—abnormal.
  - Indirect bilirubin >1.2 mg/dL.
  - Lactate dehydrogenase >60 U/L.
  - Serum AST >70 U/L.

Effects on the Fetus

1. Reduced placental function can result in low birth weight.
2. There is an increased incidence of hypoxia in both the antenatal and intrapartum period.
3. Placente fetal hypoxia; if major, intrauterine death will occur.
4. Early delivery, if the disease worsens or if abruption occurs, which will produce a preterm baby requiring resuscitation.

Complications

Immediate

1. During pregnancy:
   - Eclampsia 2% (more in acute cases)
   - Placental abruption and intrauterine fetal death
   - Oliguria and anuria
   - Dimness of vision and blindness
   - Preterm labor
   - Hemolytic anemia, elevated liver enzymes, low platelet count (HELLP) syndrome.
2. During labor:
   - Eclampsia
   - Postpartum hemorrhage may be related with coagulation failure.
3. Puerperium:
   - Eclampsia (usually occurs within 48 hour)
   - Shock (related to reduced sodium and chloride)
   - Sepsis (due to increased incidence of induction and operative delivery and low vitality).

Remote

1. *Residual hypertension:* The hypertension may persist even after 6 months following delivery in about 50% of cases.
2. *Recurrent preeclampsia:* There is 25% chance of preeclampsia to recur in subsequent pregnancies.

Preventive Measures

Preeclampsia is not a very preventable disease. However, some specific 'high-risk' factors leading to preeclampsia may be identified in individuals. These are:

1. Primigravida, especially young and elderly.
2. Poor nutrition.
3. Low level of education.
4. Presence of complicating factors like pre-existing hypertension, twins, polyhydramnios, clinical or latent diabetes and nephritis.
5. History of preeclampsia or hypertension in the family or in previous pregnancy.
6. Abnormal weight gain.
7. Rising serum uric acid level.

The following regime is enforced in such patients in an attempt to prevent or to detect early manifestations of preeclampsia:

1. Regular antenatal check-up at frequent intervals from the beginning of pregnancy to detect at the earliest, the rapid gain in weight or a tendency of rising blood pressure especially the diastolic pressure.
2. Advise to take adequate rest in bed on her left side at least for 2 hours in the afternoon from the 20th week of pregnancy onwards.
3. Low dose aspirin (60 mg) daily, beginning early in pregnancy to potentially high-risk women. It selectively reduces platelet thromboxane production.
4. Calcium supplementation (2 g/day) reduces the risk of preeclampsia.
5. Antioxidants, vitamin C and E from 16 to 22 weeks onwards.
6. Well-balanced diet, which is rich in protein.

Management and Nurse's Role

As the etiology of preeclampsia remains unclear, the management is mostly empirical and symptomatic. Objectives of care are to:

- Provide rest and a tranquil environment
- Monitor the condition

- Prevent eclampsia and other complications
- Deliver a healthy baby in optimal time with minimum maternal morbidity.

Rest

The woman should be in bed preferably in left lateral position as much as possible to lessen the effects of vena caval compression. Rest is to be continued until all the preeclamptic manifestations subside. When proteinuria develops in addition to hypertension, the risks to the mother and fetus are considerably increased. Admission to the hospital is required at this stage to monitor and evaluate the maternal and fetal condition.

Rest increases the renal blood flow causing increased diuresis, increases uterine blood flow causing improved placental perfusion and reduces the blood pressure.

Diet

As for any pregnant woman, a diet rich in protein, fiber and vitamins are recommended. Salt is neither restricted nor forced. Omission of salty food and extra salt in the dish is desirable. Fluids need not be restricted. Total calorie may be approximately 1,600 per day with about 100 g proteins. There is some evidence to suggest that prophylactic fish oil in pregnancy may act as an antiplatelet agent, thereby preventing hypertension and proteinuric preeclampsia. Calcium supplementation is also thought to be helpful as low serum calcium level is associated with hypertension.

Antihypertensive Therapy

Blood pressure usually comes down with adequate rest and sedatives. Antihypertensives have limited value in controlling the rise of blood pressure due to preeclampsia. They are used to prevent increase in blood pressure and the development of severe preeclampsia, especially when the diastolic pressure is over 110 mm Hg, and when associated with proteinuria. The common oral drugs used are either methyldopa (Aldomet) 0.5–2 g/day or an adrenoceptor antagonist (α- and β- blocker)—labetalol 200 mg 6–8 hourly. If blood pressure is not under control, nifedipine, a calcium channel blocker 10–20 mg twice a day or hydralazine 25 mg twice daily are added.

Sedatives: Mild sedatives are given to reduce the emotional factor that contributes to elevation of blood pressure. Phenobarbitone 60 mg or diazepam 5 mg at bedtime or more frequently are given.

Laxative: If the woman is constipated, a mild laxative like milk of magnesia four teaspoons at bedtime may be given.

Abdominal Examination

Abdominal examination is to be carried-out daily for women admitted to the hospital. Any discomfort or tenderness must be recorded and reported to the physician immediately as this may be indicative of placental abruption. Upper abdominal pain is highly significant and indicative of the HELLP syndrome.

Fetal Assessment

Assessment of the fetal well-being must be done by the use of kick charts, cardiotocograph monitoring and serial ultrasound scans.

Assessment of Treatment

The effect of treatment should be evaluated by maintaining records of:
- Blood pressure four times a day
- Status of edema and daily weight
- Volume of fluid intake and urinary output
- Daily examination of urinary protein
- Blood values such as hematocrit, platelet count, uric acid, creatinine and liver function test once a week
- Ophthalmoscopic examination on admission and later as needed.

Favorable Signs

In favorable cases, there is fall of blood pressure and weight with subsidence of edema. Urinary output increases with diminishing proteinuria.

Treatment

The definitive treatment for preeclampsia is termination of pregnancy. The aim of treatment is to continue the pregnancy if possible, without affecting the maternal prognosis until the fetus becomes mature enough to survive in the extrauterine environment. Thus, the duration of treatment depends on:
1. Severity of preeclampsia.
2. Duration of pregnancy.
3. Response to treatment.

Those women who respond to treatment, if pregnancy is far from term, the treatment is continued with weekly assessment. If the pregnancy is near term, the woman is kept in the hospital until completion of 37th week. Thereafter, a decision is taken either to terminate the pregnancy or to wait for spontaneous onset of labor by the due date.

For women whose blood pressure remains high, if the pregnancy is beyond 37 completed weeks, termination is considered. If less than 38 weeks, expectant treatment may be continued with careful monitoring of maternal and fetal well-being.

For those women who do not respond to treatment or develop additional symptoms, such as headache, epigastric pain and oliguria, termination of pregnancy is to be done irrespective of the period of gestation. Such patients may need prophylactic anticonvulsant therapy with magnesium sulfate. Methods of termination are:
1. Induction.
2. Cesarean section.

Indications for Induction

- Aggravation of preeclamptic symptoms in spite of medical treatment
- Persistence of hypertension in spite of medical treatment with pregnancy reaching 38 weeks or more
- Acute fulminating preeclampsia irrespective of the period of gestation
- Tendency of pregnancy to overrun the expected date
- Recurrent preeclampsia with previous history of intrauterine fetal death.

If the cervix is ripe, surgical induction with low rupture of the membranes is the method of choice. Oxytocin infusion may be added to accelerate the process in selected cases. If the cervix is unripe and the termination is not urgent, intracervical prostaglandin gel (PGE2) may be inserted to make the cervix ripe when low rupture of membranes can be performed. In severe preeclampsia, sedatives and antihypertensives are used during induction.

Indications for Cesarean Section

1. Urgent termination is indicated, but the cervix is unfavorable (unripe and closed) for surgical induction.
2. Severe preeclampsia with a tendency to prolong the induction delivery interval.
3. Associated complicating factors such as elderly primigravida, contracted pelvis, malpresentation, etc.

Management of Labor

First Stage

The midwife should remain with the pregnant women throughout the course of labor. Blood pressure tends to rise during labor and convulsions (intrapartum eclampsia) may occur. It is essential to document blood pressure and urinary output. Fluid balance should be monitored carefully. The patient should be in bed and sedatives (injection pethidine) should be given at intervals. Marked deviations should be noted and medical assistance sought. The pregnant women should be made as comfortable as possible by providing general nursing care.

Vital signs: Blood pressure and pulse are measured half hourly. Measurement of the mean arterial pressure (MAP) is recommended because of the hemodynamic changes in eclampsia. Respiratory rate and level of consciousness must be assessed periodically. Examination of the optic fundi can give an indication of cerebral edema. Cerebral irritability can be assessed by the degree of hyperreflexia or the presence of clonus.

Fluid balance: Intravenous fluids are administered using infusion pumps and the recommended infusion rate is 85 mL/h. Because of the reduced intravascular compartment in preeclampsia, poorly controlled fluid balance can result in circulatory overload, pulmonary edema, adult respiratory distress syndrome and ultimately death. A urinary catheter is inserted and urine output is measured hourly. A quantity about 30 mL/h reflects adequate perfusion. Urinalysis to detect the presence of protein, ketones and glucose is done 4 hourly.

Pain relief: Epidural analgesia may procure the best pain relief and reduce the blood pressure. If cesarean section should be done, epidural anesthesia is the best.

Fetal condition: The fetal heart rate (FHR) should be monitored continuously and deviations from the normal must be reported and acted on.

Second Stage

When the second stage commences, the obstetrician and pediatrician should be notified. The midwife will continue to care for the mother. Duration of the second stage is usually shortened by the application of a forceps or ventouse. Depending on the blood pressure reading, the woman is sedated immediately following delivery of the baby with intramuscular morphine to prevent postpartum eclampsia. Usually blood pressure drops after delivery.

Third Stage

Ergometrine and Syntometrine should not normally be used as they can cause peripheral vasoconstriction and increase blood pressure. In the presence of severe hemorrhage, Methergine intramuscularly or Syntocinon in the drip may be given.

Puerperium

The maternal condition should continue to be monitored at least every 4 hours for the next 48 hours, the period during which convulsions usually occur. Tablet phenobarbitone 60 mg in repeated doses can produce effective sedation. Hypotensive drugs may be prescribed, if the diastolic pressure is raised beyond 100 mm Hg. The woman is kept in the hospital until the blood pressure reaches a safe level and proteinuria disappears.

Signs of Impending Eclampsia

The following signs and symptoms will alert the midwife to the onset of eclampsia:

- A sharp rise in blood pressure
- Diminished urinary output which is due to acute vasospasm
- Increase in proteinuria
- Headache which is usually severe, persistent and frontal in location
- Drowsiness or confusion due to cerebral edema
- Visual disturbances such as blurring of vision or flashing lights due to retinal edema
- Epigastric pain due to liver edema and impairment of liver function
- Nausea and vomiting.

The midwife should be alert to any of these and summon medical help immediately.

Acute Fulminant Preeclampsia

Acute fulminant preeclampsia is a clinical entity where the onset of preeclamptic manifestations is acute occurring a new or there is rapid deterioration in an established case of preeclampsia over a short period. There is a constant threat of either convulsion or coma. All the features of preeclampsia generalized edema, raised blood pressure and proteinuria are intensified. Alarming symptoms, such as headache, epigastric pain, visual disturbances, etc. are evident either singly or in combination.

Treatment

Prophylactic anticonvulsant therapy with magnesium sulfate is instituted immediately in dose and schedule as outlined in the treatment of eclampsia. Blood pressure is to be stabilized by antihypertensive drugs given parenterally (*Aldomet, labetalol or hydralazine*). Response to treatment should be carefully watched by noting the blood pressure, urinary output, proteinuria and hematological parameters at regular intervals.

Obstetric Management

In cases with pregnancy beyond 37th completed week or where the condition fails to improve within reasonable period (6–8 hour), delivery should be considered irrespective of the period gestation. Termination is done depending on the Bishop's score, either by low rupture of the membranes aided by oxytocin infusion or by cesarean section.

HELLP Syndrome

The syndrome of hemolysis (H), elevated liver enzymes (EL) and low platelet count (LP) is a rare complication of PIH. The condition was first described by Weinstein in 1982. It is generally thought to represent a variant of the preeclampsia-eclampsia syndrome. This syndrome is manifested by nausea, vomiting, epigastric or right upper quadrant pain along with biochemical and hematological changes. It is observed in 10–15% of those with preeclampsia and eclampsia. Treatment is immediate delivery and management as that for acute fulminant preeclampsia.

Pregnancies complicated by HELLP syndrome have been associated with both poor maternal and poor fetal outcome. Serious maternal morbidity includes disseminated intravascular coagulation (DIC), acute renal failure, pulmonary edema, subcapsular liver hematoma and retinal detachment. Infants whose mothers have the syndrome are often small for gestational age and at risk for perinatal asphyxia. The affected lowbirth weight babies have relatively high incidences of leukopenia, neutropenia and thrombocytopenia.

Diagnosis

The variety of signs and symptoms makes diagnosis difficult. Hypertension and proteinuria may be absent or slightly elevated. Upper abdominal pain is a common manifestation of the disorder which should be investigated. Occasionally, the presence of this syndrome is associated with hypoglycemia leading to coma, severe hyponatremia and cortical blindness. Laboratory findings may show the following:
1. Hemolysis:
   - Abnormal blood picture
   - Increased bilirubin (> 20 µmol/L)
   - Increased lactic dehydrogenase (LDH) > 600 IU/L
2. Elevated liver enzymes:
   - Increased serum glutamic oxaloacetic transaminase (SGOT)/aspartate aminotransferase (AST) > 72 IU/L
   - Increased lactic dehydrogenase > 600 IU/L.
3. Low platelets: Platelet count < 100,000/µL.

Complications

Subcapsular hemorrhage of the liver is a rare, but potentially fatal complication of the HELLP syndrome. The condition usually presents with severe epigastric pain that may persist for several hours and in addition, the woman may complain of neck and shoulder pain.

Treatment

Women with HELLP syndrome should be admitted to a hospital with facilities for intensive care. In pregnancies less than 34 weeks gestation, conservative treatment is given using plasma volume expanders and vasodilators.

In term pregnancies and where there is a deteriorating maternal or fetal condition, immediate delivery is recommended.

ECLAMPSIA

Preeclampsia when complicated with convulsion and/or coma is called eclampsia. The term eclampsia is derived from a Greek word meaning 'like a flash of lightning'. It may occur quite abruptly without any warning manifestations. In majority (over 80%), the disease is preceded by features of severe preeclampsia. Thus, it may occur in women with preeclampsia or in women who have preeclampsia superimposed on essential hypertension or chronic nephritis.

Incidence

The incidence varies widely from country to country and even between different zones in the same country. In the developed countries, its prevalence is estimated to be around 1 in 2,000 deliveries. In the developing countries, particularly in the rural areas, it contributes significantly to the maternal deaths. The hospital incidence in India ranges from 1 in 500 to 1 in 30. It is more common in primigravida (75%), five times more common in twins than in singleton pregnancies and occurs between the 36th week and term in more than 50%.

Pathophysiology

Since eclampsia is a severe form of preeclampsia, the histopathological and biochemical changes are similar although intensified than those of preeclampsia.

Onset of Convulsions

Convulsions occur more frequently beyond 36th week. On rare occasions, convulsion may occur in early months as in hydatidiform mole:

1. *Antepartum (50%):* Fits occur before the onset of labor. More often, labor starts soon after and at times, it is impossible to differentiate it from intrapartum fits.
2. *Intrapartum (30%):* Fits occur for the first time during labor.
3. *Postpartum (20%):* Fits occur for the first time in puerperium usually within 48 hours of delivery.

Except on rare occasions, an eclamptic patient always shows previous manifestations of acute fulminating preeclampsia called premonitory symptoms.

Eclamptic Convulsions

The convulsions are epileptiform and consist of four stages.

1. *Premonitory stage:* The patient becomes unconscious. There is twitching of the muscles of the face, tongue and limbs. Eyeballs are rolled or turned to one side and become fixed. This stage lasts for about 30 seconds.
2. *Tonic stage:* The whole body goes into a tonic spasm. The trunk opisthotonus, limbs are fixed and hands clenched. Respiration ceases and the tongue protrudes between the teeth. Cyanosis appears. Eyeballs become fixed. This lasts for about 30 seconds.
3. *Clonic stage:* All the voluntary muscles undergo alternate contraction and relaxation. The twitchings start in the face and then involve one side of the extremities and ultimately the whole body is involved in the convulsion. Biting of the tongue occurs, breathing becomes stertorous and blood-stained frothy secretions fill the mouth. Cyanosis gradually disappears. This stage lasts for 1–4 minutes.
4. *Stage of coma:* Following the convulsion, the patient passes on to the stage of coma. It may last for a brief period or may persist until another convulsions. At times, the patient appears to be in a confused state following the fit and fails to remember the happenings. Rarely coma occurs without convulsion.

The fits usually are multiple, recurring at varying intervals. When it occurs in quick succession, it is called *status eclampticus*. Following convulsions, the temperature usually rises; pulse, respiration rates and blood pressure are also increased. The urinary output is markedly diminished, proteinuria is pronounced and the serum uric acid is raised.

Management

The patient, if at home or in the peripheral health centers, should be shifted urgently to the referral hospitals. The patient must be heavily sedated before moving her to the hospital. The aims of immediate management in the hospital are to:

- Clear and maintain the airway
- Prevent hypoxia
- Prevent injury
- Arrest convulsions
- Effect delivery in 6–8 hours.

The midwife must remain with the mother constantly. In the first instance, all effort is devoted to the preservation of the mother's life:

1. The patient should be placed in a railed cot in an isolated room, protected from noxious stimuli, which might provoke further fits. The patient is to be positioned in semiprone position in order to facilitate drainage of saliva and vomit. Side lying position helps to minimize vena caval compression. If the patient is unconscious, the position should be changed at intervals to prevent hypostatic pneumonia and bedsore. Airway is maintained and oxygen administered to prevent severe hypoxia.
2. Detailed history is to be taken from the relatives relevant to the diagnosis of eclampsia—duration of pregnancy, number of fits and the medications administered outside.
3. After the patient is properly sedated, thorough, but quick general, abdominal and vaginal examinations are done. A self-retaining catheter is introduced and the urine is tested for protein. Continuous drainage is established for measurement of the urinary output, periodic urinary analysis and for prevention of soiling of the bed due to incontinence likely to occur during fits.
4. Vital signs check (pulse, respiration and blood pressure) is to be done at every 30 minutes and recorded. Progress of labor and FHR must be monitored. Urinary output is to be noted hourly.
5. *Fluid balance:* Crystalloid solution (Ringer's lactate) is started as a first choice. Total fluids should not exceed the previous 24 hours urinary output plus 1,000 mL (insensible loss through lungs and skin). Normally, it should not exceed 2 L in 24 hours. In preeclampsia and eclampsia, although there is hypovolemia, the tissues are overloaded.
6. Anticonvulsant therapy is given to control the fit and to prevent its recurrence. Magnesium sulfate is the drug of choice. It reduces motor end-plate sensitivity to acetylcholine and thereby reduces neuromuscular irritability. Magnesium sulfate induces cerebral vasodilation, dilates uterine arteries and inhibits platelet activation. It has no detrimental effects on the neonate within therapeutic level.

Administration of Magnesium Sulfate

The regimens given below may vary between hospitals:

1. Pritchard regimen:
   – Loading dose: 4 g IV over 3–4 minutes (20 mL of 20% solution) and then 10 g deep intramuscular (IM)
   – Maintenance dose: 5 g IM in alternate buttock 4 hourly (10 mL of 50% solution).
2. Zuspan regimen:
   – Loading dose: 4 g IV over 5–10 minutes
   – Maintenance dose: 2 g/h IV infusion.

3. Sibai regimen:
   - Loading dose: 6 g IV over 20 minutes
   - Maintenance dose: 2 g/hour IV infusion.

Repeated injections are given only if the knee jerks are present, urine output exceeds 30 mL/h and the respiration rate is more than 12 per minute. The therapeutic level of serum magnesium is 4–7 mEq/L. Magnesium sulfate is continued for 24 hours after the last seizure. For recurrence of fits, further 2 g IV bolus is given over 5 minutes in the above regimens.

Magnesium sulfate is now the recommended drug of choice for routine anticonvulsant management of woman with eclampsia rather than diazepam or phenytoin. Magnesium sulfate is superior to all other drugs because it does not depress maternal or fetal respiration within the therapeutic level. The mother remains conscious and hence cooperation in childbirth and nursing are easier. Complications of deep sedation and immobilization are avoided.

High levels of the drug can be toxic and therefore the patellar reflex and respiratory rate or oxygen saturation levels (pulse oximetry) should be measured hourly. In women with oliguria, regular monitoring of serum magnesium level is necessary. Calcium gluconate is the antidote for magnesium toxicity and should be readily available.

Antihypertensives and Diuretics

In spite of anticonvulsant and sedative regimen, if blood pressure remains more than 160/110 mm Hg, antihypertensive drugs are administered. Hydralazine 5 mg IV is given slowly and repeated after 20 minutes with 10 mg, if there is no response. The blood pressure should be monitored at every 5 minutes. Hydralazine is repeated whenever the diastolic pressure rises to 110 mm Hg. Alternatively, labetalol is given by slow IV route 20 mg/h for smooth control of blood pressure. Presence of pulmonary edema requires diuretics. In such cases, frusemide is administered in doses of 20–40 mg intravenously and repeated at intervals.

Role of the Midwife

1. The woman should be placed in a sound protected room to minimize auditory stimulation.
2. Eye pads to be applied to minimize optic stimulation.
3. The room should be well-lighted so as not to miss the development of cyanosis.
4. Bed railings to be padded in order to minimize physical injury during convulsion.
5. Patient to be placed in semiprone position and the position to be changed at every 2 hours, if the patient is heavily sedated or in deep coma to avoid hypostatic pneumonia and bedsores.
6. Keep Foley's catheter in the urinary bladder and make chart of urinary output every hour.
7. Minimal handling and stimulation in order to reduce the risk of occurrence of another convulsion.
8. Maintain an IV line patent preferably in a central vein.
9. Keep a tracheotomy tray available.
10. Apply a thromboelastic stocking to prevent deep vein thrombosis.

Management during a Fit

1. In the premonitory state, a mouth gag is to be placed in between the teeth to prevent tongue bite and should be removed after the clonic phase is over.
2. The air passage is to be cleared off the mucus with a mucus sucker after convulsion.
3. The patient's head is to be turned to one side and the pillow taken off. Raising the foot end of the bed facilitates postural drainage of the upper respiratory tract.
4. Oxygen is to be given until cyanosis subsides.

The parameters to monitor are—a return to normal blood pressure, an increase in urinary output, a reduction in edema and a return to normal laboratory indices.

Complications of Eclampsia

- *Injuries:* Tongue bite, injuries due to falling out of bed
- *Cardiovascular:* Vasospasm, pulmonary embolism
- *Renal:* Oliguria, renal failure
- *Hematological:* Hypovolemia, hemoconcentration, thrombocytopenia, DIC
- *Neurological:* Cerebral edema, cerebral hemorrhage
- *Hepatic:* Subcapsular hematoma, hepatic necrosis
- *Respiratory:* Pneumonia (aspiration, hypostatic or infective)
- *Sensory:* Disturbed vision due to retinal edema or detachment (usually reversible)
- *Puerperal:* Sepsis, psychosis
- *Fetal:* Placental abruption, intrauterine growth retardation, fetal distress, intrauterine death.

Mortality

Maternal mortality is very high in India and varies from 2% to 30%, and more in rural hospitals. Causes for maternal death are:
- Cardiac failure
- Pulmonary edema
- Aspiration and/or septic pneumonia
- Cerebral hemorrhage
- Anuria
- Pulmonary embolism
- Postpartum shock
- Puerperal sepsis.

Perinatal mortality is very high to the extent of about 30–50%. The causes are:
- Prematurity
- Intrauterine asphyxia due to placental insufficiency
- Effects of drugs used to control convulsions
- Trauma during operative delivery.

Prevention

In majority of cases, eclampsia is preceded by a severe preeclampsia. Hence, the prevention of eclampsia rests on early detection and effective institutional management with judicious termination of pregnancy. However, eclampsia can occur bypassing the preeclamptic state and as such, it is not always a preventable condition. Adequate sedation and/or prophylactic anticonvulsant therapy soon after delivery of the baby in preeclampsia and meticulous observation for 24–48 hours are definite steps to prevent postpartum eclampsia.

Future Management

There is no indication that PIH causes later hypertensive disease, but it can leave an inherent disposition toward hypertension. Women with a history of preeclampsia before 32 weeks gestation have 5% risk of recurrence by this gestational age and 15% risk of recurrence overall.

Usually the blood pressure returns to normal within several weeks, but the proteinuria may persist for a longer period. The obstetrician will examine the mother for about 6 months after delivery and if all is well, she will be advised to seek medical advice as soon as a subsequent pregnancy occurs.

Summary of Nursing Process

Assessment

Assess for the following clinical manifestations of preeclampsia and eclampsia:
1. *Edema:*
   - Mild to moderate in preeclampsia
   - Severe in face, hands and pretibial area in eclampsia.
2. *Proteinuria:*
   - Trace, 1+ to 2+ in preeclampsia
   - Copious, 3+ to 4+ in eclampsia.
3. *Weight gain:*
   - 0.75–1.0 kg/week in preeclampsia
   - Sudden large increase in eclampsia.
4. *Blood pressure:*
   - In preeclampsia 140/90 to 160/110 mm Hg
   - Above 160/110 mm Hg in eclampsia.
5. *Other symptoms:*
   - Headache, blurred vision, epigastric pain and oliguria
   - Tonic-clonic seizures, cyanosis and fetal distress in eclampsia.
6. *Age and parity:* Occur more frequently in young primiparous women and multiparous women over 35 years.
7. *Predisposing factors include:*
   - Inadequate protein intake
   - Multiple pregnancies
   - Hydatidiform mole
   - Chronic renal and vascular disease.

Nursing Diagnosis

- Anxiety related to effects of the condition on pregnancy.
- Anxiety related to the fetal outcome.
- Discomforts related to the physical condition.
- Altered family process.
- Impaired rest and sleep.
- Potential for ineffective coping
- Health-seeking behavior.

Planning

- Prevent progression of PIH to convulsions
- Monitor maternal and fetal well-being
- Provide counseling and support
- Provide teaching related to diet, rest, parental care and self-care activities.

Implementation

1. Facilitate early prenatal care.
2. Assess physical parameters:
   - Blood pressure
   - Weight
   - Urine for protein
   - Edema of face, hands and pretibial area
   - Check reflexes for hyperreflexia.
3. Provide diet instructions:
   - Avoid added salt and high protein diet
   - Maintain adequate fluid intake
   - Ensure protein intake 1 g/kg/day
   - Maintain good prenatal nutrition.
4. Instruct regarding medications:
   - Antihypertensive drugs
   - Sedatives.
5. Facilitate hospitalization, if required.
6. Promote bedrest, rest on left side and quiet environment.
7. Prevent convulsions:
   - Administer magnesium sulfate as prescribed
   - Obtain magnesium sulfate blood levels every 4–6 hours
   - Monitor FHR
   - Assess urine output, proteinuria, vital signs, reflexes and respiratory effort hourly
   - Administer calcium gluconate for magnesium sulfate overdose/toxicity
   - Prepare for labor induction or cesarean birth
   - Continue magnesium sulfate for 24 hours after delivery.

Evaluation

Ensure that the expectant woman:
- Complies with treatment regimen and does not develop eclampsia
- Progresses to labor without further complications
- Verbalizes support and increased coping ability
- Verbalizes self-care measures.

GESTATIONAL HYPERTENSION

Gestational hypertension is a sustained rise of blood pressure to 140/90 mm Hg or more on at least two occasions, 4 or more hours apart beyond 20th week of pregnancy, or during the first

24 hours after delivery in a previously normotensive woman. It is associated with a much higher incidence of essential hypertension in later life than preeclampsia. Both are like the two phases of the same disorder. Essential features of this condition are:

- Absence of any evidence for the underlying cause of hypertension
- Unassociated with other evidences of preeclampsia such as edema or proteinuria
- The blood pressure returns to normal within 10 days following delivery.

The hypertension may be a stress response. Perinatal mortality remains unaffected. These patients are more likely to develop hypertension with the use of oral contraceptives or in subsequent pregnancies.

CHRONIC HYPERTENSION IN PREGNANCY

Chronic hypertensive disease is defined as the presence of hypertension of any cause before 20th week of pregnancy in the absence of hydatidiform mole or is present long after delivery.

Chronic hypertension has two possible causes:
1. It may be a long-term problem, present before the beginning of pregnancy, for example, essential hypertension
2. It may be secondary to existing medical problems, such as:
   – Renal disease
   – Systemic lupus erythematosus
   – Coarctation of the aorta
   – Cushing's syndrome
   – Pheochromocytoma (a rare tumor of the adrenal medulla).

DIAGNOSIS

Consistent blood pressure recordings of 140/90 mm Hg or more on two occasions more than 24 hours apart during the first 20 weeks of pregnancy suggest that the hypertension is a chronic problem and unrelated to pregnancy. Women with chronic hypertension tend to be older, parous and have a family or personal history of hypertension. Serial blood pressure recordings should be made in order to determine the true pattern as even normotensive women show occasional peaks. Physical examination may reveal the long-term effects of hypertension, such as retinopathy, ischemic heart disease and renal damage.

COMPLICATIONS

The perinatal outcome in mild chronic hypertension is good. However, the perinatal morbidity and mortality are increased in those women who develop severe chronic hypertension or superimposed preeclampsia. Other complications are independent of pregnancy and include renal failure and cerebral hemorrhage. In 1–2% of cases, hypertensive encephalopathy may develop if the blood pressure suddenly rises above 250/150 mm Hg.

Essential Hypertension in Pregnancy

Apart from the specific hypertensive disorder in pregnancy (PIH), essential hypertension is the most common hypertensive state in pregnancy. Its incidence varies from 1 to 3%.

Diagnosis

The diagnostic criteria of essential hypertension are:
1. Rise of blood pressure to the extent of 140/90 mm Hg or more during pregnancy prior to the 20th week.
2. Persistence of blood pressure even after 3 months following delivery.
3. Common in multipara and elderly women.
4. Presence of pre-pregnant hypertension and often family history.
5. Presence of hypertensive retinopathy.

Effects of Pregnancy on the Disease

1. There may be a midpregnancy fall of blood pressure in about 50%. However, the blood pressure tends to rise in the last trimester which may or may not reach its previous level.
2. In about 50%, the blood pressure tends to rise progressively as pregnancy advances.
3. In about 20%, it is superimposed by preeclampsia.
4. Rarely, malignant hypertension supervenes.
5. In about 30%, there is permanent deterioration of the hypertension following delivery.

Risks to Mother and Fetus

In the milder form, the maternal risk remains unaltered, but in the severe form or when superimposed by preeclampsia, the maternal risk is much increased. The babies are likely to be growth retarded due to chronic placental insufficiency. Perinatal loss is about 10% in the milder form with blood pressure less than 160/100 mm Hg. When the blood pressure exceeds 160/100 mm Hg, the perinatal loss doubles and when complicated by preeclampsia, it trebles.

Management

In mild cases with blood pressure less than 160/100 mm Hg, adequate rest, low salt diet and sedative (phenobarbital 60 mg one to three times daily) are given. Weekly or more frequent checkups are needed up to 28 weeks and thereafter weekly.

In severe cases or in cases of superimposed preeclampsia, the patient should be hospitalized and placed in the treatment protocol as described under preeclampsia. Antihypertensive drugs are given only when the blood pressure is raised beyond 160/100 mm Hg because the diminished blood pressure may reduce the placental perfusion which may be detrimental to the fetus. In cases where these drugs have been used before pregnancy, care is taken to adjust the dose during pregnancy especially during midpregnancy, when the blood pressure tends to fall.

Spontaneous labor at term is awaited in mild cases. In severe or complicated cases, termination is done after 38 weeks by low rupture of membranes with/without oxytocin drip or by cesarean section. PGE2 is used to make the cervix favorable before low rupture of membranes. Labor is managed in a manner similar to that of preeclampsia.

STUDY QUESTIONS

Short Notes

1. Definition and clinical types of pregnancy-induced hypertension.
2. Magnesium sulfate therapy.

Short Answer Questions

1. Outline the clinical features and alarming symptoms, and signs of preeclampsia.
2. Hemolysis, elevated liver enzymes and low platelet count syndrome.
3. Stages of an eclamptic convulsion.
4. Gestational hypertension.

Essay Questions

1. Describe the objectives of nursing management and care of a client with preeclamptic toxemia admitted at 37 weeks gestation.
2. Enumerate the preparation of the unit for admitting a client with 38 weeks gestation who had an eclamptic fit at home. Explain the nurse's role in the immediate management of the patient in the inpatient unit.

BIBLIOGRAPHY

1. Chesley LC. Hypertensive Disorders in Pregnancy, 1st edition. New York: Appleton-Century Crofts; 1978. pp.10-118.
2. Chesley LC. Hypertensive disorders in pregnancy. Nurse Midwifery. 1985;30(2):99-104.
3. Duley L. Magnesium sulphate regimens for women with eclampsia: messages from the Collaborative Eclampsia Trial. Bri J Obstet Gynaecol. 1996;103(2):103-5.
4. Dutta DC. Textbook of Obstetrics, 5th edition. Kolkata: New Central Book Company; 2001. pp. 234-55.
5. Harms K, Rath W, Herting E, et al. Maternal hemolysis, elevated liver enzymes, low platelet count and neonatal outcome. Am J Perinatol. 1995;12(1):1-6.
6. Hendricks CH, Brenner WE. Toxemia of pregnancy: relationship between fetal weight, fetal survival, and the maternal state. Am J Obstet Gynecol. 1971;109(2):225-33.
7. Lloyd C, Lewis VM. Hypertensive Disorders of Pregnancy. In: Bennett R, Brown L (Eds). Myles Textbook for Midwives, 13th edition. Edinburgh: Churchill Livingstone; 1999. pp. 315-27.
8. Llwellyn Jones D. Fundamentals of Obstetrics and Gynecology Obstetrics, vol. 1. London: Faber & Faber; 1990.
9. Redman CW. Eclampsia still kills. Br Med J. 1988;296(6631):1209-10.
10. Roberts JM, Redman CW. Pre-eclampsia: more than pregnancy-induced hypertension. Lancet. 1993;341(8858):1447-51.
11. Robson SC. Magnesium sulphate: the time of reckoning. BJ Obstet Gynaecol. 1996;103(2):99-102.
12. Sibai BM. The HELLP syndrome (hemolytic, elevated liver enzymes, and low platelets): much ado about nothing? Am J Obstet Gynecol. 1990;162(2):311-6.

CHAPTER 29

Medical Disorders, Gynecological Disorders and Psychiatric Disorders Associated with Pregnancy

Learning Objectives

Upon completing this chapter, the learner will be able to:
- Outline the common medical disorders.
- Describe the effects of different disorders on the woman and her fetus or the newborn.
- Outline the management of women with different medical conditions during pregnancy and labor.
- Describe the midwifery care and support required by the client and her family during pregnancy, labor and the postnatal period.

Pregnancy may be complicated by a variety of disorders and conditions that can profoundly affect the woman and her fetus. The disorders, which predate pregnancy, are important because of the way in which pregnancy affects them or the treatment for the disorders affects the pregnancy. Physical, social and psychological problems requiring nursing diagnosis and interventions are usually present.

CARDIAC DISEASE

The overall incidence of cardiac disease in pregnancy is falling in both the developed and developing parts of the world. It is less than 1% in hospital deliveries. The most common cardiac lesion is of rheumatic origin followed by the congenital disorders. Adequate treatment for rheumatic fever with appropriate antibiotics with the advancement in cardiac surgery to rectify the congenital cardiac lesions, are responsible for the change in profile over the past two decades.

Rheumatic valvular lesion predominantly includes mitral stenosis. Predominant congenital lesions include patent ductus arteriosus (PDA), atrial or ventricular septal defect (VSD), pulmonary stenosis (PS), coarctation of aorta (CoA) and Fallot's tetralogy. Rare causes are hypertensive, syphilitic or coronary heart disease (HD).

To manage pregnancy effectively in a woman with heart disease, the normal compensatory changes in the cardiovascular system that occur during pregnancy must be understood. These normal responses are only detrimental to the mother and fetus if heart disease is present.

Changes in Cardiovascular Dynamics during Pregnancy and their Effects on Heart Lesion

In normal pregnancy, the cardiovascular dynamics alter in order to meet the increased demands of the fetoplacental unit. This increases the workload of the heart quite significantly. The major cardiac changes are:
- An increase in cardiac output by 30–50%
- An increase in blood volume by 20–40%
- A rise in stroke volume by 20–40% in early pregnancy
- A fall in the blood pressure in the second trimester.

These changes commence in early pregnancy and gradually reach a maximum by the 30th week and maintained until term. Estrogens and prostaglandins are thought to be the mediators of the alterations in hemodynamics during pregnancy. A normal heart has enough reserve power so that the extra load can be tackled. A damaged heart with poor reserve may suffer cardiac failure eventually. Cardiac failure occurs during pregnancy around 30 weeks, during labor and mostly soon following delivery. Additional factors responsible for deterioration of function of the damaged heart are:

1. Advancing age.
2. Left ventricular hypertrophy.
3. Appearance of risk factors such as infection, anemia, preeclampsia excessive weight gain and multiple pregnancies, which further increase the cardiac load.
4. History of previous heart failure.
5. Inadequate supervision.

Gradings

Depending upon the cardiac response to physical activity, heart diseases are graded according to the classification of the New York Heart Association.

- *Grade I:* Uncomplicated:
  - Patients with cardiac disease, but no limitation of physical activity.
- *Grade II:* Slightly compromised:
  - Patients with cardiac disease with slight limitation of physical activity. The patients are comfortable at rest, but ordinary physical activity causes discomfort.
- *Grade III:* Markedly compromised:
  - Patients with cardiac disease with marked limitation of activity. They are comfortable at rest, but discomfort occurs with less than ordinary activity.
- *Grade IV:* Severely compromised:
  - Patients have discomfort even at rest.

Rheumatic Heart Disease

Valvular lesions predominate in rheumatic heart disease (RHD) and constitute approximately 50% of all heart diseases seen in pregnancy.

Mitral and Aortic Valve Incompetence

Pregnancy can be helpful in this case as it lowers the pressure in the arterial system, encouraging blood to flow the right way through the valves. There is however, a risk of endocarditis.

Mitral Stenosis

As the demand for cardiac output rises in pregnancy, pressure in the left atrium rises. This may lead to back pressure in the pulmonary system and pulmonary edema. The left atrium being unable to cope with the demands made upon it, begins to fibrillate and heart failure may occur.

Congenital Heart Disease

The most common congenital defects, which may remain uncorrected during the childbearing years are:
- Atrial septal defect
- Patent ductus arteriosus
- Ventricular septal defect.

All of these are openings, which allow communication between the right and left sides of the heart or in the case of patent ductus arteriosus between the pulmonary artery and the aorta. Problems arise when pulmonary vascular resistance rises, as it does in preeclampsia and blood flows from right to the left instead of passing through the lungs, leading to cyanosis. This may also happen in the third stage of labor when there is a sudden return of blood to the heart.

Risk to Mother and Fetus

Structural defects of the heart whether congenital or acquired, predispose the women to bacterial endocarditis and thromboemboli. Expert attention from obstetricians and cardiologists is needed for them.

In RHD, the maternal mortality is low and pregnancy does not affect long-term survival. The fetal outcome in RHD is usually good and little different from that in women who do not have heart disease. Maternal mortality is most likely in those conditions where pulmonary blood flow cannot be increased as in Eisenmenger's syndrome.

During pregnancy, fetuses of women with heart disease are generally growth retarded and fetal loss may be high. There is also increased incidence of congenital heart disease (CHD) in children born to mothers who have the disease themselves.

Antenatal Care

Diagnosis

Diagnosis of cardiac disease in some women may only be made during antenatal visits. Breathlessness, fatigue, swollen ankles and palpitations may all be attributable to the normal changes associated with pregnancy, but if they were present before the pregnancy began, the woman must be referred to a cardiologist. Diagnosis will be made with the aid of the clinical picture, radiography, electrocardiography (ECG) and echocardiography.

Assessment

Where there is no cardiac lesion, no further follow-up will be required. Women who have mild lesions with no hemodynamic effect may continue the pregnancy, although prophylactic antibiotic cover in labor is recommended. For those with a significant lesion with real or potential hemodynamic implications, the future of pregnancy needs to be considered and careful counseling given. If termination of pregnancy is decided upon, it is preferable that this should be done in the first trimester, as termination after 16 weeks gestation is no safer than later delivery.

General Management

Principles

1. Early diagnosis and functional grading.
2. Detection and institution of effective therapy for cardiac failure.
3. Prevention and control of additional complications such as pulmonary hypertension.
4. Mandatory hospital delivery.

Preconception Care and Advice

Women who know that they have heart disease must seek advice from both cardiologist and an obstetrician before becoming pregnant so that the risks of their condition can be discussed. In some cases preconception surgery such as initial valvotomy may be advised. The woman should be helped to control obesity and choose a diet, which will prevent anemia in order to minimize risk. It is advisable that family size should be limited, as the risks increase with each pregnancy. Contraceptive advice is therefore an important aspect of management.

Place of Therapeutic Termination

Considering high maternal deaths, cases of primary pulmonary hypertension, Eisenmenger's syndrome and pulmonary veno-occlusive diseases (PVOD) are absolute indications for termination of pregnancy. The termination should be done within 12 weeks by suction evacuation or by conventional dilation and evacuation.

Management

The aim of management is to maintain or improve the physical and psychological well-being of mother and fetus. This involves keeping a steady hemodynamic state and preventing complications. The major maternal complications are:
- Bacterial endocarditis
- Thromboemboli
- Cyanosis
- Heart failure.

The risk factors for heart failure include:
- Infections, particularly urinary tract infection
- Hypertension
- Anemia
- Multiple pregnancy
- Obesity
- Smoking.

The following advices are given to the women:
1. Adequate rest—the women should have 10 hours rest in bed at night and 2 hours in the afternoon.
2. Avoid undue strain and excitement—to limit the activities short of breathlessness.
3. Avoid caffeine, alcohol, β-mimetic drugs and high calorie or spicy diet. The diet should contain low salt, less carbohydrate, caffeine, alcohol and fat, but more protein.
4. Anemia is to be corrected by appropriate therapy.
5. Cold and infections are to be avoided as they might precipitate heart failure. Intramuscular injections of penidure 12 LA (benzathine penicillin) may be given at intervals of 4 weeks throughout pregnancy and puerperium to prevent recurrence of rheumatic fever.
6. Adequate dental care and care for such other potential sources of infection. Dental extraction if necessary, should be carried out with antibiotic cover to eliminate sources of sepsis and reduce the risk of endocarditis.

Hospitalization

Elective admission is recommended for:
1. *Grade I:* At least 2 weeks prior the expected date of delivery.
2. *Grade II:* At 28th week especially in case of unfavorable social surroundings.
3. *Grade III and IV:* As soon as pregnancy is diagnosed, the woman should be kept in the hospital throughout pregnancy.

Intrapartum Care

First Stage of Labor

The least stressful labor for a woman with cardiac disease will be spontaneous in onset and vaginal delivery. In addition to the obstetrician, the cardiologist, anesthetist and pediatrician must be informed when the woman goes into labor:
1. The woman should be confined to bed and be placed in lateral recumbent position to minimize aortocaval pressure by the gravid uterus.
2. Oxygen and resuscitation equipment must be ready and functioning. Oxygen to be administered at 5-6 L/min as and when required.
3. In the majority, analgesia is best given by epidural anesthesia.
4. Intravenous (IV) fluids should be given cautiously. As a rule, the quantity of infused fluid should not be more than 75 mL/h to prevent pulmonary edema.
5. Observation of pulse and respiratory rate should be made every 15 minutes. If the pulse rate exceeds 110 per minute between uterine contractions, rapid digitalization is done by IV digoxin 0.5 mg.
6. Cardiac monitoring (ECG) and pulse oximetry are done to detect arrhythmias and hypoxemia early. Deviations such as breathlessness and tachycardia should be reported immediately.
7. Prophylactic antibiotics are given during labor and for 48 hours after delivery, as these women are at increased risk from endocarditis. The recommended regimens include IV ampicillin 2 g and gentamicin 1.5 mg/kg (not to exceed 80 mg), at the onset, followed by repeat doses at 8 hours interval.

Women with heart disease usually have quite rapid, uncomplicated labors. The midwife should help the woman to use the techniques that she has learned for coping with stress, as she is likely to be very anxious. The mother will need encouragement to a position in which she is comfortable (lateral) and must be informed that supine position may result in marked hypotension, and maternal and fetal distress. Positions such as the lithotomy position in which the feet are higher than the trunk are best avoided because of the risk of acute heart failure resulting from the sudden increase of venous return to the heart.

Place of induction: Labor is not usually induced for uncomplicated heart disease. It is only considered safe if the benefits outweigh the disadvantages. If it is necessary to induce labor, the use of prostaglandins is advocated, but with caution as they are potent vasodilators and cause a marked rise in cardiac output.

Second Stage of Labor

Second stage of labor should be short and without undue exertion on the part of the mother. Prolonged pushing withheld breath such as the Valsalva maneuver may be dangerous for a woman with heart disease. It raises the intrathoracic pressure, pushes blood out of the thorax and impedes venous return, with the result that cardiac output falls. Midwives need to suggest to the woman that she avoids holding her breath and follows her natural desire to push; giving several short pushes during each contraction. In this way, she will also avoid facial petechiae and subconjunctival hemorrhages. Any tendency to delay in the second stage of labor is to be curtailed by forceps or ventouse under pudendal and/or perineal block anesthesia. Ventouse is preferred to forceps as it can be applied without putting the woman in lithotomy position. Some obstetricians advocate delivery in the left lateral position.

Third Stage of Labor

Conventional management is to be followed. No ergot containing preparations should be used for the third stage of labor as it causes a tonic contraction, which returns 300–500 mL of blood to the venous system. If the blood loss is excess, Syntocinon may be used as it has less effect on blood vessels than ergometrine. If the woman is in heart failure, oxytocics should be avoided. If Syntocinon is required, it is to be given by infusion accompanied by IV furosemide to prevent pulmonary edema.

Place of Cesarean Section

In general, there is no indication of cesarean section for heart disease. However, in CoA, elective cesarean section is indicated to prevent rupture of the aorta or cerebral aneurysm. The anesthesia should be epidural (preferred) or general.

Puerperium

During the first 48 hours following delivery, the heart must cope with the extra blood from the uterine circulation and it is important to monitor the woman's condition closely during this time:

1. She should be in absolute bed rest in a position comfortable to her. Intramuscular injection of morphine is given following delivery. Oxygen is administered either continuously or intermittently as required.
2. Pulse and respirations are recorded hourly and temperature 4 hourly.
3. Puerperal fever of any origin should be dealt with seriously by appropriate antibiotic therapy.
4. Breastfeeding is not contraindicated unless the woman is in heart failure. The baby needs to be examined carefully for any sign of hereditary heart disease.
5. The woman should be kept in the hospital for at least 2 weeks. In the 1st week, she should be confined to bed and allowed to move her limbs and to have breathing exercises. After a week, if everything is normal, she may be allowed to be out of bed.
6. The woman may need advice to choose a suitable method of contraception. Steroidal preparations are contraindicated as it may precipitate thromboembolic phenomenon. Intrauterine device is contraindicated due to the risk of infection, which may lead to endocarditis. Barrier method of contraception (condom) is the best recommendation. Sterilization if chosen with the completion of the family is usually delayed for 2–3 months after delivery. If the heart is not well compensated, the husband is advised for vasectomy.
7. On her return home, the woman may need extra help in the house and may need to arrange for it.

Summary of Nursing Process

Assessment

Assess for the following clinical manifestations:
- Pedal edema, progressive generalized edema
- Dyspnea on exertion
- Moist cough
- Tachycardia, irregular pulse
- Increasing fatigue
- Cyanosis of lips and nail beds
- Heart murmurs
- Severe/persistent fungal infections (*Candida*, etc.)
- Frustration as activity level is reduced
- Anxiety associated with fear of fetal and maternal demise.

Nursing Diagnosis

- Risk for fetal injury
- Risk for infection
- Ineffective airway clearance
- Actual/risk for aspiration
- Anxiety
- Anticipatory grieving
- Altered family processes
- Actual/risk for altered parenting
- Health seeking behavior.

Planning

- Protection from infection
- Promotion of graded activity with periods of rest
- Promotion of client acceptance of need for activity restriction
- Promotion and maintenance of health
- Education for self-care.

Implementation

- If no symptoms with physical activity:
  - Additional evening rest
  - Early treatment of infections.
- If comfortable at rest and with symptoms during ordinary physical activity:
  - Avoid strenuous activity
  - Administer prophylactic digitalis, diuretics and antibiotics
  - Encourage frequent rest periods
  - Anticipate forceps assisted vaginal delivery.

- If comfortable at rest with symptoms during less than ordinary activity:
  - Reduce physical activity
  - Avoid emotional stress
  - Administer digitalis, diuretics and penicillin
  - Facilitate early hospitalization and delivery
  - Anticipate recommendation of early therapeutic abortion.
  - If symptoms present at rest:
  - Anticipate recommendation of early therapeutic abortion (50% mortality associated with delivery)
  - Administer penicillin, digitalis, diuretics and rotating tourniquets
  - Prepare for vaginal delivery.

Evaluation

Ensure that the woman:
- Remains free of infection
- Follows activity and rest recommendations
- Monitors her physical response to activity
- Participates in self-care activities.

RESPIRATORY DISORDERS

Pulmonary Tuberculosis

The incidence of tuberculosis with pregnancy ranges between 1% and 2% amongst the hospital deliveries in the tropics, being confined predominantly to the underprivileged sectors of society. Incidence of tuberculosis is rising worldwide with the increasing prevalence of HIV patients.

Effects on the Woman

The onset of tuberculosis is often insidious, producing night sweats, weight loss, anorexia, coughing, purulent sputum, hemoptysis, low-grade fever and malaise. The overall effect of this is to debilitate the woman, making her less able to cope with pregnancy and her existing family.

The disease may be pre-existing or the diagnosis may be made for the first time during pregnancy. The disease may be found in the quiescent or active phase. If the patient remains under medical supervision with adequate care and treatment during pregnancy, no deleterious effect may be seen on the course of the disease, nor has the disease any adverse effect on the course of pregnancy. In active disease, fetus can be affected by transplacental route or by aspiration of amniotic fluid. Neonatal infection is mainly by postpartum maternal contact.

Management

The woman will be under the care of an obstetrician and chest physician during her pregnancy. If the disease is in the inactive or quiescent phase, periodic chest X-rays must be taken after 12 weeks and repeated at 3 monthly intervals during pregnancy and one after a month following delivery.

If the disease is in the active phase, antitubercular therapy is to be started and continued for at least 6 months following delivery or until the disease is arrested. Initial treatment includes isoniazid 300 mg per day with rifampicin 600 mg per day, both given orally for 9 months. Ethambutol 15 mg/kg/day orally is added if isoniazid resistance is suspected. Pyridoxine 50 mg per day is given routinely. None of the drugs used is teratogenic in human. *Streptomycin* is ototoxic and is avoided. Rest, both physical and emotional, and hospitalization in advanced cases is necessary.

Antenatal Care

Antenatal care is to be carried out rigidly to minimize complications like anemia or preeclampsia. The woman should be admitted at least 2 weeks prior to the expected date of delivery. If the woman is infectious, she should be in a single room. Help of a social worker will be required if she has financial and domestic difficulties. Dietary counseling to improve the nutritional status will be required.

Intrapartum Care

Problems in labor stem from fatigue and reduced lung function. Hence, the woman is kept in bed and nourishment maintained to avoid fatigue. For sedation, pethidine 75–100 mg may be given intramuscularly. Episiotomies and forceps or ventouse delivery are advocated to reduce the strain of the second stage. Blood loss in the third stage should be minimized by giving prophylactic Methergine 0.2 mg intravenously following the delivery of the anterior shoulder.

Postnatal Care

Adequate rest and good sleep are to be assured. Antituberculous therapy is to be repeated after 1 month of delivery. The baby is to be vaccinated with isoniazid resistant bacille Calmette-Guérin (BCG) vaccine whilst being protected from the disease by the use of prophylactic isoniazid syrup 20 mg/kg/day for 3 months. The vaccine becomes effective in 3–6 weeks as shown by a positive Mantoux test. If the mother has an active lesion or any of the baby's family is infected, the baby is to be separated until the baby becomes Mantoux positive.

Breastfeeding is not contraindicated with inactive or quiescent tuberculosis, if she wishes. In active lesion, however, not only is breastfeeding contraindicated but also the baby is to be separated promptly from the mother following delivery. However, if the mother has been on effective chemotherapy for at least 2 weeks, there is no need to isolate the baby. Mothers taking antitubercular therapy should be encouraged to breastfeed since the infant will receive a maximum of 20% of the normal infant dose by this route.

Caring for the baby at home makes great demands on the woman. Midwives should advice the woman and her spouse to arrange for extra help if possible. They must be explained that poor nutrition, stress and overtiredness will encourage a recurrence of active disease.

Contraception

Pregnancy is to be avoided until the disease has been quiescent for at least 2 years. When choosing a method of contraception, the woman needs to be aware that rifampicin reduces the effectiveness of oral contraception. Puerperal sterilization should be seriously considered, if the family is completed. Long-term medical follow-up is necessary in order to provide adequate help.

■ DIABETES MELLITUS

Carbohydrate Metabolism in Pregnancy

The fetus obtains glucose from its mother via the placenta by a process of facilitated diffusion. From 10th week of pregnancy, there is a progressive fall in the maternal fasting glucose level. During the third trimester, the mother begins to utilize fat stores, which were laid down during the first two trimesters. This results in a rise in free fatty acids and glycerol in the bloodstream and the woman will become ketotic more easily.

The fetoplacental unit alters the mothers' carbohydrate metabolism in order to make glucose more readily available. The placenta manufactures human placental lactogen (HPL), which produces a resistance to insulin in the maternal tissues. These results in blood glucose levels, which are higher after meals and remain raised for longer than in the nonpregnant state. Estrogen and progesterone contribute to these changes and at the end of pregnancy cortisol levels rise, which also leads to rise in blood glucose.

More insulin is produced, sometimes two or three times as much as in the nonpregnant state. The extra demands on the pancreatic β-cells can precipitate glucose intolerance or overt diabetes in women whose capacity for producing insulin was only just adequate prior to pregnancy. If a mother was already diabetic before pregnancy, her insulin needs will be increased.

Glycosuria in Pregnancy

During each antenatal visit, urine is examined as a routine for the presence of glucose. Repeat and random samples taken on one or more occasions throughout pregnancy reveal glycosuria in about 5–50% cases. Significant disturbances in carbohydrate metabolism occur in about 1% of pregnancies and the incidence of overt diabetes is about one in 300 pregnancies.

Causes of Glycosuria in Pregnancy

Renal glycosuria: During pregnancy, renal threshold is diminished due to the combined effect of increased glomerular filtration and impaired tubular reabsorption of glucose. It is present more commonly in midpregnancy. If glucose tolerance test is done, glucose leaks out into the urine even though the blood sugar level is well below 180 mg/mL (normal renal threshold). No treatment is required and the condition disappears after delivery.

Increased glomerular filtration rate: The glomerular filtration rate rises during pregnancy and glucose passes through the proximal convoluted tubule faster than it can be reabsorbed.

Impaired glucose tolerance: During pregnancy there is accelerated absorption of glucose from the alimentary tract and delayed utilization of glucose to form liver glycogen due to anti-insulin activity. These indicate that pregnancy has a diabetogenic effect, which results in glycosuria in small, but distinct group of cases especially in later months.

Renal tubular damage: This interferes with glucose reabsorption and may be revealed for the first time during pregnancy.

Glycosuria in pregnancy is not diagnostic of diabetes nor it can be used as a monitor of diabetes in the pregnant woman. Two episodes, however, are regarded as an indication for a glucose tolerance test. Glycosuria occurring any time during pregnancy with a positive family history of diabetes or past history of having a baby weighing 4 kg or more should be similarly investigated.

Gestational Diabetes

The term includes cases with abnormal carbohydrate tolerance with onset or first detected during the present pregnancy. The entity does not present until late in the second or during the third trimester. Women who are at special risk of developing gestational diabetes may be identified when the history reveals one or more of the following:

- Diabetes in a first degree relative (parents or sibling)
- Recurrent abortion
- Unexplained stillbirth
- Congenital abnormality
- A baby whose birth weight was 4 kg or more at 40 weeks
- Previous gestational diabetes or impaired glucose tolerance
- Persistent glycosuria
- Age over 30
- Obesity.

The progressive increase in insulin demand during pregnancy can make latent diabetes appear. This may resolve after the pregnancy.

Detection of Diabetes in Pregnancy

Women considered to be at risk of gestational diabetes undergo a glucose tolerance test. This will indicate whether they have normal or impaired glucose tolerance, or have developed diabetes. Before proceeding to a full glucose tolerance test, a fasting blood sample may be examined for glucose.

The methods employed for glucose tolerance tests vary slightly, but the aim is always to assess the baby's response to a glucose load. The woman is asked to fast for a period time. The fasting blood glucose level is estimated and the woman is given a measured amount of glucose in the form of a drink such as Lucozade 265 mL, which provides 75 mg glucose. Blood samples are obtained at intervals for glucose

estimation and the results compared with a normal range. The blood glucose level will rise initially, but should return to normal within a given length of time. It would be considered abnormal, if between 28 and 34 weeks of pregnancy, glucose levels in two out of four venous samples exceeded the following:
- Fasting: 90 mg
- 1 hour after ingestion of 75 g of glucose: 165 mg
- 2 hours after ingestion of 75 g of glucose: 145 mg
- 3 hours after ingestion of 75 g of glucose: 125 mg.

Effects of Diabetes on Pregnancy

When diabetes is well controlled, its effect on pregnancy is minimal. If the control is inadequate, there may be complications:
- Fertility is reduced and should conception occur, there is increased risk of spontaneous abortion and stillbirth
- Increased incidence of macrosomia and birth trauma
- Perinatal mortality rate among infants of diabetic mothers are markedly increased
- More prone to urinary tract infections and a greater susceptibility to *Candida albicans*
- The incidence of preeclampsia and polyhydramnios is increased.

Effect of Pregnancy on Diabetes

In the early stages of pregnancy, diabetic control may be complicated by nausea and vomiting. As the fetus grows, the mother needs more carbohydrate and ketosis is induced more easily, particularly in later stages of pregnancy. The diabetic, who is controlled by diet may become dependent on insulin. Women who have had diabetes since childhood and already have nephropathy or retinopathy must be monitored carefully for signs of any deterioration of their condition.

Effects on the Fetus

The effect of uncontrolled diabetes on pregnancy is due to disturbed maternal metabolism. Severe maternal ketosis can cause *intrauterine death*. Fetal blood glucose is similar to that of the mother and it is thought that congenital abnormality is caused by fetal hyperglycemia during the first trimester of pregnancy. No particular congenital abnormality is typical, but the rare combination of sacral agenesis and neurological defects are most often seen in babies of diabetic mothers. Neural tubes defects are twice as common amongst babies of diabetic mothers, and defects in the kidney and heart are seen.

Glycosylated hemoglobin (hemoglobin bound to glucose) releases oxygen poorly to the fetus and this may lead to *intrauterine growth retardation*. A compensatory fetal polycythemia develops and may result in neonatal jaundice when the excess red cells are broken down.

This is exacerbated by the relative immaturity of liver enzymes in these babies. In poorly controlled diabetes, the fetus responds to the extra glucose by producing more insulin, which increases its body fat and muscle mass resulting in *macrosomia*. Birth weight and body mass are both greater and the kidneys and adrenal cortex are larger. The head circumference and brain size are normal.

Neonatal complications include hypoglycemia, respiratory distress syndrome (RDS), hyperbilirubinemia, polycythemia, hypocalcemia, hypomagnesemia and cardiomyopathy.

Overt Diabetes

A woman with abnormal glucose tolerance test with or without symptoms and a raised fasting blood glucose level is called overt diabetes. The condition may be pre-existing or detected for the first time during present pregnancy. Diagnosis can be presumptive if:
1. The fasting plasma glucose exceeds 105 mg%.
2. The peak level exceeds 180 mg%.
3. The 2 hour value exceeds 140 mg% in glucose tolerance test.

Classification of Pregnant Diabetics

1. Group A: Gestational diabetes.
2. Group B: Overt diabetes without vasculopathy.
3. Group C: Diabetes with vasculopathy (retinopathy and/or nephropathy).

Fetal and maternal outcome of diabetic pregnancy depends on the severity of the disease and its duration.

Management

Preconceptional Counseling

Pregnancy may lead to a deterioration of the diabetes and hence the woman must be carefully examined for the presence of renal, cardiovascular or retinal changes before becoming pregnant. The woman will need to continue using some form of contraception, while improving control of her diabetes. Good control of diabetes is to be achieved before the onset of pregnancy. Appropriate advice about diet and insulin is to be given. Chances of having a diabetic child is about 1% when only the mother is diabetic, rising to 20% if both parents are diabetic.

Principles of Management

- Careful antenatal supervision and control of diabetes, to maintain the glucose level as near to physiological level as possible
- To find out the optimum time and method of delivery
- To make arrangements for the care of the newborn.

Antenatal Care

Antenatal supervision should be at monthly intervals up to 20th week and thereafter at 2 weeks intervals up to 30th week. Simultaneous consultation with a team consisting of physician, pediatrician and dietician is ideal. The *daily calorie requirement* is about 30–35 kcal/kg of body weight and an additional 200 kcal for the need of the fetus. Fat may be reduced if the woman is obese. Fiber containing food items are increased and a four-meal regimen with a bedtime snack is usually advised. Oral hypoglycemic agents are changed to insulin.

Frequent blood glucose estimation is required. Estimation of *glycosylated hemoglobin* should be done at the end of first trimester and 3 monthly thereafter. *Sonographic evaluation* is extremely helpful, not only to diagnose varieties of congenital malformations of the fetus but also to detect fetal macrosomia or growth retardation. *Assessment of the fetal well-being* is to be made from 32nd week onwards.

The midwife should alert the woman of her predisposition to urinary tract and vaginal infections so that she will seek treatment as soon as possible if symptoms develop. It is important to teach the woman about maintenance of hygiene. Examination of maternal weight and of her abdomen will help the midwife to detect polyhydramnios. In addition, the woman must be examined for any sign of diabetic complications.

Hospitalization

In uncomplicated cases, the woman is admitted in hospital at 34th to 36th week. Early hospitalization facilitates:
- Stabilization of diabetes
- Minimizes the incidence of preeclampsia, polyhydramnios and preterm labor
- Selection of the appropriate time for termination of pregnancy.

Termination of Pregnancy

Majority of intrauterine deaths of the fetus occur in the last 2 weeks of pregnancy. Hence, termination is done after 37 completed weeks. Early termination may have to be done for fetal jeopardy. Assessment of fetal lung maturity must be done beforehand and facilities of an equipped neonatal care unit should be available.

Management of Labor and Delivery

Induction of labor is done in the presence of following indications:
- Multipara with good obstetric history
- Young primigravida without any obstetric abnormality
- Presence of congenital malformation of the fetus.

Induction is done by low rupture of membranes and simultaneous oxytocin drip.

Cesarean section is indicated in the following conditions:
- Elderly primigravida
- Multigravida with bad obstetric history
- Diabetes difficult to control
- Obstetric complications like preeclampsia, polyhydramnios and malpresentation
- Presence of large baby.

About 50% diabetic women are delivered by cesarean section. Spontaneous onset of labor at term and vaginal delivery are awaited in the following conditions:
- Young primigravida or multipara with good obstetric history
- Diabetes well controlled either by diet, insulin or both, or without any obstetrical complications.

During labor, control of blood glucose is achieved through administration of IV dextrose and soluble insulin with hourly estimation of blood glucose. Epidural analgesia is preferable than strong sedatives or analgesics as they might depress the fetal respiratory center.

The midwife should monitor fetal condition throughout labor using electronic fetal monitoring. A pediatrician should be present during delivery, especially if labor has been induced, as a baby with premature lungs may require resuscitation. Polyhydramnios increases the risk of malpresentation, cord prolapse and uterine inertia during labor. Birth asphyxia is more common in both macrosomic and growth retarded babies. The large baby is prone to birth injuries. Shoulder dystocia a possible hazard. Prophylactic ergometrine is given intravenously with the delivery of anterior shoulder to minimize blood loss. The cord should be clamped immediately after delivery to avoid hypervolemia. The placenta is usually large, the cord is thick and there is increased incidence of a single umbilical artery.

Postnatal Care

Carbohydrate metabolism returns to normal very quickly after delivery of the placenta and insulin requirements will fall rapidly. The woman can resume her prepregnancy regimen. A diabetic mother who is breastfeeding should be encouraged to increase her carbohydrate intake by 50 mg a day because of the increased nutritional demands. Insulin requirements are determined according to preprandial blood glucose estimation. Although a small amount of insulin may enter breast milk, these are destroyed in the baby's stomach.

The diabetic women are more prone to infection and delayed healing. Antibiotics are given prophylactically to minimize infection. The midwife will need to advise her to change her perineal pads frequently in order to keep any wound clean and dry.

Care of the Baby

A neonatologist should be present at the time of delivery. The baby should preferably be kept in an intensive neonatal care unit and observed closely for at least 48 hours, to detect and treat any complication likely to arise:

1. Asphyxia is anticipated and to be treated effectively.
2. Birth injuries and congenital abnormalities can be present and must be looked for.
3. Hypoglycemia may occur and to prevent the babies should be fed soon after delivery. Monitoring of neonatal blood glucose needs to be done according to the protocol. If the baby is lethargic or premature and breastfeeding is a problem, 10% glucose may be given orally as the first feeding and continued with breastfeeding every 3–4 hours.

4. All babies should receive 1 mg vitamin K intramuscularly.
5. The destruction of red cells and the relative immaturity of the liver predispose the baby to jaundice.

Contraception

Barrier method of contraception is ideal for spacing of births. Low dose combined oral pills, containing third generation progestins are effective and have minimal effect on carbohydrate metabolism. The intrauterine contraceptive device (IUCD) increases the risk of pelvic infection. Tubal ligation should be seriously considered following second live birth, under local anesthesia in the puerperium.

Summary of Nursing Process

Assessment

Assess for the following clinical manifestations:
- Hyperemesis during early pregnancy
- Glycosuria, ketonuria
- Elevated blood glucose, glucose tolerance test
- Polydipsia, polyphagia, polyuria
- Rapid weight gain
- Previous large babies weighing 3,500 g or more.

Nursing Diagnosis

- Risk for fetal injury
- Risk for infection
- Ineffective airway clearance
- Actual/risk for aspiration
- Anxiety
- Anticipatory grieving
- Altered family processes
- Actual/risk for altered parenting
- Health seeking behavior.

Planning

- Regular tests for glucose levels
- Glycosuria, ketonuria
- Observing for signs of hypoglycemia and hyperglycemia
- Provision of counseling and support
- Teaching regarding disease and care activities.

Implementation

1. Obtain accurate obstetric and diet history.
2. Assess health status and report to physician regarding:
   - Hydramnios
   - Large size fetus
   - Fetal heart rate
   - Weight, blood pressure.
3. Provide instructions regarding blood glucose control:
   - Blood tests
   - Insulin injections
   - Avoidance of oral hypoglycemics
   - Management of hypoglycemia.
4. Encourage regular exercise for weight and blood sugar control.
5. Provide diet instructions:
   - Prescribed diet (2,200–2,400 kcal/day)
   - Avoid calorie restrictions
   - Eat at regularly scheduled times (3 meals and 2–4 snacks daily)
   - Observe for hypoglycemia.
6. Monitor for urinary and vaginal tract infections.
7. Prepare for delivery: Vaginal delivery is preferable to cesarean delivery.
8. Observe for the following complications:
   - Hydramnios
   - Preeclampsia and eclampsia
   - Stillbirth
   - Neonatal RDS, congenital anomalies, hyperbilirubinemia and hypoglycemia
   - Postpartum hemorrhage infection.
9. Encourage breastfeeding because breastfeeding decreases insulin requirements.
10. Provide postpartum contraceptive information:
    - Avoid oral contraceptives as it may increase the risk of deep vein thrombosis (DVT)
    - Encourage barrier contraceptives.

Evaluation

Ensure that the pregnant woman:
- Remains normoglycemic
- Shows no signs or symptoms of hypoglycemia
- Verbalizes support
- Verbalizes understanding of the disease and the implications of diabetes on pregnancy.

THYROID DYSFUNCTION IN PREGNANCY

Thyroid disease is common in women of reproductive age. The incidence of thyroid disease associated with pregnancy is varied. Hyperthyroidism occurs in about two per 1,000 pregnancies and hypothyroidism about nine per 1,000. Thyroid disease in pregnancy can have potential adverse effects on the fetus; the fetal morbidity and mortality rates in untreated women can be as high as 50%.

Hyperthyroidism

The disease should be suspected on any woman who fails to gain weight satisfactorily despite a good appetite. Other symptoms include exophthalmos, eyelid lag and persistent tachycardia. Clinical diagnosis is difficult as the physiological signs and symptoms pregnant women normally exhibit, such as heat intolerance, palpitations and mood lability may mask this condition. Hyperthyroidism when poorly controlled is associated with an increase in preterm delivery, low birth weight and fetal death. Thyroid autoimmunity is related to abortion and chromosomal abnormality with increased fetal loss. Thyroid stimulating immunoglobulins can cross the placenta and produce neonatal thyrotoxicosis with increased neonatal death.

Diagnosis

Clinical diagnosis is confirmed by measuring free T_4 and T_3 levels along with thyroid-stimulating hormone (TSH). Radioactive iodine uptake and scans should not be done during pregnancy as it will cross the placenta and damage the fetal thyroid gland permanently.

Treatment

The main form of treatment for hyperthyroidism is by means of antithyroid drugs (carbimazole, methimazole and propylthiouracil). Carbimazole is given orally with a daily dose of 20–60 mg and maintained at this dose until the woman becomes euthyroid. Then it is progressively reduced to maintenance of between 5 and 15 mg daily. Propylthiouracil is given at a daily dose of 300–450 mg and continued until the patient becomes euthyroid—the maintenance dose being 50–150 mg daily. Both the drugs may cause fetal goiter and hypothyroidism. Methimazole has been linked to a scalp defect—aplasia cutis of the neonate. Patients having marked tachycardia or arrhythmias should also have propranolol (β-blocking agent). The drugs are not contraindicated during breastfeeding provided the dose is kept relatively low and close monitoring of the neonatal thyroid functions is carried out. Propylthiouracil is the drug of choice as it crosses into the breast milk to a lesser extent. Cord blood should be taken for TSH and free T_4 at the time of delivery to detect neonatal hyperthyroidism.

Preconceptional Counseling

Considering the hazards during pregnancy, preconceptional counseling is important. Adequate treatment should be initiated to bring down the thyroid function profile to normal. Radioactive iodine therapy should not be given to women wanting pregnancy within 1 year. If pregnancy occurs inadvertently, termination should be done. Oral pill is to be withheld because of accelerated metabolism and disturbed liver function.

Hypothyroidism

Primary hypothyroidism in pregnancy is mostly related to thyroid autoimmunity. Myxedema rarely presents in pregnancy because they tend to be infertile. It is important to diagnose the condition because of the increased rate of fetal loss and reduced intelligence quotient (IQ) in these children. Complications of pregnancy like preeclampsia and anemia are high.

Diagnosis

Diagnosis may be extremely difficult. Symptoms manifest as excessive weight gain despite poor appetite, cold intolerance and a roughening of the skin. Thyroid function measurement is taken and if low, the woman is commenced on thyroxine. Therapy is started with levothyroxine, which is titrated to normalize thyroid function. The assessment is done on a monthly basis.

Antenatal Care

Women with pre-existing hypothyroidism will require monitoring of their thyroid function during pregnancy and their medication adjusted as necessary. Hypothyroid pregnant women tend to gain weight easily and the midwife needs to observe this closely for any deviation from the expected weight gain. Constipation may also be a problem because it is exacerbated by both hypothyroidism and pregnancy. Dietary advice such as increasing fiber content and fluid intake may help alleviate the problem.

Postnatal Care

After delivery, the neonate's thyroid status should be checked to identify whether there is any neonatal hypothyroidism present. There is no contraindication to breastfeeding, but the dose of thyroxine may need adjustment because of the maternal weight loss following delivery.

Postpartum Thyroiditis

About 10–15% of women develop this condition due to autoimmune thyroid disease. This is a transient disorder that occurs during the 1st year after parturition. The condition is characterized initially by symptoms of mild hyperthyroidism and may mimic postpartum psychosis. Recovery is usually spontaneous in most women, but the disorder tends to occur with subsequent pregnancies. About two-thirds will ultimately become euthyroid and the remaining one-third will become hypothyroid.

ANEMIA IN PREGNANCY

Anemia is the most common hematological disorder that may occur in pregnancy. It is a reduction in the oxygen carrying capacity of the blood, which may be due to:
- A reduced number of red blood cells (RBCs)
- A low concentration of hemoglobin
- A combination of both.

According to the standard laid down by World Health Organization (WHO), anemia in pregnancy is present when the hemoglobin concentration in the peripheral blood is 11 g/100 mL or less. However, because of prevailing socioeconomic deprivation in the developing countries, the level is brought down to 10 g/100 mL. The incidence of anemia in pregnancy ranges from 40–80% in the tropics compared to 10–20% in the developed countries.

Classification of Anemia

Anemia may be classified in various ways. A simplified classification is as follows:
- Physiological anemia
- Pathological anemia:

- Iron deficiency
- Folic acid deficiency
- Vitamin B_{12} deficiency
- Protein deficiency.
❖ Hemorrhagic anemia:
    - Acute: Following bleeding in early months of pregnancy or antepartum hemorrhage (APH)
    - Chronic: Hookworm infestation, bleeding piles, etc.
❖ Hemolytic anemia:
    - Familial: Congenital acholuric jaundice, sickle cell anemia, etc.
    - Acquired: Malaria, severe infection, etc.
❖ Bone marrow insufficiency: Hypoplasia or aplasia due to radiation, drugs or severe infection
❖ Hemoglobinopathies.

The common types of anemia, which are of concern in obstetric practice are the deficiency anemia and hemorrhagic anemia.

Physiological Anemia of Pregnancy

During pregnancy, maternal plasma volume gradually expands by 50%, an increase of approximately 1,200 mL by term. Most of the rise takes place before 32nd to 34th week's gestation and thereafter there is relatively little change. The total increase in RBCs is 25%, approximately 300 mL that occurs later in pregnancy. This relative hemodilution produces a fall in hemoglobin concentration, thus presenting a picture of iron deficiency anemia. However, it has been found that these changes are a physiological alteration of pregnancy necessary for the development of the fetus. Normal changes occurring in the blood are summarized in **Table 29.1**.

Erythropoiesis

In adults, erythropoiesis is confined to the bone marrow. Red cells are formed through stages of pronormoblasts → normoblasts → reticulocytes → mature non-nucleated erythrocytes. The average lifespan of red cells is about 120 days after which the RBCs degenerate and the hemoglobin are broken down into hemosiderin and bile pigment. For proper erythropoiesis, adequate nutrients are needed. These are minerals, vitamins, proteins and hormones. Inadequate reserve, or increased demand or deficient supply of any of the constituents interferes with the normal erythropoiesis.

Minerals: Iron is an essential element in the synthesis of hemoglobin. Traces of copper and cobalt are also required in the synthesis.

Vitamins: The specific vitamins that are required in the maturation process are vitamin B_{12}, folic acid and vitamin C.

Proteins: The proteins supply the amino acid for the synthesis of globin.

Erythropoietin: The hormone is probably responsible for increase in red cells in the bone marrow. Increased secretion of erythropoietin is brought about mostly by placental lactogen and by progesterone. Erythropoietin is produced by the kidneys (90%) and liver (10%).

Causes of Increased Prevalence of Anemia in the Tropics

Iron deficiency anemia is very much prevalent in the tropics particularly among women of childbearing age, especially in the under-privileged sector. The causes for it are:

1. *Faulty dietetic habit:* The diet rich in carbohydrate reduces the absorption of iron even when there is no deficiency of iron in the diet.
2. *Faulty absorption mechanism:* Because of the high prevalence of infestation, there is intestinal hurry, which reduces the iron absorption. Hypochlorhydria, often associated with malnutrition also hinders absorption.
3. *Iron loss:*
    a. More iron is lost through sweat to the extent of 15 mg per month.
    b. Repeated pregnancies at short intervals along with a prolonged period of lactation puts a serious strain on the iron reserve. It has been estimated that a normal healthy woman with adequate diet takes about 2 years to replenish about 1,000 mg of iron lost during childbirth and lactation.
    c. Excessive blood loss during menstruation, which is left untreated.
    d. Hookworm infestation with consequent blood depletion to the extent of 0.5–2 mg of iron daily.
    e. Chronic blood loss due to bleeding piles and dysentery also cause iron deficiency anemia.

TABLE 29.1: Normal blood values in nonpregnant and pregnant states.

Parameters	Nonpregnant state	Second half of pregnancy
Hemoglobin (Hb)	14.8/100 mL	11–14 g/100 mL
Red blood cells (RBCs)	5 million/mm^3	4–4.5 m/mm^3
Packed cell volume (PCV)	39–42%	32–36%
Mean corpuscular volume (MCV)	75–100 cubic micron (μm^3)	75–95 μm^3
Mean corpuscular hemoglobin (MCH)	27–32 pg	26–31 pg
Mean corpuscular hemoglobin concentration (MCHC)	32–36% (g/dL)	30–35% g/dL
Serum iron	60–120 μg/100 mL	65–75 μg/100 mL
Serum ferritin	20–30 mg/L (mean)	15 μg/L (mean)

(*Source:* Dutta DC. Text Book of Obstetrics, 5th edition. Kolkata: New Central Book Company; 2001).

Iron Requirements in Pregnancy

During pregnancy approximately 1,500 mg iron is needed for:
- The increase in maternal hemoglobin (400–500 mg)
- The fetus and placenta (300–400 mg)
- Replacement of daily loss through urine, stools and skin (250 mg)
- Replacement of blood lost at delivery (200 mg)
- Lactation (1 mg/day).

The woman who has sufficient iron reserve and is on a balanced diet is unlikely to develop anemia during pregnancy in spite of an increased demand of iron. But if the iron reserve is inadequate or absent, development of anemia is possible due to the following factors:
1. Increased requirements of iron.
2. Disturbed metabolism: Depressed erythropoietic function of the bone marrow.
3. Prepregnancy health status: Pre-existing anemic state.
4. Excess demand:
   a. Multiple pregnancy increases the iron demand by two folds.
   b. Rapid recurring pregnancy (within 2 year).
   c. Teenage pregnancy: The demand of iron accompanies the natural growth. At the age of 17, the additional demand is estimated to be about 270 mg during the course of pregnancy, the requirement is however, brought down to nil at the age of 21.

Routine Screening for Anemia

Pregnant women are usually screened at their first antenatal visit and thereafter at monthly intervals from the 28th week. Some physicians prescribe iron supplements for all pregnant women, while others give it to those at risk of anemia or are anemic already. Many physicians avoid giving iron during the first trimester of pregnancy owing to the gastrointestinal side effects. It may be more appropriate to administer prophylactic iron therapy in the third trimester of pregnancy. During this time the maternal iron store become depleted due to increasing fetal demand. Indications for prophylactic iron therapy include:
- Previous anemia
- Dietary conditions
- Chronic blood loss
- Low hemoglobin on booking
- Close family spacing.

Oral iron preparations given prophylactically consist of one of the iron salts, either alone or in combination with folic acid.

IRON DEFICIENCY ANEMIA

About 95% of pregnant women with anemia have the iron deficiency type. A pregnant woman is said to be anemic if her hemoglobin is less than 10 g%.

Causes

- Reduced intake or absorption of iron: This includes dietary deficiency and gastrointestinal disturbances such as morning sickness
- Excess demand such as multiple pregnancy, frequent or numerous pregnancies (more than four), chronic inflammation particularly of the urinary tract
- Blood loss from menorrhagia before conception, bleeding hemorrhoids, antepartum or postpartum hemorrhage and hookworm
- Decreased absorption due to decreased gastric acidity and dietary imbalance causing formation of insoluble salts of iron.

Signs and Symptoms

- Pallor of mucous membranes
- Lassitude and feeling of weakness
- Giddiness
- Tachycardia and palpitations
- Dyspnea
- Anorexia and indigestion
- Swelling of the legs.

Effects of Anemia on the Mother

- Reduced resistance to infection caused by impaired cell-mediated immunity
- Reduced ability to withstand postpartum hemorrhage
- Strain of even an uncomplicated labor may cause cardiac failure
- Predisposition to pregnancy-induced hypertension and preterm labor due to associated malnutrition
- Reduced enjoyment of pregnancy and motherhood owing to fatigue
- Potential threat to life: Even a minor traumatic delivery without bleeding may produce shock or a minor hypoxia during anesthesia may be become lethal.

Effects of Anemia on the Fetus/Baby

- Increased risk of intrauterine hypoxia and growth retardation
- Prematurity
- Low birth weight
- Anemia a few months after birth due to poor stores
- Increased risk of perinatal morbidity and mortality.

Investigations

The patient having a hemoglobin level below 10 g% should be subjected to a full hematological work up to ascertain the degree of anemia, the type of anemia and the cause of anemia.

By the time hemoglobin (Hb) falls, the iron store will already be depleted. The serum iron level demonstrates lack of iron, which will be usually below 30 μg/100 mL. Total iron binding capacity is elevated beyond 400 μg/100 mL. Serum ferritin level will be below 10 μg/100 mL. Midstream urine should be tested to exclude urinary tract infection, which will affect erythropoiesis. Stool examination should be done as a routine in the tropics to detect helminthic (particularly hookworm) infestation.

Prevention of Iron Deficiency Anemia

The midwife can help to identify women at risk of anemia by taking accurate history of medical, obstetric and social history. This may reveal a pre-existing problem or a lifestyle, which puts her at risk of anemia. It may also suggest that the woman is suffering from the effects of anemia.

She will be able to provide explanations appropriate to the particular woman taking into account her health and sociocultural preferences. Women need to be taught about the sources of iron and ways in which absorption can be increased. Iron intake is closely linked with calorie intake; 2,000 kcal per day will contain approximately 12–14 mg of iron, sufficient to cover the recommended daily amount of 113 mg for pregnant woman.

Management

In the tropics, majority of cases with iron deficiency anemia in pregnancy have a low socioeconomic status. The anemia is either pre-existing or is aggravated during pregnancy.

Prophylaxis

Avoidance of frequent childbirths: A minimum interval between pregnancies, should be at least 2 years, to replenish the lost iron during childbirth and lactation. This can be achieved by proper family planning guidance.

Supplementary iron therapy: After the woman becomes free of the nausea of pregnancy, daily administration of 200 mg of ferrous sulfate along with 1 mg of folic acid is a quite effective prophylactic procedure. Routine supplementation with iron and folic acid is not necessary when the hemoglobin level is high (>13 mg/dL).

Dietary advice: A balanced diet, rich in iron and protein, which is affordable by the woman and easily digestible, should be recommended.

Adequate treatments to eradicate illnesses likely to cause anemia: These are hookworm infestation, dysentery, bleeding piles, malaria and urinary tract infections.

Early detection of falling hemoglobin level: Hemoglobin level should be estimated at the first antenatal visit, at 28th and finally at 36th week.

Curative Management

Treatment of severe anemia must be preceded by an accurate diagnosis of the cause and type. Women having hemoglobin level of 7.5 mg% (ideally anyone with Hb less than 10 mg%) and those with associated obstetrical medical complications even with moderate degree of anemia should be hospitalized. Following therapeutic measures are to be instituted:

- *Diet:* A balanced diet, which is rich in protein, iron and vitamins
- Appropriate antibiotic therapy to eradicate even a minimal septic focus
- Effective therapy to cure the disease contributing to the cause of anemia
- Iron therapy to raise the hemoglobin level and to restore the iron reserve at least in part, if possible, before the woman goes into labor.

This may be oral iron or parenteral iron depending on the severity of anemia, duration of pregnancy and associated complicating factors.

Oral Iron

The daily dose of iron for treating anemia is between 120 and 180 g in divided doses. Iron is best absorbed in the ferrous form and ferrous sulfate 200 mg tablets or ferrous gluconate 300 mg tablets are generally used.

Side Effects of Oral Iron

Intolerance: This may be evidenced by epigastric pain, vomiting and diarrhea or constipation. To avoid intolerance, it is preferable to start the therapy with a smaller dose and then to increase the dose to a maximum of three tablets a day. These discomforts may be reduced by taking the iron after meals. Some women find one form of iron salts more tolerable than other form:

- The woman should be warned that her stools may turn black, but that does not mean that iron is not being absorbed.

Parenteral Iron

Parenteral iron is indicated for women who have intolerance to oral iron and those with severe anemia in advanced pregnancy (last 8–10 week of pregnancy). Parenteral iron is contraindicated for women who have liver or renal disorders.

Intramuscular Iron

Intramuscular iron is given in the form of iron dextran (imferon), which contains 50 mg of elemental iron in 1 mL and one ampule contains 2 mL. Injections should not be given in conjunction with oral iron as this enhances toxic effects such as headache, dizziness, nausea and vomiting. The injection should be given deep into the muscle to prevent staining of the skin, formation of abscess and fat necrosis.

After an initial test dose of 1 mL, the injections are to be given daily or on alternate days in doses of 2 mL intramuscularly. The injection is to be given in the buttock using the 'Z' track technique (pulling the skin and subcutaneous tissue to one side before inserting the needle).

Blood Transfusion

Blood transfusion is used rarely to treat severe iron deficiency anemia. It may be used to raise the Hb level quickly if delivery is imminent (beyond 36 week). With transfusion, improvement is seen in 3–4 days.

Precautions to be taken for blood transfusion include:

- The blood to be transfused must be fresh (collected within 24 hour) and properly grouped
- Only packed cells are transfused and the quantity should be between 80 and 100 mL at a time

- The drip should be about 10 drops per minute and transfusion should not be repeated within 24 hours
- Prior to the transfusion patient is to be sedated with 60 mg phenobarbitone
- An antihistamine (phenergan 25 mg%) and a diuretic (frusemide 20 mg) are given
- Very close monitoring of vital signs and lung sounds. Complications of transfusion are premature labor and cardiac failure. Features of transfusion reaction, if occur, are exaggerated.

Management during Labor

First Stage

The following are the special precautions to be taken when an anemic patient goes into labor:
- The patient should be in bed and should lie in a position comfortable to her
- Light analgesics are preferred for pain relief
- Oxygen administration to increase the oxygenation of maternal blood and thus diminish the risk of fetal hypoxia
- Strict asepsis to minimize the risk of puerperal infection.

Second Stage

Usually there is no problem. IV Methergine 0.2 mg should be given following the delivery of anterior shoulder.

Third Stage

Very vigilant observation is required during the third stage. Significant amount of blood loss should be replenished by fresh packed cell transfusion after taking the precautions outlined earlier. The volume of transfusion should not be more than the amount lost (to avoid overloading the heart).

Puerperium

1. The patient should be on bedrest.
2. Any sign of infection should be promptly detected and treated.
3. Predelivery antianemic therapy should be continued until the patient restores her normal clinical and hematological status. Hematinics should be continued for at least 3 months following delivery. The anemic state usually improves following delivery.
4. Dietary advice outlined earlier must be reinforced.
5. Patient and family members must be counseled for help at home for baby care and other household chores.

FOLIC ACID DEFICIENCY ANEMIA (MEGALOBLASTIC ANEMIA)

Folic acid is needed for the increased cell growth of mother and fetus, but there is a physiological decrease in serum folate levels in pregnancy. Anemia is more likely to be found toward the end of pregnancy when the fetus is growing rapidly. In India, megaloblastic anemia is usually due to a deficiency of folic acid.

Causes

- Increased demands
- Increase in maternal tissue and RBC volume
- Reduced dietary intake
- Reduced absorption
- Interference with utilization; drugs such as anticonvulsants, sulfonamides and alcohol are folate antagonists
- Infections: They reduce the lifespan of RBCs and increase cell production requiring more folic acid
- Decreased storage related to vitamin C deficiency and liver disease.

Clinical Features and Diagnosis

- The signs and symptoms are varied and may be mistaken as 'minor disorders of pregnancy' such as pallor, lethargy, weight loss, depression, nausea and vomiting, glossitis, gingivitis and diarrhea
- Examination of the red cell indices will reveal that the red cells are reduced in number, but enlarged in size (macrocytes)
- Peripheral blood smears show deficiency of iron and folic acid
- Examination of the bone marrow shows both megaloblasts and normoblasts
- Mean corpuscular volume (MCV) is either normal or raised.

The condition is generally diagnosed in the third trimester or puerperium. The patients are usually multipara and in the middle or later years of reproductive life.

Effects of Megaloblastic Anemia

Deficiency of folic acid may cause placental abruption (abruptio placentae), neural tube defects and congenital cardiac septal defects.

Management

Folic acid is administered orally in a dose of 5 mg 8 hourly. If time is short, treatment may be given with 30 mg intramuscularly for 3 days or 90 mg intravenously in 250 mL of normal saline to be followed by oral therapy. This is usually well tolerated with no side effects. Women must be taught about correct selection and preparation of foods, which are high in folic acid. Folic acid is found in leafy green vegetables such as spinach and broccoli, but is destroyed easily by prolonged boiling or steaming. Other sources include peanuts, chick peas, bananas and citrus fruits.

VITAMIN B_{12} DEFICIENCY

Deficiency of vitamin B_{12} also produces a megaloblastic anemia. Vitamin B_{12} levels fall during pregnancy, but anemia is rare because the body draws on its stores. Deficiency is most likely in vegetarians who eat no animal products at all and vitamin B_{12} supplements must be taken during pregnancy. Folic acid should not be given in case of vitamin B_{12} deficiency as it can hasten subacute degeneration of the spinal cord.

HEMOGLOBINOPATHIES

Hemoglobinopathies are inherited specific biochemical disorders where the hemoglobin is abnormal. Hemoglobin consists of a group of four molecules, each of which has a heme unit and a protein chain. The position of the amino acids in the protein chain determines the type of hemoglobin produced. Adult hemoglobin (HbA) has two α- and β-chains each, while the fetal hemoglobin (HbF) has two α- and γ-chains each. By 6 months 96% of a baby's Hb is HbA.

The type of protein is genetically determined. Defective genes lead to the formation of abnormal hemoglobin. Two common varieties are seen. *Sickle cell disease* is an inherited structural abnormality involving primarily the β-chain of HbA. *Thalassemia* is an inherited defect in the synthesis and production of globin in otherwise normal HbA. Homozygous and heterozygous forms occur. In *homozygous*, the abnormal globin chain is inherited from each parent and in *heterozygous*, the abnormal globin chain is inherited only from one parent. The later groups are not anemic, but are carriers of the defect.

SICKLE CELL DISORDERS

The sickle cell hemoglobinopathies are hereditary disorders in which defective genes produce abnormal hemoglobin β-chains; the resulting Hb is called sickle hemoglobin (HbS). In sickle cell anemia (HbSS), abnormal genes have been inherited from both parents whereas in sickle cell trait (HbAS) only one abnormal gene has been inherited. Sickle cell disorders are found most commonly in people of African or West Indian origin.

Sickle Cell Trait

Sickle hemoglobin comprises 38–45% of hemoglobin, the rest being HbA, HbA_2 and HbF. The individuals are usually asymptomatic. There is no anemia even under the stress of pregnancy. Hematuria and urinary infection are common.

If the husband is also a carrier, there is 25% chance that the infant will be homozygous sickle cell disease and 50% chance for sickle cell trait.

Sickle Cell Disease

Homozygous sickle cell disease (HbSS) is a genetically inherited disease and transmitted equally by males and females. Sickle cells have an increased fragility and shortened lifespan of 17 days resulting in chronic hemolytic anemia and causing episodes of ischemia and pain; these are known as sickle cell crises.

Diagnosis

- Identification by sickling test
- Persistent reticulocytosis
- High fasting serum iron level
- Identification of the type of hemoglobinopathy by electrophoresis.

Effects on Pregnancy

Women with sickle cell anemia are subfertile, but those who do become pregnant may suffer the following:
- Increased incidence of abortion, prematurity, intrauterine growth retardation and fetal loss
- Perinatal mortality is high
- Incidence of preeclampsia, postpartum hemorrhage and infection is increased
- Increased maternal morbidity due to infection, cerebrovascular accident and sickle cell crises
- Maternal death is increased up to 25% due to pulmonary infarction, congestive heart failure and embolism.

Effects of Pregnancy on the Disease

There is chance of sickle cell crisis, which usually occurs in the last trimester. Two types of crises are generally seen:
1. *Hemolytic crisis* is due to hemolysis with rapidly developing anemia along with jaundice. There is associated leukocytosis and fever.
2. *Painful crisis* occurs due to vascular occlusion of the various organs by capillary thrombosis resulting in infarction. Abdominal pain, vomiting, chest pain, hemoptysis or hematuria occurs depending upon the site of vascular occlusion.

Precipitating factors include psychological stress, cold climate and extreme temperature changes, strenuous physical exertion and fatigue, respiratory disease, infection and pregnancy. When subjected to low oxygen tension, HbS contracts, damaging the cell and causing it to assume a sickle shape. Damaged cells block capillaries and the resulting infarction leads to pain, affecting particularly the bones, joints and abdominal organs. Emboli may be thrown off into the circulation, which may threaten life.

Management

Preconceptional Counseling

As these conditions are inherited and in the homozygous form can be fatal, screening of the population at risk should be carried out. Blood is examined by electrophoresis, which detects the different types of hemoglobin. Prospective parents; who are known to have or carry genes for abnormal hemoglobin, need genetic counseling in order to help them make an informed decision before deciding on a pregnancy. If both parents are carriers there is a 25% chance that the fetus will be homozygous. Prenatal identification of the homozygous state of the disorder is an indication for early termination of pregnancy.

During Pregnancy

- Careful antenatal supervision
- Prophylactic folic acid 5 mg per oral (PO) daily
- Iron supplementation in proven cases of deficiency
- Regular blood transfusion at 6 weeks intervals to keep the hematocrit values above 25% and HbS concentration under 50%
- Hospitalization for any infection or appearance of unusual symptoms:
  - *Treatment* involves rest, rehydration, treatment of infection, pain relief, oxygen therapy and blood transfusion.
- Air travel is best avoided.

During Labor

- During labor, the midwife must ensure that the woman is kept well hydrated with IV fluids
- Prophylactic antibiotics, effective analgesia preferably epidural and oxygen therapy are needed
- The fetus should be monitored closely for signs of distress.

Postnatal Care

1. Antibiotic cover is continued throughout the postnatal period for prevention of puerperal sepsis.
2. Neonatal testing of all babies at risk must be done by testing the cord blood.
3. Sickle test must be done for the babies at the age of 3–4 months and those with positive results must be followed up by the hematologist. In order to prevent the high incidence of infant mortality from sickle cell anemia, early diagnosis combined with prophylaxis against infection, parental education and adequate follow-up are recommended.

THALASSEMIA SYNDROMES

The thalassemia syndromes are commonly found genetic disorders of the blood. The basic defect is a reduced rate of hemoglobin chain synthesis. This leads to ineffective erythropoiesis and increased hemolysis with resultant inadequate hemoglobin content. The syndromes are of two types—the α- and β-thalassemia depending on the globin chain synthesis affected. α- and β-thalassemia exist in both homozygous (major) and heterozygous (minor) states.

Alpha Thalassemia Major

The condition is more commonly found in South-East Asia. The child inherits abnormal genes from both parents. Rapid cell breakdown produces a severe anemia, which is incompatible with extrauterine life.

Beta Thalassemia Major

The defective genes result in severe hemoglobin deficiency, which may result in cardiac failure and death in early childhood. The use of frequent blood transfusion increases the possibility of survival. However, there is progressive hepatosplenomegaly, impaired growth, anemia, intercurrent infection and congestive cardiac failure. Chances of survival beyond teens are uncommon.

Alpha and Beta Thalassemia Minor

The heterozygous condition is the more common form of thalassemia and produces an anemia, which is more similar to iron deficiency in which the Hb, MCV and mean corpuscular hemoglobin (MCH) are lowered. Serum iron and total iron binding capacity are normal or elevated because red cells are broken down more rapidly than normal and iron is stored for future use. Serum bilirubin may be raised to about 2–3 mg%.

The diagnosis is often late when the patient fails to respond to oral iron therapy to correct anemia. There is chance for hepatic and cardiac hemosiderosis from iron overload. The reproductive performance of thalassemia minor is usually normal. They require oral iron and folate supplementation during pregnancy. If hemoglobin is low, blood transfusion is better. Parenteral iron therapy should never be given.

RENAL PROBLEMS IN PREGNANCY

Asymptomatic Bacteriuria

Asymptomatic bacteriuria (ASB) occurs in 2–10% of pregnant women owing to the physiological changes in the urinary tract during pregnancy. A diagnosis of ASB is defined as bacteriuria with more than 100,000 organisms per milliliter of urine from clean voided urine. It is important that the midwife obtains, from the antenatal mother, proper history of any previous urinary tract infection in order to make a positive prediction.

The consequences of this condition in pregnancy represent a significant risk to both mother and fetus. About 25% of these women are likely to develop acute pyelonephritis, usually in third trimester, if left untreated. The incidence of anemia and hypertension is stated high. There is increased incidence of premature and growth retarded babies.

The penicillins and cephalosporins are the drugs of choice for initial treatment and are administered for 7–14 days. A urine sample should be obtained for culture 1 week after therapy is discontinued and thereafter at regular intervals throughout the pregnancy to ensure that reinfection has not occurred.

Acute Pyelonephritis

Acute pyelonephritis occurs in 1–2% of all pregnancies. The causative organism is often *Escherichia coli* (*E. coli*). Bacteriuria in early pregnancy is a predisposing factor. The onset is acute and usually appears beyond the 16th week. The involvement is bilateral, but if unilateral, it is most frequently on the right side.

Manifestations

Acute aching pain over the loins, often radiating to the groin:
- Fever (often high) with chills and rigor
- Anorexia, nausea and vomiting

- Frequency of micturition and/or dysuria
- Flushed face and dry tongue (dehydration)
- Urine may appear cloudy.

Investigations

- Examination of midstream urine may show evidence of:
  - Acid reaction
  - Fishy smell
  - High specific gravity
  - Presence of slight proteins
  - Plenty of pus cells and RBCs.
- Urine culture and sensitivity
- Blood tests may show high leukocytosis, raised blood urea nitrogen (BUN) and creatinine depending on the extent of damage of the renal parenchyma.

Effects on Pregnancy

There may be increased fetal loss due to abortion and intrauterine fetal death caused by hyperpyrexia and low-birth-weight babies.

Treatment

Preventive
Screening of susceptible women (having history of previous urinary tract infection) at the first antenatal visit to detect significant bacteriuria.

If it is found positive, a course of nitrofurantoin 50 mg thrice daily or ampicillin 250 mg 6 hourly for 2 weeks is given. The urine should be tested at intervals of 4 weeks. The woman should be advised to pass urine frequently.

Curative
Admission to the hospital is usual. Adequate rest, easily digestible diet and plenty of fluids are given. In case of persistent vomiting, intravenous fluid therapy is started. Clean-catch midstream urine is sent for culture and sensitivity test, and pending report, antimicrobial therapy is started. If the woman is febrile, intravenous cephradine 1 g every 6 hours is administered. Once the temperature subsides, oral cephradine is started with 500 mg every 6 hours. Nitrofurantoin 100 mg thrice daily orally is the alternative. The therapy should be given for at least 10 days. After the therapy is stopped, if at least three urine cultures over the next 10 days are reported as sterile, the disease is considered cured.

Intravenous fluids may also be required to correct dehydration and an accurate record of fluid balance must be kept. During the early stages of illness, the woman will be confined to bed and the midwife should take steps to prevent complications of immobility, such as deep vein thrombosis and constipation. The midwife must monitor uterine activity, as there is a risk of labor commencing when the temperature rises. It may be necessary to reduce the temperature by tepid sponging and antipyretics. The temperature and pulse should be recorded 4 hourly.

The mother may be in considerable pain, which may be eased by the use of hot water bag to her back and Buscopan 20 mg. Antiemetics may be given to counteract nausea. Careful follow-up throughout pregnancy and especially in puerperium is mandatory. Relapses are common in puerperium (10%). The urine should be examined at monthly intervals including culture. Women should be encouraged to pass urine frequently. Any sign suggestive of urinary tract infection should be treated vigorously.

CHRONIC RENAL DISEASE

Chronic pyelonephritis may be a process from the beginning or may develop as sequelae of an incompletely treated and followed up case of acute or recurrent mild pyelonephritis. Asymptomatic bacteriuria may prove to be a resting stage in the process of development of chronic pyelonephritis. A pregnant woman with pre-existing renal disease is considered to be at risk of preeclampsia and intrauterine growth retardation. Preterm birth and perinatal mortality are increased. The woman's own condition is likely to deteriorate. Hospital delivery is essential.

During pregnancy, proteinuria tends to increase. Damage to the kidney tubules cause an activation of the renin-angiotensin system, leading to salt and water retention and a consequent rise in blood pressure. Production of erythropoietin may be reduced, leading to anemia. The presence of chronic infection predisposes the mother to superimposed acute infection. The outcome of pregnancy depends on the degree of renal dysfunction, the blood pressure and episodes of infection. Termination of pregnancy or early induction of labor may be offered if the renal condition deteriorates severely.

Examples of Pre-existing Renal Diseases

- Polycystic kidney disease
- Glomerulonephritis
- Chronic pyelonephritis
- Renal calculi and nephrotic syndrome.

Chronic hypertension is a common sequel. Anemia may develop, which become refractory to iron therapy and superimposed preeclampsia may aggravate the impaired renal function during pregnancy.

Management

The aim of management is to prevent deterioration in renal function. Renal function tests are performed at intervals throughout the pregnancy. The emergence and severity of hypertension, and preeclampsia are monitored by recording blood pressure and estimating urea, creatinine clearance and total protein excretion levels. Admission to hospital is advised if there is evidence of fetal compromise, if renal function deteriorates and proteinuria increases or if blood pressure rises. In severe cases, renal dialysis may be required.

AUTOIMMUNE DISEASES

Systemic Lupus Erythematosus

Systemic lupus erythematosus (SLE) is an autoimmune disease, which upsets the normal immunity of a person. It is characterized by the production of autoantibodies, which are antibodies, synthesized by an individual against a component of her own body. It is first diagnosed during pregnancy in 10–30% of cases.

The SLE, which is a multisystem disease, is characterized by exacerbations (flares) and remissions, but has no typical disease pattern, which often makes diagnosis difficult. It may manifest as polyarthritis, myalgia, skin rash, alopecia, pleurisy, dyspnea, pericarditis, proteinuria or anemia. Fertility rates are normal; therefore, pregnancy becomes a common management problem in these women.

Effects of Pregnancy on SLE

Long-term prognosis remains unaffected. There is chance of flare-up, especially during first half and in puerperium. Deaths occur in puerperium due to pulmonary hemorrhage and lupus pneumonia.

Effects on Pregnancy

There is increased risk of first trimester abortion, lupus nephritis, recurrent deep vein thrombosis, pregnancy-induced hypertension (PIH), intrauterine growth restriction (IUGR), prematurity and stillbirths. Neonatal lupus syndrome occurs due to crossing of maternal lupus antibodies to the fetus causing hemolytic anemia, leukopenia and thrombocytopenia. Isolated congenital heart block is seen in about one third of cases.

Investigation

Antinuclear antibodies are the standard screening test for the disease.

Management

Preconception counseling is extremely important since conception during a period of quiescence is most likely to result in a live birth. The frequency of antenatal visits is dependent on the severity of the disease and should include full hematological and immunological investigations.

Control and treatment of SLE is mainly dependent on drugs starting with analgesics, such as paracetamol and progressing to corticosteroids, immunosuppressives and cytotoxic agents in severe cases. Drug therapy is individualized and dependent upon the disease activity and organs involved. Low dose aspirin 80 mg daily is prescribed usually. It is important that the woman is made aware of the risks to herself and her baby, if SLE is left untreated, as often women are reluctant to take drugs in pregnancy.

Intrapartum Care

The timing of delivery depends upon the severity of the disease and whether there are any complications such as preeclampsia or renal involvement. Delivery should otherwise be at term. SLE patients are at risk of infection and hence, the midwife should ensure that careful handwashing and strict aseptic technique are adhered to as well as limiting the number of vaginal examinations. Observations of vital signs need to be frequent along with measurement of fluid intake and output, and assessment of urinary protein. Continuous fetal monitoring and fetal blood gas estimation are recommended. Vaginal delivery is aimed for where possible. However, because of associated problems, many fetuses are delivered by planned cesarean section. Women on long-term corticosteroid therapy should have parenteral steroid cover in labor and for 24 hours postnatally.

Postnatal Care

Following delivery of the baby, the midwife needs to encourage the woman to rest as much as possible in order to prevent exacerbation of her SLE, which is likely to occur during stressful times. Close monitoring of vital signs should continue for 24–48 hours following delivery. Breastfeeding is generally safe if the mother is receiving nonsteroid anti-inflammatory drugs (NSAIDs) or low-dose steroids. Salicylates, antimalarial and immunosuppressive agents need to be avoided. The newborn should have a careful clinical examination and undergo appropriate serological evaluation by a pediatrician in the postnatal period. The choice of contraceptives for the woman with SLE is limited to barrier methods and the midwife must educate the woman and her spouse in their proper use. Intrauterine device may predispose to infection, oral contraceptives may induce exacerbation of the disease and hence both are contraindicated.

IDIOPATHIC THROMBOCYTOPENIC PURPURA

Idiopathic thrombocytopenic purpura (ITP) is the most common tissue or organ specific autoimmune disease in women of childbearing age and accounts for 2–4% of pregnant women. This condition causes increased platelet destruction by immune processes, which may arise following viral infection or an allergic response to drugs. If the platelet count falls below 50,000/mm^3 the condition may manifest as bleeding from mucous surfaces and episodes such as epistaxis, multiple small bruises, petechiae in the skin, postpartum hemorrhage or bleeding from abdominal or perineal incisions.

Diagnosis

Diagnosis may be made following a routine full blood count of $< 100 \times 10^9/\mu L$ or when the woman presents with repeated episodes of bleeding in pregnancy.

Effects of ITP on Pregnancy and the Fetus

Postpartum hemorrhage is the major risk, which is directly related to the maternal platelet count. Maternal mortality and morbidity are now rare. The perinatal mortality can be as high as 15% in extreme cases. Complications to the fetus include gastrointestinal bleeding, hemopericardium, intraventricular hemorrhage and severe cutaneous manifestations of bleeding. Profound thrombocytopenia may develop in infants due to transplacental passage of IgG antibodies. In babies, it is a transient condition lasting between 1 week and 4 months of life.

Antenatal Care

Management of this condition during pregnancy is to be supervised by a hematologist and involves monitoring and maintaining the maternal platelet count at an acceptable level. Corticosteroid therapy is the initial treatment of choice, which will increase the maternal platelet count. If this fails, a high dose of immunoglobulin can be given intravenously.

Intrapartum Care

The objective is to plan for a vaginal delivery, avoiding an episiotomy and ensuring good control of the third stage of labor. Intravenous ergometrine is used prophylactically. A pediatrician should be present at delivery and an immediate cord platelet count is taken. Treatment may be required if the platelet count is $< 50 \times 10^9/L$ ($< 50 \times 100,000/\mu L$) or when the woman presents with repeated episodes of bleeding in pregnancy.

Postnatal Care

Following delivery, the midwife should inspect the genital tract to identify and control any bleeding sites. Strict attention to aseptic technique and careful repair of any tissue trauma is important. Breastfeeding is encouraged unless there are adverse complications. Discussion with the woman and her spouse regarding the risks of future pregnancies is important, and they should be advised that platelet levels need to be within normal limits prior to future conceptions.

EPILEPSY IN PREGNANCY

The effect of pregnancy on epilepsy is unclear. Frequency of convulsions is unchanged in about 50% and is increased in some. Increased plasma clearance of anticonvulsant drugs during pregnancy has been observed and estrogens are thought to activate the seizure foci. The adverse effects on the mother are third trimester bleeding and megaloblastic anemia, which may be related to anticonvulsant induced folate deficiency.

Birth defects are increased by two fold. Malformations include cleft lip and/or palate, mental retardation, cardiac abnormalities, limb defects and hypoplasia of the terminal phalanges. There is chance of neonatal hemorrhage, which is related to anticonvulsant-induced vitamin K dependent coagulopathy. The risk of developing epilepsy to the offspring of an epileptic mother is four fold. Preconception counseling includes:

- Initiation of monotherapy, if possible
- Administration of folic acid 1 mg daily.

Management

The dose of the chosen drug should be kept as low as possible and to be monitored regularly from the serum level. The commonly used drugs are:

- Phenobarbitone 60–180 mg daily in two to three divided doses
- Phenytoin 150–300 mg daily in two divided doses
- Carbamazepine 0.8–1.2 g daily in divided doses.

The fits are controlled by intravenous diazepam 10–20 mg. Folic acid 1 mg must be continued throughout pregnancy. There is decrease in free level of most of the anticonvulsants in pregnancy. This is due to reduced absorption and at the same time increased hepatic metabolism and renal clearance. Vitamin K 10 mg daily must be given orally in the last 2 weeks. Termination of pregnancy may be considered in consultation with a neurologist. Seizure precautions and care will be required during the postpartum period.

There is no contraindication for breastfeeding. The infant may be drowsy. By 4–6 weeks postpartum, the anticonvulsant dose must be adjusted and brought to the pre-pregnant level. Steroidal contraceptives are to be avoided due to enzyme induction.

GYNECOLOGICAL DISORDERS IN PREGNANCY

Fibroid Uterus

Description

Fibroid uterus is the common benign tumor of the uterus during pregnancy. These are benign smooth muscle tumors that occur within the uterus and is the most common tumors of the female genital tract.

Incidence

The incidence of fibroid in pregnancy is about 1 in 1,000.

Causes

- The exact cause is unknown
- Women who smoke tend to be relatively estrogen deficient and have been found to have a lower incidence of fibroid uterus.

Risk Factors

- Age 35–45 years
- Nulliparous or low parity
- Obesity
- Early menarche
- Family history of diabetes, hypertension.

Signs and Symptoms

- More than 50% asymptomatic
- Acute onset of pain over the tumor
- Malaise or even rise of temperature

- Dry, tarred tongue
- Abnormal uterine bleeding
- Pelvic pain or backache, acute pain occurs in case of torsion, infection, expulsion, red degeneration or vascular complications
- Tenderness and rigidity over the tumor
- Pressure effects on:
  - Bladder—frequency of urine, retention with overflow
  - Ureter—hydroureter, hydronephrosis
  - Bowel—constipation, tenesmus
  - Pelvic veins—edema legs
- Pelvic pressure with large fibroids.
- Leukocytosis.
- Sometimes fetal parts are not easily palpated or fetal heart sounds (FHS) are not auscultated properly.
- Size of the uterus may be more than the weeks of gestation.

Diagnosis

Confirmed diagnosis usually by an ultrasound examination.

Effects of Fibroid on Pregnancy

Pregnancy

In majority of cases, fibroids cause no problems in pregnancy. Problems occur occasionally in few women as listed below.

- Abortion: Submucous fibroid can lead to recurrent abortions. With subserous and intramural fibroids incidence of abortion is very low. Abortion occurs due to distortion of the uterine cavity, and interference with growth of uterus. Abortion may be incomplete type.
- Pressure symptoms: Growing fibroid during pregnancy affects function of surrounding organs like bladder, ureters and rectum.
- Malpresentation
- Retro-displacement of uterus
- Non-engagement of the presenting part

Labor

- Malpresentation—due to distortion of the cavity.
- Uterine inertia—due to interference with uterine contractions, particularly with multiple fibroids.
- Premature labor—due to overstretching and irritation of the uterus
- Dystocia—when fibroid is situated in isthmic or cervical region or in broad ligament, it causes obstruction for the descent of the presenting part.
- Postpartum hemorrhage—usually occurs with submucous fibroid. There is an increased chance of retained products. If placenta is implanted on fibroid, proper contraction and retraction cannot occur.
- Manual removal of placenta becomes necessary if placenta is adherent on fibroid.

Puerperium

- Subinvolution
- Secondary postpartum hemorrhage
- Puerperal sepsis
- Inversion of uterus with fundal submucous fibroid.

Effects of Pregnancy and Labor on Fibroid

Size, shape, and consistency

- As fibroid is an estrogen dependent tumor, during pregnancy there is increased secretion of estrogen which leads to increased size of fibroid.
- Microscopically, there is increased edema; hypertrophy and hyperplasia of muscle as well as increased vascularity. These changes make the fibroid soft.
- Shape of fibroid is also changed sometimes making it flat and difficult to palpate.
- Upward displacement of fibroid can occur if situated above isthmic level.

Torsion

In pedunculated subserous fibroid, torsion can occur and give rise to symptoms of acute abdomen.

Degeneration

- Red degeneration: Rate of growth of fibroid is more; blood supply cannot cope up so that surface area becomes necrosed. This usually occurs in second trimester of pregnancy.
- Obstruction to the venous outflow from the tumor is considered possible. Microscopically, there is vascular thrombosis and necrosis.
- Severe constitutional symptoms like pain, malaise, fever and vomiting can occur.
- Cystic degeneration: Due to increase in size, necrosis and hyaline degeneration occurs and ultimately fibroid becomes cystic.
- Impaction in pelvis.
- Infection: After delivery, submucous fibroid may get infected and can cause puerperal sepsis.
- Injury: During passage of fetus through birth canal, fibroid gets bruised and compressed between fetal head and pelvis and leads to PPH.
- Expulsion: With delivery of fetus and placenta, pedunculated submucous fibroid may be expelled out.
- Rupture of subserous vein of the fibroid causing intra-peritoneal hemorrhage is rare.

Treatment

In asymptomatic and uncomplicated patients, no treatment is required.

- Frequent antenatal visits and counseling of patient about possible complications.
- In complicated and symptomatic patients treatment is given according to the complication.
- In cases of impaction, manual removal of impaction is done.
- In retention of urine, self-retaining catheter may be placed.
- In red degeneration, treatment is always conservative. That is bed rest, higher antibiotics, analgesics and sedation.

- Torsion of subserous, pedunculated fibroid: It causes acute abdomen and laparotomy with myomectomy is indicated.

During labor
- Labor should be managed according to the site and size of fibroid.
- Very vigilant observation during labor for any developing complication.
- Cesarean section is indicated in cases of malpresentation, dystocia, precious pregnancy and fibroid situated in cervical canal, isthmic region or broad ligament causing mechanical obstruction.
- During cesarean section, myomectomy is avoided as blood loss is more due to increased vascularity and increased size. Cesarean hysterectomy may be required for uncontrollable PPH.
- If patient has completed child bearing, cesarean hysterectomy may be performed.
- Pedunculated subserous fibroid can be removed during cesarean section.

Uterine Prolapse

Description

Pregnancy with 1st degree uterine prolapse with mild cysto-rectocele is common; but pregnancy with 3rd degree prolapse is rare. Uterine prolapse presents a severe uterine problem in which the uterus protrudes through the pelvic floor aperture. It is usually associated with a cystocele or rectocele.

Incidence

The incidence is about 1 in 200 to 1 in 300 pregnancies.

Causes

- Previous vaginal deliveries (multiparous women)
- Obesity
- Chronic pulmonary disease
- Uterine or ovarian tumor
- Chronic cough
- Chronic constipation.

Clinical Manifestations

- Patients with first degree prolapse may report sensation of heaviness or fullness and feeling that something is coming down in the vagina.
- In more severe prolapse, when cervix protrudes at the introitus, the patient may complain of feeling like she is sitting on a ball.
- With severe prolapse, the woman is clearly aware of the mass.
- Vaginal bleeding, discharge and infection may present.
- Woman may have dyspareunia.
- A feeling of heaviness in the pelvis and backache.
- Bowel or bladder problems.
- Abortion.
- Premature labor.
- Premature rupture of membranes.
- Ascending infection.

Effects of Pregnancy on Prolapse

- Symptoms like lower abdominal pain and backache increases.
- Increased vaginal discharge and difficulty in micturition and defecation as well as symptoms of urinary infection.
- Abortion.
- Premature labor.
- Premature rupture of membranes.
- Ascending infection.
- Aggravation of changes associated with prolapse.
- Marked hypertrophy and edema of the cervix.
- Increase in uterine descend during pregnancy as well as after delivery.
- Cystocele and rectocele become pronounced.
- Uterus may become incarcerated, if it fails to rise above the pelvis by 16th week.

Labor and Puerperium

- Early rupture.
- Prolonged labor due to delayed dilatation of cervix and sagging of cysto-rectocele.
- Puerperal sepsis.
- Subinvolution.

Management

During pregnancy
- If the cervix is outside the introitus: The cervix is to be replaced inside the vagina and is kept in position by a ring pessary.
- The pessary should be kept in place until 18th–20th week of pregnancy when the body of the uterus will be sufficiently enlarged to sit on the brim of the pelvis.
- The patient is to lie in bed with the foot end raised by about 20 cm as the pelvic floor is too much lax.
- To relieve edema and congestion, the mass should be covered with gauze socked in glycerin and $MgSO_4$ powder.
- This treatment is continued till 18 to 20 weeks of pregnancy till prolapsed mass is reduced in size and replaced in vagina.
- If reposition is not possible and there is incarceration, termination of pregnancy is indicated.
- If the cervix remains outside the vaginal introitus even in the later months, it is preferable to admit the patient at 36th week.

During labor
- The patient should be in bed rest, not only to prevent early rupture of membranes but also to facilitate replacement of the prolapsed cervix inside the vagina.
- Intravaginal plugging soaked with glycerin and acriflavine not only helps in reduction of cervical edema, but also it facilitates dilatation of cervix.
- Prophylactic antibiotics, in case of premature rupture of membranes or when the cervix remains outside vagina should be administered.
- Manual stretching of the cervix or pushing up the cystocele and rectocele during contraction facilitates progressive descend of the head.
- If the head is deeply engaged with the cervix remaining thin but undilated, delivery may be facilitated by Duhrssen's incision at 2 O'clock and 10 O'clock positions followed by ventouse extraction or forceps application.
- If the head is higher up or cervix is thick, edematous and non-dilated, cesarean section is a safe procedure.

Puerperium
- The patient should lie flat on bed.
- If the mass remains outside, it should be covered with gauze soaked in glycerin and $MgSO_4$ pack is applied.
- If subinvolution is evident, a ring pessary may be put in, until involution is completed.
- Prophylactic antibiotic is administered.
- Surgery for prolapse is contraindicated in antepartum and postpartum period.
- Definitive surgery is done only after six months of delivery and preferably after the patient starts menstruating.

Ovarian Tumors in Pregnancy

Description
Benign tumors of the ovary are many and varied. The cause of most of them is unknown. The benign tumors develop from a variety of physiological imbalance.

Incidence
Ovarian tumor with pregnancy is about 1 in 2,000.

Effects of Ovarian Tumor on Pregnancy and Labor
- Pressure symptoms
- Increased chance for impaction leading to retention of urine
- Mechanical distress in presence of large tumor
- Malpresentation
- Non-engagement of the fetal head at term
- Obstructed labor.

Clinical Manifestations
- In about 50% of cases, it is asymptomatic
- Symptomatic tumors present with vague abdominal discomforts
- Retention of urine due to impaction of tumor
- Mechanical distress due to large cyst
- Acute abdomen due to complications of tumor.

Diagnosis
- Abdominal examination reveals the cystic swelling felt separated from the gravid uterus.
- Ultrasonography.

Treatment and Management
During pregnancy
- For uncomplicated tumors, the best time of elective operation is between 14th and 18th week, as the chance for abortion is less and access to pedicle is easy.
- Beyond 36 weeks: The operation is better to be withheld till delivery and the tumor is removed as early in puerperium as possible.
- If the tumor causes non-engagement of head or obstructs labor, LSCS and cystectomy or ovariotomy is performed.

During labor
- If the tumor is well above the presenting part, a watchful expectancy hoping for vaginal delivery is followed.
- If the tumor is impacted in the pelvis causing obstruction, cesarean section should be done followed by removal of the tumor in the same sitting.

Cancer Cervix with Pregnancy

Preinvasive Cancer/Cervical Intraepithelial Neoplasia (CIN)
- Cytological examination can be done during pregnancy, considering that some features of dysplasia are seen as increased cells showing mitosis are normally present during pregnancy.
- If CIN I or CIN II is detected, follow up is done till one month after delivery and then conization or hysterectomy is done as indicated.

Invasive Cancer Cervix
This is a very rare cancer (1 in 10,000) as the mean age of cancer cervix is 45–50 years and associated infection prevents conception.

Effect of Invasive Carcinoma Cervix on Pregnancy and Labor
- Abortion and preterm labor due to hemorrhage, infection and affection of general health
- Cervical dystocia, obstructed labor, cervical laceration and/or uterine rupture may occur
- Puerperal sepsis.

Effect of Pregnancy on Invasive Carcinoma

* Rapid growth of tumor
* Rapid spread if vaginal delivery is allowed

Management

* *In early pregnancy:* Wertheim's operation or hysterectomy followed by radiation therapy.
* *In late pregnancy:* Upper segment cesarean section followed by either Wertheim's operation, cesarean hysterectomy or radiation therapy.
* *During puerperium:* The tumor should be removed as early in puerperium as possible.

Displacement of Pregnant Uterus

Description

Minor variations in position of the uterus occur constantly with changes in posture with straining, with full bladder or loaded rectum. Only when the uterus rests habitually in a position beyond the limit of normal variation, should it be called displacement.

Retroverted Gravid Uterus

Retroverted uterus either congenital or acquired is considered as a normal variant of uterine position. Retroversion in pregnancy is either pre-existing or may be due to pregnancy.

Definition of Retroversion

Retroversion is the term used when the long axis of the corpus and cervix are in line and the whole organ turns backwards in relation to the long axis of the birth canal. Retroflexion signifies a bending backwards of the corpus on the cervix at the level of internal os; the two conditions are usually present together and are loosely called retroversion or retrodisplacement.

Incidence

The incidence is about 10% during first trimester of pregnancy.

Degrees

Conventionally, three degrees are described.
1. *First degree:* The fundus is vertical and pointing towards the sacral promontory.
2. *Second degree:* The fundus lies in the sacral hollow, but not below the internal os.
3. *Third degree:* The fundus lies below the level of the internal os.

Causes

Developmental
Retrodisplacement is quite common in fetuses and young children. Due to developmental defect, there is lack of tone of the uterine muscles. The infantile position is retained. This is often associated with short vagina with shallow anterior vaginal fornix.

Acquired
Puerperal: The stretched ligaments caused by childbirth fail to keep the uterus in its normal position. A subinvoluted, bulky uterus aggravates this condition.

Prolapse: Retroversion is usually implicated in the pathophysiology of prolapse which is mechanically caused by traction following cystocele.

Tumor: Fibroid, either in the anterior or posterior wall produces heaviness of the uterus and hence it falls behind.

Pelvic adhesions: Adhesions either inflammatory, operative or due to pelvic endometriosis pull the uterus posteriorly.

Anatomic changes
Favorable: In the majority, spontaneous rectification occurs. As the uterus grows, the fundus rises spontaneously from the pelvis beyond 12 weeks. Thereafter, the pregnancy continues uneventfully.

Unfavorable: In the majority, spontaneous rectification fails to occur between 12–16 weeks. The developing uterus gradually fills up the pelvic cavity and becomes incarcerated.

Changes following incarceration
Changes in the uterus: The cervix is pointed upwards and forwards and is placed even on the upper border of the symphysis pubis. Rarely, the uterus continues to grow at the expense of the anterior wall called anterior sacculation while the thick posterior wall lies in sacral hollow.

Changes in the urethra and bladder: The major brunt falls on the lower urinary tract, predominantly on the bladder. Urethral changes include marked elongation due to stretching of the anterior vaginal wall by the cervix. This causes retention of urine.

Bladder changes: As a result of retention of urine, the bladder gets distended and becomes an abdominal organ reaching even up to the umbilicus. If retention is not relieved, the following may happen:
* The bladder walls becomes thickened due to edema.
* Severe cystitis or pyelonephritis leading to uremia.
* Intraperitoneal rupture resulting in peritonitis in neglected cases.

Swelling due to full bladder disappears after catheterization.

Effects on Pregnancy

* Abortion.
* *Pregnancy:* If pregnancy continues with anterior sacculation, there is increased chance of malpresentation, non-engagement of fetal head, preterm delivery and rupture of uterus during labor.
* *Management:*
  a. Before incarceration: Periodic checkup up to 12 weeks until the uterus becomes an abdominal organ. The woman is advised to empty her bladder frequently and to lie in prone position as far as possible.

b. After incarceration
- To empty the bladder slowly by continuous drainage with a Foley's catheter.
- To put the patient in bed and advice to lie on her face or in Sim's position as far as practicable.
- Culture and sensitivity test of urine and administration of antibiotics. With this regimen, the uterus is expected to be corrected spontaneously within 48 hours.

❖ If spontaneous correction fails:
- Manual correction by pushing the uterus digitally through the posterior fornix under anesthesia. After correction, a Hodge-Smith pessary is to be inserted and to be kept up to 18th–20th week.
- In obstinate cases, when the above method fails due to adhesions, laparotomy may have to be done. Adhesiolysis may be attempted, failing which termination of pregnancy may be indicated.
- In diagnosed cases of anterior sacculation of the uterus, delivery by cesarean section is the method of choice.

❖ *Prevention:* The following guidelines are helpful during the weeks after abortion or childbirth.
- To empty the bladder at regular intervals.
- To increase the tone of pelvic muscles by regular exercise.
- To encourage lying in prone position for half to one hour once or twice daily for 4 to 6 weeks postpartum.

PSYCHIATRIC DISORDERS DURING PREGNANCY

Mood and anxiety disorders are common in women during their childbearing years. Pregnancy and postpartum periods are considered to be relatively high-risk times for women with pre-existing psychiatric illnesses, especially for depressive episodes. The prevalence of depression has been reported to be between 10 and 16% during pregnancy. For women with bipolar disorder, pregnancy and postpartum period have even higher risk. Rates of relapse are estimated at 30–50% during the postpartum period. The course of panic disorder can be variable with some studies reporting an improvement of symptoms and others reporting a worsening. In obsessive compulsive disorder, symptoms typically worsen during pregnancy. Some studies suggest an initial onset of symptoms during pregnancy. Special considerations are needed when psychotic disorders present during pregnancy.

Stress and Pregnancy

Pregnancy either induces or exacerbates pre-existing stress and in turn stress seems to have a negative effect on pregnancy, especially in the first trimester. The period of greatest stress during pregnancy, the first trimester, is also the period of highest rate of pregnancy loss. According to records, in 17th and 18th centuries, medical profession had the belief that abortion occurred as a reaction to wrath, fear, grief, joy and even disagreeable odors.

Major Depression in Pregnancy

Major depression is twice common in women than in men and frequently manifests during the childbearing years. Although pregnancy has traditionally been considered a time of emotional well-being for women conferring protection against psychiatric disorders, at least one prospective study describes rates of major and minor depression as approximately 10%. For women with past history of mood disorder, discontinuation of antidepressant medicines causes reappearance of clinically significant symptoms. It has been observed that in about one-third of depressed pregnant women, this represents the first episode of major depression.

Other risk factors of antenatal depression include marital discord or dissatisfaction, inadequate psychological supports, recent adverse life events, lower socioeconomic status, and unwanted pregnancy. High rates of relapse occur after discontinuation of maintenance pharmacological treatment in non-gravid women. In women who have been diagnosed as having recurrent depression prior to conception and in whom antidepressant medications have been discontinued, rates of relapse can be up to 75% and can be seen frequently during the first trimester. Milder forms of depression during pregnancy can be misse. Pregnant women may have many clinical signs and symptoms overlapping with those seen in major depression (e.g. sleep and appetite disturbance, decreased libido and low energy). Some medical disorders commonly seen during pregnancy, such as anemia, gestational diabetes and thyroid dysfunction, may be associated with depressive symptoms and may complicate the diagnosis of depression during pregnancy. Clinical features that may support the diagnosis of major depression include loss of pleasure, feelings of guilt and hopelessness and suicidal thoughts. Suicidal ideation and self-injurious ideation are often reported; however, the risk of self-injurious or suicidal behavior appears to be low in the population of women who develop depression during pregnancy.

Risks of untreated depression in the mother
The risks of untreated depression in the mother include:
❖ Risk of self-injurious or suicidal behavior
❖ Inadequate self-care
❖ Poor compliance with prenatal care
❖ Decreased appetite and consequently lower than expected weight gain in pregnancy leading to negative pregnancy outcomes
❖ Women with depression are also more likely to use either alcohol or illicit drugs, which are behaviors that further increase the risk to the fetus
❖ Some studies suggests that maternal depression itself may adversely affect the developing fetus.

Impact of maternal depression on the family
❖ Interpersonal difficulties
❖ Disruption in mother-baby interactions and attachment affecting infant's development
❖ Studies have also shown that depression during pregnancy significantly increases a woman's risk for post-partum depression

❖ Antenatal depression thus have significant adverse effects that may extend beyond pregnancy and have more significant long-term effects on her psychological functioning.

Bipolar Disorder

Pregnancy and especially the postpartum period are stressful periods for women and increases the risk of relapse for women with bipolar disorder. Bipolar disorder affects 0. 5–1.5% of individuals. The typical age of onset is late adolescence or early adult hood, placing women at risk for episodes throughout their reproductive years. The presentation of a woman with bipolar disorder may resemble a depressive disorder, behavioral deregulation, or general medical disorders. It is important to access history of hypomania or mania when determining diagnosis in any woman presenting with psychological symptoms. Symptoms of postpartum psychosis tend to differ from the symptoms typically seen in bipolar mania. Therefore if postpartum psychosis is actually a manifestation of bipolar disorder, accurate diagnosis depends on knowledge of these differences.

Anxiety Disorder

Hormonal changes during pregnancy such as increased prolactin, oxytocin and cortisol may contribute to the suppression of stress response that occurs during this period. Studies have suggested that women with anxiety related to pregnancy may be at greater risk for postpartum depression.

Psychotic Disorders

Women with psychotic disorders are at an increased risk of obstetric complications. Recent studies have confirmed earlier findings of low fertility in women with schizophrenia. Psychotic relapse during pregnancy is rare, but women with a history of mood disorders (affective psychosis) are at a high risk for postpartum relapse.

Treatment of Psychiatric Disorders during Pregnancy

Specific Concerns

Psychotropic medications readily cross the placenta. Therefore following factors must be considered before starting psychotropic medications.
❖ Teratogenesis.
❖ Toxicity to the neonate.
❖ Neurobehavioral sequelae.
❖ Risk of medication discontinuation.
❖ Risk of no treatment.

Treatment of Specific Psychiatric Disorders

Major Depression

❖ *Psychotherapies:* Interpersonal therapy (ITP) is useful for four major problems with respect to human psychosocial functioning—grief, interpersonal disputes, role transitions, and interpersonal deficits. This treatment is needed considering the importance of interpersonal relationships in couples expecting a baby, and the significant role of transitions take place during pregnancy and subsequent to delivery. ITP is ideal for the treatment of the depressed pregnant women.
❖ *Antidepressant therapy:* Antidepressants during pregnancy are indicated for women whose symptoms interfere with maternal well-being and functioning. Medication choice depends on prior treatment response. During pregnancy fluoxetine is usually the first line antidepressant choice. Other first line choices include nortriptyline and desipramine as they are less anticholinergic and therefore less likely to exacerbate orthostatic hypotension during pregnancy.

Bipolar Disorder

Special treatment options need to be considered due to the risk of fetal malformation when certain mood stabilizers are used during first trimester of pregnancy. Neurobehavioral teratogenicity and neonatal toxicity are also possible. Careful treatment management is necessary to reduce risks to the fetus/neonate and to effectively manage bipolar disorder in the mother.

Anxiety Disorders

Psychotherapy is found to be beneficial for panic disorder and obsessive compulsive disorder (OCD) in both pregnant and nonpregnant women. Tapering of medication may be possible with adjunctive treatment with behavior therapy during pregnancy. For mild cases of OCD, pregnant women may do well with behavior techniques. However, moderate to severe symptoms may require maintenance pharmacological treatment.
❖ *Anxiolytics:* A slow taper of antipanic medications over a period of two weeks may be possible in mild cases of panic disorder. However, maintenance medication may be necessary in patients with severe panic disorder. In such cases fluoxetine or a tricyclic antidepressant is a good treatment option. In patients who do not respond to their antidepressants, benzodiazepine may be considered. Clomipramine may also be considered but may aggravate orthostatic hypotension.

Psychotic Disorders

Neuroleptics should be considered as psychosis can be an obstetric and medical emergency.

ADOLESCENT PREGNANCY/TEENAGE PREGNANCY

Description

Teenage pregnancy is formally defined as a pregnancy in a young woman who has not reached her 20th birthday when the pregnancy ends, regardless of whether the woman is married or legally an adult (age 14 to 21 depending on the country). Usually this refers to unmarried minors who become pregnant unintentionally.

Adolescent pregnancy is pregnancy in girls age 19 or younger. Adolescent pregnancy is a complex issue with many reasons for concern. Younger adolescents (12–14 years old) are more likely to have unplanned sexual intercourse and more likely to be coerced into sex. Adolescents 18 to 19 years old are technically adults, and about half of adolescent pregnancies occur in this age group.

Causes of Teenage Pregnancy

Teenage pregnancy is defined as an unintended pregnancy during adolescence. Many teenagers do not believe that they will get pregnant if they engage in sexual activity and it happens because of peer pressure, absent parents, lack of knowledge, sexual abuse or rape and teenage drinking.

Risk factors for adolescent pregnancy
- Younger age
- Poor school performance
- Economic disadvantage
- Single or teen parents

Diagnosis

The adolescent may or may not admit to being involved sexually. If the teen is pregnant, there are usually weight changes (usually a gain, but there may be a loss if nausea and vomiting are significant). Examination may show increased abdominal girth and the health care provider may be able to feel the fundus. Pelvic examination may reveal bluish or purple coloration of vaginal walls, bluish or purple coloration and softening of the cervix, and softening and enlargement of uterus. Pregnancy test of urine and/or serum HCG are usually positive. An ultrasound examination may be done to confirm or check accurate dates for pregnancy.

Management

All options made available to the pregnant teen should be considered carefully, including abortion, adoption and raising the child with family support.
- Pregnant teens should be assessed for smoking, alcohol use and drug use and they should be offered support to help them quit.
- Adequate nutrition should be encouraged through education and family/community support. Adequate exercise and sleep should also be emphasized. Contraceptive information and services are important after delivery to prevent them becoming pregnant again. Teen mothers should be encouraged and helped to remain in school or re-enter educational programs that give them skills to be better parents and provide for the child financially and emotionally.

Prognosis

- Teen mothers are about two years behind their age group in completing their education or may even discontinue their education.
- Teen mothers who have history of substance abuse may start abusing again by about 6 months after delivery.
- They are more likely than older mothers to have a second child within two years of their first child.
- Infants born to teenage mothers are at greater risk for developmental problems. Girls born to teen mothers are more likely to become teen mothers themselves, and boys born to teen mothers have a higher than average rate of becoming criminals.

Complications

- Pregnant teens are at much higher risk of having serious medical complications such as placenta previa, pregnancy-induced hypertension, premature delivery and significant anemia.
- Infants born to teens are 2 to 6 times more likely to have low birth weight than those born to mothers age 20 or older.
- Prematurity and resultant low birth weight and intrauterine growth retardation (IUGR) are also import problems.
- Infants are at greater risk for inadequate growth, infection or chemical dependence as mothers are more likely to have unhealthy habits. It is important for pregnant teens to have early and adequate prenatal care, and counseling regarding birth control methods, prevention of sexually transmitted diseases (STD) and pregnancy risks.

Prevention

Programs for teen pregnancy prevention include:
- Knowledge-based programs that focus on teaching adolescents about their bodies and their normal functions as well as providing detailed information about contraception, and preventing STDs.
- Abstinence education programs to encourage young people to postpone sexual activity until marriage or until they are mature enough to handle sexual activity and a potential pregnancy in a responsible manner.
- Clinic focused programs to provide easier access to information, counseling by health care providers and contraceptive services. These programs are offered through school based clinics.
- Peer counseling programs which typically involve older teens to encourage adolescents to resist peer and social pressures to become sexually involved. These programs tend to use a personal approach, helping teens understand their own risks.

ELDERLY PRIMI

Women having their first pregnancy at or above the age of 30 years are called elderly primi. There are two groups of mothers, one with high fecundity—a woman may marry late but conceive soon after. Another with low fecundity—they marry early but conceive long after marriage.

Complications

During pregnancy
- Abortion
- Pre-eclampsia
- Uterine fibroid
- Medical complications like hypertension, diabetes mellitus
- Postmaturity
- Intrauterine growth retardation.

During labor
- Premature labor
- Prolonged labor
- Maternal and fetal distress
- Retained placenta
- Increased operative interference.

During puerperium
- Failing lactation
- Increased morbidity and mortality.

Management

Elderly primigravidae are considered high-risk patients. Prompt antenatal supervision and hospital delivery are essential. Maternal mortality and morbidity are high.

GRAND MULTIPARA

A commonly used definition of parity is the number of births (both live born babies and stillbirths) of at least 20 weeks of gestation that a woman has experienced. The term grand multipara refers to a pregnant mother who has had previous four or more viable childbirths. Multiparity increases the risk of pregnancy complications.

Possible Complications

During pregnancy
- Abortion
- Malpresentation
- Multiple pregnancy
- Placenta previa
- Medical disorders such as anemia, hypertension with or without preeclampsia
- Cardiac disability.

During labor
- Cord prolapse.
- Cephalopelvic disproportion.
- Obstructed labor.
- Rupture of uterus.
- Postpartum hemorrhage.
- Shock.
- Operative interferences.

During puerperium
- Subinvolution
- Failing lactation.

STUDY QUESTIONS

Short Notes

1. Common congenital defects seen in childbearing period.
2. Renal glycosuria in pregnancy.
3. Dietary advice for a prenatal client with iron deficiency anemia.

Short Answer Questions

1. Effects of diabetes in pregnancy on fetus.
2. Manifestations, investigations and management of acute pyelonephritis in pregnancy.

Essay Questions

1. Enumerate the intrapartum care of a client with grade-1 cardiac disease.
2. Describe the immediate care of the newborn of a diabetic mother.
3. Discuss the causes, manifestations and prenatal management of iron deficiency anemia in a 18-year-old primigravida.

BIBLIOGRAPHY

1. Allison JV. Lecture notes on human physiology, 2nd edition. Oxford: Blackwell Scientific Publications; 1989. pp. 132-49.
2. Becks GP, Burrow GN. Thyroid disease and pregnancy. Medical Clinics of North America. 1991;75(1):121-50.
3. Benson B. Handbook of obstetrics and gynecology, 1st edition. California: Lange Medical Publications; 1990. pp. 148-56.
4. Nima B. Midwifery and obstetrical nursing, 2nd editions. EMMES Medical Publishers; 2015
5. Bishoni A, Sachmechi I. Thyroid disease during pregnancy. American Family Physician. 1996;53(1):215-20.
6. Carpenter MW. Testing for gestational diabetes. In: Reace (Ed). Diabetes mellitus in pregnancy, 2nd edition. New York: Churchill Livingstone; 1995. pp. 453-71.
7. de Swiet M. Medical disorders in obstetric practice, 3rd edition. Oxford: Blackwell Scientific Publications; 1995. pp. 17-30.
8. Duff P. Maternal and perinatal infections. In: Gabbe SG (Ed). Obstetrics: normal and problem pregnancies, 3rd edition. New York: Churchill Livingstone; 1996.
9. Dutta DC. Textbook of obstetrics, 5th edition. Kolkata: New Central Book Company; 2001. pp. 277-323.
10. Hollingsworth DR, Resnik R. Medical counseling before pregnancy. New York: Churchill Livingstone; 1988. pp. 132-7.
11. Jowett NI, Nicol SG. Gestational diabetes—are right women being screened? Midwifery. 1986;2(2):98-100.
12. Landon MB, Samuels P. Cardiac and pulmonary disease. In: Gabbe SG (Ed). Obstetrics: Normal and Problem Pregnancies, 3rd edition. New York: Churchill Livingstone; 1996. pp. 229-35.
13. Letsky EA. Anemia in obstetrics. In: Studd J (Ed). Progress in Obstetrics and Gynecology, vol. 6. New York: Churchill Livingstone; 1987. pp. 383-90.

14. Lloyd C, Lewis VM. Common medical disorders associated with pregnancy. In: Bennet RV, Brown LK (Eds). Myles Textbook for Midwives, 13th edition. Edinburgh: Churchill Livingstone; 1999. pp. 279-314.
15. Mestman JH, Goodwin TM, Montoro MM. Thyroid disorders of pregnancy. Endocrinology and Metabolism Clinics of North America. 1995;24:41-71.
16. Nolan J. Heart disease in pregnancy. British Journal of Hospital Medicine. 1990;39(1):50-3.
17. Oates JN, Beischer NA. Gestational diabetes. In: Studd J (Ed). Progress in Obstetrics and Gynecology, vol. 6. Edinburgh: Churchill Livingstone; 1987. pp. 412-23.
18. Park K. Park's Textbook of Preventive and Social Medicine, 16th edition. Jabalpur: M/s Banarasidas Bhanot Publishers; 2000. pp. 631-46.
19. Roberton NRC. A manual of normal neonatal care. London: Edward Arnold; 1992. pp. 101-20.
20. Sala DJ. Effects of SLE on pregnancy and neonate. Journal of Perinatal and Neonatal Nursing. 1993;7(3):34-48.
21. Shabetai R. Congenital or acquired heart disease. In: Hollingsworth D (Ed). Medical counseling before Pregnancy, 1st edition. New York: Churchill Livingstone; 1988. pp. 229-35.
22. Smith JE. Pregnancy complicated by thyroid disease. Journal of Nurse-Midwifery. 1990; 35(3):143-9.
23. Snider DE Jr, Powell KE. Should women taking antituberculosis drugs breast-feed? Archives of Internal Medicine. 1984;144(3):589-90.
24. Streetly A, Dick M, Layton M. Sickle cell disease: the case of coordinated information. British Medical Journal. 1993;306(6891):1491-2.
25. Sugrue D, Drury MI. Hyperthyroidism complicating pregnancy: results of treatment by antithyroid drugs in 77 pregnancies. British Journal of Obstetrics and Gynaecology. 1980;87(11):970-5.
26. Torrance C. Absorption and function of iron. Nursing Standards. 1992;6(19):25-8.
27. Walfish PG, Chan JY. Post-partum hyperthyroidism. Clinics in Endocrinological Metabolism. 1985;14(2):417-20.
28. Wills DC, Caton D, Levelle JP, et al. Cardiac output response to prostaglandin E2-induced abortion in the second trimester. American Journal of Obstetrics and Gynecology. 1987;56(1):170-3.

Multiple Pregnancy

Learning Objectives

Upon completing this chapter, the learner will be able to:
- Describe the types of multiple pregnancies and the genesis of different varieties.
- Describe the diagnosis and management of twin pregnancy and labor.
- Describe the care of mother and babies after birth.
- Explain the problems specific to babies of multiple births and the fetal abnormalities unique to the process of multiplication.
- Explain the special needs of parents and nurses' role in management.

Multiple pregnancies are the development of more than one fetus at the same time in the gravid uterus. Simultaneous development of two fetuses is termed twins, which is the commonest. Although rare, simultaneously three fetuses (triplets), four fetuses (quadruplets), five fetuses (quintuplets) or six fetuses (sextuplets) may also develop.

INCIDENCE

The incidence varies widely. In the world, it varies from 5.6 to 46 per 1,000 births. It is highest in Nigeria, being 1 in 20 and lowest in far Eastern countries, being 1 in 200 pregnancies. In India, the incidence is about 1 in 80. While the incidence of monozygotic twins remains constant throughout the globe, being 1 in 250; it is the dizygotic twins, which are responsible for the wide variation of the incidence. Since 1980s, there has been a rise in the incidence due to the increased use of various kinds of treatments for infertility involving ovulation induction.

The number of triplets has more than trebled in the last 12 years due to the rise in infertility treatments such as in vitro fertilization (IVF) and ovulatory stimulating drugs like clomiphene citrate and gonadotropins.

TWIN PREGNANCY

Simultaneous development of two fetuses in the uterus is the most common variety of multiple pregnancies.

Varieties of Twins

1. Binovular twins: It is the most common (two-thirds) and results from the fertilization of two ova.
2. Uniovular twins (one-third) results from the fertilization of a single ovum.

Genesis of Twins

Binovular twins are also referred to as fraternal or dizygotic twins. They result from the fertilization of two ova, most likely ruptured from two different graafian follicles, usually of the same or one from each ovary, by two sperms during a single ovarian cycle. Their subsequent implantation and development differ little from those of single fertilized ovum. The babies bear only fraternal resemblance to each other (that of brothers and sisters from different births). Approximately one-third of the binovular twins may be boy pairs, one-third girl pairs and one-third boy-girl pairs.

Uniovular twins are also termed as identical or monozygotic twins. They develop from one ovum and one spermatozoon, and the twinning occurs at different periods after fertilization. The time at which the separation occurs is probably after the formation of the inner cell mass (between 4th and 8th day). Thus, two embryos will develop enclosed by a single chorion, having single placenta and two separate amniotic sacs (monochorionic, diamniotic). These twins will be of the same sex and have the same genes, blood groups and physical features such as eye and hair color, ear shapes and palm creases. However, they may be of different sizes and sometimes have different personalities.

Etiology

The cause of twinning is not known. Prevalence of binocular twins is related to:

1. *Race:* The frequency is highest amongst Negroes, lowest amongst Mongols and intermediate amongst Caucasians.
2. *Heredity:* There is hereditary predisposition likely to be more transmitted through the female.
3. *Advancing age of the mother:* Twinning increases with maternal age, peak being between 30 and 35 years.
4. *Influence of parity:* The incidence increases with parity, especially from fifth gravida onwards.
5. *Iatrogenic:* Drugs used for induction of ovulation may produce multiple fetuses to the extent of 20–40% following gonadotropin therapy and to a lesser extent (5–6%) following clomiphene citrate.

Rare Forms

Superfecundation: It is the fertilization of two different ova released in the same cycle, by separate acts of coitus within a short period of time.

Superfetation: It is the fertilization of two ova released in different menstrual cycles. The nidation and development of one fetus over another fetus is theoretically possible until the decidual space is obliterated by 12 weeks of pregnancy.

Fetus papyraceus or compressus: It is a state, which occurs if one of the fetuses dies early. The dead fetus is flattened and compressed between the membranes of the living fetus and the uterine wall. It may occur in both varieties, but is more common in uniovular twins and is discovered at delivery or earlier by sonography.

Fetus acardiacus: It occurs only in uniovular twins. Part of the fetus remains amorphous and becomes parasitic without a heart.

Vanishing twin: Occasional death of one twin and continuation of pregnancy with the surviving one. The dead fetus (if within 14 weeks) simply vanishes by resorption.

Determination of Zygosity

Determination of zygosity means determining whether or not the twins are identical.

Examination of Placenta and Membranes

Binovular twins
1. There are two placentae either completely separated or more commonly fused at the margin appearing to be one (9 out of 10). There is no anastomosis between the two fetal vessels.
2. Each fetus is surrounded by a separate amnion and chorion.
3. The intervening membranes consist of four layers—two amnions and two chorions.

Uniovular twins
1. The placenta is single. There is varying degree of free anastomosis between the two fetal vessels.
2. Each fetus is surrounded by a separate amniotic sac with the chorionic layer common to both (diamniotic, monochorionic).
3. The intervening membranes consist of two layers of amnion only **(Figs. 30.1A and B)**.

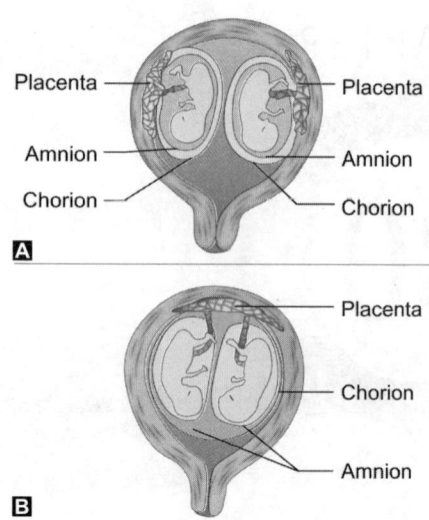

Figures 30.1A and B: Twin placentae. (A) Placenta of binovular (dizygotic) twins; (B) Placenta of uniovular (monozygotic) twins.

Sex
- Uniovular twins are always of the same sex
- Binovular twins may be of same sex or may differ.

Genetic Features (Dominant Blood Group)

If the fetuses are of the same sex and have the same genetic features (blood group), monozygosity is likely to occur.

Diagnosis of Twin Pregnancy

History
1. History of ovulation-inducing drugs, especially gonadotropins for infertility.
2. Family history of multiple pregnancies (more often in the maternal side).

Symptoms

Minor ailments of normal pregnancy are often exaggerated. Some of the symptoms are related to the abnormal enlargement of the uterus, which are:
1. Increased nausea and vomiting in early months.
2. Cardiorespiratory embarrassment in the later months such as palpitation or shortness of breath.
3. Tendency of swelling of the legs, varicose veins and hemorrhoids is greater.
4. Unusual rate of abdominal enlargement and excessive fetal movements may be noticed by an experienced parous mother.

General Examination
1. Prevalence of anemia is more, than in singleton pregnancy.
2. Unusual weight gain, not explained by preeclampsia or obesity.
3. Evidence of preeclampsia (in about 25%).

Possible Fetal Presentations in Twin Pregnancy

See **Figure 30.2**

Abdominal Examination

Inspection
1. The size of the uterus may be larger than expected for the period of gestation, particularly after the 20th week.
2. The uterus may be broad or round (barrel shape) and fetal movements may be seen over a wide area.
3. Fresh striae gravidarum may be apparent. Polyhydramnios is common.

Palpation
1. On palpation, the fundal height may be greater than expected for the period of gestation (evident from midpregnancy onwards).
2. The presence of two fetal poles (head or breech) in the fundus of the uterus.
3. Palpation of multiple fetal limbs.
4. The girth of the abdomen at the level of umbilicus is more than the normal average at term (100 cm).
5. Lateral palpation may reveal two fetal backs or limbs on both sides. Pelvic palpation may give findings similar to those on fundal palpation although one fetus may lie behind the other and make detection difficult. Location of three poles in total is diagnostic of at least two fetuses.

Auscultation
Simultaneous hearing of two distinct fetal heart sounds located at separate spots with a silent area in between two observers, gives a certain clue in the diagnosis of twins, provided the difference in the heart rates is at least 10 beats per minute.

Investigations

Ultrasound examination: Two gestational sacs can be detected as early as 10th week of pregnancy. Considering that one fetus may vanish; repeat sonar is done in second trimester. Detection of two fetal heads and their measurement of biparietal diameters can be made by the 14th week. For assessment of placentation, sonar is done between 16th and 24th week. Zygosity could be determined by identifying the intervening layers. For assessment of intrauterine growth restriction (IUGR), it should be repeatedly done at 4 weeks interval from the second half of pregnancy.

Radiography: It is done less often these days. Two fetal heads and spines could be seen on X-ray.

Duration of Pregnancy

A multiple pregnancy tends to be shorter than a single pregnancy. The average gestation for twins is 37 weeks, triplets 34 weeks and quadruplets 33 weeks.

Effects of Pregnancy

Maternal

During pregnancy
1. *Exacerbation of minor disorders:* Nausea and vomiting occurs with increased frequency and severity. Heartburn may be more persistent and troublesome than in singleton pregnancy.
2. *Anemia:* Iron deficiency and folic acid deficiency anemia are common in twin pregnancies. This is because of increased iron and folate requirements by the two

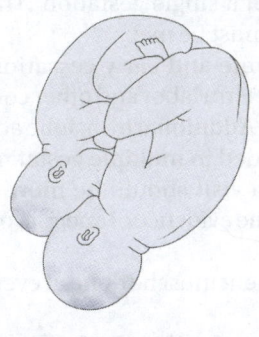
45% Vertex and vertex

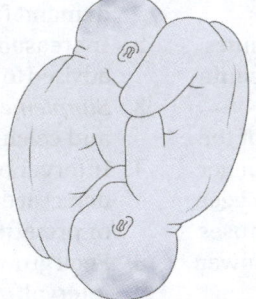
37% Vertex and breech

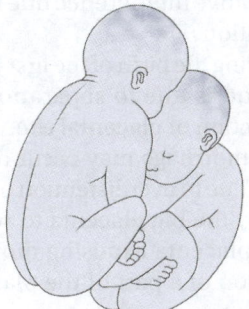
10% Breech and breech

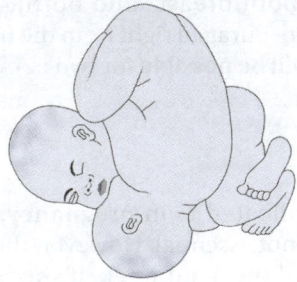
5% Vertex and transverse

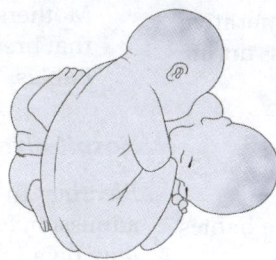
2% Breech and transverse

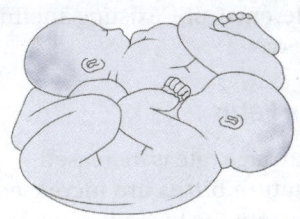
0.5% Transverse and transverse

Figure 30.2: Possible fetal presentations in twin pregnancy.

fetuses. Deficiency of folic acid (after 28th week) leads to increased incidence of megaloblastic anemia.
3. Preeclampsia (25%) is increased three times over singleton pregnancy. Overdistention of the uterus may be the possible explanation.
4. Antepartum hemorrhage may occur with slightly increased frequency. The increased incidence of placenta previa is due to the bigger size of the placenta encroaching onto the lower segment. Separation of the normally situated placenta may occur due to increased incidence of pregnancy-induced hypertension (PIH), sudden escape of liquor following rupture of the membranes of the hydramniotic sac, deficiency of folic acid and following delivery of the first baby due to sudden shrinkage of the uterine wall adjacent to the placental attachment.
5. Malpresentation is quite common in twins compared to singleton pregnancies. It is more common in the second baby.
6. Preterm labor (30%) frequently occurs and the mean gestational period for twins is 37 weeks. Overdistention of the uterus, hydramnios and premature rupture of the membranes are responsible for preterm labor.
7. Mechanical distress such as palpitation, dyspnea, varicosities and hemorrhoids may be increased. Increased weight and size of the uterus and impaired venous return from the lower limbs contribute to these discomforts. Backache and indigestion are common.

During labor
1. Early rupture of membranes and cord prolapse are likely to be increased due to increased prevalence of malpresentation. Cord prolapse is five times more common than in singleton pregnancy.
2. Increased operative interference due to high prevalence of malpresentation.
3. Bleeding following the birth of the first baby, may at times, be alarming and is due to separation of the placenta following reduction of placental site.
4. Postpartum hemorrhage may occur due to atony of the uterine muscle due to overdistention of the uterus; longer time is taken by the big placenta to separate the bigger surface of the placenta exposing more uterine sinuses and implantation of a part of the placenta in the lower segment.

During puerperium
1. There is increased incidence of subinvolution because of bigger size of the uterus.
2. Chances of infection are more because of operative interference, pre-existing anemia and blood loss during delivery.

Effects on Fetus

1. Miscarriage rate is increased.
2. Premature births are increased (80%) and the babies suffer from the hazards of prematurity.
3. *Growth problems (25%):* Weight difference of 25% or more may be seen. This may be due to twin-twin transfusion syndrome or intrauterine anomalies occurring in one fetus.
4. *Intrauterine death of one fetus:* This is increased in uniovular twin pregnancies. If a loss occurs early in gestation (before 14th week), the affected fetus simply vanishes by resorption. If the death occurs in the second trimester, a fetus papyraceus may form. If death occurs late in pregnancy, there may be death of the other fetus or it may complicate the mother with disseminated intravascular coagulation (DIC). The deaths are due to cord compression, competition for nourishment or congenital malformation.
5. Fetal anomalies are increased two folds over the singleton pregnancy, more in uniovular twins. They are in the form of anencephaly, hydrocephalus, cardiac anomalies or Down syndrome.
6. Asphyxia and stillbirth are more common due to increased prevalence of preeclampsia, malpresentation, placental abruption and increased operative interferences. The second baby is more at risk.

Antenatal Management

Early management of twin pregnancy is extremely important in order to prepare the parents by giving them the specialist support and advice they will need. This will help the mother to take additional care not only for her own benefit but also for the fetuses.

Advice

1. *Diet:* Increased dietary supplement is needed for increased energy supply to the extent of 300 kcal per day, over and above that needed in a single gestation. The increased demand for protein must be met.
2. Increased rest at home and early cessation of work is advised to prevent preterm labor and other complications.
3. *Supplement therapy:* Additional iron, folic acid, vitamins and calcium are needed in multiple gestation.
4. Interval of antenatal visit should be more frequent to detect at the earliest the evidence of anemia, preeclampsia or preterm labor.
5. Fetal growth assessment must be done at every 2–3 weeks interval.
6. *Preparation for breastfeeding:* Early in the antenatal period, the mother should be given as much information as possible about both breast- and bottle-feeding. Mothers should be encouraged right from the beginning that breastfeeding will be possible for two or even three babies.

Hospitalization

Elective: In an uncomplicated twin pregnancy, routine admission for bedrest is not essential. However, the woman may be admitted around the 32nd week, if she prefers it. Bedrest improves uteroplacental circulation. This results in increased birth weight of babies, decreased frequency of preeclampsia, decreased frequency of preterm labor and lowered perinatal mortality.

Emergency: Development of complicating factors necessitates urgent admission irrespective of the period of gestation.

Management during Labor

The higher the number of fetuses the mother is carrying, earlier the labor is likely to start. Term for twins is usually considered 37th week rather than 40 and approximately 30% of twins are born preterm that is before 37th week. As the twin pregnancy is considered a 'high-risk', the woman should be admitted in an equipped hospital preferably having an intensive neonatal care unit.

During the First Stage of Labor

1. The woman should be kept in bed and the enema withheld to prevent early rupture of membranes.
2. Use of analgesics is limited as the babies are small and rapid delivery may occur. Epidural analgesia is preferred as it facilitates manipulation of second fetus if it would become necessary.
3. Careful fetal monitoring of both babies should be done; continuous monitoring using electronic fetal monitor is better.
4. Vaginal examination should be done soon after the rupture of membranes to exclude cord prolapse.
5. An intravenous line with Ringer's solution should be set up for any urgent intravenous therapy, if required.
6. One unit of compatible and cross-matched blood should be made readily available.
7. Neonatologist should be present at the time of delivery.
8. If fetal distress occurs during labor, delivery will need to be expedited, usually by cesarean section.
9. If uterine activity is poor, the use of IV Syntocinon may be required once the membranes have been ruptured.
10. Artificial rupture of membranes may be sufficient to stimulate good uterine contractions, but may need to be used in conjunction with IV Syntocinon.
11. Throughout labor, the mother will require emotional as well as physical support from the midwife.

Management of Delivery (Second Stage)

The onset of second stage of labor should be confirmed by vaginal examination. The obstetrician, pediatrician and anesthetist should be present for the delivery because of the risk of complications. The possibility of emergency cesarean section is always present and the operating room should be ready to receive the mother at a short notice. Monitoring of both fetal hearts should continue until delivery. The delivery of the first twin should be conducted in the same manner as in normal labor if it presents by vertex. Liberal episiotomy is given to prevent intracranial damage to the fore-coming or after-coming head of the premature baby. When the first twin is born, the time of delivery and the sex are noted. The baby must be labeled as 'twin one' immediately.

After delivery of the first twin, abdominal palpation must be done to ascertain the lie, presentation and position of the second twin and to auscultate the fetal heart. A vaginal examination should be done to exclude cord prolapse, if any, and to note the status of the membranes. If the lie is not longitudinal, an attempt may be made to correct it by external cephalic version. If the presenting part is not engaged, it should be pushed into the pelvis by fundal pressure before the second sac of membranes are ruptured. If uterine activity does not recommence, IV oxytocin may be used to stimulate it.

When the presenting part becomes visible, the mother should be encouraged to push with contractions to deliver the second twin. Delivery will proceed as normal if the presentation is vertex. Delivery of the second twin must be completed within 45 minutes of the first twin as long as there are no signs of fetal distress. If there is delay, the baby is delivered, by ventouse or low forceps. If the baby presents by breech, breech extraction is done.

Methergine 0.2 mg is given intravenously with delivery of the anterior shoulder of the second baby. The baby is labeled as 'twin two' and the time of delivery and sex of the baby are noted. The risk of asphyxia is greater for the second baby and may require active resuscitation and transfer to the neonatal unit.

Management of the Third Stage

The placenta is to be delivered by cord traction applied to both cords simultaneously. It is important to deliver the placenta immediately, as emptying the uterus enables bleeding to be controlled and postpartum hemorrhage is prevented. Oxytocin drip is continued for at least 1 hour following the delivery of the second baby. The woman should be carefully watched for about 2 hours following delivery. A blood loss of more than average is often replaced by blood transfusion.

The placenta(e) should be examined and the number of amniotic sacs, chorions and placenta(e) are noted. The umbilical cords should be examined and the number of cord vessels and the presence of any abnormalities are noted.

Indications for Cesarean Section

Associated Causes

- Contracted pelvis
- Placenta previa
- Severe preeclampsia
- Previous history of cesarean section
- Cord prolapse of the first baby
- Abnormal uterine contractions.

Fetal Causes

- Both babies or even the first baby in transverse lie
- Non-vertex twins with estimated weight 2,000 g or less
- Conjoined twins
- Collision of both heads at brim preventing engagement of either head.

Complications Associated with Multiple Pregnancy

The high perinatal mortality associated with pregnancies is largely due to complications of pregnancy, such as premature onset of labor, intrauterine growth retardation and complications of delivery. The management of multiple pregnancies is concerned with prevention, early detection and treatment of these complications.

Polyhydramnios

Acute polyhydramnios may occur as early as 18th to 20th week. It may be associated with fetal abnormality and more likely due to the fetofetal transfusion syndrome (FFTS) also known as twin-to-twin transfusion syndrome (TTTS).

Fetofetal transfusion syndrome can be acute or chronic. The acute form usually occurs during labor in uniovular twins where one twin appears to bleed into the other through some kind of placental vascular anastomosis. Both fetuses may die of cardiac failure if not treated immediately.

Chronic FFTS can occur in up to 35% of monochorionic twin pregnancies. As a result, the receptor twin becomes larger, polycythemic and hypervolemic (hydrops) at the expense of the donor twin, which becomes smaller, anemic and hypovolemic. Difference of hemoglobin concentration between the two, usually exceeds 5 g% and estimated fetal discrepancy is 25% or more. The fetal and neonatal mortality is high, but some infants may be saved by early diagnosis and prenatal treatment with either amnioreduction (amniocentesis) or laser coagulation of communicating placental vessels.

The smaller twin generally has better outcome. The plethoric twin runs the risk of congestive cardiac failure and hydrops.

Fetal Abnormality

Fetal abnormality is particularly associated with monozygotic twins.

Conjoined twins (**Figs. 30.3A to C**) also called Siamese twins are twins joined in utero. The twins develop when an early embryo partially separates to form two individuals. Most conjoined twins are stillborn or die shortly after birth. Very few are born alive. Advances in surgery and technology have improved their survival rate. It is a very rare phenomenon and fewer than 5 thousand cases per year are reported in India.

Types of conjoined twins:
- Joined at thorax (Thoracopagus).
- Joined at the head (Craniopagus).

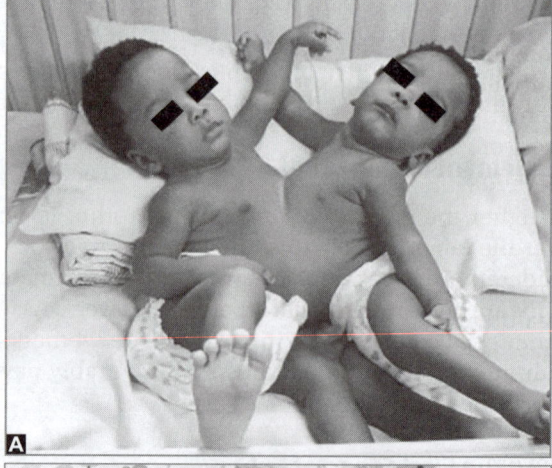
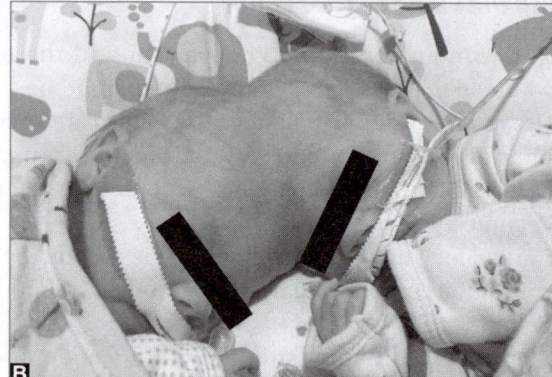
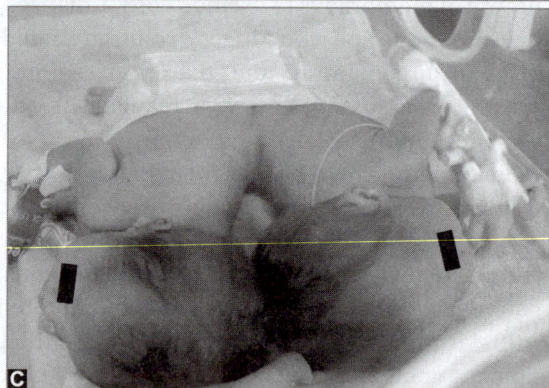

Figures 30.3A to C: Conjoined twins: (A) Joined at trunk level; (B) Heads joined; (C) Joined at heads facing opposite directions.

- Joined at the abdomen (Omphalopagus).
- Joined at the lower abdomen and pelvis (Ischiopagus).
- Joined from top of head down to umbilicus, facing each other (Cephalopagus).
- Joined at vertebral column (Rachipagus).

Acardiac formation: This occurs in about 1:30,000 deliveries. In acardia, one twin presents without a well-defined cardiac structure and is kept alive through placental anastomosis to the circulatory system of the viable fetus.

Fetus in fetu: In this, parts of a fetus may be lodged within another fetus. This can happen only in monozygotic twins.

Malpresentations

Although the uterus is large and distended, the fetuses are less mobile than may be supposed. They restrict each other's movements, which may result in malpresentations. After delivery of the first twin, the presentation of the second twin may change.

Premature Rupture of Membranes

Malpresentations due to polyhydramnios may predispose to premature rupture of the membranes.

Prolapse of the Cord

Prolapse of the cord is associated with malpresentations and polyhydramnios, and is more likely if there is a poorly fitting presenting part. The second twin is particularly at risk of cord prolapse.

Prolonged Labor

Malpresentations are a poor stimulus to good uterine action and distended uterus is likely to lead to the poor uterine activity and consequently prolonged labor.

Monoamniotic Twins

Approximately 1% of twins share the same amniotic sac. These twins risk cord entanglement with occlusion of the blood supply to one or both fetuses.

Locked Twins

Locked twins **(Figs. 30.4A and B)** is a rare, but serious complication of twin pregnancy. These are of two types. One occurs when the first twin presents by breech and the second by vertex, the other occurs when both are vertex. In both instances, the head of the second twin prevents the continued descent of the first. Interlocking occurs as the aftercoming head of the first baby is locked with the forecoming head of the second baby.

With two vertex twins, the heads get locked at the pelvic brim preventing engagement of either of the head. Cesarean section is necessary in these cases for fetal interest. Occasionally, with interlocked twins of the first type, decapitation of the first baby is done, if it is already dead. The decapitated head is pushed up, followed by delivery of the second baby and lastly, delivery of the decapitated head. This saves at least one baby.

Delay in the Birth of the Second Twin

After the birth of the first twin, uterine activity should commence within 5 minutes. Delivery of the second twin is usually completed within 45 minutes of the first birth. Delay may occur at times due to poor uterine action because of malpresentation. The risks of such delay are intrauterine hypoxia, birth asphyxia following premature separation of the placenta and sepsis as a result of ascending infection from the first umbilical cord, which lies outside the vulva.

The midwife may need to 'rub-up' a contraction and to put the first twin to the breast to stimulate uterine activity. If there appears to be an obstruction, cesarean section may be necessary. If there is no obstruction, Syntocinon infusion may be commenced and forceps delivery commenced.

Premature Expulsion of the Placenta

The placenta may be expelled before delivery of the second twin. In dizygotic twins with separate placenta, one may be delivered separately. In monozygotic twins, the shared placenta may be expelled and the risks of severe asphyxia and death of the second twin are then very high. Hemorrhage is also likely if one twin is retained in utero, as this prevents adequate retraction of the placental site.

Postpartum Hemorrhage

Poor uterine tone because of overdistention or hypotonic activity is likely to lead to postpartum hemorrhage.

Undiagnosed Twins

The possibility of an undiagnosed second baby should be considered if the uterus appears larger than expected after the delivery of the first baby, or if the baby is surprisingly smaller than expected. This is unlikely with ultrasound scanning facility. If an oxytocic drug has been given after delivery of the anterior shoulder of the first baby, the second baby is in great danger and delivery should be expedited. The baby will require active resuscitation because of severe asphyxia.

Management of Postnatal Period

Care of the Babies

Immediate care after delivery involves ensuring that both babies have clear airway. Maintenance of body temperature is vital, particularly if the newborns are small and use of overhead heater on the resuscitaire will help, if available. Proper drying and wrapping with warm baby blankets are important. Identification of the infants should be clear and parents must be given the opportunity to check the identity bracelets and cuddle their babies. The infants may have to be admitted directly to the neonatal unit from the labor

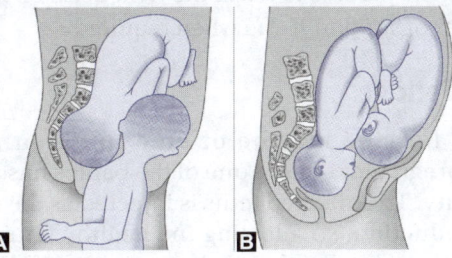

Figures 30.4A and B: Locked twins. (A) First twin breech, second twin vertex; (B) Both twins vertex.

ward and later transferred to the postnatal ward to be with the mother.

Both babies may be breastfed either simultaneously or separately. The mother may choose to feed the babies artificially. She may need help with the chosen method in the initial days. If the babies are small for dates or preterm, they may have to be fed with expressed breast milk or 'topped-up' after breastfeeding. At feeding time, the midwife must be with the mother to offer support and advice on positioning and fixing the babies as well as encouraging her to feed two babies. Using pillows to support the weight of the babies, the mother should be assisted to assume comfortable position for feeding. She might need the help of another person in the initial days whether the babies are breastfed or bottle-fed.

If the infants are of low birth weight, they are more susceptible to infection and hence the mother should be encouraged to wash her hands before handling her babies and particularly after changing their nappies.

Care of the Mother

Involution of the uterus will be slower because of its increased bulk. 'After pains' may be troublesome and analgesics must be given when she needs. If the mother is breastfeeding, a high-protein, high-calorie diet is required. She may feel hungry between meals and must be encouraged to keep snacks for such times.

In order to improve the muscle tone of the abdomen and pelvic floor, she must be instructed in postnatal exercises and encouraged to carry them out regularly. Teaching parenting skills will be important, as she will need to gain confidence in managing two babies.

One or both babies may sometimes remain in the nursery for few days. Mothers in such situations need assistance with visiting the babies, feeding and bonding. Postnatal depression has been shown to be slightly higher in twin mothers. Stress, isolation and exhaustion are all significant precipitants of depression, and mothers of twins are more bound to be vulnerable.

TRIPLETS AND HIGHER ORDER BIRTHS

Triplets may develop from fertilization of a single ovum or two, or even three ova; similarly with quadruplets and quintuplets. Female fetuses usually outnumber the male ones. The diagnosis is often accidental following sonography, radiography or during births. Clinical course and complications are intensified compared to twins. Perinatal loss is markedly increased due to prematurity. Preterm delivery is common (50%) and usually occurs by 22nd to 34th week. Discordance of fetal growth is more common than in twins. Perinatal loss is related to low birth weight.

The mode of delivery for triplets or more is nearly always by cesarean section. The midwives must be prepared to receive several small babies within a very short time span. The special dangers associated with these births are asphyxia, intracranial injury and perinatal death.

All mothers of triplets or more must arrange for extra practical help well before the babies are born. The emotional stress and anxiety of the birth, having babies in the neonatal unit, and worries or practical and financial help will all seem overwhelming, if no previous arrangements have been made.

DISABILITY AND BEREAVEMENT

Perinatal mortality and long-term morbidity are both more common among multiple births than singletons. The perinatal mortality rate for twins is about four times that of singletons and for triplets is about 12 times.

The grief of parents following the death of one of a multiple set, should not be underestimated. They often have conflicting emotions as they will feel and grieve for the child who has died, whilst wanting to rejoice at the birth of the healthy twin. They may need help in relating to the surviving baby. When one or more of a multiple set is disabled, often the healthy child needs special attention. As the healthy baby grows up, he/she may feel guilt for the disability of the other one, or feel resentful for the attention the other one needs or even the loss of twinship. Any of these may lead to emotional and behavioral problems if not addressed early on.

EMBRYO REDUCTION/SELECTIVE REDUCTION

Embryo reduction is the reduction of an apparently higher order multiple pregnancy down to two or even one embryo, so that the chances of survival are much higher.

This may be offered to parents who have conceived triplets or more, whether spontaneously or because of infertility treatment. The procedure is usually carried out between the 10th and 12th week of pregnancy. It is done by inserting a needle under ultrasound guidance via the vagina or more commonly through the abdominal wall into the fetal thorax. Potassium chloride or saline is used. All embryos remain in the uterus until delivery. Usually the pregnancy is reduced to two embryos, but in some cases to three or even one. Parents who are offered this treatment, must be offered counseling, which should include:

- ❖ The advantages and disadvantages of reducing pregnancy
- ❖ The risks of continuing with a higher multiple pregnancy
- ❖ The risks of embryo reduction
- ❖ The effects on the surviving children
- ❖ How parents may feel afterwards
- ❖ Help for the parents to reach the right decision for them
- ❖ The offer of support if and when required.

Selective Feticide

Selective feticide may be offered to parents with a multiple pregnancy, where one of the babies has a serious abnormality. The affected fetus is injected as described in embryo reduction, so allowing the healthy fetus to grow and develop normally. Counseling must be offered to the parents as for embryo reduction. The full impact of the procedure and their bereavement will not often be felt until the birth of their remaining baby/babies, many weeks later. At the time of delivery, the parents must be offered appropriate care and understanding in their bereavement.

STUDY QUESTIONS

Short Notes

1. Varieties of twins.
2. Fetofetal transfusion syndrome.
3. Conjoined twins.

Short Answer Questions

1. List the rare forms of multiple gestations.
2. Features for determination of zygosity on placenta and membranes.
3. Abdominal palpation findings suggestive of a twin pregnancy.

Essay Questions

1. Describe the nursing management of a client with twin pregnancy during labor and delivery (first, second and third stages).
2. Explain the types of locked twins and dangers of the condition.
3. Describe the immediate care of newborns following twin birth and special assistance to the mother.

BIBLIOGRAPHY

1. Dutta DC. Textbook of obstetrics, 5th edition. Kolkata: New Central Book Company; 2001. pp. 216-25.
2. Fisk N. Scientific basis of fetofetal transfusion syndrome and its treatment. In: Ward RH, Whittle M (Eds). Multiple Pregnancy. London: RCOG Press; 1995. p. 235.
3. Margie D. Multiple pregnancy. In: Bennet R, Brown K, Myles (Eds). Textbook for midwives, 13th edition. Edinburgh: Churchill Livingstone; 1999. pp. 351-8.
4. Moore TR, Gale S, Benirschke K. Perinatal outcome of forty-nine pregnancies complicated by acardiac twinning. American Journal of Obstetrics and Gynecology. 1990;163(3):907-12.
5. Parulekar SV. Textbook for midwives, 2nd edition. Bombay: Vora Medical Publications; 1998. pp. 385-92.
6. Thorpe K, Golding J, MacGillivray I, et al. Comparison of prevalence of depression in mothers of twins and mothers of singletons. British Medical Journal. 1991;302(6781):875-8.

CHAPTER 31

Preterm Labor, Premature Rupture of Membranes and Intrauterine Fetal Death

Learning Objectives

Upon completing this chapter, the learner will be able to:
- Describe the factors that contribute to premature labor.
- Describe the management of women during the different stages of preterm labor.
- Discuss the immediate care of preterm neonates.
- Describe the diagnosis and management of preterm rupture of membranes in different stages of pregnancy.
- Describe the diagnosis, management and care of woman who have intrauterine fetal death.

PRETERM LABOR

Definition

Preterm labor is defined as labor occurring before 37th completed week of pregnancy counting from the 1st day of the last menstrual period. The lower limit of gestation is not uniformly defined. In the developed countries, it has been brought down to 20 weeks; whereas in the developing countries, it is 28 weeks.

Causes

In more than 50% of cases, the cause of preterm onset of labor is not known. The following are however, related with increased incidence of preterm labor.

History
- Previous history of induced or spontaneous abortion or preterm delivery
- Asymptomatic bacteriuria or recurrent urinary tract infection
- Smoking habits
- Low socioeconomic and nutritional status.

Complications in Previous Pregnancy

Maternal
1. Pregnancy complications such as preeclampsia, antepartum hemorrhage, premature rupture of membranes and polyhydramnios.
2. Medical and surgical illnesses like acute fever, acute pyelonephritis, diarrhea, acute appendicitis, toxoplasmosis and abdominal operation.
3. Chronic diseases such as hypertension, diabetes, decompensated heart lesion, severe anemia.
4. Genital tract infections such as bacterial vaginosis, β-hemolytic *Streptococcus, Chlamydia, Mycoplasma*.

Fetal
Multiple pregnancy, congenital malformations, intrauterine death.

Placental
Infarction, thrombosis, placenta previa or abruption.

Idiopathic (majority)
Premature effacement of the cervix with a hyperirritable uterus and early engagement of the head. It is presumed that there is premature activation of the same system involved in initiating labor at term.

Presentation of the Woman

- Regular uterine contractions with or without pain (at least one in every 10 minute)
- Dilatation (>2 cm) and effacement (90%) of the cervix
- Pelvic pressure, backache and/or vaginal discharge.

Objectives of Management

The objectives of management are:
- To minimize the risk of perinatal mortality and morbidity
- To preserve maternal health.

Management Approaches

- To prevent preterm onset of the labor if possible
- To arrest preterm labor if not contraindicated
- Appropriate management of labor
- Effective neonatal care.

Prevention

In about 50% of cases, the cause remains unknown. For the remaining group, decision has to be taken whether to allow the pregnancy to continue or not. The risk of delivery of a low-birth-weight baby has to be weighed against the risks to the unborn or to the mother if pregnancy continues.

Preventive Measures

1. Identification of risk factors from the history and employing measures for rectification such as adequate rest, nutritional supplement, avoidance of smoking and encirclage operation, if required.
2. Premature effacement of cervix: The women are to be put to bedrest and tocolytic agents may be administered.
3. Selective continuation of complicated pregnancies such as twins, polyhydramnios, placenta previa, preeclampsia, etc. with rest and appropriate therapy. These patients are to be admitted in the hospital for close observation.
4. Confirming the gestational age before induction.

Investigations

- Full blood count
- Urine for routine analysis, culture and sensitivity
- Endocervical swab for any kind of causative organism
- Ultrasonography for fetal well-being, cervical length and placental location
- Serum electrolytes and glucose levels when tocolytic agents are to be used.

To Arrest Preterm Labor

Attempts to arrest preterm labor may be taken in about 10–20% of women where the fetus is not compromised, the maternal condition remains good and membranes are intact. The following regime may be instituted in an attempt to arrest premature labor:

- Adequate rest in bed; the woman is to lie preferably in left lateral position
- Adequate sedation is ensured with diazepam 5 mg orally or phenobarbitone 30–60 mg orally twice or thrice daily
- Adequate hydration is maintained
- Antibiotics are given if infection is evident or culture report suggests
- Tocolytic agents are administered to inhibit uterine contractions. Tocolytic agents can be used as short-term (1–3 day) or long-term therapy.

Short-term Therapy

Short-term therapy is used:
1. To delay delivery for at least 24 hours, glucocorticoid therapy for mother to enhance fetal lung maturation, if premature labor starts before 34th week.
2. To enable transfer of the woman with the baby in utero to a unit more able to manage a preterm neonate.

Long-term Therapy

Long-term therapy is instituted if pregnancy is to be prolonged for at least 1 week following established onset of labor prior to 34th week.

Glucocorticoid therapy
Maternal administration of glucocorticoids is advocated where the pregnancy is less than 34 weeks. This helps in fetal lung maturation, so that the incidence of respiratory distress syndrome can be minimized. Either betamethasone (Betnesol) 12 mg IM at every 12 hours for two doses or dexamethasone (Decadron) 8 mg IM at every 12 hours, three doses is given. If the delivery is delayed for more than 7 days after the injection, treatment must be repeated.

Management of Preterm Labor

Labor is judged to have started when the woman experiences regular, painful uterine contractions accompanied by either bloody show, rupture of membranes or complete effacement of the cervix. The principles in the management of preterm labor are:
1. To prevent asphyxia, which makes the neonate more susceptible to respiratory distress syndrome (RDS).
2. To prevent birth trauma.

First Stage

1. The woman is put to bed to prevent early rupture of membranes.
2. Oxygen is given by mask to ensure adequate fetal oxygenation.
3. Strong sedatives or acceleration of labor is to be avoided. Epidural analgesia is the choice.
4. Progress of labor should be monitored clinically or (preferably) by electronic monitoring.
5. In case of delay or anticipating a tedious traumatic vaginal delivery, it is better to deliver by cesarean section.

Second Stage

1. The birth should be gentle and slow to avoid rapid compression and decompression of fetal head.
2. Liberal episiotomies should be done under local anesthesia, especially in primigravida to minimize head compression.
3. Tendency to delay must be curtailed by low forceps.
4. The cord must be clamped immediately at birth to prevent the development of hypervolemia and hyperbilirubinemia.

5. Place the baby in intensive neonatal care unit under the care of a neonatologist.

Preterm fetuses before 34th week presented by breech, are generally delivered by cesarean section.

Immediate Management of the Preterm Baby Following Birth

1. The cord is to be clamped quickly to prevent hypervolemia and development of hyperbilirubinemia.
2. The cord length should be about 10–12 cm in case exchange transfusion will be required due to hyperbilirubinemia.
3. The air passage should be cleared of mucus promptly and gently. The stomach contents are also to be sucked out.
4. Adequate oxygenation must be provided.
5. The baby should be wrapped in a sterile warm blanket or towel, or laid in the warmer with the head slightly lowered (temperature 36.5°C–37.5°C).
6. Vitamin K 1 mg to be injected intramuscularly to prevent hemorrhagic manifestations.
7. Bathing is not appropriate for the preterm baby.

Preterm babies are functionally immature and need special care for their survival.

Support for the Mother

The attendance of a support person throughout labor is crucial. This is usually the midwife who will monitor the maternal and fetal well-being as well as provide psychological support. An individual approach to care and instructions during labor will be required. It is quite important to communicate with the woman effectively, evaluate whether labor is progressing as expected and listen to her requests. Once the baby is born, the mother will be anxious about the baby's condition and appropriate communication must be maintained. The mother must be given the opportunity to see the baby prior to transfer to the nursery.

PREMATURE RUPTURE OF MEMBRANES

Synonym: Prelabor rupture of membranes.

Definition

Spontaneous rupture of membranes any time beyond 28th week of pregnancy and before the onset of spontaneous uterine activity resulting in cervical dilation is called 'premature rupture of membranes' (PROM). When rupture of membranes occurs beyond 37th week, but before the onset of labor, it is called term 'premature rupture of membranes' and when it occurs before 37 completed weeks, it is called 'preterm premature rupture of membranes' (PPROM).

Incidence

Premature rupture of membranes occurs in approximately 10% of all pregnancies.

Causes

In majority, the causes are not known. Possible causes are:
- Increased friability of membranes
- Decreased tensile strength of membranes
- Polyhydramnios
- Cervical incompetence
- Multiple pregnancies
- Infection such as chorioamnionitis, urinary tract infection and lower genital tract infection.

Manifestations

The only manifestation is the escape of watery discharge per vagina either in the form of a gush or slow leak.

Confirmation of diagnosis is done by employing the following methods:
1. Speculum examination to inspect the liquor escaping out through the cervix.
2. Examination of the fluid collected from the posterior fornix (vaginal pool) for:
   a. Detection of pH by litmus or nitrazine paper. The pH becomes 6–6.2 (normal vaginal pH during pregnancy is 4.5–5.5, whereas that of liquor amnii is 7–7.5).
   b. To note the characteristic ferning pattern when a smeared slide is examined under microscope.

Risks of PROM

The implications are less serious when the rupture occurs near term than earlier in pregnancy:
1. In 'term PROM', labor starts in 80%–90% of cases within 24 hours. PROM is one of the important causes of preterm labor and prematurity.
2. Chances of ascending infection are more if labor fails to start within 24 hours. Liquor gets infected (chorioamnionitis), which may be followed by fetal and maternal systemic infection.
3. Increased incidence of cord prolapse, especially when associated with malpresentation.
4. Continuous escape of liquor for long duration may lead to dry labor.
5. Fetal pulmonary hypoplasia, especially in preterm PROM when associated with oligohydramnios.
6. Primary antepartum hemorrhage.

Ultrasonography is done to assess the fetal well-being.

Management

If PROM is suspected, the woman is admitted to the labor room:
1. Careful history is taken.
2. A sterile speculum examination is done to check the pooling of liquor in the posterior fornix, to note the state of the cervix and to detect any cord prolapse.
3. Patient is put to bedrest and sterile vulval pad is applied to look for leakage.

4. A digital vaginal examination should be avoided to reduce the risk of infection.
5. Fetal heart rate is checked to assess the fetal condition (an infected fetus may have a tachycardia).
6. Maternal pulse, temperature, uterine tenderness and any offensive smelling discharge are observed, and noted.

Once the diagnosis is confirmed, management depends on:
- Gestational age of the fetus
- Whether the woman is in labor or not
- Any evidence of sepsis
- Prospect of fetal survival if delivery occurs.

Term PROM

If the pregnancy is 38 weeks, the woman is not in labor and there is no evidence of fetal distress, she is observed in the hospital. Generally, in 90% of cases, spontaneous labor starts in 24 hours. If labor does not start in 24 hours, induction of labor is commenced with oxytocin. Cesarean section is performed for obstetric reasons (non-cephalic presentations).

Preterm PROM

If the pregnancy is less than 34 weeks, the fetus appears to be uncompromised and antepartum hemorrhage (APH), and labor have been excluded, she will be managed expectantly for fetal maturity.

If the gestational age is 34 weeks or more, spontaneous labor is awaited for 24–48 hours. If labor does not commence, induction with oxytocin is instituted. For presentations other than cephalic, cesarean section is chosen. On rare occasions, the leak seals spontaneously (especially if it is hind water leak) and the pregnancy continues.

If the membranes rupture before 24 weeks of gestation, the outlook is not good; the fetus is likely to succumb either to the problems caused by oligohydramnios or to those caused by preterm birth. Prophylactic antibiotics are given to minimize maternal and perinatal risks of infection. Oral ampicillin 500 mg is given 6 hourly for 3 days. Infection is evident by maternal tachycardia, rise in temperature, uterine tenderness, leukocytosis and bacterial growth from vaginal swab. Intravenous ampicillin or cephradine along with metronidazole is administered in case of chorioamnionitis.

Psychological consideration of the woman and her spouse must be considered vital, as it is an extremely disturbing situation for them. Understanding care, adequate explanations and support from caregivers are required as the decisions for management are taken and executed.

INTRAUTERINE FETAL DEATH

Intrauterine fetal death (IUD) includes antepartum deaths occurring beyond 28th week of gestation and usually results in the delivery of a macerated fetus.

Etiology

Fetal deaths during pregnancy are related to a number of maternal and/or fetal complications, which produce either chronic or acute placental insufficiency. However, in about 20–30% of cases, the cause remains unknown.

Pregnancy Complications

1. *Preeclampsia:* Spasm of the uteroplacental vessels leads to reduction of placental blood flow and placental insufficiency.
2. *Antepartum hemorrhage:* Both placenta previa and abruptio placentae can cause fetal death by producing acute placental insufficiency. Abruptio placentae will cause more deaths than placenta previa with identical area of separation because of frequent association with preeclampsia.

Pre-existing Medical Diseases and Acute Illnesses during Pregnancy

1. *Chronic hypertension:* It produces chronic placental insufficiency and is usually less lethal, unless preeclampsia supervenes.
2. *Diabetes:* Long-standing diabetes with atherosclerotic changes in the pelvic blood vessels may lead to chronic placental insufficiency and death of fetus. Associated preeclampsia, polyhydramnios, congenital malformation and maternal ketosis are some of the factors responsible.
3. *Chronic nephritis:* Continuation of pregnancy beyond the period of viability is rare and fetal death occurs due to massive placental infarction.
4. *Syphilis:* Though it is rare nowadays, but produces fetal deaths by the spirochete affecting the placenta and the fetus.
5. *Hyperpyrexia (malaria):* Acute fever of the mother over 39.4°C can kill the fetus directly.
6. Severe anemia may cause fetal death in some cases through maternal anoxemia.
7. *Other rare causes:* Hepatitis (viral), toxoplasmosis, malaria, poliomyelitis, mumps, etc.

Fetal Causes

1. *Congenital malformation:* A fetus with gross congenital malformations, incompatible with extrauterine independent existence is more vulnerable to die in utero.
2. *Rh-incompatibility:* Excessive hemolysis of fetal blood by antibodies formed in the mother produces fetal anemia, anoxia and heart failure.
3. *Postmaturity:* Unexpected death may occur during pregnancy due to placental insufficiency, however, the risk is more during labor.

Iatrogenic

1. *External version:* It may result in a true knot of the cord or entanglement of the cord round the neck or limbs of the fetus.
2. Quinine group of drugs if administered in higher than therapeutic doses.

Idiopathic

1. In about 20–30% cases, the cause remains undetermined and is attributed to placental insufficiency.
2. Sometimes intrauterine fetal deaths recur in subsequent pregnancies.

Signs and Symptoms

Repeated examinations are often required to confirm the diagnosis:
1. Absence of fetal movements, which were previously experienced by the woman.
2. Retrogression of the breast changes that occur during pregnancy.
3. Gradual retrogression of the height of the uterus, so that it becomes smaller than the period of amenorrhea.
4. Uterine tone is diminished and the uterus feels flaccid. Braxton-Hicks contractions are not easily felt.
5. Fetal movements are not felt during palpation.
6. Fetal heart sounds, which were audible before, is absent. Doppler effect of ultrasound is a better alternative to ordinary stethoscope.
7. Eggshell crackling like feel of fetal head, if elicited is more indicative of the diagnosis.

Investigations

1. *Sonography:* Evidences of fetal death are lack of fetal movement (including cardiac) during a 10-minute period of careful observation, oligohydramnios and collapsed cranial bones.
2. Straight X-ray abdomen may reveal the following features in varying degree either singly or in combination:
   a. Spalding sign (*refer* **Fig. 16.2**): The irregular overlapping of the cranial bones one on another due to liquefaction of the brain matter and softening of the ligamentous structures supporting the vault. It usually appears 7 days after death.
   b. Hyperflexion of the spine and in some cases hyperflexion of the neck are seen.
   c. Crowding of the ribs shadow with loss of normal parallelism.
   d. Appearance of gas shadow (Robert's sign) in the chambers of the heart and great vessels may be seen as early as 12 hours after death.

Complications

1. *Extreme psychological upset of the woman:* She will need enormous amount of support to deal with the problem.
2. *Infection:* As long as the membranes remain intact, infection is unlikely, but once the membranes rupture, infection, especially by gas-forming organisms like *Clostridium perfringens* may occur.
3. *Blood coagulation disorders:* If the fetus is retained for more than 4 weeks (as occurs in 10–20% cases), there is possibility of defibrination from silent DIC. It is due to gradual absorption of thromboplastin, liberated from the dead placenta and decidua into the maternal circulation.
4. *During labor:* Uterine inertia, retained placenta and postpartum hemorrhage.

Prevention

While IUD cannot be totally prevented, prenatal care and monitoring can help to reduce the incidence:
1. Regular antenatal care to prevent and detect early conditions that contribute to IUD and instituting effective therapy.
2. Screening the 'at-risk mothers' for fetal well-being and to terminate the pregnancy at the earliest evidences of fetal compromise.

Management

Expectant Management (Noninterference)

In about 80% of cases, spontaneous expulsion occurs within 2 weeks of fetal death. The woman may remain at home with the advise to come to the hospital for delivery. If spontaneous expulsion fails to occur within 2 weeks, the woman is to be admitted. Fibrinogen estimation is done every week and a falling fibrinogen level, approaching 150 mg%, should be arrested by infusion of heparin. The woman and her family are likely to be upset psychologically and should be assured of safety of noninterference.

Interference

Indications of interference are:
- Manifestations of uterine infection
- Falling fibrinogen level
- Tendency of prolongation of pregnancy beyond 2 weeks.

Early termination is now preferred as reliable diagnosis could be made with ultrasonography and prostaglandins are available for effective induction.

Termination of pregnancy is done by medical induction. Vaginal administration of prostaglandin (PGE_2) gel in the posterior fornix is used effectively where the cervix is unfavorable. The procedure may be repeated after 6–8 hours. The procedure may be supplemented with oxytocin infusion.

Oxytocin infusion is widely practiced and effective in cases where the cervix is favorable. To begin with 5–10 units of oxytocin in 500 mL of Ringer's solution is administered through intravenous drip. Consecutive two bottles may be administered at a time. In case of failure, a higher dose is administered on the following day. Oxytocin of 20 units in 500 mL of Ringer's solution are run at 30 drops per minute (80 mU/min). The strength of the drip may be increased to 40 units after the first bottle, if contractions fail to start. More than two bottles should not be administered at one time because of the risk of antidiuretic effect. If the uterus still does not respond, the procedure is repeated after vaginal administration of prostaglandins.

Cesarean section is done only for those with major placenta previa, transverse lie or two or more previous cesarean sections.

Bereavement Management

The mother who has given birth to a dead baby suffers a great deal of emotional burden. This may be compounded by the process of maceration having changed the baby's appearance. The midwife should provide all the support and sympathy to the bereaved couple. Lactation is usually suppressed with bromocriptine (Parlodel) 2.5 mg twice daily for 10 days. Counseling for future pregnancies is to be done at the time of postpartum checkup after 6 weeks.

STUDY QUESTIONS

Short Notes

1. Preterm labor.
2. Premature rupture of membranes.
3. Preventive measures for intrauterine fetal death.

Short Answer Questions

1. Important measures in the immediate care of a preterm baby.
2. Causes of the premature rupture of membranes.

Essay Questions

1. A 28-year-old client has started labor contractions at 35 weeks gestation. Describe the management measures in first and second stages of labor.
2. Describe the risks of premature rupture of membranes and management of a client admitted in labor room with the condition.
3. Explain the manifestations of intrauterine fetal death and management of a client, and family facing the situation.

BIBLIOGRAPHY

1. Dutta DC. Textbook of obstetrics, 5th edition. Kolkata: New Central Book Company; 2001. pp. 334-47.
2. Gunn GC, Mishell DR, Morton DG. Premature rupture of the fetal membranes: a review. American Journal of Obstetrics and Gynecology. 1970;106(3):469-83.
3. Hameed C, Tejani N, Verma UL, et al. Silent chorioamnionitis as a cause of preterm labor refractory to tocolytic therapy. American Journal of Obstetrics and Gynecology. 1984;149(7):726-30.
4. Kappy KA, Cetrulo CL, Knuppl RA, et al. Premature rupture of the membranes: a conservative approach. American Journal of Obstetrics and Gynecology. 1979;134(6):655-61.

CHAPTER 32

Post-term Pregnancy, Induction of Labor, Prolonged Labor and Disorders of Uterine Action

> **Learning Objectives**
>
> Upon completing this chapter, the learner will be able to:
> - Discuss the diagnosis and management of post-term pregnancy.
> - Review the indications for induction of labor and the various methods used.
> - Describe how uterine dysfunction may result in a prolonged labor or a precipitate labor.
> - Discuss the serious complications of obstructed labor, which may result in morbidity or mortality of mother or baby or both.
> - Describe the role of the midwife in the care and management of such situations.

POST-TERM PREGNANCY

Synonym: Prolonged pregnancy.

Post-term pregnancy is defined as one that exceeds 294 days calculating from the 1st day of the last menstrual period. The pregnancy continues beyond 2 weeks of the expected date of delivery. The terms 'prolonged pregnancy' and 'post-term pregnancy' are used synonymously, and relate to the duration of pregnancy. 'Postmaturity' and 'postmature' are terms that relate to the neonate, and refer to features and conditions of the baby.

Incidence

The incidence of post-term pregnancy averages about 10%.

Etiology

The exact cause of the prolonged pregnancy is not clear, but certain factors are seen related:
1. Hereditary factors: The condition often runs in family and often manifests in consecutive pregnancies in the same individual.
2. High standards of living with sedentary habits often tend to prolong pregnancy.
3. Elderly primigravida or elderly multiparae are more likely to have prolonged pregnancy.
4. Anencephaly without polyhydramnios.

Diagnosis

Menstrual History

If the woman is sure about her date with previous history of regular cycles, it is a reliable diagnostic aid in the calculation of the period of gestation. However, in cases of pregnancy occurring during lactational amenorrhea or soon following withdrawal of the pill, difficulty arises. In such cases previously documented antenatal records of first visit may help.

Clinical Findings

Clinical findings, which are evident when an otherwise uncomplicated pregnancy overrun the expected date by 2 weeks are:
1. *Weight loss*: The regular periodic weight checking shows stationary or even falling weight.
2. *Girth of the abdomen*: The normally, the girth of the abdomen at the level of umbilicus increases steadily up to the completion of 38th week and then remains steady up to term. Thereafter, the girth gradually diminishes because of diminishing liquor amnii.
3. *History of false pain*: Appearance of false pain followed by a subsidence with continuation of pregnancy is suggestive. The false pain is presumed to coincide with the expected date.
4. *Abdominal palpation*: As liquor amnii diminishes there may be changes in the height of the fundus, size of the fetus and hardness of the skull bones. The uterus 'full of fetus' is a feature usually associated with post-term pregnancy.
5. *Internal examination*: Feeling of hard bones either through the cervix or through the fornix usually suggests maturity.

6. *Ultrasonography*: In early pregnancy, this can be used to assess the duration of pregnancy and fetal age. Measurements taken in the first or second trimesters have been found to be accurate within 5 days in 95% cases. Crown-rump length (CRL), biparietal diameter (BPD) and femur length (FL) are the measurements of choice for assessment of fetal age. Composite biometry is of more value in the assessment of maturity of the fetus.
7. *Straight X-ray abdomen*: Overall fetal shadow, thickness and density of the skull bone shadow, appearance, and density of the ossification centers in the upper end of the tibia and lower end of the femur are taken together to assess the maturity.

Clinical Presentation for Retrospective Diagnosis

In addition to the increased length of gestation at which the baby is delivered, the following criteria have been used to establish the diagnosis of post-term pregnancy retrospectively, i.e. after the birth of the baby:
1. *General appearance:* Baby looks thin and old. There is absence of vernix caseosa. Body and the cord are stained with greenish yellow color. Head is hard without much evidence of molding. Nails are protruding beyond the nail beds.
2. *Liquor amnii:* Scanty and may be saffron colored with meconium.
3. *Placenta:* There is evidence of aging of the placenta manifested by excessive infarction and calcification.
4. *Cord:* There is diminished quantity of Wharton's jelly, which may precipitate cord compression.
5. *Macrosomia:* Birth weight of 4 kg or more occurs in about 10% cases.

Dangers of Post-term Pregnancy

During Pregnancy

There is chance for fetal hypoxia due to placental insufficiency, as the pregnancy overruns the expected date. Placental aging leads to diminished placental function with resultant fetal hypoxia. The hypoxic state may be aggravated by such associated factors as elderly woman, hypertensive disorders in pregnancy and history of bleeding during pregnancy.

During Labor

There is increased incidence of asphyxia and intracranial damage due to:
1. Aggravation of pre-existing hypoxia leading to increased fetal distress.
2. Increased incidence of difficult labor due to big size baby, nonmolding of the head due to hardening of the skull bones and occasional shoulder dystocia.
3. Increased incidence of operative delivery.
4. Cord compression related to scanty liquor amnii and less Wharton's jelly in the cord.

Following Birth

1. Meconium aspiration syndrome and atelectasis as the result of intrauterine anoxia and consequent inhalation of meconium containing liquor amnii.
2. Low Apgar scores.
3. Hypoglycemia and polycythemia occur in growth retarded post-term babies.

All these factors lead to increased perinatal loss, the magnitude of which is doubled at 43rd week and tripled at 44th week compared to that delivered at term.

There is increased maternal morbidity related to hazards of induction, instrumental and operative delivery.

Management of Post-term Pregnancy

The management of post-term pregnancy takes into account, the increased risk to the fetus as pregnancy lengthens. Two forms of care are generally offered, expectant management with fetal surveillance or elective induction of labor before 42nd week of gestation. Both aim to diminish the jeopardy to the fetus.

Expectant Management

1. *Biophysical profile*: Ultrasound assessment of fetal breathing, fetal movement, fetal tone, reactivity of the heart rate and amniotic fluid volume could be used to predict fetal well-being in a high-risk pregnancy.
2. *Cardiotocography (CTG) or non-stress testing*: Fetal heart rate (FHR) is monitored weekly and the monitor strip is assessed for the presence of reactivity and whether the baseline rate is within the normal range.
3. *Amniotic fluid measurement*: Measurements are taken in several perpendicular planes to make the diagnosis of oligohydramnios. Intervention is indicated if the amniotic fluid volume falls below 30 mm.

Elective Induction

The active approach to post-term pregnancy or one approaching the upper limits of term is for the mother to have labor induced. It is done between 10 and 14 days, and a little earlier in primigravida.

If the cervix is favorable (ripe), induction is done by stripping the membranes by low rupture of the membranes. If the liquor amnii is found clear, oxytocin infusion is added to make it more effective. Careful fetal monitoring is mandatory. If the liquor amnii is thickly meconium stained, suggestive of chronic placental insufficient, cesarean section is performed.

If the cervix is unripe, it is made favorable by vaginal administration of prostaglandins (PGE_2 gel). This is followed by low rupture of membranes (LRMs). Oxytocin infusion is added when required.

When postmaturity is associated with complicating factors like contracted pelvis, postcesarean pregnancy, malpresentation, elderly primigravida, etc. an elective cesarean section is done.

Associated complications of pregnancy that are likely to produce placental insufficiency such as preeclampsia, history of bleeding during pregnancy, diabetes and Rh-negative pregnancy should not be allowed to go beyond the expected date and termination to be done either by induction or cesarean section as appropriate.

Care during Labor

Whether spontaneous or induced, the labor may be prolonged because of a big baby and poor molding of the head. More analgesia is required for pain relief. Possibility of shoulder dystocia is present. Careful fetal monitoring must be done with available gadgets. If fetal distress appears, prompt delivery either by cesarean section or by forceps is to be done. Psychological care and measures to prevent maternal exhaustion must be taken.

INDUCTION OF LABOR

Induction of labor is the stimulation of uterine contractions before the onset of spontaneous labor. It is an obstetric intervention that should be used when elective birth will be beneficial to mother and baby. The purpose of induction is to effect the birth of the baby. Successful induction depends on adequate contractions, which are effective in bringing about progressive dilatation of the cervix. The procedure is more likely to be successful when the cervix is ripe, i.e. it has undergone structural changes to produce softening, dilatation and effacement.

Indications for Induction

Induction is indicated when the benefits to the mother or the fetus outweigh those of continuing the pregnancy and it is associated with the following maternal, fetal or combined factors.

Maternal Indications

1. *Prolonged or post-term pregnancy:* This is the main indication for induction of labor.
2. *Previous history of unexplained intrauterine death:* Timely intervention provides an opportunity to avert the repetition of the disaster.
3. *Medical problems:* Woman with concurrent renal, respiratory or cardiac disease may require induction of labor.
4. Intrauterine death of the fetus.
5. Chronic polyhydramnios with maternal distress.
6. *Congenital malformation of the fetus:* For psychological reasons and to minimize the complications, termination is preferable to continuation of pregnancy. However, the pregnancy should be continued until such time when the induction is more likely to be successful.

Fetal Indications

- Chronic placental insufficiency leading to growth retardation of the fetus

- Rh isoimmunization
- Unstable lie—after correcting into longitudinal lie
- Diabetes mellitus
- Postmaturity.

Combined Indications

Continuation of pregnancy may adversely affect both the mother and the baby:
1. Preeclampsia and eclampsia.
2. Minor degree of placenta previa.
3. Abruptio placentae: Early termination saves the mother from untoward complications like blood coagulation disorders and anuria. The baby can also be saved.
4. Premature rupture of membranes.
5. Chronic hypertension.

Contraindications to Induction of Labor

- Contracted pelvis and cephalopelvic disproportion
- Persistent malpresentation such as transverse or compound presentations
- Pregnancy with previous cesarean section
- Elderly primigravida especially associated with obstetric or medical complicating factors
- High-risk pregnancy with compromised fetus
- Cord presentation or cord prolapse
- Placenta previa
- Pelvic tumor.

In these circumstances, if delivery is imperative, it should be effected by cesarean section.

Dangers of Induction

Apart from the inherent hazards of the methods employed, the following are the dangers of induction. The hazards are however, to be weighed against the possible risks of continuation of pregnancy to the mother and/or the fetus due to the complication for which induction is contemplated.

Maternal

1. Psychological upset, more so when there is failure for which cesarean section is contemplated.
2. Tendency of prolonged labor due to abnormal uterine action.
3. Increased need of analgesia during labor.
4. Increased operative interference.
5. Increased morbidity.

Fetal

1. Iatrogenic prematurity.
2. The hypoxia due to disordered uterine action, prolonged labor and operative interference.

Methods of Ripening of the Cervix

The cervix is normally two centimeters long, firm and closed throughout pregnancy. Its shape is tubular with a rigid structure designed to retain the fetus within the uterus until term. Maturation of the cervix is the result of physiological processes that soften, efface and dilate the cervix prior to the onset of labor. This begins as much as 5–6 weeks prior to labor.

The ripeness of the cervix can be effectively achieved by employing the following methods:
1. Prostaglandin (PGE_2) used either in the form of gel 500 µg intracervical or 1–2 mg in the posterior fornix, or in the form of a pessary 3 mg in the posterior fornix. The application may have to be repeated after 6–8 hours. Loosening of the cervical collagen fibers occurs following its application. Labor will start in 30%–50% of cases.
2. *Stripping of the membranes:* It is possible if one finger can be introduced through the cervix. In order to carry-out the procedure, a vaginal examination with some cervical stretching is needed.
3. Oxytocin infusion may be used with some success. However, on occasion, labor starts following the use of any of the method.

Assessment of the Cervix

In order to decide on the method of induction, assessment of the cervix is required. A preinduction score using the Bishop's score is done **(Table 32.1)**. Key elements in the assessment are dilatation, effacement, position, consistency and station of the presenting part. Five different features are considered and each is awarded a score of between 0 and 3. When a score of 6 or over is reached, the prognosis for induction is good.

Labor Induction and Bishop score

The Bishop score is used primarily as a "preinduction" cervical assessment tool. For a woman to have a successful vaginal birth, her cervix must be soft, effaced and dilated. Bishop score is known as a "cervical scoring system" developed by Dr E Bishop in 1964 to determine if a woman is a good candidate for labor induction (cervical favorability).

Indications of the Bishop's Score Measurement

1. The fetal station measures the baby's descent in the pelvis. A fetus is said to be at "zero station", when it has reached the zero line—an imaginary line between the two ischial spines of pelvic bone. The baby's position above the zero line is always a "minus" station and its positions below the zero lines are "plus stations". Stations go from – 5 at the pelvic inlet (entrance to the true pelvis) to + 4 at the pelvis outlet (inferior opening of the pelvis).
2. Cervical dilatation is measured in centimeters (some health professionals express it in fingers). A pregnant woman's cervix is fully open when it is dilated to 10 centimeters. The cervix begins to dilate days before a woman goes in to labor. Normally, once active labor sets in, dilation proceeds at a much faster pace. Cervical dilation measurements go from "0" centimeters (closed cervix) to 10 centimeters.
3. Cervical effacement refers to the thinning and shortening of the cervix, which changes the "shape" of the birth canal from a tube into a flaring tunnel. Effacement is measured in percent. The cervix of a woman who is not pregnant is "0 percent" effaced. When a pregnant woman's cervix is 50% effaced, it is half its original thickness. When 100% effaced, the cervix is completely thinned out and the mother is ready for vaginal delivery.
4. Position refers to position of the cervix. During pregnancy, the mother's cervix points backwards (it is in posterior position). Towards the end of pregnancy the cervix will come forward (anterior position). An anterior position is more favorable for vaginal delivery than a posterior position.
5. *Cervical consistency:* The softer the cervix is, the better the chance of vaginal delivery. Consistency is measured on a scale of firmness (firm, medium and soft). To determine a woman's Bishop Score, each of the five components listed above is given a score of 0 to 2 or 0 to 3. The highest possible score is 13.

Methods of Induction

- Medical
- Surgical
- Combined.

Medical Induction

1. Oxytocin induction.
2. Prostaglandin induction.

Indications for medical induction are:
- Intrauterine death of fetus
- Premature rupture of membranes

TABLE 32.1: Bishop's preinduction scoring system.

Score	Dilatation	Effacement	Station	Position	Consistency
0	Closed	<30%	-3	Posterior	Firm
1	1–2 cm	40–50%	-2	Mid-position	Moderately firm
2	3–4 cm	60–70%	-1	Anterior	Soft
3	5 + cm	80 + %	+ 1	–	-

Total score = 13, Favorable = 6 – 13, Unfavorable = 0 – 5

- Along with surgical induction, to shorten the induction—delivery interval
- In cases of failure of surgical induction.
  Drugs used:
  - Oxytocin
  - Prostaglandins.

Oxytocin induction

The synthetic preparation (Syntocinon) is widely used as intravenous infusion, which is diluted in isotonic solution such as normal saline. The infusion should be controlled through a pump to enable accurate assessment of volume and rate. Manual counting of the drops per minute may be followed carefully. The rate of infusion must be titrated against the assessment of strength and frequency of uterine contractions. As labor becomes established, the uterus becomes more sensitive to oxytocin and the infusion rate may need to be reduced as labor progresses. The midwife should aim to administer the lowest dose required to maintain, well-spaced uterine contractions, typically occurring every 3 minutes, lasting for 45–50 seconds. The objective of oxytocin administration is not only to initiate effective contraction but also to maintain the normal pattern of uterine activity until delivery and at least 30–60 minutes beyond that.

Calculation of the infusion dose

The infusion is expressed (recorded) in terms of milliunits per minute. This can give an accurate idea about the exact amount administered per minute irrespective of the concentration of the solution **(Table 32.2)**.

In majority of cases, a dose of less than 16 milliunits per minute (2 units in 500 mL of Ringer's solution with drop rate of 60 per minute) is sufficient. Conditions where fluid overload is to be avoided, infusion with high concentration and reduced drop rate is used. The interval for escalating the drop rate is 15–30 minutes. The total dose required for initiating labor ranges from 600 to 12,000 milliunits with an average of 4,000 milliunits.

Observations during oxytocin induction
1. The pregnant woman should never be left alone when the oxytocin infusion is running.
2. Rate of flow of the infusion should be maintained accurately, especially when the drip is regulated by counting the drops per minute.
3. Response to uterine contraction should be meticulously observed in the absence of an electronic monitoring device. The number of contractions in 10 minutes and the tonus of the uterus in between contractions (using fingertip palpation) should be noted.
4. Fetal heart rate should be noted every 15 minutes.
5. Continuous electronic fetal monitoring is ideal, especially for high-risk cases. CTG equipment can record FHR and uterine contractions simultaneously.
6. *Maternal condition:* Pulse rate and blood pressure are to be checked hourly. The amount of urine should be noted when larger doses are administered (in excess of 20 mU/min). Any untoward symptoms like precordial pain or uneasiness should be detected promptly.
7. *Progress of labor:* Progressive descent of the head and the rate of cervical dilatation are to be noted. The color of the liquor amnii should be inspected periodically.

Indications for stopping the infusion
1. Nature of uterine contractions:
   a. Abnormal uterine contractions occurring frequently (every 2 minute or less) or lasting more than 60 seconds.
   b. Increased tonus (tension) in between contractions.
2. Evidences of fetal distress.
3. The appearance of untoward maternal symptoms.

Side effects of oxytocin
1. Hyperstimulation of the uterus: Oxytocin exposes the mother and fetus to the risk of hyperstimulation of the uterus, which could cause fetal hypoxia and uterine rupture. Hyperstimulation may cause the uterus to contract continuously for several minutes (contractions lasting longer than 60 second and more frequently than every 2 minute). The relaxation between contractions is inadequate. If this occurs, the midwife should turn off the infusion and inform the obstetrician. The uterus recovers from the hyperstimulation rapidly as the infusion is discontinued. Oxytocin should not be given as a bolus injection during labor because of the risk of hyperstimulation.
2. Prolonged use may contribute to uterine atony postpartum.
3. Water retention and water intoxication can occur with prolonged use, due to its antidiuretic effect.

Effectiveness

The drug is effective in most of the cases either with single or repeated infusions. However, oxytocin is less effective in cases of intrauterine death, elderly primigravida or early gestational period with unfavorable cervix **(Box 32.1)**.

Prostaglandin induction

Prostaglandin E2 (Dinoprostone):
- Dinoprostone preparations include dinoprostone gel (prepidil gel), dinoprostone vaginal suppository (prostin) and dinoprostone vaginal insert (cervidil).
- Cervical ripening with these agents is accomplished through cervical softening, cervical smooth muscle relaxation and stimulation of uterine contractions.

TABLE 32.2: Calculation of the dose of oxytocin delivered in milliunits (mU).

Units of oxytocin mixed in 500 mL Ringer's solution or normal saline	Drops per minute		
	15	30	60
1 unit = 1,000 mU	Milliunits per minute		
1	2	4	8
2	4	8	16
3	16	32	64

Note: 1 unit (1,000 mU) of oxytocin in 500 mL IV solution:
- At 15 drops/min gives 2 mU/min
- At 30 drops/min gives 4 mU/min
- At 60 drops/min gives 8 mU/min.

BOX 32.1: Nursing alert.

Oxytocin use
An accidental bolus of oxytocin can be life-threatening for both the mother and fetus. To avoid this potential hazard, oxytocin should always be administered through an infusion pump and inserted by piggyback through the main intravenous line at the port closest to the client.

Interventions for uterine hyperstimulation include:
- Turn off the pitocin
- Change the client's position (lying on left side is best)
- Administer oxygen
- Notify the physician

❖ A speculum examination is needed insert prepidil (gel) and the patient should remain in recumbent position for a minimum of 30 minutes after insertion.
❖ Prostin gel is inserted transcervically, after a vaginal speculum examination. Cervidil is inserted vaginally and does not require a speculum examination before insertion. After insertion, it is recommended that the patient remain in a supine position for two hours. Uterine contractions may begin several hours after insertion.

Prostaglandin F_1 (Misoprostol):
❖ Its use for cervical ripening has been supported by American College of Gynecology (ACOG).
❖ This medication may be administered via the following routes: vaginal, oral, buccal, and sublingual and rectally. The peak action may vary. Oxytocin should not be initiated until a minimum of four hours after the last dose. Misoprostol has been associated with an increased risk of uterine tachysystole and meconium staining, although oral misoprostol administered every four hours appears to be as effective as vaginal administration with a low incidence of uterine tachysystole, no increase in side effects, a lower cesarean section rate and a higher degree of patient satisfaction.
❖ In general cervical ripening is not recommended for women attempting a vaginal birth after cesarean (VBAC) delivery.

Advantages
❖ Effective method for use in cases of intrauterine death or in cases of unfavorable cervix.
❖ No antidiuretic effect.

Drawbacks
❖ More systemic side effects when used orally or intravenously, but vaginal administration has minimal side effects.
❖ The adverse uterine effect (hyperstimulation) if occurs, usually lasts for a longer period compared to oxytocin.
❖ Systemic side effects include pyrexia, diarrhea and vomiting.

Other Drugs used for Induction

Nitric oxide donors (Glyceryl trinitrate, isosorbide mononitrate).
❖ It has been suggested that nitric oxide compounds which stimulate cervical ripening without stimulating uterine contractions and may be used as an effective outpatient cervical ripening method.
❖ They have been found to be less effective than prostaglandins, but have fewer safety concerns and higher patient satisfaction.
❖ Used in combination with prostaglandins (inpatients), their use may be synergistic resulting in shorter induction to vaginal delivery time and reduced uterine tachysystole.

Surgical Induction

Methods are:
1. Artificial rupture of membranes (ARMs).
2. Stripping of the membranes.

Artificial rupture of membranes or amniotomy
Amniotomy is performed to induce labor when the cervix is favorable or during labor to augment contractions. A well-fitting presenting part is essential, to prevent cord prolapse. ARM may also be done to visualize the color of the liquor amnii or to attach a fetal scalp electrode for continuous electronic monitoring of the FHR.

Rupture of the membranes allows the presenting part to descend with improved application to the cervical os. This increased stimulation results in stronger contractions as levels of prostaglandins rise. Reduction of amniotic fluid volume causes the onset of labor.

Amniotomy may be used on its own or in association with oxytocin and may be either low rupture, involving rupture of the forewaters, or less commonly, high rupture, which requires the hindwater to be ruptured.

Hazards of amniotomy
❖ The intrauterine infection, particularly iatrogenic from digital or instrumental contamination
❖ Chance of umbilical cord prolapse: The chance is minimized in cases with an engaged head
❖ Bleeding from the following sources:
  – Fetal vessels in the membranes (vasa previa)
  – The friable vessels in the cervix
  – A low lying placental site (placenta previa)
  – Liquor amnii embolism.

Immediate beneficial effects of amniotomy
❖ Lowering of the blood pressure in preeclampsia and eclampsia
❖ Relief of the maternal distress in polyhydramnios
❖ Control of bleeding in antepartum hemorrhage (APH)
❖ Release of tension in abruptio placentae thereby minimizing uterorenal reflex.

Types
1. **Low rupture of membranes:** Low rupture of membranes (LRMs) method of amniotomy is widely practiced with high degree of success. The membranes below the

presenting part overlying the internal os are ruptured using a Kocher's artery forceps to drain some amount of amniotic fluid.

Contraindication: In chronic polyhydramnios the gush of amniotic fluid is difficult to control and sudden decompression may precipitate early separation of the placenta and accidental hemorrhage.

Observations: As the membranes rupture, the following are to be noted:
- Color of amniotic fluid
- Status of the cervix
- Station of the head
- Presence or absence of cord prolapse
- Quality of FHR.

Hazards: Same as mentioned for ARM.

2. **High rupture of membranes:** High rupture of membranes (HRMs) is a procedure where the puncture of the hindwater above the presenting part is made with a special instrument called Drew-Smythe catheter.

This method is almost obsolete now. It was used in chronic hydramnios associated with congenital malformations of the fetus or with floating head, where regulated escape of liquor amnii facilitates settling down of the presenting part. Slow decompression also prevents premature placental separation.

Conditions to be fulfilled:
- Cervix should be at least one finger dilated
- Vertex must be presenting
- Forewaters must be present.

Contraindications:
- Antepartum hemorrhage
- Severe preeclampsia or eclampsia.

Hazards:
- Injury to the placenta
- Accidental injury to the uterine wall
- Injury to the fetal parts specially to the eye
- Accidental low rupture of membranes
- Displacement of the presenting part
- Intra-amniotic infection
- Longer induction—delivery interval compared to LRM.

While forewaters preservation is maintained and chance of cord prolapse is minimized with HRM, the LRM is widely practiced, as it is a more effective method of surgical induction.

Stripping the membranes

Stripping the membranes off its attachment from the lower uterine segment is used as an effective procedure for induction provided the cervical score is favorable. It is used as a preliminary step prior to rupture of membranes. Prostaglandins are rapidly produced as the fetal membranes are detached from the decidua. Stretching and ripening of the cervix or at times initiation of labor results.

In order to carry out the procedure a vaginal examination with some cervical stretching is needed. This provides additional stimulus for prostaglandin release. This method is employed as an alternative to medical induction in post-term pregnancy.

Combined Method

The combined medical and surgical methods are commonly used to increase the efficacy of induction by reducing the induction delivery interval. The oxytocin infusion is started either prior to or following rupture of membranes depending mainly upon the state of the cervix and head-brim relation. With the head engaged, it is preferable to induce with prostaglandin gel or to start oxytocin infusion followed by ARM.

Advantages of combined methods
1. More effective than any single method.
2. Shortens the induction delivery interval and thereby minimizes the risk of infection, and lessens the period of observation.

PROLONGED LABOR

The labor is said as prolonged when the combined duration of the first and second stage is more than the arbitrary time limit of 18 hours. The prolongation includes prolonged cervical dilatation in the first stage and/or inadequate descend of the presenting part during the first and second stage of labor.

A latent phase that exceeds 20 hours in primigravida and 14 hours in multiparae is abnormal. The causes include unripe cervix, malposition and presentation, cephalopelvic disproportion, and premature administration of excessive sedation.

Causes of Prolonged Labor

Anyone or combination of the basic elements in labor could be responsible to create the situation.

First Stage

Failure to dilate the cervix:
1. Fault in power includes abnormal uterine contraction such as uterine inertia or in coordinate uterine action.
2. Fault in the passage includes contracted pelvis, cervical dystocia, pelvic tumor or even full bladder.
3. Fault in the passenger includes malposition and malpresentation, congenital anomalies of the fetus such as hydrocephalus.
4. *Others:* Injudicious early administration of sedatives and analgesics before the actual active labor begins.

Second Stage

Sluggish or nondescend of the presenting part due to:
- Fault in the power:
  - Uterine inertia
  - Inability to bear down
  - Epidural analgesia
  - Constriction ring.

- ❖ Fault in the passage:
  - Contracted pelvis and disproportion
  - Undue resistance of the pelvic floor or perineum due to spasm or old scarring
  - Soft tissue pelvic tumor.
- ❖ Fault in the passenger:
  - Malposition
  - Malpresentation
  - Big baby
  - Congenital malformation of the baby.

Diagnosis

Prolonged labor is a manifestation of an abnormality, the cause of which should be detected by a thorough abdominal and vaginal examination supplemented by partographic analysis of labor. Intranatal radiography is useful in determining the fetal station and position as well as pelvic shape and size.

First Stage

If the first stage of labor lasts more than an arbitrary period of 12 hours or if the cervical dilatation arrests more than 2 hours, it is considered as abnormal.

Rate of cervical dilatation is sluggish to less than 1 cm/h in nullipara and less than 1.5 cm/h in multipara. There may be slow descending of the head (normal 1 cm/h in primipara and 2 cm/h in multipara).

The first stage of labor is divided into a latent and an active phase. During latent phase, the uterus contracts regularly and the mother experiences discomfort, and pain. The cervix effaces and dilatation occurs. The duration of latent phase varies according to each individual and with parity. The average duration of latent phase in nulliparous women is 8.6 hours.

The active phase is distinguished by an increased rate of dilatation of cervix with descend of the presenting part. A prolonged active phase is caused by a combination of factors including the cervix, the uterus, the fetus and the mother's pelvis.

Second Stage

The second stage is considered prolonged if it lasts for more than 2 hours in primigravida and 1 hour in multipara. The diagnostic features are:

1. Sluggish or nondescend of the presenting part even after full dilatation of the cervix (failure of the head to descend within 1 hour is called arrest).
2. Variable degrees of molding and caput formation in cephalic presentation.

Dangers of Prolonged Labor

Fetal

The fetal risk is increased due to the combined effect of:

1. Hypoxia due to diminished uteroplacental circulation specially after rupture of the membranes.
2. Intrauterine infection.
3. Intracranial stress or hemorrhage following prolonged stay in the perineum and/or increased molding of the head.
4. Increased operative delivery.

All these result in increased perinatal loss due to asphyxia, intracranial hemorrhage and neonatal sepsis.

Maternal

There is increased incidence of:

1. Maternal distress.
2. Postpartum hemorrhage.
3. Trauma to the genital tract—concealed (undue stretching the perineal muscles, which may cause prolapse of uterus at a later stage) or revealed such as cervical tear, rupture of uterus.
4. Increased operative delivery.
5. Puerperal sepsis.
6. Subinvolution.

Management

The management of a mother experiencing a prolonged labor will be the responsibility of the obstetric team. Midwives must seek medical advice on recognizing any aberration from normal:

1. When progress is slow, attempts should be made to determine the cause before deciding on management. An expectant management for inefficient uterine action is to encourage ambulation to produce a return to normal activity. When mobility was encouraged, oxytocics were less frequently required to improve contractions..
2. The upright position for the laboring mother improves the application of the presenting part on to the cervix and triggers the neuroendocrine reflex. This would make the contractions less painful although stronger and more efficient than when remaining recumbent. Upright position or one where the woman adopts a forward leaning posture are helpful in encouraging an anterior rotation of the occiput.
3. When poor progress of labor is due to hypotonic, inefficient contractions, oxytocin increases the strength and frequency of the contractions. Cephalopelvic disproportion should be excluded before attempts are made to speed up the contractions. Correction of ineffective uterine contractions includes *amniotomy and administration of oxytocin or administration of oxytocin* in the presence of the previously ruptured membranes. When labor is induced or augmented with oxytocin, the midwife must be vigilant and aware of the risk of hyperstimulation of the uterus.
4. *Comfort and analgesia:* Adequate analgesia should be offered to the mother. Where labor is prolonged intramuscular injection of pethidine or an epidural block affords complete pain relief in most of the cases. They should be helped to adopt the most comfortable position. General hygiene is important, especially where

the membranes have been ruptured. Soiled pads and linen should be changed as necessary.
5. *Observations:* All observations are to be recorded on the partogram. Infection may develop where there has been prolonged rupture of membranes. Temperature should be taken 4 hourly. Vaginal swabs may be taken and broad-spectrum antibiotics commenced when infection is suspected. Pulse and blood pressure are recorded hourly or more frequently as the woman's condition requires.
6. *Fluid balance:* An accurate record should be kept. The woman should be encouraged to empty her bladder 2 hourly. If she is unable to void, a catheter should be inserted, as a full bladder may affect the uterine action in labor. Recording output is important when oxytocin is administered because of its antidiuretic effect. Fluid overload can occur, which causes hyponatremia, affecting mother and baby.
7. *Assessment of progress:* Vaginal examination is carried out usually every 4 hours. Progress is noted by increasing dilatation along with the consistency of the cervix and application of the cervix to the presenting part. The degree of molding should be noted, and any increase over successive examinations reported. Descend of the presenting part must be assessed by noting the station of the presenting part on vaginal examination. The color of the amniotic fluid needs to be noted and if meconium is present, this should be reported.
8. *Fetal well-being:* Fetal heart rate must be monitored carefully by frequent auscultation or continuously, using electronic fetal monitor. Fetal blood sampling may be used to support a decision to continue with labor or intervene.

The presence of meconium-stained liquor amnii and an abnormal fetal heart tracing is suggestive of fetal hypoxia. A pediatrician should be present at the birth and precautions to be taken to prevent aspiration of meconium. If the mother is in labor at home, it may be necessary to transfer her to a hospital with facilities for operative delivery and care of the neonate.

Prolonged Second Stage of Labor

A lengthy second stage may result from ineffective contractions, poor maternal effort and loss of, or absence of, a desire to push caused by epidural analgesia. A full bladder or a full rectum can also impede progress. A large fetus, malpresentation or malposition may account for delay and an assisted birth may be necessary.

A reduced pelvic outlet in association with an occipitoposterior position may result in deep transverse arrest.

Management of a Prolonged Second Stage

A vaginal examination should be carried out to confirm position, attitude and station of the presenting part. The fetal heart should be auscultated after every contraction or electronic monitoring used.

In the presence of inefficient uterine contractions, an infusion of oxytocin should be commenced. The usual observations for the use of oxytocin are to be followed. Mothers with related factors, such as preeclampsia or prematurity, management of the second stage, will be assessed constantly.

Options for Delivery

Delivery may be expedited where the conditions alter or mother or fetus becomes distressed. Ventouse or forceps will be used where the pelvic outlet is adequate and vaginal birth can be safely carried out. Cesarean section may be necessary where there is evidence of cephalopelvic disproportion.

Maternal Distress

The following are the evidences of maternal distress:
- Anxious look with sunken eyes
- Dry tongue
- Acetone smell in mouth
- Rising pulse rate of 100 per minute or more
- Hot, dry vagina often with the offensive discharge
- Scanty, high-colored urine with presence of acetone.

DISORDERS OF UTERINE ACTION

Precipitate Labor (Over-efficient Uterine Action)

A labor is called precipitate when the combined duration of the first and second stage is less than 2 hours. It is common in multiparae and may be repetitive. Rapid expulsion is due to the combined effect of hyperactive uterine contractions associated with diminished soft tissue resistance.

Maternal Risks

- Extensive laceration of the cervix, vagina and perineum (to the extent of complete perineal tear)
- Postpartum hemorrhage
- Inversion of uterus
- Infection.

Fetal Risks

- Intracranial stress and hemorrhage because of rapid expulsion without time for molding of the head
- The baby may sustain serious injuries if delivery occurs in standing position due to bleeding from the torn cord and direct hit on the skull.

Management

The woman with previous history of precipitate labor should be hospitalized prior to labor. The uterine contractions may be suppressed by administering ether during contractions **(Box 32.2)**. Delivery of the head should be controlled. Episiotomy should be done liberally. Elective induction of labor by LRM and careful conduction of controlled delivery may be done.

> **BOX 32.2:** Nursing alert.
>
> **Nursing interventions during precipitous delivery**
> - Instruct the woman to pant with contractions if the fetal head is crowning
> - With gloved hand, apply gentle pressure against the fetal head occiput or vertex to maintain flexion and prevent it from popping out quickly. Support perineum with the other hand
> - When the fetal head is born, instruct the woman to pant and not to push. Suction the fetal mouth and nares with a bulb syringe
> - Insert two fingers along the back of the fetal neck for Nuchal cord. If present, pull it over the infant's head, clamp twice and cut between the clamps. Unwind the cord from around the neck
> - While requesting the woman to push gently, place one hand on each side of the infant's head over the ears and exert gently downward pressure on the head to assist in the birth of the anterior shoulder. Then exert gentle upward pressure to assist with the delivery of posterior shoulder. Support the rest of the infant's body as he or she is born
> - Check the firmness of the fundus and observe for vaginal bleeding
> - Watch for signs of placental separation and receive the placenta when expelled.

Cervical Dystocia

Cervical dystocia is one where despite effective contractions the cervix (external os) fails to dilate, although it may efface. Cervical dystocia may be primary or secondary. The primary type of dystocia occurs predominantly during the first birth. The nondilatation may be due to the presence of excessive fibrous tissue or spasm of circular muscle fibers surrounding the os. The secondary cervical dystocia results usually from the effect of scarring or rigidity of cervix from the effect of previous operation, or disease.

The cervix becomes very much thinned out and well applied to the head. Initially, the uterine contractions remain good, but ultimately become ineffective. On occasion, edema of the anterior lip may occur and delivery may be accomplished by avulsion (tearing away) of the anterior lip or annular detachment of the cervix.

Management

In the presence of associated complications, where vaginal delivery is found unsafe, cesarean section is performed.

If the head is sufficiently low down with only a thick rim of cervix left behind, the rim may be pushed up manually during contraction or traction given by Ventouse. In others, where the cervix is very much thinned out, but only half dilated a Dührssen's incision at 2 and 10 O'clock positions may be given followed by Ventouse or forceps application.

Generalized Tonic Contraction (Uterine Tetany)

In generalized tonic contraction, pronounced retraction occurs involving whole of the uterus, up to the level of internal os. There is no physiological differentiation of the active upper segment and the passive lower segment of the uterus. The uterine contraction ceases after a period and the whole uterus undergoes a sort of tonic muscular spasm holding the fetus inside.

Causes

- Failure to overcome the obstruction by powerful contractions of the uterus
- Irritability caused by repeated unsuccessful attempts at artificial delivery
- Injudicious administration of oxytocics, especially following intramuscular administration of oxytocin.

Clinical Manifestations

- The woman is in prolonged labor with severe and continuous pain
- Evidences of dehydration and ketoacidosis
- On abdominal examination:
  - The uterus is somewhat smaller in size
  - Tense and tender
  - Fetal parts are not well defined
  - Fetal heart sound (FHS) is not audible on auscultation.
- On vaginal examination:
  - Jammed head with big caput
  - Dry and edematous vagina.

Treatment

1. Deep sedation by intramuscular morphine 15 mg or pethidine drip.
2. Correction of dehydration and ketoacidosis by administering Ringer's solution in rapid infusion.
3. Administration of antibiotics.
4. Active management: After a period of rest, the abnormal uterine action may subside when spontaneous delivery is possible, if there is no obstruction. In the presence of obstruction, however, operative procedure may be required to deliver the fetus.

Tonic Uterine Contraction and Retraction (Bandl's Ring)

Tonic uterine and retraction type of uterine contraction is predominantly due to obstructed labor. There is gradual increase in intensity, duration and frequency of uterine contraction. The relaxation phase becomes less and less, ultimately a state of tonic contraction results. Retraction, however, continues.

The lower segment elongates and becomes progressively thinner to accommodate the fetus driven from the upper segment. *A circular groove encircling the uterus is formed between the active upper segment and the distended lower segment, called pathological retraction ring or Bandl's ring.* In normal labor, a ridge forms between the upper and lower segments, which is termed as the *retraction ring*. In obstructed labor, this phenomenon becomes exaggerated and is visible above the symphysis pubis as Bandl's ring (**Figs. 32.1A to C**). Due to pronounced retraction, there is marked reduction of blood flow to the placenta, leading to fetal jeopardy and even death.

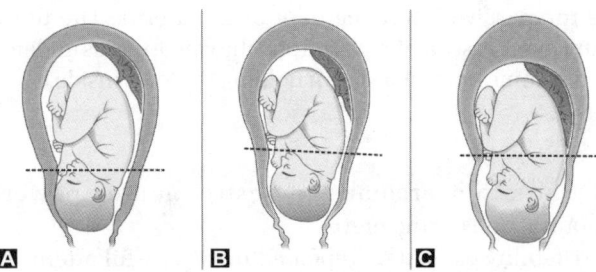
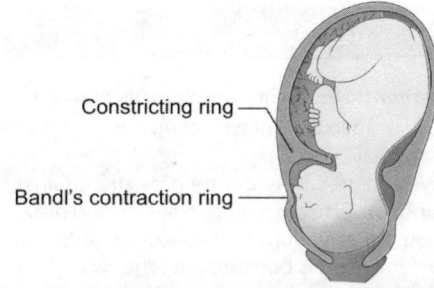

Figures 32.1A to C: Pathogenesis of retraction ring (Bandl's ring). (A) Normal labor; (B) Early obstruction; (C) Late obstruction.

Figure 32.2: Representation of constriction ring and Bandl's ring.

In primigravida, further retraction may cease in response to obstruction and labor may come to a standstill as a state of exhaustion. Contractions may recommence after a short period of rest with renewed vigor. In multiparae, retraction continues with progressive circumferential dilatation and thinning of the lower segment. There is progressive rise of the Bandl's ring, moving nearer and nearer to the umbilicus and ultimately, the lower segment ruptures.

Clinical Features

- Patient is in agony from continuous pain and discomfort
- Features of exhaustion and ketoacidosis
- On abdominal palpation:
  - Upper segment is hard, uniformly convex and tender, lower segment is distended and tender
  - The pathological retraction ring is placed obliquely between the umbilicus and symphysis pubis, and rises upwards as time passes
  - Fetal parts may not be well-defined
  - Fetal heart sound is usually absent.
- Pelvic examination reveals:
  - Dry, hot vagina
  - Fully dilated cervix
  - Membranes absent.

Prevention

Tonic uterine contraction is a preventable condition. The abnormality either in the passage (bony or soft tissue) or in the passenger (malpresentation or malformation of the fetus) can be detected during antenatal, or early intranatal period and appropriate treatment solves the problem.

Management

- Morphine 15 mg is given intramuscularly
- Intravenously 5% dextrose and Ringer's solution to correct fluid volume deficit and ketoacidosis
- Vaginal delivery followed by exploration of the uterus to exclude rupture of the uterus
- Cesarean section is rarely indicated.

Constriction Ring (Contraction Ring)

Contraction ring is one form of incoordinate uterine action where there is localized spastic contraction of a ring of circular muscle fibers of the uterus. It is usually situated at the junction of the upper and lower segment around a constricted part of the fetus usually around the neck in cephalic presentation. It may appear in any stage of labor and is usually reversible.

Its occurrence is associated with injudicious administration of oxytocics, premature rupture of membranes and premature attempts at instrumental delivery (**Fig. 32.2**).

Diagnosis

Diagnosis is difficult. Failure of the presenting part to advance even with effective contractions with the cervix lying loose is suspicious. It is revealed during:
- Cesarean section in the first stage
- During forceps application in the second stage
- During manual removal of placenta in the third stage.

It is then referred to as *hour glass contraction*. The labor is prone to be delayed. Maternal condition is not much affected, but the fetus may be in danger because of the hypertonic state.

Management

1. *First stage:* The diagnosis is made during cesarean section. The ring may have to be cut vertically to deliver the baby.
2. *Second stage:* Diagnosed when correct application of forceps fails to deliver the baby. Conformation is done by palpating the ring after removing the forceps. If the baby is in good condition, cesarean section is done even at this stage. If the baby is dead, forceps may be reapplied after relaxing the uterus by administering adrenaline subcutaneous and amyl nitrate by inhalation alternatively. If these fail to relax the uterus in 5 minutes, general anesthesia is given to complete the forceps delivery.
3. *Third stage:* The diagnosis is made during attempted manual removal of the placenta. Deepening the anesthesia is usually effective. Alternatively, adrenaline or amyl nitrate may be administered.

Obstructed Labor

Obstructed labor is one where in spite of good uterine contractions, the progressive descend of the presenting part is arrested due to mechanical obstruction. This may result either from the faults in the fetus or in the birth canal or both.

Incidence is about 1–2% in the developing countries.

Causes

1. Fault in the passage:
   a. Contracted pelvis and cephalopelvic disproportion are the common causes.
   b. *Soft tissue obstructions*: These include cervical dystocia, cervical or broad ligament fibroid and impacted ovarian tumor.
2. Fault in the passenger:
   a. Brow presentation
   b. Congenital malformations such as hydrocephalus, fetal ascites, conjoined twins
   c. Big baby associated with deflexed head and occipitoposterior position
   d. Impacted mentoposterior
   e. Compound presentation
   f. Locked twins.

Signs of Obstructed Labor

The presenting part does not enter the pelvic brim despite good contractions. The midwife should exclude the reasons such as full bladder, loaded rectum, or excessive liquor amnii volume as factors contributing to the failure in descent.

As the presenting part does not descend, cervical dilatation is slow. The cervix hangs loosely like 'an empty sleeve' as the presenting part is not applied to it. Early rupture of membranes or formation of a large elongated sac of forewaters is seen.

Late signs

Clinical signs include pyrexia and a rapid pulse rate. Urinary output is poor and hematuria may be present. Profound fetal bradycardia or fetal demise may follow.

The uterus becomes molded round the fetus and it fails to relax properly between contractions. Uterus goes into tonic contraction. A visible retraction ring or Bandl's ring may be seen above the symphysis pubis. This is similar in appearance to a full bladder. Uterine exhaustion, in which contractions may cease for a while before recommencing with renewed vigor, may occur in primigravida.

Vagina may feel hot and dry. The presenting part is high and feels wedged and immovable. There is excessive molding of the fetal skull and a large caput succedaneum present. Little urine is obtained on catheterization of the bladder.

Effect on the mother

1. Exhaustion due to constant agonizing pain and anxiety.
2. Dehydration due to increased muscle activity.
3. Metabolic acidosis due to accumulation of lactic acid produced by the contractile uterine and voluntary muscles.
4. Intrauterine infection may follow prolonged rupture of membranes.
5. Injury to the genital tract including rupture of uterus due to thinning of the lower uterine segment, which may be spontaneous in multiparae or may be traumatic following instrumental delivery.
6. Postpartum hemorrhage and shock due to the effects of traumatic delivery and blood loss or because of dehydration, and ketoacidosis.
7. Bladder injury due to trauma: The base of the bladder and urethra, which may be nipped in between the presenting part and symphysis pubis, may undergo pressure necrosis. The devitalized tissue may become infected and later on slough off resulting in the development of vesicovaginal fistula.
8. Remote effects are variable degrees of vaginal atresia, rectovaginal fistula and secondary amenorrhea.

All these lead to increased maternal morbidity and mortality.

Effect on the fetus

1. Asphyxia results from tonic uterine contraction, which interferes with uteroplacental circulation or due to cord prolapse, especially in shoulder presentation, leading to permanent brain damage.
2. Acidosis as the result of maternal acidosis.
3. Intracranial hemorrhage due to supermolding of the head or due to traumatic delivery.
4. Ascending infection can cause neonatal pneumonia.

All these effects lead to increased perinatal loss.

Management of Obstructed Labor

Management includes prevention of obstructed labor in the first instance. Risk factors such as history of prolonged labor and difficult births must be noted in the antenatal period. Malpresentations or signs of cephalopelvic disproportion must be identified by abdominal examination and after confirmation; elective cesarean section may be advocated.

During labor, careful assessment of the progress will help to detect lack of descent before labor becomes obstructed. Correlation of findings from abdominal examination and vaginal examination helps to confirm descend of the presenting part through the pelvis. This is aided by observation of both maternal and fetal condition and assessment of the length, strength and frequency of contractions. If the midwife suspects that labor is obstructed, she must seek appropriate medical aid immediately.

Measures of management

1. Sedate the woman with the pethidine 75–100 mg.
2. Correct dehydration and ketoacidosis by rapid infusions of appropriate solution.
3. Parenteral antibiotics are administered to overcome any infection that may be present.
4. Accurate record of observations of maternal and fetal conditions.

Obstetric management

If obstructed labor is recognized in the first stage of labor as when the head is extended to brow presentation, cesarean section is done. In the second stage of labor, failure to progress and descend may be caused by deep transverse arrest. If obstruction cannot be overcome by rotation and assisted birth, cesarean section should be performed as soon as possible.

If the mother is laboring at home, she must be transferred to a hospital with facilities for immediate cesarean and resuscitation of the neonate. If the labor is obstructed and the fetus has died, this will still be the mode of delivery, as vaginal birth cannot be achieved. Following the birth of the baby and prior to repair of the uterus and abdomen, exploration of the uterus is done to exclude uterine rupture or tear.

The fetus is likely to be delivered in a shocked and asphyxiated condition, and facilities for resuscitation and expert care should be available. The pediatrician should be present at birth and the parents need to be informed that the baby may need special care after birth.

STUDY QUESTIONS

Short Notes

1. Post-term pregnancy.
2. Successful induction of labor.
3. High rupture of membranes.
4. Stripping of membranes.
5. Precipitate labor.
6. Obstructed labor.

Short Answer Questions

1. Signs of obstructed labor.
2. Development and clinical manifestations of retraction ring.
3. Development, diagnosis and management of constriction ring.

Essay Questions

1. Explain the methods of medical induction of pregnancy and monitoring of a client during oxytocin induction.
2. Describe the methods of surgical induction of labor, its hazards, benefits and nurses responsibilities in caring for a client following artificial rupture of membranes.
3. Enumerate the effects of obstructed labor on mother and baby, and measures of management.

BIBLIOGRAPHY

1. Caldeyro Barcia R. The influence of maternal position on time of spontaneous rupture of membranes, progress of labor and fetal head compression. Birth and Family Journal. 1979;6(1):7-15.
2. Crowley P, O'Herlihy C, Boylan P. The value of ultrasound measurement of amniotic fluid volume in the management of prolonged pregnancies. British Journal of Obstetrics and Gynaecology. 1984;91(5): 444-8.
3. Dutta DC. Textbook of Obstetrics, 5th edition. Kolkata: New Central Book Company; 2001. pp. 334-47, 432-541, 558-67.
4. Flynn AM, Kelly J. Ambulation in labor. British Medical Journal. 1978;2:591-3.
5. Mackenzie IA. The therapeutic role of prostaglandins in obstetrics. In: Studd J (Ed). Progress in Obstetrics and Gynecology, vol. 8, 1st edition. Edinburgh: Churchill Livingstone; 1990. pp. 8-14.
6. Shiers CV. Prolonged pregnancy and disorders of uterine action. In: Bennel RV, Brown KL (Eds). Myles Textbook for Midwives, 13th edition. Edinburgh: Churchill Livingstone; 1999. pp. 489-506.

CHAPTER 33

Malpositions and Malpresentations

Learning Objectives

Upon completion of this chapter, the learner will be able to:
- Discuss the midwife's diagnosis and management of clients in labor with malpositions and malpresentations.
- Enumerate the risks for mother and baby with different malpositions and malpresentations.
- Describe the possible outcome for mother and baby for different conditions.

The midwife must know how to manage certain deviations from normal and obstetric complications until they are resolved or until the physician arrives. Occasionally she is confronted with these deviations from normal, because a patient arrives in second stage with no prenatal care or record, or because of an emergency. Theoretically and ideally, all of these deviations from normal and complications should have been diagnosed; these should be anticipated before delivery and before their occurrence. Situational circumstances with women in India, however, dictate that this will not be the case always. The conditions included in this chapter are:
- Occipitoposterior position
- Face presentation
- Brow presentation
- Breech presentation
- Shoulder presentation
- Compound presentation
- Shoulder dystocia
- Unstable lie.

OCCIPITOPOSTERIOR POSITION

Occipitoposterior position is a malposition of the head and occurs in about 13% of all head positions. The presenting part is vertex and the denominator is the occiput. Right occipitoposterior position (ROP) is three times as common as left occipitoposterior position (LOP).

Postulated Causes of Occipitoposterior Positions

- Pendulous abdomen common in multiparous women
- Anthropoid pelvic brim
- The transverse diameter of the brim being nearer the sacrum encourages the biparietal diameter to accommodate posteriorly
- A flat sacrum with a poorly flexed head leads to further deflexion and occipitoposterior position
- The placenta on the anterior uterine wall tends to encourage the fetus to flex around it.

Palpation

The fetal back is found to one side in early labor before descend of head. Fetal head is in the posterior position in early labor with descent of head. The limbs are to the front and give a hollowing above the head. This is particularly notable after rupture of membranes.

Auscultation

The fetal heart is heard best in the flank, but descends to just above the pubis as the head rotates and descends.

Vaginal Examination

The membranes tend to rupture early, often before labor is well-established. If the membranes are intact, they may protrude through the cervix. The head is deflexed so the anterior fontanel is readily felt in the anterior part of the pelvis near the iliopectineal eminence. The sagittal suture is directed towards the right sacroiliac joint (in ROP). The posterior fontanel is not readily felt till the head is in the lower pelvic cavity.

Course of Labor

Occipitoposterior position may lead to disorganized labor especially in the primigravida. Initially the contractions are sustained and irregular, accompanied by marked backache. Analgesia may be required to ease the discomfort. Engagement of the head is encouraged if the woman lies on the side which the fetus faces. Walking about after rest also helps.

Labor tends to be long and contractions become more normal as labor progresses. Retention of urine is common in occipitoposterior labor and catheterization may be required.

The woman may feel the need to bear down before the second stage is reached probably due to pressure on the sacrum and rectum. Dilatation must be confirmed before she is encouraged to bear down.

Mechanisms of Labor in Occipitoposterior Position

In the occipitoposterior position, the head engages in the right oblique diameter for the ROP and in the left oblique diameter for the LOP. The engaging transverse diameter is biparietal (9.5 cm) and anteroposterior diameter is either suboccipitofrontal (10 cm) or occipitofrontal (11.5 cm).

Possible courses of labor
Long arc rotation
In favorable circumstances, with increasing flexion, the occiput reaches the pelvic floor and rotates 3/8th of a circle (135°) forward (a long arc rotation) to an occipitoanterior position. Mechanisms will then continue as in an anterior position (ROA or LOA). In about 90%, delivery occurs in thin manner.

Posterior rotation of the occiput
With severe deflexion, posterior rotation of the occiput of 1/8th of a circle (45°) occurs as sinciput reaches the pelvic floor and rotates posteriorly. With posterior rotation, the possible outcomes are:
- Face-to-pubis delivery with a spacious gynecoid pelvis
- Persistent occipitoposterior position in which the occiput goes into the hollow of the sacrum.

Short arc rotation
In unfavorable circumstances, as with an android or anthropoid pelvis and weak uterine contractions, deflexion of the head persists. The occiput reaches the pelvic floor and rotates 1/8th of a circle (45°) anteriorly and sagittal suture comes to lie in the transverse diameter of the pelvis. Further rotation is unlikely and the condition ends up as *deep transverse arrest*.

Nonrotation of the occiput
As the fetal head descends, deflexion continues. There is nonrotation of the occiput resulting in an *oblique posterior arrest*.

Mechanism of Labor in Right Occipitoposterior Position

- The lie is longitudinal
- The attitude of the head is deflexed
- The presentation is vertex
- The position is right occipitoposterior
- The presenting part is the middle or anterior area of the left parietal bone
- The occipitofrontal diameter (11.5 cm) lies in the right oblique diameter of the pelvic brim
- The occiput points to the right sacroiliac joint and the sinciput to the left iliopectineal eminence.

Positional movements
1. *Engagement:* Takes place in the right oblique diameter of the pelvis.
2. *Flexion:* Descent occurs with increasing flexion, the occiput becomes the leading part.
3. *Internal rotation of the head:* The occiput reaches the pelvic floor first and rotates forwards 3/8th of a circle (135°) along the right side of the pelvis to lie under the symphysis pubis. The shoulders turn 2/8th of a circle (90°) and reach the right oblique diameter (long internal rotation).
4. *Crowning:* The occiput impinges beneath the symphysis pubis and the head is crowned.
5. *Extension:* The head (sinciput, face and chin) is born by extension.
6. *Restitution:* The occiput turns 1/8th of a circle (45°) to the right and the head re-aligns itself with the shoulders.
7. *Internal rotation of the shoulders:* The anterior shoulder rotates 1/8th of a circle (45°) to the right.
8. *External rotation of the head:* At the time of internal rotation of the shoulders, the occiped turns a further 1/8th of a circle (45°) to the right.
9. *Lateral flexion:* The anterior shoulder escapes under the symphysis pubis. Posterior shoulder sweeps the perineum and the body is born by lateral flexion. After the long internal rotation of 135°, further mechanisms continue as in a ROA delivery.

Mechanism of Labor with Posterior Rotation of the Occiput

With a spacious gynecoid pelvis, the baby may be born from a persistent occipitoposterior position as *face to pubis* (**Fig. 33.1**):
1. *Engagement:* Takes place in the right oblique diameter of the pelvis.
2. *Flexion:* With increasing flexion, the occiput becomes the leading part.

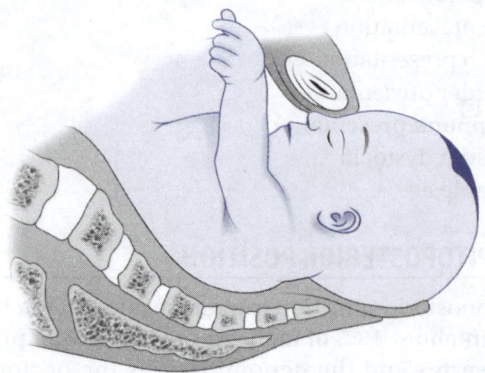

Figure 33.1: Face-to-pubis delivery, occipitofrontal diameter emerges out of the introitus.

3. *Internal rotation:* The occiput turns 1/8th of a circle (45°) backwards and sagittal suture comes to lie in the anteroposterior diameter of the mother's pelvis.
4. *Crowning:* Further descend occurs until the root of the nose impinges under the symphysis pubis.
5. *Birth of the baby's head* is by a double mechanism of flexion and extension. The sinciput impinges beneath the symphysis pubis and becomes the pivotal point for delivery of head. The head stays in flexion as the occiput distends the perineum and is born to the nape of the neck. The remainder of the head is then born by extension as the head falls back toward the rectum with the face looking upward.
6. *Restitution:* The head moves 1/8th of a circle to the right.
7. *External rotation* of further 1/8th of a circle to the right.
8. Birth of a shoulders and body by lateral flexion.

FACE PRESENTATION

When the attitude of the head is one of extension, the occiput of the fetus will be in contact with its spine and the face will present.

The incidence is about 1:500 and the majority develops during labor from vertex presentations with the occiput posterior; this is termed as secondary face presentation. Less commonly, the face presents before labor; this is termed as primary face presentation. There are six positions in a face presentation **(Figs. 33.2A to F)**; the denominator is the mentum and presenting diameters are the submentobregmatic (9.5 cm) and bitemporal (8.2 cm).

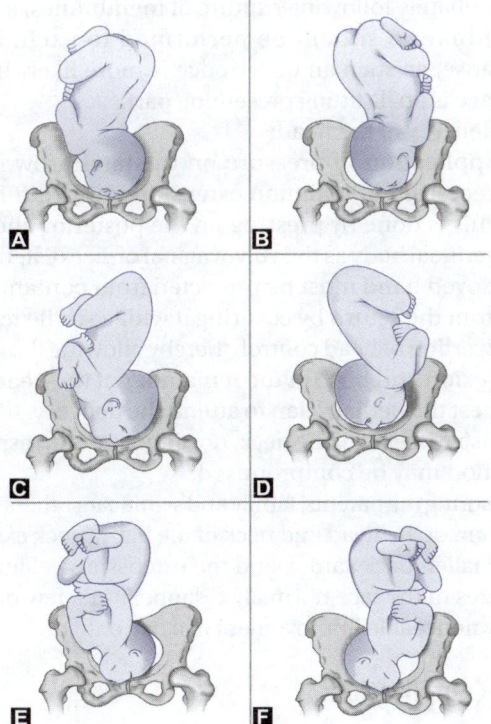

Figures 33.2A to F: Six positions of face presentation. (A) Right mentoposterior; (B) Left mentoposterior; (C) Right mentolateral; (D) Left mentolateral; (E) Right mentoanterior; (F) Left mentoanterior.

Causes

Contracted pelvis: In the flat pelvis, the head enters in the transverse diameter of the brim, the head becomes extended and a face presentation develops. In an android pelvis, the occiput does not descend; the head becomes extended and face presentation results.

Polyhydramnios: If the vertex is presenting and the membranes rupture spontaneously, the resulting rush of fluid may cause the head to extend as it sinks into the lower uterine segment.

Congenital abnormality: An anencephalic fetus in cephalic presentation ends up as face presentation, because the vertex is absent. Face is thrust forward. In very rare instances, a tumor of the fetal neck may cause extension of the head.

Diagnosis of Face Presentation

Antenatal diagnosis is rare because face presentation develops during labor in the majority of cases. A known anencephalic fetus in a cephalic presentation may be presumed to be a face presentation. Palpation in the intrapartum period may reveal the following:

❖ Occiput may feel prominent with a groove between head and back
❖ The limbs may be palpated on the side opposite to the occiput
❖ Fetal heart is best heard through the chest on the same side as the limbs.

In a mentoposterior position, fetal heart is difficult to hear because the fetal chest is in contact with the maternal pelvis. Many babies with face presentation begin labor either in brow presentation or with a hyperextended head and convert to a face during descent.

On vaginal examination, the fetal part is high. It may feel soft and irregular (lumpy) similar to a breech. When the cervix is fully dilated, orbital ridge, eyes, nose and mouth may be felt. Confusion between the anus and mouth could arise. The hard gums are diagnostic and the fetus may even suck the examining finger as it approaches the mouth.

Mechanisms of Labor

❖ The lie is longitudinal
❖ The attitude is one of extension of head and back
❖ The presentation is face
❖ The position is one of the following:
  – Left mentoanterior (LMA), left mentoposterior (LMP), left mentotransverse (LMT)
  – Right mentoanterior (RMA), right mentoposterior (RMP), right mentotransverse (RMT).
❖ The denominator is mentum
❖ The presenting part is the left malar bone.

Engagement

Engagement takes place when the submentobregmatic diameter has passed through the pelvic inlet (about 70% of all face presentations engage as either mentum anterior or mentum transverse varieties. The remaining 30% engages as a posterior variety).

Extension

Descend takes place with increasing extension. The mentum (chin) becomes the leading part because the head is extended.

Descent Occurs Throughout

Internal rotation of the head occurs when the chin reaches the pelvic floor and rotates.
1. Rotation of the chin anteriorly:
   – 45° (1/8th of a circle) for RMA and LMA to MA
   – 90° (2/8th of a circle) for RMT and LMT to MA
   – 135° (3/8th of a circle) for RMP and LMP to MA.
2. Rotation of the chin posteriorly:
   – 45° (1/8th of a circle) for RMP and LMP to MP.

Mentum Anterior Position

In mentum anterior position, birth of the head is by double mechanism of extension and flexion. Extension is maintained until the chin is born by escaping beneath the symphysis pubis. The submental area beneath the chin impinges beneath the symphysis pubis and becomes the pivotal point for the delivery of the rest of the head by flexion (**Figs. 33.3A and B**). The remaining head is born sequentially starting with the sinciput, vertex and occiput as the head flexes.

If the chin rotates posteriorly into a mentum posterior position, the mechanisms of labor cease at this point because the baby cannot deliver vaginally from this position—*persistent mentoposterior position*. This is because the length of the neck of the fetus is only about half as long as the length of the sacrum. Therefore, it is not possible for the chin to escape from the vaginal floor over the perineum, thereby allowing the remainder of the head to be born by flexion. This condition must be recognized before impaction of the head takes place with its extremely poor prognosis for the baby. Delivery must be affected by immediate cesarean section.

Restitution

Restitution takes place when the chin turns 45° (1/8th of a circle) in the direction from whence the head rotated during internal rotation. For example, if the rotation was from an RMT to an MA, the restitution is 45° to an RMA (to the woman's right) position.

Internal Rotation of the Shoulders

The shoulders enter the pelvis in the oblique diameter and the anterior shoulder reaches the pelvic floor first and rotates forward 45° (1/8th of a circle) along the left side of the pelvis in the RMA position and along the right side in LMA position.

External Rotation of the Head

External rotation of the head occurs simultaneously. The chin moves further 45° (1/8th of a circle) in the same direction as restitution.

Birth of the Shoulders and Body by Lateral Flexion

The anterior shoulder escapes under the symphysis pubis, the posterior shoulder sweeps the perineum and the body is born by a movement of lateral flexion.

Midwifery Management of a Face Presentation

1. Recognition of the face presentation and notification of the physician of the malpresentation.
2. A fetal scalp electrode must not be applied, and care should be taken not to infect or injure the eyes during vaginal examination.
3. Close monitoring of the mechanism of labor or internal rotation and immediately informing the physician if rotation is to a direct mentum posterior position.
4. Immediately following rupture of membranes, a vaginal examination should be performed to exclude cord prolapse, as such an occurrence is more likely because the face is an ill-fitting presenting part.
5. For delivery of the head:
   a. Application of pressure on the fetal brow may be necessary to maintain extension until chin is born. This is done by pressing on the posterior end of the perineal body as the vulvovaginal orifice distends. The gloved hand must be protected from contamination from the return by covering it with a sterile towel.
   b. Exertion of head control, thereby allowing the gradual flexion and birth of the remainder of the head.
6. Request the pediatrician to attend the delivery. If there is extensive edema of the neck, nose and mouth, respiratory function may be compromised.
7. Reassuring the parents, family and significant others that the position of the head and neck of the baby (neck extended, head fallen backwards), and the extensive swelling of the features of the face normally disappear in a few days and show noticeable improvement in a day or two.

Possible Complications

Obstructed Labor

Because the face, unlike the vertex does not mold, a minor degree of pelvic contraction may result in obstructed labor.

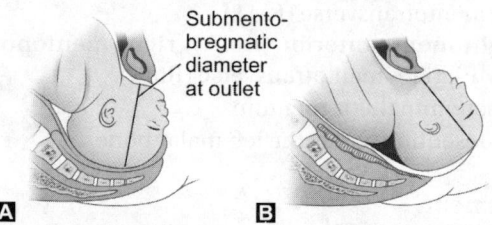

Figures 33.3A and B: Birth of head in mentoanterior position. (A) Chin escapes under symphysis pubis; (B) Head is born by a movement of flexion.

In a persistent mentoposterior position, the face becomes impacted and cesarean section is necessary.

Cord Prolapse

A cord prolapsed is more common when the membranes rupture because the face is an ill-fitting presenting part. The midwife should always perform a vaginal examination when the membranes rupture in order to detect such an occurrence.

Facial Bruising

The baby's face is always bruised and swollen at birth with edematous eyelids and lips. The head is elongated and the baby will initially lie with the head extended.

Cerebral Hemorrhage

The lack of molding of the facial bones can lead to intracranial hemorrhage caused by excessive compression of the fetal skull or by rearward compression in the typical molding of the fetal skull found in this presentation **(Fig. 33.4)**.

Maternal Trauma

Extensive perineal laceration may occur at the time of delivery due to the large submentovertical and biparietal diameters distending the vagina and perineum. There is an increased incidence of operative delivery, either forceps or cesarean section, both of which increase maternal morbidity.

■ BROW PRESENTATION

In the brow presentation, the fetal head is primarily extended with the frontal bone lying at the pelvic brim. The presenting part is bounded by the anterior fontanel and orbital ridges. The presenting diameter is mentovertical (13.5 cm) **(Fig. 33.5)** which exceeds all diameters in an average size pelvis. The incidence of this presentation is 1 in 1,000 deliveries.

Causes

Causes are the same as for a face presentation.

Diagnosis

Brow presentation is not usually detected before the onset of labor.

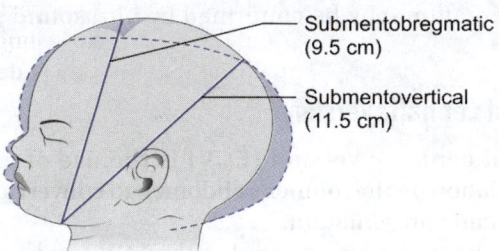

Figure 33.4: Molding in a face presentation (dotted line).

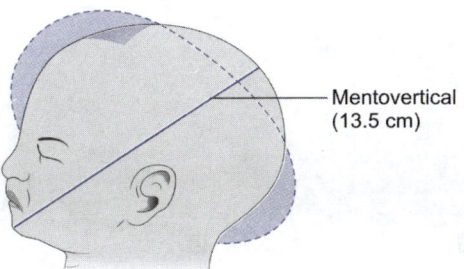

Figure 33.5: Molding in a brow presentation (dotted line).

Abdominal Palpation

The head is high, appears unduly large and does not descend into the pelvis in spite of good uterine contractions.

Vaginal Examination

The presenting part may be high and difficult to reach. The anterior fontanel may be felt on one side of the pelvis and orbital ridges on the other. A large caput succedaneum may mask these landmarks if the woman has been in labor for some time.

Management

The obstetrician must be informed immediately if brow presentation is suspected. Obstructed labor usually results unless cesarean section is done immediately. In extremely rare cases, vaginal delivery may be possible with a large pelvis and a small baby, though the midwife should never expect such a favorable outcome.

If there is no fetal distress, the physician may allow labor to continue for a short, while in case further extension of the head converts the brow presentation to a face presentation. Occasionally spontaneous flexion may occur resulting in a vertex presentation.

■ BREECH PRESENTATION

In a breech presentation, the fetus lies longitudinally with the buttocks in the lower pole of the uterus. The presenting diameter is the bitrochanteric (10 cm) (measured at the level of the hip joint) and the denominator is the sacrum. This presentation occurs in approximately 3% pregnancies at term.

Positions of Breech Presentation

There are six positions for a breech presentation which are illustrated in **Figures 33.6A to F**.

Types of Breech Presentation (Figs. 33.7A to D)

Breech with Extended Legs (Frank Breech)

The breech presents with the hips flexed and legs extended on abdomen. About 70% of breech presentations are of this type. It is particularly common in primigravida whose good uterine muscle tone inhibits flexion of the legs and free turning of the fetus.

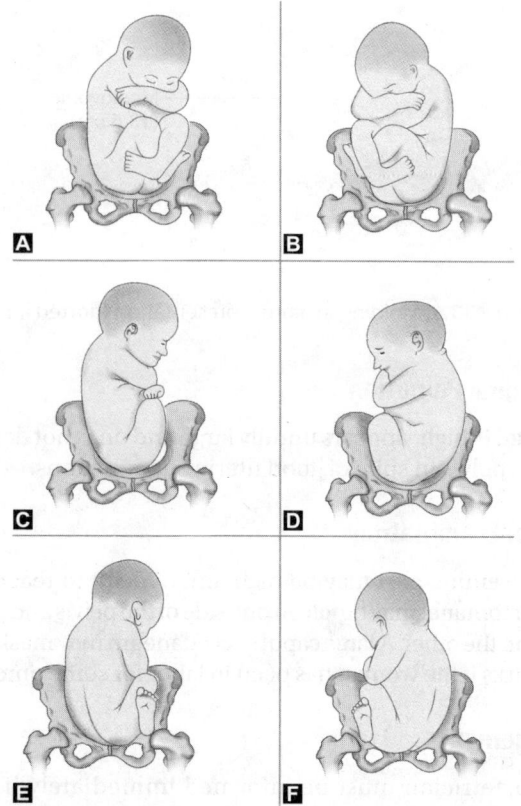

Figures 33.6A to F: Six positions in breech presentation. (A) Right sacroposterior; (B) Left sacroposterior; (C) Right sacrolateral; (D) Left sacrolateral; (E) Right sacroanterior; (F) Left sacroanterior.

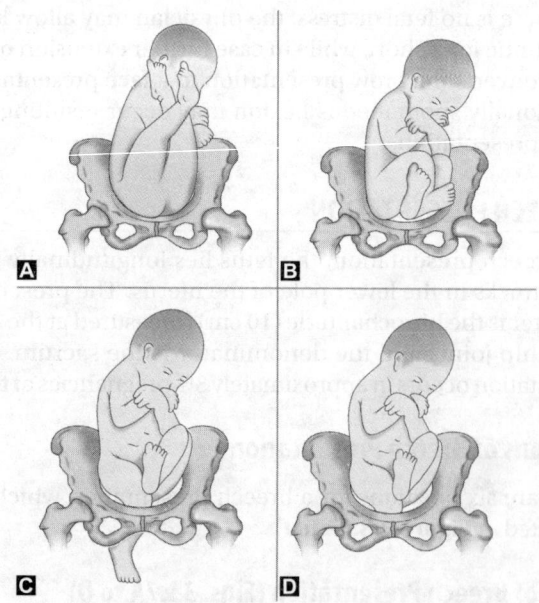

Figures 33.7A to D: Types of breech presentation. (A) Frank breech; (B) Complete breech; (C) Footing presentation; (D) Knee presentation.

Complete Breech

The fetal attitude is one of complete flexion, hips and knees are both flexed and the feet tucked in behind the buttocks.

Footling Breech

One or both feet present because neither hips nor knees are fully flexed. The feet are lower than the buttocks which distinguish this presentation from the complete breech.

Knee Presentation

One or both hips are extended with the knees flexed. This is very rare.

Diagnosis

Antenatal Diagnosis

On palpation, the lie is longitudinal with a soft presentation, which more easily felt during Pawlik's grip. The head can be felt in the fundus as a round hard mass which may be made to move independently of the back by balloting it with one or both hands. If the legs are extended, the feet may prevent such nodding. When the breech is anterior, and the fetus is well-flexed, it may be difficult to locate the head, but a combined grip of upper and lower poles may aid diagnosis. The woman may complain of discomfort under her ribs especially at night due to pressure of the head on the diaphragm.

Auscultation

When the fetus has not passed through the pelvic brim, the fetal heart is heard above the umbilicus. When the legs are extended, the breech descends into the pelvis easily. The fetal heart is then heard at a lower level.

An ultrasound examination may be used to confirm a breech presentation. X-ray examination may be used for the purpose of diagnosis and pelvimetry.

Diagnosis during Labor

Breech presentation may be diagnosed by abdominal palpation on admission in labor.

On vaginal examination, the breech feels soft and irregular with no sutures palpable. The anus may be felt and fresh meconium on the examining finger is usually diagnostic. If the legs are extended, the external genitalia are very evident, but it must be remembered that these become edematous.

If a foot is felt, the midwife should differentiate it from the hand by noting that the toes are all of the same length and the big toe cannot be opposed to other toes. The foot is at right angles to the leg and the heel has no equivalent in the hand.

Presentation may be confirmed by ultrasound scan or X-ray.

External Cephalic Version

External cephalic version (ECV) is the use of external manipulation on the mother's abdomen to convert a breech to a cephalic presentation.

It has been demonstrated that the ECV can reduce the number of babies presenting by the breech at term by two-third and therefore reduce the cesarean section rate for breech presentations.

Turning the fetus from a breech to a cephalic presentation before 37th week of gestation does not reduce the incidence of breech birth or rate of cesarean section, as it is likely to turn itself back spontaneously.

Method

An ultrasound scan is performed to localize the placenta, and to confirm the position and presentation of the fetus. A 30 minute cardiotocography (fetal heart monitoring) is performed to establish that the fetus is not distressed at the start of the procedure and maternal pulse and blood pressure are recorded.

The woman is asked to empty her bladder. The midwife then assists the woman to a comfortable supine position. The foot of the bed may be elevated to help free the breech from the pelvic brim. The abdomen is dusted with talcum powder to prevent pinching of the mother's skin during the procedure. The ECV may be uncomfortable for the mother, but may not be painful. The breech is displaced from the pelvic brim and iliac fossa. With one hand on each pole, the obstetrician makes the fetus perform a forward somersault. If this is not successful, then a backward somersault is attempted.

If the fetus does not turn easily, then the procedure is abandoned, but may be tried again after few days. The fetal heart should be auscultated after the procedure or a cardiotocogram performed.

Version may be performed immediately prior to the onset of labor. If the woman is Rh-negative, an injection of anti-D immunoglobulin is given as prophylaxis against isoimmunization caused by any placental separation.

Complications

1. Knotting of the umbilical cord should be suspected if bradycardia occurs and persists. The fetus is immediately turned back to a breech presentation. The woman is admitted for observation and if necessary, cesarean section is performed.
2. *Separation of the placenta:* Pain or vaginal bleeding during and after the procedure must be reported and taken care of.
3. *Rupture of the membranes:* If this occurs, the cord may prolapse because neither the head nor the breech is engaged.

Contraindications

- Preeclampsia or hypertension because of the increased risk of placental abruption
- Multiple pregnancy
- Oligohydramnios
- Ruptured membranes
- A hydrocephalic fetus
- Any condition, which would require delivery by cesarean section.

Assessment for Vaginal Delivery

The capacity of the pelvis to accommodate the fetal head must be assessed before the buttocks are delivered and the head attempts to enter the brim. The fetal size in relation to maternal pelvis must also be assessed by an ultrasound examination to avoid fetal hypoxia as the head enters the pelvic brim after the buttocks are delivered.

Mechanism of Labor for Left Sacroanterior Position

1. Lie is longitudinal.
2. Attitude is one of the complete flexion.
3. Presentation is breech.
4. Position is left sacroanterior (LSA).
5. Denominator is the sacrum.
6. Presenting part is the left (anterior) buttock.
7. Bitrochanteric diameter (10 cm), enters the pelvis in the left oblique diameter of the brim.
8. Sacrum points to the left iliopectineal eminence:
   a. Descend takes place initially with increasing compaction, owing to increased flexion of the limbs. Descend then occurs throughout.
   b. Engagement of the hips takes place in an LSA position with the sacrum in the left anterior portion of the mother's pelvis and bitrochanteric diameter in the left oblique diameter of the mother's pelvis.
   c. *Internal rotation of the buttocks:* The anterior buttock reaches the pelvic floor first and rotates forwards 45° (1/8th of a circle) along the right side of the pelvis to lie underneath the symphysis pubis. The bitrochanteric diameter is now in the anteroposterior diameter of the outlet.
   d. *Birth of the buttocks by lateral flexion:* The anterior buttock escapes under the symphysis pubis, the posterior buttock sweeps over the perineum and the buttocks are born by a movement of lateral flexion.
   e. *Restitution of the buttocks:* The anterior buttock turns slightly to the mother's right side.
   f. *Internal rotation of the shoulders:* The shoulders enter the pelvis in the same left oblique diameter. The anterior shoulder rotates 45° (1/8th of a circle) along the right side of the pelvis and escapes under the symphysis pubis.
   g. *External rotation of the buttocks:* With the internal rotation of the shoulders, the delivered body also rotates and sacrum returns to a left sacrotransverse (LST) position from an LSA position.
   h. *Birth of the shoulders takes place by lateral flexion:* When born spontaneously, the anterior shoulder impinges beneath the symphysis pubis and serves as the pivotal point for the lateral flexion necessary for the delivery of the posterior shoulder via the curve of Carus. Birth of the anterior shoulder then follows as the body straightens out.
   i. *Internal rotation of the head:* The head enters the pelvis with the sagittal suture in the transverse diameter of the brim. The occiput rotates forward

along the left side and suboccipital region (nape of the neck) impinges on the under surface of the symphysis pubis.

j. External rotation of the body takes place simultaneously. The body turns so that the back of the baby is upward and the baby is facing down.

k. *Birth of the head by flexion:* The chin, face and sinciput sweep over the perineum and the head is born in a flexed attitude.

Types of Breech Delivery

1. *Spontaneous breech delivery*: The delivery occurs with little assistance from the attendant.
2. *Assisted breech delivery*: The buttocks are born spontaneously, but some assistance is provided for delivery of extended legs or arms and the head.
3. *Breech extraction*: This is a manipulative delivery performed by an obstetrician to hasten delivery in an emergency, such as the fetal distress.

Management of Delivery

Before the actual delivery begins, the following should have taken place:

1. Complete dilatation of the cervix.
2. Elimination of any question about the adequacy of the pelvis.
3. Emptying of the bladder.
4. Adequate explanation to mother for effective pushing effort.
5. Readiness for a full-scale newborn resuscitation effort.
6. Positioning so, there is plenty of room for lateral flexion and downward traction that is lithotomy position.
7. Notification and presence or immediate availability of the consulting physician anesthesiologist and pediatrician.

When the buttocks are distending the perineum, the woman is placed in the lithotomy position and the vulva is swabbed and draped with sterile towels. The bladder is usually catheterized at this stage. An epidural anesthesia, pudendal block or local infiltration is carried out by the physician:

1. The woman is encouraged to push with the contractions and the buttocks are delivered spontaneously.
2. If the legs are flexed, the feet disengage at the vulva and the baby is born up to the umbilicus.
3. A loop of cord is gently pulled down to avoid traction on the umbilicus. If the cord is being nipped behind the pubic bone, it should be moved to one side.
4. Feel for the elbows, which are usually on the chest. If so, the arms will escape with the next contraction. If the arms are not felt, they are extended. There is no need for facilitation of the progress of the mechanisms of labor until the baby is born up to the umbilicus. After that, the remainder of the baby is to be born in 3–5 minutes to avoid any anoxia with resulting possible brain damage. Traction exerted on the baby prior to birth, up to the umbilicus may cause:

   a. The arms to fly up in a reflex action, thereby extending them above, over or behind the head and causing later difficulties in the delivery.
   b. The head to deflex, which may cause problems with delivery of the head.

5. Place a warm towel around the baby from just below the umbilicus down. This would keep the baby warm as well as give a non-slippery hold on the baby, which is essential to exert traction.

Delivery of the Shoulders

The uterine contractions and the weight of the baby will bring the shoulders down onto the pelvic floor where they rotate into the anteroposterior diameter of the outlet:

1. The obstetrician now grasps the baby by the hips with thumbs on either sacroiliac region and fingers on the corresponding iliac crest **(Fig. 33.8)**.
2. The baby is then tilted towards the maternal sacrum in order to free the anterior shoulder.
3. When the anterior shoulder has escaped, the buttocks are lifted toward the mother's abdomen to enable the posterior shoulder and arm to pass over the perineum.

If the arm has become extended, it is delivered first by inserting the fingers of the hand in vagina (the hand other than the one holding the baby's feet) to reach the elbow and sweeping it across the baby's chest downwards to delivery.

In order to do this, the feet of the baby is grasped in one hand with the index finger between the legs, and middle finger and thumbs each encircling a leg **(Fig. 33.9)**.

Care must be taken in holding the baby at an angle so that the head will enter the pelvis in the transverse diameter. The back must remain lateral until this has happened.

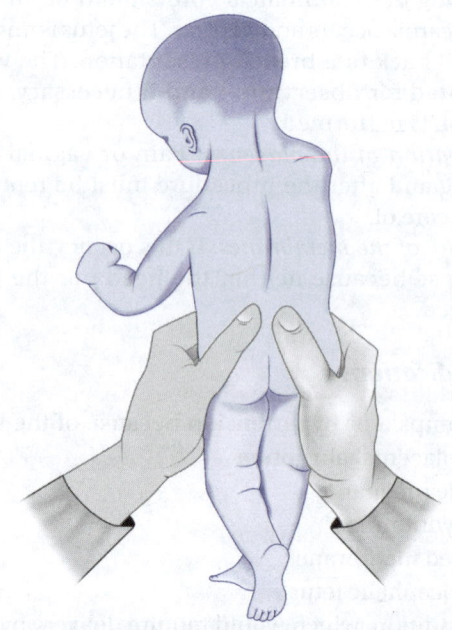

Figure 33.8: Correct grasp of baby on the hips in Løvset maneuver.

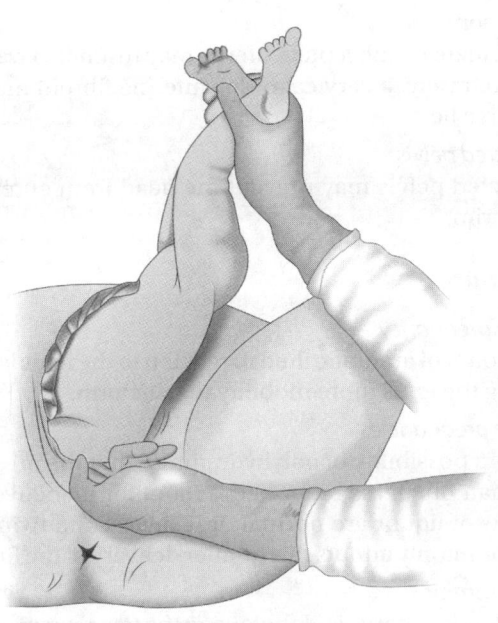

Figure 33.9: Delivery of the posterior shoulder in a breech presentation.

Delivery of the Head

When the back has been turned, the infant is allowed to hang from the vulva without support for 1–2 minutes. The baby's weight brings the head onto the pelvic floor on which the occiput rotates forwards. The sagittal suture is now in the anteroposterior diameter of the outlet. Gradually, the neck elongates, the hairline appears and the suboccipital region can be felt. Controlled delivery of the head is vital to avoid any sudden change in intracranial pressure and subsequent cerebral hemorrhage.

Methods of delivering the aftercoming head
Forceps delivery
The obstetrician usually applies forceps to the aftercoming head to achieve a controlled delivery.

Burns-Marshall method
The obstetrician grasps the baby's ankles from behind with forefinger between the two. The baby is kept on the stretch with sufficient traction to prevent the neck from bending backwards. The occipital region and not the neck should pivot under the apex of the pubic arch. The feet are taken up through an arc of 180° until the mouth and nose are free at the vulva. The right hand may guard the perineum in order to prevent sudden escape of the head. An assistant may now clear the airway and the baby will breathe. The mother should be asked to take deliberate, regular breaths, which allow the vault of the skull to escape gradually, taking 2 or 3 minutes.

Mauriceau-Smellie-Veit maneuver
(jaw flexion and shoulder traction)
The method is used when there is delay in descend of the head because of extension (excessive shoulder traction is avoided as it may cause Erb's palsy).

The baby is laid astride the right arm with the palm supporting the chest. Two fingers are inserted well back into the mouth to pull the jaw downwards and flex the head (two fingers may be placed on the malar bones and the middle finger in the mouth, if they can be accommodated). Two fingers of the left hand are hooked over the shoulders with the middle finger pushing up the occiput to aid flexion. Traction is applied to draw the head out of the vagina and when the suboccipital region appears, the body is lifted to assist the head to pivot around the symphysis pubis. Once the face is free, the airway may be cleared and the vault delivered slowly **(Fig. 33.10)**.

Delivery of Extended Legs

The baby can be born with the legs extended (frank breech) and assistance is usually required. When the popliteal fossae appear at the vulva, two fingers are placed along the length of one thigh with the fingertips in the fossa. The leg is swept to the side of the abdomen (abducting the hip) and the knee is flexed by the pressure on its undersurface. As this movement is continued, the lower part of the leg will emerge from the vagina. This process should be repeated in order to deliver the second leg.

Complications of Breech Presentation

Apart from the difficulties already mentioned, other complications can arise, most of which affect the fetus:
1. *Impacted breech:* Labor becomes obstructed when the fetus is disproportionately large for the size of the maternal pelvis.
2. *Cord prolapse:* This is common in a flexed (complete) or footling breech, as these have ill-fitting presenting parts.
3. *Birth injury:* Superficial tissue damage. Edema and bruising of the baby's genitalia may be caused by pressure on the cervix. In a footling breech, a prolapsed foot which lies in the vagina or at the vulva for a long time, may become edematous and discolored.

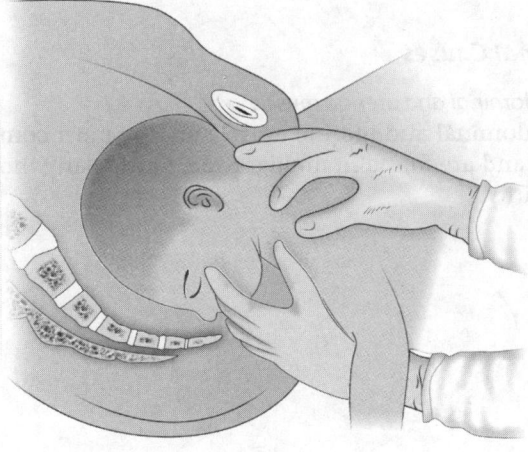

Figure 33.10: Delivery of head after flexing the head (Mauriceau-Smellie-Veit grip).

4. *Fracture of humerus*, clavicle, femur, or dislocation of shoulder or hip caused during delivery of extended arms or legs.
5. Erb's palsy caused by the brachial plexus being damaged by the twisting of the neck.
6. *Trauma to the internal organs:* A ruptured liver or spleen may be produced by grasping the abdomen.
7. *Damage to the adrenals:* This also happens by grasping the abdomen. Adrenalin release can cause shock.
8. Spinal cord damage or fracture of the spine caused by bending the body backwards over the symphysis pubis, while delivering the head.
9. Intracranial hemorrhage caused by rapid delivery of the head which has had no opportunity to mold. Hypoxia may also cause intracranial hemorrhage.
10. *Fetal hypoxia:* This may be due to cord prolapse or cord compression or to premature separation of the placenta.
11. *Premature separation of the placenta:* Retraction of the uterus takes place, while the head is still in the vagina and the placenta begins to separate. Excessive delay in the delivery of the head may cause severe hypoxia in the fetus.
12. *Maternal trauma:* The maternal complications of breech delivery are the same as found in other operative vaginal deliveries.

SHOULDER PRESENTATION

When the fetus lies with its long axis across the long axis of the uterus (transverse), the shoulder is most likely to present. Occasionally the lie is oblique, but this does not persist, as the uterine contractions during labor make it either longitudinal or transverse.

Shoulder presentation **(Figs. 33.11A and B)** occurs in approximately 1 in 300 pregnancies. Only 17% of these remain as transverse at the onset of labor. The head lies on one side of the abdomen with the breech at a slightly higher level on the other. The fetal back may be anterior or posterior.

Causes

Maternal Causes

Lax abdominal and uterine muscle
Lax abdominal and uterine muscle are the most common causes and are found in multigravida, particularly those of high parity.

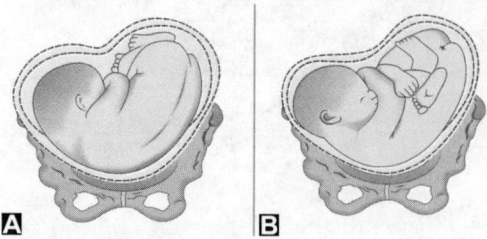

Figures 33.11A and B: Shoulder presentations.
(A) Dorsoanterior; (B) Dorsoposterior.

Uterine abnormality
A bicornuate or subseptate uterus may result in a transverse lie. More rarely, a cervical or low uterine fibroid may cause transverse lie.

Contracted pelvis
Contracted pelvis may prevent the head from entering the pelvic brim.

Fetal Causes

Preterm pregnancy
The amount of amniotic fluid in relation to the fetus is greater, allowing the fetus more mobility than at term.

Multiple pregnancies
There is a possibility of polyhydramnios, but the presence of more than one fetus reduces the room for maneuver when amounts of liquor are normal. It is the second twin, which more commonly adopts this lie after delivery of the first fetus.

Polyhydramnios
The distended uterus is globular and the fetus can move freely in the excessive liquor.

Macerated fetus
Lack of muscle tone causes the fetus to slump down into the lower pole of the uterus.

Placenta previa
Placenta previa may prevent the head from entering the pelvic brim.

Diagnosis

Antenatal

On abdominal palpation, the uterus appears broad and the fundal height is less than expected for the period of gestation. On pelvic and fundal palpation neither head nor breech is felt. The mobile head is found at one side of the abdomen and the breech at a slightly higher level at the other. Ultrasound examination may confirm the lie and presentation.

Intrapartum

The findings on abdominal palpation are as above when the membranes are intact. After the membranes have ruptured, the irregular outline of the uterus is more marked. If the uterus is contracting strongly and becomes molded around the fetus, palpation is very difficult. The shoulder is wedged into the pelvis.

Vaginal examination should not be performed without first excluding placenta previa. The membranes usually rupture early because of the ill-fitting presenting part with a high-risk of cord prolapse.

If the labor has been in progress for some time, the shoulder may be felt as a soft mass and ribs with their gridiron pattern. With further progress of labor, an arm may prolapse, and this should be differentiated from a leg by checking the characteristics and differences.

Possible Outcome

There is no mechanism of labor for a shoulder presentation. Delivery must be by cesarean section to avoid obstructed labor and subsequent uterine rupture.

Management

In the Antenatal Period

In the antenatal period, if placenta previa or contracted pelvis is detected as a cause, an elective cesarean section is required. Once such causes are excluded, an external version may be attempted. If this fails or if the lie changes to transverse after an external version, the woman is admitted in the hospital until delivery because of the risk of cord prolapse, if the membranes rupture.

In the Intrapartum Period

If transverse lie is detected early in labor, when the membranes are still intact, the physician may attempt an external version followed by a controlled rupture of membranes. If the membranes have ruptured spontaneously, a vaginal examination must be performed immediately to detect possible cord prolapse.

Immediate cesarean section should be performed:
- If the cord prolapses
- When the membranes have already ruptured
- When external version is unsuccessful
- When labor has already been in progress for some hours.

Complications
- Prolapse of cord when the membranes rupture
- Prolapse of arm when the shoulder has become impacted
- Obstructed labor and rupture of uterus
- Fetal death.

Management
Immediate cesarean section under general anesthesia, regardless of whether the fetus is alive or dead.

COMPOUND PRESENTATION

Compound presentation (**Figs. 33.12A and B**) is one in which hand or occasionally a foot, lies alongside the head. On rare occasions, head, hand and foot are felt in the vagina. This is a serious situation which may occur with a dead fetus.

Compound presentation tends to occur with a small fetus or a roomy pelvis. If diagnosed during the second stage of labor, the midwife should try to hold the hand back to allow delivery of the head.

SHOULDER DYSTOCIA

Shoulder dystocia by definition, is difficulty in the birth (or delivery) of the shoulders. In practice, this refers to cephalic presentations in which the shoulders have become impacted. Shoulder dystocia occurs when one shoulder (usually

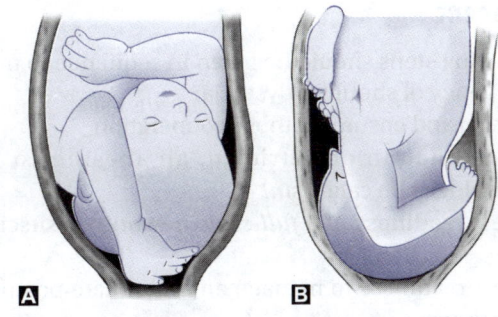

Figures 33.12A and B: Compound presentation. (A) Head with hand alongside; (B) Head with hand behind it.

the anterior) or both shoulders (rarely) impact above the pelvic brim. The problem occurs if the shoulders attempt to enter the true pelvis with the bisacromial diameter in the anteroposterior diameter of the pelvic brim, instead of either in the left or right oblique diameter of the pelvic brim, which is the normal method of entry during the normal mechanism of labor (the oblique diameter is larger than the anteroposterior diameter).

Incidence

The incidence of shoulder dystocia is not accurately known. It is reported as varying from 0.37 to 1.1%.

Risk Factors

The possibility of shoulder dystocia should be anticipated anytime when any of the following conditions exist:
- Maternal diabetes
- Obstetric history of large babies (over 4,000 g)
- Family history of large siblings
- Maternal obesity (over 90 kg)
- Large fetus (fetal macrosomia, over 4,000 g)
- Any estimated fetal weight 500 g or more greater than the woman's largest previous baby
- Maternal age over 35 years
- High parity.

Warning Signs and Diagnosis

The delivery of the head with or without forceps may have been quite easy, but more commonly the head may have advanced slowly and the chin may have had difficulty sweeping over the perineum. Once the head is delivered, it may look as if it is trying to return to the vagina. It is caused by shoulder traction and is called the *turtle sign*.

Shoulder dystocia is diagnosed when the maneuvers normally used by the midwife fails to accomplish delivery. It is important for the midwife to know how to manage this situation because, even with anticipation, diagnosis cannot be made until after the head is born. This gives little time to resolve the problem before the baby is either damaged or dead.

Management

The following steps should be taken in sequence to manage the emergency of shoulder dystocia:

- Stay calm and ensure mother's cooperation
- Request that an obstetrician, an anesthetist and a neonatologist be called *stat*
- Request readiness of a *full-scale* newborn resuscitation effort
- Request readiness to manage an immediate postpartum hemorrhage.

The obstetrician may try the following maneuvers to dislodge the shoulders and deliver the baby:

1. Check the position of the shoulders and rotate them into one of the oblique diameters of the pelvis. Instruct the mother not to push. Rotation is accomplished by placing all the fingers of one hand on one side of the baby's chest, and all the fingers of the other hand on the baby's back on the opposite side and pressing with the amount of force necessary to move the baby. It is necessary that the entire hand is used and not just two fingers for maximum strength. Under no circumstances, the baby's head should be moved as this would result in injury to the brachial or cervical nerve plexus or fracture of the cervical vertebrae.
2. Downward and outward pressure is applied on the sides of the baby's head, while another person applies suprapubic pressure.

   Suprapubic pressure is most effective if the person applying it stands on a footstool in order to get greater force behind the downward push. In mild dystocia, the baby may be delivered with this step.

   Under no circumstances, allow the fundal pressure to be applied erroneously. This will only further impact the shoulders, waste time, possibly cause injury to the fetus and possibly rupture the uterus with disastrous sequelae to both mother and baby.
3. If the baby is not delivered:
   a. Cut or enlarge the episiotomy. A deep mediolateral episiotomy will allow more room for manipulation.
   b. Catheterize the woman to empty her bladder.
   c. Place the woman in an exaggerated lithotomy position.
   d. Do a vaginal examination to rule out causes of shoulder dystocia (after the head is born) other than impacted shoulders. This requires the insertion of the entire hand as far as it can be in. Other causes to be ruled out at this stage are:
      - Short umbilical cord (relative or absolute)
      - Enlargement of the thorax or abdomen of the fetus might be caused by tumors or severe edema
      - Locked twins
      - Conjoined twins
      - Bandl's retraction ring.
4. If the dystocia is diagnosed as resulting from shoulder dystocia, attempt is made again to deliver the baby by the application of suprapubic pressure, while the obstetrician uses firm downward and outward pressure on the side of the baby's head. The baby may be delivered after this step if the condition was a moderate shoulder dystocia.

Other Manipulative Procedures

McRoberts Maneuver

The maneuver involves helping the woman to lie flat and to bring her knees up to her chest as far as possible. This will rotate the angle of the symphysis pubis superiorly and use the weight of the mother's legs to create gentle pressure on her abdomen releasing the impaction of the anterior shoulder. This maneuver is associated with the lowest level of morbidity and requires least force to accomplish delivery.

Suprapubic Pressure

Suprapubic pressure should be exerted on the side of the fetal back and toward the fetal chest. This may help to adduct the shoulders and push the anterior shoulder away from the symphysis pubis.

Rubin's Maneuver

The maneuver requires the midwife/obstetrician to identify the posterior shoulder on vaginal examination, then to push the posterior shoulder in the direction of the fetal chest, thus rotating the anterior shoulder away from the symphysis pubis. By adducting the shoulders, this maneuver reduces the 12 cm bisacromial diameter.

Wood's Maneuver

The maneuver requires the obstetrician to insert her/his hand into the vagina and identify the fetal chest. Then, by exerting pressure on to the posterior fetal shoulder, rotation is achieved. This maneuver abducts the shoulders, rotates them into a more favorable diameter and enables the completion of the delivery.

Zavanelli Maneuver

If the maneuvers described above have not been successful, the obstetrician may consider the Zavanelli maneuver as a last hope for delivery of a live infant.

This requires the reversal of the mechanisms of delivery so far and reinsertion of the fetal head into the vagina. Delivery is then completed by cesarean section.

Complications Following Shoulder Dystocia

Maternal Complications

- Hemorrhage
- Rupture of uterus.

Fetal Complications

- Neonatal asphyxia
- Erb's palsy from brachial plexus injury
- Neonatal death.

UNSTABLE LIE

An unstable lie is a condition in which at any time after 36 completed weeks of pregnancy, the fetal lie is oblique or transverse and the presentation changes from one examination to another.

Causes

Any condition in late pregnancy that increases the mobility of the fetus or prevents the head from entering the pelvic brim may cause this:
- Lax uterine muscles in multigravida
- Contracted pelvis
- Polyhydramnios.

Management

The woman is admitted to the hospital to avoid unsupervised onset of labor with a transverse lie.

After hospitalization, the lie may stabilize. If it does not, labor may be induced after 38th week of gestation, provided there is no placenta previa. The woman's bladder and rectum are emptied, and an external cephalic version is done if the fetus is in a malpresentation. When the fetus is in a vertex presentation, labor is induced with an oxytocin infusion. Fetal presentation is checked in every 5 minutes. Once regular contractions are established, a vaginal examination is done to rule out cord presentation. The membranes are then stripped and a high rupture of membranes is done, removing as much of amniotic fluid as possible, so that the head enters the pelvis. Oxytocin infusion is continued and the woman is encouraged to empty her bladder frequently. Forewater is not ruptured until the head is deeply engaged and labor is well-advanced. Labor is regarded as a trial.

STUDY QUESTIONS

Short Notes

1. Causes of occipitoposterior position.
2. Features of brow presentation.
3. Footling presentation.
4. Complete breech.
5. Shoulder dystocia.

Short Answer Questions

1. Face presentation and its causes.
2. Types of breech presentation.
3. External cephalic version.
4. Burns-Marshall method of delivering the aftercoming head.

Essay Questions

1. Describe the mechanism of labor in occipitoposterior position with a long arc rotation.
2. Describe the mechanism of labor in left mentoanterior position.
3. Enumerate the mechanism of labor in left sacroanterior position.
4. Enumerate the possible complications in a breech delivery, which the midwife should be aware of and take measures to prevent.

BIBLIOGRAPHY

1. Bahar AM. Risk factors and fetal outcome in cases of shoulder dystocia compared with normal deliveries of a similar birth-weight. British Journal of Obstetrics and Gynaecology. 1996;103(9):868-72.
2. Bennett RV, Brown LK. Myles Textbook for Midwives, 13th edition. Edinburg Churchill Livingstone; 1999. pp. 507-38.
3. Coates T, Shiers CV. Midwifery and obstetric emergencies. In: Myles (Ed). Textbook for Nurses, 13th edition. Edinburgh: Churchill Livingstone; 1999.
4. Dutta DC. Textbook of Obstetrics, 5th edition. Kolkata: New Central Book Company; 2001. pp. 390-431.
5. Hofmeyr GJ. Breech presentation and abnormal lie in late pregnancy. In: Chalmers I, Enkin MW, Heirse MJNC (Eds). Effective Care in Pregnancy and Childbirth. Oxford: Oxford University Press; 1997.
6. Resnik R. Management of shoulder girdle dystocia. Clinical Obstetrics and Gynecology. 1980;23(2):559-64.
7. Rubin A. Management of shoulder dystocia. Journal of the American Medical Association. 1964;189:835-7.
8. Sandberg EC. The Zavanelli maneuver: a potentially revolutionary method for the resolution of shoulder dystocia. American Journal of Obstetrics and Gynecology. 1985;152(4):479-84.
9. Woods CE. A principle of physics as applied to shoulder delivery. American Journal of Obstetrics and Gynecology. 1943;45:796-804.
10. Zhang J, Bowes WA Jr, Fortney JA. Efficacy of external cephalic version: a review. Obstetrics and Gynecology. 1993;82(2):306-12.

CHAPTER 34

Obstetric Operations

Learning Objectives

Upon completing this chapter, the learner will be able to:
- Describe the indications for the procedure of evacuation of uterus.
- Describe forceps and ventouse deliveries and management of women undergoing the procedure.
- Discuss the indications and preparation of the mother for cesarean section.
- Discuss the different types of destructive operations.
- Describe the care and support to mothers undergoing different procedures.

DILATATION AND EVACUATION

The procedure consists of dilatation of the cervix and evacuation of the products of conception from the uterine cavity. It may be done as a one-stage operation of dilatation and evacuation in the same sitting or a two-stage operation in which the first phase is slow dilatation of the cervix and the second phase is rapid dilatation of the cervix and evacuation.

One-stage Operation

Indications

- Incomplete abortion (most common)
- Inevitable abortion
- Medical termination of pregnancy (6–8 week)
- Hydatidiform mole in the process of expulsion.

Preparation for the Operation

Local preparation, perineal care and catheterization are done once the decision is made for evacuation. The woman and her spouse are given adequate explanation and psychological support.

Procedure

The procedure is done under general anesthesia. Internal examination is done by the obstetrician to note the size and position of the uterus and the state of dilatation of the cervix.

If the cervix is not sufficiently dilated to admit one finger, it is dilated up to the desired extend by the graduated metal dilators. The products are removed by an ovum forceps. The uterine cavity is then curetted gently by a blunt curette. Injection Methergine 0.2 mg is administered intravenously during the procedure.

The uterus is massaged bimanually and when it is found firm and the bleeding is minimal, the vagina and perineum are cleaned and the woman is sent back to her bed.

Two-stage Operation

Indications

- First trimester abortion
- Missed abortion (8–10 week uterus)
- Hydatidiform mole with unfavorable cervix (long, firm and closed os).

Procedure

First phase (Figs. 34.1A to C)
First phase consists of introduction of laminaria tents into the cervical canal to effect its slow dilatation or introduction of intravaginal prostaglandin E_2 gel 2 mg or pessary 3 mg into the posterior fornix at least 12 hours beforehand.

Prior to insertion of the tent, the woman is asked to empty her bladder, the tent of appropriate size is selected and the threads attached to one end are tied to the roller gauze.

Steps
1. Internal examination is done to note the size and position of the uterus and state of the cervix.

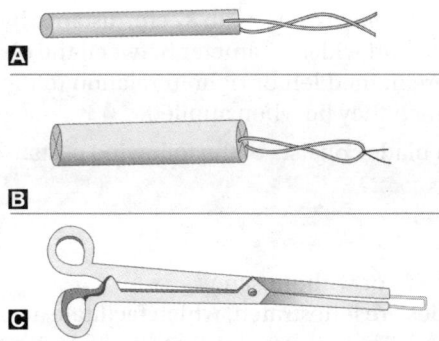

Figures 34.1A to C: Laminaria tents. (A) Prior to introduction; (B) Swollen, while kept in the cervical canal; (C) Held by tent introducing forceps.

2. A vaginal speculum is introduced. The anterior lip of the cervix is grasped by an Allis forceps to steady the cervix.
3. The cervical canal may have to be dilated, especially in primigravida, by one or two metal dilators to facilitate the introduction of tents.
4. The tents are introduced one after the other, holding it by tent introducing forceps. The tents are introduced for at least 4 cm (1.5 inch) so that the tips are placed beyond the internal os.
5. The upper vagina is packed with roller gauze to prevent the displacement of tents.
6. The patient is returned and preferably confined to bed.
7. Prophylactic antibiotic is usually administered. No anesthesia is required for the procedure.

Second phase
Second phase consists of further dilatation of the cervix by graduated metal dilators followed by evacuation of the uterus. The woman is brought to the operating room usually after 12 hours. Preparation of the patient for the procedure is same as for the first stage evacuation. The operation maybe performed under local paracervical block or under general anesthesia.

Steps of the evacuation procedure
1. The posterior vaginal speculum is introduced after removing the vaginal packing. The tents are removed with a sponge holding forceps. The vagina and cervix are swabbed with an antiseptic solution and the speculum is removed.
2. Vaginal examination is done to note the size and position of uterus and the state of dilatation of the cervix.
3. A retaining speculum (Auvard speculum) is introduced and the anterior lips of the cervix are held by an Allis forceps to steady it. A uterine sound is introduced into the uterine cavity to ascertain the length of the cavity and position of the uterus.
4. The cervix is dilated with the graduated metal dilators up to the desired extent to facilitate introduction of the ovum forceps.
5. The products of conception are removed by introducing the ovum forceps. Intravenous (IV) Methergine 0.2 mg is given during this stage to minimize blood loss.
6. The uterine cavity is thoroughly curetted by a flushing (blunt) curette.
7. The speculum and Allis forceps are removed and the uterus massaged bimanually. After confirming a well-contracted uterus with minimal bleeding, the vulva is cleaned and a perineal pad is placed.
8. Intramuscular (IM) Methergine is repeated postoperatively and prophylactic antibiotic may be given.

Dangers of Dilatation and Evacuation Operation

Immediate Dangers

❖ Hemorrhage due to incomplete evacuation or atonic uterus
❖ Injury such as cervical laceration or uterine perforation
❖ Shock due to excessive blood loss, uterine perforation or anesthetic complications
❖ Increased morbidity.

Late Dangers

❖ Pelvic inflammation
❖ Infertility
❖ Cervical incompetence
❖ Uterine adhesions.

FORCEPS DELIVERY

Forceps delivery is a means of extracting the fetus with the aid of obstetric forceps when it is inadvisable or impossible for the mother to complete the delivery by her own efforts. Forceps are also used to assist the delivery of the aftercoming head of the breech and on occasion to withdraw the head up and out of the pelvis at cesarean section.

Ever since the invention of obstetric forceps around 1600 AD by the Chamberlen family, many designs were invented and modified. Forceps deliveries were formerly classified by the level of the head at the time the forceps were applied, i.e. high cavity, midcavity and low cavity. Low-cavity forceps is the one frequently performed, as cesarean section is usually preferred to the more traumatic high- and mid-cavity operations.

Low-cavity forceps can be divided into *rotational* and *nonrotational*. Rotational forceps delivery refers to a maneuver of the fetal head from a malposition into a more favorable position with the aid of specially designed forceps, usually Kielland's. Examples of non-rotational forceps are:
❖ Wrigley's forceps and Simpson's forceps (low cavity)
❖ Neville-Barnes and Haig Ferguson's forceps (high- and mid-cavity forceps).

Basic Construction of the Forceps (Fig. 34.2)

Obstetric forceps consist of two separate blades, each with a handle. Each blade is marked 'L' (left) or 'R' (right). They are inserted separately on either side of the fetal head and locked together by English or Smellie lock (rotational forceps have a sliding lock). The blades are spoon shaped

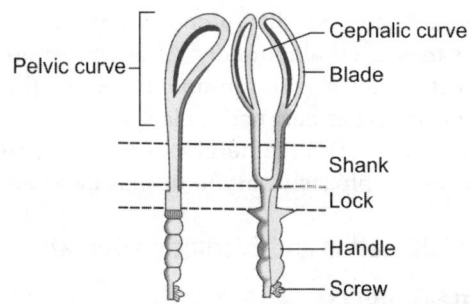

Figure 34.2: Different parts of a long curved obstetric forceps.

to accommodate the fetal head and fenestrated to minimize trauma, and for lightness. The spoon shape of the blade is called *cephalic curve*. When the blades are articulated, it holds the fetal head. The blades are attached to the handle at an angle, which corresponds to the curve of Carus (curve on the axis of birth canal). This is termed as the *pelvic curve* of the blade. When the blades are correctly placed on the fetal head, the handles will be neatly aligned.

Types of Currently Used Obstetric Forceps

Only three varieties are commonly used in present day obstetrics **(Figs. 34.3A to C)**. They are:
- Long curved forceps with or without axis traction device
- Short curved forceps
- Kielland's forceps.

Long Curved Obstetric Forceps

The long curved obstetric forceps is relatively heavy and is about 37 cm (15 inch) long. In India, Das's variety (named after Sir Kedarnath Das) is commonly used. It is comparatively lighter and slightly shorter than its western counterpart, and is quiet suited for the comparatively small pelvis and small baby of Indian women.

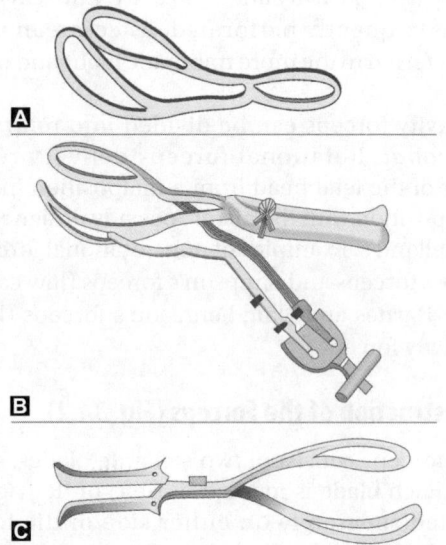

Figures 34.3A to C: Different types of obstetric forceps. (A) Short curved forceps; (B) Axis traction forceps; (C) Kielland's forceps.

Forceps measurements are length 37 cm, distance between the tips is 2.5 cm and widest diameter between the blades 9 cm.

Blades are named left or right in relation to the maternal pelvis in which they lie when applied.

Parts: Each blade consists of the following parts:
- Blade
- Shank
- Lock
- Handle with or without screw.

The blades are fenestrated, which facilitate a good grip of the fetal head. There is usually a slot in the lower part of the fenestrum of the blades to allow the upper end of the axis traction rod to be fitted.

Blade: It has two curves. The 'pelvic curve' is designed to fit the curve on the axis of the birth canal (curve of Carus). The front of the forceps is the concave side of the 'pelvic curve'. The 'cephalic curve' on the flat surface, which when articulated, grasps the fetal head without compression.

Shank: It is the part between the blade and the lock, and usually measures 6.25 cm (2½ inch). It increases the length of the instrument and thereby facilitates locking of the blades outside the vulva. When the blades are articulated, the shanks are not apposed together.

Lock: The common method of articulation consists of a socket system located on the shank at its junction with the handle (English lock).

Handle: The handles are apposed when the blades are articulated. It measures 12.5 cm (5 inch). A screw may be attached usually at the end (or at the base) of one blade, commonly left, to keep the blades in position.

Axis traction device: It can be applied with advantage in midforceps operation, especially following manual rotation of the head. It provides traction in the correct axis of the pelvic curve and as such, less force is necessary to deliver the head. It consists of traction rods and traction handle.

Short Curved Forceps (Wrigley's Forceps)

The instrument is lighter, shorter and stubby handled. It is short due to reduction in the length of the shanks and handles. It has a marked cephalic curve with a slight pelvic curve. The instrument is used for very low forceps deliveries for the aftercoming head of a breech delivery or at cesarean section.

Kielland's Forceps

Kielland's forceps is a long, almost straight (very slight pelvic curve) obstetric forceps without any axis traction device. It has a sliding lock. Kielland's forceps is used when the head is in an occipitolateral or occipitoposterior position. After the blades are applied, the head is rotated to an occipitoanterior position. It facilitates grasping and correction of asynclitic head because of its sliding lock.

In the hands of an expert, it is a useful and preferred instrument. It can be used in an un-rotated vertex or face presentation. Grasping and correction of an asynclitic head is facilitated because of its sliding lock.

The blades are named anterior and posterior. The anterior blade is to be inserted first. Application of the blade is done either by wandering method or direct method. Wandering method is usually applied in deep transverse arrest. Anterior blade is introduced laterally over the baby's face. Then it is gently moved around the face to be placed over the anterior parietal bone. Posterior blade is introduced between the head and the sacrum. Rotation of the head can be achieved at the same level or at a lower level, after pulling the head down. Epidural anesthesia is generally preferred for this procedure.

Limitations

Because of the complexity in the technique of its application, there are chances of injuries to the vagina or perineum. Deep mediolateral episiotomy is mandatory.

Classification According to the Level of the Fetal Head at which the Forceps are Applied

1. *High forceps operation:* The application of forceps on a fetal head where the biparietal diameter has not yet passed the pelvic brim (non-engaged head). Cesarean section is preferred to this type of forceps application.
2. *Mid forceps operation:* Refers to the application of the forceps where the biparietal diameter has passed the brim of the pelvis, but not passed the level of ischial spines.
3. *Low forceps operation:* Refers to the application of the forceps where the biparietal diameter has passed the level of ischial spines.
4. *Outlet forceps:* The forceps are applied on the fetal head lying on the perineum and is visible at the introitus in between contractions. The sagittal suture should lie in the anteroposterior diameter of the outlet. In the present day practice, 90% of forceps applications are the low forceps categories. All outlet forceps are low forceps, but not all low forceps are outlet forceps.

Indications of Forceps Operation

Delay in the second stage due to uterine inertia. If the head is on the perineum for 20–30 minutes without advancement, forceps application may be decided:
- Maternal indications:
  - Maternal distress
  - Preeclampsia, eclampsia
  - Vaginal birth after cesarean section (VBAC)
  - Heart disease
  - Failure to bear down during the second stage of labor due to regional blocks, paraplegia or psychiatric disturbance.
- Fetal indications:
  - Appearance of fetal distress in the second stage
  - Cord prolapse
  - Aftercoming head of breech
  - Low-birth-weight baby
  - Postmaturity.

Prerequisites for Forceps Delivery

There are certain conditions, which must exist before forceps delivery can be performed:
- The cervix must be fully dilated and effaced
- Membranes must be ruptured
- Presentation and position must be suitable to apply the blades correctly to the sides of the head (sagittal suture in anteroposterior diameter of pelvic outlet)
- The head must be engaged with no parts of the head palpable abdominally
- No appreciable cephalopelvic disproportion
- The bladder must be emptied
- Presence of good uterine contractions as a safeguard to postpartum hemorrhage.

Preparation of the Woman

The woman should be prepared in advance for the possibility of a forceps delivery if this looks likely. Full explanation of the procedure and the need for it must be given to the woman.

Once the decision has been made, adequate and appropriate analgesia must be offered. When analgesia has been instituted and the obstetrician is ready to proceed, the woman's legs are placed in lithotomy position. Both legs must be placed simultaneously to avoid strain on the woman's back and hips.

The woman should be tilted toward the left at an angle of 15° by the use of a pillow or a rubber wedge under the mattress to prevent aortocaval occlusion.

Preparations must also be done for the baby including equipment for resuscitation. In some hospitals a pediatrician will also be present.

Procedure

Procedure of Low Forceps Operation

1. The woman's vulval area is thoroughly cleaned and draped with sterile towels using aseptic technique. The bladder is emptied using a straight catheter.
2. A vaginal examination is performed by the obstetrician to confirm the station and exact position of the fetal head.
3. A pudendal block, supplemented by perineal and labial infiltration with 1% lignocaine hydrochloride, is given to produce effective local anesthesia.
4. An episiotomy may be done prior to introduction of the blades or during traction when the perineum becomes bulged and thinned out by the advanced head.
5. The forceps are identified as left or right by assembling them briefly before proceeding **(Fig. 34.4)**.
6. The left blade is passed gently between the perineum and fetal head with the first two fingers of the operator's right hand lying alongside the fetal head protecting the maternal tissue. The tip of the forceps blade slides lightly over the head, into the hollow of the sacrum and is then 'wandered' to the left side of the pelvis where it should sit alongside the head.

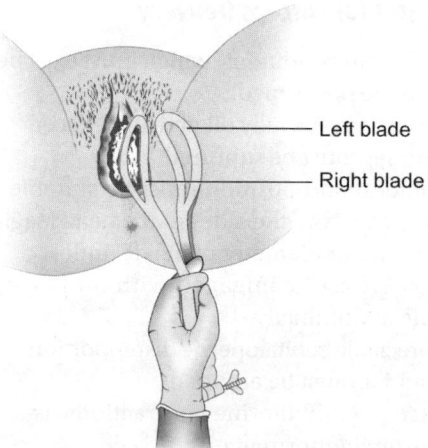

Figure 34.4: Identification of the forceps blades.

7. The procedure is repeated with the right blade until it sits on the right of the pelvis. It should then be easy to lock the two blades and there should be little or no gap between the handles. A significant gap suggests that the forceps are wrongly positioned and they should be reapplied after carefully checking the position of head.
8. During the application stage of the forceps, the woman should be given full support and attention by the midwife.
9. The fetal heart rate is to be monitored throughout.
10. As soon as the operator is ready and the uterus contracts, the woman is encouraged to push. To supplement her efforts, the obstetrician exerts steady, downward traction on the forceps. Traction is released between contractions. Intermittent traction is continued in a downward and backward direction until the head comes to the perineum. The pull is then directed horizontally straight toward the operator until the head is almost crowned. The direction of pull is gradually changed toward the mother's abdomen to deliver the head by extension **(Figs. 34.5A to D)**.
11. The blades are removed one after the other, the right one first.
12. Following the birth of the head, usual procedures are to be followed as in normal delivery. IV Methergine 0.2 mg is to be administered with the delivery of the anterior shoulder. Episiotomy is repaired as quickly as possible and the woman is made comfortable.

Manual Rotation of the Fetal Head Followed by Midforceps Operation

Some obstetricians prefer to rotate the fetal head manually in cases of occipitoposterior position, as this is likely to be less traumatic than instrumental rotation. The exact position of the fetal head must be determined. The obstetrician grasps the head usually by sinciput and rotates it, encouraging the flexion.

The commonly used forceps is the long curved one with or without axis traction device. Kielland's forceps is useful in the hands of an expert.

General anesthesia is preferable. The blades are introduced as in the low forceps operation. An assistant is required to hold the left handle after its introduction. If axis traction rod is used, this must be already attached to the blade. During introduction of the right blade, the traction rod must be held forward otherwise it will prevent locking of the blades.

The direction of the pull is first downward and backward, then horizontal or straight and finally upward and forward. With axis traction device, the traction handle is to be attached to the traction rods. During traction, the traction rods should remain parallel to the shanks. When the base of the occiput comes under the symphysis pubis, the traction rods are to be removed.

Difficulties in Forceps Operation

The difficulties are mainly due to faulty assessment before the operative delivery is undertaken. However, there is hardly any difficulty with low forceps operation.

Difficulties in the application of blades are caused by incompletely dilated cervix and unrotated or non-engaged head. Difficulty in locking are caused by:
- Application on unrotated head
- Improper insertion of the blade (not for enough in)
- Failure to depress the handle against the perineum
- Entanglement of the cord or fetal parts inside the blades

Causes of Failure

The causes of failure to deliver with traction are:
- Undiagnosed occipitoposterior position
- Faulty cephalic application
- Wrong direction of traction
- Mild pelvic contraction
- Constriction ring.

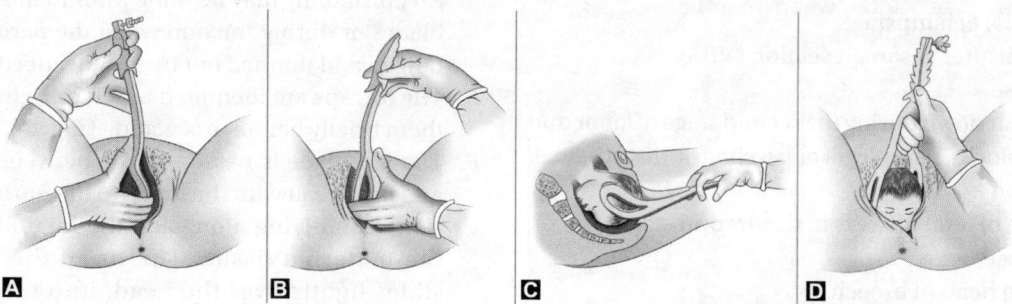

Figures 34.5A to D: Steps of forceps application. **(A)** Introduction of the left blade; **(B)** Introduction of the right blade; **(C)** Traction of the head; **(D)** Change of the grip in the final stage.

Complications of Forceps Operation

The hazards of the forceps operation are mostly related to the faulty technique and to the indications for which the forceps are applied.

In the Mother

Immediate complications
- Injury:
  – Extension of the episiotomy towards rectum or upwards up to the vault of vagina
  – Vaginal lacerations
  – Cervical tear especially when applied through an incompletely dilated cervix
  – Bruising and trauma to the urethra.
- Postpartum hemorrhage due to trauma or atonic uterus related to prolonged labor or effect of anesthesia
- Shock due to blood loss, prolonged labor and dehydration
- Sepsis due to devitalization of local tissues and improper asepsis.

Late complications
- Chronic low backache due to tension imposed on softened ligaments of lumbosacral or sacroiliac joints during lithotomy position
- Genital prolapse or stress incontinence.

In the Infant

Immediate complications
- Asphyxia due to intracranial stress out of prolonged compression
- Intracranial hemorrhage due to malapplication of the blades
- Cephalhematoma
- Facial palsy due to damage to facial nerve
- Abrasions on the soft tissues of the face and forehead by the forceps blade, severe bruising will cause marked jaundice
- Tentorial tear from compression of the fetal head by the forceps.

Prophylactic Forceps (Elective)

Prophylactic forceps refers to forceps delivery only to shorten the second stage of labor when maternal and/or fetal complications are anticipated. The indications are:
- Eclampsia
- Heart disease
- Previous history of cesarean section
- Postmaturity
- Low-birth-weight baby
- Patients under epidural anesthesia
- To curtail the painful second stage.

Prophylactic forceps application is done only after the criteria of low forceps are fulfilled.

Trial Forceps

Trial forceps is a tentative attempt of forceps delivery in a case of suspected midpelvic contraction with a preamble declaration of abandoning it in favor of cesarean section, if moderate traction fails to overcome the resistance. The procedure is conducted in an operating room keeping everything ready for cesarean section. If moderate traction leads to progressive descend of the fetal head, the delivery is completed vaginally, if not, cesarean section is done immediately.

Failed Forceps

When a deliberate attempt in vaginal delivery with forceps has failed to expedite the process, it is called failed forceps. It is predominantly due to lack of obstetric skill with poor clinical judgment. Failure in the operative delivery may be due to improper application or failure of descend of the head even with forcible contraction.

Causes for Failed Forceps

- Incompletely dilated cervix
- Unrotated occipitoposterior position
- Undiagnosed brow or hydrocephalus or fetal ascites
- Constriction ring
- Large baby with the shoulders impacted at the brim.

Management

- Assess the effect on mother and fetus
- Start IV infusion with 5% dextrose if one is not already in place
- Administer parenteral antibiotic
- Exclude rupture of uterus and plan for other modes of delivery
- The woman should be shifted to an equipped hospital.

VACUUM EXTRACTION (VENTOUSE DELIVERY)

Ventouse is an instrumental device designed to assist delivery by creating a vacuum between it and the fetal scalp.

Equipment

The ventouse or vacuum extractor (**Fig. 34.6**) consists of the following basic components:
1. Suction cup (4 sizes—30, 40, 50 and 60 mm).
2. A vacuum pump.
3. Traction rod device.

Various modifications of the earlier instrument, introduced in 1956 by Mulmström, are now available. Modern vacuum extractors use an electrical pump, which has sensitive controls. The vacuum is built up steadily and is maintained efficiently, so that the cup is less likely to come off.

A metal or Silastic (firm rubber) cup is applied to the fetal head; a vacuum is created inside this cup, which is connected to the pump by rubber tubing and traction is then applied.

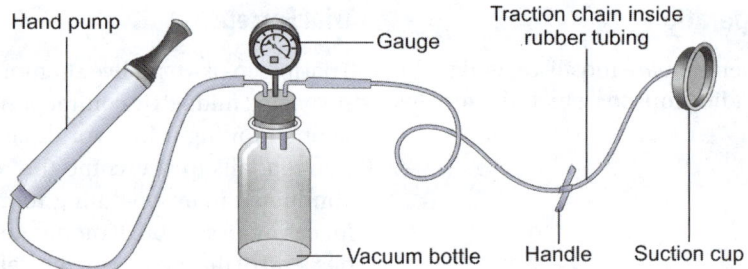

Figure 34.6: Ventouse or vacuum extractor.

Inside the rubber tubing is a metal chain designed to take the strain of traction, with a metal handle to give the operator a good grip.

Indications

- Deep transverse arrest with adequate pelvis
- Delay in descend of the high head in case of the second baby of twins
- Malpositions—occipitolateral and occipitoposterior
- Delay in the second stage of labor or late first stage
- As an alternative to forceps operation except in:
  – Face presentation and aftercoming head of breech
  – Fetal distress or prematurity.
- Maternal exhaustion.

Advantages of Ventouse over Forceps

- Ventouse can be used in unrotated or malrotated occipitoposterior position of the head
- It can be applied even through an incompletely dilated cervix
- It is not a space-occupying device like the forceps blades
- Lesser traction force is needed (10 kg)
- It can be used safely even when the head remains at a high level in second baby of twins
- It is comfortable and injuries to the mother are less
- Requires less technical skill for the operator.

Advantages of Forceps over Ventouse

- Forceps operation can quickly expedite the delivery in case of fetal distress, where ventouse will be unsuitable as it takes longer time
- Forceps is safe for a premature baby; the fetal head remains inside the protective cage
- It can be employed in anterior face or in aftercoming head of breech
- In suspected pelvic contraction, where moderate traction is required, ventouse will be ineffective.

Contraindications for Ventouse

- Fetal distress, where urgent delivery is needed
- Face presentation
- Prematurity, chance of scalp avulsion or subaponeurotic hemorrhage is more
- Fetal bleeding disorder.

Conditions to be Fulfilled

- There should not be any bony resistance below the head
- The head of a singleton baby should be engaged
- Cervix should be at least 6 cm dilated.

Procedure (Fig. 34.7)

The prerequisites are as for forceps delivery. The operator must be completely familiar with the technique appropriate to the particular cup design. The woman is positioned and prepared as for forceps delivery. The position of the fetal head is determined and an appropriate size and type of cup selected. Pudendal block or perineal infiltration with 1% lignocaine is done. The instrument is assembled and the vacuum is tested prior to its application.

Step 1: Application of the Cup

The cup is introduced after retraction of the perineum with two fingers of the hand. The cup is placed against the fetal head nearer to the occiput with the 'knob' of the cup pointing toward the occiput. This will facilitate flexion of the head.

A vacuum of 0.2 kg/cm^2 is induced by hand pump slowly, taking at least 2 minutes. A check is made with fingers round the cup to ensure that no cervical or vaginal tissue is trapped inside the cup. The pressure is gradually raised at the rate of 0.1 kg/cm^2/min until the effective vacuum of 0.8 kg/cm^2 is reached in about 10 minutes time. The scalp is sucked into the cup and an artificial caput succedaneum (chignon) is produced. The chignon usually disappears within few hours.

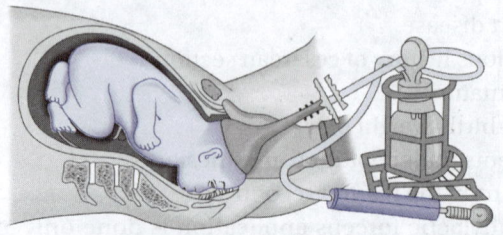

Figure 34.7: Application of vacuum extractor.

Step 2: Traction

Traction is exerted using one hand in the direction of the curve of Carus. Traction must be at right angles to the cup and synchronous with the uterine contractions; while applying traction, fingers of the other hand are to be placed against the cup to note the correct angle of traction, rotation and advancement of the head. Ventouse delivery may take slightly longer than forceps delivery. However, if there is no advancement during four successive uterine contractions, it should be abandoned. On no account, traction should exceed 30 minutes.

As soon as the head is delivered, the vacuum is reduced by opening the screw—release valve and the cup is then detached. The delivery is then completed in the normal manner. Silicon rubber cups (silc cups) are currently used, as they are soft and can be smoothly applied over the contour of the fetal head. They could be folded and introduced into the vagina before being placed over the fetal head.

Silicone/Silastic Rubber Cup (Fig. 34.8)

The silicone rubber cup can be used in place of the metal cup of Malmström vacuum extractor. The cup is used when the mother is cooperative, the baby is average sized and there is minimal caput.

The silicone rubber cup is used in the following manner—it is folded and gently inserted into the vagina with one hand from above downwards, while the other hand parts the labia. A gentle twist may help it to unfold into place in the vagina and thereafter it is essentially not maneuverable being larger in diameter than the metal cup and having a relatively inflexible handle.

With the pressure at 0.2 kg/cm^2, a check is made to ensure that no maternal tissue is caught under the cup and then the pressure is raised to 0.6–0.8 kg/cm^2 depending on the size of the baby or weeks of gestation. Gentle to moderate traction along the pelvic axis for the duration of next two to three contractions should deliver the head.

One hand should rest on the bell of the cup while the other applies traction. The hand on the cup detects any early detachment and also indicates whether the head moves downwards with each pull. The fingers on the head can promote flexion of the head.

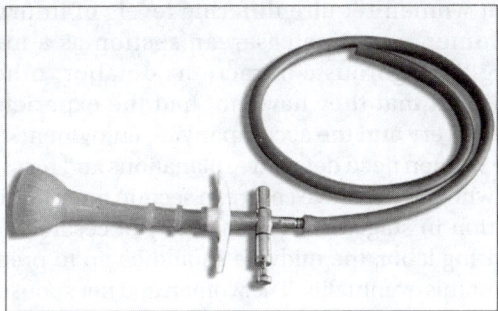

Figure 34.8: Silicone/silastic rubber cup.

Complications

Fetal

1. Sloughing of the scalp.
2. Cephalhematoma.
3. Cerebral trauma, such as tentorial tear.
4. *Chignon:* This is an area of edema and bruising where the cup was applied; all babies delivered by ventouse will have a chignon. These normally subside uneventfully, but may occasionally become infected.

Maternal

Trauma to the mother is rare. Injuries may occur due to inclusion of the soft tissues such as the cervix or vaginal wall inside the cup.

Failure

An attempted vacuum extraction may be unsuccessful. Exerting too much traction will result in the cup coming off. The cup is likely to come off in unskilled or impatient hands.

CESAREAN SECTION

Cesarean section is an operative procedure whereby the fetuses after the end of 28th week are delivered through an incision on the abdominal and uterine walls. The first operation performed on a woman is referred to as a primary cesarean section. When the operation is performed in subsequent pregnancies, it is called repeat cesarean section.

Incidence

The incidence of cesarean section is steadily rising. During the last decade, there has been two-to-three-fold rise in the incidence from the initial rate of about 10%. Factors responsible are—increased safety of the operation due to improved anesthesia, availability of blood transfusion and antibiotics. Increased awareness of fetal well-being and identification of risk factors have caused reduction of difficult operative or manipulative vaginal deliveries. Obstetricians as well as women choose not to take even slightest risk of abnormal labor.

Indications for Cesarean Section

Elective Cesarean Section

The term, elective, indicates that the decision to deliver the baby by cesarean section has been made during the pregnancy and before the onset of labor. While some indications are absolute, others will depend on a combination of factors.

Absolute (definite) indications include:
- Cephalopelvic disproportion
- Major degrees of placenta previa
- Multiple pregnancies with three or more fetuses
- Advanced carcinoma of cervix
- Pelvic tumors such as cervical fibroid.

In all these cases, there is possibility of insuperable obstruction for vaginal delivery and cesarean section may have to be performed even if the fetus is dead.

Relative (possible) indications include:
- Malpresentation:
  - Persistent transverse lie, brow or mentoposterior
  - Big breech or average breech with associated complicating factors.
- Pregnancy-induced hypertension:
  - Acute fulminating preeclampsia
  - Eclampsia with uncontrolled fits and the woman is not in labor.
- Medical gynecological conditions:
  - Chronic hypertension, chronic nephritis
  - Diabetes—uncontrolled with previous history of fetal wastage
  - Heart disease—uncorrected coarctation of aorta or organic heart lesions.
- Previous scar following classical cesarean section or hysterotomy
- Antepartum hemorrhage
- Bad obstetric history of recurrent fetal wastage.

If the indication for cesarean section pertains specifically to one pregnancy, such as placenta previa, vaginal delivery may be expected on subsequent occasions. However, certain conditions, such as cephalopelvic disproportion due to contracted pelvis, will recur and a uterus that has been scarred twice or more, carries a greater risk of uterine rupture and requires to repeat cesarean operation.

Emergency Cesarean Section

Emergency cesarean section is performed when adverse conditions develop during labor:
1. Cord prolapse.
2. Uterine rupture (acute) or scar dehiscence.
3. Cephalopelvic disproportion diagnosed in labor.
4. Fulminating pregnancy-induced hypertension.
5. Eclampsia.
6. Failure to progress in the first or second stage of labor.
7. Fetal distress, if delivery is not imminent. Fetal distress in the first stage is more likely in previously compromised baby of intrauterine growth restriction (IUGR), hypertensive disorder, postmaturity or in hypertonus state following oxytocin induced or augmented labor and incoordinate uterine action.
8. Abnormal uterine contractions: Prolongation of labor due to incoordinate uterine action.

Contraindications

In the absence of maternal interest, the following are the contraindications for cesarean section:
- Dead fetus
- Baby, too premature to survive outside the uterus
- Presence of blood coagulation disorders.

Types of Operations

Lower Segment Cesarean Section

In lower segment cesarean section (LSCS), the extraction of the baby is done through an incision made in the lower segment through a transperitoneal approach. The lower segment of the uterus forms after about 32 week's gestation and is less muscular than the upper segment of the uterus. In a lower segment cesarean section, a transverse incision is made in the lower segment; this heals faster and successfully than an incision in the upper segment of the uterus. There is less muscle and more fibrous tissue in the lower segment, which reduces the risk of rupture in a subsequent pregnancy. It is the only method practiced in present day obstetrics and unless specified, cesarean section means lower segment operation. It is commonly performed through a transverse incision on the abdomen, the *pfannenstiel* or *bikini line* incision.

Classical Cesarean Section

In classical cesarean section, the baby is extracted through an incision made in the upper segment of the uterus. Its indications in the present day practice are very much limited and are rarely performed.

Indications
1. Gestation of less than 32 weeks before the lower segment has formed.
2. Placenta previa, which is situated anteriorly, in order to avoid incision of the placenta.
3. Hourglass constriction.
4. Lower segment approach is difficult due to dense adhesions from previous operation or severely contracted pelvis (osteomalacic or rachitic) with pendulous abdomen.
5. Lower segment approach is risky due to big fibroid in the lower segment or carcinoma cervix.
6. Postmortem section: Contemplating to have a live baby.
7. A classical section is always performed through a midline incision.

Preparation of the Mother

Psychological Preparation

Different women require differing levels of information. Some women welcome cesarean section as a means of escaping the rigorous contractions of labor; others feel disappointed that they have not had the experience of a normal delivery and the accompanying enjoyment.

Some women need detailed explanations and reassurance. Women who have elective cesarean section, may be given the information in stages. If the possibility of cesarean section arises during labor, the midwife should begin to prepare the woman for this eventuality. The woman and her spouse should be kept informed of the events and progress during labor as well as assured of assistance.

Physical Preparation

1. Intravenous infusion is started if one has not already been established.
2. Abdomen is prepared as for laparotomy.
3. A non-particulate antacid (0.3 molar sodium citrate 30 mL) is given orally before transferring the woman to operating room. It is given to neutralize the existing gastric acid.
4. If the cesarean section is an elective procedure, ranitidine (H_2 blocker) 150 mg is given orally the night before and repeated (50 mg IM or IV), 1 hour before surgery to raise the gastric pH.
5. Metoclopramide (Reglan) 10 mg IV is given to increase the tone of the lower esophageal sphincter as well as to reduce the stomach contents. It is administered about 3 minutes of preoxygenation in the operating room.
6. The stomach should be emptied, if necessary by a stomach tube (emergency procedure).
7. Bladder must be emptied by passing a catheter before or after induction of anesthesia and left in place.
8. Bowel preparation is done the evening before (two glycerin suppositories) for elective cesarean section clients.
9. The woman is dressed in clean operation gown and any valuables are either placed in safekeeping or given to the family. Any rings or bracelets, which cannot be removed, are covered with adhesive strapping.
10. Premedication sedatives must not be given.

Procedures in Cesarean Section

Anesthesia

A method, which is considered safe by the anesthetist is employed. General, epidural or spinal anesthesia may be used.

Position

The woman is placed in dorsal position. In susceptible cases, to minimize any adverse effects of vena caval compression, an angle of 15° tilt to her left using sand bags until delivery of baby is beneficial.

Incision on the Abdomen

A low transverse incision is made about two fingers breadth above the symphysis pubis (modified pfannenstiel) or above the symphysis pubis (pfannenstiel or bikini line incision). Some obstetricians make a vertical infraumbilical or paramedian incision, which extends from about 2.5 cm below the umbilicus to the upper border of the symphysis pubis. The anatomic layers incised are:

- Fat
- Rectal sheath
- Muscle (rectus abdominis)
- Abdominal peritoneum
- Uterine muscle.

The surgeon usually incises the rectus sheath by a scalpel, but divides the rectus muscle digitally, splitting it transversely. This method minimizes blood loss. Alternatively, the incision may be extended on either side using a pair of curved scissors to make it a curved incision of about 10 cm (4 inch) in length, the concavity directed upwards.

Delivery of the Head

The uterine cavity is then opened, the membranes are ruptured and the amniotic fluid is aspirated. The head is delivered by hooking the head with the fingers, which are carefully inserted between the lower uterine flap and the head until the palm is placed below the head. As the head is drawn to the incision line, the assistant is to apply pressure on the fundus. Obstetric forceps (Wrigley's forceps) are often used to extract the head from the pelvis.

Delivery of the Trunk

As soon as the head is delivered, the mucus from the mouth, pharynx and nostrils is to be sucked out using rubber catheter attached to an electric sucker. When the baby is born, an oxytocic drug (Methergine 0.2 mg) is administered before the placenta and membranes are delivered. The cord is cut between two clamps and the baby is given to the nurse.

Removal of the Placenta and Membranes

The placenta is extracted by traction on the cord with simultaneous pushing on the fundus toward the umbilicus (controlled cord traction). The placenta and membranes are removed intact.

Suturing of the Uterine Wound

The margins of the wound are picked up by Allis tissue forceps or Green-Armytage hemostatic clamps. The uterine muscle is sutured in two layers using continuous running sutures, the second of which tends to align the cut edges of the pelvic peritoneum. Repair of the rectus sheath brings the rectus abdominis into alignment. The subcutaneous fat is sometimes sutured and finally the skin is closed with sutures or clips.

Postoperative Care

Immediate Care (4–6 Hours)

In the immediate recovery period, the blood pressure is recorded every 15 minutes. Temperature is recorded every 2 hours. The wound must be inspected every half an hour to detect any blood loss. The lochia are also inspected and drainage should be small initially. Following general anesthesia, the woman is nursed in the left lateral or 'recovery' position until she is fully conscious, since the risks of airway obstruction or regurgitation and silent aspiration of stomach contents are still present. Analgesia is given as prescribed.

First 24 Hours

Intravenous fluids (5% dextrose or Ringer's lactate) are continued. Blood transfusion is helpful in anemic mothers for speedy postoperative recovery. Injection Methergine 0.2 mg IM may be repeated. Parenteral antibiotic is usually given for the first 48 hours. Analgesics in the form of pethidine 75–100 mg are administered as required. Ambulation is encouraged on the day following surgery and baby is brought to her.

After 24 Hours

The blood pressure, pulse and temperature are usually checked every 4 hours. Oral feeding is started with clear liquids and then advanced to light and regular diet. Intravenous fluids are continued for about 48 hours. Urinary catheter may be removed on the following day when the woman is able to get up to the toilet. The woman is helped to get out of bed as soon as possible and encouraged to become fully mobile.

The mother must be encouraged to rest as much as possible and needed help is to be given with care for the baby. This should preferably take place at the mother's bedside and should include support with breastfeeding.

The mother is usually discharged with the baby after the abdominal skin stitches are removed by the 4th or 5th day.

Complications of Cesarean Section

The complications are related either to the operation (inherent hazards) or to the indications for which the operation is done. Thus, the complications are more following emergency rather than elective operations:

1. Postpartum hemorrhage related to uterine atony and rarely blood coagulation disorders.
2. *Shock related to blood loss:* It might occur when the operation is done following prolonged labor.
3. *Anesthetic hazards:* Mostly associated with emergency operations and related to aspiration of gastric contents.
4. *Sepsis:* The common sites of infection are urinary tract, abdominal wound, uterus, peritoneal cavity and lungs.
5. Intestinal obstruction may be mechanical due to adhesions or bands, or paralytic following peritonitis.
6. *Thrombosis:* Leg vein thrombosis and pulmonary embolism are likely to occur following cesarean section.
7. Wound complications such as wound sepsis, hematoma, dehiscence and burst abdomen may happen.

Late complications include menstrual irregularities, chronic pelvic pain or backache. Remote surgical complications may be incision hernia and intestinal obstruction due to adhesions and bands.

The risk of scar rupture is a possible complication in future pregnancies. Babies born by cesarean section have increased risk of respiratory distress syndrome (RDS) compared to those delivered vaginally.

Cesarean Hysterectomy

Cesarean hysterectomy refers to an operation where cesarean section is followed by removal of the uterus. The common conditions are:

- Atonic uterus and uncontrolled postpartum hemorrhage
- Morbid adherent placenta
- Big fibroid
- Extensive lacerations due to extension of tears with broad ligament hematoma
- Grossly infected uterus
- Rupture of uterus with fetus inside.

DESTRUCTIVE OPERATIONS (EMBRYOTOMIES)

The destructive operations are designed to diminish the bulk of the fetus to facilitate easy delivery through the birth canal. It may occasionally be necessary to destroy the fetus in the interest of saving the mother's life. There are four types of operations.

Craniotomy

Craniotomy is an operation to make a perforation on the fetal head to evacuate the contents followed by extraction of the fetus. The various instruments used for craniotomy are shown in **Figures 34.9A to C**.

Indications

1. Cephalic presentation producing obstructed labor with a dead fetus. This is the most common indication of craniotomy in the referral hospitals of the developing countries.
2. Hydrocephalus even in a living fetus: This is applicable to the forthcoming and aftercoming head.
3. Interlocking heads of twins.

For the procedure to be done safely, the cervix must be fully dilated.

Sites of Perforation

- *Vertex:* On the parietal bone, on either side of the sagittal suture.

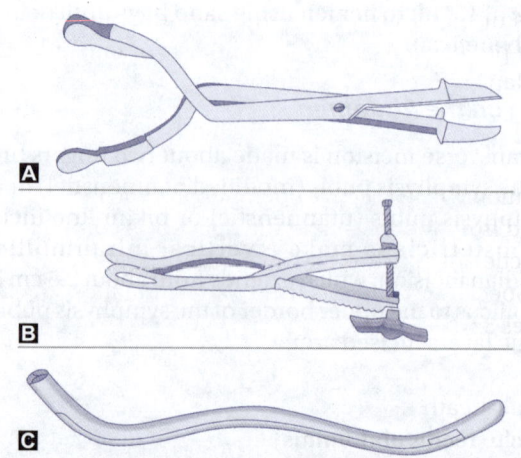

Figures 34.9A to C: Instruments for craniotomy. (A) Oldham's perforator; (B) Cranioclast; (C) Budin's cannula.

* *Face:* Through the orbit or hard palate.
* *Brow:* Through the frontal bone.

Suture is avoided to prevent collapse of the bone thereby preventing escape of brain matter.

Procedure

The obstetrician introduces two fingers (index and middle) into the vagina and the fingertips are placed on the proposed site of perforation. If the suture line cannot be defined because of a big caput, the perforation is done through the dependent part.

An assistant fixes the head suprapubically, while the operator introduces the perforator with the blades closed, protecting the anterior vaginal wall and the bladder with the fingers in the vagina. When the tip reaches the site of perforation, the skull is perforated using rotating movements. After the skull is perforated, the instrument is advanced further and the handles are approximated so as to allow separation of the sharp blades, which will extend the perforation. The blades are then apposed and brought out keeping the tip of blades still inside the cranium. The perforator is then rotated at right angles and the above step is repeated to make the perforated area look like a cross.

The instrument with the blades closed is again thrust beyond the guard, to churn the brain matter. After the brain matter is churned, the perforator is brought out under the guidance of two fingers still placed in the vagina.

Similar procedure could be performed using a sharp-pointed Mayo scissors. With the fingers, the brain matter is evacuated in order to make the skull collapse as much as possible.

When the skull is found sufficiently compressed, the extraction of the fetus is achieved either by using a cranioclast or by two giant vulsella. Traction is now exerted in the same direction as in forceps operation. After the delivery of the placenta, the vaginal canal and uterus are explored for evidence of any tear or rupture. Injection Methergine is given and rest of the delivery is completed as in normal delivery.

In aftercoming head of breech, the perforation is done through the occipital bone, while the baby is being pulled forwards or backwards to fix the head during perforation. After the perforation, the brain matter is evacuated and the skull collapsed. Delivery is completed by traction on legs.

Decapitation

Decapitation is a destructive operation in which the fetal head is severed from the trunk and the delivery is completed with the extraction of the trunk and then of the decapitated head per vagina. Special instruments used for decapitation are shown in **Figures 34.10A to D**.

Indications

* Neglected shoulder presentation with dead fetus where the neck is easily accessible
* Interlocking head of twins.

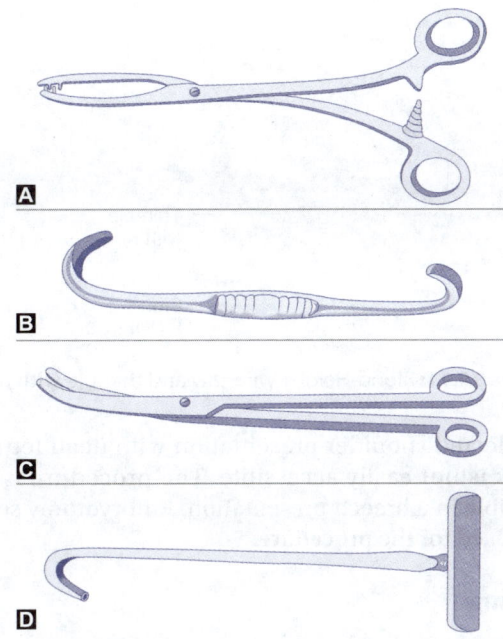

Figures 34.10A to D: Special instruments for decapitation. (A) Giant vulsellum; (B) Hook with crochet; (C) Embryotomy; (D) Decapitation hook with knife.

Procedure

If the fetal hand is not prolapsed, a hand is brought down. For this, a roller gauze is tied on the wrist and an assistant gives traction toward the side away from the fetal head to make the neck more accessible and fixed. Two fingers of the hand (index and middle) are then introduced into the vagina with the palmar surface downwards and the fingertips are placed on the superior surface of the neck. The decapitation hook with knife is introduced under the guidance of the fingers in the vagina, the knob pointing toward the fetal head. The hook is pushed above the neck and rotated about the angle of 90° to place the knife firmly against the neck.

By upward and downward movement of the hook with knife, the vertebral column is severed. The rest of the soft tissue may be severed by the same instrument or by an embryotomy scissors. The decapitated head is pushed up and the trunk is delivered by traction of the prolapsed arm.

The decapitated head is delivered by using the crochet (blunt hook) or forceps. Decapitation may be performed using a Blond-Heidler wire (**Fig. 34.11**) saw and thimble. The neck is severed by the wire saw after passing the wire loop around the fetal neck.

Evisceration

The operation consists of removal of thoracic and abdominal contents piecemeal through an opening on the thoracic or abdominal cavity at the most accessible site. The objective is to diminish the bulk of the fetus, which facilitates the extraction.

Indications

1. Gross fetal malformations such as fetal ascites or hugely distended bladder.

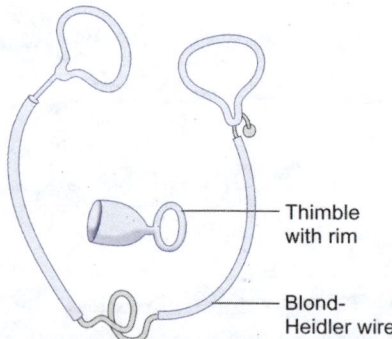

Figure 34.11: Blond-Heidler wire saw and thimble with rim.

2. Neglected shoulder presentation with dead fetus and neck is not easily accessible. The procedure is more feasible in a breech presentation. Embryotomy scissors are used for the procedure.

Cleidotomy

The operation consists of reduction of the width of the shoulder girdle by division of one or both the clavicles. The operation is done only on dead fetus with shoulder dystocia. The clavicles are divided by the embryotomy scissors or long straight scissors introduced under the guidance of two fingers of left hand placed inside the vagina.

Postoperative Care Following Destructive Operations

1. A self-retaining (Foley's) catheter is inserted following craniotomy and maintained for 3–5 days or until bladder tone is regained.
2. Intravenous drip is to be continued until dehydration is corrected. Blood transfusion maybe given if required.
3. Antibiotic is given either parenterally or orally.

Complications

- Injury to the uterovaginal canal
- Postpartum hemorrhage—atonic or traumatic
- Shock due to blood loss and/or dehydration
- Puerperal sepsis
- Subinvolution of uterus
- Injury to the adjacent viscera—vesicovaginal fistula or rectovaginal fistula.

STUDY QUESTIONS

Short Notes

1. Dilatation and evacuation operation.
2. Outlet forceps.
3. Failed forceps.
4. Ventouse delivery.

Short Answer Questions

1. Basic construction of (parts of) obstetric forceps.
2. Maternal and fetal indications of forceps application.
3. Possible complications of forceps operation for an infant.
4. Indications for an emergency cesarean section.
5. Craniotomy as a destructive operation.

Essay Questions

1. Enumerate the prerequisites for forceps delivery and preparation of a client for forceps application.
2. Enumerate the indications for ventouse delivery and its advantages over forceps delivery.
3. Describe the preparation of a mother for lower segment cesarean section.

BIBLIOGRAPHY

1. Ruth Bennett V. Obstetric anesthesia and operations. In: Myles (Ed). Textbook for Midwives, 13th edition. Edinburgh: Churchill Livingstone; 1999. pp. 552-62.
2. Depp R. Cesarean delivery and other surgical procedures. In: Gabbe SG, Niebyl JR, Simpson JL (Eds). Obstetrics: Normal and Problem Pregnancies, 2nd edition. Edinburgh: Churchill Livingstone; 1991. pp. 292-315.
3. Dutta DC. Textbook of obstetrics, 5th edition. Kolkata: New Central Book Company; 2001. pp. 609-41.
4. Mac Donald R. Indications and contraindications for epidural blockade in obstetrics. In: Reynolds S (Ed). Epidural and spinal blockade in obstetrics. 1st edition, London: Baillière Tindall; 1990. pp. 94-9.

CHAPTER 35

Obstetric Emergencies

Learning Objectives

Upon completing this chapter, the learner will be able to:
- Describe the emergency situations in midwifery including vasa previa, cord prolapse and shoulder dystocia with possible causes and actions to be taken.
- Describe the conditions of uterine rupture.
- Discuss the causes, detection and management of amniotic fluid embolism.
- Discuss the different types of shock in obstetric clients and management.
- Describe the procedure of basic life support.

VASA PREVIA

Vasa previa, this term is used when a fetal blood vessel lies over the os in front of the presenting part. This usually occurs when fetal vessels from a velamentous insertion of the cord cross the area of the internal os to the placenta. However, vasa previa may also occur when there is a succenturiate placenta since the vascular connections to the succenturiate lobe are also unprotected vessels coursing between the chorion and amnion. With fetal descent and rupture of the membranes, the vessels are subject to compression and rupture with resulting exsanguination and anoxia of the fetus.

Vasa previa occurs in less than 0.2% of pregnancies. While extremely rare it should be thought of as a possibility, any time the midwife is not positive of what she feels presenting at the cervical os.

Diagnosis

1. Vasa previa may sometimes be palpated on vaginal examination, when the membranes are still intact. Pulsations felt may be synchronous with the fetal heart rate.
2. A speculum examination may be done to visualize the blood vessel.
3. It may also be visualized on ultrasound.
4. Fresh vaginal bleeding, which commences at the time of rupture of membranes, may be due to ruptured vasa previa.

Management

Immediate consultation with the physician is mandatory when the midwife believes the presenting part to be abnormal. The fetal heart rate should be monitored. If in the first stage of labor and the fetus is alive, an emergency cesarean section is carried out. If the mother is in the second stage of labor, delivery should be expedited and a vaginal birth may be achieved. The mode of delivery will be dependent on parity and fetal condition.

A pediatrician should be present at delivery and, if the baby is alive, hemoglobin estimation is necessary after resuscitation. The baby will require a blood transfusion, but the mortality rate is high with this emergency.

PRESENTATION AND PROLAPSE OF THE UMBILICAL CORD (FIGS. 35.1A AND B)

There are three clinical types of abnormal descend of the umbilical cord by the side of the presenting part. All these are included under the heading cord prolapse:
1. *Occult prolapse:* The cord lies alongside, but not in front of the presenting part and is not felt by the fingers on internal examination.
2. *Cord presentation:* The cord is slipped down below the presenting part and lies in front of it in the intact bag of membranes.
3. *Cord prolapse:* The cord lies in front of the presenting part inside the vagina or outside the vulva following rupture of the membranes.

Incidence

The incidence of cord prolapse is about 1 in 300 deliveries. It occurs mostly in parous women especially in higher parities.

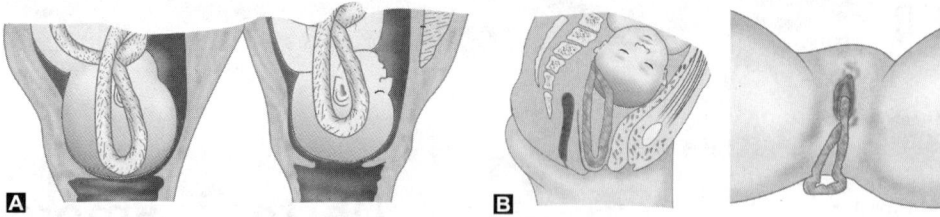

Figures 35.1A and B: Cord presentation and prolapse. (A) Cord presentation; (B) Cord prolapse.

Predisposing Factors

Predisposing factors are same for both presentation and prolapse of cord. Any situation where the presenting part is neither well applied to the lower uterine segment nor well down in the pelvis may make it possible for a loop of cord to slip down in front of the presenting part. Such situations include:
- Malpresentations
- Prematurity
- Multiple pregnancy
- Polyhydramnios
- High head
- Multiparity.

Malpresentations

The commonest malpresentation associated with cord prolapse is transverse followed by breech, especially complete (legs flexed) or footling. This relates to the ill-fitting nature of the presenting part and the proximity of the umbilicus to the buttocks. In this situation, the degree of compression will be less than with a cephalic presentation, but there is still a danger of asphyxia. Face and brow presentations are less common causes of cord prolapse.

Prematurity

The size of the fetus in relation to the pelvis and the uterus allows the cord to prolapse. Babies of very low birth weight, less than 1,500 g, are particularly vulnerable.

Multiple Pregnancy

Malpresentation of the second twin is common in multiple pregnancy.

Polyhydramnios

The cord is liable to be swept down in a gush of liquor if the membranes rupture spontaneously. Controlled release of liquor with artificial rupture of membranes is sometimes performed to prevent this.

High Head

If the membranes rupture spontaneously when the fetal head is high, a loop of cord may pass between the uterine wall and the fetus resulting it lying in front of the presenting part.

Multiparity

The presenting part may not be engaged when the membranes rupture and malpresentation is more common.

Diagnosis

Occult Prolapse

Occult prolapse is difficult to diagnose. The possibility should be suspected if there is:
1. Persistence of variable deceleration of fetal heart rate pattern detected on continuous fetal monitoring in an otherwise normal delivery.
2. Persistent fetal souffle with irregular heart sounds.

Cord Presentation

The diagnosis of cord presentation is made by feeling the pulsation of the cord through the intact membranes. It is however, rarely detected, but may also be associated with aberrations in fetal heart monitoring, such as decelerations.

Cord Prolapse

The cord is felt below or beside the presenting part on vaginal examination. A loop of cord may be visible at the vulva. The cord is more commonly felt in the vagina or in cases where the presenting part is high; it may be felt at the cervical os. Pulsation can be felt between contractions if the fetus is alive.

Risks to Mother and Fetus

Maternal

The maternal risks are incidental due to emergency operative delivery, which involves the risk of anesthesia, blood loss and infection.

Fetal

The fetus is at risk of anoxia due to acute placental insufficiency from the moment cord is prolapsed. The blood flow is occluded either due to mechanical compression by the presenting part against the incompletely dilated cervix/pelvic wall or due to vasospasm of the umbilical vessels due to exposure to cold or irritation, when exposed outside the vulva or as a result of handling. The danger is more in vertex presentation, especially when the prolapse is through the anterior segment of the pelvis or when the cervix is partially dilated.

Management of Cord Presentation

The aim is to preserve the membranes and to expedite the delivery:
- The midwife should discontinue vaginal examination in order to reduce the risk of rupturing the membranes
- Medical help should be summoned immediately
- Fetal heart should be auscultated as frequently as possible or obtained through continuous electronic monitoring
- Cesarean section is the most likely method of delivery
- During the time of preparing the woman for operative delivery, she is kept in exaggerated Sims' position to minimize cord compression.

Management of Cord Prolapse

Immediate Action

1. When diagnosis of cord prolapse is made, the midwife calls for urgent assistance.
2. The mother and her family must be given explanation about the findings and the emergency measures that will be needed.
3. If oxytocin infusion is in progress, it should be stopped.
4. If the baby is alive, the aim of immediate management is to minimize pressure on the cord until such time when the woman is prepared for assisted delivery or is transferred to an equipped hospital. For this, the gloved fingers are to be introduced into the vagina to lift the presenting part of the cord. The fingers should be placed inside the vagina until definitive treatment is instituted.
5. Postural treatment is given until the delivery of the baby, either vaginally or by cesarean section. The woman is placed in exaggerated elevated Sims' position with pillow under the hip. The foot end of the bed may be elevated. High Trendelenburg or knee-chest position, which has been traditionally mentioned, is very tiring and distressing to the woman.
6. If the cord lies outside the vagina, it should be replaced into the vagina to minimize vasospasm due to irritation and to maintain the temperature.
7. If much of the cord is outside the vulva, it should be covered with sterile wet gauze, to prevent spasm of the umbilical vessels due to draughts.

Definitive Management

1. Cesarean section is the ideal management when the baby is sufficiently mature enough to survive. Where the fetus is confirmed alive and delivery is not imminent, the birth must be expedited with the greatest possible speed to reduce the mortality and morbidity associated with this condition.
2. If immediate cesarean section is not possible or the baby is too premature, reposition of the cord may be an alternative. The cervix must be at least half dilated and the cord wrapped in a large piece of sterile roller gauze, is manually pushed above the presenting part under general anesthesia. This is followed by stimulation of uterine contraction with oxytocin drip, if necessary. When the cervix is about three-fourth dilated, ventouse traction may be applied to deliver the baby. This is possible only with vertex presentation and carries high fetal risks.
3. If the head is engaged, delivery is completed by forceps. With a breech engaged, a breech extraction is done.
4. If the fetus is confirmed dead, labor is allowed to proceed, awaiting spontaneous termination.

DYSTOCIA CAUSED BY FETAL ANOMALIES

Fetal Macrosomia (Generalized Fetal Enlargement)

Birth weight of more than 4 kg is considered overweight. The causes are hereditary, size of parents, particularly the mother, poorly controlled maternal diabetes and gestational diabetes, postmaturity and multiparity. Diagnostic evidence includes disproportionate increase in uterine size, feeling the fetus big and firm, and ultrasonographic evaluation of the dimensions of the head, thorax and abdomen.

Dangers of macrosomia are dystocia due to cephalopelvic disproportion and shoulder dystocia. Fetal risks include asphyxia, birth trauma and meconium aspiration syndrome leading to increased perinatal loss. Management includes selective preterm induction of labor and wider use of cesarean section.

Shoulder Dystocia

The term shoulder dystocia is used to describe failure of the shoulders to spontaneously traverse the pelvis after delivery of the head.

The anterior shoulder becomes trapped behind or on the symphysis pubis, whilst the posterior shoulder may be in the hollow of the sacrum or high above the sacral promontory.

Shoulder dystocia is not a common emergency. The incidence varies between 0.37 and 1.1. Risk factors, diagnosis and management are explained in Chapter 33: Malpositions and Malpresentations.

Hydrocephalus

Excessive accumulation of cerebrospinal fluid in the ventricles with consequent thinning of the brain tissue and enlargement of the cranium occurs in about 1 in 2,000 deliveries. It is associated with other congenital malformations in one third of cases. Recurrence rate is about 5% and breech presentation occurs in about 25% cases.

Diagnosis

Minor degree may escape attention in the antenatal period, but the severe degree presents with the following features:
- The head is felt larger, globular and softer than the normal head
- The head is high-up and impossible to push down into the pelvis

- ❖ The sensation felt is comparable to that obtained when a ping-pong ball is squeezed
- ❖ Fetal heart sound is situated high-up above the umbilicus
- ❖ X-ray will reveal:
  - Cranial shadow as globular rather than normal ovoid
  - Fontanels and sutures are wide
  - Vault bones may show irregular thinning.
- ❖ Ultrasonography may show dilatation of the lateral ventricles and thinning of the cerebral cortex
- ❖ Internal examination during labor reveals:
  - Gaping sutures and fontanels
  - Crackling sensation on pressing the head.

In breech presentation, however, the diagnosis is not made until the after-coming head is arrested at the brim.

Management

The pregnancy is continued until a stage when induction can be performed, usually beyond 36th week. Induction is done by rupture of membranes and oxytocin when the cervix is 3–4 cm dilated; decompression of the head is done using a sharp-pointed scissors or a perforator.

In breech presentation, the arrested head is decompressed by perforating the suboccipital region. Exploration of the uterus is done after delivery of the head. If an open spina bifida is present, a uterine dressing forceps or a Drew-Smythe catheter is passed through the opening into the ventricle to drain the fluid.

Outcome

Fetal outlook is extremely poor. The fetus either is delivered stillborn or dies in the neonatal period. Babies, who survive, may be mentally defective. Maternal prognosis is favorable in diagnosed cases. In undiagnosed cases, obstructed labor with its consequences may occur. Rupture of membrane occurs even before the cervix is fully dilated because of too much distension of the lower segment by the head.

Neural Tube Defects

Anencephaly and spina bifida comprise 95% of neural tube defects (NTDs) and the remaining 5% is encephalocele. It is more common in lower socioeconomic group.

Anencephaly

The incidence of anencephaly is about 1 in 1,000 births. The anomaly develops from deficient development of the vault of the skull and brain tissue, but the facial portion is normal. The pituitary gland is often absent or hypoplastic.

About 70% of anencephalic fetuses are females. It is more prevalent in first birth, and in young and elderly mothers.

Diagnosis

In the first half of pregnancy, the diagnosis is made by detecting elevated α-fetoprotein in amniotic fluid and confirmed by ultrasonography. In the latter half of pregnancy, the diagnosis is difficult, especially when associated with hydramnios. On internal examination, face presentation is diagnosed and confirmed by ultrasonography or X-ray.

Complications

- ❖ Hydramnios
- ❖ Malpresentation—face and breech
- ❖ Premature labor, specially when associated with hydramnios
- ❖ Tendency of postmaturity
- ❖ Shoulder dystocia
- ❖ Obstructed labor, if the head and neck try to engage together because of short neck.

Management

If confirmed before, in the antenatal period, termination of pregnancy is to be done. During labor, if shoulder dystocia occurs, it should be managed by cleidotomy.

Prevention

Pre-pregnancy counseling is essential for future pregnancies. Folic acid supplementation beginning 1 month before conception to about 12 weeks conception has reduced the incidence of NTD significantly.

Enlargement of Fetal Abdomen

Enlargement of fetal abdomen sufficient to produce dystocia, may be due to ascites, distended bladder or enlargement of kidney by a tumor or an umbilical hernia.

Antenatal diagnosis may be made accidentally by X-ray or by ultrasonography. Fetal appearance on X-ray resembles 'Buddha position'. The diagnosis is usually made when there is difficulty in the delivery of the trunk following birth of the head. Confirmation is done by introducing the hand and palpating the hugely distended abdomen. Decompression of the abdomen is done by simple puncture with a trocar, which is soon followed by spontaneous delivery.

Conjoined Twins

The varieties of incomplete twinning result in the development of conjoined twins. The condition is extremely rare and often causes surprise dystocia.

AMNIOTIC FLUID EMBOLISM

Amniotic fluid embolism condition occurs when amniotic fluid enters the maternal circulation through a tear in the membranes or placenta. The body responds in two phases. The initial phase is one of vasospasm causing hypoxia, hypotension and cardiovascular collapse. The second phase is the development of left ventricular failure with hemorrhage and coagulation disorder followed by pulmonary edema. Mortality and morbidity are very high.

The presence of thromboplastin rich liquor amnii in the maternal circulation blocks the pulmonary arteries and triggers the complex coagulation mechanism leading to disseminated intravascular coagulation (DIC). There will be severe clotting defect with profuse bleeding per vagina or through the venipuncture sites due to consumption of coagulation factors.

Predisposing Factors

Amniotic fluid embolism can occur at any stage in gestation. It is mostly associated with labor, though cases in early pregnancy and postpartum have been reported. Factors are the following:
1. Transfer of amniotic fluid from the uterus to the maternal circulation can be insidiously associated with a tear in the membranes.
2. Amniotic fluid under pressure may enter maternal circulation in the first phase of hypoxia during hypertonic uterine activity.
3. Procedures such as insertion of an intrauterine catheter and artificial rupture of membranes are associated with the condition.
4. In cases of placental abruption, the placental bed is disrupted, and the barrier between the maternal circulation and amniotic sac may be breached.
5. It can occur during a cesarean section, termination of pregnancy or in association with ruptured uterus.
6. Trauma may occur during intrauterine manipulation such as internal podalic version.

The condition is difficult to predict and equally difficult to prevent.

Clinical Features

- Sudden onset of maternal respiratory distress; the woman becomes severely dyspneic and cyanosed
- There is maternal hypotension and uterine hypertonia
- Fetal distress in response to hypoxia caused by hypertonia
- Cardiopulmonary arrest follows quickly in minutes
- Many mothers present with convulsions immediately preceding the collapse.

Emergency Management

Any one of the above symptoms is indicative of an acute emergency. The mother may be in a state of collapse and resuscitation must be started at once. Specific management of the condition is life support and high levels of oxygen are required. Mothers who survive may suffer neurological impairment.

Complications

Disseminated intravascular coagulation is likely to occur within 30 minutes of the initial collapse.
Acute renal failure occurs due to heavy bleeding and the prolonged hypovolemic hypotension. Transfer to an intensive therapy unit for specialized care is indicated.

Effect on the Fetus

Perinatal mortality and morbidity are high, where amniotic fluid embolism occurs before the birth of the baby. Delay in the time from initial maternal collapse to delivery needs to be minimal if fetal death is to be avoided.

SHOCK

Shock is defined as a state of circulatory inadequacy with poor tissue perfusion resulting in generalized cellular hypoxia leading to dysfunction of organs and cells.

Shock can be acute, but prompt treatment results in recovery with little detrimental effect on the mother. However, inadequate treatment or failure to initiate effective treatment can result in chronic multisystem organ failure, which may be fatal.

Classification of Shock

Based on the basic pathophysiology of shock and its clinical correlation, shock may be classified as follows:
1. *Hypovolemic shock:* The result of a reduction in intravascular volume:
   a. Hemorrhagic shock: Associated with postpartum or postabortal hemorrhage, ectopic pregnancy, placenta previa, abruptio placentae, rupture of uterus and obstetric surgery.
   b. Fluid loss shock: Associated with excessive diarrhea, vomiting, diuresis or too rapid removal of amniotic fluid.
   c. Supine hypotensive syndrome: Associated with compression of inferior vena cava by pregnant uterus.
   d. Shock associated with disseminated intravascular coagulation: Intrauterine dead fetus syndrome and amniotic fluid embolism.
2. *Cardiogenic shock:* Impaired ability of the heart to pump blood:
   a. Failure of the left ventricular ejection in cardiac arrest and myocardial infarction.
   b. Failure of left ventricular filling associated with cardiac tamponade and pulmonary embolism.
3. *Neurogenic shock:*
   a. Chemical injury: Associated with aspiration of gastrointestinal contents during general anesthesia, especially in cesarean section (Mendelson's syndrome).
   b. Drug induced: Associated with spinal anesthesia.
4. *Septic shock (endotoxic shock):* Typically associated with septic abortion, chorioamnionitis, pyelonephritis and rarely postpartum endometritis. This type of shock may be hypovolemic, but has primary cardiogenic and cellular components also. In this section, hypovolemic shock and septic shock are discussed as either of which may occur because of childbearing.

Hypovolemic Shock

The body reacts to the loss of circulating fluid in stages as follows:

1. *Initial stage:* The reduction in fluid or blood decreases the venous return to the heart. The ventricles of the heart are inadequately filled, causing a reduction in stroke volume and cardiac output. As cardiac output and venous return fall, the blood pressure is reduced. The drop in blood pressure decreases the supply of oxygen to the tissues and cell function is affected.

2. *Compensatory stage:* The drop in cardiac output produces a response from the sympathetic nervous system through the activation of receptors in the aorta and carotid arteries. Blood is redistributed to the vital organs. Vessels in the gastrointestinal tract, kidneys, skin and lungs constrict. The response is seen by the skin becoming pale and cool. Peristalsis slows, urinary output is reduced and exchange of gas in the lungs is impaired. The heart rate increases in an attempt to improve cardiac output and blood pressure. Pupils of the eyes dilate. The sweat glands are stimulated and the skin becomes moist and clammy.

    Adrenaline and aldosterone from adrenal glands and antidiuretic hormone from posterior pituitary gland are secreted causing vasoconstriction, an increased cardiac output and a decrease in urinary output. Venous return to the heart will increase, but unless the fluid loss is replaced, this will not be sustained.

3. *Progressive stage:* This stage leads to multisystem failure. Compensatory mechanisms begin to fail with vital organs lacking adequate perfusion. Volume depletion causes further fall in blood pressure and cardiac output. The coronary arteries suffer lack of supply. Peripheral circulation is poor, with weak or absent pulses.

4. *Late stage (irreversible):* Hypotension continues and cannot be reversed by replacement of fluid because of stagnation of blood at the microvascular level. Color of skin becomes ashen gray. Metabolic acidosis starts and for elimination of accumulated carbon dioxide, the respiratory rate becomes rapid. Imperceptible low volume pulse, oliguria and mental confusion occur. Multisystem failure and cell destruction are irreparable. Treatment of any kind is practically useless in this phase. Death ensues.

Management

Urgent resuscitation is needed to prevent the mother's condition from deteriorating and causing irreversible damage. The priorities are to:

1. *Maintain the airway:* If the mother is severely collapsed, she should be turned on to her side and oxygen administered at a rate of 6–8 L/min. If she is unconscious, endotracheal intubation may be necessary.

2. *Replace fluids (infusion and transfusion):* Blood should be taken for crossmatching prior to commencing intravenous fluids. A plasma expander or fresh frozen plasma is given until whole blood is available.

3. *Avoid warmth:* Constriction of the peripheral blood supply occurs in response to the shock and keeping the mother warm may interfere with this response, causing further deterioration in her condition.

4. *Control of hemorrhage:* Specific surgical and medical treatment for control of hemorrhage should start along with the general management of shock.

Clinical observations for the mother in shock (monitoring)

- Assess the level of consciousness; signs of restlessness and confusion are to be noted
- Monitor blood pressure every 30 minutes or continuously
- The cardiac rhythm may be monitored continuously
- Assess skin color and temperature hourly
- Assess central venous pressure and fluid balance for adequacy of circulating volume
- Watch for occurrence of any further bleeding.

Detailed observation charts are to be maintained and the mother may be transferred to a critical care unit.

Septic Shock

There is an overwhelming infection, commonly from gram-negative organisms such as *Escherichia coli*, *Proteus* or *Pseudomonas pyocyaneus*. These organisms are common pathogens in the female genital tract and have endotoxins present in their cells. Endotoxins release components that trigger body's immune response. Septic shock can less commonly be caused by gram-positive bacteria or by multiple organisms.

The placental site is the main point of entry for an infection associated with pregnancy and childbirth. This may occur following septic abortion, prolonged rupture of membranes, obstetric trauma or in the presence of retained placental tissue.

The body's primary response to infection is alteration in the peripheral circulation. Cells damaged by the infecting organisms release histamine and enzymes that contribute to vasodilatation and increased permeability of the capillaries. Mediators are also reduced that have the opposite action of vasoconstriction. The overall response, however, is one of vasodilatation, which reduces the systemic vascular resistance.

Clinical signs

1. In the initial phase, there is marked flushing of the face and the skin feels warm.
2. Temperature rise varies from 101°F to 105°F.
3. Tachycardia, tachypnea and rigors occur.
4. Hemorrhage may be present, which either could be due to the events of childbearing or because of disseminated intravascular coagulation.
5. As vasodilatation continues, hypotension leads to kidney damage with reduced glomerular filtration and acute tubular necrosis and oliguria.
6. If the shock condition does not improve, the patient passes clinically to the stage of 'irreversible shock'. She remains cold and clammy with ashen gray cyanotic appearance.

7. Anuria, cardiac or respiratory distress and coma may supervene.
8. Disseminated intravascular coagulation is also a feature of septic shock.
9. Multisystem organ failure will result as an effect of the continued hypotension and myocardial depression. Failure of the liver, brain and respiratory systems follows, and death results.

Management

Management is based on preventing further deterioration by restoring circulatory volume and eradication of the infection. A full infection screening should be carried out including a high vaginal swab, midstream urine and blood cultures. Retained products of conception if detected on ultrasound should be removed.

Measures of management include intravenous administration of antibiotics, intravenous fluids, adjustment of acid-base balance, steroids, prevention and treatment of intravascular coagulation and toxic myocarditis, administration of oxygen and elimination of the source of infection. These are as follows:

1. *Antibiotics:* Broad-spectrum antibiotics are given to start with and after confirming the sensitivity, specific antibiotics are given intravenously.
2. *Intravenous fluids and electrolytes:* Septic shock associated hemorrhagic hypotension is treated with liberal infusion and blood transfusion. Oliguria with high specific gravity is an indication for liberal fluid administration, whereas a low specific gravity indicates fluid restriction. Impairment of renal function contraindicates administration of electrolytes.
3. *Correction of acidosis:* Bicarbonate is administered to correct metabolic acidosis.
4. *Maintenance of blood pressure:* Inotropic agents such as adrenaline, noradrenaline, dopamine and dobutamine are administered to increase the cardiac contractility. Vasodilator drugs such as sodium nitroprusside, nitroglycerin and diuretics are used in selected cases to reduce the after load and pulmonary edema.
5. Corticosteroids are given to exert an antiendotoxin effect and to counteract anaerobic oxidative mechanism.
6. As a prophylactic measure for DIC, heparin may be given. Fresh frozen plasma or whole blood transfusion may be used.
7. In unresponsive septic shock following septic abortion or puerperal sepsis, hysterectomy may be done to eliminate the source of infection.

The mother may require care and management in a critical or intensive care unit. The family should be kept informed of progress.

RUPTURE OF UTERUS

Definition

A break in the continuity of the uterine wall any time beyond 28 weeks of pregnancy is called rupture of the uterus.

The rupture is described as complete rupture when it involves a tear in the wall of the uterus including the peritoneal coat and with or without expulsion of the fetus.

Incomplete rupture is tearing of the uterine wall without involving the perimetrium. Life of both mother and fetus may be endangered in either situation.

Rupture during Pregnancy

Rupture that occurs during pregnancy is usually complete, involves the upper segment and usually occurs in later months of pregnancy.

Rupture during Labor

Spontaneous rupture, which occurs in an otherwise intact uterus during labor as an end result of obstructed labor. This type of rupture is then termed as obstructive rupture. The rupture involves the lower segment and usually extends through one lateral side to the upper segment.

Non-obstructive rupture occurs in grand multipara and usually occurs early in labor. Weakening of the uterine walls due to repeated previous births may be the responsible factor. The rupture usually involves the fundal area and is complete.

Scar Rupture

Dehiscence of an existing uterine scar may also occur. This involves rupture of the uterine wall, but the fetal membranes remain intact. The fetus is retained within the uterus and is not expelled into the peritoneal cavity. Lower segment scars rarely rupture during pregnancy. Classical or hysterotomy, scar is likely to give way during later months of pregnancy.

Causes of Rupture of the Uterus

Spontaneous rupture of the uterus can be precipitated in the following circumstances:
- High parity
- Injudicious use of oxytocin, particularly where the mother is of high parity
- Obstructed labor: The uterus ruptures due to excessive thinning of the lower segment
- Neglected labor, where there is previous history of cesarean section
- Extension of cervical laceration upwards into the lower uterine segment
- Trauma as a result of accident or injury
- Perforation of a non-pregnant uterus may result in rupture in a subsequent pregnancy, usually in the upper uterine segment
- Antenatal rupture of the uterus may occur where there has been a history of previous classical cesarean section.

Signs of Intrapartum Rupture of the Uterus

A complete rupture of a non-scarred uterus may be accompanied by:
- Sudden collapse of the mother who complains of severe abdominal pain

- Increase of maternal pulse rate
- Alteration of fetal heart rate including the presence of variable decelerations on the monitor strip
- Fresh vaginal bleeding
- Uterine contractions may stop and the contour of abdomen alters
- Fetal heart sounds may be lost
- The fetus becomes palpable in the abdomen as the presenting part regresses
- The mother goes into shock, the degree of which depends on the extent of the rupture and the blood loss.

Signs of Incomplete Rupture

Incomplete rupture may have an insidious onset or may be silent and usually discovered after delivery or during a cesarean section. This is more commonly associated with previous cesarean section.

Blood loss associated with incomplete rupture can be scanty as the rupture occurs along the fibrous scar tissue.

Incomplete rupture may also manifest as postpartum hemorrhage following vaginal delivery. Whenever shock during third stage is more severe than the blood loss warrants or the mother fails to respond to treatment given, the possibility of incomplete rupture should be considered.

Management

Depending upon the state of the clinical condition, resuscitation needs to be done followed by laparotomy, or in acute conditions; resuscitation and laparotomy are to be done simultaneously. Following laparotomy any of the following procedures may be adopted:

- Hysterectomy in spontaneous obstructive rupture; a quick subtotal hysterectomy is usually done
- Repair is mostly applicable in cases of scar rupture where the margins are clean
- Repair and sterilization (tubal ligation) is mostly done in patients with a clean cut scar rupture having desired number of children.

The mother will be unprepared for the events that have occurred and therefore may be totally opposed to hysterectomy. Explanation and preparation of both mother and family are important though this is an emergency situation.

BASIC LIFE SUPPORT/ CARDIOPULMONARY RESUSCITATION

Basic life support (BLS) is the emergency treatment of a victim of cardiac or respiratory arrest through cardiopulmonary resuscitation (CPR) and emergency cardiac care until more definitive medical treatment is available. CPR is an emergency procedure in which the heart and lungs are forced to work by manually compressing the chest overlying the heart and forcing air into the lungs. CPR is often used to maintain circulation and respiration when the heart or lung has stopped functioning.

The objective is to ensure oxygenation of the brain, heart and other vital organs until appropriate definite medical treatment (advanced life support) can restore normal circulatory and respiratory actions.

Sequence of Basic Life Support

The new guidelines by American Heart Association (AHA) (2010) have changed the sequence of CPR from ABC (airway breathing, circulation) to CAB (chest compressions first, than airway and breathing):

1. *Determine unresponsiveness:* If a mother is found collapsed, her level of consciousness is to be determined by gently shaking a shoulder and enquiring 'are you alright' **(Figs. 35.2A to C)**.
2. *Determine pulselessness:* Check for carotid pulse on one side of neck for not more than 5 seconds.
3. *Call for help:* If no response, call for help and request someone to get an automated external defibrillator (AED), if available. Do not leave the patient to get help.

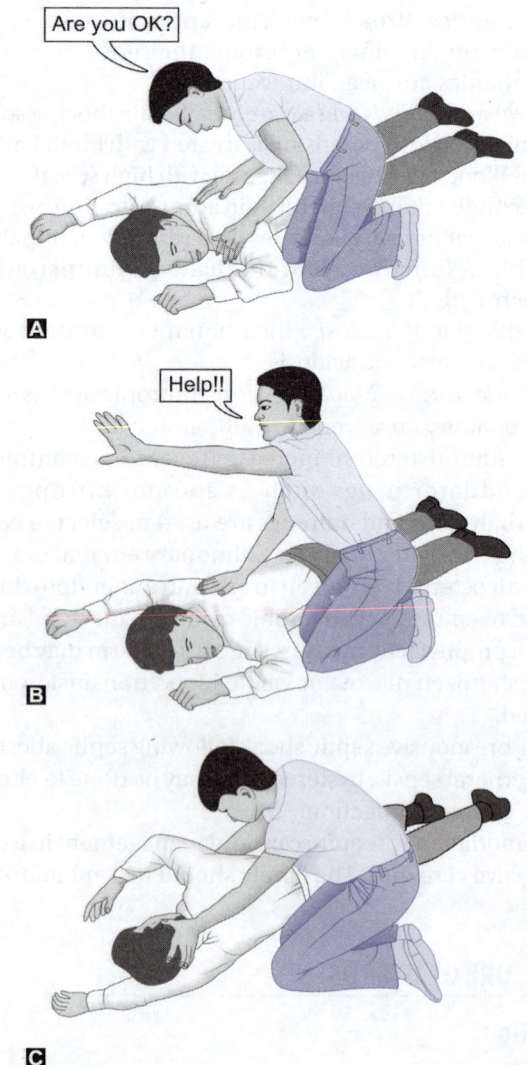

Figures 35.2A to C: Determining unresponsiveness.

4. *Position the victim (mother):* Position the patient on an arrest board or on a flat firm surface on her back. Remove pillows and place victim's arms alongside the body.
5. *Rescuer position (midwife):* To provide BLS, the midwife must stand at a suitable height by the victim's side near her chest or have the victim on the floor and kneel at the side, at the level of the victim's shoulders.

Circulation

Chest compressions (Figs. 35.3A and B)

Start chest compressions at a rate of at least 100 compressions per minute. Using the index finger nearest to the legs of the patient, locate the lower rib margin and move the fingers up where the ribs connect to the sternum. Place the middle finger of this hand on the notch and index finger next to it. Place the heel of the opposite hand next to the index finger on the sternum. Ensure that the long axis of the heel of hand is parallel to the long axis of the sternum. Remove first hand from the notch and place on top of the hand that is on the sternum. Extend or interlace fingers, do not allow them to touch the chest. Keep arms straight, shoulders directly over the hands on sternum and lock elbows.

Compress the chest 2 inches (5 cm) and compression depth of one third of the chest.

Release the external chest compression completely and allow the chest to return to its normal position after each compression. The time allowed for release should be equal to the time required for compression. Do not lift hands off the chest.

The rate of compressions should be 30 compressions to 2 ventilations. Re-evaluate the patient after four cycles (use the mnemonic 1, 2, 3...) to keep rhythm and timing. For CPR performed by one or two rescuers the compression rate is 100 per minute.

Airway (Figs. 35.4A to C)

Open the victim's airway by using one of the following maneuver:
1. *Head tilt-chin lift maneuver:* Place one hand on the victim's forehead and apply firm backward pressure with the palm to tilt the head back. Then place the fingers of the other hand under the bony part of the lower jaw near the chin and lift up to bring the jaw forward.
2. *Jaw-thrust maneuver:* Grasp the angles of the patient's lower jaw and lift with both hands, one on each side, displacing the mandible forward.
3. Place an airway if available.

Breathing

1. Occlude nostrils with thumb and index finger of the hand on the forehead that is tilting the head back. Form a tight

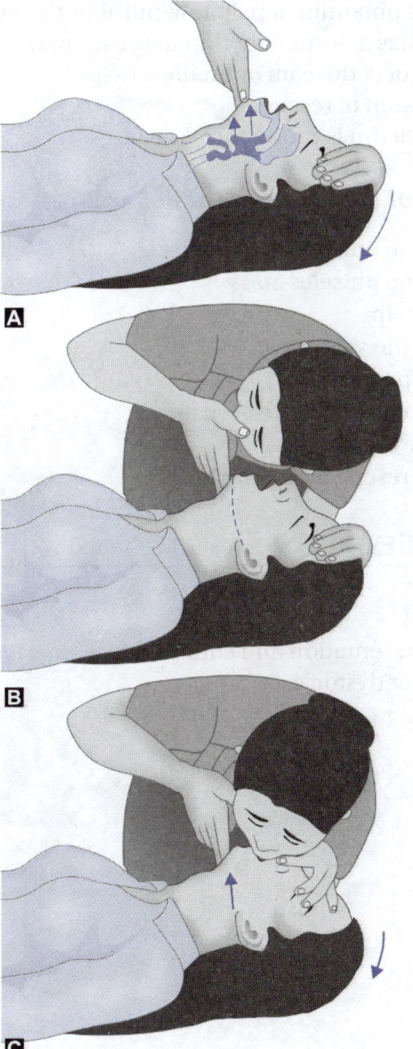

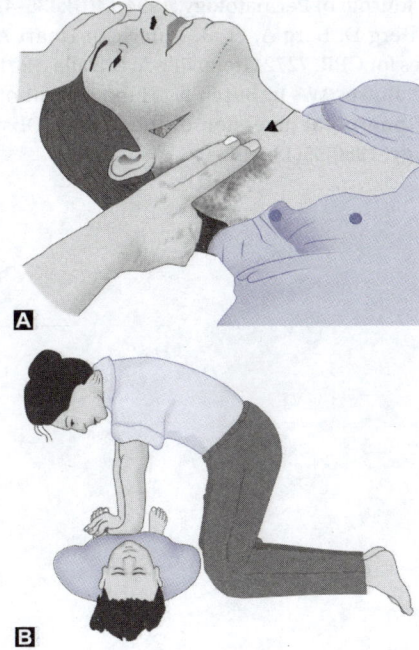

Figures 35.3A and B: Chest compression. (A) Checking for carotid pulse; (B) Positioning hands for chest compressions.

Figures 35.4A to C: Airway support. (A and B) Head tilt-chin lift maneuver; (C) Providing mouth-to-mouth respiration.

seal over the patient's mouth or place an appropriate respiratory arrest device (Ambu bag and mask) and give two full breaths of approximately 0.5–2 seconds allowing time for both inspiration and expiation.
2. Observe for rise and fall of chest.
3. Perform two rescue breathing after 30 compressions (the ratio remains the same for single or two person rescuers).

Using special resuscitation equipment automated external defibrillator (AED): While resuscitation proceeds, simultaneous efforts must be made to obtain and use special resuscitation equipment to manage breathing and circulation and to provide definitive care. Definitive care includes defibrillation, pharmacotherapy for dysrhythmias and acid-base disturbances, and ongoing monitoring and skilled care in an intensive care unit.

When to Stop CPR?

Cardiopulmonary resuscitation can be stopped when the following situations occur:
1. Return of spontaneous circulation as evidenced by the rescuer obtaining a palpable pulse in the victim or the victim has a normal rhythm in the monitor.
2. Arrival of code team or medical help.
3. Exhaustion of rescuer.
4. When victim is pronounced dead.

Summary of the Sequence of BLS

- Determine unresponsiveness
- Determine pulselessness
- Call for help
- Position the victim
- Rescuer position
- Perform chest compressions
- Open the airway
- Perform rescue breathing.

STUDY QUESTIONS

Short Notes

1. Cord presentation and cord prolapse.
2. Shoulder dystocia.
3. Chest compression first, then airway and breathing (CAB) of basic life support.

Short Answer Questions

1. Vasa previa.
2. Fetal macrosomia.
3. Anencephaly.
4. Hydrocephaly.

Essay Questions

1. A 34-year-old client, Mrs S is in labor for 5 hours. At the time of rupture of membranes, the umbilical cord has become visible at the vulva. Describe the measures of management.
2. Explain what is amniotic fluid embolism, its causes, clinical features and management.
3. Define septic shock, explain its clinical manifestations and management.

BIBLIOGRAPHY

1. Bahar AM. Risk factors and fetal outcome in cases of shoulder dystocia compared with normal deliveries of a similar birthweight. British Journal of Obstetrics Gynaecology. 1996;103(9):868-72.
2. Clark SL. New concepts of amniotic fluid embolism: a review. Obstetrical and Gynecological Survey. 1990;45(6):360-8.
3. Dutta DC. Textbook of Obstetrics, 5th edition. Kolkata: New Central Book Company; 2001. pp. 441-6.
4. Gonik B, Held B, Allen SC. An alternate maneuver for management of shoulder dystocia. American Journal of Obstetrics and Gynecology. 1983;145(7):882-3.
5. Naef RW, Morrison JC. Guidelines for management of shoulder dystocia. Journal of Perinatology. 1994;14(6):435-41.
6. Sayre R, Berg D, Berg A, et al. American Heart Association Guidelines for CPR. 7272 Greenville Ave, Dallas; 2010. pp. 1-12.
7. Watson P, Bowes WA Jr, Besch N. Management of acute and subacute puerperal inversion of the uterus. Obstetrics and Gynecology. 1980;55(1):12-6.

CHAPTER 36

Complications of Third Stage of Labor

Learning Objectives

Upon completing this chapter, the learner will be able to:
- Describe the causes and management of postpartum hemorrhage.
- Discuss the diagnosis and management of placenta accreta.
- Describe the varieties and dangers of inversion of uterus.
- Describe the measures to prevent inversion of uterus and management if the problem occurs.

Of all the stages of labor, third stage is the most crucial for the mother. Dangerous complications may appear unexpectedly in an otherwise uneventful first or second stage.

POSTPARTUM HEMORRHAGE

Definition

Postpartum hemorrhage is defined as excessive bleeding from the genital tract at any time following the baby's birth up to 6 weeks after delivery. A quantitative definition is related to the amount of blood loss in excess of 500 mL following birth of the baby.

While the quantitative definition may be useful for statistical purposes, the effect of the blood loss is more important rather than the amount of blood lost. Hence, the clinical definition states, "Any amount of bleeding from or into the genital tract following birth of the baby up to the end of the puerperium, which adversely affects the general condition of the mother, evidenced by rise in pulse rate and falling blood pressure is called postpartum hemorrhage".

Incidence

The incidence varies widely because lack of uniformity in the criteria used in definition. The incidence is about 1% amongst hospital deliveries.

Classification

Depending on the time of occurrence, postpartum hemorrhage is classified as:
1. *Third stage hemorrhage:* Bleeding that occurs before expulsion of placenta.
2. *Primary postpartum hemorrhage or true postpartum hemorrhage:* Bleeding that occurs subsequent to expulsion of placenta and within 24 hours.
3. *Secondary postpartum hemorrhage:* Bleeding occurs subsequent to the first 24 hours following birth up to until the 6th week postpartum. This is also termed as delayed or late puerperal hemorrhage.

Postpartum hemorrhage is one of the most alarming and serious emergencies, which a midwife may face and is especially terrifying if it occurs immediately following a normal delivery. It may also prove a frightening experience for the mother. The midwife is often the first and may be the only professional person present when a hemorrhage occurs. Her prompt and competent action will be crucial in controlling blood loss and reducing the risk of maternal morbidity or even death.

Causes

There are several causes for third stage bleeding and primary postpartum hemorrhage, which include atonic, traumatic and blood coagulopathy.

Atonic Uterus

Atonicity of the uterus is the most common cause (80%) of postpartum hemorrhage. This is a failure of the myometrium at the placental site to contract and retract, and to compress torn blood vessels and control blood loss by a living ligature action. When the placenta is attached, the volume of blood flow at the placental site is approximately 500–800 mL/min. The following are the conditions, which often interfere with the retraction of the uterus as a whole and of the placental site in particular:

1. *Incomplete separation of the placenta:* If the placenta remains fully adhered to the uterine wall, it is unlikely to cause bleeding. However, once separation has begun, maternal vessels are torn. If placental tissue remains partially embedded in the spongy decidua, efficient contraction and retraction is interrupted.
2. Retained cotyledon, placental fragments or membranes will similarly impede efficient uterine action.
3. *Precipitate labor:* When the uterus has contracted vigorously and frequently resulting in duration of labor, that is less than 1 hour, then the uterine muscle may have insufficient opportunity to retract.
4. *Prolonged labor:* In a labor where the active phase lasts more than 12 hours, uterine inertia (sluggishness) may result due to muscle exhaustion.
5. *Over distension of the uterus:* In multiple pregnancy, polyhydramnios and large baby, the myometrium becomes excessively stretched and therefore less efficient.
6. *Placenta previa:* The placental site is partly or wholly in the lower segment where the thinner muscle layer contains few oblique fibers. This results in poor control of bleeding.
7. *Placental abruption:* Blood may have seeped between the muscle fibers, interfering with effective action. When severe, this results in a Couvelaire uterus.
8. *General anesthesia:* Anesthetic agents may cause the uterine relaxation, particularly in inhalational agents like halothane.
9. *Mismanagement of the third stage of labor:* 'Fundus fiddling' or manipulation of the uterus may precipitate arrhythmic contractions, so that the placenta only partially separates and retraction is lost.
10. *A full bladder:* If the bladder is full, its proximity to the uterus in the abdomen on completion of the second stage may interfere with the uterine action.
11. *Initiation or augmentation of delivery by oxytocin:* Postdelivery uterine atonicity is likely to develop, as oxytocin will increase the power of contraction without improving the retraction power of the uterine muscle.
12. *Constriction ring:* Hour-glass constriction formed in the upper segment across the partially separated placenta or at the junction of upper and lower segments with the fully separated placenta trapped in the upper segment, may produce excessive bleeding.
13. *Etiology unknown:* A precipitating cause may never be discovered. Predisposing factors, which might increase the risk of atonic postpartum hemorrhage include:
    a. Previous history of postpartum hemorrhage or retained placenta: In such women there is a risk in subsequent pregnancies.
    b. High parity: With each successive pregnancy, fibrous tissue replaces muscle fibers in the uterus, reducing its contractility and the blood vessels become more difficult to compress. Women who have had five or more deliveries, are at increased risk.
    c. Fibroids: These benign tumors may impede efficient uterine action.
    d. Anemia: Women who enter labor with reduced hemoglobin concentration (below 10 g/dL) may succumb more quickly.

Traumatic Hemorrhage in Third Stage

Causes
- Perineal, vaginal and cervical tears
- Lower segment tears
- Uterine rupture
- Vulvar injuries.

If bleeding occurs despite a well-contracted uterus, it is almost certainly the consequence of trauma. Trauma to the genital tract usually occurs following operative delivery, though it may occur even after spontaneous delivery. Trauma involves usually the cervix, vagina, perineum (episiotomy wound and lacerations), paraurethral region and rarely ruptures the uterus. The bleeding is usually revealed, but can rarely be concealed (vulvovaginal or broad ligament hematoma).

In order to identify the source of bleeding, the mother is placed in lithotomy position under a good directional light. The external injuries are usually identified and torn vessels are clamped and ligated. A speculum is inserted to visualize internal trauma (vagina and cervix). Tissue or artery forceps may be used to obtain hemostasis prior to suturing under general anesthesia.

If bleeding persists when the uterus is well contracted and no evidence of trauma can be found, uterine rupture must be suspected. Following a laparotomy, this is repaired, but if bleeding remains uncontrolled, a hysterectomy may become inevitable.

Blood Coagulation Disorders

Causes
- Disseminated intravascular coagulation
- Excessive fibrinolysis
- Inherited coagulation disorders
- Idiopathic thrombocytopenic purpura.

Postpartum hemorrhage may be the result of coagulation failure. The failure of the blood to clot may be due to diminished procoagulants (washout phenomenon) or increased fibrinolytic activity. It can occur following severe preeclampsia, abruptio placentae, amniotic fluid embolism, hemolysis elevated liver enzymes, low platelet count (HELLP) syndrome, intrauterine death or sepsis.

Fresh blood is usually the best treatment, as this will contain platelets and the coagulation factors V and VIII. Fresh frozen plasma and fibrinogen may also be infused.

Signs of Postpartum Hemorrhage

1. Vaginal bleeding is visible outside, either as slow trickle or rarely a copious flow. Rarely, the bleeding is concealed either remaining inside the uterovesical canal or in the surrounding tissue space resulting in hematoma.
2. Pallor.

3. Rising pulse rate.
4. Falling blood pressure.
5. Altered level of consciousness may become restless or drowsy.
6. Enlarged uterus, as it fills with blood or blood clot. It feels boggy on palpation, i.e. soft and distended lacking tone.
7. Maternal collapse.

The effect of blood loss depends on pre-delivery hemoglobin level, degree of pregnancy-induced hypervolemia and the speed at which blood loss occurs. Alteration of pulse and blood pressure appears only after substantial amount of blood loss and as such is a comparatively late manifestation. On occasion, blood loss is so rapid and brisk that death may occur within a few minutes.

The state of the uterus, as felt per abdomen, gives a reliable clue as regards the cause of bleeding. In traumatic hemorrhage, the uterus is well contracted. In atonic hemorrhage, the uterus is flabby and becomes hard on massaging. However, both the atonic and traumatic may coexist.

Prophylaxis

Postpartum hemorrhage cannot always be prevented. However, the incidence and magnitude can be reduced substantially if following guidelines are followed.

Antenatal

1. Improvement of the health status of women, especially to raise their hemoglobin level as near to normal as possible, so that they can withstand the blood loss.
2. Screening of high-risk women, such as those with twins, hydramnios, grand multipara, antepartum hemorrhage (APH), history of previous third stage complications and severe anemia for delivery in a well-equipped hospital.
3. Blood grouping and typing should be done for the high-risk mothers, so that no time is lost during an emergency.

During Labor

Prevent prolonged labor and ketoacidosis by following good management practices:
1. Prophylactic administration of oxytocic drugs for the third stage.
2. Baby should be pushed out by the retracted uterus and not be pulled out. One should take 2–3 minutes to deliver the trunk after the head is born.
3. Temptation of fiddling with or kneading the uterus, pulling the cord or Crede's expression of placenta to be avoided.
4. In all cases of induced or accelerated labor by oxytocin, the infusion should be continued for at least 1 hour after the delivery and prophylactic ergometrine should be given with the delivery of the anterior shoulder.
5. For any woman known to have placenta previa, two units of crossmatched blood should be kept available.
6. The woman should be observed for about 2 hours after the delivery and after being satisfied that the uterus is hard and contracted. The pulse and blood pressure should be within normal limits before transferring the woman to the ward/postpartum floor.

Management of Third Stage Bleeding

Three basic principles apply in the management of postpartum hemorrhage in the third stage:
1. Call the obstetrician when the midwife thinks that the bleeding is more than expected.
2. Stop the bleeding by employing the following measures:
   a. Rub up a contraction. The fundus is felt gently with the fingertips to assess its consistency. If it is soft and relaxed, the fundus is massaged with a smooth circular motion without applying undue pressure. When a contraction occurs, the hand is held still.
   b. Give an oxytocic to sustain the contraction. Ergometrine 0.2 mg is given intravenously.
   c. Empty the uterus. If the placenta is still inside, it should be delivered. If it has been born, any clots should be expelled by firm, but gentle pressure on the abdomen.
3. Resuscitate the mother:
   a. Start a dextrose saline drip and arrange for blood transfusion, if necessary.
   b. The mother's legs may be lifted up in order to allow blood flow from them up to the central circulation (the foot of the bed should not be raised as this encourages pooling of blood in the uterus, which prevents the uterus contracting).
   c. The bladder is to be catheterized in order to minimize trauma, should an operative procedure be necessary and to exclude a full bladder as a precipitating cause for further bleeding.
   d. The woman may be sedated with morphine 10–15 mg intramuscularly. The placenta and membranes must be re-examined for completeness since retained fragments are often responsible for uterine atony.

Manual Removal of Placenta (Figs. 36.1 and 36.2)

When the placenta remains undelivered even 30 minutes following the birth of the baby, it is considered a retained placenta requiring manual removal. The procedure is done by the physician under anesthesia. General anesthesia is used if the mother's condition permits. Epidural or spinal anesthesia offers an alternative depending on the situation.

Manual removal is performed with full aseptic precautions. The vulva and vagina are swabbed with antiseptic solution and sterile leggings are placed as in other vaginal operations. The bladder is catheterized.

With the left hand, the umbilical cord is held taut, while the right hand is coned and inserted into the vagina and uterus following the direction of the cord. Once the placenta is

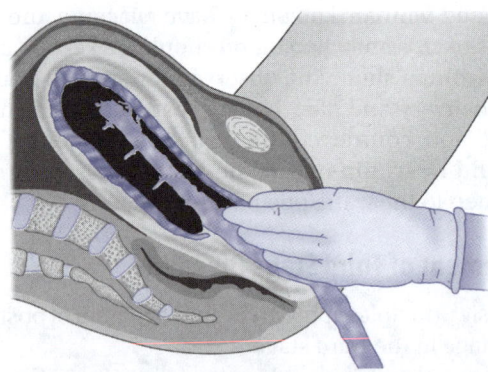

Figure 36.1: Introduction of the hand into the uterus in a cone-shaped manner.

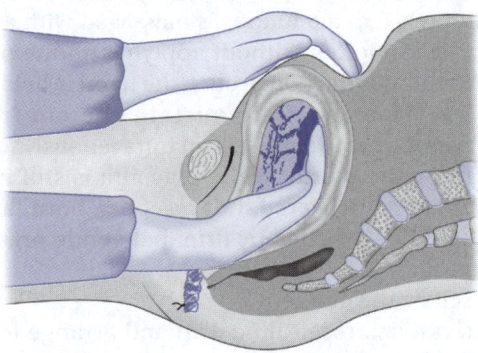

Figure 36.2: Manual removal of placenta.

located, the cord is released, so that the left hand may be used to support the fundus abdominally.

The operator will feel for a separated edge of the placenta. The fingers of the hand are extended and the border of the hand is gently eased between the placenta and the uterine wall with the palm facing the placenta. With a sideways slicing movement, the placenta is carefully detached. When the placenta is completely separated, it is extracted by traction of the cord by the left hand. The right hand is still inside the uterus for exploration of the cavity to be sure that nothing is left behind. The placenta should be checked immediately for completeness, so that any further exploration, if needed, may be carried out immediately.

After the completion of manual removal, inspection of cervicovaginal canal is made to exclude any injury. Intravenous ergometrine 0.25 mg is given and the uterus is massaged to make it hard.

Difficulties
- Hour-glass contraction leading to difficulty in introducing the hand
- Morbid adherent placenta, which may cause difficulty in getting to the plane of cleavage of placental separation.

Complications
- Hemorrhage due to incomplete removal
- Injury to the uterus
- Shock
- Infection
- Inversion
- Subinvolution
- Thrombophlebitis
- Embolism.

Observation of the Mother Following Third Stage Hemorrhage

Once the bleeding is controlled:
1. Total blood volume lost must be estimated as accurately as possible.
2. Maternal pulse and blood pressure are recorded quarter hourly and temperature taken 4 hourly.
3. The uterus should be palpated frequently to ensure that it remains well contracted and lochia lost must be observed.
4. Intravenous fluid replacement should be carefully calculated and administered to avoid circulatory overload. Monitoring the central venous pressure will provide an accurate assessment of the volume required, especially if blood loss has been severe.
5. Fluid intake and urinary output are recorded as indicators of renal function. The output should be measured on an hourly basis by the use of a selfretaining catheter.
6. The woman should remain in the labor ward until her condition is stable for close monitoring.
7. All records should be meticulously completed and signed as soon as possible.
8. Continued vigilance will be important for 24–48 hours.
9. Provision should be made for the woman to have a quiet period of recuperation.

PRIMARY POSTPARTUM HEMORRHAGE

Principles
- To diagnose the cause of bleeding—atonic or traumatic
- To take prompt and effective measures to control bleeding
- To correct hypovolemia.

Immediate Measures

The following immediate measures are taken by the attending physician, when the amount of blood loss is more than a liter:
- Calls for additional help
- Puts in one or two large bore (16 gauge) intravenous cannula
- Sends blood for group and crossmatching (if not done before) and requests for two units of blood
- Starts rapid infusion with normal saline (crystalloid) or plasma substitutes like Haemaccel (colloids) to reexpand the vascular bed. Monitoring of pulse, blood pressure, fluids infused, urinary output, drugs given and central venous pressure (when cited) are important.

Management Steps

Step 1: Palpation of Fundus

The first step is to feel the uterus for its consistency to determine the likely cause of bleeding. If the uterus is found atonic:
- Massage the fundus to make it hard and express the blood clot.
- Methergine 0.2 mg is to be given intramuscularly.
- Empty the bladder if it is found full (by inserting a self-retaining catheter).
- Examine the expelled placenta and membranes, if available, for evidence of missing cotyledons or pieces of membranes.

Step 2: Exploration of Uterus

If the uterus fails to remain firm and relaxes again with more bleeding:
- The uterus is to be explored under general anesthesia. Simultaneous inspection of the cervix, vagina and paraurethral region is done to exclude coexistent bleeding sites. Another dose of ergometrine is given. In refractory cases, 0.25 mg of 15-methyl-PGF2 is administered either intramuscularly or transabdominally into the myometrium to bring back the uterine tone. This may be repeated every 1–1.5 hours whenever necessary. If the uterus remains atonic, the next step is taken.

Step 3: Bimanual Compression (Fig. 36.3)

Bimanual compression is done to apply pressure to the placental site. The fingers of the right hand are inserted into the vagina like a cone; the hand is formed into a fist and placed into the anterior vaginally fornix, the elbow resting on the bed. The left hand is placed behind the uterus abdominally, the fingers pointing toward the cervix. The uterus is brought forward and compressed between the palm of the left hand and the first in the vagina. If bleeding persists, a clotting disorder must be excluded before exploration of the vagina and uterus.

During this period, the resuscitative measures are to be continued unless the general condition improves. With oxytocics and blood transfusion, most cases respond well. Uterine contraction and retraction regain and bleeding stops. However, in rare cases, when the uterus fails to contract, the following measures may be tried as an alternative to hysterectomy.

Step 4: Hot Intrauterine Douche

Hot intrauterine douche is an effective method to stimulate the uterus to regain its tone. The temperature of the fluid should be about 108°F (47.8°C) and some antiseptic lotions are mixed in the douche. If the method fails, the next step may be tried.

Step 5: Tight Intrauterine Packing

Intrauterine packing is done under general anesthesia. A 5 m long and 8 cm wide strip of gauze soaked in antiseptic solution is used. The gauze is placed high up and packed into the fundal area, while the uterus is steadied by the external hand. Gradually, the rest of the uterine cavity is packed, so that no empty space is left behind. A separate pack is used to fill the vagina. An abdominal binder is placed. The intrauterine packing exerts direct hemostatic pressure to the open uterine sinuses and stimulates uterine contraction. Antibiotic is given and the plug should be removed after 24 hours under morphine premedication. Intrauterine packing is useful in uncontrolled postpartum hemorrhage, where other methods have failed and the patient is being prepared for transfer to a tertiary care center.

Last Step: Hysterectomy

If, in spite of the above measures, the uterus fails to contract and blood coagulopathy is excluded, then hysterectomy may have to be performed.

Prognosis

Postpartum hemorrhage is one of the life-threatening emergencies in the third stage. It is responsible for maternal deaths in about 1%, especially in the developing countries. Prevalence of malnutrition and anemia, inadequate antenatal care and lack of blood transfusion facilities are some of the important contributing factors. There is also increased morbidity. These include shock, puerperal sepsis, failing lactation, pulmonary embolism, thrombosis and thrombophlebitis. Late sequelae include Sheehan's syndrome (selective hypopituitarism) or rarely diabetes insipidus.

Breaking of the Cord

Breaking of the cord is an occasional occurrence during completion of the third stage of labor. It is crucial to check that

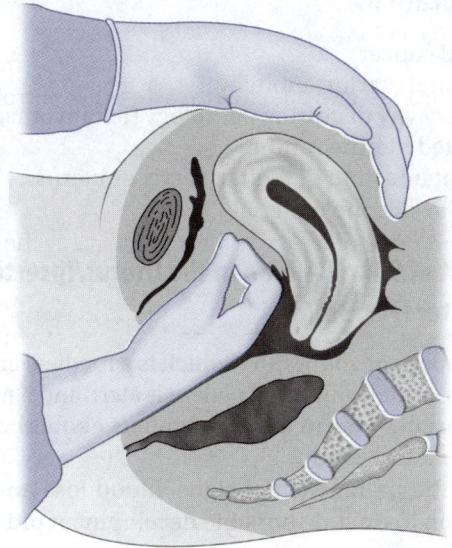

Figure 36.3: Bimanual compression of the uterus.

the uterus remains firm before further action is taken. If the placenta remains adherent, manual removal of the placenta is to be done by the obstetrician. If the placenta is palpable in the vagina, it is probable that separation has occurred. The mother may be encouraged to push with the next contraction and fundal pressure may be used. Great care must be taken not to exert undue pressure on the fundus. It may cause considerable pain and discomfort to the mother. If fundal pressure is performed without good uterine contraction, acute inversion may occur.

INTRAUTERINE TAMPONADE USING BAKRI BALLOON

The Bakri balloon is a medical device invented by Dr Younes Bakri, a French obstetrician in 1992 for the treatment of obstetric hemorrhage during cesarean delivery. Later it was used to manage hemorrhage from lower uterine segment due to placenta previa and placenta accreta. As per WHO recommendations, the use of intrauterine balloon tamponade (UBT) is recommended for treatment of postpartum hemorrhage (PPH) due to uterine atony, if the woman does not respond to uterotonics.

Definition

Bakri balloon insertion is a procedure used for temporary control or reduction of postpartum hemorrhage when conservative management of uterine bleeding is warranted after bleeding from genital tract laceration and retained products of conception have been excluded.

Description of the Bakri Balloon

The device consists of a 24 French, 54 cm long silicon catheter that contains a large central lumen and a balloon around it at the proximal end below the tip **(Figs. 36.4 and 36.5)**.

The collapsed balloon is inserted into the uterus. When filled with the fluid, the balloon adapts to the configuration of the uterine cavity to tamponade endometrial bleeding. The central lumen of the catheter allows drainage and aids to monitor ongoing bleeding above the level of the balloon.

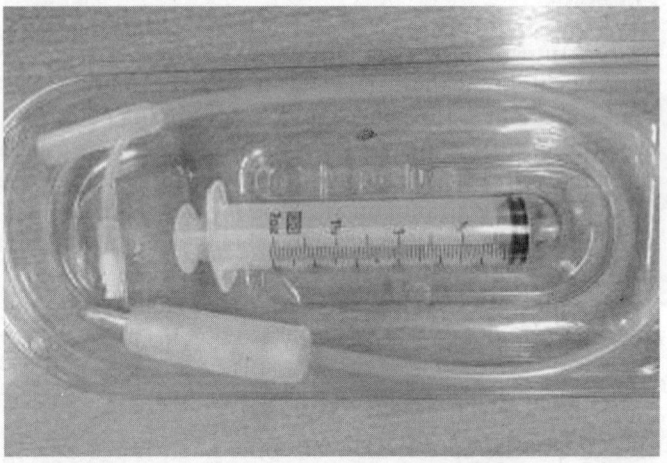

Figure 36.4: Bakri balloon.

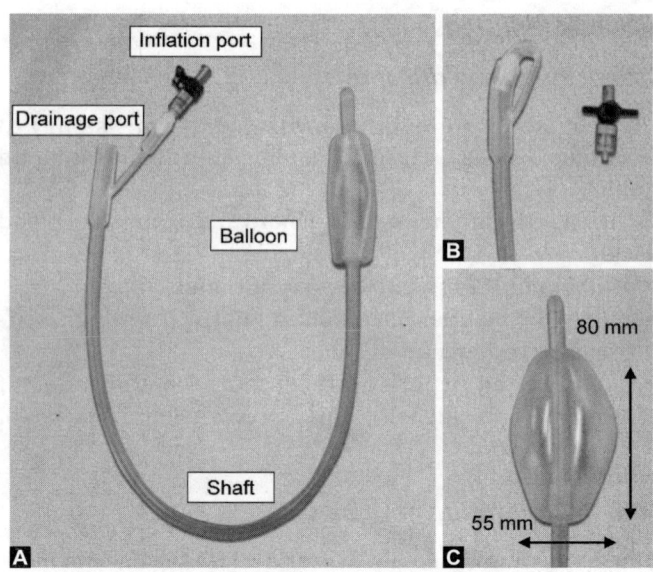

Figures 36.5A to C: Parts of Bakri balloon.

Mechanism of Action of the Balloon in the Control of Bleeding

The balloon is believed to act by exerting inward to outward pressure against the uterine wall resulting in a reduction in persistent capillary and venous bleeding from the endometrium and the myometrium.

Indications for Balloon Use

- For temporary control or reduction of PPH when conservative management of bleeding is warranted
- Failure to cause sustained control of hemorrhage after vaginal delivery, secondary to uterine atony
- As a temporary measure to decrease hemorrhage while waiting and preparing for other definitive treatment such as abdominal uterine surgery or uterine artery embolization.

Contraindications

- Cervical cancer
- Congenital uterine anomaly
- Uterine cavity distorting pathology (leiomyomas)
- Suspected uterine rupture
- Purulent infection of vagina, cervix or uterus
- Allergy to silicone material

Placement of Bakri Balloon in the Uterus/Insertion of the Catheter (Fig. 36.6)

Explain to patient about PPH, which is a medical emergency and obtain written consent if patient is alert, and if not a quick verbal consent. Inform family members about the need for immediate intervention.

- Assess the patient's vital signs, blood loss and general condition to exclude possible development of shock
- Place the patient in lithotomy position, drape and clean the perineum with antiseptic solution to avoid infection

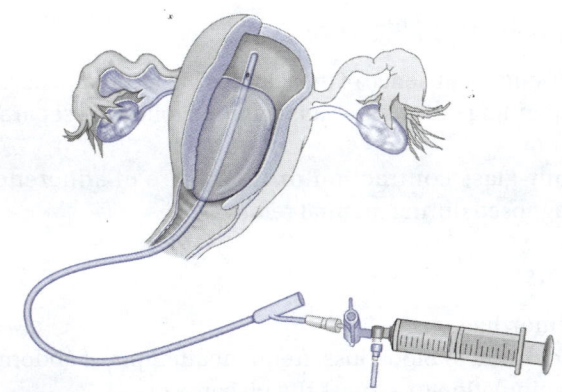

Figure 36.6: Bakri balloon inserted in the uterus and inflated.

- Insert a Foley's catheter to empty the bladder.
- Cleanse vagina and cervix with povidone iodine to maintain asepsis.
- Assist the doctor who will inspect the uterine cavity and visualize the cervix.
- The deflated balloon is then inserted into the uterine cavity under ultrasound guidance, making sure that the entire portion of the balloon passes the cervical canal above the internal os.
- Once the placement is confirmed, the balloon will be inflated with the recommended amount of 500 mL of sterile normal saline. A vaginal pack may be placed if needed to maximize the effect of tamponade.

Transabdominal Placement: Postcesarean Delivery

- The balloon is inserted through the uterine incision to the cervix and then into the vagina.
- The uterine incision is then closed, taking special care not to damage the balloon by the suture needle.
  An alternative approach used is to close the uterus first and then to insert the balloon from the vagina and inflate it while the surgeon watches from above.

Precautions

- Never inflate the balloon with air, carbon dioxide or any other gas which may cause complications.
- Do not fill the balloon with more than 500 mL. Overinflation may result in the balloon getting displaced into the vagina
- Insert and leave a Foley's catheter in the bladder to collect urine and monitor urine output
- Always confirm proper placement of the balloon using an ultrasound after inflating it to the predetermined volume.

Postprocedural Care

- Connect the drainage port of the balloon to a collection bag to monitor hemostasis
- Monitor the patient for signs of increased bleeding and uterine cramping
- The device should not be kept indwelling for more than 24 hours
- Closely monitor bleeding, fundal height and vital signs of the patient
- After 6 hours and up to 24 hours, if the patient is stable with no virginal bleeding and her fundal height is at the same level. Start to slowly remove the fluid from the balloon
- Use antibiotics if recommended to avoid the risk of iatrogenic infection
- Use of oxytocin or other uterotonics such as Methylergometrine and prostaglandins are generally recommended.

SECONDARY POSTPARTUM HEMORRHAGE

Secondary postpartum hemorrhage is bleeding from the genital tract more than 24 hours after delivery of the placenta and may occur up to 6 weeks after delivery. It is most likely to occur between 8th and 14th day after delivery.

Causes

- Retained bits of cotyledons, membranes or a large uterine blood clot
- Separation of slough over a deep cervicovaginal laceration
- Subinvolution of the placental site due to delayed healing process because of low-grade infection
- Secondary hemorrhage from cesarean section wound
- Withdrawal bleeding following estrogen therapy for suppression of lactation
- Other causes are chorion epithelioma, carcinoma cervix, placental polyp or fibroid polyp.

Clinical Features

- The lochia is heavier than normal and will consist of a bright red loss
- The lochia may be offensive, if infection is a contributing factor
- Subinvolution of uterus and often a patulous os
- Pyrexia and tachycardia
- Varying degrees of anemia: Proportionate to the blood loss.
  As this is an event most likely to occur at home, women should be alerted to the possible signs of postpartum hemorrhage prior to discharge from the postnatal ward.

Management

The principles of management are:
- To assess the amount of loss and to replace the lost blood.
- To find out the cause and to take appropriate steps to rectify it.

Supportive Therapy

- Resuscitative measures including blood transfusion, if the bleeding is heavy
- Ergometrine 0.5 mg intramuscularly, if the bleeding is uterine in origin
- Antibiotics as a routine.

Conservative Therapy

Bedrest and observation for 24 hours, if the bleeding is mild.

Active Management

- Exploration of the uterus under general anesthesia, if retained bits of placenta or membranes is the cause
- Gentle curettage is done and the materials removed are to be sent for histopathological examination
- Ergometrine 0.5 mg is given intramuscularly.

Secondary bleeding following cesarean section may at times require laparotomy for applying hemostatic sutures. Rarely, ligation of internal iliac artery or hysterectomy may become necessary.

Nursing Considerations

- If the uterus is still palpable, massaging the uterus and expressing the clots may help
- The mother must be encouraged to empty her bladder
- All the pads and linen must be assessed for the volume of blood lost
- Vital signs and general condition must be monitored
- Hemoglobin estimation, iron treatment and teaching about iron-rich foods
- Help to breastfeeding mothers to save the milk for the baby.

RETAINED PLACENTA

The placenta is said as retained when it is not expelled out even after 30 minutes of the birth of the baby.

Causes

There are three physiological phases involved in the normal expulsion of the placenta:
1. Separation through the spongy layer of the decidua.
2. Descend into the lower uterine segment and vagina.
3. Expulsion to outside.

Interference with any of these physiological processes results in its retention in the following manner:
1. Placenta completely separated, but retained. This is due to poor voluntary expulsive efforts specially following prolonged and exhaustive labor.
2. Simple adherent placenta due to uterine atonicity in case of grand multipara, over distention of uterus, prolonged labor, bigger placental surface area or uterine malformation. The commonest cause of retention of non-separated placenta is atonic uterus.
3. Placenta becomes incarcerated following partial or complete separation due to constriction ring (hourglass contraction). This may be due to intravenous ergometrine given at the delivery of anterior shoulder, premature attempts to deliver the placenta before it is separated and unnecessary kneading or fiddling of the uterus.
4. Morbid adherent placenta—partial or rarely complete.

Signs of Retained Placenta

- Presence or absence of the features of placental separation depending on whether it is retained following separation or not
- Hour-glass contraction or the nature of adherence is diagnosed during manual removal.

Dangers

- Hemorrhage
- Shock due to blood loss, frequent attempts of abdominal manipulation to express the placenta out
- Puerperal sepsis
- Risk of its recurrence in subsequent pregnancies.

Management

- A separated placenta that is retained, is expressed by controlled cord traction
- An unseparated retained placenta is removed manually under general anesthesia as described earlier. During manual removal, complications such as hour-glass contraction or morbid adherent placenta may be detected, which are managed as follows.

Hour-glass Contraction

The ring should be made to relax by:
1. Deepening the plane of anesthesia.
2. Subcutaneous injection of 0.5 mL of 1 in 1,000 adrenaline hydrochloride.
3. Inhalation of two amyl nitrate capsules of 5 minimum each.

If the ring is too tight and bleeding is absent, the operation is to be postponed. The woman is to be sedated with morphine 15 mg intramuscularly. After 4–6 hours of observation, manual removal is done.

If the ring is not too tight and bleeding is continuing, the ring is to be manually stretched by the cone-shaped hand, beginning at the upper border of the placenta in order to minimize bleeding.

Morbid Adherent Placenta

Diagnosis is made during attempted manual removal. On rare occasions, no cleavage between the placenta and the uterine wall is noted and a diagnosis of a total placenta accreta is made.

Complications Accompanying Retained Placenta and Management

1. *Retained placenta with shock, but not hemorrhage:* To treat the shock and when the condition improves, manual removal is to be done, if not already separated.
2. *Retained placenta with hemorrhage:* Same management as outlined for third stage hemorrhage.

3. *Retained placenta with sepsis:* The woman is usually delivered outside and is admitted in the referral hospital after few hours or even days after delivery. Sepsis is a potential risk or may already be present. Intrauterine swabs are taken for culture and sensitivity test and broad-spectrum antibiotic is given. Blood transfusion is usually required. On examination, if the placenta is found separated, it is expressed out. If found retained, manual removal is to be carried out as soon as the patient's general condition permits.
4. *Retained placenta with an episiotomy wound:* The bleeding points of the episiotomy wound are to be secured by artery forceps. A manual removal is done without delay followed by repair of episiotomy wound

PLACENTA ACCRETA

Placenta accreta is an abnormal partial or total adherence of the placenta to the uterine wall. The placenta is directly adhered to the myometrium with either defective decidua or no decidua in between. When the chorionic villi extent further than contact with the myometrium and actually penetrate the uterine wall, the condition is called placenta increta. Placenta percreta occurs when the chorionic villi invade through the entire uterine wall to the serosa layer. These conditions are rare complications.

The probable cause is defective decidual formation. The condition is usually associated with placenta previa. It may also occur when the placenta is situated over injured sites as following cesarean section, dilation and curettage operation, manual removal or myomectomy.

Diagnosis

1. A partial placenta accreta is first seen as an acute third stage hemorrhage resulting from a partially separated placenta. Clinical diagnosis is made when the placenta's adherence is discovered during attempted manual removal of the retained placenta.
2. A complete placenta accreta has no signs and symptoms since there is no partial separation and, therefore, no hemorrhage. It is discovered during attempted manual removal of the retained placenta.
3. Definitive diagnosis of placenta accreta is made by microscopic examination. Pathological confirmation includes absence of decidua basalis, absence of fibrinoid layer and varying degrees of penetration of the villi into the muscle bundles.

Placenta accreta is an obstetric disaster. Any suspicion that a retained placenta is due to placenta accreta requires that the midwife immediately place an urgent call for the physician. While waiting, the midwife must do all she can to maintain the woman and prepare her for immediate surgery.

Management

1. In partial placenta accreta, where major separation is possible, the adherent area is separated manually leaving behind bits of placental tissue with the uterine wall. Oxytocin is administered for uterine contraction and intrauterine plugging to achieve hemostasis. If the uterus fails to contract, hysterectomy is done.
2. In complete placenta accreta, hysterectomy is done in parous women. In women desiring to have another child, conservative management may be undertaken. This consists of cutting the umbilical cord as high as possible and leaving behind the placenta, which is expected to be autolyzed in due course of time. Appropriate antibiotics are given.

Risks of placenta accreta include hemorrhage, shock, infection and rarely inversion of uterus.

INVERSION OF THE UTERUS

Inversion of the uterus is a rare, but potentially life-threatening situation in which the uterus is turned inside out partially or completely. The incidence is about 1:20,000 deliveries. The obstetric inversion is usually an acute one and usually complete.

Classification of Inversion (Figs. 36.7A to C)

1. *First degree:* There is dimpling of the fundus, which remains above the level of the internal os.
2. *Second degree:* The uterus is inverted and the fundus passes through the cervix, but lies inside the vagina.

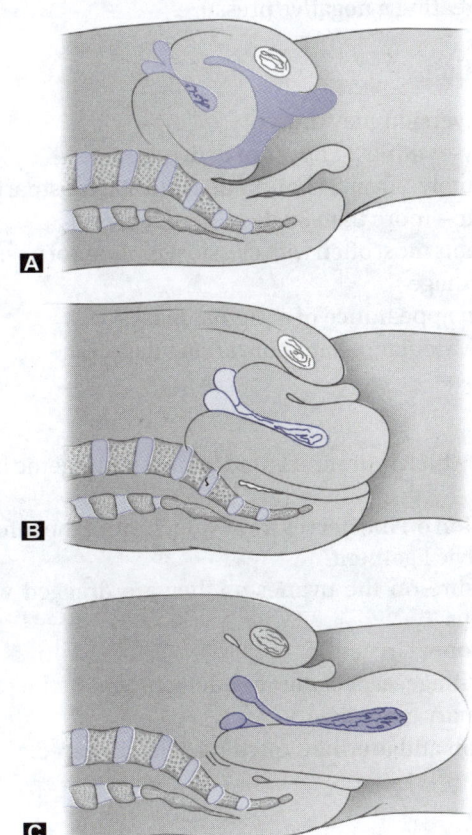

Figures 36.7A to C: Acute inversion of the uterus. (A) First degree; (B) Second degree; (C) Third degree.

3. *Third degree (complete):* The endometrium with or without the attached placenta is visible outside the vulva. The uterus, cervix and part of the vagina are inverted and visible.

Causes

The inversion may be spontaneous or more commonly induced.

Spontaneous (40%)

Spontaneous is brought about by local atony of the placental site over the fundus associated with sharp rise of intra-abdominal pressure as in coughing, sneezing or bearing down effort. Fundal attachment of the placenta, short cord and placenta accreta are often associated.

Induced (60%)

Induced is due to mismanagement of third stage of labor:
- Pulling the cord when the uterus is atonic specially when combined with fundal pressure
- Crede's method of placental expression, while the uterus is relaxed
- Faulty technique in manual removal: Pulling the partially separated placenta, or firmly pressing on the atonic uterus by the external hand or rapidly withdrawing the internal hand thereby creating a negative pressure.

Presentation

Uterine inversion may present:
- Acutely—within 24 hours of delivery
- Sub acutely—over 24 hours and up to 30th postpartum day
- Chronic—more than 30 days after delivery
- It presents most often with classic symptoms of postpartum hemorrhage
- Sudden appearance of a vaginal mass
- Cardiovascular collapse of varying degree.

Dangers

- Shock, which is profound and mainly neurogenic in origin due to:
  - Tension on the nerves from stretching of the infundibulopelvic ligament
  - Pressure on the ovaries as they are dragged with the fundus
  - Peritoneal irritation.
- Hemorrhage, especially after detachment of the placenta
- Pulmonary embolism
- Infection and uterine sloughing, if left uncared.

Diagnosis

- Acute lower abdominal pain with bearing down sensation
- Varying degree of shock
- On abdominal examination:
  - Dimpling or cupping of the fundal surface
  - Fundus cannot be palpated.
- Incomplete variety, a pear-shaped mass protrudes outside the vulva with the broad end pointing downwards and looking reddish purple in color.

Management

Before Shock Develops

Immediate medical support must be summoned. Urgent manual replacement (even without anesthesia if not easily available) must be done as outlined below:
1. To push the fundus with the palm of the hand, along the direction of the vagina toward the posterior fornix.
2. To apply counter support with the other hand placed on the abdomen.
3. After replacement, the hand should remain inside the uterus until the uterus becomes contracted by parenteral oxytocics.
4. The placenta is to be removed manually only after the uterus becomes contracted; a partially separated placenta may be removed prior to replacement to reduce the bulk, which facilitates replacement.
5. Usual treatment of shock including blood transfusion should be arranged as and when required.

After Shock Develops

1. The treatment of shock should be instituted vigorously. Morphine 15 mg intramuscularly, dextrose saline drip and arrangements for blood transfusion to be made.
2. To push the uterus inside the vagina if possible and to pack the vagina with antiseptic roller gauze.
3. Foot end of the bed to be raised.
4. Replacement of the uterus under general anesthesia to be done along with resuscitative measures.

If manual replacement fails, the method of hydrostatic replacement is instituted. This involves the instillation of warm saline through a douche nozzle. The pressure of the fluid builds up as several liters are run into the vagina and restores the uterus to the normal position, while the operator seals off the introitus by one hand inserted into the vagina.

If the inversion cannot be manually replaced it may be due to the development of a cervical constriction ring. Drugs can be utilized to relax the constriction ring and facilitate the return of the uterus to its normal position.

Throughout the procedure, the woman and her husband and/or family should be kept informed of what is happening. Assessment of vital signs and level of consciousness is of great importance.

Prevention

- Do not employ any method to expel the placenta out when the uterus is relaxed
- Avoid pulling the cord simultaneous with fundal pressure.

STUDY QUESTIONS

Short Notes
1. Postpartum hemorrhage.
2. HELLP syndrome.
3. Inversion of uterus.

Short Answer Questions
1. Classification of postpartum hemorrhage.
2. Causes of atonic uterus.
3. Causes of traumatic hemorrhage in third stage of labor.
4. Bimanual compression of uterus.
5. Placenta accreta.

Essay Questions
1. A postpartum client has developed secondary postpartum hemorrhage 2 days after delivery with subinvolution of uterus. Explain the possible management measures and nursing considerations.
2. A client has not expelled the placenta 40 minutes after delivery of the fetus. The condition is determined as 'retained placenta'. Explain the possible management measures and nursing care.

BIBLIOGRAPHY
1. Bonnar J, McNicol GP, Douglas AS. Coagulation and fibrinolytic mechanisms during and after normal childbirth. Br Med J. 1970;2(5703):200-3.
2. Dutta DC. Textbook of Obstetrics, 5th edition. Kolkata: New Central Book Company; 2001. pp. 441-53.
3. Levy V, Moore J. The midwife's management of the third stage of labour. Nurs Times. 1985;81(39):47-50.
4. McDonald S. Physiology and management of the third stage of labor. In: Bennett RV, Brown KL (Eds). Myles Textbook for Midwives, 13th edition. Edinburgh: Churchill Livingstone; 1999. pp. 471-85.
5. Newton M, Mosey LM, Egli GE, et al. Blood loss during and immediately after delivery. Obstet Gynecol. 1961;17:9-18.

CHAPTER 37

Injuries to the Birth Canal

Learning Objectives

Upon completing this chapter, the learner will be able to:
- Describe the causes of perineal lacerations and management including perineal repair.
- Describe the perineal management at delivery and perineal care following delivery.
- Discuss the causes, detection and management of women in the event of uterine rupture.

LACERATIONS OF PERINEUM

Injuries to the birth canal commonly occur during childbirth and contribute significantly to maternal morbidity. The maternal genital tract injuries occur in both natural and instrumental deliveries. Avoidance, early detection and effective management can minimize the morbidity and prevent gynecological problems in future.

Injuries to Vulva

Lacerations tear of the vulval skin posteriorly and the paraurethral tear on the inner aspect of the labia minora are common sites. Paraurethral tears often bleed briskly as the labia are highly vascular. Prompt repair may be necessary to secure hemostasis.

Perineal Tears/Lacerations

The perineum may be torn due to several factors:
1. Over stretching of the perineum due to large baby, face delivery, outlet contraction with narrow pubic arch, shoulder dystocia and forceps delivery.
2. Rapid stretching of the perineum due to rapid delivery of the head during uterine contraction, precipitate labor and breech delivery.
3. Inelastic perineum as in rigid perineum in elderly primigravida, scar in the perineum following previous operations, such as episiotomies or perineorrhaphy and vulval edema.
4. Unattended delivery and inability of the woman to stop bearing down.

Classification

Spontaneous tears are usually classified in degrees that are related to the anatomical structures, which have been traumatized. The classification only serves as a guideline because it is often difficult to identify the structures precisely.

First degree
Involves lacerations of the fourchette (lower end of the posterior vagina) only.

Second degree
Involves the fourchette and the superficial perineal muscles, namely the bulbocavernosus and the transverse perineal muscles, and in some cases the pubococcygeus.

Third degree (complete tear)
Involves in addition to the above structures and the anal sphincter.

Fourth degree (central tear)
The tear extends to the rectal mucosa.

Prevention

Conduct of second stage of delivery with due care in those with increased likelihood of laceration:
1. Maintain flexion of the head until the occiput comes under the symphysis pubis, so that lesser suboccipitofrontal (10 cm) diameter emerges out of the introitus.
2. Assure the woman not to bear down during contractions to avoid forcible delivery of the head.
3. Deliver the head in between contractions.
4. Perform timely episiotomies.
5. Take care during delivery of the shoulders.

Management

Tears must be repaired immediately following the delivery of the placenta in order to minimize blood loss and to reduce the chance of infection. In case of delay beyond 24 hours, the repair is to be withheld. Antiseptic dressing and antibiotics are given and the wound allowed to heal by granulation tissue or repaired after the infection is controlled. Complete tears (third degree) that are delayed beyond 24 hours are repaired after 3 months.

Repair

The woman is placed in lithotomy position. A good source of light is essential. Vagina, vulva and perineal region are swabbed with antiseptic solution, and the area is draped. Perineal infiltration is carried out by the physician with 1% lignocaine hydrochloride (10–20 mL). Infiltration is not required, if the delivery is conducted under pudendal block or epidural anesthesia. In complete tear, general anesthesia may be administered.

In the first and second degree tears, the vaginal mucosa is sutured first. The first suture is placed at or just above apex of the tear. Thereafter, the vaginal walls are apposed by interrupted sutures with chromic catgut number '00' using curved, round body needle from above downwards until the fourchette is reached.

In third degree perineal tear, the rectal and anal mucosa are sutured first from above downwards with chromic catgut number '00' by interrupted stitches using curved atraumatic needle. Muscle walls and facia are then sutured by interrupted stitches using the same materials. The torn ends of the sphincter ani are then reconstituted with a figure of eight stitch using number '00' chromic catgut.

Repair of the perineal muscles is done in two layers by interrupted sutures using number '00' chromic catgut.

The perineal skin is apposed by interrupted sutures either with chromic catgut, nylon or silkworm gut using a cutting needle. The sutured area should be inspected in order to confirm hemostasis before the vaginal pack is removed. A vaginal examination is made to ensure that the introitus has not been narrowed. Upon completion, a rectal examination is done in order to ensure that no sutures have penetrated the rectal mucosa. Any such sutures if found must be removed to prevent fistula formation.

The area is cleaned and a sterile, sanitary pad placed over the vulva and perineum. The woman's legs are then removed gently and simultaneously from the lithotomy supports and she is made comfortable.

Aftercare

1. The mother should be explained about the nature of trauma and repair, and information given on whether or not the sutures will need to be removed.
2. A low residue diet is given from the 2nd day onwards.
3. Stool softeners, such as mild milk of magnesia are given twice daily. If the woman does not pass stool and has discomfort, a small quantity enema (fleet enema or oil enema) is given.
4. Intestinal antiseptics, such as metronidazole are given for 5–7 days.

Vaginal Tears

Vaginal lacerations without involvement of the perineum or cervix sometimes occur. The most common site is the lower third of the vagina. The lower end of the vagina may be torn transversely from its junction with the perineum, leaving a deep cavity behind an intact perineum. Injuries of the upper and lower third of the vagina are rare. These are usually seen following instrumental or manipulative delivery. In such cases, the tears are extensive and often associated with active bleeding.

Management

A vaginal tear is sutured by interrupted or continuous sutures using chromic catgut number '00'. In case of extensive lacerations, in addition to sutures, hemostasis may be achieved by intravaginal plugging by roller gauze soaked with glycerin and acriflavine. The plug should be removed after 24 hours.

Colporrhexis

Rupture of the vault of the vagina is called colporrhexis. It may be primary where only the vault is involved or secondary when associated with cervical tear (more common). It is said to be complete when the peritoneum is opened up. The tear may be traumatic or spontaneous especially in multiparae.

Treatment is exploration and repair from below, if the tear is limited to the vault and accessible part of the cervix. If however, the tear extends high up into the lower segment, laparotomy is to be done simultaneously with resuscitative measures.

Cervical Tears

Minor degrees of cervical tears often occur during first delivery. Major extensive tears requiring attention is also common. This is the most common cause of traumatic postpartum hemorrhage.

Causes

1. Iatrogenic: Attempted forceps delivery or breech extraction through an incompletely dilated cervix.
2. Rigid cervix: This may be congenital or due to scarring from previous operations on the cervix.
3. Strong uterine contractions as in precipitate labor.
4. Extremely vascular cervix as in placenta previa.
5. Detachment of the cervix: Annular detachment of the cervix may occur following prolonged labor in primary cervical dystocia.

6. Partial detachment may occur when the cervix is caught between the head and the pelvic wall.
7. Failure to remove a cerclage suture.
8. Congenital elongation of the cervix or vaginouterine prolapse.

Signs

Excessive vaginal bleeding following delivery in the presence of a hard and contracted uterus is suggestive of cervical tear. Exploration of the uterovaginal canal under good light is essential to confirm the diagnosis and assess the tear.

Management

Minor tears require no treatment. Deep cervical tears associated with bleeding should be repaired soon after delivery of the placenta. The repair should be done under general anesthesia in lithotomy position with a good light.

PELVIC HEMATOMAS

Collections of blood anywhere in the area between the pelvic peritoneum and the peritoneal skin are called pelvic hematoma.

Anatomical Types

Depending upon the location of the hematoma, whether below or above the levator ani muscle, it is termed as:
- Infralevator hematoma
- Supralevator hematoma.

Infralevator Hematoma

Vulval hematoma is the most common in this type.

Causes

1. Trauma of spontaneous labor, prolonged labor and forceps operations resulting in rupture of paravaginal venous plexus.
2. Improper hemostasis during repair of vaginal or perineal tears or episiotomy wound.
3. Rough uterine massage for controlling postpartum hemorrhage may cause development of small hematomas in the supraperitoneal connective tissue and in the broad ligaments.

Manifestations

- Persistent, severe pain in the perineal region
- Rectal tenesmus or bearing down efforts, when extension occurs to the ischiorectal fossa
- Retention of urine
- Variable degrees of shock or collapse
- Tense swelling at the vulva, which becomes dusky and purple in color and tender to touch
- Pallor, rapid pulse and low blood pressure
- A tender pelvic lump on palpation.

Treatment

A small hematoma (<5 cm) is treated conservatively with cold compress. When it is larger than 5 cm or increasing in size, it needs to be evacuated. The patient is given blood and narcotic analgesics are administered for pain.

The hematoma is drained under general anesthesia and bleeding points are secured. The dead space is to be obliterated by deep mattress sutures and a closed suction drain may be kept for 24 hours. Prophylactic antibiotic is to be administered.

Supralevator Hematoma

Causes

- Extension of cervical laceration or primary vault rupture (colporrhexis)
- Lower uterine segment rupture
- Spontaneous rupture of paracervical venous plexus adjacent to the vault.

Diagnosis

- Unexplained symptoms with features of shock following delivery
- Abdominal examination reveals swelling above the inguinal ligament pushing the uterus to the opposite side
- Vaginal examination reveals occlusion of the vaginal canal by a bulge or a bogy swelling felt through the fornix
- Ultrasonography may show the exact localization of the hematoma.

Management

- Treatment of shock
- Exploratory laparotomy and drainage of the hematoma (blood clots are scooped out)
- The bleeding points, if seen, are to be secured and ligated
- Any injury to the uterus and/or cervix is repaired
- The broad ligament is drained extraperitoneally using corrugated rubber drain
- Bilateral internal iliac artery ligation may be required to control bleeding.

RUPTURE OF THE UTERUS

Rupture of the uterus is an uncommon injury and when it happens, it can be a catastrophic event, as it places the mother and fetus at high risk for morbidity and mortality (**Fig. 37.1**).

Definition

A rupture is defined as an abrupt tearing of the uterus and can be complete or incomplete.

Classification of Rupture

Scar Rupture and Dehiscence

1. In scar rupture disruption of the entire length of the scar occurs. With classical scars, rupture occurs late in

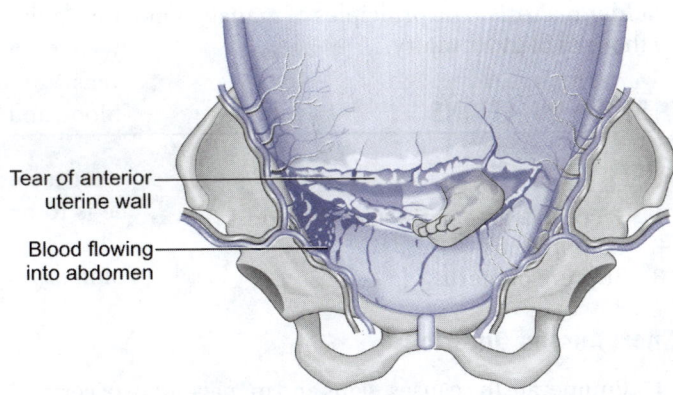

Figure 37.1: Uterine rupture.

pregnancy or early labor. Bleeding is slight, unless the placenta is lying underneath. Rupture in lower segment scars occur with obstructed labor. It is accompanied by a 'tearing pain'. Bleeding may not be heavy.
2. Dehiscence is disruption of part of the scar and not the entire length. It tends not to cause any bleeding and is without clinical significance.

Complete and Incomplete Rupture

1. Complete uterine rupture extends through the entire wall and peritoneum with the entire contents spilling into the abdominal cavity.
2. An incomplete uterine rupture extends through the endometrium and myometrium without involving the peritoneum.

Spontaneous and Traumatic Rupture

1. A spontaneous rupture is one that occurs during labor owing to a myometrium weakened by a previous scar.
2. A traumatic uterine rupture may be caused by trauma resulting from obstetric instruments, obstetric interventions or accidents such as fall or blow on the abdomen.

Risk Factors

- A tumultuous labor resulting from oxytocin induction when not controlled carefully
- Multiparity combined with use of oxytocin
- Obstructed labor such as with absolute cephalopelvic disproportion
- Accidents such as falling face downwards
- Trauma due to forceps, breech extraction or internal version late in labor
- Excessive fundal pressure
- Shoulder dystocia.

Signs and Symptoms

1. *Exquisite abdominal pain:* When the rupture is complete, the woman experiences a transient relief from pain followed by cessation of contractions.
2. Vaginal bleeding.
3. Intra-abdominal bleeding, which may lead to rapid collapse. Blood may be confined retroperitoneally as a broad ligament hematoma.
4. Lack of progress in labor.
5. Shock from hemorrhage (hypovolemic shock).
6. Alteration in shape of abdominal swelling.
7. The uterus contracts and may be mistaken for a fetal head in the suprapubic region.
8. *Palpation of fetal parts outside the uterine wall (superficial fetal parts):* The fetus is wholly or partly extruded into the abdominal cavity and quickly dies whether or not the tear is complete or incomplete (complete when the peritoneum is also torn through).
9. Rapid onset of fetal distress progressing to absence of fetal heart sounds.
10. Restlessness and anxiety.
11. An empty pelvis on vaginal examination.

Dehiscence of a lower segment scar may cause virtually no bleeding or shock and is described as silent rupture. The injury is discovered only on section for delay in labor.

Management

- Emergency cesarean delivery with repair of the rupture, if the woman is undelivered and the symptoms are not severe
- Cesarean hysterectomy, if the tear is severe and cannot be repaired.

Nursing Care

1. Continuous assessment of the woman who is predisposed to develop a rupture. In those with classical cesarean scar, the rupture is likely to occur even before labor begins.
2. Monitor the progress of labor carefully in order to facilitate early identification or abnormal symptoms.
3. Cautious use of oxytocin in women with uterine scar.

Once a Rupture is Diagnosed

- Monitor maternal and fetal vital signs and fluid status
- Administer oxygen for the benefit of both woman and fetus
- Urinary catheterization to be done and mother to be prepared for surgery
- Provide information to the woman and her family of the situation, interventions being planned and the prognosis
- Emotional support to the woman and her immediate family members.

VISCERAL INJURIES

Injury to Bladder

Causes

Injury to bladder may be due to:
1. Trauma:
   a. During instrumental vaginal delivery such as forceps delivery or destructive operations.

b. Abdominal operation, such as hysterectomy for rupture of uterus or repeat cesarean section.
2. Sloughing fistula: This results from prolonged compression of the bladder between the fetal head and symphysis pubis in obstructed labor.

Clinical Manifestations

1. Traumatic:
   a. Urine dribbles out following the operative surgery.
   b. Blood-stained urine following cesarean section or hysterectomy.
2. Sloughing fistula:
   a. Dribbling of urine occurs after varying interval following prolonged labor (5–7 day).
   b. Missing of a chunk of tissue seen on examination.

Management

Immediate repair is preferable for traumatic fistula, if the woman's general condition is good and facilities are available.

In unfavorable condition, a self-retaining catheter is introduced and kept for 10–14 days. Urinary antiseptics are given and bladders wash done daily. Spontaneous closure may occur and if it does not, repair is done after 3 months.

Injury to the Rectum

Rectal injury is rare because the middle third of the rectum is protected by the curved sacral hollow and the upper third is protected by the peritoneal lining. Prolonged compression of the rectum by the head in midpelvic contraction with a flat sacrum predisposes to ischemic necrosis of the anterior rectal wall and results in rectovaginal fistula. The repair in such cases should be postponed for at least 3 months.

Injury to the Urethra

Urethral injury may be traumatic resulting from instrumental delivery or during pubiotomy. It may occur due to ischemic sloughing, the mechanism of which is similar to that of bladder necrosis. The principles of management are similar to those of bladder injury.

■ STUDY QUESTIONS

Short Notes

1. Second degree perineal laceration.
2. Colporrhexis.
3. Rupture of uterus.

Short Answer Questions

1. Enumerate the causes, signs and management of cervical tears.
2. Enumerate the manifestations and management of pelvic hematoma.

Essay Question

1. Define rupture of uterus; describe the types of rupture, signs and symptoms, management and nursing care.

■ BIBLIOGRAPHY

1. Dutta DC. Textbook of obstetrics, 5th edition. Kolkata: New Central Book Company; 2001. pp. 454-7.
2. Grant A. Repair of episiotomies and perineal tears. British Journal of Obstetrics and Gynaecology. 1986;93(5):417-9.
3. Grant A. Repair of perineal trauma after childbirth. In: Chalmers I, Enkin M (Eds). Effective care in pregnancy and childbirth. Oxford: Oxford University Press; 1989.
4. Harrison RF, Brennan M, North PM, et al. Is routine episiotomies necessary? British Medical Journal. 1984;288(6435):1971-5.
5. Helen V. Nurse-Midwifery, 2nd edition. Boston: Jones and Bartlett Publishers; 1999. pp. 293-94.
6. Hillan EM. Physiology and management of the second stage of labor. In: Bennel RV, Brown KL (Eds). Myles textbook for midwives, 13th edition. Edinburgh: Churchill Livingstone; 1999. pp. 447-63.

CHAPTER 38

Complications of Puerperium

Learning Objectives

Upon completing this chapter, the learner will be able to:
- Describe the infections in the postnatal period and nurses' role in prevention and management.
- Describe the breast problems and venous complications that occur in postnatal women.
- Explain the different types of psychological disturbances seen in the puerperium and their management.

PUERPERAL PYREXIA

An elevation in temperature to 38°C (100.4°F) or more occurring on two separate occasions at 24 hours apart (excluding the first 24 hour) within the first 10 days following delivery is called puerperal pyrexia.

Causes

- Puerperal sepsis
- Urinary tract infection (UTI): Cystitis, pyelonephritis
- Breast infection
- Infection of laparotomy wound (cesarean section)
- Intercurrent infection: Acute bronchitis, pneumonia, influenza, acute appendicitis and enteric fever
- Thrombophlebitis
- Deep vein thrombosis (DVT)
- Flaring up of tuberculosis.

Puerperal sepsis is thought to be due to genital tract infection unless proved otherwise.

PUERPERAL SEPSIS

Definition

Puerperal sepsis is an infection of the genital tract, which occurs as a complication of delivery.

Conditions that Favor the Development of Sepsis

The vaginal flora in late pregnancy and during labor consists of the organisms such as Döderlein's bacillus, *Candida albicans*, *Staphylococcus albus* or *aureus*, *Streptococcus*, *Escherichia coli* and *Clostridium welchii* on occasion. These organisms remain dormant and are harmless during normal delivery, conducted in aseptic condition. However, the following conditions favor the development of sepsis in puerperal women:

- Damage to the cervicovaginal mucous membrane
- The open wound created by the cleavage of the decidua, which takes place when the placenta is separated (placental site)
- The blood clots at the placental site are an excellent media for the growth of bacteria.

Predisposing Factors of Puerperal Sepsis

Antepartum Factors

- Malnutrition and anemia
- Preeclampsia
- Premature rupture of membranes
- Chronic debilitating illness
- Sexual intercourse during late pregnancy.

Intrapartum Factors

- Introduction of organisms into the upper genital tract during vaginal examinations, especially after rupture of membranes during manipulative delivery
- Dehydration and ketoacidosis during labor (prolonged labor)
- Traumatic operative delivery
- Hemorrhage antepartum or postpartum
- Retained bits of placental tissue or membranes
- Placental site lying close to vagina (placenta previa).

Causative Organisms

The organisms responsible for puerperal sepsis are the following:
1. *Aerobic: Staphylococcus pyogenes, E. coli, Klebsiella, Pseudomonas, S. aureus* and non-hemolytic *Streptococcus*.
2. *Anaerobic: Streptococcus, C. welchii, C. tetani* and *Bacteroides*.

Mode of Infection

Puerperal sepsis is essentially a wound infection. Placental site (being a raw surface), lacerations of the genital tract or cesarean section wounds may be infected in the following ways:
1. *Endogenous:* Organisms present in the genital tract before delivery become pathogenic.
2. *Autogenous:* Organisms present elsewhere in the body migrate to the genital organs either through bloodstream or by droplet infection, are conveyed to the site by the woman herself, or her attendants. Common sites from where organisms are transferred include septic throat, feces and skin infection.
3. *Exogenous:* Infection is contracted from sources outside the client. The organisms are usually introduced from the respiratory tract of attendants, physicians or nurses. The infection may be dust borne or as droplet and may occur during vaginal examination, or from contaminated linen.

Pathology

Puerperal infection is a wound infection. The primary sites of infection are perineum, vagina, cervix and uterus:
1. *Perineum:* Lacerations of the perineum are likely to be infected. The wound edges become red and swollen. There may be collections of sanguinopurulent discharge or pus resulting in complete disruption of the wound.
2. *Vagina:* The vaginal lacerations are infected directly or by extension from the perineal infection. The mucosa is swollen and hyperemic resulting in necrosis and sloughing.
3. *Cervix:* The cervical lacerations become the site of infection.
4. *Uterus:* The uterus is the most common site of infection. The decidua over the placental site is the common site to be infected first. The infection usually manifests between 3rd and 6th day of delivery. Uterine infection is termed as *endometritis*. In *putrid endometritis,* the decidua becomes infected and necrosed and sloughs off. The infection to the deeper myometrium is prevented by a zone of leukocytic barrier. The discharge becomes offensive.

Invasion to the myometrium and spread to the distant sites may occur when the infection is severe by organisms like beta (β)-hemolytic streptococci.

Spread of infection to other sites may lead to the following:
1. *Pelvic cellulitis (parametritis):* Infection of the pelvic peritoneum and levator ani muscle.
2. *Salpingitis:* Infection of the fallopian tubes and ovaries with formation of tubo-ovarian mass.
3. *Peritonitis:* Localized pelvic abscess or generalized infection.
4. *Thrombophlebitis:* Ovarian vein of one side is usually involved. Uterine veins may also be involved.
5. *Septicemia and pyemia:* These may lead to endocarditis, pericarditis, renal abscess, lung abscess and meningitis or arthritis. These are rare nowadays with the advent of potent antibiotics.

Clinical Features

Local Infection

- Slight rise in temperature, generalized malaise or headache
- Redness and swelling of the local wound
- Pus formation and disruption of wound.

Uterine Infection

- Pyrexia of variable degrees and tachycardia
- Red, copious and offensive lochia
- Subinvoluted, tender and soft uterus.

Severe Infection

- Fever with chills and rigor
- Rapid pulse
- Scanty, odorless lochia
- Involuted uterus.

Parametritis

- Sustained rise in temperature (7–10 days)
- Constant pelvic pain
- Tenderness on either side of the hypogastrium
- Unilateral, tender mass felt on vaginal examination
- Leukocytosis.

Pelvic Peritonitis

- Pyrexia with increased pulse rate
- Lower abdominal pain and tenderness
- On vaginal examination, tenderness of the fornix and with movement of the cervix
- Collection of pus in the pouch of Douglas.

General Peritonitis

- High fever with rapid pulse
- Vomiting
- Generalized abdominal pain
- Tender and distended abdomen.

Thrombophlebitis

- Swinging temperature with chills and rigor
- Features of pyemia according to the organs involved.

Septicemia

- High temperature associated with rigor
- Rapid pulse
- Headache, insomnia or mental confusion
- Positive blood culture
- Signs and symptoms of metastatic infection in the lungs, meninges or joints.

Investigations

1. Bacteriological study:
   - Smear
   - Culture and antibiotic sensitivity of purulent material
   - High vaginal and cervical swabs
   - Peritoneal fluid
   - Blood culture as appropriate.
2. Urine:
   - Routine and microscopic examination
   - Culture, if infection is suspected.
3. Complete blood count (CBC).
4. Ultrasonography: For diagnosis of pelvic masses, pelvic abscess, pelvic peritonitis, retained bits of placenta and/or membranes.
5. Other specific investigations as per clinical condition such as chest X-ray or blood for malaria parasites.

Prevention

Antenatal

- Improvement of general condition
- Treatment of septic foci
- Abstinence from sexual intercourse in the last 2 months
- Care about personal hygiene—use clean water for bathing
- Avoiding contact with people having infection such as cold and boils
- Avoiding unnecessary vaginal examinations and douches in the later months.

Intrapartum

1. Staff (physicians and nurses) attending on labor clients should be free of infections.
2. Full surgical asepsis to be taken, while conducting delivery.
3. Women having respiratory tract infection or skin infection should be admitted in single room or separate ward.
4. Membranes should be kept intact as long as possible and vaginal examination should be restricted to minimum.
5. Traumatic vaginal delivery and intrauterine manipulation should be preferably avoided. If required, should be done using fresh (sterile) gloves with liberal use of strong antiseptic solutions.
6. Lacerations of the genital tract should be repaired promptly and meticulously with perfect hemostasis.
7. Excessive blood loss during delivery should be replaced promptly by transfusion to improve the general body resistance.
8. Prophylactic antibiotics must be administered in cases of premature rupture of membranes, prolonged labor or following traumatic delivery.

Postpartum

- Nurses to take aseptic precautions, while dressing the perineal wound
- Restriction of visitors in the postpartum ward
- Mothers to be instructed to use sterile sanitary pads and to change them frequently
- Vulva and perineum to be washed/cleaned with mild antiseptic solution following urination and defecation
- Infected mothers and babies are to be isolated
- To keep the floor of the inpatient ward dust free by frequent mopping (wet swabbing).

Treatment

- The woman should be placed in a separate room/ward with adequate light and ventilation
- Complete rest is to be given in head high position, which helps in drainage of lochia and localization of infection to the pelvis, if there is pelvic peritonitis
- Analgesics and sedatives are administered to enforce rest
- Broad-spectrum antibiotics are given intravenously until antibiotic sensitivity reports are available, followed by specific antibiotics
- Stool softeners are administered (milk of magnesia at bedtime) to keep the bowels open
- Anemia to be corrected by blood transfusion
- Infected wounds of perineum, vulva and vagina are laid open for drainage, cleaned and dressed with antiseptic preparations.

Surgical Treatment

- The stitches of the perineal wound may have to be removed to facilitate drainage of pus and relieve pain; after the infection is controlled, secondary sutures may be given later
- Infected retained products should be removed as early as possible under cover of antibiotics by digital exploration of the uterine cavity
- Pelvic abscess should be drained by colpotomy
- Abscess above the Poupart's ligaments should be incised and the pus drained.

Nursing Process for Mothers with Puerperal Sepsis

Assessment

Assess for the following clinical manifestations:
- Elevation in temperature to 38°C (100°F) or above with chills
- Foul-smelling lochia
- Abdominal tenderness and pelvic pain

- Pain and burning on urination
- Tachycardia
- Increased white blood cells (WBCs)
- Presence of predisposing:
  - Traumatic birth
  - Prolonged difficult labor
  - Dehydration
  - Excessive vaginal discharge
  - Pronged rupture of membranes
  - Anemia
  - Retained placental fragment
  - Hemorrhage.
- Mother frustrated due to extreme fatigue
- May appear uncooperative and uninterested.

Nursing Diagnosis

- Risk for injury
- Knowledge deficit
- Interrupted breastfeeding
- Fluid deficit
- Impaired gas exchange
- Fear
- Body image disturbance
- Ineffective individual coping
- Self-care deficit
- Altered family process
- Risk for altered mother-baby attachment.

Planning

- Provide teaching regarding hygienic measures
- Administer treatment specific to infection
- Provide opportunities to express feelings
- Provide education for self-care.

Implementation

- Assess vital signs every 2–4 hours
- Obtain cultures, blood and urine samples
- Evaluate pain and lochia
- Provide routine postpartum care
- Use meticulous handwashing techniques
- Teach handwashing techniques to mother
- Provide warm sitz baths, hot compress application or heat lamp exposure
- Provide reassurance and support
- Isolate woman as indicated.

Evaluation

Ensure that woman:
- Demonstrates handwashing and verbalizes understanding of hygienic measures
- Continue ordered medications to full recovery
- Verbalizes feelings and increased ability to cope
- Verbalizes understanding of self-care measures to treat and prevent infection, and increase comfort.

SUBINVOLUTION OF THE UTERUS

Subinvolution of the uterus is impaired and deficient involution of the uterus following delivery.

Causes of Subinvolution

Predisposing Factors

- Grand multiparity
- Overdistension of uterus as in twins and hydramnios
- Maternal ill health
- Cesarean section
- Prolapse of the uterus
- Uterine fibroids (leiomyomas)
- No sucking by the baby.

Aggravating Factors

- Retained products of conception
- Uterine sepsis
- Retention of lochia (lochiometra).

Clinical Features

- Excessive or prolonged discharge of lochia
- Irregular or excessive uterine bleeding
- Irregular cramp-like pain
- Uterine height more than normal for the particular day of postpartum.

Subsequently, the patient may suffer from conditions such as uterine prolapse or retroversion, which is the cause of subinvolution.

Management

Subinvolution is managed by treating the cause:
- Antibiotics for sepsis
- Exploration of the uterus for retained products
- Pessary in prolapse or retroversion.

BREAST COMPLICATIONS (FIG. 38.1)

The common breast complications in puerperium are breast engorgement, cracked and retracted nipple, mastitis, breast abscess and failing lactation.

Breast Engorgement (Box 38.1)

Breast engorgement may occur due to excessive production of milk, obstruction to outflow of milk or poor sucking of milk by the baby. It usually manifests after the milk secretion starts (3rd or 4th postpartum day).

Chapter 38: Complications of Puerperium

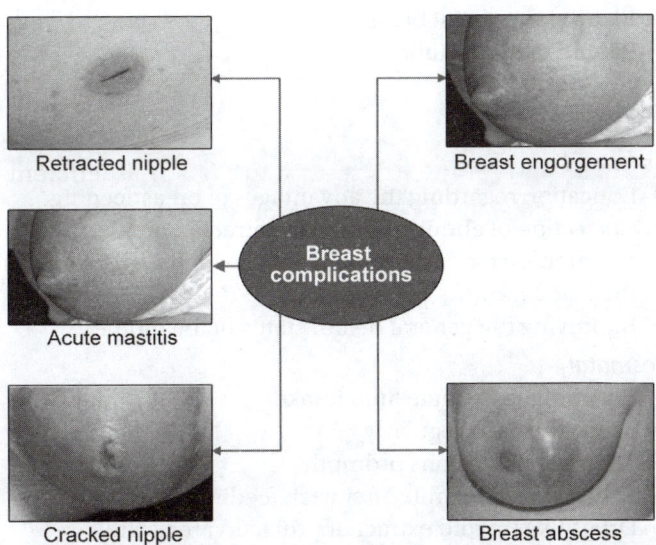

Figure 38.1: Breast complications *(For color version, see Plate 4).*

BOX 38.1: Client education.

1. **Prevention of breast engorgement**
   Teach client to:
   - Breast feed the infant frequently, 8–10 times in 24 hours to prevent discomfort and mastitis
   - Avoid supplements of water or formula for the first 3 to 4 weeks (exclusive breastfeeding on demand)
   - Express milk when feedings are missed
   - Wear a well-fitting supportive bra
2. **Treatment for breast engorgement**
   - Apply hot, moist towels to the breasts for 3 to 5 minutes; or take a hot shower before nursing
   - Hand expresses some milk to soften the areola after using moist heat
   - Use gentle breast massage before and during breast feeding
   - Avoid bottles, pacifiers and nipple shields during this period which can cause nipple confusion for the infant
   - Apply cold compress to breasts after feeding to relieve discomfort
   - When the baby will take only one breast at a feeding, use a breast pump or hand express milk from the other breast
   - Use a breast pump or hand express milk to soften the areola when the baby cannot latch on to the nipples because the breasts are full

---

Symptoms

- Both breasts feel tender, tense and firm
- Nipples become edematous and flushed
- The veins over the breasts become engorged and prominent
- Generalized malaise and rise in temperature
- Painful breastfeeding.

Preventive Measures

- To initiate breastfeeding early and feeding at frequent intervals
- Exclusive breastfeeding on demand
- Feeding in correct position (sitting).

Management

- Support the breasts with a binder or brassiere
- Manual expression of milk after each feeding and keeping the interval short between feeds
- Analgesics for pain
- The cause of poor sucking by the newborn should be corrected.

Cracked Nipple

The nipple may become painful due to loss of surface epithelium with the formation of a raw area on the nipple or due to a fissure situated at the tip, or the base of the nipple. These two conditions often co-exist, which are referred to as the cracked nipple.

Causes

- Inadequate hygiene resulting in the formation of a crust over the nipple
- Retracted nipple
- Vigorous sucking and an inadequate milk flow.

The woman experiences soreness and pain at the site of the fissure. The fissure may become infected and the infection may spread to the deeper tissue producing mastitis and hence, it should be treated vigorously.

Prophylaxis includes local cleanliness during pregnancy and in the puerperium before and after each breastfeeding to prevent crust formation over the nipple.

Treatment

- Application of tincture of benzoin after the night feeding and the fissure is likely to be healed in 8–12 hours
- The nipple is to be kept dry and exposed to air
- Breast milk should be removed by manual expression or pump
- If infected, an antiseptic cream is applied locally
- If it fails to heal, breastfeeding from the affected breast is stopped for 24 hours.

Retracted Nipple

Retracted nipple is common in primigravida. If left uncorrected, it may lead to difficulty in breastfeeding and predispose to cracked nipple. Manually pulling out the retracted nipple during the last 2 months of pregnancy is useful to rectify the defect. After delivery, the nipple is pulled out by the suction action of a disposable syringe. The procedure may have to be repeated for few days.

Acute Mastitis

There are two types of mastitis:
1. Infection follows a cracked nipple to involve the breast parenchymal tissues leading to cellulitis. The lacteal system remains unaffected.
2. Infection reaches the lactiferous ducts leading to the development of primary mammary adenitis.

In either type, the responsible organism is predominantly *S. aureus*. In superficial cellulitis, the onset is acute during the 1st week of puerperium. In mammary adenitis, the onset is insidious and usually occurs near the end of the 2nd week. The infection may occur even several weeks after the delivery.

Clinical Features

- Generalized malaise and headache
- Fever (102°F or over) with chills
- Severe pain and swelling in one quadrant of the breast with its apex at the nipple
- The overlying skin is hot and flushed and feels tense and tender.

If not treated adequately, it can lead to destruction of breast tissues with the formation of a breast abscess.

Treatment

1. Prophylactic: Antenatal care to nipple, prevention of engorgement and isolation of the infected baby.
2. Curative:
   - Isolation of mother and baby
   - Suspension of breastfeeding on the affected side until the infection is controlled
   - Manual expression of milk to relieve engorgement
   - Suppression of lactation by bromocriptine (Parlodel) 2.5 mg orally for 14 days
   - Antibiotic therapy for at least 10 days
   - Analgesics and sedatives as required.

Breast Abscess

Features of breast abscess are flushed breasts, brawny edema, marked tenderness and swinging temperature. If an abscess is formed, it is to be drained under general anesthesia. The cavity is packed with gauze, which should be replaced after 24 hours by a smaller pack. The procedure is continued until it heals up.

Failing Lactation

Causes

- Debilitating state of the mother
- Elderly primigravida
- Failure to suckle by the baby regularly
- Depression or anxiety state in the puerperium
- Reluctance or apprehension to nursing
- Premature baby who is too weak to suck
- Ill development of breasts
- Painful breast lesion.

Treatment

Antenatal
- Education regarding the advantages of breastfeeding
- Correction of abnormalities like retracted nipple
- Maintenance of adequate breast hygiene especially in the last 2 months of pregnancy
- Improving the general health status of the mother.

Postnatal
- Encourage adequate fluid intake
- Nurse the baby regularly
- Treat painful lesions promptly
- Express residual milk after each feeding
- Drugs like thyroid extract or prolactin are useful.

VENOUS THROMBOSIS

Thrombosis of the leg and pelvic veins is one of the common and important complications in the puerperium. The prevalence is low in Asian and African countries compared to western countries.

Causes

1. Stasis of blood in the pelvic and leg veins as in cases, where the woman has been on prolonged bedrest during pregnancy and following operative delivery.
2. Alteration in the blood constituents: Continuation of hypercoagulable state.
3. Infection: Pelvic cellulitis, which causes inflammation of the venous wall to which a thrombus may be attached.
4. Traumas to the venous wall: Pelvic veins are traumatized during labor due to the pressure of the fetal head.
5. Other high-risk factors such as advancing age, high parity, use of estrogen, obesity, anemia and heart disease.

Types

The puerperal venous thrombosis is classified as:
- Phlebothrombosis: Superficial and deep
- Thrombophlebitis.

In *phlebothrombosis*, the initial event is intravascular thrombosis. In *thrombophlebitis*, the initial event is inflammation of the venous wall to which the thrombus is attached.

Superficial Vein Thrombosis

Superficial thrombosis usually occurs in pre-existing varicose veins in the legs. It usually remains localized. On rare occasion, it may spread upwards to involve the long saphenous vein and thence to the femoral vein. Detachment of the thrombus, if occurs leads to *pulmonary embolism*. The onset is within the 1st week. There is pain and tenderness on the affected area. There may be slight rise in temperature and pulse rate. The overlaying skin looks red due to reaction of the clot. The condition subsides within a week with obliteration of the vein.

Deep Vein Thrombosis

Deep vein thrombosis may develop as a primary condition or the deep vein may be involved secondarily as an extension of superficial venous thrombosis. Occasionally, superficial and DVT occurs simultaneously.

Symptoms
Symptoms include pain in the calf or sole, swelling in the leg and often slight rise of temperature and pulse rate between the 7th and 10th day of postpartum.

On examination, there is calf tenderness on deep pressure and a positive Homans' sign—pain in the calf on dorsiflexion of the foot and edema of the leg.

Investigations
- Doppler ultrasound to detect the changes in the velocity of blood flow in the femoral vein
- Phlebography to note the filling defect in the venous lumen
- Isotopic venography to detect radioactivity.

Management
In high-risk situations, the following preventive measures are to be adopted:
- Leg movement and exercises
- Elastic stockings
- Active breathing exercises
- Avoiding sitting with legs dangling down
- Intermittent calf muscle compression such as pneumonic cuff, passive dorsiflexion
- Prophylactic anticoagulant therapy
- Avoiding the use of estrogens for suppression of lactation.

Management measures for the client with DVT include:
- Bedrest with the foot end raised above the heart level
- Analgesics to relieve pain in the affected area and sedatives to ensure sleep
- Antibiotics
- Heparin therapy—15,000 units intravenous (IV) followed by 10,000 units 4–6 hourly and heparin is continued for 7–10 days or even longer then *warfarin* orally is commonly used in addition to heparin and may be continued for 3–6 months as maintenance therapy
- Gentle movement in bed to be started when the pain subsides about a week
- Caval filter may be inserted, if there is a free-floating thrombus detected by scan or phlebogram.

Thrombophlebitis

Postpartum thrombophlebitis originates in the thrombosed veins at the placental site by organisms such as anaerobic streptococci or *Bacteroides fragilis*. When localized in the pelvis, it is called *pelvic thrombophlebitis*. There is no specific clinical feature for pelvic thrombophlebitis, but it is suspected when pyrexia continues for more than a week in the absence of any other cause in postnatal mothers.

Phlegmasia alba dolens
Extrapelvic spread may reach to the lungs or kidney (left). Retrograde extension to ileofemoral vein produces the clinicopathological condition of *phlegmasia alba dolens* or *white leg*.

Clinical features
- Usually develops in the 2nd week of postpartum
- Mild fever prior to local manifestations and at times fever with chills
- Headache, malaise and rising pulse rate
- Affected leg is painful, swollen, white and cold
- Tenderness and induration along the course of the femoral vein
- Polymorphonuclear leukocytosis seen on blood count.

Prevention and management
Preventive and curative measures are the same as those outlined for DVT.

PULMONARY EMBOLISM

Pulmonary embolism occurs when part of a clot breaks away from a vessel wall and enters the systemic circulation. It causes an obstruction once it reaches a vessel with a lumen smaller than it and usually a pulmonary artery.

While DVT in the leg or in the pelvis is most likely, the cause of pulmonary embolism in 80–90%, it occurs without any previous clinical manifestations of DVT. The predisposing factors are those already mentioned in venous thrombosis.

Signs and Symptoms

Small Pulmonary Embolism

The clinical features depend on the size of the embolus and on the preceding health status of the mother. The classic symptoms of small emboli are:
- Chest pain
- Dyspnea, coughing, slight hemoptysis
- Pyrexia
- Tachycardia.

Any of the above symptoms, however slight, must be reported to the physician immediately. The woman should be offered reassurance and oxygen, if required, until medical assistance is obtained.

Major Pulmonary Embolism

- Sudden acute chest pain
- Marked distress, shock or sudden collapse
- Dyspnea, cyanosis
- Pyrexia, tachycardia/bradycardia and hypotension
- Distension of jugular veins.

This constitutes an obstetric emergency. If a major pulmonary artery becomes blocked, sudden acute chest pain will occur immediately followed by respiratory collapse, cardiac failure and possibly death. Death usually occurs within a short time from shock and vagal inhibition.

Diagnostic Procedures

- X-ray of the chest
- Lung scan
- Pulmonary angiography.

Treatment and Management

- Resuscitation—cardiac massage, oxygen therapy and IV heparin
- The IV fluid support
- Blood pressure (BP) to be maintained by dopamine or adrenaline
- Thrombolytic therapy with streptokinase
- Tachycardia is counteracted with digitalis
- Pain may be relieved by IV morphine.

If the woman does not respond to this therapy or if repeated attacks occur, surgical treatment like embolectomy, placement of caval filter or ligation of inferior vena cava and ovarian veins may have to be done. Surgical treatment is done following pulmonary angiography.

PSYCHOLOGICAL DISTURBANCES IN THE PUERPERIUM

The events of pregnancy, labor and delivery together with the peak experience of giving birth, all contribute to a mixture of emotional reactions in the mother during the 1st week of puerperium. There are three distinctive types of psychological disturbances seen in the puerperium—postpartum blues (baby blues), postpartum depression and puerperal psychosis.

Postpartum Blues

Postpartum blues is a mild, benign and transient mood change that begins within 3–4 days after delivery and peaks on the 4–5 day. It affects nearly 7 in 10 mothers.

The most common symptom is unprovoked weeping and spikes of elation. Other symptoms include irritability, anger, hostility, headache, feelings of unreality, exhaustion, sleep deprivation and restlessness. Baby blues generally disappear without medical intervention within 2 weeks. If the symptoms persist longer, another diagnosis may be identified.

Social interventions such as a relative babysitting for few hours, so that the mother can get some sleep or assistance with household chores, or providing instruction on newborn care can often help significantly. Women who have this condition are likely to have it recur with subsequent pregnancies.

Postpartum Depression

The onset of postpartum depression is gradual developing after the 2nd week. The condition may last for 3–6 months and in some cases, it will persist throughout the 1st year of the baby's life. Such depression is disabling for the mother. It causes much disruption of family life and mother-baby relationships.

Causes

Postnatal depression is a reactive illness provoked by demand overload. A specific etiology is not known, however, certain contributory factors identified are:
- Experiencing stress-inducing life events around the time of childbirth such as bereavement or relationship disharmony
- Low self-esteem, lack of support and stress associated with postnatal care
- Severe 'maternal blues' later developing to depression
- Demands of motherhood and loss of personal freedom.

Diagnosis

Symptoms of postpartum depression are similar to those of depression occurring at any other time. Characteristic symptoms include bouts of crying, sadness and emotional liability, guilt, loss of appetite or anorexia, profound sleep disturbances, poor concentration and memory, irritability and feelings of inadequacy to care for the newborn or other children.

In postpartum depression, there is the tendency to experience difficulty falling asleep, but once asleep, the woman will sleep for long periods. They often feel well in the morning, but deteriorate as the day goes on. In most other depression, early waking is the pattern with symptoms more acute in the morning. The woman may feel constantly tired in spite of adequate periods of rest and may appear over anxious about her baby in spite of evidence that the baby is well and thriving.

Some women may not communicate or admit their feelings. They conceal their depression so well that the condition may not be diagnosed for months. Knowledge of the individual woman and awareness of her body language may help to identify potential risk.

Management

Early detection and initiation of appropriate treatment brings the best prognosis. If the midwife suspects a woman is depressed, this should be reported to the physician.

In less severe cases, treatment with mild sedation or antidepressants may be prescribed. Counseling is known to be helpful, particularly if initiated at an early stage. Involvement of the spouse and other family members may also be advantageous. When the depression is more advanced, admission to a hospital will be necessary. Untreated or undiagnosed depression can evolve into a psychotic illness.

Puerperal Psychosis

The onset of puerperal psychosis is usually rapid occurring within the first few days of delivery and rarely beyond the first 2–3 weeks. The condition is more common in primiparous women and in those who have suffered previous psychosis. No defined cause has been identified.

Diagnosis

Puerperal psychosis may have an acute onset. The woman may appear to be experiencing normal emotional adaptive responses to childbirth and may exhibit symptoms similar to those of maternal blues, which is a psychological phenomenon manifested as unexplainable sadness and frequent bouts of crying.

These become more profound with extreme mood swings during which feelings of guilt or anxiety may be expressed. The euphoria following childbirth is seen extended and exaggerated in puerperal psychosis. The onset of symptoms may be heralded by a time of acute restlessness and inability to sleep. Subsequently, the behavior of the woman may become bizarre. She may do or say inappropriate things, or react out of character. She may experience delusions or hallucinations and become detached from the reality of her situation. She may state that her baby is abnormal, believe it to be possessed and may avoid the baby.

There may be periods of normal behavior and at other times, she may appear depressed. She may experience suicidal impulses or desires to harm her baby.

Treatment

Because of extreme nature of the illness, medical help is required as a matter of emergency. The woman must be kept under constant observation until appropriate psychiatric help is obtained.

Heavy sedation is given at the time of onset. Early treatment with antipsychotic drugs under the care of a psychiatric team is usually instituted. Admission to a psychiatric unit and treatment with lithium and/or electroconvulsive therapy is given. Psychosis may persist for 8–10 weeks even with prompt treatment, especially when the woman has a pre-existing history of schizophrenia or manic depressive illness **(Box 38.2)**.

Prognosis

Whilst complete recovery is often achieved, it is possible that further episodes of illness will occur throughout the woman's life and there is an increased risk of recurrence in subsequent pregnancies.

Role of the Midwife

The community midwife should continue to visit both mother and baby to undertake the non-psychiatric aspects of postnatal care. Family support also needs consideration. The midwife needs to offer advice and support to women during subsequent pregnancies and to alert the physician regarding psychiatric care when appropriate in order to initiate prompt referral, should it become necessary.

The community midwife should be able to help the mother to re-establish the mother-baby relationship and to rebuild self-esteem by encouraging care of the baby within a safe environment.

> **BOX 38.2:** Nursing alert.
>
> **Warning signs of illness after delivery**
> - Fever greater than 38° C (100.4° F)
> - Severe pain, redness or swelling in the episiotomy or cesarean section incision
> - Foul smelling vaginal discharge
> - Increased bleeding; soaking of a sanitary pad more than once in an hour or larger amount of bright red lochia after discharge
> - Passing of several large clots
> - Backache or severe abdominal pain or cramping or pain in the episiotomy or perineal area
> - Reddened, tender, swollen breasts that may have hardened lumps
> - Pain, redness and swelling of the legs
> - Burning on urination or frequent urination
> - The blues or crying that lasts for several days
> - Depression that is severe or does not go away
> - Thoughts of harming the baby
> - Suicidal thoughts
> - Insomnia
> - Loss of energy
> - Impaired concentration
> - Feeling of worthlessness

STUDY QUESTIONS

Short Notes

1. Puerperal pyrexia.
2. Breast engorgement.
3. Endometritis.
4. Autogenous infection of perineum.

Short Answer Questions

1. Subinvolution of the uterus.
2. Acute mastitis.
3. Breast abscess.
4. Thrombophlebitis.

Essay Questions

1. Explain pulmonary embolism, signs and symptoms, and management. Enumerate the possible nursing diagnoses and plan of care.
2. Explain the psychological disturbances that can occur in the puerperal period and their management.

BIBLIOGRAPHY

1. Calhoun BC, Brost B. Emergency management of sudden puerperal fever. Obstetrics and Gynecology Clinics of North America. 1995; 22(2):357-67.
2. Donnica M. Postpartum Depression, article 154. [online]. Available from www.drdonnica.com [Accessed 2005].
3. Dutta DC. Textbook of obstetrics, 5th edition. Kolkata: New Central Book Company; 2001. pp. 467-78.
4. Hynes L. Physiology, complications and management of the puerperium. In: Bennett RV, Linda KB (Eds). Myles Textbook for Midwives, 13th edition. Edinburgh: Churchill Livingstone; 1999. pp. 589-614.
5. Llewellyn Jones D. Fundamental of Obstetrics and Gynecology, 6th edition. London: Mosby; 1994. pp. 86-7.
6. McKenzie CAM, Vestal KW. High-risk Perinatal Nursing. St Louis: WB Sounders; 1983.
7. Neeson JD. Clinical manual of maternity nursing. Philadelphia: JB Lippincott; 1987.
8. Ridgway LE. Puerperal emergency: Vaginal vulvar hematomas. Obstetrics and Gynecology Clinics of North America. 1995;22(2):275-82.

SECTION VIII

NORMAL NEONATE

Section Outline

39. Baby at Birth
40. Physiology, Screening, Daily Care and Observation of the Newborn
41. Infant Feeding
42. High-risk Neonates—Low Birth Weight, Preterm and Intrauterine Growth Restricted Babies

CHAPTER 39

Baby at Birth

Learning Objectives

Upon completing this chapter, the learner will be able to:
- Identify the physiological changes that must occur for the newborn at the birth to adapt to extrauterine life.
- Identify the normal characteristics of the newborn.
- Describe the care of the baby during and immediately after birth.
- Identify factors to be considered when the baby fails to establish respiration at birth and describe the goals and methods of neonatal resuscitation.

The transition from intrauterine to extrauterine life presents a number of challenges for the newborn. To leave the nurturing environment of the mother's womb, it must endure intense contractions of the uterus and pass through the birth canal or the mother's abdomen to the waiting world. Upon birth, the newborn's body must establish circulation, initiate respiration and maintain its own metabolism, i.e. all tasks that were previously managed by the mother through the placenta. Incredible and formidable, as all these tasks sail through this transition smoothly. Yet, when difficulty is encountered, an astute midwife is often the first to note the changes and alert the pediatrician so that prompt intervention can begin (Fig. 39.1).

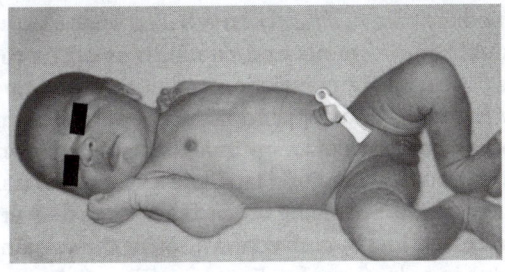

Figure 39.1: Healthy newborn *(For color version, see Plate 4)*.

EXTRAUTERINE ADAPTATION

In order to care for newborns, the midwife requires the knowledge of transition from the fetus to the newborn. All the systems in the non-distressed full-term neonate are adequate to adapt to extrauterine life immediately after birth. This complex process of change and instability is known as the transitional period. The midwife must know, understand and be aware of, as well as assess the changes that take place as the neonate goes through its transitional period.

Respiratory Changes

The respiratory system is the most challenged in the change from intrauterine to extrauterine environment. Upon arrival into an atmospheric environment, there is an immediate demand on the neonate for respiration. The organ responsible for fetal respiration prior to delivery is the placenta. Upon delivery, the lungs change from a fluid-filled state to a system well-prepared for and capable of respiration.

The phenomenon that occurs to stimulate the neonate to take the first breath is believed to be a combination of biochemical changes and a number of physical stimuli to which the neonate is subjected such as cold, gravity, pain, light and noise, which causes excitation of the respiratory center. The first active breath of air once taken and sustained set in motion and a nearly inexorable chain of events that:
- Converts the fetal circulation to adult circulation
- Empties the lung of fluid
- Establishes the neonatal lung volume and the characteristics of pulmonary functions.

The primary concern at the time of delivery is the establishment of respiration. The prompt onset of breathing is essential for subsequent mental and physical development.

When the head is delivered, mucus drains from the nares and mouth. Many neonates gasp and even cry at this time. Therefore, suctioning the mouth and nares with a bulb syringe or mucus sucker to prevent aspiration of mucus, or amniotic fluid may be necessary as soon as the head is accessible.

More mucus will be noted as the body is compressed during delivery. This release of fluid allows air to be taken into the lungs.

Gentle rubbing of the neonates back, flicking the sole of the foot or vigorous drying of the infant to reduce heat loss are sufficient aids in stimulation of respiration. If stimulation is too vigorous such as slapping or exposure to extreme cold, it becomes distressful and tends to inhibit respiration.

Sustained regular respirations are established normally within 60 seconds of delivery and are accompanied by simultaneous changes occurring in the cardiovascular system.

Circulatory Changes

With the initiation of respiration, the fetal circulation undergoes changes that allow the newborn to sustain extrauterine existence. These begin with the clamping of the umbilical cord and the first breath taken by the newborn. Korones (1986) identified five attributes of fetal circulation that must be altered for the infant to make the switch from the fetal to mature circulation:
- Closure of the ductus arteriosus
- Closure of the foramen ovale
- Closure of the ductus venosus
- Decreased pulmonary vascular resistance
- Increased aortic blood pressure (BP).

These changes are initiated in the normal infant by the clamping of the cord and the first breath. This eliminates the placental supply of oxygen and forces the neonate to obtain oxygen from the lungs. This alters the path of blood flow and causes changes in blood volume, pressure and chemical composition. The onset of respiration increases the arterial oxygen pressure (pO_2). This increase in oxygen causes vasodilatation of pulmonary arterioles and an abrupt decrease in pulmonary resistance. The anatomic changes then follow.

A much larger amount of blood is pumped into the pulmonary arteries by the right ventricle and a smaller amount through the ductus arteriosus. The ductus arteriosus begins to atrophy and eventually is known as the *ligamentum arteriosum*.

As the pulmonary circulation increases, more blood is returned from the lungs to the left atrium. Increase in pressure in the left atrium causes the foramen ovale to close. Placental circulation ceases to function when the umbilical cord is clamped. The ends of the hypogastric arteries atrophy are known as the *hypogastric ligaments*.

The ductus venosus becomes occluded and is known as the *ligamentum venosus*. The umbilical vein becomes obliterated and is known as the *ligamentum teres*. These interdependent cardiopulmonary adaptations, which take place at birth are essential to survival.

Other Systems

The newborn must begin to manufacture, breakdown and excrete substances on its own. Disorders of metabolism such as hypocalcemia or hypoglycemia may result if the newborn is not up to the challenge. The neurological system must begin the functions that protect and preserve life. The urinary system must be patent and excrete urine, and the gastrointestinal system must become functional.

Thermal Regulation

The neonate loses heat instantly at birth because of large body surface area, especially the head, which comprises 25% of the neonates size. Specific ways in which the neonate loses heat are:
1. *Evaporation:* Whenever the skin becomes wet in a relatively dry room or incubator.
2. *Radiation:* When heat is transferred from the body to cooler objects in the environment (surfaces not in contact with the body).
3. *Convection:* With the movement of cool air passing over the surface of the body (skin).
4. *Conduction:* When heat is lost from the surface of the body to other objects in direct contact with the skin.

The newborn will attempt to conserve energy by peripheral vasoconstriction and adoption of a flexed posture. However, the neonate is capable of producing heat through both general and brown fat (adipose tissue) metabolism. Brown fat is located in the upper thorax, axillae and beneath the skin in the upper part of the back. This fat is different from white fat. If the neonate is cold, the autonomic nervous system triggers the brown fat deposits to release and metabolize the stored fat. The white fat or the ordinary adipose tissue, which acts as a reservoir for potential energy cannot be utilized as readily as brown fat. Brown fat is a limited resource, which is rapidly depleted during periods of cold stress.

The neonate uses up energy at the time of delivery. If the delivery room is cooler than the intrauterine temperature, the neonate will lose heat through evaporation, conduction, convection and radiation. Bathing and placing the baby in an unwarmed crib causes further heat loss. Heat loss can be minimized by having the room (where the baby is born) warm, drying the neonate as soon as possible after delivery, wrapping the baby in a warm blanket and placing him/her in a warm crib next to the mother. Particular care must be taken to prevent heat loss from the head, which represent 25% of neonates surface area.

IMMEDIATE CARE OF THE BABY AT BIRTH

The immediate care of a newborn is based on the knowledge, transitional requirements and capabilities of the midwife. Chances of heat loss by convection, radiation and evaporation are very high and hence appropriate preparations must be made for the provision of an optimal thermal environment in the delivery room. This would facilitate a successful transition to extrauterine life. Switching off the fan prior to delivery helps to minimize heat loss by convection. Closing the curtains in the room helps in reduction of radiant heat loss.

Initial Care

As the baby's head is born, excess mucus may be wiped gently from his/her mouth taking care not to touch the nares as it may cause reflex inhalation. The baby is to be handled gently, while he/she will be drawn up towards the mother's abdomen. The time of baby's birth and the sex are noted, and recorded soon after the baby is expelled from his/her mother.

Clearing the Airway

In normal births, clearing the airway usually involves:
1. Holding or placing the baby, so that the head is lower than the body and is turned somewhat to the side for drainage.
2. Wiping of the baby's face and fluid from the nose and mouth.
3. Suctioning the nasal and oral passages with a soft rubber bulb syringe or mucus sucker.

If necessary, the airway may be cleared with the aid of a mucus extractor or soft suction catheter attached to low-pressure (10 cm H_2O) mechanical suction. It is important to aspirate the oropharynx prior to the nasopharynx, so that when the baby gasps, as his/her nasal passages are aspirated, mucus or other material is not drawn down into the respiratory tract.

Clamping and Cutting the Cord

Separation of the baby from the placenta is achieved by cutting the umbilical cord between two clamps, which should be applied approximately 8–10 cm from the umbilicus with enough space between them to allow easy cutting. Application of a gauze piece (4 × 4) over the cord, while cutting with scissors will avoid blood spraying the delivery field. There is no pain for either the baby or the mother at the site of the cutting of the umbilical cord.

The timing of clamping of the cord is not crucial unless asphyxia, prematurity or Rhesus (Rh) incompatibility is present. Some centers advocate delay of clamping until respiration is established and cord pulsation has ceased, thus ensuring that the infant receives placental transfusion of about 70 mL of blood.

Leboyer (1976) advocated delayed cord clamping for an entirely different reason. He believed that this allowed the newly born baby to have two sources of oxygen during transition:
1. From the lungs.
2. From the placenta through the umbilical cord.

Then, when the gradual transition from dependence on the placenta to dependence on the lungs is completed, as evidenced by cessation of cord pulsations, the umbilical cord is clamped and cut. The process is completed by approximately 4–5 minutes after birth.

There is also the view that the placental circulation so acquired may predispose to neonatal jaundice. Name bands are to be applied to the infant and mother before the cord is cut.

Identification

When babies are born in the hospital, it is essential that they are identifiable from one another. Name bands are used in most places for this purpose, usually one on the infant's wrist and one on the ankle, each of which should indicate legibly the mother's name (family name), sex of the infant and date and time of birth. The midwife should ensure that the name bands are fastened securely and are neither too tight to excoriate the skin nor impede circulation or too loose risking loss. The identification bands should remain on the baby until his/her discharge from the hospital.

Evaluation of the Newborn at Birth

After the baby is seen making respiratory effort, the midwife can proceed to dry the infant in order to avoid evaporative heat loss, while attending to the assessment procedure also. At 1 minute, after the baby's birth, the midwife will assess the baby's general condition and will repeat this for 5 minutes. The factors assessed are heart rate, respiratory effort, muscle tone, reflex response to stimulus and color **(Figs. 39.2 and 39.3)**. A score of 0, 1 or 2 is awarded to each of the signs in accordance with the guidelines in **Table 39.1**. This scoring system, the Apgar score is recognized and used universally. Of the five signs, the heart rate and the respiratory rate are the most important.

The color of babies with pigmented skin is best assessed by inspecting the color of the mucous membrane. Of the five signs, color is least important and some centers have discontinued recording this part of the score making the maximum score 8 rather than 10. Documentation of this modified system when used, requires to be specified in the baby's birth record, e.g. 'Apgar minus color score equal seven'.

A normal infant in good condition at birth will achieve an Apgar score of 7–10. Medical aid should be sought, if the score is less than seven. For an Apgar minus color scoring, a score of less than six requires medical aid **(Box 39.1)**.

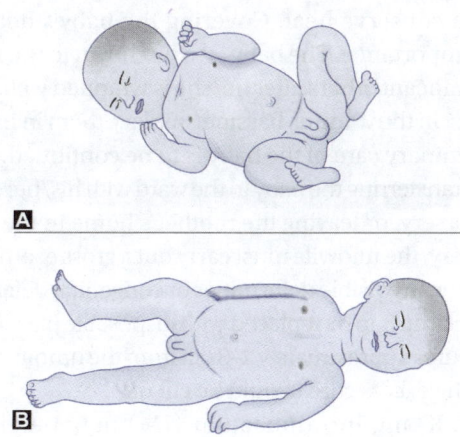

Figures 39.2A and B: Newborn. (A) With good muscle tone and Apgar score 2; (B) With poor muscle tone and Apgar score 0.

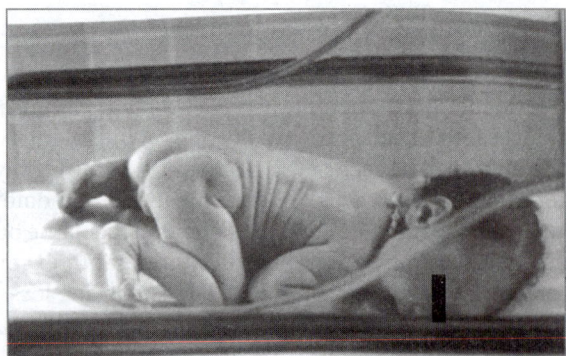

Figure 39.3: Acrocyanosis.

TABLE 39.1: Apgar score.

Signs	Score 0	Score 1	Score 2
Heart rate	Absent	Less than 100 beats per minute (bpm)	More than 100 bpm
Respiratory effort	Absent	Slow, irregular	Good or crying
Muscle tone	Limp	Some flexion of limbs	Active
Reflex response to stimulus	None	Minimal grimace	Cough or sneeze
Color	Blue, pale	Body pink, extremities blue	Completely pink

Prevention of Heat Loss (Fig. 39.4)

It is important to keep the baby warm. This is initiated by wiping off and drying the baby, so that body heat is not lost. Subsequent actions vary, but may include use of:
- Bodily contact with the mother
- Radiant warmer or 200 watt bulb
- Warmed blankets.

The wet towel must be removed before wrapping the baby in warm blankets. Skin-to-skin contact with the mother assists the baby to conserve heat. Covering the baby's head is of particular importance. The baby is to be shown to the mother and her significant others after he/she is wrapped well. After a period of rest in the warmer, bassinet or place them in mother's arms, preliminary care of the baby is to be continued.

Prior to transferring the baby to the ward with his/her mother or to the nursery, or leaving the mother's home in the case of home delivery, the midwife must carry out a gross examination of the baby for any visible deformities or congenital defects. The initial cord clamp is to be replaced with disposable plastic clamp or cord ligatures approximately 2–3 cm from the umbilicus (skin edge) and the excess cord should be cut off.

Vitamin K_1 mg intramuscular (IM) may be given as prophylaxis against bleeding disorders. Erythromycin or gentamicin eye ointment is applied as prophylaxis against gonococcal infection within 1 hour of birth.

BOX 39.1: Nursing alert.

Newborn evaluation at delivery

Assess	Normal findings
Respirations	Rate 30–60 bpm, irregular No retractions No grunting
Apical pulse	Rate 120–160 bpm
Temperature	37.5°C (97.5°F)
Skin color	Body pink with bluish extremities
Umbilical cord	Two arteries, one vein
Gestational age	Should be above 37 weeks

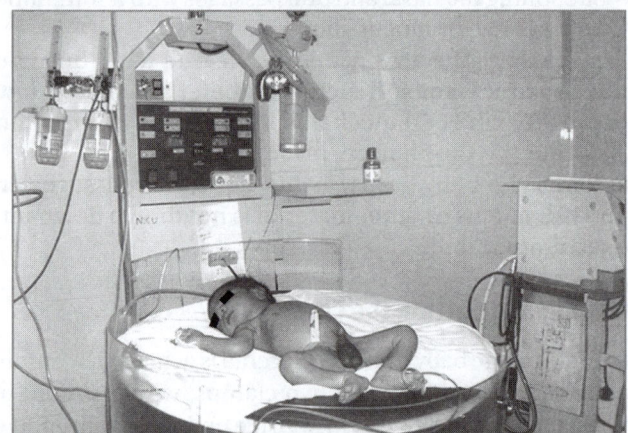

Figure 39.4: Newborn in radiant warmer
(*For color version, see Plate 4*).

NORMAL CHARACTERISTICS AND PHYSICAL FEATURES OF A HEALTHY NEWBORN

A healthy neonate born at term (between 38th and 42nd week) has an average birth weight (above 2,500 g) cries immediately following birth, establishes independent rhythmic respiration and quickly adapts to the changed environment.

The weight is variable from country to country. In India, the weight varies from 2.7 to 3.1 kg with a mean of 2.9 kg. The length is 50–52 cm. Head circumference measures about 35 cm and the biparietal diameter measures about 9.5 cm.

Posture

The newborn assumes the attitude of its intrauterine life, i.e. extremities flexed and fists clenched. However, the extended attitude of the head in face presentation or legs in frank breech persists for few days more.

Skin

Slight peripheral skin cyanosis (acrocyanosis) is common, but soon becomes pinkish with the establishment of cardiopulmonary function. Vernix caseosa covers the skin, particularly the back and creases. Lanugo is present over the face, back and extremities. Mongolian spots (benign bluish pigmentation) are present over the sacrum and they disappear by 4 years of age.

Head

Head is larger in relation to the rest of the body. Evidences of varying degrees of molding are present in vaginally delivered babies with cephalic presentation. Varying degrees of caput may be evident (cephalohematoma is not present at birth).

Face

The face is comparatively smaller in relation the head. The eyes remain closed most of the time. The gums are smooth. The cartilages of the ears and nose are well-formed and the cheeks are full.

Neck

The neck is short.

Trunk

The chest is barrel shaped. The circumference is less than that of the head. Breathing pattern is abdominal. Heart rate is usually 120–140 per minute. Respiration rate is usually 30–60 per minute. Abdomen is usually soft and may be protuberant or flat. Bowel sounds are audible.

Genitalia

In male, the foreskin will cover the glans, an orifice is present at the tip. The testes can usually be palpated in the scrotum. In female, the labia minora and clitoris are covered by labia majora.

Extremities

Symmetrical and proportionate to the rest of the body.

Temperature

Normal body temperature for a neonate is 97.7°F–99.5°F (36.5°C–37.5°C).

Urine

Small amount of urine of low specific gravity is passed.

Stool

Meconium may be passed soon after birth or within the first 24 hours.

Hematological Findings

The total blood volume is about 300 mL a few hours after birth. The average blood volume is estimated to be 85 mL/kg and body weight consisting 41 mL of plasma and 44 mL of red blood cell (RBC) mass.

The normal newborn's glucose levels are 50–60 mg/100 mL, RBCs 6.8 million/mm^3, and platelets 350,000/mm^3. Clotting power may be poor because of deficient vitamin K. Newborn reflexes are present at birth.

INITIAL ASSESSMENT OF THE NEWBORN

During the early hours of life, the newborn should receive a complete assessment. According to Phibbs (1982), there are three general goals when assessing the newborn:
1. To detect significant medical problems so that they can be treated appropriately.
2. To protect the newborn from harmful processes such as chilling or nosocomial infections.
3. To promote good health by facilitating the normal adaptations to extrauterine life.

At delivery and before the initial assessment takes place, some obstetricians or midwives elect to place the apparently normal neonate on the mother's abdomen, where she and the baby glimpse at each other for the first time. Others immediately hand the infant to the obstetric or neonatal nurse for assessment and care. In either case, after the mother has seen the infant, the midwife places the baby on the baby bed in the delivery room, briefly examines it, suctions the mouth and nose if necessary, obtains footprints (if it is a requirement), applies identifying bands to the extremities and cleans the baby superficially.

Much of the newborn's physical examination can be conducted without awakening him/her although the baby must be fully exposed at intervals for a complete and accurate examination. The neonate must be recovered as soon as possible after the examination to avoid chilling. Scrupulous handwashing is essential before touching the newborn to avoid transferring microorganisms. The infant must be examined systematically, but speedily beginning from the head followed by inspecting the whole body to detect any congenital abnormality. It is important to determine whether the newborn appears of normal size and development for the estimated gestational age. From there, many examiners take a head-to-toe or systems approach to the examination.

General Appearance

The overall appearance of the newborn must be noted. The following should be found in the normal baby:
- Body symmetrical and cylindrical in contour
- Head large in proportion to the rest of the body
- Small hips
- Narrow chest
- Protruding abdomen.

Measurements

Variations in measurements may occur, but relationships are consistent. The following are the average measurements:
- Head circumference: 35 cm
- Chest measurement: 32 cm

❖ Crown-rump length: 35 cm
❖ Crown-heel length: 51 cm.

Activity

General body movements are symmetric and include sneezing, yawning, sucking, rooting, swallowing, grasping, responding to sound, blinking and crying. Variations in the infant's cry indicate the following:
1. *Persistent weak cry:* The infant is sick.
2. *Persistent high-pitched cry:* Possible intracranial injuries.
3. *Persistent inconsolable cry:* The infant is sick.
4. *Cry stops when the baby is picked up*: Normal.
5. Any type of cry that is not normal must be reported to the pediatrician.

Color

Melanin pigmentation is present in varying degrees at birth. The color of the epidermis darkens with exposure to light in infants of dark-pigmented parents. If the infant is pink with bluish nail beds, palms, soles and extremity and color improves with activity and the infant is normal. However, if this coloring becomes worse with activity, watch for cyanosis around the mouth and fingernail beds. It may be due to intracranial hemorrhage, cardiac problems or central nervous system involvement.

Skin

The normal full-term infant is covered with vernix caseosa. The skin has a velvet softness and elastic texture because of subcutaneous fat. Premature newborn's skin is thin, red, shiny due to lack of subcutaneous fat and covered by plentiful lanugo and vernix caseosa. Post-term babies will have less vernix caseosa on the body and the skin may be wrinkled and peeling. Other observations to be made on the skin are:
1. *Vascular nevi:*
   - Stork beak mark (stork bite) **(Fig. 39.5)**: Dilatation of capillary vessels and minute arteries; found at the nape of the neck and extending over the lower occipital area between the eyebrows, on upper eyelids and around the nose.
   - Strawberry mark **(Fig. 39.6)**: Bright red spot. It may be seen anywhere on the baby's body.

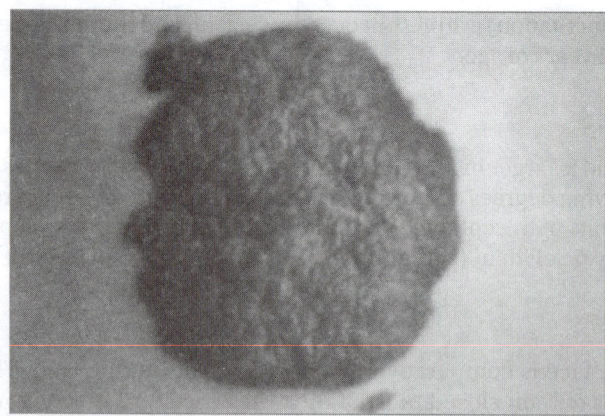

Figure 39.6: Strawberry mark.

   - Port-wine stain **(Fig. 39.7)**: Smooth, flat, superficial angioma and varies in size from a few millimeters to an area that covers most of the face and neck.
2. *Pigmented nevi:* Moles from light brown to black.
3. *Mongolian spots* **(Fig. 39.8)**: Bluish or slate-colored pigmentation over sacral area.

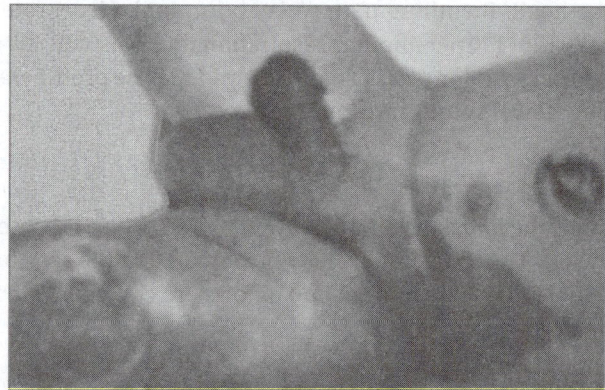

Figure 39.7: Port-wine stain.

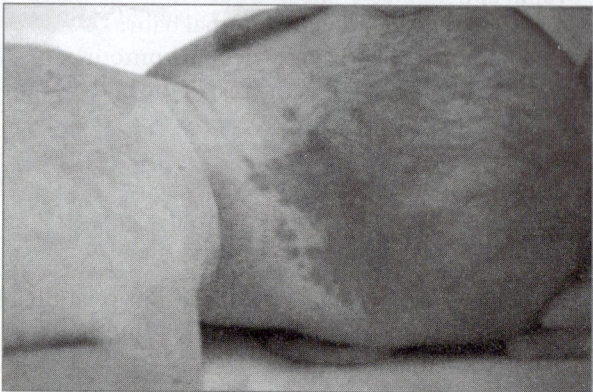

Figure 39.5: Stork beak mark.

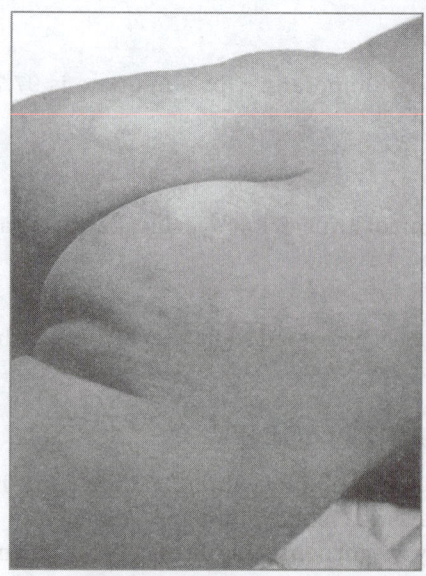

Figure 39.8: Mongolian spots.

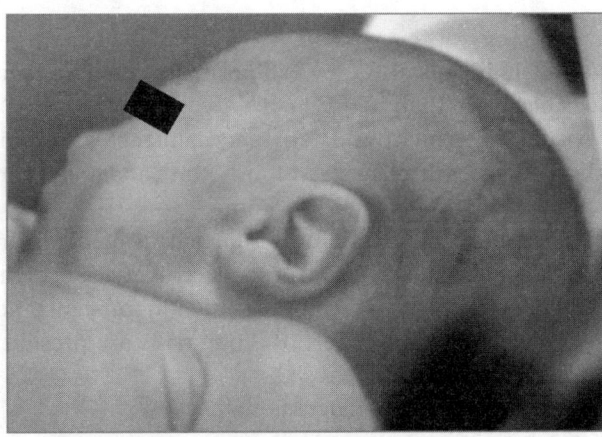

Figure 39.9: Forceps marks.

4. *Trauma:* Firm areas of indurations in subcutaneous tissue. The skin may be reddened or purplish mainly caused by forceps injuries **(Fig. 39.9)**.
5. Deep blue face with pink body is noticed following tight nuchal cord.

Head

The head is to be examined for the following:
1. Temporary asymmetry because of molding and overlapping of cranial bones should be noted.
2. *Fontanels*:
   - Anterior: Diamond shaped
   - Posterior: Triangle shaped
   - Bulging fontanels indicate intracranial pressure
   - Depressed fontanels indicate dehydration.
3. *Caput succedaneum:* Swelling on the scalp resulting from pressure of the cervix.
4. *Cephalohematoma*: Subperiosteal bleeding, does not cross suture lines and has hard edges around the soft center.

Eyes

The eyes should not be forced open for the examination. The following observations should be made:
1. *Puffy*: Common after forceps delivery.
2. Minor drainage after eye prophylaxis drops is instilled.
3. Pupils react to light. Unequal size may be due to brachial plexus paralysis. Ptosis may also be present.
4. *Opaqueness*: Suggest cataract formation.
5. Almond-shaped eyes if present concomitantly with other signs, suggests Down syndrome.
6. *Subconjunctival hemorrhage*: Small patch or patches of red within the sclera.
7. *Ptosis of the eyes or lids*: May indicate nerve damage.

Nose

Newborns breathe through the nose. Any flaring of the nostrils may indicate respiratory distress.

Ears

The ears of the term infant are well-formed. Preterm infants lack cartilage and their ears are very soft and flexible. Check the ears for the following:
1. Presence of canal.
2. The awake infant reacts with a startle to a sudden noise.
3. Size and shape.
4. Deformed ear lobes with the upper margin of the pinna-rolled down and thickened as in Down syndrome (trisomy 21).
5. Low-set ears: Autosomal chromosome abnormalities (trisomy 15 and 18).

Mouth

The following should be noted when examining the mouth:
1. Cleft lip or palate.
2. *Epstein pearls*: Tiny cysts found on the palate at the junction of the hard and soft palate.
3. *Facial nerve paralysis*: Asymmetry of the mouth when open, especially when crying.
4. Natal teeth or macroglossia.
5. *Circumoral cyanosis*: A bluish tinge of the lips in the first few hours of life.
6. *Pooling of saliva*: First symptom of tracheoesophageal fistula and first feeding must be observed.

Neck

Check the neck for the following:
1. Head is freely movable.
2. Neck webbed on shoulders may indicate Down syndrome or Turner's syndrome.
3. Tightness of muscles on one side may indicate torticollis.
4. Brachial palsy or fractured clavicle: Reflexes absent on the side of fracture, arm remains extended when lying on back and immobilization of affected side.

Chest

The newborn has a barrel chest and check for the following features:
1. *Respiration*: After the first period of activity, respiration should be quiet and free of adventitious sounds like rales or rhonchi; both sides of the chest should expand equally with inspiration. A grunding sound on expiration or a gasping, shrill sound on inspiration indicates respiratory distress. If the chest appears to be pulled back towards the spine on inspiration, retractions-associated respiratory distress is indicated and the pediatrician should be notified immediately.
2. *Heart*: Normal heart rates are 120–160 beats per minute (bpm).
3. Clavicles should be palpated. One or both may be fractured during delivery.

4. *Breasts (supernumerary nipples)*: Extra nipples are relatively common, but glandular tissue does not usually accompany the nipples.

Abdomen

1. Should look round and protruding.
2. Umbilical cord stump: Two arteries and one vein should be present. If three vessels are not found, congenital malformations should be investigated.
3. Masses: Umbilical or inguinal hernias, or other abnormal masses are sometimes seen.
4. Bowel sounds are generally active.

Genitalia

The genitals of the full-term newborn should appear to be normally formed.

Male

1. The foreskin will cover the glans.
2. Urethral meatus should be at the tip. Deviations indicate hypospadias or epispadias.
3. The testes can usually be palpated in the scrotum.

Female

1. Labia minora is prominent, but should be covered by labia majora.
2. Some vaginal discharge in response to maternal hormones is normal. In breech infants, the genitals may be edematous and discolored from passage through the vagina.

Back

Hold the infant prone and evaluate the spine. It should not have abnormal curvatures or lesions. Observe for the following:
1. A dimple in the coccygeal-sacrococcygeal area may denote a pilonidal cyst, sinus opening or spina bifida.
2. Tufts of hair may indicate fistula.

Anus

Presence of a perforate anus must be verified. A soft rubber catheter is gently inserted in the rectum, if no stools have been passed.

Upper Extremities

Note the proportion to the rest of the body, the symmetry and spontaneous movement of the arms and hands.

Arms

Arms should be of equal length when extended. Infant should resist having arms extended.

Hands

Hold fingers in fists and they will normally grasp fingers or objects placed in their hands:
1. A single deep, sharp and transverse palmar crease (simian line) along with a flat and stubby thumb and a short little finger is found in Down syndrome.
2. Fingers may show webbing (abnormal fusion of fingers), polydactylism (extra digits) or syndactylism (fewer digits).
3. Nails: Fingernails are well-developed in most instances extending beyond fingertips. Long nails are present in post-term infants.
4. Skin tags may be seen occasionally.

Lower Extremities

Check the legs for symmetry, range of motion and proportion to the rest of the body:
1. Should be of equal length when extended.
2. With knees flexed, legs should abduct to table in frog-like position. Dislocated hip is suspected, if abduction is asymmetrical and if hip click is present.
3. If legs are persistently limp (flaccid), it is indicative of spinal cord lesion.

Feet

Soles of the full-term neonate are normally wrinkled. Wrinkles may be absent in preterm infants:
1. Acrocyanosis (blue discoloration of the hands and feet) is common immediately after birth.
2. Congenital malformations such as talipes equinovarus, talipes calcaneovalgus and bowing of legs must be noted.
3. Toes may show webbing and polydactylism or syndactylism.
4. The first and second *toes* are widely separated in Down syndrome.

Neurologic Examination

The normal newborn exhibits the following reflexes such as the Moro or embracing reflex, the tonic neck reflex, the stepping reflex, the palmar grasp reflex and the rooting or sucking reflex. The newborn that appears jittery or exhibits jerky movements of the extremities may suffer from low blood sugar, disturbances of calcium metabolism or may, in fact, be having seizures.

Cardiovascular Examination

After quieting the baby with a pacifier or finger, auscultate the heart sounds and feel for pulses in the upper and lower extremities. Although cardiac murmurs are common as the newborn makes the transition from intrauterine to extrauterine life, they should be documented and should be informed to pediatrician. Congenital heart defects may or may not be obvious in the first day of life.

BIRTH ASPHYXIA/ASPHYXIA NEONATORUM

Birth asphyxia is clinically defined as failure to initiate and maintain spontaneous respiration following birth. Perinatal asphyxia is the most appropriate term. Perinatal asphyxia is the state of decreased oxygen delivery (hypoxia) to the fetus or neonate resulting in inadequate tissue perfusion (ischemia). It is manifested by low Apgar score and metabolic acidosis. Often it is the continuation of an antepartum or intrapartum event. Although majority of infants gasp and establish respirations within 60 seconds of birth, asphyxiated neonates fail to initiate and sustain respirations at birth. In developing countries 3% of all newborn babies develop moderate to severe asphyxia.

Cause of Perinatal Asphyxia

About 90% of asphyxia events occur in the antepartum or intrapartum periods as a result of placental insufficiency and the rest as postnatal occurrence.
- Maternal lack of oxygen due to placental insufficiency, antepartum hemorrhage or premature separation of placenta
- Obstruction of the baby's airway by mucus, blood, liquor or meconium
- Intranatal pneumonia developed when membranes have been ruptured for some time
- Immaturity of the infant causing mechanical dysfunction because of immaturity of lungs and lack of surfactant
- Congenital abnormalities such as tracheal atresia
- Depression of respiratory center due to maternal medicines such as narcotics given to mother, within one hour prior to delivery
- Cerebral damage during traumatic forceps or vacuum delivery causing intracranial hemorrhage
- Cord prolapsed, true knot in the cord or cord around the neck
- Major congenital anomalies, e.g. congenital heart defect, abnormalities of central nervous system or abnormalities within the respiratory tract.

Etiology

- Causes in the respiratory center.
- Paralysis due to cerebral hemorrhage.
- Depression by drugs such as morphine, pethidine or anesthesia.
- Causes in the lungs:
  - Congenital atelectasis
  - Respiratory distress syndrome due to deficient lung surfactant
  - Causes in the respiratory passage
  - Obstruction by meconium, liquor, blood, mucus.

Diagnosis

Diagnosis is based on the degree of asphyxia—mild, moderate or severe, manifested as clinical features.

Clinical Features

Table 39.2 summarizes clinical features and types of asphyxia.

Management

As soon as the baby is born, assessment of respiratory efforts must be done. The APGAR score is assessed within a minute.

Dry and Position the Baby

Absence of any effort, resuscitation measures are taken immediately.
- The baby's upper airway should be cleaned by gentle suction of the oropharynx and nasopharynx.
- The baby is dried quickly and transferred to a well facilitated resuscitation area.
- The baby's shoulders may be elevated on a small rolled towel to straighten the trachea by slight extension of head.

Clear the Airway

If meconium is present in the airway, suction under direct vision should be performed by passing a laryngoscope and visualizing the larynx. If the baby does not respond to clearing of his airway, further steps of neonatal resuscitation to be started.

RESUSCITATION OF THE NEWBORN

Rationale for Resuscitation

The goals of resuscitation are to establish and maintain a clear airway, to ensure effective circulation to correct acidosis and to prevent hypothermia, hypoglycemia and hemorrhage. Careful intrapartum assessment of the fetal heart rate can alert the midwife to the probable need for resuscitation. The fetus undergoing prolonged period of asphyxia may make gasping attempts followed by apnea in utero (primary apnea). At birth, weaker gasps may be followed by a last gasp and *secondary period of apnea*. The heart rate falls dramatically and without intervention the infant dies. The infant born in secondary apnea cannot be revived with suctioning and

TABLE 39.2: Clinical features of asphyxia and its types.

	Asphyxia livida	*Asphyxia pallida*
Degree	Mild (early stage)	Severe (late stage)
Skin color	Blue	Pale white
Respiratory efforts	May be present	Absent
Heart beats	Strong, 8 – 120/min	Weak < 80/min
Eyes	Reactive pupils	Dilated pupils
Muscle tone	A degree of muscle tone	Flaccid
Reflexes	Present	Absent
Prognosis	Good, easy resuscitation	Bad, difficult resuscitation

tactile stimulation; ventilation and perhaps cardiac massage are required.

The asphyxiated infant has low oxygen levels, elevated carbon dioxide and lower blood pH (acidosis). This condition contributes to vasospasm of pulmonary arterioles and increased resistance to blood flow in the lungs after birth. The weak gasp of the asphyxiated newborn cannot overcome this resistance and establish adequate respiration. As the hypoxia continues, the heart rate slows and the myocardium contracts ineffectively. The BP drops and systemic circulation slows, leading to organ damage.

Degrees of Resuscitation (Fig. 39.10)

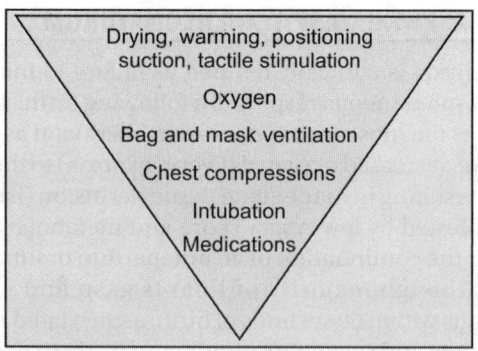

Figure 39.10: Inverted pyramid reflecting the degrees of neonatal resuscitative efforts.

Resuscitative requirements vary with the infant's condition at 1 minute of age:
1. The baby with an Apgar score of 7–10 has a blood pH of 7.20–7.40. This baby has minimal depression and a normal transition period can be expected:
   a. Suction the oropharynx and then the nose to clear the airway and provide tactile stimulation (Fig. 39.11).
   b. Dry the infant and provide warmth: Apply warm blankets to the baby on the mother's abdomen or use radiant warmer (warmer may not be required in the tropics).
   c. Continue to observe transition closely.
2. The baby with an Apgar score of 4–6 has a blood pH of 7.09–7.19 (moderate acidosis). This baby has moderate depression probably reflecting a period of primary apnea:
   a. Dry the infant.
   b. Place infant under radiant heat source.
   c. Suction the oropharynx and then the nose to clear the airway and provide tactile stimulation; give free-flow oxygen by face mask.

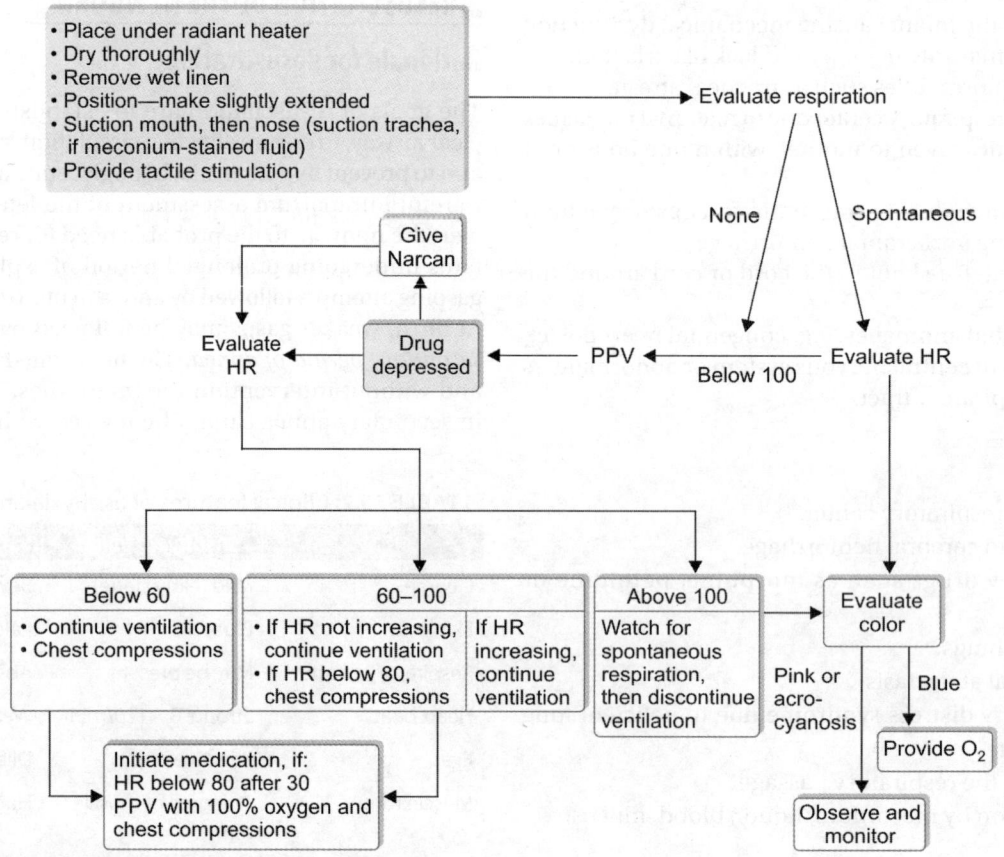

Figure 39.11: Resuscitation of the newborn in the delivery room.
(HR: heart rate; O$_2$: oxygen; PPV: positive pressure ventilation)
(*Source*: Textbook of Neonatal Resuscitation, © 1990 American Heart Association and the American Academy of Pediatrics, recommended by the National Neonatology Forum, India).

d. If infant is still apneic or has a heart rate below 100, begin positive pressure ventilation by face mask attached to an anesthesia bag or self-inflating bag with an oxygen reservoir; for both give nearly 100% oxygen.
e. Continue free-flow oxygen after infant has established good respiratory effort.
3. The infant with an Apgar score of 0–3 has a blood pH of 7.00 or below (severe acidosis). This baby has severe depression reflecting secondary apnea:
   a. Suction the infant to clear the airway.
   b. Dry the infant.
   c. Place the infant in the work area under radiant heat source.
   d. Begin positive pressure ventilation.
   e. If positive pressure ventilation does not ensue with bag and mask, perform endotracheal intubation.
   f. If heart rate is less than 60 after 30 seconds of adequate ventilation, begin cardiac massage. Continue massage until infant can sustain heart rate over 80 with ventilation alone.

Supplies and Equipment

Though the need for resuscitation can be anticipated in some situations, there are occasions when a baby is born in poor condition without forewarning. It is essential that resuscitation equipment are always available and in working order in the delivery room and nursery area in close proximity to oxygen and suction outlets. The equipment and medications should include those that will provide adequate ventilation or resuscitation, thermoregulation, correction of hypoglycemia, fluids and electrolytes, plasma expanders and cardiac stimulants. The personnel in attendance at the delivery of a baby must be familiar with the equipment and resuscitation techniques. A list of essential equipment includes the following.

Suctioning Equipment

- Bulb syringe
- DeLee mucus trap with No. 10 French (Fr) catheter or mechanical suction
- Suction catheters No. 6, 8 and 10
- Feeding tube No. 8 Fr and 20 mL syringe.

Bag and Mask Equipment

- Infant resuscitation bag with pressure release valve or pressure gauge with a reservoir capable of delivering 90–100% oxygen
- Face masks with cushioned rims: Newborn and premature sizes
- Oral airways: Newborn and premature sizes
- Oxygen with flow meter and tubing.

Intubation Equipment

- Laryngoscope with straight blades No. '0' (premature), No. '1' (newborn)
- Extra bulbs and batteries for laryngoscope
- Endotracheal tubes—sizes 2.5, 3.0, 3.5 and 4.0 mm internal diameter
- Stylet
- Scissors.

Medications

- Epinephrine 1:10,000 ampules (1 mL ampule of 1:1,000 available in India)
- Naloxone hydrochloride (neonatal Narcan 0.02 mg/mL)
- Volume expander (one or more)
- Albumin solution of 5%
- Normal saline
- Ringer's lactate
- Sodium bicarbonate 4.2% (1 mEq/2 mL) (7.5% strength available in India approximately 0.9 mEq/mL)
- Dextrose 10% concentration 250 mL
- Sterile water 30 mL
- Normal saline 30 mL.

Miscellaneous

- Radiant warmer
- Stethoscope
- Adhesive tapes
- Syringes 1 mL, 2 mL, 5 mL and 20 mL sizes
- Needles No. 21, 22 and 26
- Umbilical cord clamp
- Umbilical catheters 3.5 and 5 Fr sizes
- Umbilical artery catheterization tray
- Gloves.

Initial Steps

Preventing Heat Loss

- Place infant under a warmer
- Quickly dry off amniotic fluid
- Replace wet sheets with a dry one.

Positioning

- Place the baby on his/her back with head slightly down (15° tilt)
- Neck slightly extended.

Suctioning

- Suction the mouth first and then nose
- Tactile stimulation
- If infant does not breathe immediately give tactile stimulation, but only twice (flick or tap the sole of foot twice or rub the back).

Evaluation

1. After the above steps evaluate the baby's vital signs:
   – Respirations

- Heart rate
- Color.
2. If respiration is normal, go on evaluating heart rate.
3. If baby is apneic, begin positive pressure ventilation.
4. If heart rate is over 100 bpm, go on evaluating color.
5. If less than 100 bpm, initiate positive pressure ventilation.
6. If infant is pink, no further action is necessary.
7. If there is central cyanosis, administer free flow oxygen (tip of the tube held 1.25 cm from nares delivers approximately 90% oxygen).

Bag and Mask Ventilation/Positive Pressure Ventilation (Figs. 39.12A to C)

Indications

- Infant apneic
- Heart rate less than 100 bpm.

Procedure

The newborn should be on his/her back with neck slightly extended.

A tight seal to be formed over the infant's mouth and nose:
- Ventilate at the rate of 40–50 per minute with 20–25 cm H_2O pressure
- Ventilate for 15–30 seconds and evaluate
- Have an assistant to evaluate, listen to the heart rate for 6 seconds and multiply by 10.

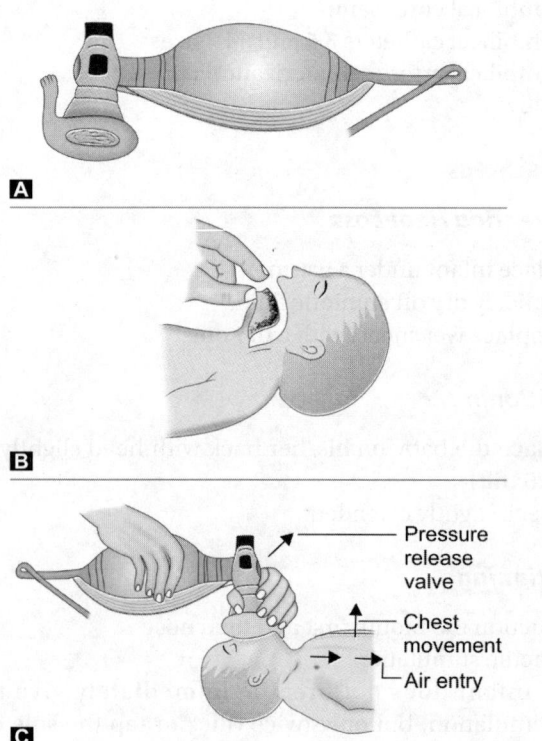

Figures 39.12A to C: Bag and mask ventilation. (A) Bag and mask for ventilation; (B) Correct position (sniffing position) of the baby's head for ventilating; (C) Bag squeezed to move the chest with each squeeze.

Evaluation

1. Heart rate above 100 bpm and spontaneous respiration—discontinue bagging.
2. Heart rate 60–100 bpm and increasing—continue ventilation.
3. Heart rate 60–100 bpm and not increasing—continue ventilation.
4. Check whether chest is moving adequately.
5. Heart rate below 80 bpm—start chest compressions.
6. Heart rate below 60 bpm—in addition to bagging and chest compressions, consider intubation and initiate medications.

Signs of Improvement

- Increasing heart rate
- Spontaneous respiration
- Improving color.

Continue to provide free flow oxygen by face mask after respiration has established.

If the baby deteriorates, check the following:
- Placement of face mask for tight seal
- Head position and presence of secretions
- Pressure being used
- Presence of air in the stomach preventing chest expansion
- Oxygen being delivered (100% or not).

For bagging lasting for more than 2 minutes insert an orogastric tube to vent the stomach.

Chest Compressions

Chest compressions (**Figs. 39.13A and B**) consist of rhythmic compressions of the sternum that compresses the heart against the spine, increases the intrathoracic pressure and circulates blood to the vital organs.

Chest compressions must always be accompanied by ventilation with 100% oxygen to assure that the circulating blood is well oxygenated.

Indications

1. Heart rate less than 60 bpm after bagging with 100% oxygen for 15–30 seconds.
2. Heart rate 60–80 bpm and not increasing after bagging with 100% oxygen for 15–30 seconds.

Procedure

Site: Lower third of the sternum below an imaginary line between the two nipples.

Depth: Depress the sternum to a depth of ½–¾ inch at a rate of 100–120 bpm.

Rate: 100–120 bpm. Coordinate heart compression with ventilation.

Discontinue when infant can maintain heart rate above 80 by ventilation alone.

volume expanders (for hypovolemia) and dopamine (for hypotension). Naloxone is given if needed to reverse the effects of maternal narcotics given in the preceding 3 hours **(Table 39.3)**.

Changes Recommended in the 2010 AHA Guidelines for Neonatal Resuscitation

Anticipation of the Need to Resuscitate: Elective Cesarean Section

Infants without antenatal risk factors, who are born by elective cesarean section performed under regional anesthesia at 37–39 weeks of gestation have decreased requirement for intubation, but have a slightly increased need for mask ventilation compared with infants after normal vaginal delivery.

Assessment of Heart Rate, Respiratory Rate and Oxygenation

Once positive pressure ventilation or supplementary oxygen administration has begun, assessment should consist of simultaneous evaluation of three clinical characteristics such as heart rate, respiratory rate and evaluation of the state of oxygenation. State of oxygenation is optimally determined by a pulse oximeter rather than by simple assessment of color.

Supplementary Oxygen Administration

Pulse oximetry with the probe attached to the right upper extremity should be used to assess any need for supplementary oxygen. For babies born at term, it is best to begin resuscitation with air rather than 100% oxygen. Administration of supplementary oxygen should be regulated by blending oxygen and air and the amount to be delivered should be guided by an oximetry monitored from the right upper extremity (i.e. usually the wrist or palm).

Suctioning

Suctioning immediately after birth (including suctioning with a bulb syringe) should be reserved for babies who have an obvious obstruction to spontaneous breathing or require positive pressure ventilation.

Compression-to-ventilation Ratio

The recommended compression-to-ventilation ratio remains 3:1. If the arrest is known to be of cardiac etiology, a higher ratio (i.e. 5:2) should be considered.

Delayed Cord Clamping

There is increasing evidence of benefit of delaying cord clamping for at least 1 minute in term and preterm infants not requiring resuscitation.

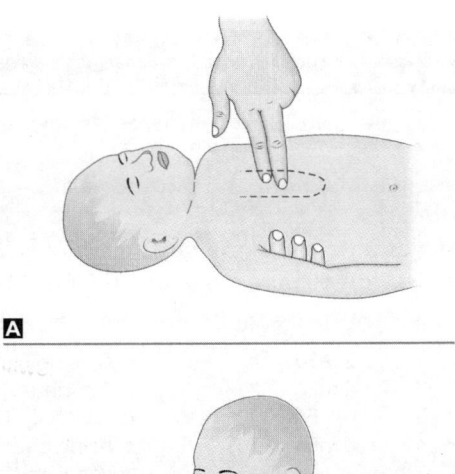
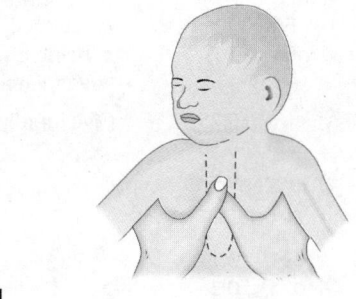

Figures 39.13A and B: External cardiac massage. (A) Two-finger technique; (B) Thumb technique.

Endotracheal Intubation

Indications

1. Heart rate below 60 bpm in spite of bagging and chest compressions.
2. Presence of meconium in the amniotic fluid.

Procedure

1. Place infant with head lightly extended with a rolled towel under the shoulder.
2. Introduce laryngoscope over the baby's tongue at the right corner of the mouth.
3. Advance 2–3 cm, while rotating it to midline, until the epiglottis is seen. Elevation of the epiglottis by the tip of the laryngoscope reveals the vocal cord.
4. Suction secretions, if needed.
5. Pass the endotracheal tube to a distance of 1.5–2 cm into the trachea, hold it firmly, but gently place and withdraw the laryngoscope slowly.
6. Attach the endotracheal tube to the adapter on the bag.
7. Ventilate with oxygen by bag. An assistant should check for adequate ventilation of both lungs with stethoscope.

Medications

Medications should be administered, if despite adequate ventilation with 100% oxygen and chest compressions, the heart rate remains 80 bpm. Medications used are adrenalin (for hypotonia), sodium bicarbonate (to correct acidosis),

TABLE 39.3: Medications for neonatal resuscitation.

Medications	Concentration	Preparation (in mL)	Dosage/Route	Weight (in kg)	Total dose	Total (in mL)	Rate/Precautions
Epinephrine (adrenaline)	1:10,000	1	0.1–0.3 mL/kg IV or IT	1 2 3 4		0.1–0.3 0.2–0.6 0.3–0.9 0.4–1.2	Give rapidly
Volume expanders	Whole blood Albumin 5% Normal saline Ringer's lactate	40	10 mL/kg IV	1 2 3 4		10 20 30 40	Give over 5–10 minute
Sodium bicarbonate	0.5 mEq/mL (4.2% solution)	20	2 mEq/kg IV	1 2 3 4	2 mEq 4 mEq 6 mEq 8 mEq	4 8 12 16	• Give slowly, at least 2 minute • Give only if infant being effectively ventilated
Naloxone (Narcan)	0.4 mg/mL	1 1	0.25 mL/kg IV, IM, SQ, IT	1 2 3 4		0.25 0.50 0.85 1.00	Give rapidly
	1.0 mg/mL		0.1 mL/kg IV, IM, SQ, IT	1 2 3 4		0.1 0.2 0.3 0.4	
Dopamine	$\dfrac{6 \times \text{Weight (kg)} \times \text{Desired dose (µg/kg/min)}}{\text{Desired fluid (mL/h)}}$ = mg of dopamine per 100 mL of solution		Begin at 5 µg/kg/min may increase to 20 µg/kg/min (if necessary) IV	1 2 3 4		In µg/min: • 5–20 • 10–40 • 15–60 • 20–60	• Give as a continuous infusion using an infusion pump • Monitor HR and BP Seek consultation

(IV: intravenous; IT: intratracheal; IM: intramuscular; SQ: subcutaneous; HR: heart rate; BP: blood pressure).
(*Source:* Textbook of Neonatal Resuscitation, 1990 © American Heart Association, recommended by the National Neonatology Forum, India.)

STUDY QUESTIONS

Short Notes

1. Acrocyanosis.
2. Vernix caseosa.
3. Port-wine stain.
4. Cephalohematoma.
5. Caput succedaneum.

Short Answer Questions

1. Apgar scoring.
2. Fontanels.
3. Respiratory changes in newborn at birth.
4. Thermoregulation in newborn at birth.

Essay Questions

1. Explain the initial assessment to be performed on a newborn.
2. A newborn with Apgar score 7 is in minimal depression and needs basic resuscitation. Explain the steps of resuscitation.

BIBLIOGRAPHY

1. Apgar V. The newborn (Apgar) scoring system. Reflections and advice. Pediatric Clinics of North America. 1966;13(3): 645-50.
2. Arnold HW, Putnam NJ, Barnard BL, et al. Transition to extrauterine life. American Journal of Nursing. 1975;81(3):65-77.
3. Dutta DC. Textbook of obstetrics, 5th edition. Kolkata: New Central Book Company; 2001.
4. Helen V. Nurse midwifery, 2nd edition. Boston: Jones and Bartlett Publishers; 1996.
5. Karpen M, Conrad L, Chitwood L. Essentials of maternal-child nursing, 2nd edition. Massachusetts: Western Schools Press; 1995.
6. Korones SB. High risk newborn infants: the basis for intensive nursing care, 3rd edition. Mosby: St Louis; 1981.
7. Leboyer F. Birth without violence. New York: Knopf; 1976.
8. Michie MM. The baby at birth, In: Bennet RV, Brown KL (Eds) Myles. Textbook for midwives, 13th edition. Edinburgh: Churchill Livingstone; 1999.
9. Moore ML. The newborn and the nurse. Philadelphia: Saunders; 1972.
10. Phibbs RH. Evaluation of the newborn. In: Rudoph AM, Hoffman J (Eds). Pediatrics. Norwalk, CT: Appleton-Century-Crofts; 1977.

Physiology, Screening, Daily Care and Observation of the Newborn

Learning Objectives

Upon completing this chapter, the learner will be able to:
- Describe the external features of the normal newborn baby.
- Describe the functioning of different body systems in relation to their stage of maturity.
- Describe the behavior of the baby during the 1st week of life.
- Describe the daily examination and observations of the newborn baby.
- Discuss the role of the midwife in providing guidance and assistance to mothers in the care of their babies.

Extrauterine life presents a challenge to the newborn infant. The most important changes taken place are in the heart and lungs at birth. However, continued adaptations are necessary in the 1st week of life as the infant assumes independence from the maternal and placental nurturing, which the body enjoyed before birth. The newborn remains dependent on the mother or caregiver for nutrition and protection, but is responsible for his/her own metabolism, homeostasis and other functions essential for survival.

PHYSIOLOGY

Respiratory System

At birth, the respiratory system is developmentally incomplete, growth of new alveoli continuing for several years. Respiration rate is usually 30–60 breaths per minute. The breathing is diaphragmatic, chest and abdomen rising and falling synchronously. Breathing pattern is erratic. Respirations are shallow and irregular, being interspersed with brief 10–15 seconds of apnea. This is known as periodic breathing. The pattern of respiration alters during sleeping and waking states. Babies are obligatory nose breathers and do not convert automatically to mouth breathing when nasal obstruction occurs. Respiratory difficulties can occur because of neurological, metabolic, circulatory or thermoregulatory dysfunction as well as infection, airway obstruction or abnormalities of airway tract itself.

The baby has a lusty cry, which he/she uses to evoke a response from the attendants with a view to control the environment. The cry is normally loud and of medium pitch unless neurological damage, infection or hypothermia is present, when it may be high pitched or weak. Transient cyanosis may arise in the first few days when the baby is crying.

Cardiovascular System

The heart rate is rapid with 120–160 breaths per minute and fluctuates in accordance with the baby's respiratory function and activity or sleep rate. Peripheral circulation is sluggish. This results in mild cyanosis of hands and feet and circumoral areas, and in generalized mottling when the skin is exposed. Blood pressure fluctuates according to activity and ranges from 80/50 to 85/55 mm Hg in the first 10 days of life.

The total circulating blood volume at birth is 80 mL/kg body weight. However, this may be raised if there is delay in clamping the umbilical cord at birth. The hemoglobin levels are high (18–20 g/dL) of which 50%–80% is fetal hemoglobin. Conversion from fetal to adult hemoglobin is completed in the first 1–2 years of life. Hemoglobin, red cell count and hematocrit levels decrease gradually during the first 2–3 months of life during which time erythropoiesis is suppressed. The white cell count is high initially and decreases rapidly.

Breakdown of excess red blood cells in the liver and spleen predisposes to jaundice in the 1st week. Because delayed of colonization of the intestine, by the bacteria that synthesize vitamin K is delayed until feeding is established, vitamin K-dependent clotting factors II (prothrombin), VII, IX and X are low. This inhibits blood clotting. During the 1st week, platelet levels equal those of the adult, but there is a reduced capacity for adhesion and aggregation.

Thermal Regulation

Thermal control in the neonate remains poor for some time. Owing to the immaturity of the hypothalamus, temperature regulation is inefficient and the infant remains vulnerable to hypothermia, particularly when exposed to cold or draughts, wet, unable to move about freely or when deprived of nutrition. As a baby, who is cold and unable to shiver; will attempt to maintain the body heat by adopting flexed posture, increasing his/her respiratory rate and activity. The body may also cry. These activities increase calorie consumption and may result in hypoglycemia, which in turn will compound the effects of hypothermia.

The infant's normal core temperature is 36°C–37°C. A healthy, clothed, term infant will maintain this body temperature satisfactorily if the environment is not cold, his/her nutrition is adequate and the movements are not restricted by tight swaddling. An unstable temperature may indicate infection.

Renal System

The kidneys are functionally immature at birth. Glomerular filtration rate is low and tubular resorption capabilities are limited. The infant is not able to concentrate or dilute urine very well in response to variations in fluid intake. The ability to excrete drugs is also limited and the baby's renal function is vulnerable to physiological stress.

The first urine is passed at birth or within the first 24 hours and thereafter with increasing frequency as fluid intake rises. The urine is dilute, straw colored and odorless. Cloudiness caused by mucus and urates may be present initially until fluid intake increases. Urine is voided by reflex emptying of the bladder. As the neonatal pelvis is small, the bladder becomes palpable abdominally when full.

Gastrointestinal System

The gastrointestinal tract of the neonate is structurally complete though functionally immature. The mucous membrane of the mouth is pink and moist. The teeth are buried in the gums and ptyalin secretion is low. Small epithelial pearls (Epstein's pearls) are sometimes present at the junction of the hard and soft palates. Sucking pads in the cheek give them a full appearance. Sucking and swallowing are coordinated.

The stomach has small capacity (15–30 mL) at birth, which increases rapidly in the 1st week of life. The cardiac sphincter is weak, which gives rise to regurgitation or posseting. Gastric emptying time is normally 2.5–3 hours. Enzymes are present though there is a deficiency of amylase and lipase, which diminishes the infant's ability to digest compound carbohydrates and fat.

When food enters the stomach, a gastrocolic reflex results in increased peristalsis, often accompanied by reflex emptying of the bowel. Bowel sounds are present within 1 hour of birth. Meconium present in the large intestine from 16th week's gestation is passed within the first 24 hours of life and is totally excreted within 48–72 hours. This first stool is blackish green in color, is tenacious and contains bile, fatty acids, mucus and epithelial cells. From 3rd to 5th day, the stools undergo a transitional stage and are brownish yellow in color. Once feeding is established, yellow feces are passed. The consistency and frequency of stools reflect the type of feeding. Breast milk results in loose, bright yellow and inoffensive acid stools. The baby may pass 8–10 stools a day. The stools of the bottle-fed infant are paler in color, semiformed, less acid and have a slightly sharp smell. The bottle-fed baby passes four to six stools a day and there is increased tendency to constipation.

Physiological immaturity of the liver results in low production of glucuronyl transferase for the conjugation of bilirubin. This together with a high level of red cell breakdown may result in a transient jaundice, which is manifest on the 3rd–5th day (physiological jaundice). Glycogen stores are rapidly depleted after birth and hence early feeding is required to maintain normal blood glucose levels. Feeding stimulates liver function and colonization of the gut, which assists in the formation of vitamin K.

Reproductive System

Spermatogenesis in boys does not occur until puberty, but the total complement of primordial follicles containing primitive ova is present in the ovaries of girls at birth. In both sexes, withdrawal of maternal estrogens results in breast engorgement, sometimes accompanied by secretion of 'milk' by the 4th or 5th day. Female infants may develop pseudomenstruation for the same reason.

Musculoskeletal System

The muscles are complete at birth with growth occurring by hypertrophy. The long bones are incompletely ossified to facilitate growth at the epiphyses. The bones of the vault of the skull also reveal lack of ossification. This is essential for growth of the brain and facilitating molding during labor. Molding is resolved within a few days of birth. The posterior fontanel closes at 6–8 weeks. The anterior fontanel remains open until 18 months of age, making assessment of hydration and intracranial pressure possible by palpation of fontanel tension.

Immunological Adaptations

Neonates are susceptible to infections, particularly those gaining entry through the mucosa of the respiratory and gastrointestinal systems. Minor infections become generalized very easily.

The baby has some immunoglobulins at birth. There are three main immunoglobulins IgG, IgA and IgM, and of these only IgG is small enough to cross the placental barrier. It affords immunity to specific viral infections during the first few months of life.

IgM and IgA do not cross the placental barrier. Levels of IgM at term are 20% of those of the adult and takes 2 years to attain the adult levels. This relatively low level of IgM is thought to render the infant more susceptible to enteric infections. IgA levels are also very low and increase slowly. IgA protects against infection of the respiratory tract, gastrointestinal tract and eyes. Breast milk, especially colostrum provides the infant with passive immunity in the form of *Lactobacillus bifidus*, lactoferrin, lysozyme and secretory IgA.

The thymus gland, where lymphocytes are produced, is relatively large at birth and continues to grow until 8 years of age.

Neurological System

The nervous system is remarkably immature both anatomically and physiologically at birth. This results in predominantly brainstem and spinal reflex activity with minimal control by the cerebral cortex in the early months. After birth, brain growth is rapid, requiring constant and adequate supplies of oxygen and glucose. The immaturity of the brain renders it vulnerable to hypoxia, biochemical imbalance, infection and hemorrhage. Temperature instability and uncoordinated muscle movement reflect the incomplete development of brain.

The neonate is equipped with a wide range of reflex activities, the presence of which at varying ages provides indication of the normality and integrity of neurological and musculoskeletal systems.

Moro Reflex or Embracing Reflex (Fig. 40.1)

Moro reflex occurs in response to a sudden stimulus. Acceptable ways to elicit a Moro reflex include the following:
- Holding the baby at 45° angle and then permitting the head to drop 1 or 2 cm
- The examining table is struck near the head of the baby
- The table is jarred suddenly
- A loud noise or handclap is utilized.

The infant responds by abducting and extending the arms and fanning the fingers, sometimes accompanied by a tremor. The arms then flex and embrace the chest. A similar response may be seen in the legs, which, following extension flex onto the abdomen. The reflex is symmetrical and is present for the first 8 weeks of life. Absence of Moro reflex may indicate brain damage or immaturity. Persistence of the reflex beyond the age of 6 months is suggestive of mental retardation.

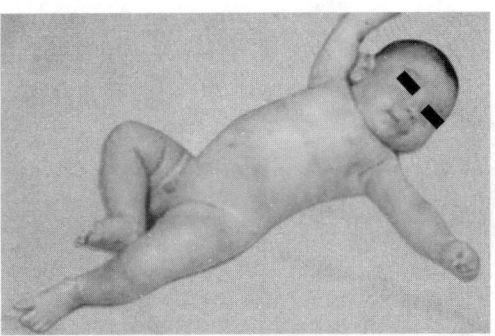

Figure 40.2: Tonic neck reflex.

Tonic Neck Reflex (Fig. 40.2)

The infant is placed on his/her back and the head is turned to the side. The arm and leg on the same side extend and the opposite arm and leg flex; thus the infant assumes a fencing position. The head is turned to the opposite side and the same reaction should occur. The response may be present in the newborn for about 2–3 months. If it persists longer than this time, it usually indicates neurological dysfunction.

Palmar Reflex/Grasp Reflex (Fig. 40.3)

With the baby in supine and the head in midline, the finger of the examiner or a thin object such as a pencil is placed in the baby's hand. The newborn shows palmar reflex by wrapping the palm and the fingers around it. Normally, there should be flexion of all the infant's fingers around the examiner's finger.

When fingers of the examiner are placed in both the hands, if the newborn holds so tightly that they can be picked up and held by their grasp alone, this may present a hyperkinetic reaction. This reflex diminishes, weakens and disappears after 3 months. Complete absence of the reflex may be found in brain damage.

Plantar Reflex (Fig. 40.4)

The examiner's thumb or a thin object such as a pencil is pressed against the ball of the infant's foot. There should be flexion of all toes. The absence of this response is correlated with defects of the lower spinal cord. This reflex disappears in 2–3 years.

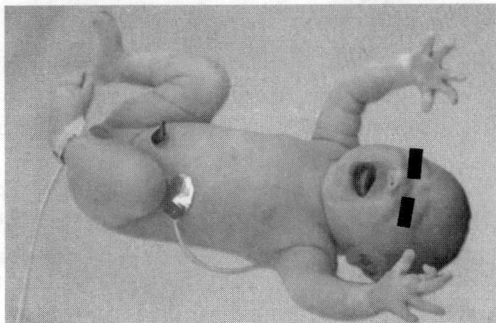

Figure 40.1: Moro reflex *(For color version, see Plate 5)*.

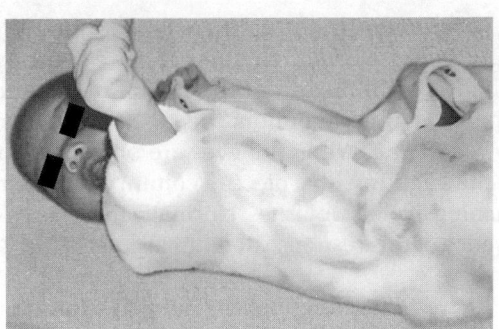

Figure 40.3: Palmar reflex *(For color version, see Plate 5)*.

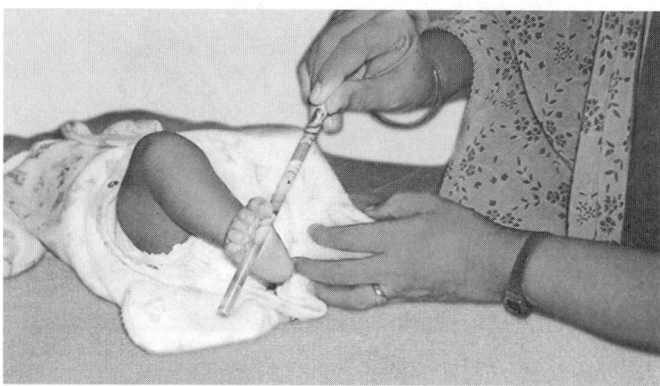

Figure 40.4: Plantar reflex *(For color version, see Plate 5).*

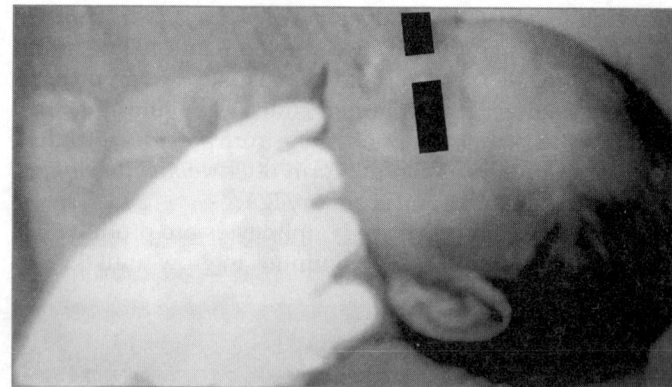

Figure 40.6: Eliciting rooting reflex.

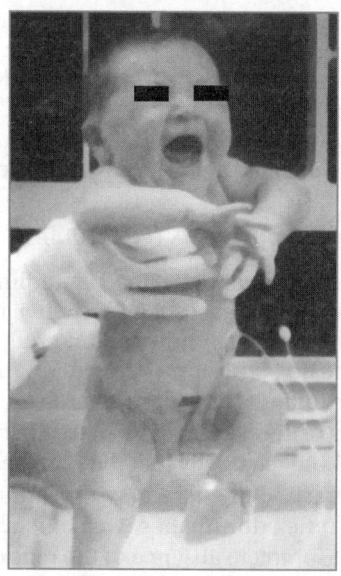

Figure 40.5: Stepping reflex *(For color version, see Plate 5).*

Walking/Stepping Reflex (Fig. 40.5)

The baby is held so that the sole of the foot touches a flat surface. This should stimulate a stepping or dancing movement with both legs. This reflex is present at birth and gradually disappears after 3–4 weeks.

Reflexes of the Eyes

1. *Blink reflex:* A bright light is shone suddenly at the infant's eyes. Normally a quick closure of the eyes and a slight dorsal flexion of the head are elicited. With impaired light perception, this response is absent.
2. *Corneal reflex:* When the eyes are open, the cornea is touched lightly with a piece of cotton, with care to avoid touching eyelids or lashes. Normally the eyes close. The absence of this response denotes lesions of the V cranial nerve.
3. *Doll's eye reflex:* Keeping the baby in supine position, move the head slowly to left or right. Eyes lag behind and do not immediately adjust to the new position of head.

Reflexes of the Mouth

1. *Rooting reflex:* The corner of the baby's mouth, the upper lip and the lower lip are touched in turn with the finger (**Fig. 40.6**). Upon stimulation, the head turns toward the stimulated side, the mouth opens, the tongue moves to the point of stimulation and infant tries to suck on the stimulating object. Rooting reflex is elicited when the baby is alert. A baby whose hunger has been satisfied will turn away from the stimulation.
2. *Sucking and swallowing reflex* (**Fig. 40.7**): If the examiner's index finger is placed in the infant's mouth, rhythmical sucking movements will be felt. Sucking is often less intense and less regular during the first 3–4 days. Poor sucking may be noted in apathetic or hyperactive babies and is the first indication of problems such as sepsis.
3. *Gag, cough and sneeze reflexes:* These protect the infant from airway obstruction.
4. *Babinski's reflex:* The lateral aspect of the sole of the infant's foot is scratched, going from heel to toes. This must be more than pressure; if not, a plantar reflex instead of a Babinski's reflex will be elicited. The Babinski's reflex shows a dorsal flexion of the big toe. It is present in the newborn until 9–10 month. A poor response may be due to nervous system immaturity; absence of the response may be due to defects in the lower spinal cord.

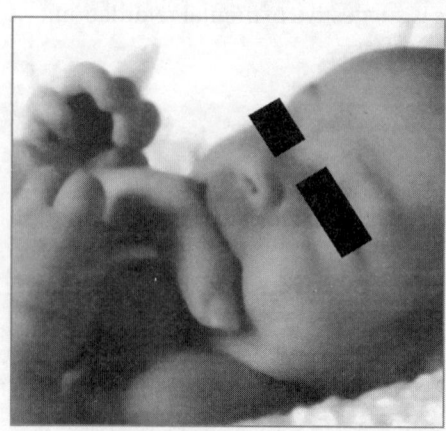

Figure 40.7: Sucking and swallowing reflex.

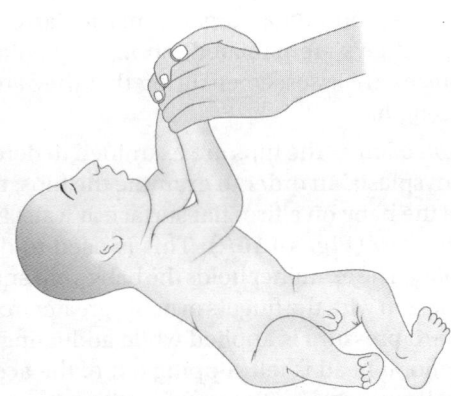

Figure 40.8: Traction response (head lag).

Body Reflex

1. *Traction response (head lag):* When pulled upright by the wrists to a sitting position the head will lag initially, then right itself momentarily before falling forward onto the chest **(Fig. 40.8)**.
2. *Ventral suspension:* When held prone, suspended over the examiner's arm, the baby shortly holds the head level with the body and flexes the limbs **(Fig. 40.9)**.
3. *Incurvation of trunk/Perez reflex/Galant reflex:* Hold the baby suspended ventrally and stroke the sides of spine alternatively. The baby would turn the pelvis to the side stimulated. This response indicates general muscle tone as the baby is suspended. No response indicates central nervous system (CNS) deficit. The reflex disappears in 1 month.

Special Senses and Behavior Pattern

Vision

The structures necessary for vision are present and functional at birth although immature. The baby is sensitive to bright lights, which cause him/her to frown or blink. The body demonstrates a preference for black and white patterns and the shape of human face. His/her focusing distance is about 15–20 cm, which allows him/her to see the mother's face when being nursed. He/she can track a moving object briefly within the first 5 days. His/her ability to establish eye contact with the mother helps to enhance bonding. By 2 weeks of age, the body can differentiate his/her mother's face from that of a stranger.

Hearing

The baby turns the eyes towards sound, comforted by low-pitched sounds. High-pitched sounds make him the body. A sudden sound elicits a startle or blink reflex. He/she prefers the sound of the human voice to other sounds. The baby can discriminate between voices and prefers the mother's. This too, promotes mother-baby interaction.

Smell and Taste

Babies prefer the smell of milk to that of other substances and show a preference for human milk. Within a few days, the baby can differentiate the smell of his/her mother's milk. The baby turns away from unpleasant smells. His/her preference for sweet taste is demonstrated by vigorous and strong sucking and a grimacing response to bitter, salty or sour substances.

Touch

Infants are acutely sensitive to touch, enjoys skin-to-skin contact, immersion in water, stroking, cuddling and rocking movements. A puff of air on baby's face induces an inspiration or gasp reflex. His curving response to touch and the gasp reflexes enhance his/her relationship with the mother. The baby withdraws from painful stimuli, bulges his brow and nasolabial furrow and may cry vigorously.

Sleeping and Waking

Following the initiation of respiration at birth, the baby remains alert and reactive for a period of approximately 1 hour after which the baby relaxes and sleeps. The length of this first sleep varies from a few minutes to several hours. Subsequent sleeping and waking rhythms show marked variations and the baby takes some time to settle into his/her individual pattern. Initially, waking periods are related to hunger, but within a few weeks, the waking periods last longer and meet the need for social interaction.

Two sleep states are identifiable

- *Deep sleep* in which the baby's eyes are closed, respirations are regular, no eye movements are present, response to stimuli is delayed and is quickly suppressed. Jerky movements may occur at intervals.
- *Light sleep* in which eye movements could be observed through the closed eyelids. Respirations are irregular and sucking movements occur intermittently. Response to stimuli occurs more readily and may result in alteration of sleep state. Random movements are noted.

Awakening states

A wider range of awakening states is observed, ranging from drowsiness to crying.

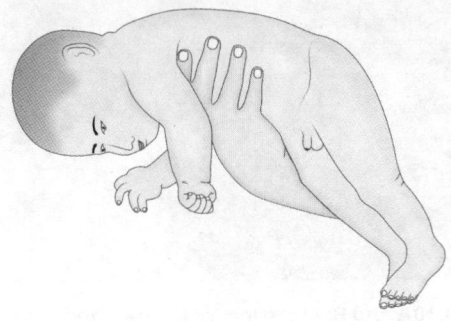

Figure 40.9: Ventral suspension.

- *Drowsy state:* The baby's eyes may be open or closed with some fluttering of the eyelids. Smiling may occur. Limb movements are generally smooth, but are interspersed by startle responses.
- *Quiet alert state:* Motor activity is minimal, the baby is alert to visual and auditory stimuli.
- *Active alert state:* The baby is generally active and reactive to the environment.
- *Active crying state:* The baby cries vigorously and may be difficult to console. Muscular activity is considerable.

The amount of time that the baby spends in which state varies and influences the way in which he responds to stimuli, whether visual, auditory or tactile.

Crying

Crying is the way in which the baby communicates discomfort and summons assistance. With experience, it is possible to differentiate the cry and identify the need, which may be hunger, thirst, pain general discomfort (for example, wanting a change of position or feeling too cold or too warm), boredom, loneliness or a desire for physical and social contact. The mother needs to learn how to comfort her baby. Rocking induces sleep, swaddling and upright position appear to be soothing.

Growth and Development

Because of physical limitations, the baby is dependent on the mother (or other caregiver) for his/her continued growth, development and survival. These will progress satisfactorily only if the baby is in a safe environment, the nutritional needs are met and the psychological development is promoted by appropriate stimulation and loving care. Abnormality of the baby's body systems, inadequate nutrition or emotional deprivation will compromise the baby's ability to grow and develop to his/her full potential. His relatively immature organ functions and vulnerability to infection and hypothermia demand that care must be designed to meet the needs and capabilities.

PHYSICAL EXAMINATION (SCREENING)

All newborn babies are routinely examined by a pediatrician within the first 24 hours of life and again prior to discharge home. Some of the examination duplicates what has been described earlier under initial assessment and hence only additional aspects are considered here. A general appraisal of the baby's color, overall appearance, muscular activity and response to handling are made throughout the examination.

Neurological assessment: The baby's reflex responses are elicited in order to establish normality of the nervous system. These are tested when the baby is in quiet alert state. Absent or weak responses may indicate immaturity, cerebral damage or abnormality.

Auscultation: The heart and lung sounds are auscultated. A heart murmur may be present for some days after birth.

Palpation: The abdominal organs, particularly the liver, spleen and kidneys are palpated, noting any enlargement. Femoral pulses are assessed ensuring that they are full and of equal strength.

Examination of hips: The hips are examined to detect developmental dysplasia. In order to examine the hips, the examiner places the baby on a firm flat surface at waist height:

1. *Barlow's test* (**Fig. 40.10A**): This is used to detect hip instability. The examiner holds the baby's hip and knees at 90° of flexion with the fingers over the greater trochanters. Backward pressure is applied while adducting the hips. The femoral head is felt slipping out of the acetabulum posterolaterally when the test is positive.
2. *Ortolani's test* (**Fig. 40.10B**): This sign is present when the hip is dislocated. The maneuver relocates the femoral head. With the examiner's fingers on the baby's greater trochanters, the hips and knees are flexed to 90°. The hips are then abducted while applying upward pressure over the greater trochanters. A positive sign is detected when a 'click' is felt as the femoral head renters the acetabulum.

GESTATIONAL AGE ASSESSMENT

The American Academy of Pediatrics (AAP) recommended since 1967 that all newborns be classified by birth weight and gestational age, and the Dubowitz scoring system by Ballard et al (1991) remains the most popular method for determining gestational age. The examination provides a score of neuromuscular and physical maturity that can be mathematically projected onto a corresponding age, to reveal the gestational age in weeks.

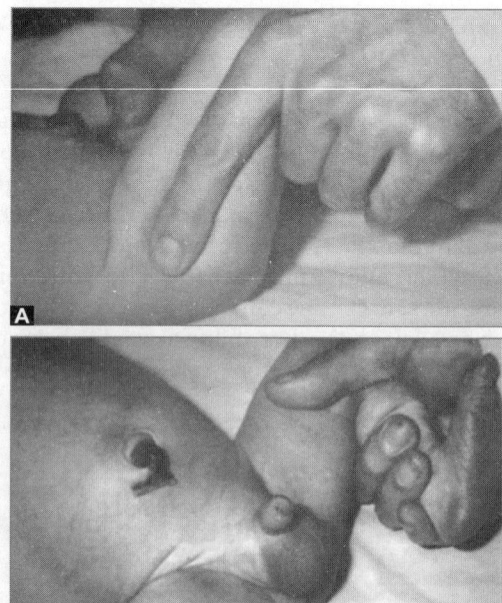

Figures 40.10A and B: Assessing for Barlow's and Ortolani's signs. (A) Barlow's sign; (B) Ortolani's sign.

The Ballard gestational age by maturity rating consists of two scoring systems **(Fig. 40.11)**. Physical maturity and neuromuscular maturity of six to seven characteristics each; scores from each system are added together and mathematically projected on the maturity rating scale to determine the gestational age by examination. The systems scored reflect the decreasing flexibility of muscles and joints in prematurity and the return to original positioning after movement indicative of a mature term infant. This examination is usually performed within the first 12 hours of life and is more accurate when done on term infants between 10 and 36 hours of life when the baby has had sufficient opportunity to rest following birth and when he/she is awake.

Gestational age and birth weight are considered jointly and marked on centile chart. The baby's birth weight is plotted against the gestational age. A baby whose weight lies between the 10th and 90th percentile this is described as appropriate for gestational age (AGA); if the birth weight is greater than 90th percentile this is described as large for gestational age (LGA) and a baby whose weight is below the 10th percentile is described as being small for gestational age (SGA).

Assessment of Neuromuscular Maturity

The assessments are done in the following manner:
1. *Posture:* Posture is the natural position that the newborn assumes on its back. It is observed with the infant quiet and in supine position.
   - Score:
     - 0: Arms and legs extended
     - 1: Beginning of flexion of hips and knees, arms extended
     - 2: Stronger flexion of legs, arms extended
     - 3: Arms slightly flexed, legs flexed and abducted
     - 4: Full flexion of arms and legs.
2. *Square window:* The examiner uses his/her thumb to gently press the infant's wrist and palm toward the infant's forearm. Either the angle that the wrist and the third and fourth fingers make against the forearm or the angle that the wrist and thumb make against the forearm is used for scoring.
3. *Arm recoil:* With the infant in supine position both the forearms are flexed at chest level for 5 seconds,

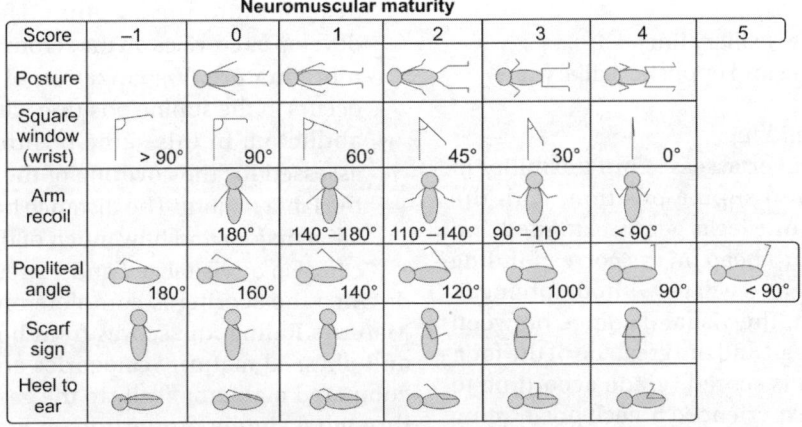

Figure 40.11: New Ballard score (NBS).
(*Source:* Ballard J. New Ballard, expended to include extremely premature infants. Journal of Pediatrics. 1991;119:417).

then fully extended by pulling on the hands and then released. After release from extension, the amount of return to original position is observed and scored. The sign is fully positive (4) if the arms return briskly to full flexion. If the arms return to incomplete flexion or the response is sluggish, it is graded less (1–3). If they remain extended or only followed by random movements, the score is 0.

4. *Popliteal angle:* This is the assessment of the angle created when the knee is extended. The infant is assessed in the supine position with the pelvis flat and the thigh of one leg resting on the abdomen while the knee is extended by exerting upward pressure on the heel of the leg with the examiner's right index finger behind the angle until resistance is met. The popliteal angle is measured.
5. *Scarf sign:* In the supine position, the infant's hand is grasped between the thumb and first finger of the nurse's hand and, in one sweeping movement, the nurse attempts to place the hand on the opposite shoulder. Using a finger, the nurse marks on the infant's chest where the elbow of the infant falls and the scores in this category is made accordingly:
   - Elbow reaches opposite axillary line
   - Elbow between midline and opposite axillary line
   - Elbow reaches midline
   - Elbow will not reach midline.
6. *Heel to ear:* This maneuver assesses hip flexibility in infants. With the baby in supine position, with the pelvis on a flat surface, one leg is gently extended and moved toward the infant's head on the corresponding side as near to the head as it will go without forcing it. When resistance is met, the visual distance between the ear on the infant's head and the great toe of the foot, along with leg position is scored (grade according to diagram). Infants who experienced breech positioning or who are suspected of having developmental dysplasia of the hip may show a great amount of flexibility (**Fig. 40.11**).

Assessment of Physical Maturity

1. *Skin:* Scoring in this category is based on palpation and visual inspection. Skin texture, transparency, relative thickness and flaking and peeling of the epidermis are noted. Transparency, defined as skin through which veins can be seen, is evident in premature (preterm) infants and disappears with increasing maturity. Flaking of skin and peeling with wrinkles occur in post-term infants.
2. *Lanugo:* Lanugo is the fine hair seen mostly on the back and arms of premature infants. It eventually thins out in the lumbar region and disappears, leaving small traces on shoulders. Lanugo is lighter in color and softer than body hair and curls at the end.
3. *Palmar surface:* Creases on the soles of both feet are scored according to the extent to which the creases cover the soles. The best way to visualize the extent of plantar creases is to gently curl the infant's toes toward the heel and determine the score.
4. *Breast:* The amount of breast tissue is approximated by gently measuring the tissue present on the infant using a measuring tape in millimeters or by grasping the tissue between the examiner's thumb and forefinger. In addition, the bud and areola are inspected for size and stippling (shade of color). Lastly, the area of breast tissue is palpated to determine its elevation from the chest wall.
5. *Eye and ear:* Eyelids should be open and should open easily in the mature infant. Ears are inspected for incurving of the pinna and palpated for a determination of the thickness of cartilage. The upper lobe recoil is performed bilaterally to validate the return to the posterior upright position when moved anteriorly and inferiorly.
6. *Genitalia:* Both male and female genitalia are assessed with the infant in the supine position and the legs abducted. At about 35 weeks' gestational age, the testes descend into the scrotum. Deep creases gradually develop as crevices on the scrotum as the infant becomes more mature. Visualization of a pendulous scrotum occurs in the supine position with the lower extremities abducted. In this same position, female infants are assessed for the covering of the clitoris and the size of the labia majora. The distance between the edges of the labia majora and how much of the genitalia are covered can also be visualized and scored.

Once the scoring is complete on the Ballard Newborn Maturity Rating, the scores from both the neuromuscular and physical maturity categories are totaled. This score is compared mathematically to the gestational age (in weeks) through a simple proportionate formula that equates the score range with the gestational age in weeks and calculates the exact position of score within that range. An infant determined to be less than 37 weeks' gestational age is called preterm or premature. An infant whose score falls between 37 weeks and 42 weeks' gestational age is called term, and an infant that has scored beyond 42 weeks' gestation is called post-term.

DAILY CARE AND OBSERVATION OF THE NEWBORN

The daily assessment is important for identification of early problems. If the initial assessment supports that the infant is normal, the following should be done daily.

Minor disorders that are most common among newborns are detected during daily observations and assessment is discussed in **Table 40.1**.

Check Vital Signs

1. Respirations are to be regular, smooth and quiet, the rate about 40 breaths per minute.

TABLE 40.1: Minor disorders of newborn.

Sl. No.	Minor problem	Treatment
1.	**Erythema toxicum (newborn rash).** Skin rashes consisting of small, red, flat or raised lesions seen on chest, abdomen, back and buttocks of newborn (**Fig. 40.13**)	No specific treatment needed. It will disappear within first two weeks
2.	**Milia** Yellow, pin-point size lesions seen on the bridge of the nose, chin or cheeks. These are distended sebaceous glands in the skin	The lesions will disappear after few weeks. No treatment needed
3.	**Telangiectic nevi (stork bite/angel kisses)** Dilation of capillary vessels and minute arteries; seen at the nape of neck, extending over to the lower occipital area, between the eye brows, on upper eyelids and around the nose (*refer* **Fig. 39.5**)	The lesion blanches when pressed and gradually fades when the baby grows
4.	**Mongolian spots** Aggregations of melanin rich dark cells. Purple or bluish dark areas of discoloration mostly present over the sacrum and coccygeal area of a large percentage and seen over back, buttocks, and extremities (*refer* **Fig. 39.8**)	No treatment needed. The discoloration disappears as the child grows
5.	**Nevus flammeus (port-wine stain)** Smooth, flat, superficial angioma (dilated blood vessels) that vary in size from a few millimeters to an area that covers most of the face and neck, things or abdomen (*refer* **Fig. 39.7**)	These do not fade with time
6.	**Epstein epithelial pearls** Small epithelial inclusion cysts. These appear as whitish spots on the hard palate or along the alveolar ridge	No treatment is required
7.	**Bednar's aphthae** Small ulcers on mucus membrane, usually located in hard palate posteriorly and generally bilateral. May be caused by rigorous sucking	Condition will disappear by itself
8.	**Conjunctivitis (sticky eyes)** Eyes red with purulent exudates. Eyelids are swollen. Onset occurs within 24 hours of birth and lasts for about 24 days. It may occur due to silver nitrate drops instilled after birth or bacterial conjunctivitis	Cleaning the eyelids with cotton balls socked in warm saline solution and use of erythromycin (0.5%) every 6 hours for 7–10 days will cure the condition
9.	**Stuffy nose** Mouth breathing and excessive air swallowing which in turn may lead to abdominal distension and vomiting	The nostrils may be cleaned with cotton socked with normal saline
10.	**Napkin rash (ammonium dermatitis)** The perianal skin becomes red, indurated and excoriated due to the dermatitis. More common in artificially fed babies	Frequent care and attention to the napkin area and changing of napkin at regular intervals
11.	**Perianal dermatitis** Seen around the anal opening. Occurs due to the alkalinity of the stool and is common in artificially fed babies	Use of lactose instead of glucose in feed
12.	**Oral thrush** It manifests as white patches with erythematous margins distributed over tongue and buccal mucosa. The patches of thrush are adherent and they often bleed if attempted to remove (**Fig. 40.12**)	Local application of 0.5% aqueous solution of gentian violet or nystatin suspension (100,000 units/ml) applied to each side of mouth with a cotton tipped swab 3–4 times a day is effective
13.	**Congenital hydrocele** Collection of fluid in the testicular structure. This is due to hormone withdrawal	No specific treatment is needed. It will usually disappear. Incision and drainage can be done
14.	**Genital crisis** This include mastitis neonatorum, hydrocele, vaginal bleeding, and vaginal mucoidal secretions due to withdrawal of maternal hormone after birth	It does not need any treatment. It will disappear with local aseptic cleaning of genitalia. If breast engorgement is present, there is no need to squeeze or to express milk

2. Temperature to be taken in the axilla, ear (tympanic membrane) or in the groin every 4–6 hours.

Weight

Weight is to be checked daily and evaluated according to birth weight. Weight loss is normal in the first few days, but more than 10% body weight loss is abnormal. Most babies regain birth weight in 7–10 days, thereafter gaining weight at a rate of 150–200 g per week.

General Changes in Color and Activity

Any cyanosis should be reported to the pediatrician immediately. Jaundice may be noted from the 3rd day and is abnormal if it rises earlier, deepens or persists beyond the 7th day.

Feeding Status

The amount taken and difficulties, if any, are to be observed and recorded.

Head

Assessment of the anterior fontanel, which should be level, resolution of caput succedaneum and molding, and identification of any new swelling such as cephalohematoma to be done.

Mouth

Should be clean and moist. Adherent white plaques indicate oral thrush infection **(Fig. 40.12)**.

Umbilical Cord

The umbilical cord base is inspected and cleaned daily.

Elimination

The stools are observed and compared with expectations in relation to the baby's age and feeding method. Constipation, loose stools or sore buttocks may be observed and noted. The frequency of passing urine and stools in the past 24 hours should be noted.

Bath

Cleansing the skin may be done daily or as frequently as required, specially the face, skin flexures and napkin area, to prevent excoriation. A daily bath is recommended if the baby is at home. As the baby is undressed, the skin is inspected for rashes, septic spots or abrasions. Skin rashes, such as erythema toxicum may alarm the mother, although it is of little significance **(Fig. 40.13)**.

Parent-infant Interaction

The baby is kept in a cot/crib by the bedside of the mother (rooming-in). This practice helps to establish the mother-baby relationship and to become conversant with the art of baby care when she goes home with the baby.

■ VACCINATION AND IMMUNIZATION

Immunization is essential as it is important for prevention of childhood diseases and disabilities and is thus a basic need for all children. This starts in the early neonatal period itself where early protection is desirable.

Immunization or vaccines are an important way to protect babies from life-threatening diseases. Vaccines are among the safest and most effective preventive measures. The National Immunization Schedule (NIS) for Infants, Children and Pregnant mothers, published in 2022 is given in **Table 40.2**.

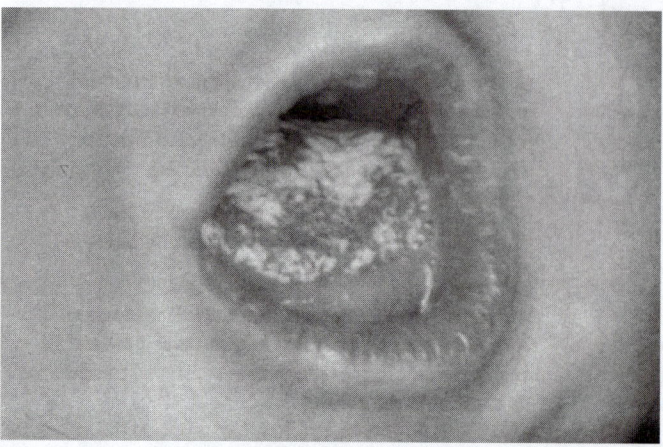

Figure 40.12: Oral thrush *(For color version, see Plate 5)*.

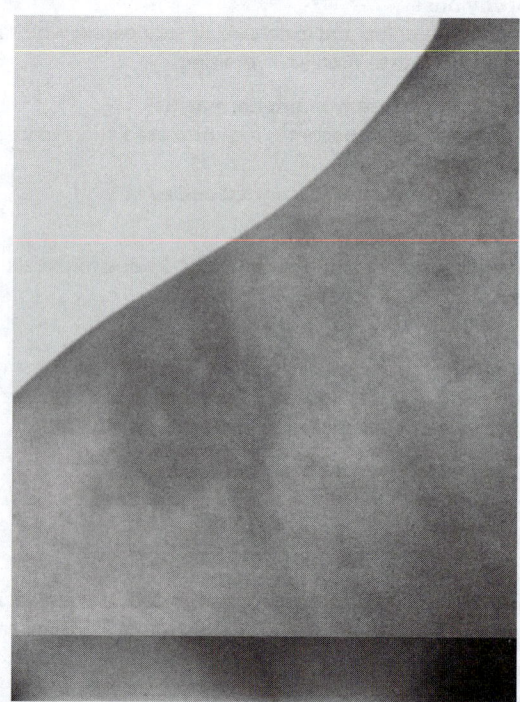

Figure 40.13: Erythema toxicum *(For color version, see Plate 5)*.

TABLE 40.2: National Immunization Schedule (NIS) for Infants, Children and Pregnant Women, 2022.

Vaccine	When to give	Dose	Route	Site
For pregnant women				
TT-1	Early in pregnancy	0.5 mL	Intramuscular	Upper arm
TT-2	4 weeks after TT-1	0.5 mL	Intramuscular	Upper arm
TT- Booster	If received 2 TT doses in a pregnancy within the last 3 years	0.5 mL	Intramuscular	Upper arm
For infants				
BCG	At birth or as early as possible till one year of age	0.1 mL (0.05 mL until 1 month age)	Intradermal	Left upper arm
Hepatitis B - Birth dose	At birth or as early as possible within 24 hours	0.5 mL	Intramuscular	Antero-lateral side of mid-thigh
OPV-0	At birth or as early as possible within the first 15 days	2 drops	Oral	Oral
OPV 1, 2 and 3	At 6 weeks, 10 weeks and 14 weeks (OPV can be given till 5 years of age)	2 drops	Oral	Oral
Pentavalent 1, 2 and 3	At 6 weeks, 10 weeks and 14 weeks (can be given till one year of age)	0.5 mL	Intramuscular	Antero-lateral side of mid-thigh
Rotavirus	At 6 weeks, 10 weeks and 14 weeks (can be given till one year of age)	5 drops	Oral	Oral
IPV	Two fractional dose at 6 and 14 weeks of age	0.1 mL	Intra dermal two fractional dose	Intradermal: Right upper arm
Measles /MR (1st dose)	9 completed months–12 months (can be given till 5 years of age)	0.5 mL	Subcutaneous	Right upper arm
JE - 1	9 completed months–12 months	0.5 mL	Subcutaneous	Left upper arm
Vitamin A (1st dose)	At 9 completed months with measles Rubella	1 mL (1 lakh IU)	Oral	Oral
For children				
DPT booster-1	16–24 months	0.5 mL	Intramuscular	Antero-lateral side of mid-thigh
Measles/ MR (2nd dose)	16–24 months	0.5 mL	Subcutaneous	Right upper arm
OPV Booster	16–24 months	2 drops	Oral	Oral
JE-2	16–24 months	0.5 mL	Subcutaneous	Left upperarm
Vitamin A (2nd to 9th dose)	16–18 months. Then one dose every 6 months up to the age of 5 years.	2 mL (2 lakh IU)	Oral	Oral
DPT Booster-2	5–6 years	0.5 mL	Intramuscular	Upper arm
TT	10 years and 16 years	0.5 mL	Intramuscular	Upper arm

(Source: www:/nhm.gov.in)

Nursing Responsibilities for Child Immunization

Nursing personnel are mostly responsible for administration of immunization and its related activities in collaboration with other health team members. The nursing personnel should shoulder the responsibility to organize the immunization sessions and to ensure the achievement of universal immunization. Administration of vaccine is the main assignment but other related activities are also vital for success of immunization program. The nursing responsibilities at various levels can be summarized as follows:

- Motivation of people about the importance of immunization and its benefits
- Estimation of beneficiaries of the area and identification of nonparticipants and drop outs of immunization
- Assessment of problems and reasons for non-acceptance of immunization and intervening to solve their problems
- Providing information, health education and communication sessions regarding time, place, available vaccines and other health facilities related to immunization

- Organization of immunization clinics at different institutions, immunization camps, out-reach and home-based services
- Arrangements and maintenance of required amount of vaccines and other necessary equipment and materials for the particular immunization center/clinic
- Maintenance of cold-chain system at immunization center/during transportation of vaccines to home/clinics with necessary precautions to preserve the efficiency and potency of vaccines
- Administration of vaccines in accordance with the basic nursing skills and instructions related to use of specific vaccines
- Observation of possible reactions after vaccination and providing necessary instructions about care of the child following immunization, to the parent and family
- Providing information about the next date of visit to complete the immunization as per schedule and dangers of default
- Maintenance of immunization card with required information and next date of visit
- Reporting about immunization coverage and problems of the particular area
- Updating own knowledge regarding advancement of immunization practices and changing attitudes.

STUDY QUESTIONS

Short Notes

1. Moro reflex.
2. Tonic neck reflex.
3. Palmar reflex.
4. Stepping reflex.
5. Babinski's reflex.

Short Answer Questions

1. Reflexes of the mouth in a newborn.
2. Sleeping and awakening status in a newborn.

Essay Question

1. Explain the daily care and observation of a newborn baby.

BIBLIOGRAPHY

1. Ballard JL, Khoury JC, Wedig K, et al. New Ballard Score expanded to include extremely premature infants. Journal of Pediatrics. 1991;119(3):417-23.
2. Blackburn ST, Loper DL. Maternal, Fetal and neonatal physiology: a clinical perspective. Philadelphia: WB Saunders; 1992.
3. Brazelton TB. Neonatal behavioral assessment scale, 2nd edition. Spastics International Medical Publications. London: Blackwell Scientific; 1984.
4. Clausen, Flook, Ford. Maternity nursing today. New York: McGraw-Hill Book Co; 1973.
5. De Casper A, Fifer W. Of human bonding: newborns prefer their mother's voices. In: Oates J (Ed). Cognitive Development in Infancy. Hove: Lawrence Erlbaum Associates; 1987.
6. Downey J, Bidder RT. Perinatal information on infant crying. Child Care Health and Development. 1990;16(2):113-21.
7. Lynna LY, John EC. Maternity nursing care. New York: Thomson, Delmar Learning; 2007.
8. Michie MM. The normal baby. In: Bennett RV, Linda KB (Eds). Myles Textbook for Midwives, 13th Edition. Edinburgh: Churchill Livingstone; 1999. pp. 685-704.
9. National Immunization Schedule, National Health Mission. https://nhm.gov.in.
10. Perry SE. The newborn. In: Bobak IM (Ed). Maternal Child Nursing Care, 4th edition. St Louis: Mosby; 1995.
11. Rushforth JA, Levene MI. Behavioural response to pain in healthy neonates. Archives of disease in Childhood. 1994;70(3):F174.

CHAPTER 41

Infant Feeding

Learning Objectives

Upon completing this chapter, the learner will be able to:
- Describe the structure and functions of female breast.
- Outline the properties and components of breast milk.
- Describe the role of midwife in ensuring successful breastfeeding.
- Discuss the different causes of difficulty with breast-feeding.
- Discuss the principles of bottle feeding and the foods used.

BREASTS AND LACTATION

The breasts are secreting glands, composed of 15–24 *lobes*, separated from one another by fatty tissue. These lobes are divided into lobules, each lobule containing a certain number of *alveoli* and ducts. The alveoli contain *acini cell*, which produce milk and are surrounded by myoepithelial cells, which propel the milk out into small ducts. These ducts connect with larger ones called *lactiferous ducts*. One large duct leaves each lobe and widens to form a *lactiferous sinus* or *ampulla* which acts as a temporary reservoir for milk. A *lactiferous tubule* from each sinus opens on the surface of the nipple **(Fig. 41.1)**.

The nipple which is composed of erectile tissue is covered with epithelium contains plain muscle fibers and have sphincter-like action in controlling the flow of milk. Surrounding the nipple is an area of pigmented skin called *areola*, which contains the Montgomery's glands. These produce a sebum-like substance, which acts as a lubricant during pregnancy and throughout breastfeeding. Breasts, nipples and areolae are varying considerably in size from one woman to another.

The mechanism of milk production and ejection, called *let-down*, is determined hormonally. During pregnancy, estrogens and progesterone induce alveolar and ductal growth as well as stimulate the secretion of colostrum. Other hormones are also involved and they govern a complex sequence of events, which prepare the breasts for lactation. The production of milk is held in abeyance until after delivery, when the levels of placental hormones fall. Immediately after the delivery of the placenta, these hormones diminish, thereby activating the anterior lobe of the pituitary to release prolactin which acts on the acini cells stimulating them to produce milk. This process which takes from 2 to 4 days, is enhanced by the sucking stimulus of the baby.

Prolactin is more important to the initiation of lactation than to its continuation. As lactation progresses, the prolactin response to suckling diminishes and milk removal (by the baby feeding or breast expression) becomes the driving force behind milk production. Oxytocin causes contraction of the myoepithelial cells as well as the uterine myometrial cells. In the early days of lactation, the let-down or milk ejection reflex is unconditioned and therefore likely to be inhibited by emotions. Later, it becomes a conditioned reflex responding to the baby's cry or other circumstances associated with the baby or feeding. Negative emotions such as fear, anger, anxiety and embarrassment as well as the presence of pain may inhibit the let-down reflex.

PROPERTIES AND COMPONENTS OF BREAST MILK

Breast milk is bluish white in color and appears to be very watery. It is high in both lactose and fat, but low in protein and phosphate. The composition is reversed in its precursor, colostrum, which is normally found in the alveoli during the later phase of pregnancy. Colostrum, a yellowish fluid, which is high in antibodies, is an excellent food for the baby during 2–3 days before the milk comes in.

Breast milk varies in its composition with the time of day, the stage of lactation and in response to maternal nutrition. It meets all the nutritional requirements of the new baby and has many other important properties as well.

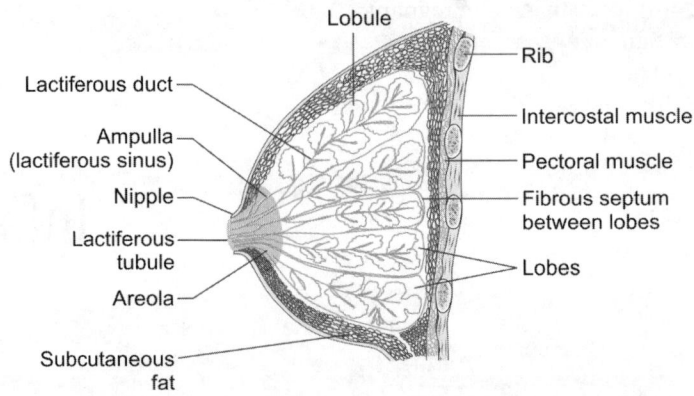

Figure 41.1: A cross-section of the lactating breast.

Fat

Fat in breast milk provides the baby with more than 50% of caloric requirements. The fat content is lowest in the morning and highest in the afternoon, and the proportion increases during the course of the feed. It is utilized very rapidly due to the action of the enzyme lipase which is present in the milk.

Lactose

Lactose in breast milk is converted into galactose and glucose by the action of the enzyme lactase, and these sugars provide energy to the rapidly growing brain. Lactose enhances the absorption of calcium and promotes the growth of lactobacilli which increase the intestinal acidity.

Protein

Protein in breast milk is much less compared to any other mammalian milk, which makes it thinner. Breast milk is whey dominant and forms soft, flocculent curds when acidified in the stomach. This provides a continuous flow of nutrients to the baby. Colostrum contains nearly three times the amount of protein that is present in mature milk and contains all amino acids. It also contains secretory immunoglobulin A (IgA) and lactoferrin.

Fat-soluble Vitamins

Mature breast milk contains vitamin A, D, E and K. For bloodclotting factors vitamin K is essential and the baby's gut flora synthesizes adequate amounts only after 2 weeks of birth. All babies are given vitamin K soon after birth to meet the need until colonization of the gut occurs.

Water-soluble Vitamins

All of the B vitamins are present at levels necessary for daily requirement. Vitamin C which is required for collagen synthesis is also present in adequate quantity if the mother eats a good diet.

Minerals and Trace Elements

Although the amounts of iron are less than those found in formula, the bioavailability of iron found in breast milk is very much higher; 70% of iron found in breast milk is absorbed, whereas only 10% is absorbed from formula. Babies who are fed on fresh cow's milk or formula need iron supplements to prevent anemia. Preterm babies do not have good iron stores and may need supplementation with oral iron. Breast milk contains zinc, calcium, phosphorus, sodium and potassium in quantities lesser than in formula. However, the higher bioavailability of these minerals and trace elements ensure that the infant's needs are met.

Anti-infective Factors

Breast milk has the following anti infective agents which are protective for the newborn:

1. Leukocytes (macrophages and neutrophils) that surround and destroy harmful bacteria by their phagocytic activity.
2. Secretory IgA and interferon produced by lymphocytes in breast milk.
3. Immunoglobulin IgA, IgG, IgM and IgD are all found in breast milk. It 'paints' the intestinal epithelium and protects the mucosal surface against entry of pathogenic bacteria and enteroviruses.
4. Lysozyme, a general anti-infective agent.
5. Lactoferrin that prevents pathogenic *Escherichia coli* from obtaining the iron which they need for survival.
6. The bifidus factor promotes the growth of gram-positive bacilli in the gut flora particularly, *Lactobacillus bifidus*, which discourages the multiplication of pathogens.

MANAGEMENT OF BREASTFEEDING

Antenatal Preparation

The majority of women decide when they conceive that they want to breastfeed their babies. Some may not take a decision early. However, it is important to teach all pregnant women about the benefits of breastfeeding. Preparation for breastfeeding must begin when pregnancy starts altering the breasts and nipples. A comfortable brassiere that does not compress the breast may be worn to support the increasing weight. Daily cleansing with water and a soft clean cloth followed by careful drying must be done. If nipples are inverted or flat, the procedure of nipple rolling must be explained to the mother. With lightly lubricated thumb and index finger, the mother will need to roll the nipple of each breast for approximately 30 seconds everyday in the 9th month. If the mother understands how the milk is produced and how much her baby will be benefited from breastfeeding, she may well succeed with feeding her baby.

Commencement of Breastfeeding

The first feed is a profoundly important experience for the mother and her baby. Unless individual circumstances indicate otherwise, the mother should have her baby with her immediately after delivery and breastfeeding should begin as soon as possible. The time of first feed, depend largely on the needs of the baby. Some babies demonstrate a need to feed almost as soon as they are born. Other babies show no interest until they are an hour or so old.

Whenever the first feed takes place, the quality of that experience is of utmost importance for the mother and baby. The early feedings might best consist of approximately 5–10 minutes suckling on each breast, while the nipples are accustomed to it. This frequent suckling stimulates the production and let-down of lactation and reduces the potential severity of engorgement. Therefore, it is essential that there be no missed feedings, including those at night.

Preparation and Position of the Mother

The mother should be prepared for each feeding. She should be:
1. In a comfortable position, this means any position that is comfortable for her and allows for proper positioning of her baby. This can be accomplished in a side lying, reclining or sitting position **(Figs. 41.2A to E)**. Generous use of pillows for support and comfort is most useful.
2. Without discomfort or pain. Her bladder should be empty. Any pain such as afterbirth pains, episiotomy or laceration repair pain should have received comfort measures prior to breastfeeding time.
3. Rested and relaxed.
4. Assured of available help as necessary.
5. Her hands should be washed and nipples cleansed with plain water.

Preparation and Position of the Baby

The baby's immediate preparation for breastfeeding is to have a clean, dry diaper and if necessary, to be swaddle wrapped. Swaddle wrapping **(Figs. 41.3A to D)** when properly done, may be comforting rather than confining to babies because they feel held close and secure rather than bound. The wrapping is to be loose enough for freedom of motion of the legs. What has to be achieved is control of waving arms. For new mothers who will need this initially, it will be just a few feedings before they can cope without swaddle wrapping their baby.

Position the baby so that he/she will not be doubled up or have a twisted neck when sucking and that the head and body are supported. In bringing the baby and breast together, the following are helpful:

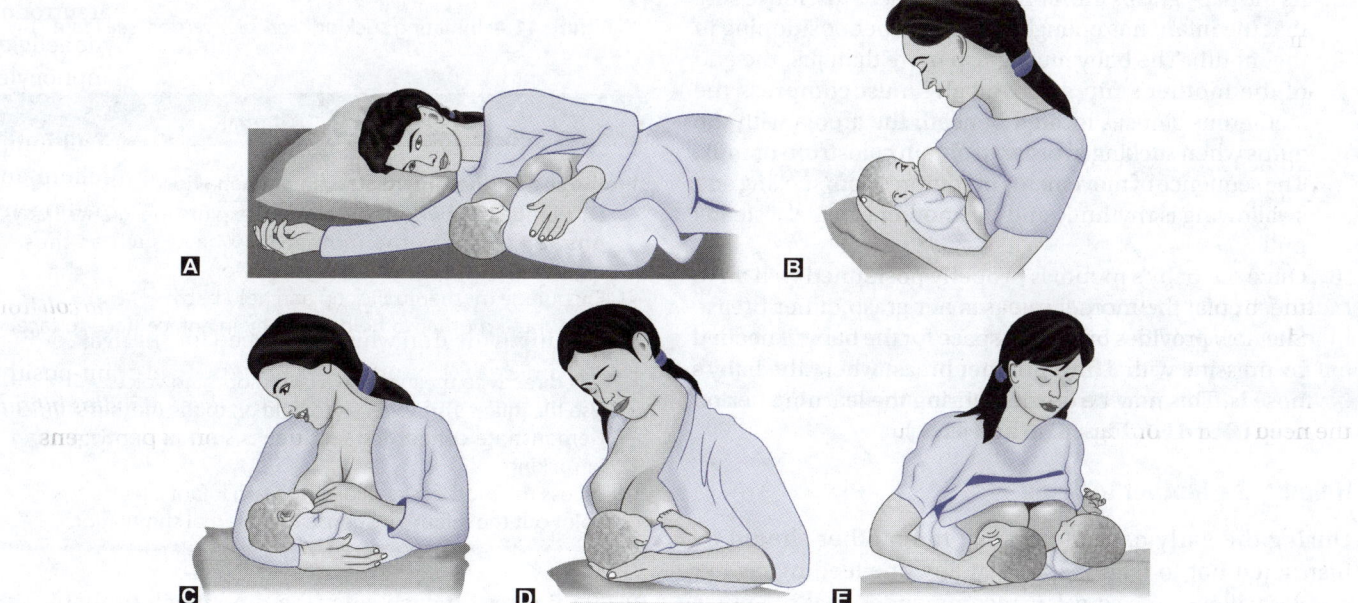

Figures 41.2A to E: Feeding positions. (A) Feeding lying down; (B) Holding baby across the lap supporting with opposite arm; (C) Holding baby across the lap supporting with same side arm; (D) Holding baby underarm, sitting on side of bed; (E) Positioning twin babies underarm. *(For color version, see Plate 6).*

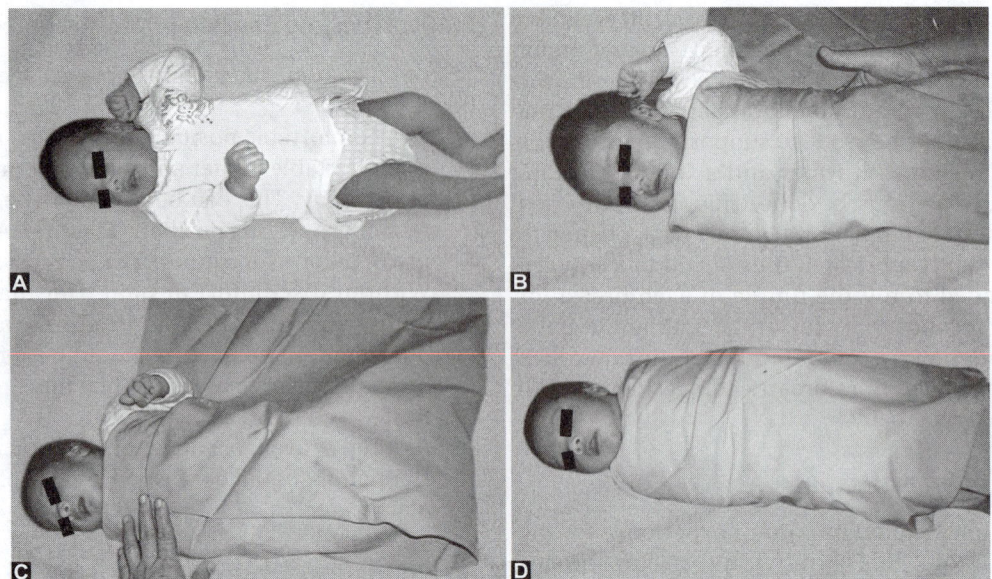

Figures 41.3A to D: Swaddle wrapping. (A) Baby placed on a baby sheet corner to corner with head end of the sheet folded at neck level; (B) One end of sheet taken over body to opposite side and tucked with one arm inside; (C) Foot end of sheet folded over baby's body; (D) Remaining end of sheet taken over body and tucked with second arm inside *(For color version, see Plate 6)*.

1. Let the baby find the breast and grasp the nipple. Do not thrust the breast in the baby's face, as this is frightening to the baby.
2. Help the mother learn to hold her breast in such a way as to guide and control the breast and facilitate the baby's grasping of it.
3. Touch the baby's cheek with the nipple so the baby will turn towards the breast (use of the rooting reflex).
4. Express a few drops of colostrum/milk so they are on the surface of the nipple. This provides the baby with instant gratification and reinforces learning **(Fig. 41.4)**.
5. As the baby grasps the nipple, the mother must make sure that the infant has enough of it for proper positioning in the mouth. The baby must grasp more than just the end of the mother's nipple. The baby must compress the lactiferous sinuses located beneath the areola with the gums when sucking in order to obtain colostrum or milk. The sequence of movements of compression, sucking and swallowing is rhythmic and the mother can feel a steady pull.
6. Once the baby's mouth is properly positioned well on to the areola, the mother releases her grasp of her breast. She now provides breathing space for the baby, if needed by pressing with a finger on her breast where the baby's nose is. This may be needed during the learning period only **(Box 41.1, Figs. 41.5 and 41.6)**.

Helping the Mother to Begin

During the early days of nursing, the mother should be instructed not to feed too long at any one feeding, as her nipples will become sore. It is recommended that she nurse from 3 to 5 minutes at every feeding during the 1st day, from 5 to 7 minutes during the 2nd day, and from 7 to 10 minutes during the 3rd day. In a week, she should be able to nurse

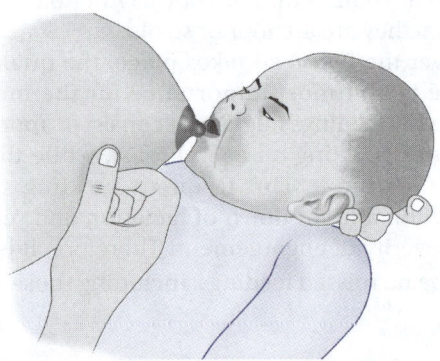

Figure 41.4: Initiating sucking *(For color version, see Plate 7)*.

BOX 41.1: Nursing alert.

Promoting mother-infant attachment behavior
- Encourage to unwrap the infant and explore the infant's body
- Answer concerns the mother may have such as those regarding cord care or feeding behavior
- Encourage mother to pick up and hold baby
- Encourage mother to hold her baby in enface (face to face) position
- Talk directly to the infant in a calm, soothing voice
- Use the infant's grasp reflex to hold on to the mother's finger.
- Demonstrate comforting techniques such as gentle patting or rocking
- Assess the mother's readiness to learn infant care
- Point out the infant's response to maternal stimulation

10–20 minutes on each side (the time it will probably take to empty it).

If the infant is crying hard when she wants to start breastfeeding, she should first calm the baby by holding firmly

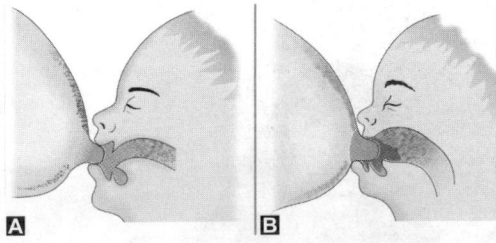

Figures 41.5A and B: Technique of breastfeeding. (A) Baby feels the nipple at his lips; (B) Nipple is sucked into the mouth.

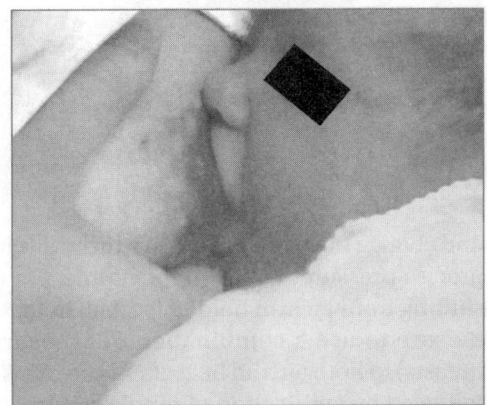

Figure 41.6: Baby's lips in contact with areola
(For color version, see Plate 7).

and closely, and by talking gently to him/her. An upset baby who is put to breast does not realize the nipple is in the mouth and will continue to cry loudly which may upset the mother and frustrate the baby. Once the baby is calm, he will be able to grasp the nipple and begin sucking.

The mother should nurse from both breasts at each feeding, alternating the side on which she begins. A suggestion to help the mother remember which side to start on at the next feeding is to have her put a safety pin in the bra strap on the side on which she will begin to nurse the next time. The baby should nurse on both sides because he sucks hardest on the first side and gets about 90% of the milk in that breast during the first 5–10 minutes of nursing. Using both breasts provides the necessary stimulus to keep up a sufficient amount of milk production in the breasts. This is especially important during the early weeks of nursing.

Feeding Behaviors

Babies usually will suck a bit; rest a bit (maintaining their hold on the nipple, while they rest) and then suck some more. Some babies go to sleep once they get little food in their stomach and feel warm and comfortable next to the mother. The mother should be prepared for this, so she does not get upset. She can loosen the blankets around the baby, so that he is not quite so warm and drowsy during feeding. If this does not work, she may try any of the following—rub the soles of the baby's feet, stroke the abdomen or change the position. The mother should also be prepared for the strong uterine contraction; she will feel when the baby first latches on to her breast.

Suction must be broken before trying to remove the baby from the breast. Pulling the baby off causes injury to the nipple. Suction is broken by slipping a finger into the corner of the baby's gums. Once the suction is broken, the baby is easily removed from the breast without injury to the nipple. The baby is then burped and put to the other breast **(Figs. 41.7 and 41.8)**.

Lactation is established and maintained by a combination of the following:
- Starting breastfeeding as soon as possible after delivery
- Frequent feedings during the first few days using both breasts
- No missed feedings or supplementary feedings
- Rotation of breasts as the starting and ending breasts to provide for complete emptying of both breasts
- Rested, relaxed and pain-free mother during feeding times
- Baby properly positioned on the breast.

The baby's neck should be slightly extended and the chin should be in contact with the breast. A generous portion of areola should be taken in by the lower jaw.

Timing and Frequency of Feeding

It is usual in the 1st or 2nd day for the baby to have 6–8 hours gaps between good feeds. This is normal and provides an excellent opportunity for the mother to rest. As the milk volume increases, the feeds become more frequent and a little shorter. After the first few days, the baby will settle into his/her individual pattern of feeding frequency. This is described as 'self-demand feeding' or 'baby-led feeding' (i.e. feeding the baby when he/she is hungry). It is unusual for a healthy baby to feed less often than six times in 24 hours from the 3rd day. If he demands fewer feeds, the reasons should be investigated. Individual mother-baby pairs develop their own unique pattern of feeding and provided the baby is thriving, there is no need to change it.

Care of the Breasts

1. Daily washing is necessary for breast hygiene. The normal skin flora is beneficial to the baby. Using soap, alcohol or other drying agents can lead quickly to cracking of the

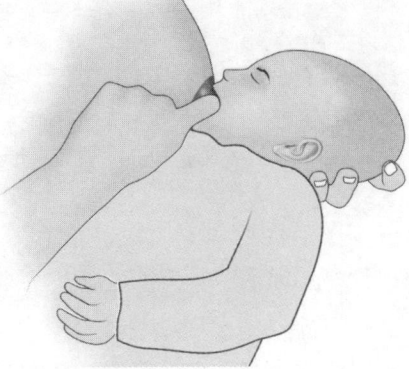

Figure 41.7: Breaking suction before removing the baby from breast
(For color version, see Plate 7).

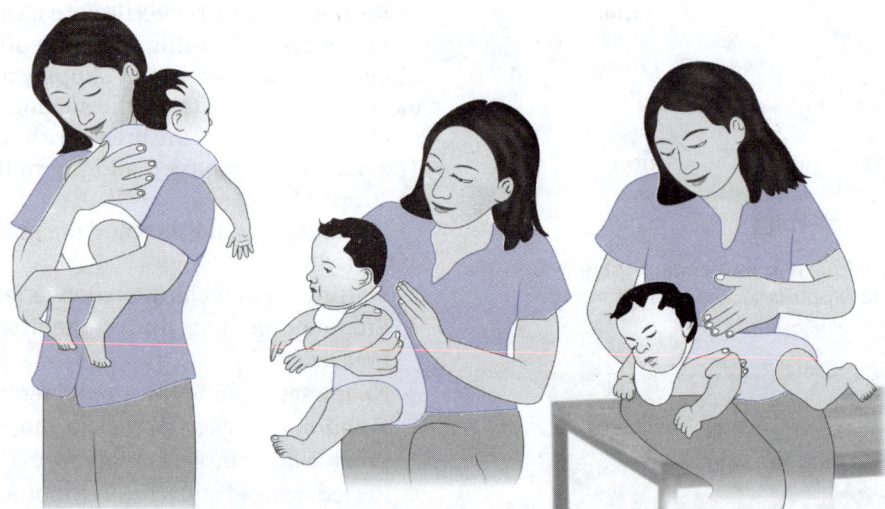

Figure 41.8: Burping positions *(For color version, see Plate 7).*

nipples. Providing good support to breasts is important to avoid discomfort.

2. If the breasts become engorged, apply warmth to breasts, prior to each breastfeeding, to promote milk flow. This can be accomplished with warm washcloths or warm showers **(Fig. 41.9)**.
3. If there is areolar enlargement; manual expression of the milk to soften the area prior to nursing the baby will help the baby latch on to the nipple properly and easily.
4. Use manual expression of milk to empty the breasts after the baby has nursed, if they are still uncomfortably full and engorged after the feeding.
5. Ice bags may be applied to breasts between feedings to reduce swelling and pain.
6. If the nipples become tender:
    a. Nurse on the less sore nipple first until there is let-down, then switch the baby to the sore nipple to empty that breast and meet the baby's sucking needs.
    b. Use a pacifier rather than the end of feedings on the nipples to meet the baby's sucking needs until the nipples are not sore.
    c. Breastfeed more frequently for shorter periods.
    d. Be sure the baby is properly positioned on the breast and change the baby's position which will change the precise pressure points on the nipple. For example, shifting from an arm hold to football hold.
    e. Be sure to use a combination of exposure (of the breasts) to both air and heat after each breastfeeding, followed by application of nipple cream.
7. Be sure to break the suction before removing the baby from the breast.

Benefits of Breastfeeding

To the Mother

There are well known and documented physiological benefits to the breastfeeding mother:

1. Studies conducted on women of various cultures have shown that women who breastfeed have markedly decreased chance of developing breast cancer.
2. The incidence of thrombophlebitis is lower in breastfeeding mothers.
3. Postpartum uterine involution is more rapid in mothers who breastfeed. Therefore, delayed postpartum hemorrhage is also less common.
4. Lactation has been shown to suppress ovulation for about 75 days postpartum in almost 100% of women who do not supplement their infants with bottle. Thus, breastfeeding for a short time is a preferred contraceptive.

To the Baby

1. Breast milk is of ideal composition for easy digestion with low osmotic load.
2. Colostrum and breast milk provide antibody protection (passive immunity) against several types of viruses.
3. Breastfed babies show a marked decrease in respiratory infections and gastroenteritis. Lysozyme, an enzyme present in breast milk destroys invasive organisms, especially *E. coli*. Additional resistance to the gut from invading organisms is given by lactoferrin and bifidus factor and secretory IgA contained in breast milk.

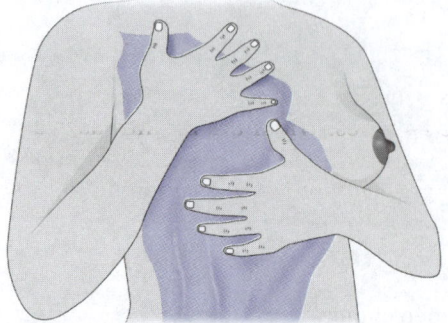

Figure 41.9: Applying warm towel to engorged breast *(For color version, see Plate 7).*

4. Allergic disorders, such as infantile eczema, asthma and hay fever are much less common in breastfed babies.
5. Since the weight gain of a breastfed baby is less than that of a bottle-fed one, obesity is less common.
6. Breastfeeding offers a psychological benefit by establishing healthy mother-baby relationship.
7. Breast milk is readily available for the baby at the right temperature.

Volume of the Feed

Well-grown infants are born with good glycogen reserve and high levels of antidiuretic hormone. Consequently, they do not need large volumes of milk or colostrum any sooner than they are made available physiologically. In the first 24 hours, the baby takes an average of 5 mL per feed; in the second 24 hours, this increases to 14 mL per feed.

The average requirement of milk is about 100 mL/kg/24 h on the 3rd day and is increased to 150 mL/kg/24 h by the 10th day.

Difficulties in Breastfeeding and Management

At times, breastfeeding causes some problems.

Difficulties due to Mother

* *Inadequate supply of milk:* The mother who says she does not have enough milk for her baby probably is not nursing often enough. The nurse should instruct the mother that the oftener the baby nurses, the more milk she will have. The milk supply is directly related to the frequency of nursing—the more often the baby nurses, the more milk is produced.
* *Baby who will not suck:* An infant who refuses to suck at the breast or who thrusts the tongue toward the roof of the mouth presents special problem. These babies will usually suck beautifully from a bottle nipple and therefore it is important not to supplement them with an artificial nipple. Expressed milk may be given by spoon or eyedropper. Milk can be dribbled down over the breast into the baby's mouth which might help baby to begin sucking from the breast.
* *Breast ailments such as engorgement of breast, cracked nipple, depressed nipple and mastitis:* For mastitis, she should consult the physician. Once treatment has begun, she will be able to nurse the baby (management of each condition is discussed earlier in this Chapter).
* *Anxiety and stress:* Anxiety, upset or emotional trauma influences milk ejection; therefore a mother who is not able to relax prior to nursing may find that her milk will not let-down. If possible, she should be encouraged to lie down, while nursing and concentrate on relaxing her baby. If lying down is not possible, she could sit down, put her feet up and perhaps read something. Her goal must be gearing her thoughts toward something other than the cause of upset.
* *Blistered nipple:* A blistered nipple is usually an indication of improper sucking by the baby. It most often is caused by the infant grasping only the nipple and not the areolar area. These blisters may bleed when they are broken. Ultraviolet light and resting the nipple for 24–48 hours are preferred methods of treatment.
* *Poor attachment of breast:* It leads to quick, shallow sucks instead of slow and deep. Areola remains outside the mouth. This causes nipple pain. Assistance and instructions from the midwife can improve the technique of breastfeeding. Proper placement of the nipple is on top of the baby's tongue with as much of the areolar space as possible in mouth.
* *Short nipples:* As the baby has to form a teat from both the breast and nipple, short nipples can cause problems and the mother should be reassured of this.
* *Abnormally large nipples:* If the baby is small, his/her mouth may not be able to get beyond the nipple and on to the breast. Lactation could be initiated by expressing the milk. As the baby grows and the breast and nipple become more protractile, breastfeeding may become possible.
* *Inverted and flat nipples:* Many babies are able to attach to the breast, even if the nipple is considered unfavorable. In difficult cases, it may be necessary to initiate lactation by expressing and delay attempting to attach the baby to the breast until lactation is established and the breasts have become soft and the breast tissue more protractile.

Difficulties due to Baby

* *Low birth weight baby:* The baby is too small or too feeble to suck. Tube feeding of expressed milk and artificial feeding are given until the baby becomes able to suck from breasts.
* *Temporary illness:* Such as cerebral irritation, respiratory tract infection and nasal obstruction due to congestion and lethargy due to jaundice or oral thrush may all lead to improper suckling. Due to lack of proper nipple stimulation and improper emptying, the milk may dry up. This must be recognized early and prevented.
* *Overdistention of the stomach with swallowed air:* The problem can be prevented by burping the baby several times during feeding.
* *Cleft palate:* The baby is unable to form a vacuum and thus form a teat out of the breast and nipple. Feeding expressed milk using special teat device can be done until the baby has had a surgical repair. Feeding with spoon can be another method.

Contraindications to Breastfeeding

1. Drugs used for cancer, certain hormones and radio-active isotopes. When the mother uses any of these, breastfeeding should be suspended.
2. The human immunodeficiency virus (HIV) infection may be transmitted in breast milk. In cases where artificial feeding is difficult, the mother may be counseled as regard the risks and benefits and helped to make an informed choice.
3. Chronic medical illness, such as decompensated organic heart lesion and pulmonary tuberculosis.

4. Puerperal psychosis.
5. Women receiving high doses of antiepileptic, anticoagulant and antithyroid drugs.
6. Breastfeeding may be suspended when the mother is treated with metronidazole and chloramphenicol.

Underfeeding and Overfeeding

Normal progress of feeding is evidenced by:
1. General condition—happy baby sleeps between feeds and at night, does not vomit and passes urine at least six times in 24 hours.
2. Vigor which is manifested by movements of the limbs and cry.
3. Expected level of weight gain.

Features of Underfeeding

- Failure of the infant to gain weight as per schedule, evidenced from the weight curve
- Dissatisfied baby evidenced by cry in between feeds and at night
- Constipation
- Scanty, high-colored urine.

Management is to substitute the lesser amount of milk by artificial feed.

Features of Overfeeding

Overfeeding usually occurs at the end of st week. The features are **(Box 41.2)**:
- Vomiting soon after feeding
- Frequent, loose, bulky stools with undigested curds and fat
- Excoriation over the buttocks
- Variable weight curve—excess, stationary or at times falling.

Management is to put the baby to breast for shorter periods. It may be helpful to give little sterile water prior to each feed.

BOX 41.2: Client education.

Breastfeeding for adequate milk supply
- Remember that the more milk the baby removes from the breasts, the more will be produced
- Expect to breast feed every 2–3 hours until the milk supply is established
- Do not skip feedings or supplement feedings. Night feedings are necessary to establish adequate milk supply for the first few weeks after delivery
- Breast feed for at least 15–20 minutes so that the baby will receive the rich hind milk
- Try to relax as often as possible and accept offers from family and friends for help
- Offer both breasts to the infant at every feeding
- Eat adequate healthy diet and drink plenty of fluid

Suppression of Lactation

If a mother chooses not to breastfeed or if has a late miscarriage; or stillbirth, lactation needs to be suppressed. The woman may experience discomfort for a day or two, but if unstimulated, the breasts will naturally cease to produce milk. In order to reduce discomfort the breasts must be supported with a breast binder. Suppression with hormones is effective, but carried the risk of thrombosis.

Complementary and Supplementary Feeds

Complementary feeds are given after giving the baby breastfeeds. Complementary feeds may become necessary for babies who are small for dates, lethargic, jaundiced or difficult to attach. Mothers may be instructed to give their expressed milk by bottle.

Supplementary feeds are given in place of breastfeeds. This is justified only in cases where the mother has severe illness, because each breastfeed missed by the baby will interfere with the establishment of lactation and damage the mother's confidence.

Baby-friendly Hospital Initiative

In 1992, United Nations International Children's Emergency Fund (UNICEF) and World Health Organization (WHO) launched the baby-friendly initiative amongst doctors, nurses, health workers and parents in hospitals and maternity centers to promote, protect and support breastfeeding. The objective is to re-establish the superiority of breastfeeding in order to protect the newborn's health by becoming baby friendly. In order to fulfill the initiative, the UNICEF and WHO laid down 10 steps to create the baby-friendly environment. These are:
- There must be a written breastfeeding policy
- All healthcare workers must be trained to implement this policy
- All pregnant women must be informed about the benefits of breastfeeding
- Mothers must be helped to initiate breastfeeding within half an hour of birth
- Mothers are shown the best way to breastfeed
- Unless medically indicated, the newborn should be given no food or drink other than breast milk
- To practice 'rooming in' by allowing mothers and babies to remain together 24 hours a day
- To encourage demand of breastfeeding
- To encourage exclusive breastfeeding
- No artificial teats should be given to babies
- Breastfeeding support groups are to be established and mothers must be referred to them on discharge.

A baby-friendly hospital should also provide other preventive health cares, e.g. infant immunization, rehydration salts against diarrheal dehydration and child's growth and development surveillance.

ARTIFICIAL FEEDING

When the infant is fed by any preparation other than breast milk, it is called artificial feeding. As artificial feeding is commonly accomplished by using a bottle, it is often called bottle feeding.

Indications of Artificial Feeding

- Contraindications of breastfeeding either temporary or permanent (as mentioned earlier)
- Inadequate quantity of breast milk
- Changing lifestyle of women (expressed breast milk may be an alternative).

Food Used

The kind of formula used varies. In general, boiled, diluted cow's milk, dried milk and milk formulas are commonly used. In some countries, goat's milk and buffalo's milk are used. Ready-to-use formulas in single use bottles are used in developed countries. However, there is no perfect substitute for breast milk.

Cow's Milk

Cow's milk when compared with human milk contains more protein and minerals, and less lactose and about the same amount of fat **(Table 41.1)**.

Qualitative differences

Though, the quantitative differences shown above can be rectified, some of the qualitative differences are difficult to approximate. *Sugar* content in both human and cow's milk is in the form of lactose, but as the concentration is higher in human milk, it is sweeter. *Fat proportion* in both milks is same, but the fat globules in the cow's milk are coarser and hence more difficult to digest than human milk. Protein of human milk contains two-third lactalbumin which is soluble and easily digestible and one-third caseinogen. The caseinogen content of the breast milk can be digested by the gastric juice with formation of flocculent curd (woolly), whereas in cow's milk, it is converted into heavy, tough casein curd causing indigestion. The sodium content of cow's milk is about four times higher than that of human milk which may lead to hypernatremia and the resulting thirst causes baby to cry.

Modification of cow's milk

Quantitative changes in the constituents in the cow's milk can be done by dilution followed by addition. One part of milk is added to one part of water. This reduces the protein content to half, while fat and sugar contents are reduced greatly. Sugar is added in the form of glucose or cane sugar to bring about readjustment in sugar content. Boiling changes the caseinogen and makes it easily digestible.

Preparation of a feed

Preparation of a feed for the infant should preferably be done each time prior to feeding. A formula that can be used is to divide the weight of the baby in pounds by two, which gives the amount of feed in ounces; 1½ ounces should be water and the remainder cow's milk. One teaspoon of cane sugar is to be added.

Example of preparation of a feed for an infant weighing 8 lbs:

Amount of feed = 4 ounces, which is made up of water 1½ ounces, milk 2½ ounces and cane sugar 1 teaspoon full.

The mixture is to be boiled in a clean saucepan to be followed by cooling before the baby is fed.

Dried Milk

Three varieties of dried milk are commercially available. Full cream dried milk, half cream dried milk and humanized dried milk. If full strength is to be used, one level scoop measure is added to 30 mL (1 ounce) of water. This gives the same composition and calorie value as that of cow's milk. When half strength is required, one level scoop measure is to be added to 60 mL.

Babies may be fed either by spoon from the bowl/cup or by feeding bottle. The cup and spoon are easy to clean. The feeding utensils (cup and spoon or bottle and teat) should be cleaned prior to and after each feeding. The rubber teat and bottle should be boiled once a day.

Preparation of the Mother for Artificial Feeding

1. Mothers who choose to feed their babies artificially should be shown how to prepare a bottle feed safely. If the mother and baby are at home, this demonstration should take place in her house, using her own articles. If she is in the hospital, she may be shown there.
2. Clear instructions about the volumes of milk/powder, water and sugar must be given so that she understands accurate measurements.
3. Effective cleaning of utensils must be explained. For boiling, full immersion is essential and the contents of the pan must be boiled for at least 5 minutes.
4. Rinsing of the bowl and spoon or bottle prior to feeding must be done using recently boiled water.
5. The mother should try to stimulate breastfeeding conditions for the baby by holding close and maintaining eye-to-eye contact.
6. The size of the hole in the teat should be of correct size. A useful test for the correct hole-size is to turn the bottle

TABLE 41.1: Composition of human and cow's milk.

Milk	Sugar	Fat	Protein	Minerals	Water	Calories
Human	7	3.5	1.2	0.4	89	67
Cow	4.5	3.5	3.4	0.8	88	67

upside down; the feed should drip at a rate of about one drop per second.
7. Burping of the baby should be done in the middle and at the end of each feed.
8. Not more than 20 minutes should be spent for each feed.
9. The mother should be warned about the dangers of 'bottle propping' and told that the baby must never be left unattended while feeding from a bottle.

WEANING FROM THE BREAST

Weaning is the period during which the baby gets accustomed to food other than its mother's milk. This period extends from 6th month to 1 year. During this period, the baby's demand is more, breast milk cannot supply the necessary need and as such, additional foods are required.

Breastfeeding should be stopped gradually. The mother may eliminate one breastfeeding a day and offer cup or bottle feeding at that time. In a few days, the mother may eliminate another nursing and feed the baby twice by cup or bottle or additional food. She should continue in this manner until her milk has dried up. Weaning may be completed by 10 months to 1 year.

Semi-solid foods, such as rice, dal, boiled fish, boiled egg and fruits such as banana are incorporated in the tropical countries. Problems usually encountered during the weaning period are nutritional disturbances and weaning diarrhea due to altered composition of the food.

STUDY QUESTIONS

Short Notes

1. Breast engorgement.
2. Complementary feeding.
3. Supplementary feeding.

Short Answer Questions

1. Preparation and position of mother for breastfeeding.
2. Benefits of breastfeeding to a baby.
3. Baby-friendly hospital initiative.
4. Underfeeding and overfeeding.

Essay Questions

1. Enumerate the preparation, positioning and related instructions to be given to a new mother for successful breastfeeding of her newborn.
2. Prepare a list of nursing diagnoses appropriate for breastfeeding mothers. Write a plan of care for any two.

BIBLIOGRAPHY

1. Applebaum RM. The modern management of successful breast feeding. Pediatr Clin North Am. 1970;17(1):203-25.
2. Clausen JP, et al. Maternity Nursing Today, 1st edition. New York: McGraw Hill; 1973. pp. 116-24.
3. Dutta DC. Textbook of Obstetrics, 5th edition. Kolkata: New Central Book Company; 2001. pp. 479-89.
4. Fisher C. Feeding. In: Bennett RV, Linda KB (Eds). Myles Textbook for Midwives, 13th edition. Edinburgh: Churchill Livingstone; 1999. pp. 685-706.
5. Helen V. Nurse-Midwifery, 2nd edition. Boston: Jones and Bartlett Publishers; 1996. pp. 411-22.
6. Moody J, Britten J, Hogg K. Breastfeeding your baby. A National Childbirth Trust Guide. HMSO, London; 1996.
7. Saarinen UM, Siimes MA. Iron absorption from breast milk, cow's milk and iron-supplemented formula: an opportunistic use of changes in total body iron determined by hemoglobin, ferritin, and body weight in 132 infants. Pediatr Res. 1979;13(3):143-7.

CHAPTER 42

High-risk Neonates—Low Birth Weight, Preterm and Intrauterine Growth Restricted Babies

Learning Objectives

Upon completing this chapter, the learner will be able to:
- Describe the different classes of low birth weight babies.
- List the characteristics of low birth weight babies.
- Discuss the appropriate care for these babies.

HIGH-RISK NEONATES

A high-risk neonate can be defined as a newborn regardless of birth weight, size or gestational age who has a greater than average chance of morbidity or mortality especially within the first 28 days of life. A high-risk newborn may appear well and clinically normal at birth but has a much greater chance than most infants of developing clinical problems such as hypothermia, apnea, and infection in the newborn period. Morbidity develops because of conditions superimposed on normal course of events associated with birth and the adjustments to extra uterine life.

LOW BIRTH WEIGHT BABIES

The internationally accepted definition of a lowbirth weight (LBW) baby is one whose weight at birth is 2,500 g or less. Further classification within the LBW group include the very lowbirth weight (VLBW) baby weighing 1,001–1,500 g and extremely lowbirth weight (ELBW) baby who weighs 1,000 g or less.

In order to assess a LBW baby's needs or likely progress, in addition to the birth weight, an assessment of the gestational age is important. Because, infants born at term or post-term may weigh less than 2,500 g and occasionally the baby of a diabetic mother may weigh much more than 2,500 g even before 37 weeks. When gestational age is considered, a *term infant* is one born after 37 completed weeks of gestation. A preterm infant is one born before 37 completed weeks of gestation.

A classification of LBW babies is done after correlating both the birth weight and gestational age (**Fig. 42.1**).

Centile charts have been devised on which the baby's birth weight is plotted against his gestational age. A baby whose weight lies between the 10th and 90th centile is considered *appropriate for gestational age (AGA)*. The growth potential of this baby is normal. If birth weight is greater than the 90th percentile, this is described as a *large for gestational age (LGA)* and a baby whose weight is below the 10th percentile is described as being *small for gestational age (SGA)*. It follows that a baby born at term may be AGA, SGA or LGA; similarly, a preterm baby may be AGA, LGA or SGA.

Incidence of Low Birth Weight

The incidence of LBW is generally higher in those countries where the mean birth weight is low and as such varies from about 5–40% of live births. In India about a third of the infants weigh less than 2,500 g.

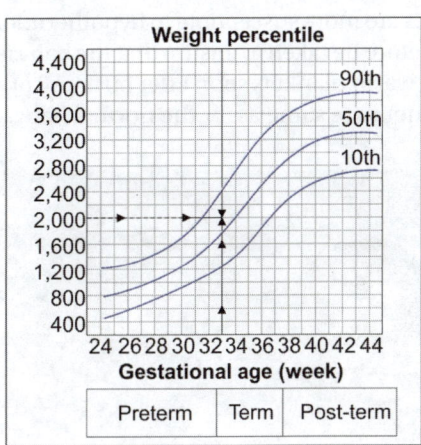

Figure 42.1: Correlation of birth weight and gestational age in percentile.

The factors influencing the LBW of the baby include short gestational period, socioeconomic standard, nutritional and environmental factors. Ethnic background and genetic control are also significant.

▮'SMALL FOR GESTATIONAL AGE' TERM INFANT

Clinical Appearance

Typically, the body is long and thin with a disproportionately large head. The skin is often dry and peeling, and there are abundant palmar and plantar skin creases. These babies are described as having the look of 'worried old men'. In behavior, they are active and indicate from an early age that they are hungry. These babies show an asymmetrical growth pattern. Their length is less affected and occipitofrontal head circumference may well be within the normal range for a term infant **(Figs. 42.2A and B)**.

A second group of SGA babies shows symmetrical growth retardation in utero. These are likely to be very normal babies whose size is compatible with ethnic and genetic expectations. Multiple gestation babies are frequently of this type—symmetrically growth retarded.

A third group of babies with stunted growth in utero is by the teratogenic effects of infection, drug or alcohol abuse. In these babies, all three parameters, weight, length and occipitofrontal circumference are compromised. These babies are likely to present a variety of problems in the neonatal period.

Causes of Intrauterine Growth Retardation

These include maternal disease such as hypertensive disorders which lead to poor placental perfusion, reduced availability of nutrients or placental transfer of substances, which have a teratogenic effect. Extremes of maternal age, socioeconomic factors, parity and the number of fetuses in utero may all affect the normal growth pattern.

Management at Birth

These babies are more susceptible to hypothermia. Extra care should therefore be taken to ensure that the baby is dried and wrapped in warm blankets soon after birth. All other aspects of management are same as for the normal baby.

Feeding

In order to meet the needs of a baby who has been starved in utero, early and frequent feeding must be instituted. These babies are hungry and mothers who choose to breastfeed may start as soon as possible. Breast milk from mothers of SGA babies has increased proteins and immunoglobulins for the first few days.

The SGA babies have a higher metabolic rate and higher energy expenditure than AGA babies and require more calories than AGA babies. Lack of subcutaneous fat and liver glycogen stores further compromise their nutritional reserves. For formula fed babies, feeds are therefore calculated at a rate of 9 mL/kg/day, increasing by 10–15 mL/kg/day. Blood glucose levels should be monitored at least 6 hourly for the first 48 hours. These babies loose minimal amounts of weight before gaining weight rapidly.

Temperature Control

Small for gestational age babies have relatively mature temperature control mechanism. However, due to lack of subcutaneous fat, they are more susceptible for hypothermia from fluctuations in environmental temperature.

The temperature should therefore be monitored regularly and maintained at optimum level.

Skin Care

Babies whose skin is dry, peeling or cracked require special attention. They must be kept clean and dry to prevent infection. An emollient may be applied to skin after bath.

▮PRETERM BABY

A baby born before 37 completed weeks of gestation calculating from the 1st day of last menstrual period is arbitrarily defined as a preterm baby. Babies born before 37 weeks (premature) usually weigh 2,500 g or less.

Less than 5% of preterm babies may weigh more than 2,500 g.

Incidence

The incidence of preterm babies is about 20–25% and constitutes two-third of LBW babies.

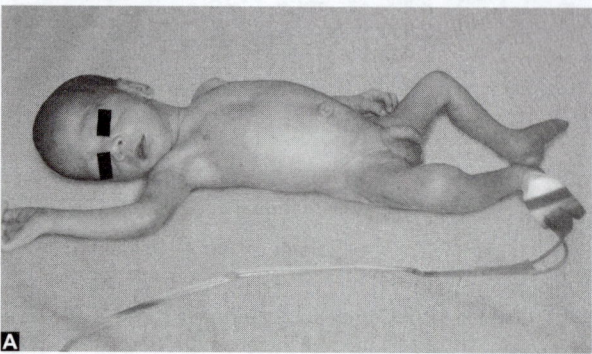
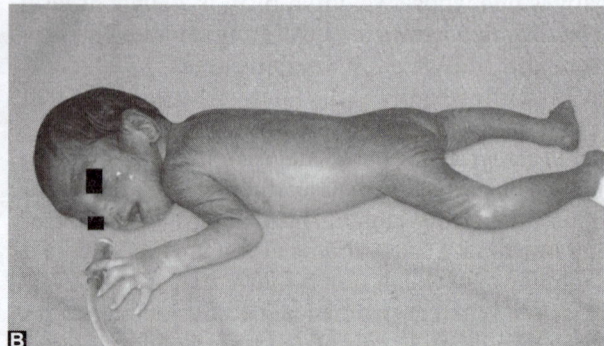

Figures 42.2A and B: Appearance of a newborn. (A) Small gestational age newborn; (B) Preterm newborn *(For color version, see Plate 8)*.

Causes of Prematurity

The causes of preterm birth remain unknown although several factors are considered to predispose to shortened pregnancy.

Multiple Pregnancy

Overdistension of the uterus frequently results in spontaneous preterm labor especially when there are more than two babies.

Maternal Disease in Pregnancy

Preeclampsia, polyhydramnios or antepartum hemorrhage due to either placenta previa or placental abruption may prompt the decision to terminate the pregnancy early.

Previous Obstetric History

There is increased incidence of preterm labor in women who give history of previous induced or spontaneous abortion or preterm delivery.

Low Socioeconomic and Nutritional Status

Women in low socioeconomic group appear to have shorter gestation period though there may be other compounding factors such as maternal illness.

Uterine Anomalies

Uterine anomalies, such as cervical incompetence and malformation of uterus.

Infections

Infection's, such as pyelonephritis, acute appendicitis or genital tract infections.

Chronic Diseases

Chronic diseases associated with pregnancy, such as hypertension, diabetes, severe anemia and decompensated heart lesions.

Fetal Causes

- Conditions where fetal well-being may be seriously compromised if pregnancy were continued, such as placental insufficiency and Rhesus disease
- Presence of congenital abnormalities possibly complicated by growth retardation.

Clinical Appearance

The weight is 2,500 g or less and length is usually less than 44 cm. Relative to his size, the preterm baby has a big head, small thoracic area and large abdomen. The skull bones are soft, wide sutures and large fontanels. Pinnae of ears are soft and flat. The eyes are kept closed.

The skin is thin, red, shiny, due to lack of subcutaneous fat and covered by plentiful lanugo and vernix caseosa. Muscle tone is poor. Plantar creases are not visible before 34th week. The testicles are undescended; the labia minora are exposed because the labia majora are not in contact. The nails are not grown up to the fingertips.

Risks Associated with Prematurity

Asphyxia

The babies are likely to be asphyxiated because of anatomical and functional immaturity.

Hypothermia

A LBW baby has reduced subcutaneous as well as brown fat. Preterm babies often fail to maintain normal range of temperature.

Pulmonary Problems

The deficient lung surfactant in preterm babies born before 34th week predisposes to pulmonary problems such as respiratory distress syndrome (RDS) and atelectasis.

Cerebral Hemorrhage

The causes are soft skull bones which allow dangerous degree of molding, fragile capillaries and hypoprothrombinemia.

Infection

Protective passive immunity is usually acquired from the mother during the later months of pregnancy. As the protective immunoglobulin transferred from the mother is less, the incidence of infection is increased by 3-10 folds.

Jaundice

Physiological jaundice is exaggerated in preterm babies. Because of hepatic insufficiency, the bilirubin produced by the excessive hemolysis cannot be conjugated adequately for excretion as bile leading to rise in unconjugated bilirubin which is responsible for jaundice.

Anemia

Lack of stored iron, hypofunction of the bone marrow and excessive hemolysis all contribute to anemia.

Retrolental Fibroplasia (Retinopathy of Prematurity)

The cause is related to the liberal administration of high concentration of oxygen (above 40%) for a prolonged period (1-2 day) following birth. Blindness occurs usually within 6 months due to the formation of an opaque membrane behind the lens. Other factors like extreme prematurity, hypoxia, lactic acidosis, vitamin E deficiency and bright light have been implicated as causes of blindness.

Care of the Preterm Baby at Birth

In the absence of problems during labor, the preterm baby will frequently establish respiration successfully and require no active resuscitation. It is important to be sure that optimum conditions surround his immediate care. Specific aspects of care are the following:

1. The cord is to be clamped quickly to prevent hypervolemia and later development of hyperbilirubinemia.
2. Adequate oxygenation must be provided through mask in concentration not exceeding 35%.
3. The baby should be wrapped including head in a warm blanket or towel and laid on the side with the head slightly lowered. Temperature must be maintained at 36.5–37.5°C.
4. The baby should be handled with extreme gentleness. Bathing is not appropriate for the preterm baby.

Preterm babies are functionally immature and 'special care' is needed for their survival. Transfer to special baby care unit or neonatal intensive care unit may be needed in order to maintain their health status.

Principles of Care

- To maintain a relatively stable body temperature and adequate humidification
- To prevent or treat atelectasis
- To prevent infection
- To maintain adequate nutrition.

Body Temperature

Premature babies have difficulties in maintaining temperature due to their:

- Large surface area to body mass ratio
- Lack of subcutaneous fat
- Lack of brown fat deposits—these are normally laid down after 36th week
- Comparatively thin skin with increase in transepidermal water loss and consequent heat loss from evaporation
- Lack of glycogen stores to use in heat generation by increasing metabolic rate
- Inability to reduce temperature by sweating.

In order to preserve and maintain thermal homeostasis, the preterm infant should be nursed in a neutrothermal environment. Failure to do so will cause an increase in metabolic rate, increase in oxygen requirements and may lead to respiratory difficulty.

Smaller babies are to be nursed in an incubator to maintain their temperature within normal limits. Alternatively, the baby can be managed under radiant warmer. The skin temperature should be maintained at 36–37°C with surrounding humidity at 50% **(Fig. 42.3)**.

If it is not possible to maintain the temperature and humidity of the room, the baby should be kept in a warm crib or baby cot. Rubber hot water bottles, filled with hot

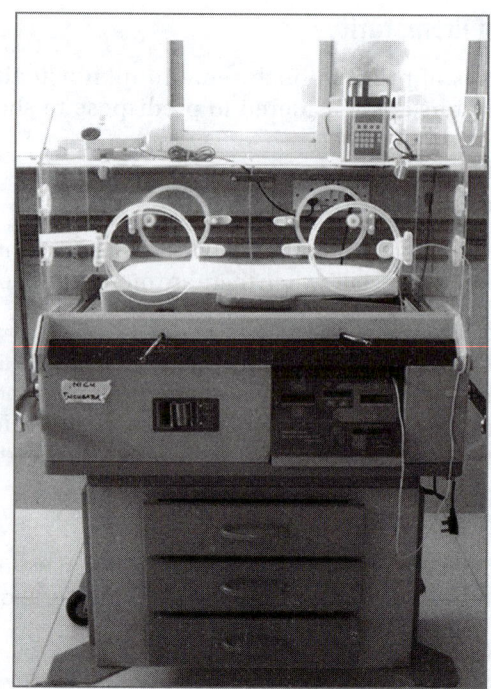

Figure 42.3: An Isolette/incubator for care of preterm baby
(For color version, see Plate 8).

(not boiling) water may be used to warm the crib. Care should be taken to see that the bottles are stoppered and well covered with clothing. The temperature of the crib should be maintained at 30°C (85°F).

Respiratory Support

Baby's air passages are to be cleared and oxygen administered with the baby in the incubator. Continuous oxygen monitoring by pulse oximeter (90–92%) and periodic blood gas sampling are required.

Desirable levels are:
- PaO_2: 55–65 mm Hg
- $PaCO_2$: 35–45 mm Hg
- pH 7.35–7.45.

Surfactant replacement therapy may be required for some babies.

Prevention of Infection

As the transfer of protective immunoglobulins from the mother to a preterm baby is less, the incidence of infection is increased 3–10 fold. The most common types of infection are bronchopneumonia, meningitis and gastroenteritis. Great care should be taken to minimize risk factors. All caregivers should follow correct handwashing techniques. Use of bactericidal soaps or antiseptic solutions is recommended. Drying the hands properly is also important. While in the hospital, separate articles must be used for the baby and use of disposable articles must be encouraged to reduce the risk of nosocomial infection.

Nutritional Needs

Breast milk is the first choice of nutrition for all LBW babies. Colostrum, foremilk, hindmilk and preterm milk help faster growth of the body. Lucas et al. (1994) have demonstrated that babies who were breastfed had a higher intelligence quotient (IQ) at the age of 5 and 8 years than their formula-fed counterparts. A further advantage of breast milk for the preterm baby is improved gastric emptying.

The sucking swallowing reflex is developed by the preterm baby around 34th week's gestation, but the babies must be individually assessed. For babies who are able, direct feeding from the breast between 1 and 2 hours of birth eliminates hypoglycemia, lowers serum bilirubin and neurological sequelae. It should be remembered however, that a preterm baby may tire easily and not be able to sustain the effort long enough to obtain his necessary fluid requirements. In addition, the energy expended in sucking may leave insufficient calories to support growth and development. Hence, regular breastfeeding may be offered, if this does not overtire the baby. For smaller babies, it is preferable to offer complementary and/or supplementary feeds from a cup or spoon. Those babies who are too immature to meet their nutritional needs by breastfeeding may still be put to the breast for short periods, as this will help to establish lactation. If unable to put the baby directly to the breast, the mother may improve lactation by expressing milk.

Feeding intervals depend on the birth weight of the baby and range from hourly in extreme prematurity to 3 hourly feeds in babies born after 36th week.

Feeding Methods

The methods used for feeding depend on the size and vigor of the infant and his ability to suck and swallow. Thus, while comparatively bigger babies can be put to breast right from the beginning; smaller babies should be fed by any of the following methods:
- Tube feeding (gavage)
- Dropper, bowl and spoon
- Bottle feeding
- Intravenous fluid therapy.

Generally, babies weighing less than 1,200 g or less than 30 weeks gestational age are started on intravenous fluids first. Tube feeding is initiated after 2–3 days followed by spoon feeding after 2–4 weeks and thereafter breastfeeding. Babies weighing 1,200–1,800 g with gestational age 30–34 weeks may be started on tube feeding and gradually move on to spoon feeding and breastfeeding. Whereas babies weighing over 1,800 g or above 34 weeks gestation may be started on breastfeeding straight away.

Tube Feeding or Gavage

Nasogastric or orogastric feeding may be given using a size five French gauge catheter (0.5 mm internal diameter). Preference for the oro- or nasogastric route may vary in institutions. An orogastric tube may be easier to pass, but it is more likely to be dislodged. Hence, care should be taken to ensure that the tube is correctly positioned before instilling milk. The baby's position must be maintained in a head-up tilt. Measurement of the tube must be made from the root of the nose to the xiphisternum with the baby's head in a position of slight extension plus 2.5 cm. The tube must be aspirated and checked for the acidity of gastric aspirate prior to giving the milk. Expressed milk may be started with a small amount and is gradually built up. The ordered amount of fluid may be given by gravitation or by pressure.

Dropper or Spoon Feeding

Dropper is used when the baby can swallow, but fails to suck.

Bottle Feeding

Bottle feeding is used when the baby can suck and swallow, but cannot manage to express the milk out from the breast.

Intravenous Fluid Therapy

Babies nursed within the incubator or under radiant warmer have increased fluid requirement due to the increased insensible water loss. Monitoring of fluid is done by measuring body weight, urine output, urine specific gravity and serum sodium.

Nature of Food

Breast milk expressed from the mother is ideal. If this is not available, diluted cow's milk in a proportion of 1:1 (milk:water) for the 1st month and 2:1 during the 2nd month is an alternative substitute. One teaspoonful of glucose should be added to 50 mL of prepared milk for the first 10 days and thereafter reduced to one teaspoonful to 100 mL of formula. Premature infants require more calories than mature babies because of relatively greater loss of heat from the body surface. To meet the calorie requirements, the amount of milk given is progressively increased until the baby is receiving 200 mL/kg of body weight. This may be achieved by 2 weeks. Because of small stomach capacity, weak cardiac sphincter and poor cough reflex, the feeds should be small and are to be given at shorter intervals. Thus, initially a much smaller volume is to be given.

All premature babies should receive additional supplement of vitamins and minerals which should be started after 2 weeks.

Skin Care

A newborn preterm baby is not bathed for the first few days. Depending on the gestational age of the baby, the epidermal layer of the skin may be more or less keratinized and therefore, afford variable protection against invading organisms. In the neonatal period, there is accelerated maturation of the epidermal layer of the preterm baby's skin. This process of keratinization may, however, be hampered if the baby is regularly immersed in a bath of water and toweled dry. Bathing will also alter the naturally low pH of the skin provided by normal skin flora, especially if alkaline or bactericidal soaps are used. Keeping the baby socially clean by removing milk or vomit debris and keeping the napkin area clean and dry will suffice.

Promotion of Growth and Development

Promotion of growth and development is one of the important objectives in caring for the LBW infant. One of the ways in which this can be done is by positioning the baby correctly. Encouraging the baby to adopt a flexed position will reduce heat loss and conserve energy. This can be achieved by using rolled blankets or sheets in the incubator to prevent the baby roaming around inside. Mother should be allowed to see her baby in the nursery. Stroking or caressing and interacting with the baby must be encouraged. They would then find it easier to pluck up courage to pick up and hold the baby. Macedo and Attree (1994) described that touching increases the production of growth hormone and strengthens the immune system. Parents may also enjoy the contact and feel that they are doing something possible and helpful for the baby. However, it should be remembered that each baby is an individual and some may be less responsive to this stimulation than others may. Close observation is necessary to pick up the behavioral cues that suggest the baby is unhappy.

Kangaroo Care

Placing the baby in skin-to-skin contact with mother or father is called kangaroo care. It was first described in Columbia. The idea has since then spread to other parts of the world. This involves placing the naked baby (wearing only a napkin) against the mother's chest inside her blouse or dress. The baby's back may be covered with a blanket if necessary. Both mother and baby were found to enjoy the experience; the baby goes to quiet sleep which is most beneficial for his growth and development.

Favorable Signs of Progress

Preterm babies who thrive well show the following favorable signs:
- Skin color remains pink all the time
- Smooth and regular breathing
- Increasing vigor evidenced by movements of limbs and cry
- Progressive gain in weight; baby loses 1–1.5% of birth weight everyday for the first 5–7 days. Thereafter, the baby gains birth weight by 10–14 days.

Preterm babies are discharged when they attain sufficient weight (about 2,000 g in tropics), have good vigor and able to suckle the breast successfully.

Advice to Mother on Discharge

Wherever possible, supervision of the baby to be continued at home by public health nurses or health visitors. The following advices are to be given to the mother:
- Feeding instructions, if formula feeding, all aspects of preparation of feeds and sterilizing of equipment
- Clothing, to prevent heat loss
- Bedding, to place the baby on his side to prevent aspiration and no pillows to be used in order to reduce the risk of suffocation
- Multivitamin and iron supplementation as prescribed
- Immunization and check up.

INTRAUTERINE GROWTH RESTRICTED BABIES

Intrauterine growth restriction (IUGR) is present in those babies whose birth weight is below the tenth percentile of average for the gestational age. Growth retardation can occur in preterm, term or post-term babies.

Other terms used are *intrauterine growth restriction, dysmaturity and small for date.*

Incidence

Dysmaturity comprises about one-third of LBW babies. The incidence among term babies is about 5% and that among post-term babies is about 15%.

Types of IUGR Fetuses

Based on the clinical evaluation and ultrasound examination, the small fetuses are divided into two types:
1. *Fetuses that are small and healthy:* The birth weight is less than tenth percentile for their gestational age. They have normal subcutaneous fat and usually have uneventful neonatal course.
2. *Fetuses whose growth is restricted by pathological processes (true IUGR):* Depending upon the relative size of their head, abdomen and femur, the fetuses are subdivided into:
   a. The *symmetrical type or type I* of growth retardation is most often caused by structural or chromosomal abnormalities or congenital infection (TORCH). The pathologic process is intrinsic to the fetus and involves all the organs including the head.
   b. In the *asymmetrical type or type II,* the fetus is affected in later months during the phase of cellular hypertrophy. The total cell mass remains the same, but size is smaller than normal. Maternal disease alters the fetal size by reducing uteroplacental blood flow restricting the oxygen and nutrient transfer or by reducing the placental size.

Causes of IUGR

Maternal

1. Constitutional: Small women have small babies. Genetic and racial factors may be associated.
2. Maternal nutrition before and during pregnancy: As most of the fetal weight gain occurs beyond 24th week of pregnancy, malnutrition, anemia and hypertension in the second half of pregnancy play significant role in the reduction of the birth weight.
3. Low blood oxygen as in cyanotic disease.
4. Malabsorption syndrome.
5. Toxins: Alcohol, smoking, chronic renal failure, chronic urinary tract infection, etc.

Fetal

- Congenital anomalies either cardiovascular, renal or others
- Chromosomal abnormalities, such as trisomy 21, trisomy 18, trisomy 16, trisomy 13 and Turner's syndrome
- Accelerated fetal metabolism due to TORCH agents ('TORCH' stands for toxoplasmosis, rubella, cytomegalovirus and herpes simplex)
- Multiple pregnancy.

Placental

Poor blood flow to the placental site which leads to chronic placental insufficiency with inadequate substrate transfer. This occurs in conditions, such as preeclampsia, essential hypertension, chronic nephritis, organic heart disease, placental infarction, chronic placental abruption, circumvallate placenta, velamentous insertion of cord, etc.

Physical Features of the Baby at Birth

1. Weight deficit at birth about 600 mg below the minimum percentile standard.
2. Length is unaffected.
3. Head circumference is relatively larger than the body.
4. Physical features show dry and wrinkled skin because of less subcutaneous fat, scaphoid abdomen, and thin meconium stained vernix caseosa and thin umbilical cord. Pinna of ears has cartilaginous ridges. Plantar creases are well-defined.
5. The baby is alert, active and has normal cry. Eyes are open.
6. Reflexes are normal.

Neonatal Complications

- Asphyxia (intrauterine and neonatal)
- Hypoglycemia due to shortage of glycogen reserve in the liver because of hypoxia
- Meconium aspiration pneumonia
- Hypothermia
- Pulmonary hemorrhage
- Polycythemia
- Necrotizing enterocolitis (NEC) due to reduced intestinal blood flow
- Hyperviscosity syndrome.

Symmetrical growth retarded baby is likely to grow slowly after birth, whereas the asymmetrical baby is more likely to grow faster after birth. The fetuses having retardation of growth evidenced before third trimester are likely to have retarded neurological and intellectual development in infancy. The worst prognosis is for IUGR caused by congenital infection, congenital abnormalities and chromosomal defects.

When a small for gestational age fetus is suspected prenatally careful search is made to determine the presence of growth retardation with the help of sonography. If it is present, the type of IUGR and the possible causes are investigated. If a fetus is symmetrically growth retarded, tests are done to detect fetal anomalies including fetal blood sampling and karyotyping, to prevent unnecessary cesarean section for a malformed baby.

After exclusion of the possible structural and chromosomal abnormalities and congenital infections, the woman with growth retarded fetus is hospitalized. Termination of pregnancy is done after 38th week in an equipped hospital where intensive intranatal monitoring is possible and having facilities for intensive neonatal care. Precautions during labor are those required for preterm delivery. During labor, the woman should preferably be in left lateral position. Any slight evidence of hypoxia should be urgently dealt with by cesarean section in the first stage and forceps in the second stage.

Immediate Care of the Baby at Birth

A pediatrician should be available at the time of delivery. All precautions as outlined for premature delivery are to be taken. The baby should be placed preferably in the intensive neonatal care unit. All the protocols of management of preterm babies are to be followed. Special care is to be taken to prevent and treat hypoglycemia.

Early feeding within 1–2 hours is to be started with 5–10 mL of 10% glucose. The feeding is to be repeated at 2 hourly intervals. If the baby tolerates it, expressed milk or humanized milk may be given 2 hourly in small amounts for 48 hours.

Blood glucose is checked using 'dextrostix screening test' 2 hourly after birth and before each feeding for 48 hours. If the blood glucose level falls below 30 mg, 10% glucose is to be given intravenously.

LARGE FOR GESTATIONAL AGE/HEAVY FOR DATES INFANT

Introduction

A baby whose birth weight is greater than 90th percentile on the intrauterine growth chart is known as large for gestational age. It is also known as macrosomia. According to gestational age the baby may be born at term or preterm.

Assessment findings

- Weight generally more than 4,000 g.
- Plump and full faced. Fractures or intracranial hemorrhage due to exposure to trauma during vaginal delivery.
- Hemorrhage due to exposure to trauma during vaginal delivery.
- Possible asymmetry of chest secondary to diaphragmatic paralysis occurring from edema of phrenic nerve.
- Immature reflexes.

Causes

- LGA may result from a genetic factor where male neonates tend to be larger than females.
- Neonates of large parents tend to be larger.
- Neonates of multiparous women tend to be larger.
- Neonates of diabetic mothers tend to be larger as high glucose levels provide a stimulus for continued insulin production in the fetus leading to excessive growth and fat deposition.

Risks Associated with LGA

- Increased incidence of cesarean deliveries, birth trauma and injury.
- Hypoglycemia.
- Polycythemia.

Management

- Close observation and supportive care. Although large in size, the neonate is immature requiring care similar to that of premature neonate.
- Anticipate the need for endotracheal intubation and mechanical ventilation at birth.
- Administer oxygen as needed and monitor transcutaneous oxygen levels (pulse oximetry readings).
- Have emergency resuscitation equipment and medications readily available.
- Institute measures to maintain a neutral thermal environment, anticipate the need for radiant warmer or incubator.
- Use firm but gentle touch when handling neonate and avoid vigorous stroking and rubbing.
- Monitor glucose levels and fluid and electrolyte balance.
- Provide education, support and guidance to parents and family.
- Explain all procedures and treatments to parents and family.

STUDY QUESTIONS

Short Notes

1. Kangaroo care.
2. Retrolental fibroplasia.
3. Physiological jaundice.

Short Answer Questions

1. Low birth weight babies.
2. Small for gestational age babies.
3. Instructions to the mother of a preterm baby prior to discharge from the hospital.

Essay Questions

1. Explain the principles of care and management of a preterm baby.
2. Describe the state of intrauterine growth retardation, types of IUGR and care of the baby at birth.

BIBLIOGRAPHY

1. Blackburn ST, Loper DL. Maternal, Fetal and Neonatal Physiology: A Clinical Perspective. Philadelphia: WB Saunders; 1992.
2. Davies PS, Clough H, Bishop NJ, et al. Total energy expenditure in small for gestational age infants. Arch Dis Child Fetal Neonatal Ed. 1995;75(1):F46-48.
3. Dutta DC. Textbook of Obstetrics, 5th edition. Kolkata: New Central Book Company; 2001. pp. 490-501.
4. Ewer AK, Durbin GM, Morgan ME, et al. Gastric emptying in preterm infants. Archives of Diseases in Child Fetal Neonatal Edition. 1994;71(1):24-7.
5. Halliday AC. The healthy low birth weight baby. In: Bennett RV, Brown LK (Eds). Myles Textbook for Midwives, 13th edition. Edinburgh: Churchill Livingstone; 1997. pp. 731-48.
6. Hema KR, Johnson R. Management of Growth-restricted Fetus. The Obstetrician and Gynecologist. 2000;2(6):13.
7. Kattiwinkel J. University of virginia. (1995). Newborn assessment and resuscitation.virginia.[online]. Available from www.vital.com/doctor/drJohn-Kattiwinkel
8. Lucas A, Morley R, Cole TJ, et al. A randomised multicentre study of human milk versus formula and later development in preterm infants. Arch Dis Child Fetal Neonatal Ed. 1994;70(2):F141-6.
9. Nima B. Midwifery and obstetries, 2nd edition. EMMES Medical Publishers; 2015.
10. Whitelaw A. Kangaroo baby care: just a nice experience or an important advance for preterm infant? Pediatrics. 1990;85(4):604-5.

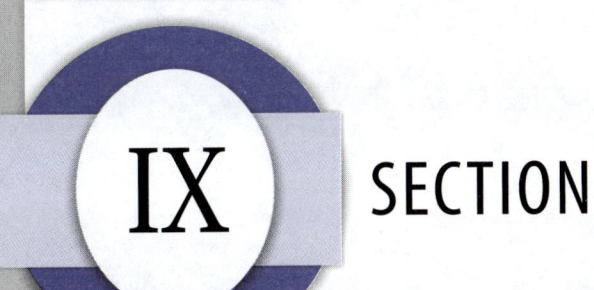

SECTION IX

ILL BABY

Section Outline

43. Recognizing the Ill Baby
44. Respiratory Problems of the Newborn
45. Birth Trauma, Hemorrhage and Convulsions
46. Congenital Abnormalities, Genetic Screening and Genetic Counseling
47. Jaundice and Infections in the Newborn
48. Metabolic and Endocrine Disorders in the Newborn
49. Neonatal Intensive Care Unit

CHAPTER 43

Recognizing the Ill Baby

Learning Objectives

Upon completing this chapter, the learner will be able to:
- Assess and identify the ill neonate.
- Provide an overview of the potential or presenting problems of the neonate.
- Outline the needs of the family in the care of the newborn.

INTRODUCTION

The transition from intrauterine to extrauterine life ordinarily proceeds smoothly and the majority of newborn babies are born normal and healthy. These babies require no intervention after delivery except to be dried and then to be given back to their mothers. However, even though the labor and delivery may have been uneventful, the baby still needs to be observed at this time to ensure that the respirations are normal, that there is good color, the body temperature is stable and that the baby is active and responsive.

The midwife must be able to recognize the signs and signals caused by illness, some of which may be subtle and nonspecific. The labor and delivery have an obvious effect on the well-being of the infant. Korones (1986) stated it well as "The events that follow birth have their origins in those that proceeded it." It is therefore critical that the nurse be aware of the mother's prenatal course and labor history to understand what has happened and prepare for what is to come.

ASSESSMENT OF GESTATIONAL AGE

Immediately following stabilization of respiration and temperature, the newborn should be examined for any gross congenital abnormalities or evidence of birth trauma. They should also have their weight and gestational age plotted on a standard growth chart. Infants can be classified as:

1. *Appropriate for gestational age (AGA):* Between the 10th and 90th percentile.
2. *Small for gestational age (SGA):* Below the 10th percentile.
3. *Large for gestational age (LGA):* Above the 90th percentile.
4. *Preterm:* Born before 37th week of gestation.

This classification allows the midwife to assess infants who may require specialized care. Newborns, who are SGA, LGA or preterm, are at increased risk for respiratory distress, hypoglycemia, polycythemia and disturbed thermoregulation. In the recent years, it is increasingly being recognized that race, sex and maternal height have important effects on classification. Female babies have a lower neonatal mortality than males, blacks were found to have a higher survival rate than whites.

Decreasing morbidity and mortality is the goal of all those involved in the care of the newborn. Hence, early recognition of existing or potential problems is vital if the appropriate treatment is to be initiated as soon as possible. Reviewing the maternal health history is an essential starting point. Both prenatal and perinatal complications can affect the health of the neonate.

Maternal Conditions, Which can Affect the Newborn

- Pregnancy-induced hypertension
- History of epilepsy
- Diabetes
- Substance abuse
- Sexually transmitted diseases (STDs).

Factors Related to Labor and Delivery, Which may have Effects on the Newborn

- Prolonged rupture of membranes
- Abnormal fetal heart rate pattern
- Meconium staining in amniotic fluid
- Difficult or rapid delivery
- Cesarean section and the reason for it.

Problems may become manifest in the newborn over a period of few hours as the baby adapts to living without placental support. The midwife needs to be able to recognize the warning signs and initiate prompt action if deterioration of the baby's condition is to be prevented.

WARNING SIGNS

Most of the information the midwife requires for the assessment of an infant's well-being comes from observation. The baby must be examined systematically commencing at the head and working gradually to the feet.

Pallor

The presence of underlying problems is often manifested in the skin. The presence of meconium on the skin, usually seen in the nail beds and around the umbilicus, is frequently associated with infants who have cardiorespiratory problems. A pale, mottled color of the skin is an indication of poor perfusion. The anemic infant's appearance is usually pale pink, white or in severe cases where there is vascular collapse, gray.

Cause of Anemia

Cause of anemia in the newborn period are:
- Hemolytic disease
- Twin-to-twin transfusion in utero (which causes one infant to be anemic and the other polycythemic)
- Maternal ante- or intrapartum hemorrhage.

Causes of Pallor other than Anemia

- Hypothermia and hypocalcemia
- Shock
- Respiratory disorders
- Cardiac anomalies
- Sepsis.

Plethora

Plethoric babies are usually described as beetroot in color. Their color may indicate an excess of circulating red blood cells (polycythemia)—venous hematocrit greater than 70%. Newborn infants can become polycythemic if they are recipients of:
- Twin-to-twin transfusion in utero
- A large placental transfusion.

Contributing factors are delayed clamping of the umbilical cord or holding the infant below the level of the placenta, thereby allowing blood to flow into the baby and giving a greater circulating blood volume.

Other infants seen plethoric are:
- Small for gestational age babies
- Infants of diabetic mothers (hypoglycemia)
- Those with Down syndrome.

Cyanosis

Central cyanosis is a serious condition. The mucous membranes are the most reliable indicators of central color in all babies. If the tongue and mucous membranes appear blue, this indicates low oxygen saturation levels in the blood, usually of respiratory or cardiac origin. Episodic central cyanotic attacks may be an indication that the infant is having convulsions. Peripheral cyanosis of the hands and feet is common during the first 24 hours of life and is a non-specific sign of illness. Central cyanosis always demands urgent attention.

Jaundice

Early onset of jaundice (occurring in the skin and sclera within the first 12 hour of life) is abnormal and needs investigating. If a jaundiced baby is unduly lethargic, is a poor feeder, vomits or has unstable body temperature, this may indicate infection and steps should be taken to exclude this.

Other Factors that Affect the Appearance of the Skin

Preterm infants have thinner and reddish skin compared to term infants. In post-term infants, the skin is often dry and cracked. The SGA infant may have folds of loose skin over joints due to the lack of subcutaneous fat. This can predispose the infant to hypoglycemia and hypothermia. If the infant is dehydrated, the skin may be pale, dry and cool to touch. Other signs of dehydration are pallor or mottled skin, sunken fontanel or eyeball sockets and tachycardia.

SYSTEM-WISE ASSESSMENT

Integumentary System

Skin Rashes (Fig. 43.1)

Skin rashes are quite common in newborn babies and most are benign, and self-limiting.
- *Milia* are white or yellow papules seen over the chin, nose and forehead. These disappear spontaneously over the first few weeks of life.
- *Miliaria* also called heat rash is a skin condition caused by blocked sweat ducts and trapped sweat beneath the skin. Heat rash is common during hot, humid weather. The treatment is to nurse the infant in light clothes and to keep in cooler environment.
- *Petechiae or purpuric rash* occur in neonatal thrombocytopenia. The petechial rash may appear over

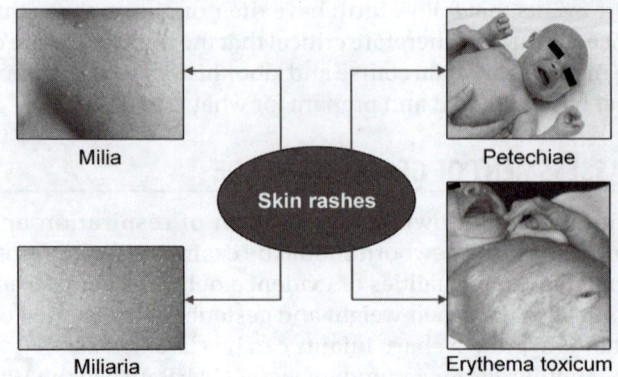

Figure 43.1: Skin rashes *(For color version, see Plate 8).*

the whole body. There may also be prolonged bleeding from the umbilicus, puncture sites and into the gut. Thrombocytopenia may be found in infants with:
- Congenital infections
- Maternal idiopathic thrombocytopenia
- Severe Rhesus (Rh) hemolytic disease.

Bruising can occur following breech extractions, forceps deliveries and ventouse extractions. The bleeding can lead to decrease in circulating blood volume predisposing the infant to anemia or hypotension.

Erythema toxicum or urticaria neonatorum is a rash that consists of white papules on an erythematous base and occurs in about 30–70% of infants. This condition is benign and can be confirmed by examination of smear of aspirate from a pustule, which will show numerous eosinophils (white blood cells, indicative of allergic response).

Infectious Lesions (Figs. 43.2A to F)

- *Oral thrush* **(Fig. 43.2A)**: It is a fungal infection of the mouth and throat. It is very common in neonates, especially if they have been on antibiotics. It presents as white patches seen over the tongue and mucous membranes and as a red rash on the perineum.
- *Bullous impetigo* **(Fig. 43.2B)**: It is a condition, which makes the skin look as though, it has been scalded and is caused by streptococci or staphylococci. It presents a widespread tender erythema, followed by blisters, which break, leaving raw areas of skin. It is particularly noticeable around the napkin area, but can also cause umbilical sepsis, breast abscess and conjunctivitis, and in deep infections, there may be involvement of bones and joints.
- *Neonatal conjunctivitis* **(Fig. 43.2C)**: Sticky eyes are common during the first 2–3 days after birth. Unilateral conjunctivitis is often due to *Chlamydia trachomatis*. Purulent conjunctivitis is generally due to gram-positive cocci. It is treated with antibiotic drops.
- *Herpes simplex virus* **(Fig. 43.2D)**: The infection usually occurs during delivery, 70% of infected newborns will produce a rash, which appears as vesicles or pustules. It is a serious viral infection. Mortality depends on the severity of the illness.
- *Umbilical sepsis* **(Fig. 43.2E)**: It can be caused by a bacterial infection. Periumbilical redness or discharge may occur and antibiotic therapy is required to prevent an ascending infection.
- *Pyoderma* **(Fig. 43.2F)**: Pustules are seen on the scalp, neck, groin and axillae. These are more common in summer. Spread of infection may lead to formation of abscess and septicemia. Hexachlorophene skin care is adequate in most cases. If the lesions are spreading, antibiotics are administered.

Respiratory System

Respiratory distress in the newborn can be a presentation of number of clinical disorders and is the major cause of morbidity and mortality in the neonatal period.

It is important to observe the infant's breathing when infant is at rest and when baby is active. The midwife should always start by observing the skin color and then carry out a respiratory inspection, taking into account whether the child is making an extra effort or insufficient effort to breathe.

- *Breathing*: Respiration should be counted by watching the lower chest and abdomen rise and fall for a full minute. The rate should be between 40 and 60 breaths per minute, but will vary between levels of activity. The chest should expand symmetrically. If the child's respiratory

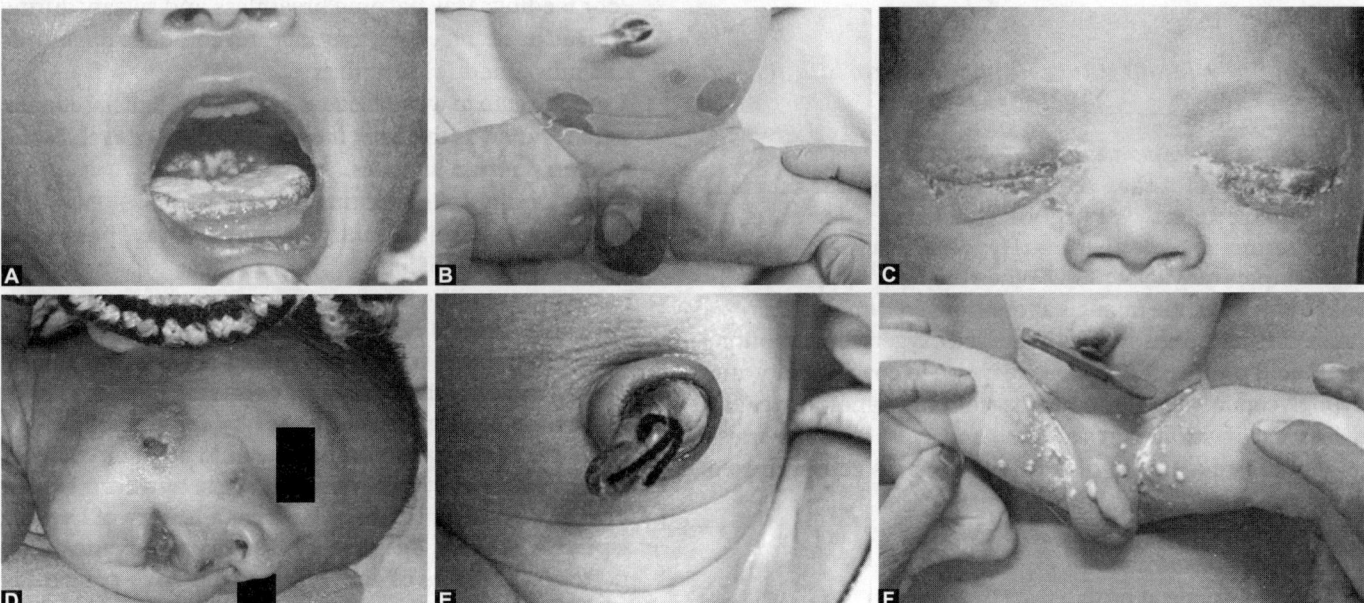

Figures 43.2A to F: Infectious lesions: (A) Oral thrush; (B) Bullous impetigo; (C) Neonatal conjunctivitis; (D) Herpes simplex virus; (E) Umbilical sepsis; (F) Pyoderma. *(For color version, see Plate 8).*

rate is above 60 breaths per minute, this is described as tachypnea. An infant with tachypnea may be described as having respiratory distress and further observations should be made of the quality of respirations to identify if there is any inspiratory pulling in the chest wall above, and below the sternum or between the ribs (retraction). If nasal flaring is also present, this may indicate that there has been a delay in the clearance of lung fluid or that a serious respiratory problem is developing.

- *Grunting:* Heard either with a stethoscope or audibly, is an abnormal expiratory sound. These infants require help with their breathing by either intubation or continuous positive airway pressure ventilation.
- *Apnea:* It is cessation of breathing for 20 seconds or more. It is associated with pallor, bradycardia, cyanosis, oxygen desaturation or a change in the level of consciousness (Fanaroff and Martin, 1987). The most common cause of apnea in preterm babies is pulmonary surfactant deficiency or immaturity of the central nervous system. Other disorders that may produce apnea in the newborn are hypoxia, pneumonia, aspiration, pneumothorax, metabolic disorders (hypoglycemia, hypocalcemia, acidosis) and maternal drugs. Neurological problems such as intracranial hemorrhage, developmental disorders of the brain and congenital anomalies of the airway may also cause apnea. Apnea may be induced by stimulation of the posterior pharynx by suction catheter.

Body Temperature

Thermoregulation is a critical physiological function in the newborn that is closely related to the survival of the infant. "A neutral thermal environment is defined as the ambient air temperature at which oxygen consumption or heat production is minimal with body temperature in the normal range".

Normal Body Temperature Range for Term Infants

- *Axillary:* 36.5–37°C
- *Rectal (core temperature):* 36.7–37.2°C.

Environments that are outside the neutral thermal environment may result in the infant developing hypothermia or hyperthermia. Hypothermia is defined as a core temperature below 36°C. When the body temperature is below this level, the infant is at risk from cold stress. This can cause complications such as increased oxygen consumption, lactic acid production, apnea, decrease in coagulability and hypoglycemia. In preterm infants, cold stress may also cause a decrease in surfactant secretion and synthesis. The stress of hypothermia can be disastrous in infants compromised at birth as with:

- Severe asphyxia
- Extensive resuscitation
- Delayed drying at birth
- Respiratory distress
- Hypoglycemia
- Sepsis
- Preterm or small gestational age (due to poor glucose stores, decreased tissue and little or no brown fat stores).

When the neonate is exposed to cold the baby will at first become very restless, then as body temperature falls, the infant adopts a tightly flexed position to try to conserve heat. The sick or preterm infant will tend to lie supine in a frog-like position. The baby often looks pale or mottled and uninterested in feeding. Hypoglycemia is common in infants who develop hypothermia and this can cause them to have jittery movements of limbs.

Hyperthermia

Hyperthermia is an axillary temperature above 37.5°C. The usual cause of hyperthermia is overheating of the environment. It can also be a clinical sign of sepsis, brain injury or drug therapy. If the infant is too warm, he/she may become restless and may have bright red cheeks. The respiratory rate will be increased. Problems caused by hyperthermia are hypernatremia, jaundice and recurrent apnea. Variability in body temperature may be the first and only sign that a baby is unwell.

Cardiovascular System

The normal heart rate for term infants is 120–160 beats per minute and for preterm infant's 130–170 beats per minute. Heart rate persistently outside this range may suggest an underlying cardiac problem. Warning signs suggestive of congenital heart disease are:

- Cyanosis, which is out of proportion to the degree of respiratory distress.
- Persistent tachypnea.
- Persistent tachycardia at rest.
- Poor feeding: May become breathless and sweaty during the feed or after feeding; they may not complete their feeds and subsequently fail to thrive.
- A sudden gain in weight leading to clinical signs of edema; usually noted as the baby having puffy feet or eyelids and swollen scrotum in males.
- A very loud systolic murmur.
- Evidence of cardiac enlargement on X-ray, persisting beyond 48 hours of life.
- Enlargement of the liver.

Cardiovascular dysfunction should be suspected for infants who present with lethargy and restlessness during feeding. Problems that occur in neonatal cardiovascular functions are usually caused either by congenital defects or by failure of the transition from fetal to adult circulation. Persistent pulmonary hypertension of the newborn is seen in term or post-term infants who have a history of hypoxia or asphyxia at birth. Respiratory distress and cyanosis are seen before 12 hours of age. Infants who have congenital heart disease will be asymptomatic in the neonatal period. Infants who are breathless may have heart disease. The first indication of an underlying cardiac lesion may be the presence of a murmur, heard on routine examination. However, a soft localized systolic murmur with no evidence of any symptoms of cardiac disease is usually of no significance.

Central Nervous System

Assessment of an infant's neurological status is usually carried out when the baby is awake and not crying. Abnormal postures, which include neck retraction, frog-like postures, hyperextension or hyperflexion of limbs, jittery or abnormal involuntary movements, high pitched or weak cry could be indicative of neurologic impairment.

Neurological Disorders

Neurological disorders found at or soon after birth, may be either prenatal or perinatal in origin and include:

1. Congenital abnormalities such as hydrocephaly, microcephaly, encephalocele, chromosomal anomalies.
2. Hypoxic or ischemic cerebral injuries.
3. Birth traumas, skull fractures, spinal cord and brachial plexus injuries, subdural and subarachnoid hemorrhage.
4. Infections passed on to the fetus (toxoplasmosis, rubella, cytomegalovirus, syphilis).

Neurological disorders that appear in the neonatal period need to be recognized promptly in order to minimize brain damage.

- *Infection:* Meningitis, encephalitis, etc.
- *Hypoxia:* Birth asphyxia, respiratory distress, apneic episodes.
- *Metabolic:* Acidosis, hypoglycemia, hyponatremia, hypernatremia, hypothermia, hypocalcemia.
- *Drug withdrawal:* Narcotics, barbiturates, general anesthesia.
- *Hemorrhage:* Intracranial hemorrhage, intraventricular hemorrhage.
- *Secondary bleeding:* Intracranial hemorrhage from thrombocytopenia or disseminated intravascular coagulation.

Manifestations of neurological disorders

1. *Jitteriness:* The baby has tremors that are rapid movement of the extremities or fingers that are stopped when the limb is held or flexed. This is seen in infants who are affected by drug withdrawal or in infants with hypoglycemia.
2. Irritability.
3. *Jerking activity:* Movement of one body part.
4. *Seizures:* These are often very subtle and easily missed. Common causes are asphyxia, metabolic disturbance, infection, intracranial hemorrhage and genetic defects.
5. Twitching.
6. *Hypotonia (floppiness):* Poor muscle tone or loss of body tension. As a result of this, the infant adopts an abnormal position. Causes of hypotonia are:
   – Maternal sedation
   – Birth asphyxia
   – Prematurity
   – Infection
   – Down syndrome
   – Metabolic problems, e.g. hypoglycemia, hyponatremia, inborn errors of metabolism
   – Spinal cord injuries
   – Hypothyroidism
   – Neuromuscular disorders.

Genitourinary System

Urinary infections in the newborn period are quite common, especially in males. The baby typically presents with lethargy, poor feeding, increasing jaundice and vomiting. Urine may be cloudy in appearance or smelly.

Renal problems may present as a failure to pass urine. The normal infant usually passes urine 4–10 hours after birth. Normal urine output for a term baby in the 1st day of life should be 2–4 mL/kg/h. Urine output less than 1 mL/kg/h (oliguria) should be investigated.

Common Causes of Reduced Urinary Output

- Inadequate fluid intake
- Increased fluid loss due to hyperthermia related to the use of radiant heaters and phototherapy units
- Congenital abnormalities
- Infection
- Birth asphyxia.

Gastrointestinal Tract

Gastrointestinal problems commonly seen in newborns are gastroschisis or omphalocele, esophageal atresia, malrotation of the gut, volvulus, meconium ileus, necrotizing enterocolitis (NEC), imperforate anus, rectal fistulas and Hirschsprung's disease.

Omphalocele can be diagnosed prenatally by ultrasound, which provides time for parents to be prepared for the events that will follow birth. Esophageal atresia can be diagnosed when the mother presents with polyhydramnios, because the fetus is unable to swallow the amniotic fluid. Newborn usually presents with copious saliva, which causes gagging, choking, pallor or cyanosis. If not careful with feeding, the baby may aspirate the milk and develop severe respiratory arrest.

Vomiting and Diarrhea

Vomiting in the newborn can occur due to obstruction, malformations or structural damage anywhere below the stomach. Gastrointestinal disorders often present with vomiting, abdominal distension, a failure to pass fecal matter, or diarrhea with or without blood in the fecal matter. Vomiting can also occur due to overfeeding, infection or intestinal abnormalities. The midwife should distinguish between posseting that occurs with winding and over handling after feeding, and vomiting due to overfeeding, infection or intestinal abnormalities. Early vomiting may be caused by the infant swallowing meconium or maternal blood at delivery. This can cause a gastritis, which will eventually settle.

The normal full-term infant usually passes stools about eight times a day. Breastfed babies' feces are often looser and more frequent than those of bottle fed and the color varies. The infant who has infection can often display signs of gastrointestinal problems, usually poor feeding, vomiting and/or diarrhea. Diarrhea caused by gastroenteritis is usually very watery and may sometimes resemble urine. Babies with bacterial or viral gastroenteritis must be isolated. Loose stools can also be a feature of infants being treated for hyperbilirubinemia with phototherapy.

Duodenal Atresia

Duodenal atresia condition usually presents with bile-stained vomiting within 24 hours of birth. Abdominal distension is not usually present, but often visible peristalsis is seen over the stomach. Insertion of a nasogastric tube may reveal large amount of bile in the stomach and usually there is a history of polyhydramnios and a delay in passing meconium. The most common associated anomaly is Down syndrome, which occurs in nearly 30% of cases.

Malrotation of the Gut

Malrotation may present as a mechanical bowel obstruction caused by the abnormal attachments (Ladd's bands). The infant usually has no problems in the first few days of life, then presents with bilious vomiting and abdominal distension.

Volvulus

Volvulus can occur in infants who have an incomplete rotation of the gut. Because of venous impairment and mucosal injury, there may be blood passed per rectum. Bilious vomiting also occurs. These infants are commonly very ill.

Meconium Ileus

Meconium ileus is usually seen in babies with cystic fibrosis. Meconium is usually not passed, but occasionally small pellet-like stools, pale in color may be passed. This must not be mistaken for a bowel movement. Vomiting occurs and gradually increases. Initially the vomitus may contain gastric secretions and feed, but later becomes bilious.

Necrotizing Enterocolitis

Necrotizing enterocolitis is an acquired disease of the small and large intestines caused by ischemia of the intestinal mucosa. It occurs more often in premature babies who have been asphyxiated at delivery or SGA babies who suffer from polycythemia and hypothermia. Vomiting is the common manifestation. Gastric aspirate is large and bile stained. The abdomen becomes distended, stools are large and blood stained. Non-specific signs include temperature elevation, unstable blood glucose, lethargy and poor peripheral circulation in the early stages. As the illness progresses, the infant becomes apneic and bradycardic, and may require ventilating.

Imperforate Anus

Imperforate anus anomaly is seen in some babies. All infants should be checked for this at birth.

Rectal Fistulas

Presence of meconium in the urine is diagnostic of this condition. In female infants, meconium may be passed through the vagina.

Hirschsprung's Disease

Hirschsprung's disease condition should be suspected in babies with delayed passage of meconium, i.e. beyond 24 hours of life. It is caused by an absence of ganglion cells in the distal rectum, colon and sometimes in the small intestine. An incomplete obstruction occurs above the affected segment. Abdominal distension and vomiting are present. The vomit becomes bile stained if meconium is not passed.

Metabolic Disorders

Metabolic disorders commonly seen are galactosemia and phenylketonuria. Infants present with vomiting, weight loss, jaundice and lethargy.

NURSING MANAGEMENT OF THE HOSPITALIZED NEWBORN AND THE FAMILY

Admission of a newborn into a neonatal unit interrupts the normal course of events that surrounds a birth. This can seriously damage the parent-infant bond. In the care of the baby, the midwife should try to normalize the environment of the neonatal unit as much as possible so that the neonate, who is separated from his/her mother and subjected to multiple caregivers, will have reduced stress. Specific measures to reduce stress for which she must pay special attention are minimizing handling of the baby and reducing noise levels. At the start of the shift, the midwife should determine the needs of the infant and carry out the required care, all at one time, instead of repeatedly disturbing the baby. Lester and Tronick (1990) have stated that the best care for the sick infant is rest.

A lot of noise that occur in neonatal units are unnecessary and can be eliminated if thought is given. Staff may talk in normal speaking voice. Noise produced by banging of feeding bottles, closing of incubator doors or dropping items on the incubators are to be avoided. Day and night cycles should be recognized and lights should be dimmed at nighttime and noise further reduced.

Involvement of Parents of the Hospitalized Baby

Following the delivery, if a baby is to be admitted to the neonatal unit, the parents should be allowed to touch or hold the baby, even if it is just for a few moments, before the baby is taken to the neonatal unit.

Parents should be encouraged to visit their baby in the neonatal unit as soon as they are able. They should be given explanation about the baby's condition and the equipment being used. Any questions the parents may have should be answered in a positive manner.

The premature infant may require a lengthy stay in a neonatal unit in which parenting roles may be difficult to establish owing to the physical condition of the baby who may be in a ventilator, being fed intravenously, or be under phototherapy light. All these may be barriers between the infant and the parents, which affect their confidence. Parents should be encouraged to communicate with the baby even if it has to be through the porthole window of the incubator.

As soon as the baby's condition and tolerance to handling permits, the parents should be encouraged to involve in the baby's care. This early involvement will strengthen their understanding of the baby belonging to them and increase their confidence in their ability to provide care. This is of fundamental importance to the general well-being of the baby. Encouraging the mother to breast or bottle feed the baby in the nursery or to express the milk may make her feel she is contributing to her baby's care in a way that nobody else can.

Parents should be allowed to hold and cuddle their babies as soon as possible, based on the baby's condition. Skin-to-skin contact (kangaroo care), where the baby is placed naked (apart from a nappy) between the mother's breasts has been shown to be most beneficial. It can improve oxygenation and breathing rates, have a calming effect, and in the infant, reduce stress levels; it may also increase breast milk supply and boost the mother's confidence.

Discharge planning should commence long before the baby is ready for home. Encouraging parents to participate in the care of their baby from the beginning enables them eventually to be the sole caregivers and resume total charge. Every mother should learn how to feed, bathe, dress and generally care for her child. If the baby has special needs related to feeding or observation, the mother/parents must be given needed training, so that she will feel comfortable about caring for their baby before going home.

CONCLUSION

Nursing care of the family who has a sick newborn is extremely demanding and must involve a multidisciplinary team approach. The care must address the rehabilitative needs of the infant and the educational, psychosocial and financial needs of the family. In the early postpartum period, it is particularly challenging to work with the parents. At this time, parents are going through the shock of having an ill baby. They must be given the time and support to go through the grief process. Nurses can make the passage through the process easier by being accessible and keeping the lines of communication open between the parents and staff. Nurses should educate the family about the disorder and their infant's present and future care needs. When they are ready, parents should be encouraged to become involved in their infant's care.

STUDY QUESTIONS

Short Notes

1. Plethora.
2. Cyanosis in newborns.
3. Jaundice in newborns.
4. Grunting.
5. Apnea.
6. Meconium ileus.

Short Answer Questions

1. Skin rashes in newborns.
2. Infectious lesions in newborns.
3. Hypoglycemia in newborns.
4. Hypothermia in newborns.
5. Hirschsprung's disease.
6. Necrotizing enterocolitis.

BIBLIOGRAPHY

1. Bain JE. Recognizing the ill baby. In: Bennett RV, Linda KB (Eds). Myles Textbook for Midwives, 13th edition. Edinburgh: Churchill Livingstone; 1999. pp. 731-48.
2. Davis CF, Young DG. Gastroenterology. In: Roberton NRC (Ed). Textbook of Neonatology, 2nd edition. New York: Churchill Livingstone; 1992. pp. 170-8.
3. Dutta DC. Textbook of Obstetrics, 5th edition. Kolkata: New Central Book Company; 2001. pp. 502-34.
4. Fanaroff AA, Martin JM. Neonatal Perinatal Medicine, 1st edition. St Louis: Mosby; 1987. pp. 619-20.
5. Halliday HL. Handbook of Neonatal Intensive Care, 1st edition. London: Bailliere Tindall; 1989. pp. 10-38.
6. Korones SB. High Risk Newborn Infants, 4th edition. St Louis: Mosby; 1986. pp. 208-12.
7. Lester BM, Tronick EZ. Guidelines for stimulation with preterm infants. Clin Perinatol. 1970;17(1):XV-XVII.
8. Mayfield SR, Bhatiya J, Nakamura KT, et al. Temperature measurements in term and preterm neonates. J Pediatr. 1984;104(2):271-5.
9. Whitelaw A, Sleath K, Heisterkamp, et al. Skin to skin contact for very low birthweight babies and their mothers. Arch Dis Child. 1988;63(11):1377-81.

CHAPTER 44

Respiratory Problems of the Newborn

Learning Objectives

Upon completing this chapter, the learner will be able to:
- Review the anatomy and physiology of the respiratory system.
- Describe the clinical signs of respiratory problems in the newborn.
- Outline the causes of respiratory problems in the neonatal period.
- Describe the management of common respiratory problems.
- Describe the principles of caring for a baby with respiratory problems.

Respiratory problems are the most common cause of morbidity and mortality in the neonatal period. Problems can occur in term as well as in premature infants. The midwife in managing labor and giving direct care to the newborn baby is able to recognize the first signs of respiratory distress.

ANATOMY AND PHYSIOLOGY OF THE RESPIRATORY SYSTEM

The lungs in utero are nonfunctional as the placenta oxygenates the fetus and carries away waste products. They are bathed in fluid, which is expelled by pressure during the process of labor. Ultrasonographic studies have shown that some respiratory movements occur in utero. It has also been proved that such movements are essential for the normal growth of the lungs.

The basic requirements for initiation and maintenance of pulmonary respiration are:
- Intact neurological and respiratory apparatus
- Clear airway
- Adequate alveolar area and stable expanded alveoli
- Sufficient pulmonary perfusion
- Satisfactory lymphatic drainage
- Oxygen diffusion and dissociation capacity
- Carbonic anhydrase activity of blood.

With the completion of the second stage, the following events play a major role in the initiation of respiration:
1. The clamping of the umbilical cord results in a fall in arterial oxygen and a slight rise in carbon dioxide tension. These factors taken together stimulate the respiratory center directly and via chemoreceptors in the carotid body.
2. Sensory impulses from changes in skin temperature and proprioceptive impulses from joints directly stimulate the respiratory center.
3. With the inflation of the lungs, there is augmentation of respiratory effort.

The first cry, gasp or breath (short inspiration followed by long expiration) establishes a functional residual capacity and brings about a huge increase in pulmonary perfusion and subsequent normal pattern of breathing. A negative intrathoracic pressure of 15 cm water is needed to establish regular respiration. This should also be sufficient to overcome the surface tension. With the first breath the lungs are inflated with air and the placenta is replaced as the organ of respiration. After birth, the baby develops additional conductive airways and alveoli. The lungs are not fully developed until the age of 8 years.

Anatomical and Physiological Difference Between the Baby and Adult

The main differences are:
1. The baby is an obligatory nose breather because of the high, anterior position of the larynx, which produces a direct airway to the lungs from the nasal cavity.
2. The narrowest part of the baby's airway is below the vocal cords at the level of the cricoid cartilage, which increases the risk of obstruction (in adults and older children the narrowest part of the airway is above the vocal cords).
3. The infant's airways are smaller in diameter and become easily blocked by inflammation and secretions.

4. The infant has fewer alveoli for exchange of gases and to maintain air reserves (resting volume) in the lungs, making him/her more sensitive to hypoxia.
5. The muscles in the chest wall are weak and the ribs are more pliable than in the adult, providing less support to keep the lungs expanded.
6. The ribs are more horizontally placed, so that contraction of the diaphragm in breathing draws in the lower ribs. In addition, a baby's breathing movement is more diaphragmatic.
7. Because of the weaker chest muscles and pliable ribs, the baby is at great risk of respiratory fatigue than an adult.
8. The baby has a greater metabolic rate than an adult. Oxygen consumption in the baby is 6–8 mL/kg/min compared to 3–4 mL/kg/min in adult.

CLINICAL SIGNS OF RESPIRATORY PROBLEMS

Common signs found in most respiratory problems are as follows:
1. Increased work of breathing causing:
   a. Recession of intercostals and subcostal muscles and retraction of the sternum; the chest wall appears to be caving in.
   b. The chin appear to pull down the head to move up and down, and the nostrils to flare as the baby tries to draw in as much air as possible, using accessory muscles in the upper body.
   c. Grunting caused by the baby breathing out against a partially closed glottis in an effort to keep as much air as possible in the lungs.
2. Hypoxia causing pallor or cyanosis of the skin and mucous membrane.
3. Alteration in general appearance and behavior:
   a. A tense worried appearance and distorted chest because of the increased work of breathing.
   b. The baby may be restless and unable to feed adequately because of breathing difficulties.
   c. The baby will become lethargic with more severe respiratory difficulties in struggling with the effort of breathing. An exhausted baby may become apneic.
4. *Tachypnea:* The respiratory rate will be increased (beyond 60 breaths per minute) in an effort to achieve adequate gaseous exchange.

CAUSES OF RESPIRATORY PROBLEMS

Breathing problems have many causes, which are not necessarily respiratory in origin. The causes include:
- Infection
- Aspiration
- Lung immaturity
- Transient tachypnea of the newborn
- Pneumothorax
- Congenital problems
- Central nervous system disorders
- Cardiovascular and circulatory problems
- Apnea of prematurity.

Infection

Generalized Infection

A baby having generalized infection may present with signs of respiratory distress. The baby may have a respiratory rate greater than 60 breaths per minute and be pale or cyanosed because of hypoxia.

Congenital or Acquired Pneumonia

A baby may be born with pneumonia that will be present soon after birth. If the membranes have been ruptured for longer than 24 hours, the baby is at greater risk of developing pneumonia. In order to prevent serious neonatal infection the midwife needs to be vigilant for signs of sepsis in the mother, such as purulent vaginal discharge, maternal pyrexia or offensive smelling liquor. When maternal sepsis is suspected an intravenous antibiotic is administered to mother before delivery. When the membranes are ruptured for longer than 18–24 hours, the baby is screened for infection. If the baby shows signs of sepsis such as raised or suppressed white cell count or the baby exhibits signs of infection, such as poor temperature control, poor feeding, respiratory signs, or hypoglycemia, then intravenous antibiotics may be prescribed. Organisms such as group B *Streptococcus*, which may be commensal to the mother's vagina, can cause congenital pneumonia and generalized septicemia. A baby with severe group B streptococcal sepsis will be critically ill.

After birth, the baby is exposed to organisms in the environment, which can cause pneumonia. Common organisms that are commensal to the skin of adults, such as *Staphylococcus epidermidis,* can cause serious respiratory infection in the newborn.

Aspiration

At the time of delivery, it is possible for the baby to inhale any of the fluids that are present when he/she takes the first breath.

Meconium Aspiration

During labor, if there is fetal distress, hypoxia can stimulate peristalsis and relaxation of the anal sphincter and meconium is then released into the amniotic fluid. If the fetus becomes very distressed, he/she may start to make gasping movements in utero before birth, taking in surrounding amniotic fluid. If the amniotic fluid is heavily stained with thick meconium, this can cause the baby breathing difficulties after delivery. In delivering a mother with meconium stained liquor, arrangements must be made for immediate resuscitation of the baby. The person responsible for resuscitation will visualize the vocal cords using a laryngoscope; if meconium is present around the cords, meconium aspiration is unlikely. However, if meconium is present below the vocal cords, the baby will be intubated and the trachea suctioned to remove any inhaled meconium that is accessible. Because meconium is thick and tenacious, it blocks the airways. Meconium is alkaline and irritant to lung tissues, and can lead to a chemical pneumonitis.

Clinical presentation: Meconium aspiration syndrome is typically seen in term and post-term infants, particularly the intrauterine growth restricted group. A baby with meconium aspiration syndrome will present with signs of respiratory distress, which can range from mild to severe (clinical signs of respiratory problems). The chest may appear barrel shaped or hyperinflated. There may also be yellow-green staining of the skin and nail beds. A baby with severe meconium aspiration will need mechanical ventilation, intravenous antibiotics and chest physiotherapy to help clear the lungs.

Other Aspiration Problems

The baby inhales maternal blood or amniotic fluid at delivery, which can result in similar problems to meconium aspiration. In addition, a baby may inhale milk resulting in aspiration pneumonia. This may occur because of vomiting or when there is a fistula between the airway and the esophagus.

Lung Immaturity: Respiratory Distress Syndrome/ Hyaline Membrane Disease

Respiratory distress syndrome (RDS) occurs commonly in preterm neonates, babies of diabetic mothers and infants delivered by cesarean section or breech delivery. It is the commonest cause of respiratory disease and one of the most common causes of neonatal mortality. The pathologic finding is widespread atelectasis. A homogeneous eosinophilic membrane (hyaline membrane) is found plastering the alveolar ducts and terminal bronchioles. Hyaline membrane is made up of proteins that are exuded into the alveoli and airways of a baby with RDS. It is caused by deficiency of surfactant in the baby's lungs. Surfactant is made by cells in the alveolar walls. Its production slowly increases from 20th weeks of gestation, with a surge at 30th to 34th week and at term with the onset of labor.

A number of factors cause surfactant deficiency in the neonate, which include:
- Gross lowering of the surface tension reducing factor (lecithin)
- Hypoperfusion of the pulmonary vascular bed
- Alteration in the fibrinolytic mechanism within the lung.

In cases with deficient surfactant (lecithin), as in premature baby, the pressure needed to open up and expand the alveoli are very high and much beyond the ability of the baby. Hence, there is collapse of the lung (atelectasis) and the clinical manifestations of RDS appear.

Hypoxia reduces surfactant synthesis, which in preterm with low reserves of surfactant has more impact than in the healthy term baby. With maternal diabetes, it is thought that surfactant maturation is delayed, particularly when the prenatal control of diabetes has been poor. In elective cesarean section delivery, the stimulus of labor, which increases surfactant production, is absent.

Course of Development of RDS

Neonates are as follows:
- Preterm
- Diabetic mother
- *Cesarean section:* Deficient surfactant
- *Breech delivery:* Pulmonary atelectasis
- *Hypothermic:* Hypoxia and acidosis
- *Hypovolemic:* Formation of hyaline membrane.

The infant develops both respiratory and metabolic acidosis. pCO_2 may rise to even 80 mm Hg in a severe case.

Clinical Features

The clinical manifestations usually appear abruptly, 4–6 hours after birth as follows:
- Recession of intercostal and subcostal muscles, and retraction of the sternum
- Tachypnea with a breathing rate greater than 60 breaths per minute
- Expiratory grunt
- Cyanosis.

On X-ray examination, the lung field has a white 'ground glass' (non-transparent glass) appearance as the alveoli are collapsed and not filled with air. The main airways that are air filled, stand out as dark areas. The severity ranges from mild transient distress to rapidly progressing fatal illness causing death within a few hours. The more premature and sick the baby is at the onset of RDS, the more complicated the recovery will be.

Preventions

1. Administration of betamethasone (steroid) before preterm delivery, especially to women who go into labor before 34th week of gestation. Crowley et al (1990) suggested The use of antenatal steroids reduce the incidence of RDS by 50% and the mortality by 35%.
2. Administration of prophylactic artificial surfactant into the baby's lungs after delivery.
3. Assessment of lung maturity before premature induction of labor and to delay the induction as much as possible to avoid risk to the fetus.
4. Prevention of fetal hypoxia in diabetic mothers.

Management

The overall aim of managing the treatment of RDS is to support the baby's breathing and to maintain the baby in as good condition as possible as given below:
1. The baby should be in the intensive neonatal care unit and nursed in a warm incubator with high humidity. Air passage is to be cleaned periodically through endotracheal suction. Minimum disturbance and handling are to be ensured.
2. Adequate warmed and humidified oxygen therapy in concentration of 35–40% under positive pressure is to be administered through endotracheal intubation to relieve hypoxia and acidosis.
3. Prevention and treatment of infection.

4. Correction of hypovolemia with albumin or other colloid solution.
5. Correction of anemia and electrolyte imbalance, if any.
6. Frequent monitoring of pO_2, pCO_2, pH and base excess to detect metabolic and respiratory acidosis and rectification accordingly. Acidosis is corrected by intravenous administration of sodium bicarbonate.
7. Surfactant therapy to reduce surface tension and to stabilize the alveolar air-water interface; direct tracheal instillation is done.
8. *Feeding:* Intragastric feeding is the preferred method. If there is chance for vomiting and aspiration, intravenous administration of 10% glucose may be given through a catheter inserted into the umbilical or peripheral vein.

Complications

Complications of hyaline membrane disease are:
- Intraventricular hemorrhage
- Bronchopulmonary dysplasia
- Pulmonary hemorrhage
- Pneumothorax
- Retrolental fibroplasia
- Neurological abnormalities.

About one-third of the babies with RDS die. Infants with mild affection may survive with prompt and effective management.

Transient Tachypnea of the Newborn

Transient tachypnea occurs mostly in term infants, although it can affect the preterm group as well. It is caused by the delayed clearing of lung fluid after birth. It is more common in babies born by cesarean section. The baby with transient tachypnea of the newborn (TTN) will present with tachypnea (sometimes the respiratory rate will be over 100 breaths per minute), mild grunting and slight subcostal and intercostal recession. The baby may also be cyanosed. The baby with TTN is treated with oxygen therapy and may even require ventilation, if the condition is severe. Prophylactic antibiotic therapy is likely to be started, as it is difficult to differentiate the condition from serious infection. The baby's condition improves as the lung fluid clears, usually within 24 hours.

Pneumothorax

Pneumothorax may occur spontaneously after delivery or may result from overvigorous bag and mask ventilation.

Clinical Signs of Pneumothorax

- Pallor or cyanosis
- Difficulty in breathing
- An asymmetrical appearance of the chest
- The abdomen may appear distended as the pneumothorax can push the diaphragm down
- The breath sounds will not be equal on auscultation.

A diagnosis will be made by chest X-ray. Treatment may require the pneumothorax to be drained with a chest drain. If the pneumothorax is not severe and the baby is not distressed, the baby may be treated with oxygen therapy and intravenous fluids until the air from the pneumothorax is reabsorbed.

Pneumothoraces are most common in babies who require mechanical ventilation. This type of air leak may also involve air trapped in the lung tissue and this is known as pulmonary interstitial emphysema.

Congenital Problems

Several congenital problems can cause respiratory difficulties. These may involve a mechanical obstruction of the respiratory tract and an abnormality of development in the chest and its structures.

Upper Airway Problems

1. Choanal atresia: Nasal obstruction allowing the baby to breath only through the mouth.
2. Cleft palate, which allows the tongue to fall to the back of the pharynx causing obstruction.
3. Laryngeal obstruction: Presence of cysts or laryngomalacia when the baby has a 'floppy larynx' causing laryngeal stridor.

Lower Airway Problems

1. Tracheoesophageal fistula, providing an abnormal passage between the trachea and esophagus.
2. Hypoplastic lungs: Lung tissue that has not developed adequately.
3. Diaphragmatic hernia, where the gut herniates up into the chest cavity through a defeat in the diaphragm.

Central Nervous System Disorders

The newborn may show signs of respiratory distress with problems affecting the central nervous system. The most common among them is hypoglycemia, which results in deprivation of energy to brain tissue, which can cause convulsions. Apnea may be the only outward sign of a convulsion in the neonate, as the neurological system is immature. Intracranial hemorrhage may also result in signs of respiratory distress. This is most common after perinatal asphyxia.

Cardiovascular and Circulatory Problems

Because of the changes in circulation at birth, certain cardiovascular problems will be present with some respiratory signs in the neonatal period. Among the problems presenting at birth are those which involve failure of the fetal circulation to change fully to the postnatal pattern and congenital malformation of the heart and major blood vessels.

Patent Ductus Arteriosus

In patent ductus arteriosus (PDA), the ductus arteriosus fails to close causing blood to be diverted from the lungs. In normal neonates, the ductus arteriosus is functionally closed by about

12 hours of age. Closure may be delayed by hypoxia, RDS and cyanotic heart disease. The ductus arteriosus secretes prostaglandins from cells in its walls, which encourage it to stay open in utero. In preterm babies, these cells remain active after delivery and encourage the duct to remain open.

Persistent Pulmonary Hypertension of the Newborn/Persistent Fetal Circulation

Persistent pulmonary hypertension can be present in babies without apparent cause and in babies who have conditions such as RDS, polycythemia, hypoglycemia due to maternal gestational diabetes, postmaturity and meconium aspiration syndrome.

A baby with persistent pulmonary hypertension will present with signs of respiratory distress and cyanosis. The aim of treatment is to maintain the general condition of the baby until the pulmonary vascular resistance falls, allowing normal circulation to be established.

Structural Heart Defects

Congenital heart defects will present in the neonatal period with signs of respiratory distress and include:
- Transposition of the great arteries
- Atrial and ventricular septal defects
- Valve stenosis
- Hypoplastic heart
- Coarctation of aorta.

Some conditions such as *tetralogy of Fallot* are a combination of several defects. In addition, congenital heart disease is common in the presence of other congenital abnormalities such as Down syndrome.

Apnea of Prematurity

Apnea is a common problem found in babies of less than 34 weeks' gestation. It occurs because of immaturity of the respiratory center in the brain and respiratory fatigue. Cardiorespiratory monitoring and use of therapeutic respiratory stimulants help to prevent prolonged apnea. Physical stimulation of the baby, when he/she is apneic, may be sufficient stimulus to 'remind' him/her to breathe. Alternatively, if he/she does not respond to tactile stimulation, a bag and mask without oxygen may be used to ventilate until the baby breathes spontaneously.

PRINCIPLES OF CARING FOR A BABY WITH RESPIRATORY PROBLEM

Objectives of caring for a baby with respiratory problems are to provide support to relieve the work of breathing and detect signs of deterioration. The principles, which are to be applied by the midwife caring for a baby with respiratory problems are:
- Positioning
- Observation
- Oxygenation
- Nutrition and hydration
- Basic physical care needs
- Meeting the emotional and psychological needs of the baby and family.

Positioning

A baby with breathing difficulties will breathe more easily in the prone position or supported on either side in a symmetrically flexed position and with the head slightly elevated. The neonate is more likely to block the airway if the chin is too far upwards or downwards because the neck is short in comparison to that of the adult or older child.

The baby should be nursed on a soft sheet to give him/her tactile warmth and comfort. Newborn babies are not comfortable with the feel of wide-open spaces and need to feel secure. Rolled soft blankets or sheets can be kept on the sides to provide boundaries. Care must be taken that the support does not impede breathing. It is important to instruct mothers that the prone or supported side position is contraindicated at home because of the danger of suffocation and cot death.

Observation

A baby with any type of breathing difficulty needs to be closely monitored for signs of deterioration in his/her condition. A baby with noisy breathing due to secretions in the airway and no sign of respiratory distress is to be kept warm and fed early. The noisy breathing often settles as the secretions disperse.

A respiratory rate over 60 breaths per minute is indicative of respiratory distress. Color of the baby and the work of breathing should also be noted. Continuous cardiopulmonary monitoring should be used in a baby showing signs of respiratory distress because it allows for close monitoring without disturbing him/her. The baby is then able to rest, conserving energy for breathing.

Oxygenation

The baby with breathing difficulties is provided with oxygen according to the needs as assessed by the color, rate and work of breathing and measurement of blood oxygenation. The need for oxygen is determined by the blood gas results and by the clinical assessment. Oxygen can be provided to babies by the following methods.

Ambient or Head Box Oxygen

Warmed and humidified oxygen can be provided either into an incubator or enclosed cot or by head box/hood (a clear Perspex dome that is placed over the baby's head into which oxygen is delivered). It is essential that the concentration of oxygen be assessed accurately by means of an oxygen analyzer placed near the baby's head.

Nasal Cannula

Nasal cannula method can be used when the baby's condition improves and the baby can be nursed out of the incubator. Low flow oxygen can be delivered by this method. With the cannula, the baby can be handled more easily.

Mechanical Ventilation

When a baby is unable to support his/her own respiratory effort, intubation followed by mechanical ventilation is

used. Neonatal ventilators, which are pressure controlled are generally used. This mode of ventilation allows the lungs to inflate and gaseous exchange to occur. Methods of ventilation commonly used are:
- Intermittent mandatory ventilation (IMV)
- Intermittent positive pressure ventilation (IPPV)
- Trigger ventilation
- Continuous positive airway pressure (CPAP)
- High frequency oscillation ventilation (HFOV).

In babies with severe respiratory disease HFOV is used. It is thought that the lower volumes of gas given at lower pressures, at rates of 400–1,000 or more breaths per minute, reduce trauma to vulnerable lung tissue.

Nutrition and Hydration

A baby who has breathing problem will be either unable to feed or find sucking difficult. A full stomach will also impede breathing and intestinal peristalsis slows down in a sick infant. Gastric tube feeding is given to meet the nutritional needs and hydration requirements if the baby's breathing difficulty is minimal and short-lived. However, most babies with breathing difficulties will initially require an intravenous infusion of 10% dextrose, calculated according to weight.

If the baby's respiratory problem is not predicted to be resolved in 48 hours and if total parenteral nutrition is available, it will be administered especially in low birth weight and intrauterine growth restricted babies. Milk feeding is introduced as early as possible, as it is the most natural form of feeding. A small volume, such as 0.5–1.0 mL/h of expressed breast milk may be fed by gastric tube to even very sick and preterm babies in order to stimulate natural enzyme activity in the gut.

As the baby develops the ability to suck, more sucking feeds can be introduced and orogastric or nasogastric feeds may be reduced gradually. For a baby with respiratory problem, it is important to assess the hydration status by maintaining accurate intake and output record. Urine output may be assessed by weighing the nappies before and after the baby has worn them. Weight of the baby must be taken daily. Blood electrolytes are measured daily for infants on intravenous fluids.

Mothers who wish to breastfeed their babies need all possible support and encouragement to maintain the milk supply through the stressful period. It is the midwife's role to educate the mother to express and store the milk and to feed the baby as the baby progresses with his/her sucking ability.

Basic Physical Care Needs

Babies who are preterm and critically ill have reduced ability to maintain normal body temperature. Incubators, heated cots and added humidity are generally used to assist in the maintenance of temperature.

The baby with breathing difficulty, receiving assistance for maintenance of body temperature may not tolerate the handling required for activities such as nappy changing. Midwives must therefore practice minimal handling and coordination of activities where possible.

Meeting the Emotional and Psychological Needs of the Baby and Family

The baby in the neonatal (intensive care) unit with breathing difficulties is separated from the family and deprived of physical contact with the family. The machinery surrounding the baby imposes barriers to his/her family, especially the mother who must provide the physical comfort of contact.

The midwife caring for the baby must be aware of the impact of this separation and involve the mother in the care of the baby whenever possible. Activities such as touching, stroking and talking to the baby must be encouraged whenever the mother and/or father will be in the unit.

Parents need to be provided with consistent and accurate information about their baby's condition.

STUDY QUESTIONS

Short Note

1. Basic requirements for initiating respiration at birth.

Short Answer Questions

1. Meconium aspiration.
2. Transient tachypnea of newborn (TTN).

Essay Question

1. Describe the occurrence, clinical features and management of newborns having respiratory distress syndrome (RDS).

BIBLIOGRAPHY

1. Clark RH. High-frequency ventilation. Journal of Pediatrics. 1994;124:661-70.
2. Crowley P, Chalmers I, Keirse MJ. The effects of corticosteroid administration before preterm delivery: an overview of the evidence from controlled trials. British Journal of Obstetrics Gynaecology. 1990;97(1):11-25.
3. Dutta DC. Text Book of Obstetrics, 5th edition. Kolkata: New Central Book Company; 2001. pp. 509-10.
4. Livingstone A. Respiratory problems. In: Bennett RV, Linda KB (Eds). Myles Textbook for Midwives, 13th edition. Edinburgh: Churchill Livingstone; 1999. pp. 765-76.
5. Northway WH, Rosan RC, Porter DY. Pulmonary disease following respiratory therapy for hyaline-membrane disease. Bronchopulmonary dysplasia. New England Journal of Medicine. 1967;276(7):357.
6. Roberton NRC. Disorders of the respiratory tract. In: Roberton NRC (Ed). A manual of Neonatal Intensive Care, 3rd edition. London: Edward Arnold; 1993.

Birth Trauma, Hemorrhage and Convulsions

Learning Objectives

Upon completing this chapter, the learner will be able to:
- Describe the trauma, which may occur during birth to various structures.
- Describe the major types of hemorrhages in the newborn due to trauma, hypoxia, coagulopathies and other causes.
- Discuss convulsions in the newborn.
- Outline the preventive strategies, which will reduce the incidence of complications.
- Describe the measures for effective management.
- Describe the interventions with parents.

Birth trauma remains an important cause of perinatal mortality and morbidity in countries where comprehensive antenatal and intranatal care is inadequate.

TRAUMA DURING BIRTH

Trauma or injury during birth occurs to:
- Skin and superficial tissues
- Muscles
- Nerves
- Bones.

Trauma to Skin

Damage to the skin is often iatrogenic and results from forceps blades, vacuum extractor cups, scalp electrodes and scalpels. Poorly applied forceps blades or vacuum extractor cups can result in abrasions of the scalp and bruising of the face. Scalp electrodes and fetal blood sampling techniques can cause puncture wounds. Occasionally, during incision of the uterus at cesarean section, laceration of the baby's skin can occur.

All of these injuries are detected during the physical examination of the baby after birth. Abrasions and lacerations should be kept clean and dry. If there is any indication of infection, medical advice should be sought and antibiotics may be required. Deeper lacerations may need closure with Band-aid or suture material.

Trauma to Superficial Tissues

Trauma to soft tissues involves edematous swellings and/or bruising. During labor, the part of the fetus overlaying the cervical os can be subjected to pressure from a 'girdle of contact'. This leads to obstruction of the venous blood return resulting in congestion and edema. The edema usually consists of serum and blood (serosanguineous fluid).

Caput Succedaneum (Figs. 45.1A to C)

Caput succedaneum is the formation of a swelling due to stagnation of fluid in the layers of the scalp beneath the girdle of contact. In occipitoanterior position, a single caput succedaneum may be present. If the occiput rotates anteriorly in occipitoanterior position, a second caput succedaneum can develop. If there is delay in the second stage of labor, the perineum acts as another 'girdle of contact' to form a second caput succedaneum. A false caput succedaneum can occur when a vacuum extractor cup is used. Because of its distinctive shape, the resulting edematous swelling is known as a 'chignon'.

Caput usually forms after rupture of the membranes and is present at birth. The swelling does not tend to enlarge and, if double, is unilateral. It is likely that the baby will experience some discomfort, therefore, gentleness when handling or dressing the baby is important. The caput succedaneum usually resolves by 36 hours of life with no long-term consequences.

Other Injuries

The cervical os may restrict venous blood return, when the fetal presentation is other than cephalic. If the face is the presenting part, it will become congested and bruised, and the eyes and lips edematous. In a breech presentation, the fetus will develop bruising and edema to the genitalia.

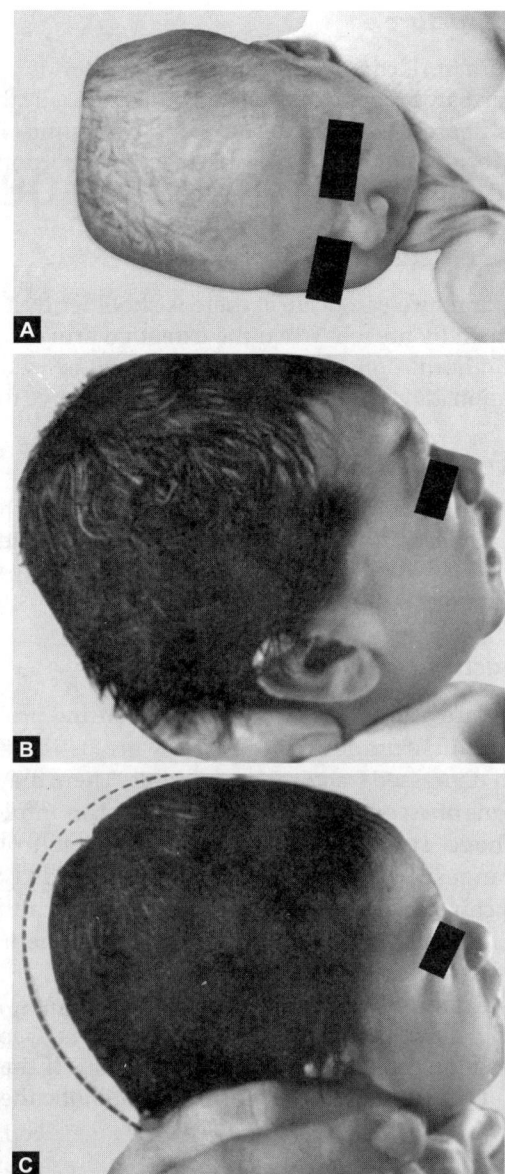

Figures 45.1A to C: Birth injuries on fetal head. (A) Cephalohematoma; (B) Caput succedaneum; (C) Caput succedaneum resolved.

born by the breech. The damage causes torticollis, which means a twisted neck. Torticollis presents as a small lump of approximately 2 cm diameter over the sternomastoid muscle on the affected side of the neck. The lump consists of blood and fibrous tissue, and appears to be painless for the baby.

Stretching of the muscle can be achieved by laying the baby to sleep on the affected side and by using muscle stretching exercises. The swelling will resolve over several weeks.

Nerve Trauma

Trauma occurs commonly to the facial nerve or the brachial nerve plexus.

Facial Nerve Palsy

Damage to the facial nerve usually results from its compression against the ramus of mandible by a forceps blade, resulting in unilateral 'facial palsy'. A unilateral facial weakness is seen with the eyelid of the affected side remaining open even during sleep and the mouth drawn over to the normal side on crying **(Fig. 45.2)**. There may be difficulty with the early feedings, if the baby cannot form an effective seal on the nipple or teat. There is no specific treatment. As the eyelid remains open, the eyeball must be kept lubricated by instilling antibiotic eyedrops or ointment. Feeding difficulties are usually overcome by the baby's own adaptation. Spontaneous resolution of the condition usually occurs within 7–10 days.

Brachial Palsy

Trauma to the brachial plexus (group of nerves) usually results from stretching or effusion due to excessive lateral flexion, rotation or traction of the head and neck during birth by breech or when shoulder dystocia occurs. Unilateral involvement is common. There are three main injuries, i.e. Erb's palsy, Klumpke's palsy and total brachial plexus palsy.

Erb's palsy

This is the commonest type when the V and VII cervical nerve roots are involved. The resulting paralysis causes the arm to lie on the side with extension of the elbow, pronation of the

This type of trauma is immediately apparent at birth. As it is very likely, the baby will experience pain, the midwife must take extreme care when handling or dressing the baby. With the swollen genitalia, excoriation of the overlying skin is likely and care should be taken to keep the area clean and dry to prevent infection.

Muscle Trauma

Injuries to muscle can occur when it is torn or when its blood supply is disrupted.

Torticollis

The sternomastoid muscle can be damaged during the birth of the anterior shoulder when the fetus presents by vertex or during rotation of the shoulders when the fetus is being

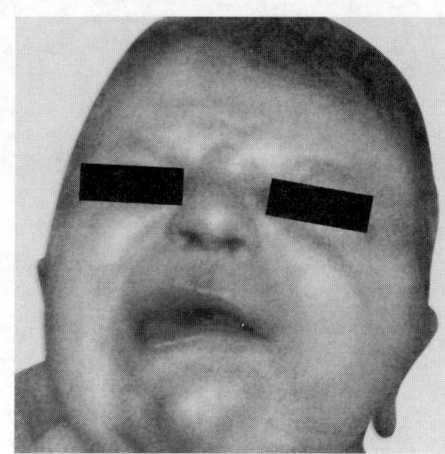

Figure 45.2: Facial palsy (mouth drawn over to the normal side).

forearm and flexion of the wrist. The hand is partially closed and the arm is inwardly rotated **(Fig. 45.3)**. This is commonly known as the 'waiter's tip' position. Moro reflex and biceps jerks are absent on the affected side. Treatment consists of the use of a splint to hold the arm abducted to a right angle and externally rotated; the forearm is flexed at right angle and supinated and the hand is dorsiflexed. Massage and passive movements are advocated. Full recovery may take several weeks or even months. Severe injury may produce permanent damage.

Klumpke's palsy

This type of palsy is due to the affection of the lower cords of the plexus involving VII and VIII cervical or even the I thoracic nerve root. The upper arm has normal movement, but the lower arm, wrist and hand are affected. The arm is flexed at elbow, the wrist extended, the hand flaccid and the fingers flexed. Grasp reflex is absent. When the I thoracic nerve is involved; there may be homolateral ptosis with small pupil due to sympathetic nerve involvement. Treatment consists of splinting the arm with the forearm pronated and the fingers extended. Prognosis is good when the injury is due to stretching. If it is due to hemorrhage or tear, the deformity may be permanent.

Total brachial plexus palsy

There is damage to all the brachial plexus nerve roots. There is complete paralysis of the arm and hand with a lack of sensation and circulatory problems. If there is bilateral paralysis, spinal injury should be suspected. Investigations include X-ray or ultrasound examination of the clavicle, arm, chest and cervical spine and assessment of joints. Passive movements of joints and limb should be initiated under the direction of a physiotherapist.

Spontaneous recovery within days to weeks is expected. For babies who do not recover spontaneously within 4–6 months, surgical repair has been effective.

Bone Trauma

Fractures are rare, but the most commonly affected bones are the clavicle, humerus, femur, and those of the skull. With all fractures, a 'crack' may be heard during the birth.

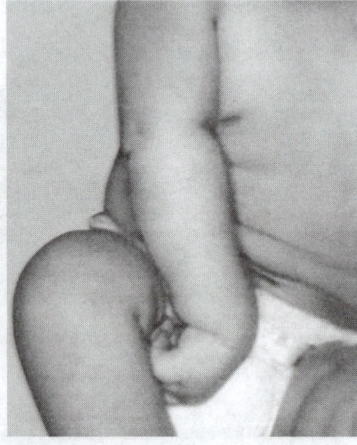

Figure 45.3: Erb's palsy (affected arm rotated inwardly).

Clavicle Fracture

Clavicle fracture can occur if there is shoulder dystocia or during birth by breech. The affected bone is usually the one, which is nearest to the maternal symphysis pubis. During neonatal examination, it is possible to feel a distortion in the bone and crepitus or callus formation.

Humerus Fracture

Midshaft fracture can occur if there is shoulder dystocia or during birth by breech, when the extended arm is brought down and born. Considerable deformity will be evident on examination and the baby will be reluctant to move the arm.

Femur Fracture

Midshaft fractures can occur during birth by the breech, when the extended legs are brought down and born. Considerable deformity is evident on examination and the baby will be reluctant to move the leg owing to pain.

Skull Fracture

Skull fractures, although rare, can occur during prolonged or difficult instrumental births. They are usually linear, although depressed fractures are possible. There may be no signs. Signs of associated complications such as intracranial hemorrhage, raised intracranial pressure, neurological disturbances, leakage of cerebrospinal fluid (CSF) or seizures can sometimes lead to the detection of a fracture. A cephalohematoma may sometimes overlie the fracture leading to its detection.

X-ray examination can confirm the diagnosis. Linear fractures of the skull usually require no treatment. Depressed fractures may require surgical intervention. If there is a leakage of CSF through the ear or nose, antibiotic therapy is indicated.

Treatment

In case of suspected fracture, X-ray examination is done to confirm the diagnosis. Fractures of limbs are usually green-stick type, but may be complete. Fracture of the clavicle requires no treatment. In fracture of the humerus, immobilization of the arm is achieved by placing a pad in the axilla and splinting the arm to the chest with a bandage. In fracture of the femur, immobilization of the leg is achieved by using a splint and bandage. Rapid reunion occurs with callus formation. Union of the clavicle occurs in 7–10 days, while the humerus and femur take 2–3 weeks. Deformity is rare even where the bone ends are not in good alignment.

DISLOCATIONS

The common sites of dislocations of joints are shoulder, hip, jaw and V–VI cervical vertebrae. Confirmation is done by radiology, and the help of an orthopedic surgeon should be sought.

VISCERAL INJURIES

Liver, kidneys, adrenals or lungs are occasionally injured mainly during breech delivery. The commonest result of the injury is hemorrhage. Severe hemorrhage is fatal. In minor hemorrhage, the baby presents features of blood loss in addition to the disturbed function of the organ involved. Treatment is directed to correct the hypovolemia and anemia, and specific management to tackle the injured viscera.

HEMORRHAGE

Hemorrhage in the newborn can be due to trauma or hypoxia, or it can be related to coagulopathies and other causes. Blood volume in the term baby is approximately 80–100 mL/kg and in the preterm baby 90–105 mL/kg body weight; therefore, even a small hemorrhage can be potentially fatal. Hemorrhage in the newborn can be classified according to the principal cause.

Hemorrhage due to Trauma

Cephalohematoma (Figs. 45.4A and B)

Cephalohematoma is the effusion of blood under the periosteum, which covers the skull bones. During a vaginal birth, if there is friction between the fetal skull and the bones of the maternal pelvis, such as in cephalopelvic disproportion or precipitate, the periosteum is torn from the bone, causing bleeding underneath. It may be caused by forceps delivery and may be associated with fracture of the skull bone. Because the skull bones are not fused in the newborn and as the periosteum is adherent to the edges of the skull bones, cephalohematoma is confined to one bone.

However, more than one bone may be affected; therefore double or multiple hematomas may develop.

Cephalohematoma is never present at birth, but gradually develops after 12–24 hours, grows larger over the subsequent few days and can persist for weeks. The swelling is circumscribed, soft, fluctuant and incompressible, and does not cross a suture line.

No treatment is necessary; the blood is absorbed and the swelling subsides in 6–8 weeks leaving an entirely normal skull. Precautions to prevent infection and avoidance of trauma are important.

Subaponeurotic Hemorrhage (Fig. 45.5)

Subaponeurotic type of hemorrhage is rare. The epicranial aponeurosis under the scalp is pulled away from the periosteum of the skull bones and bleeding occurs with resultant swelling. It can occasionally result from an otherwise normal birth, but more often, it is associated with vacuum extraction.

The swelling is present at birth, increases in size, and is a firm, fluctuant mass. The swelling can cross suture lines and can extend into the subcutaneous tissue of neck and eyelids. Bruising may be present for days and sometimes weeks. The blood is reabsorbed and the swelling resolves over 2–3 weeks. Normally no treatment is required. If the hemorrhage is severe, the baby will show signs of shock. Supportive care including blood transfusion may be required. In rare cases, the hemorrhage is massive and the baby may die.

Subdural Hemorrhage

Normally, molding of the fetal skull bones and stretching of the underlying structures during birth is well tolerated by the fetus. When there is trauma to the fetal head involving excessive compression, abnormal stretching and eventually tearing of the dura can occur, leading to rupture of the venous sinuses and the development of a subdural hemorrhage. Predisposing traumatic circumstances include those in which the molding is rapid, abnormal or excessive such as precipitate or rapid birth, malpositions, malpresentations, cephalopelvic disproportion and undue compression during forceps maneuvers. A tentorial tear is the most common lesion and is most often experienced by term babies.

Slight hemorrhage produces hematoma, which may remain stationary or increase in size. Neurological symptoms may appear acutely or may have insidious onset, like vomiting, irritability and failure to gain weight. Hydrocephalus and mental retardation may be late sequelae.

Large subdural hemorrhage usually results from:
1. Tear of the tentorium cerebelli thereby opening up the straight sinuses or rupture of the vein of Galen.

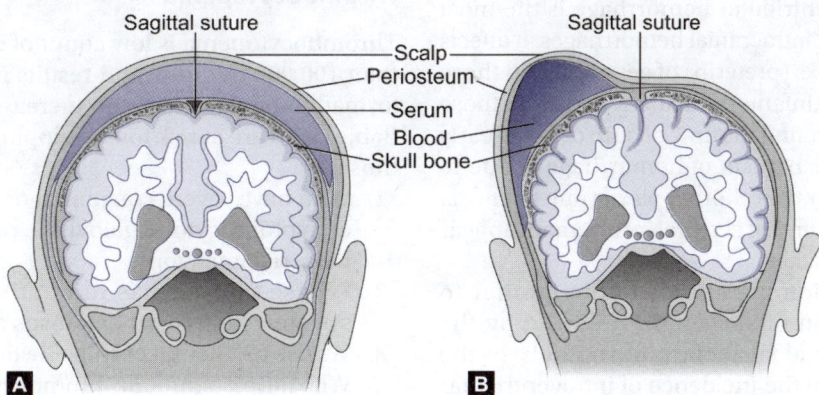

Figures 45.4A and B: Hemorrhage due to trauma. (A) Caput succedaneum; (B) Cephalohematoma *(For color version, see Plate 9).*

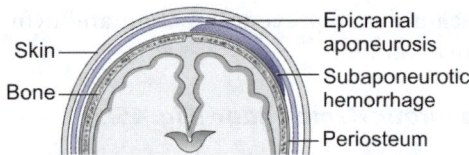

Figure 45.5: Subaponeurotic hemorrhage.

2. Injury to the superior *sagittal* sinus; the baby is likely to suffer severe asphyxia and will be difficult to resuscitate or delivered stillborn. In lesser affection, the baby recovers from the respiratory depression. Gradually the features of cerebral irritation appear, such as frequent high pitch cry, neck retraction, incoordinate ocular movements, convulsion, vomiting and bulging of the anterior fontanel.

Diagnosis is confirmed by cranial ultrasound scan. Supportive treatment is geared toward controlling the consequences of asphyxia and raised intracranial pressure. Subdural taps may be required to drain large collections of blood. This type of hemorrhage can be fatal.

Hemorrhage Due to Hypoxia

Subarachnoid Hemorrhage

Subarachnoid hemorrhage occurs when small amounts of capillary or venous bleeding takes place in the subarachnoid space due to tear of some small veins running from the brain to one of the sinuses. Preterm babies, who suffer hypoxia and term babies who suffer traumatic births are vulnerable.

It often goes unnoticed, as many babies show no sign in the 1st week of life. After a week, the baby may show signs of twitching of the extremities, incoordinated eye movements and generalized convulsions. The baby becomes listless. Preterm babies may have apneic spells.

Diagnosis can be confirmed by computerized tomography scanning. When lumbar puncture is performed, the CSF will be uniformly bloodstained. Management involves the control of the consequences of asphyxia and the control of convulsions. Recovery is usually favorable.

Periventricular or Intraventricular Hemorrhage

Periventricular or intraventricular hemorrhage is the most common and serious of all intracranial hemorrhages. It affects infants of less than 32 weeks (preterm) of gestation and those weighing less than 1,500 g. Infants particularly at risk are those who experience hypoxia around the time of birth or in the early postnatal period. The mechanism of hemorrhage is due to intense congestion of the fragile choroid plexus due to anoxia leading to rupture. The features of cerebral involvement appear abruptly and usually end fatally.

Prenatal administration of steroids to the mother to stimulate the maturation of surfactant followed by the administration of artificial surfactant postnatally to the preterm baby has reduced the incidence of intraventricular hemorrhage in the recent years.

Hemorrhage Related to Coagulopathies

These hemorrhages occur because of temporary disruption in the baby's blood-clotting abilities.

Hemorrhagic Disease of the Newborn

Hemorrhagic disease of the newborn (HDN) is due to temporary deficiency of the specific clotting factors, factor II (prothrombin), factor VII (proconvertin), factor IX (plasma thromboplastin component) and factor X (thrombokinase). These factors are proteins, which require vitamin K to convert them into active clotting factors.

The babies who are more susceptible to developing HDN are those suffering birth trauma, asphyxia, postnatal hypoxia and those who are preterm, of low birth weight or who are receiving antibiotic therapy. Babies who have been exclusively breastfed or who have been feed poorly are also considered to be at risk. After the neonatal period, infants who have liver disease or cystic fibrosis are more likely to develop late HDN due to disruption of vitamin K absorption from the bowel. Manifestations of HDN are bleeding from the umbilicus, puncture sites, the nose and the skin due to bruising.

Gastrointestinal bleeding is manifested as melena and hematemesis. In early and late HDN, serious extracranial and intracranial bleeding can also occur. Diagnosis is confirmed if blood tests reveal prolonged prothrombin time (PT) and partial thromboplastin time (PTT). The platelet count is normal.

With any form of HDN, the baby will require administration of vitamin K, 1–2 mg intramuscularly. In severe cases, when coagulation is grossly abnormal and there is active bleeding into vital structures, replacement of deficient clotting factors is essential and will involve transfusion of fresh-frozen plasma and/or transfusion of the specific clotting factor. If circulation collapse and severe anemia have occurred, a transfusion of red cell concentrate will be required in addition to fresh-frozen plasma. Affected babies may also require other supportive therapy to assist in their recovery. Prophylactic administration of vitamin K, 1 mg intramuscularly to all babies, within the 1st hour after birth is an effective measure for preventing HDN.

Thrombocytopenia

Thrombocytopenia is low count of circulating platelets, less than 100,000 per mm^3 and results from a decreased rate of formation of platelets or an increased rate of consumption. Babies who are at risk for developing thrombocytopenia are those:

1. Who have severe congenital or acquired infection such as syphilis, cytomegalovirus, rubella, toxoplasmosis or bacterial infection.
2. Whose mother has idiopathic thrombocytopenia, systemic lupus erythematosus or thyrotoxicosis.
3. Whose mother takes thiazide diuretics.
4. Who have isoimmune thrombocytopenia.
5. Who have inherited thrombocytopenia.

In mild cases, localized petechial rash appear soon after birth. In severe cases, there is widespread and serious hemorrhage from multiple sites. Diagnosis is based on history, clinical examination and the presence of a reduced platelet count. It is differentiated from other hemorrhagic disorders because coagulation time, fibrin degradation products (FDPs) and red blood cell morphology are normal. In mild cases, no treatment is required, in severe cases where there is hemorrhage and very low platelet counts, a transfusion of platelet concentrate may be required.

Disseminated Intravascular Coagulation

Disseminated intravascular coagulation (DIC) is an acquired coagulation disorder, which is associated with the release of thromboplastin from damaged tissue, stimulating abnormal coagulation and fibrinolysis. The consequences include widespread deposition of fibrin in the microcirculation and excessive consumption of clotting factors and platelets.

The DIC occurs secondary to other primary conditions. Maternal causes include preeclampsia, eclampsia and placental abruption. Fetal causes include severe fetal distress, the presence of a dead twin in the uterus and a traumatic birth. Neonatal causes include conditions resulting in hypoxia and acidosis, severe bacterial or viral infections, hypothermia, hypotension and thrombocytopenia. As the clotting factors and platelets are depleted and fibrinolysis is stimulated, the baby will develop a generalized purpuric rash and will bleed from multiple sites including pulmonary and intracranial hemorrhage. With the stimulation of the clotting cascade, multiple microthrombi appear in the circulation. These can occlude vessels, leading to organ and tissue ischemia and damage, particularly affecting the kidneys, resulting in hematuria and reduced urinary output. The baby will become anemic due to the hemorrhage and fragmentation of red cells.

Laboratory findings will show a low platelet count, low fibrinogen level, distorted and fragmented red blood cells, and low hemoglobin and raised FDPs with PT and PTT.

Treatment includes the correction of underlying cause, if possible, and full supportive care. In order to control the DIC, transfusions of fresh-frozen plasma, cryoprecipitate, concentrated clotting factors and platelets are required. When the baby has anemia, transfusion of whole blood or red cell concentrate is required. Occasionally an exchange transfusion of fresh heparinized blood may be performed, removing FDPs and at the same time replacing the clotting factors.

If treatment of the primary disorder and/or replacement of clotting factors do not lead to resolution, heparin may be administered to try to reduce fibrin deposition. The prognosis depends on the severity of the primary condition as well as of the DIC and the response to treatment.

Inherited Coagulation Factor Deficiencies

The X-linked recessive conditions such as hemophilia (factor VIII deficiency), rarely causes problems in the neonatal period, but may present with excessive bleeding after birth trauma or surgical intervention such as circumcision. Diagnosis is confirmed by a prolonged PTT and a normal PT with decreased levels of specific factors. Replacement transfusions are required.

An affected baby will require continuing follow-up by hematologists after discharge at home. Education, genetic counseling and support will be required for the family if they lack experience of the condition.

Hemorrhage Related to Other Causes

Umbilical Hemorrhage

Umbilical hemorrhage usually occurs because of poorly applied ligatures. Tampering with partially separated cords before they are ready to come off, can also cause bleeding. Cord hemorrhage is a potential cause of death. The use of plastic cord clamps has almost eliminated this type of hemorrhage. In places where plastic clamps are not used, care must be taken to tie the cord well using a reef knot. If umbilical bleeding does not stop after 15–20 minutes, a purse string suture should always be inserted.

Hematemesis and Melena

These signs are usually seen when the baby has swallowed maternal blood during delivery or from cracked nipples during breastfeeding. The diagnosis must be differentiated from hemolytic disease of the newborn, esophageal and gastric or duodenal ulceration, from other causes of melena such as intestinal duplications, hemangiomas within the gut, necrotizing enterocolitis and anal fissure.

If the cause is swallowed blood, no specific treatment is required. If the cause is cracked nipples, appropriate treatment must be given to the mother.

Hematuria

Hematuria can be associated with coagulopathies, urinary tract infections and structural abnormalities of the urinary tract. Birth trauma may cause renal contusion and hematuria. Occasionally, after suprapubic aspiration of urine, mild hematuria may occur. Treatment of the primary cause usually resolves the hematuria.

Umbilical arterial and venous catheters, central venous lines, radial and femoral artery lines, and peripheral venous infusion sites all carry potential danger of severe hemorrhage resulting from dislodgement of the catheter from the vessel or from accidental disconnection of the catheter from the infusion administering set.

Close observation and careful handling of these infants and their infusion lines are imperative to prevent these potentially fatal hemorrhages. If such a hemorrhage does occur, continuous pressure should be applied to the site or, especially for the umbilicus, it should be squeezed between the fingers until hemostasis occurs naturally or hemostatic sutures can be applied. A replacement transfusion of whole blood or packed red cells may be required.

PREVENTION OF TRAUMA IN THE NEWBORN

Comprehensive antenatal and intranatal care is the key to success in the reduction of birth trauma and consequently in the reduction of perinatal mortality and neonatal morbidity.

Antenatal Period

Careful screening to identify babies likely to be traumatized during vaginal delivery in order to employ elective cesarean sections. Mothers with contracted pelvis, cephalopelvic disproportion, malpresentations like breech or transverse lie are to be included for cesarean section.

Intranatal Period

1. Continuous fetal monitoring, if available, to detect early evidences of fetal distress.
2. Determination of pH by fetal blood sampling to detect early sign of distress in order to prevent traumatic fetal anoxia.
3. Careful cutting of the episiotomies after placing two fingers between the head and the stretched perineum to prevent injury to the scalp.
4. Undue stretching of the neck to be avoided to minimize injuries to the brachial plexus or sternomastoid muscle.

Preterm Delivery

- Avoidance of strong sedation
- Prevention of anoxia
- Liberal episiotomies and use of forceps to prevent intracranial compression
- Administration of vitamin K, 1 mg intramuscularly to prevent or minimize hemorrhage from the traumatized area.

Instrumental Delivery

1. Difficult forceps to be withheld in preference to cesarean section.
2. Traction to forceps blades to be applied only after correct placement of blades (over the biparietal plane) is confirmed.

Vaginal Breech Delivery

1. Proper selection of cases and utmost care and gentleness to be executed, while conducting breech delivery.
2. Episiotomies to be given as a routine.
3. After-coming head to be delivered without haste and by forceps preferably.
4. Acute bending at neck to be prevented, while applying forceps.
5. The trunk should not be pulled to one side too much (injury to the brachial plexus and sternomastoid muscle occur due to stretching).
6. Care to be taken while performing different maneuvers to prevent fractures, dislocations and visceral injuries.

CONVULSIONS IN THE NEWBORN

A convulsion in the newborn is a sign of a neurological disturbance. Convulsions (seizures, fits) can present quite differently in a neonate than those of later infancy, childhood or adulthood due to the lack of development of neuronal contacts and myelination.

Manifestations

Neonatal convulsions are always visible manifestations of some underlying pathology. *It is manifested as abnormal sudden or repetitive movements of any part of the body.* Convulsive movements are to be differentiated from jitteriness or tremors in which the movements are rapid, rhythmic and equal, which are often stimulated or made worse by disturbance and can be stopped by touching or flexing the affected limb. They are normal in an active, hungry baby and are usually of no consequences. *Convulsive movements tend to be slower, less equal, not essentially stimulated by disturbance, cannot be stopped by restraint and are always pathological.*

Types of Neonatal Convulsions

Ballweg (1991) suggested that the types of movement a baby has, can help classify the convulsions as either subtle, tonic, focal, clonic or myoclonic.

Subtle Convulsions

Subtle convulsions include movements such as blinking or fluttering of the eyelids, staring, clonic movements of the chin, horizontal or downward movement of eyes, sucking, drooling and sticking the tongue out, cycling movements of the tongue and apnea. Both term and preterm infants can experience subtle convulsions.

Tonic Convulsions

If the baby has tonic convulsions, there will be extension or flexion of limbs, altered patterns of breathing and maintenance of eye deviations. Tonic convulsions are more common in preterm babies.

Multifocal Clonic Convulsions

Multifocal clonic convulsions are seen in term babies and the movements include random jerking movements of extremities. Term babies also experience *focal clonic convulsions*, which are localized, repetitive, clonic jerking movements. An extremity, a limb or a localized muscle group can be affected.

Myoclonic Convulsions

Myoclonic convulsions are the least common, but affect both term and preterm babies. The movements are single or multiple flexion jerks of the feet, legs, hands or arms, which should not be confused with similar movements a sleeping baby can demonstrate.

During a convulsion, the baby may have tachycardia, hypertension, raised cerebral blood flow and raised intracranial pressure.

Causes of Convulsion in the Newborn

1. Central nervous system causes:
   - Intracranial hemorrhage
   - Intracerebral hemorrhage
   - Hypoxic ischemic encephalopathy
   - Kernicterus.
2. Metabolic:
   - Hypo- and hyperglycemia
   - Hypo- and hypercalcemia
   - Hypo- and hypernatremia
   - Hypomagnesemia
   - Inborn errors of metabolism.
3. Infective:
   - High fever
   - Meningitis
   - TORCH infection ('TORCH' stands for toxoplasmosis, rubella, cytomegalovirus and herpes simplex)
   - Tetanus.
4. Iatrogenic:
   - Respiratory stimulants
   - Analeptic drugs
   - Drug toxicity, e.g. theophylline.
5. Others:
   - Cerebral malformations
   - Drug withdrawal.

Investigations

- Full blood count
- Blood, urine and CSF cultures
- Serum IgM- and IgG-specific TORCH titers.
- Biochemical estimation of glucose, calcium, magnesium, bilirubin and electrolytes
- Blood gas levels to detect acidosis and hypoxemia
- Ultrasonography and computed tomography (CT) scan of the head to detect intraventricular and/or subarachnoid hemorrhage or congenital malformations.

Management

Control of Convulsions

Immediate treatment of a convulsion includes getting the assistance of a pediatrician/neonatologist, while ensuring that the baby has a clear airway and adequate ventilation either spontaneously or mechanically. It also includes turning the infant to the semiprone position with the head neither hyperflexed nor hyperextended. Gentle oral and nasal suctioning to remove any milk or mucus if required. If the baby is breathing, but cyanosed, facial oxygen is to be given at a flow rate of 2–3 L/min. If apnea occurs and cyanosis persists, resuscitation may be required. The baby should be handled minimum. If the baby is nursed in an incubator without covering blankets, yet dressed and well supported, observation and maintenance of neutral thermal environment can be achieved.

Intravenous administration of phenobarbitone 10 mg/kg body weight slowly over a period of 3–5 minutes is effective. A maintenance dose of 5 mg/kg body weight per day is administered intramuscularly for a period of 4 weeks or longer. In resistant cases IV phenytoin (Dilantin), 15 mg/kg at the rate of 0.5 mg/kg/min, followed by maintenance dose of 5 mg/kg/day is administered.

Treatment of the Underlying Pathology

- *Hypoglycemia:* Glucose infusion, 2 mL/kg of 10% glucose is given over a period of 2–3 minutes. Glucose infusion is continued at a rate of 6–8 mg/kg/min. Blood glucose must be maintained at 40–60 mg/dL.
- *Hypomagnesemia:* Magnesium sulfate 0.2 mEq/kg is given IV every 6 hours until magnesium level is normal.
- *Infection:* Appropriate antibiotic therapy following septic work-up.
- *Hypocalcemia:* Intravenous administration of 2 mL/kg of 10% calcium gluconate over 5 minutes. This is to be followed by oral calcium chloride 250 mg with each feed for few days.
- *Raised intracranial tension:* 10 mL of 20% mannitol to be given intravenously over 30–60 minutes.

Observation and Recording

It is important that observations of convulsion are documented, noting the type of movement, the areas affected, the length, any color change, any change in heart rate, respiratory rate or blood pressure and any immediate sequel.

The outcome for babies who have convulsions depends on the cause of the convulsion, the type of convulsion and the electroencephalogram (EEG) tracing. Babies who have congenital malformations of the brain, hypoxic ischemic encephalopathy or bacterial meningitis tend to have higher mortality or poor neurological outcome. Babies who have late hypocalcemia, hyponatremia or primary subarachnoid hemorrhage are more likely to survive neurologically intact.

Babies, who experience subtle, generalized tonic and myoclonic convulsions, tend to have poorer neurological outcome than babies experiencing the other types of convulsions do. Abnormal EEG tracings generally indicate a poor prognosis.

Managing Parents

When babies suffers trauma during birth, or hemorrhage or convulsions, parents are likely to be extremely shocked. Although the extent of parental contact with the baby will depend on the nature of the birth injury, all parents are entitled to be given honest and clear information about their baby's condition as soon as possible after detection. It is recommended that parents receive this type of bad news when they are together and from someone who is known to them. The neonatologist giving the information will need to give time for parents to clarify their questions. Follow-up explanations by nursing personnel and encouragement for parental interactions are essential. Continuing supportive care will also be required for them to deal with the stressful situation.

STUDY QUESTIONS

Short Notes

1. Caput succedaneum.
2. Torticollis.
3. Facial nerve palsy.
4. Erb's palsy.
5. Klumpke's palsy.
6. Total brachial plexus palsy.

Short Answer Questions

1. Cephalohematoma.
2. Subaponeurotic hemorrhage.
3. Subdural hemorrhage.
4. Measures to prevent trauma in newborns during intranatal period.

Essay Question

1. Describe the manifestations, types, causes and management of neonatal convulsions.

BIBLIOGRAPHY

1. Ballweg DD. Neonatal seizures: an overview. Neonatal Network. 1991;10(1):15-21.
2. Blackburn ST. Assessment and management of neurological dysfunction. In: Kenner C, Brueggemeyer A, Gunderson LP (Eds). Comprehensive Neonatal Nursing, 1st edition. Philadelphia: WB Saunders; 1993. pp. 341-6.
3. Brucker J, Laurent JP, Lee R, et al. Brachial plexus birth injury. Journal Neuroscience Nursing. 1991;23(6):374-80.
4. Dutta DC. Textbook of Obstetrics, 5th edition. Calcutta: New Central Book Company; 2001. pp. 515-6.
5. Greig C. Trauma during birth, hemorrhage and convulsions. In: Bennett RV, Linda KB (Eds). Myles Textbook for Midwives, 13th edition. Edinburgh: Churchill Livingstone; 1999. pp. 777-92.
6. Jobe AH, Mitchell BR, Gunkel JH. Beneficial effects of the combined use of prenatal corticosteroids and postnatal surfactant on preterm infants. American Journal of Obstetrics and Gynecology. 1993;168(2):508-13.
7. McCulloch M. Neurological disorders. In: Beachy P, Deacon J (Eds). Core Curriculum for Neonatal Intensive Care Nursing, 1st edition. Philadelphia: WB Saunders; 1993. pp. 314-28.
8. Richards C, Reed J. Child health Your baby has Down's syndrome. Nursing Times. 1991;87(46):60-1.

CHAPTER 46

Congenital Abnormalities, Genetic Screening and Genetic Counseling

Learning Objectives

Upon completion of this chapter, the learner will be able to:
- Discuss congenital abnormalities and their identifiable causes.
- Describe the major clinical manifestations of selected autosomal and X-linked disorders.
- Describe the major features of selected disorders that result from numerical and structural chromosomal abnormalities.
- Discuss the methods and significance of genetic screening.
- Discuss the various elements of genetic counseling.

A congenital abnormality is any defect in form, structure or function present in a neonate. The incidence of significant congenital malformations is about 2–5% at birth. A lower incidence of 1 in 500 is however reported from the hospital statistics in India. In the western countries, major fetal abnormalities account for about 20% of perinatal deaths and many survivors are physically and/or mentally handicapped.

CAUSES OF CONGENITAL ABNORMALITIES

Identifiable defects can be categorized as:
- Chromosome and genetic disorders abnormalities
- Teratogenic causes
- Multifactorial causes
- Unknown causes.

Chromosome Abnormalities and Genetic Disorders

Each human cell carries a blueprint for reproduction in the form of 44 chromosomes referred to as autosomes and 2 sex chromosomes. Each chromosome comprises a number of genes. A fertilized zygote should have 22 autosomes and 1 sex chromosome from each parent. If a fault occurs in the formation of the gametes or following fertilization, an excess, or deficit of chromosomal material will result. Each abnormal chromosomal pattern has a different clinical presentation. Common forms of chromosomal abnormalities are trisomy 21 (Down syndrome), trisomy 18 (Edwards' syndrome) and trisomy 13 (Patau syndrome).

Genes are composed of deoxyribonucleic acid (DNA) and each is concerned with the transmission of one specific hereditary factor. Genetically, inherited factors may be *dominant* or *recessive*. A dominant gene will produce its effect even if present in only one chromosome of a pair. An autosomal dominant condition can usually be traced through several generations. A recessive gene needs to be present in both chromosomes before producing its effect.

Teratogenic Causes

A teratogen is any agent that raises the incidence of congenital abnormality. The list of known and suspected teratogens is the following:
1. Prescription drugs:
   - Anticonvulsants
   - Anticoagulants
   - High concentrations of vitamin A (for gene treatment).
2. Drugs used in substance abuse:
   - Heroin
   - Alcohol
   - Nicotine.
3. Environmental factors:
   - Radiation
   - Chemicals (digoxins, pesticides).
4. Infective agents:
   - Rubella
   - Cytomegalovirus
   - Varicella
   - *Toxoplasma*.
5. Maternal diseases:
   - Diabetes
   - Epilepsy.

Several factors influence the effect(s) produced by any one teratogen such as gestational age of the embryo or fetus at the time of exposure, length of exposure and toxicity of the teratogen.

Multifactorial Causes

These are due to genetic effect in addition to one or more teratogenic influences. These include neural tube defects, congenital heart defects, cleft palate and cleft lip.

Advancing maternal age increases the incidence of Down syndrome (mongolism) to the extent of 1 in 100 births at the age of 40. Increasing parity is associated with high incidence of malformation except anencephaly or spina bifida, which is common in first birth. Maternal malnutrition is associated with increased incidence of fetal malformations.

Unknown Causes

In spite of a growing body of knowledge, the specific cause of large number of abnormalities (90%) remains unspecified.

COMMON MALFORMATIONS AND SYNDROMES OF GASTROINTESTINAL TRACT

Most of the abnormalities affecting gastrointestinal (GI) system call for prompt surgical intervention, e.g. atresia, gastroschisis and exomphalos. If prenatal diagnosis has been made, the parents will be at least partially prepared. After the baby is delivered and prior to obtaining their consent for surgery, they should be permitted to hold the baby and the pediatric surgeon must provide adequate explanation.

Gastroschisis and Exomphalos (Figs. 46.1A and B)

Gastroschisis is a paramedian defect of the abdominal wall with extrusion of bowel, which is not covered by peritoneum, thus making it very vulnerable to injury and infection. A surgical closure of the defect is usually possible.

Exomphalos or omphalocele is the condition in which the bowel or other viscera protrude through the umbilicus. Very often these babies have other abnormalities such as heart defects, which could be contraindication to surgery in the neonatal period. Closure of the defect may consequently be delayed as long as 1 or 2 years.

Immediate management of both the above conditions is to cover the herniated abdominal contents with warm sterile gauze or a saline silastic bag. Stomach contents should be aspirated. Transfer of the baby to a surgical neonatal intensive care unit (ICU) is then expedited.

Atresias

Esophageal Atresia (Fig. 46.2)

Esophageal atresia occurs when there is incomplete canalization of the esophagus in early intrauterine development. It is commonly associated with tracheoesophageal fistula,

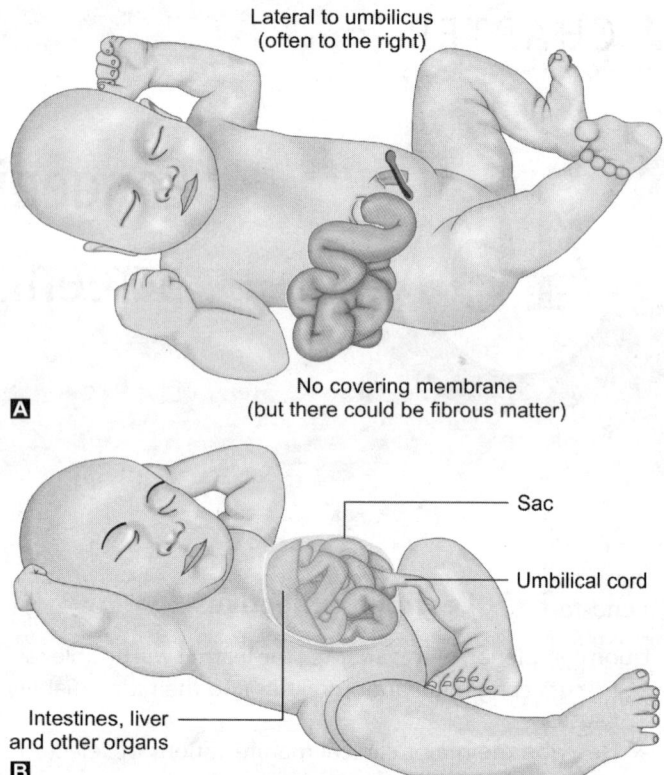

Figures 46.1A and B: (A) Gastroschisis; (B) Exomphalos.

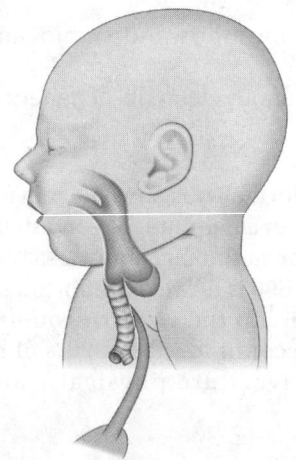

Figure 46.2: Esophageal atresia.

which connects the trachea to the upper or lower esophagus or both. The most common type of abnormality is where the upper esophagus terminates in a blind pouch and the lower esophagus connects to the trachea. The abnormality should be suspected in the presence of maternal polyhydramnios. At birth, the baby has copious amounts of mucus coming from the mouth. An orogastric tube may travel less than 10–12 cm. Radiography will confirm the diagnosis.

The baby must be given no oral fluid. He/she should be transferred immediately to a pediatric surgical unit. It may be possible to anastomose the blind ends of the esophagus. If the distance is too large, a series of bouginages may be

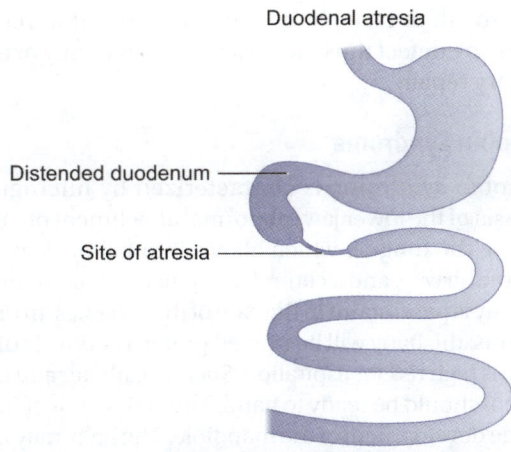

Figure 46.3: Duodenal atresia.

carried out in an attempt stretch the ends of the esophagus, stimulate growth and thereby eventually facilitate repair of end-to-end anastomosis. Alternatively, a Teflon graft or transplant of a section of colonic tissue will be needed later. If the repair is delayed, a cervical esophagostomy may be performed to allow drainage of secretions. Meanwhile, the baby will require feed via a gastrostomy tube.

Duodenal Atresia (Fig. 46.3)

If duodenal atresia has not already been diagnosed in the prenatal period, persistent vomiting within the first 24–36 hours of birth will be the first features encountered. The vomit will often contain bile, unless the obstruction is proximal to the entrance of the common bile duct. Abdominal distension may not be present and the baby may pass meconium. A characteristic double bubble of gas may be seen on radiological examination. Treatment is by surgical repair. Outcome is good, if the baby is otherwise healthy.

Rectal Atresia and Imperforate Anus (Figs. 46.4A and B)

Imperforate anus is often obvious at birth on examination of the baby, but a rectal atresia might not become apparent until it is noted that the baby has not passed meconium. Where, the first temperature is taken by rectal thermometer, the problem may be noted earlier. Both conditions require the baby to have surgical intervention.

Other possibilities that should be considered if a baby fails to pass meconium in the first 24 hours are:
- *Malrotation:* This is a developmental abnormality, where incomplete rotation of the gut has taken place, giving rise to signs of obstruction. Surgical correction is necessary.
- *Cystic fibrosis:* This is an autosomal recessive condition. Majority of cases are not diagnosed until later in infancy or childhood when the child fails to thrive or have repeated chest infections. In this condition, the meconium is particularly viscous and causes intestinal obstruction. There is accompanying abdominal distension and bile-

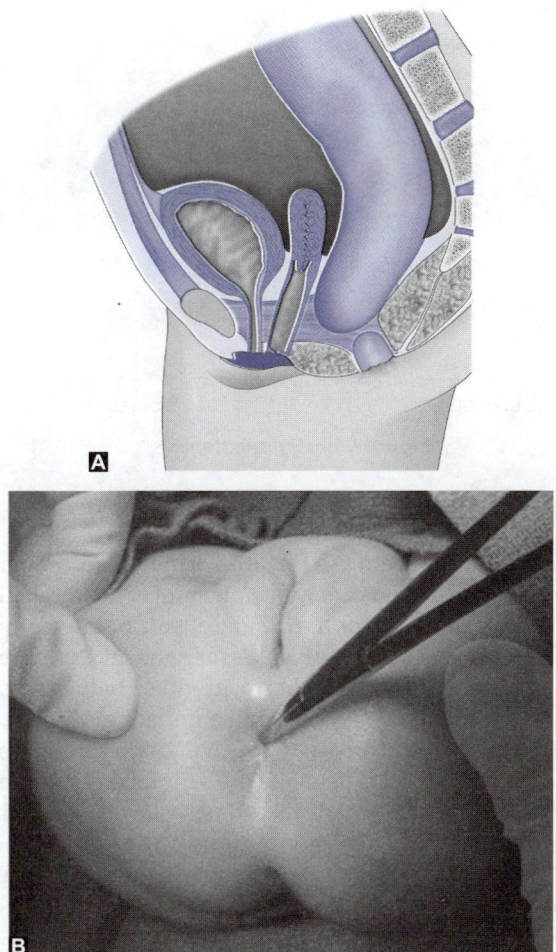

Figures 46.4A and B: (A) Rectal atresia; (B) Imperforate anus.

stained vomiting. Definite diagnosis will be by identifying a raised immunoreactive trypsinogen (IRT) level. Treatment is supportive rather than curative and involves intravenous (IV) therapy and gastrografin enema to relieve obstruction, administration of pancreatin and chest physiotherapy.
- *Hirschsprung's disease:* In this disease, the bowel has an aganglionic section. The incidence is about 1 in 5,000 births. Due to the presence of the aganglionic section, peristalsis does not occur and the bowel therefore becomes obstructed. The baby develops abnormal distension and bile-stained vomiting. Definite diagnosis is made by doing a colonic biopsy. Resection of the aganglionic section of the bowel and anastomosis is indicated.

Pyloric Stenosis (Fig. 46.5)

Pyloric stenosis arises from a genetic defect, which causes hypertrophy of the muscles of the pyloric sphincter. The characteristic clinical presentation is projectile vomiting usually around 6 weeks of age, but it may occur earlier in some babies. Boy babies are usually affected and surgical repair is by Ramstedt's operation.

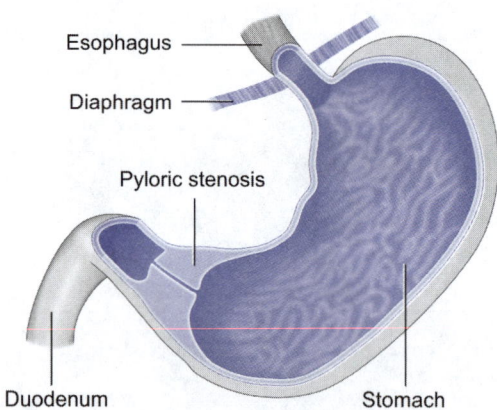

Figure 46.5: Pyloric stenosis.

Cleft Lip and Cleft Palate (Fig. 46.6)

Cleft in the lip may occur as a single deformity or accompanied by cleft palate. The defect may be unilateral or bilateral. Clefts in the palate may affect hard palate, soft palate or both. Some defects will include alveolar margins and sometimes the uvula. The greatest problem with these babies initially is feeding. If the defect is limited to a unilateral cleft lip, the mother may be able to breastfeed the baby. Where, there is the additional problem of cleft palate presents feeding problems. Feeding with specially made teats or spoon will be required.

Middle ear infection is common in these babies and repeated infections could impede hearing and subsequent development of speech. Mother should be encouraged to feed with expressed breast milk and assisted with the task of feeding as it will require lot of patience.

Surgical repair of the cleft lip may be performed at the age of 3–4 months. Closure of the palate defect is often suggested at around the age of 12–15 months. The delay is to allow normal growth to take place, which may result in reducing the size of the defect thus increasing the possibility of a more satisfactory repair.

Pierre Robin Syndrome

Pierre Robin syndrome is characterized by micrognathia (hypoplasia of the lower jaw) abnormal attachment of muscles controlling the tongue, which allows it to fall backward and occlude the airway, and a central cleft palate. Maintenance of a clear airway is paramount in the care of these babies. In order to achieve this, the baby will be nursed prone. Feeding is difficult and there is high risk for aspiration. Suction catheter and oxygen equipment should be ready to hand. The action of sucking may encourage development of the mandible. The baby may have to be kept in the hospital until the lower jaw has grown sufficiently.

ABNORMALITIES RELATING TO RESPIRATORY SYSTEM

Any abnormality of the respiratory tract or accessory respiratory muscles is likely to hamper the process of successful transition from fetus to neonate.

Diaphragmatic Hernia (Fig. 46.7)

In diaphragmatic hernia condition, there is defeat in the diaphragm, which allows herniation of abdominal contents into the thoracic cavity. The extent to which lung development is compromised as a result, depends on the size of the defect and the gestational age at which herniation first occurred. The condition may be suspected at birth if the baby is cyanosed and difficulty is experienced in resuscitation. Since, the majority of such defects are left sided, heart sounds will be displaced. The abdomen may have a scaphoid appearance. Chest X-ray will confirm the diagnosis. Immediate surgical repair of the defect is necessary. Prognosis relates to the degree of pulmonary hypoplasia. Coexistent abnormalities such as cardiac defects or chromosomal anomalies are usually seen.

Choanal Atresia (Fig. 46.8)

Choanal atresia is a unilateral or bilateral narrowing of the nasal passage(s) with a web of tissue, or bone occluding the

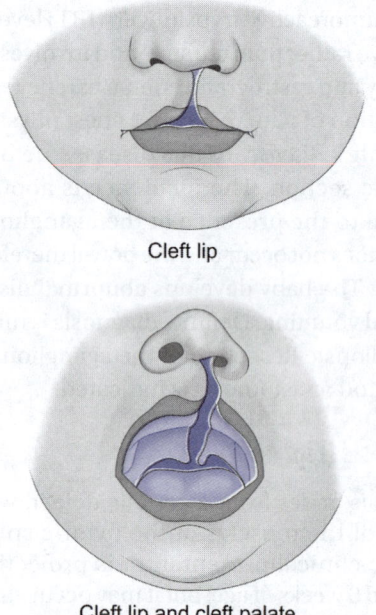

Figure 46.6: Cleft lip and palate.

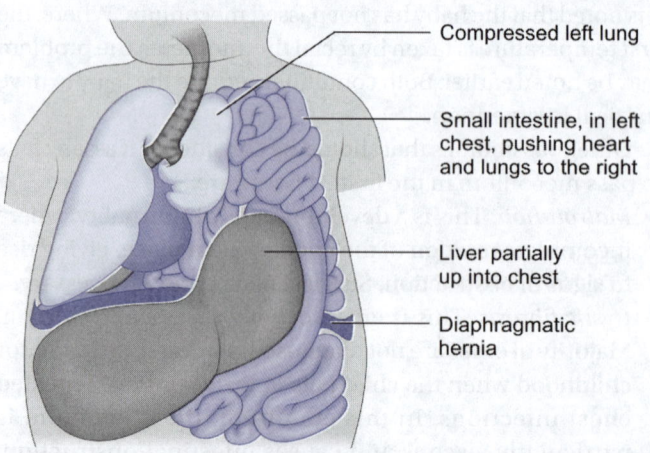

Figure 46.7: Diaphragmatic hernia.

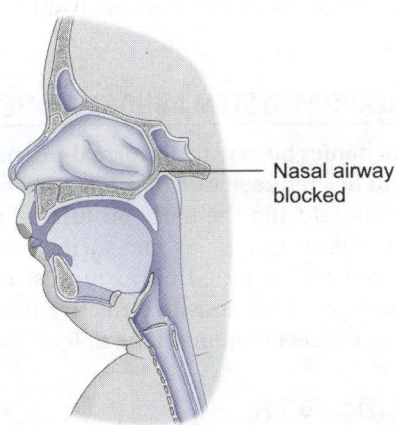

Figure 46.8: Choanal atresia.

CONGENITAL CARDIAC DEFECTS

Babies born with congenital defects comprise the second largest group of babies, born with abnormalities. The underlying mechanisms that produce cardiac defects are thought to be either abnormal cell migration or disordered intracardiac blood flow. Majority of the defects cannot be attributed to a single cause. About 10% of the defects occur due to chromosomal and genetic factors or caused by teratogens.

Detection of Cardiac Defects

An increasing number of problems are now being identified by ultrasound scanning. However, most defects are identified during the neonatal examination. Congenital cardiac anomalies of the newborn can be divided into two groups, (1) cyanotic heart disease and (2) acyanotic heart disease.

Cyanotic Cardiac Defects

Cyanotic cardiac defects include:
- Transposition of great arteries
- Total anomalous pulmonary venous drainage
- Tricuspid atresia
- Tetralogy of Fallot
- Pulmonary atresia
- Univentricular heart.

The first signs that a cardiac defect is present are the persistence of central cyanosis, tachypnea and tachycardia. Administration of oxygen to these babies will be ineffective in improving their color. Chest X-ray should be performed to exclude anomalies of the respiratory tract disease and diaphragmatic hernia. Echocardiography may be done to explore the precise nature of the defect.

Transposition of great arteries

This is a condition where the aorta arises from the right ventricle and the pulmonary artery from the left ventricle. Consequently, oxygenated blood circulates back through the lungs and deoxygenated blood back into the systemic circuit. Unless lifesaving intervention is instituted immediately, the baby will die. Prostaglandin infusion may be commenced to maintain patency of the ductus arteriosus, which may be followed by a Rashkind septostomy. This procedure involves creating an artificial septal defect to allow oxygenated blood to access the systemic circulation. Corrective surgery is then carried out later.

Some of the other defects do not initially present with marked cyanosis. These babies for a time may be considered healthy **(Figs. 46.10A and B)**.

Acyanotic Cardiac Defects

Anomalies included in acyanotic cardiac defects group are:
- Left heart hypoplasia
- Coarctation of the aorta
- Patent ductus arteriosus
- Atrial or ventricular septal defects.

nasopharynx. Tachypnea and dyspnea are cardinal features particularly when a bilateral lesion is present. The baby's color will improve with crying. Maintaining clear airway is obviously essential and an oral airway may have to be used to affect this. A unilateral defect may not be noticed until the baby feeds for the first time, when respiratory difficulty and cyanosis occur. Surgery will be required to remove the obstructing tissue. Occasionally, choanal atresia is associated with other abnormalities.

Laryngeal Stridor (Fig. 46.9)

Laryngeal stridor is a noise made by the baby usually on inspiration and exacerbated by crying. Most commonly, the cause is laryngomalacia due to laxity of the laryngeal cartilage. With stridor, the baby is generally not in distress though it may sound distressing. Parents often require repeated reassuring. The condition may resolve overtime perhaps by 2 years. If however, there are other accompanying signs of dyspnea or feeding problems, further investigations would be necessary to rule out additional abnormalities.

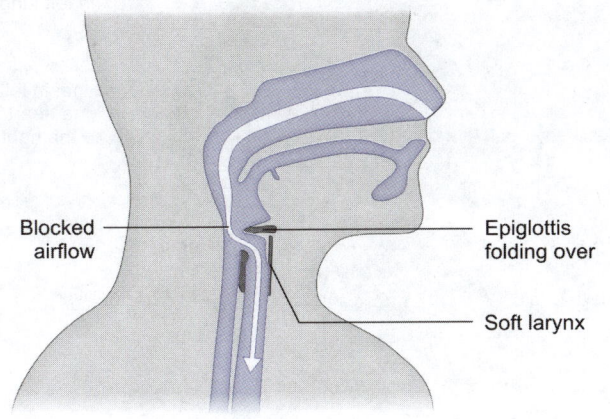

Figure 46.9: Laryngomalacia.

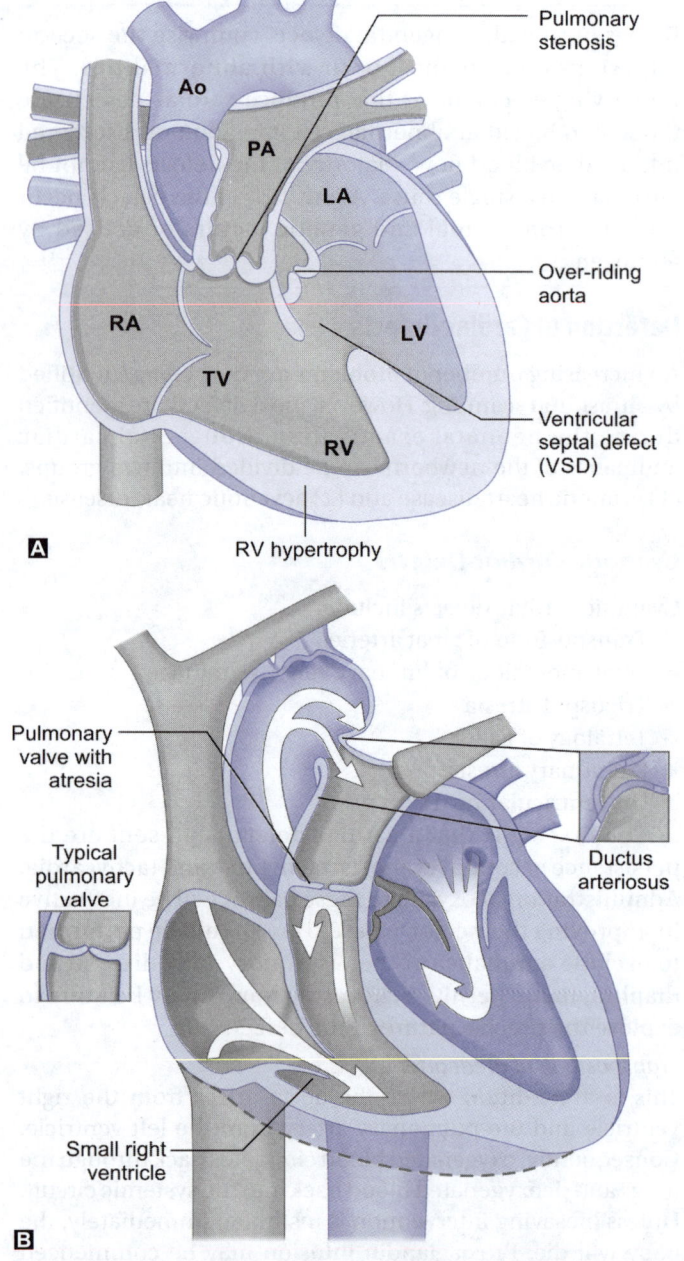

Figures 46.10A and B: (A) Tetralogy of Fallot; (B) Pulmonary atresia. (Ao: arota; PA: pulmonary artery; LA: left atrium; LV: left ventricle; RV: right ventricle; TV: tricuspid valve; RA: right atrium)

These babies may manifest signs of cardiac failure such as tachypnea, tachycardia and cyanosis following the exertion of crying or feeding. Detailed examination may reveal heart murmurs and diminution or absence of femoral pulse.

Corrective surgery is sometimes possible for coarctation of the aorta depending on the extent of the stricture. Babies with hypoplastic heart disease have a poor prognosis. It is important that each baby is examined thoroughly before discharge from the hospital. It is equally important to realize, however, not all heart murmurs heard at this time are significant. Parents must be instructed to seek medical advice for any change in the baby's behavior such as breathlessness or cyanosis.

CENTRAL NERVOUS SYSTEM ABNORMALITIES

The number of babies born with abnormalities of the central nervous system has reduced due to the mothers taking folic acid supplements during the early months of pregnancy. Prenatal screening tests such as measuring the alpha (α)-fetoprotein levels and detailed ultrasound scanning have resulted in some parents choosing selective termination of pregnancies, where severe neural tube defects are found.

Anencephaly (Fig. 46.11)

Anencephaly is characterized by the absence of the forebrain and vault of the skull. It is a condition, which is incompatible with sustained life, but occasionally such a baby is born alive. It is important for the midwife to wrap the baby (the head) carefully before showing to the mother. Parents may however want to hold the baby and see the full extent of the abnormality. Though unpleasant, it may facilitate their grieving process and will help them to accept the reality of the situation.

Spina Bifida Aperta

Spina bifida aperta condition results from failure of fusion of the vertebral column. There are various forms of the spina bifida.

Meningocele

Meningocele (**Fig. 46.12**) is a sac-like protrusion of either the cerebral or spinal meninges through a congenital defect in the skull, or the vertebral column. It forms a cystic hernia that is filled with cerebrospinal fluid, but does not contain neural tissue. The anomaly is designated as cranial meningocele or spinal meningocele depending on the site of the defect.

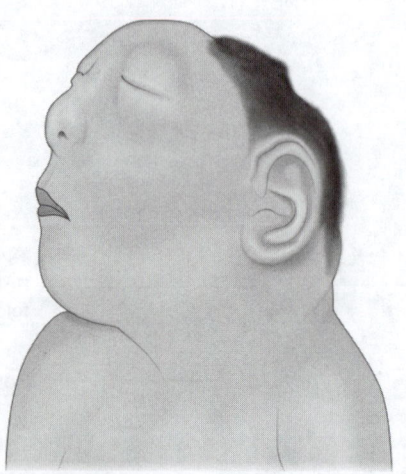

Figure 46.11: Anencephaly.

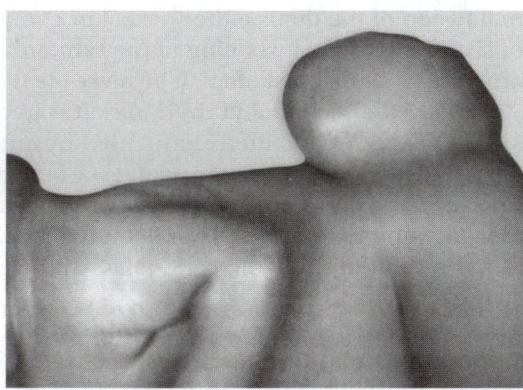

Figure 46.12: Meningocele.

Meningomyelocele

Meningomyeocele **(Fig. 46.13)** involves the spinal cord. This lesion may be enclosed or the meningocele may rupture and expose the neural tissue. Meningomyelocele usually gives rise to neural damage producing paralysis distal to the defect and impaired function of urinary bladder and bowel. The lumbosacral area is the most common site for these to present, but they may appear at any point in the vertebral column.

When the defect is at the base of skull level, it is known as encephalocele. The added complication with encephalocele is that the sac may contain varying amounts of brain tissue. Normal progression of the brain may be impeded by a large lesion of this type.

Immediate management involves covering open lesion with a non-adherent dressing. Babies with enclosed lesions should be handled with great care in order to preserve the integrity of the sac, thus reducing the risk of meningitis. Surgical closure is possible for meningocele.

Spina Bifida Occulta

Spina bifida occulta is the minor type of defect, where the vertebra is bifid. There is usually no spinal cord involvement. A tuft of hair or sinus at the base of the spine may be noted on first examination of the baby. Ultrasound examination will confirm the diagnosis and rule out any associated spinal cord involvement.

Hydrocephalus

Hydrocephalus is a condition, which arises from a blockage in the circulation and absorption of cerebrospinal fluid. The lateral ventricles increase in size and eventually compress the surrounding brain tissue. Hydrocephaly may either be present at birth or develop following surgical closure of a meningomyelocele. The risk of cerebral impairment may be minimized by the insertion of a ventriculoperitoneal shunt. As the baby grows, this will need to be replaced. Risks with the shunt devices are that the line blocks and the shunt becomes a portal for infection leading to meningitis. Signs of increased intracranial pressure to be watched for include:
- Large, tense anterior fontanel
- Splayed (spread out) skull bones
- Inappropriate increase in occipitofrontal circumference
- Sun-setting appearance to the eyes
- Irritability or abnormal movements.

Microcephaly (Fig. 46.14)

Microcephaly is the condition where the occipitofrontal circumference is more than two standard deviations below normal for gestational age. The disproportionately small head may be the result of intrauterine infection such as rubella, a feature of fetal alcohol syndrome or part of a number of defects in some trisomic disorders. The baby invariably will be mentally impaired.

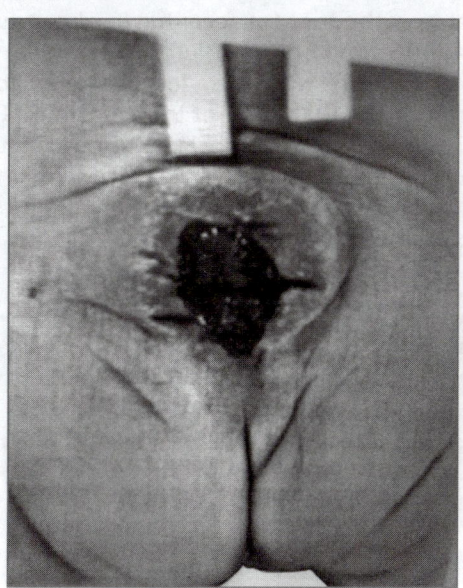

Figure 46.13: Meningomyelocele.

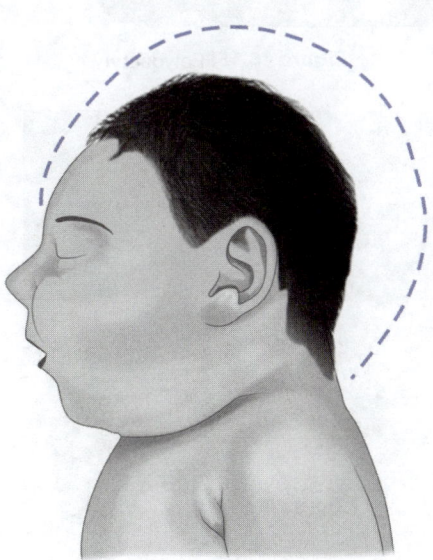

Figure 46.14: Microcephaly.

MUSCULOSKELETAL DEFORMITIES

Musculoskeletal deformities vary from relatively minor anomalies as an extra digit to major deficits such as absence of a limb.

Polydactyly and Syndactyly

Polydactyly (supernumerary digits) **(Fig. 46.15)** occur either on the hands or on the feet. In fact, their occurrence on the hands is sufficiently frequent to make this the most common congenital anomaly of the upper extremity. In some families, it occurs as a hereditary trait. Most frequently, it appears as an accessory and often hypoplastic appendage, sometimes no more than a simple skin tag on the ulnar surface of the little finger. Alternatively, the thumb may be duplicated. Polydactyly is occasionally seen in conjunction with other congenital malformations.

With the exception of a simple skin tag, which may be ligated and allowed to slough, surgical intervention is almost invariably indicated. In cases that are more complex, the operation may be delayed until the age of 2 or 3 years, when phalangeal and metacarpal ossification centers are present and the anatomic status can be more precisely defined.

Syndactyly **(Fig. 46.16)** second only in incidence to polydactyly as an abnormality of the upper extremity is an abnormal fusion of the digits either partial or complete. It may consist of interdigital webbing of the skin only or the bony structure, or both. Most often, it involves the third and fourth fingers or the second and third toes. It is frequently a hereditary characteristic unaccompanied by any other abnormality. However, it can appear as a feature of a syndrome such as Apert's syndrome, which is a genetically inherited condition in that there is premature fusion of the sutures of the vault of the skull, cleft palate and complete syndactyly of both hands and feet.

Treatment is by surgical operation. Since, premature intervention may lead to a poor result, surgery is best performed shortly before the child enters school.

Careful examination including separation and counting of the baby's fingers and toes during the physical examination is important in order not to miss anomalies such as polydactyly and syndactyly.

Limb Reduction Anomalies

Limb reduction anomalies comprise a wide range of possibilities. In some, either a hand or a foot will be completely missing, while in others a normal hand or foot will be present at the end of a shortened limb. Thalidomide, an antiemetic has been a proven teratogenic in this context.

The child is not ill and will not be upset by the defect. However, the parents of a child with limb defect will grieve the loss of their perfect child. Children usually prove themselves most adaptable and able to cope.

Talipes Equinovarus

Talipes equinovarus **(Fig. 46.17)** is a common congenital anomaly occurring once in 1,000– 1,600 births and accounts for more than 95% clubfoot. It affects males twice commonly as females. In this condition, the foot is turned downward and inward so that the sole is directed medially. In some instances, the condition may be attributable to an unusual fetal posture—the foot (or feet) having been held in an abnormal position within the uterus. In such cases, the position of comfort, which the foot assumes postnatally will often indicate the origin of the deformity. If the foot can be passively placed in a normal position without force, correction will almost certainly take place spontaneously or with a conservative mode of treatment. Treatment should be started as early as possible.

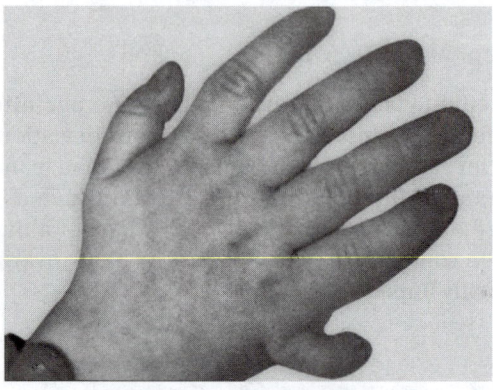

Figure 46.15: Polydactyly.

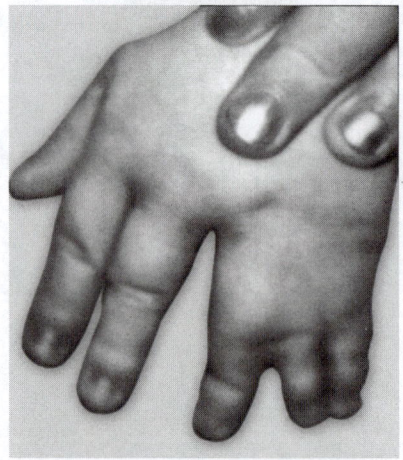

Figure 46.16: Syndactyly.

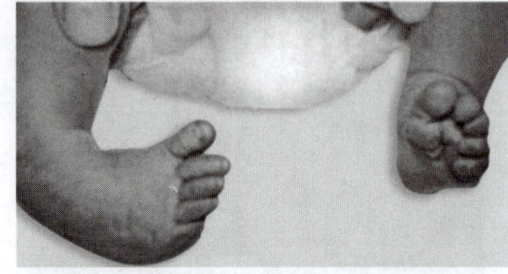

Figure 46.17: Talipes equinovarus.

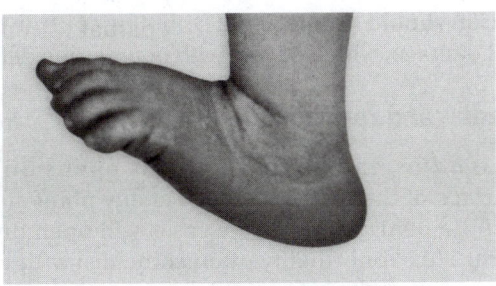

Figure 46.18: Talipes calcaneovalgus.

When the condition is mild, it may be completely corrected within 6–10 weeks. When force is required to place the foot in normal position, this indicates that shortening of the ligaments and tendon is present are more involved and prolonged orthopedic treatment will be required.

Talipes Calcaneovalgus

Like talipes equinovarus, talipes calcaneovalgus **(Fig. 46.18)** deformity may stem from an abnormal intrauterine position. The foot is held in dorsiflexion and deviated laterally. Shortening of the soft tissues on the dorsum of the foot, limits the degree of plantar flexion and inversion.

Generally, the condition is positional and the only treatment required is regular passive stretching. Less frequently, correction by exercise and application of plaster cast is required. When the foot cannot be passively corrected, the causative structural abnormality should be sought and appropriate orthopedic treatment instituted.

Congenital Hip Dysplasia

Congenital dysplasia of the hip is a condition in which there is an abnormal development of the hip joint and related ligaments and soft tissues **(Figs. 46.19A and B)**. The head of the femur may be in proper position although susceptible to dislocation by appropriate maneuvering. Alternatively, it may be either partially or totally dislocated. Characteristic clinical signs of hip abnormalities in the infant are asymmetry of the skin folds and creases on the dorsal surfaces together with apparent shortening or lengthening of the affected leg. For example, in congenital abduction contracture of the hip, the skin folds of the thighs and popliteal creases are asymmetrical, and the affected leg appears to be longer. In a dislocated hip, where the head of the femur is displaced upward and laterally, the affected extremity appears shorter and the inguinal crease is deeper, and more cephalad on the affected side.

The condition affects females six to eight times as frequently as males and the left hip three times more than the right hip. In 25% of cases, the condition is bilateral. The fundamental cause of the defect is still controversial.

Limitation of abduction, present at birth or developing within the first few weeks of life is a cardinal sign of congenital subluxation (partial dislocation or displacement). Early evidence of the condition may be obtained by the Ortolani's maneuver. In this maneuver, the infant's thighs are flexed to a right angle and fully abducted. The thigh under suspicion is then adducted, while still in the flexed position and pressure is applied along the long axis of the femur in the direction of the posterior lip of the acetabulum. As dislocation occurs, a click (the click of exit) is felt when the femoral head passes over the posterior lip. A similar click (the click of exit) is noted on reversal of the maneuver as the hip slips back into the joint. X-ray examination may help in the diagnosis.

In congenital dysplasia with dislocation, the femoral head is usually dislocated posteriorly and a reverse Ortolani's sign may be detected, i.e. a click of entry is felt on abduction and a click of exist on adduction. With lateral and upward displacement of the femoral head, there is an apparent shortening of the affected leg together with a 15°–20° external rotation of the limb and limitation of passive abduction with the hip flex at 90°. The inguinal crease is deeper and more cephalad on the affected side and there is an asymmetry of the thigh. When the infant is placed in a prone position, the

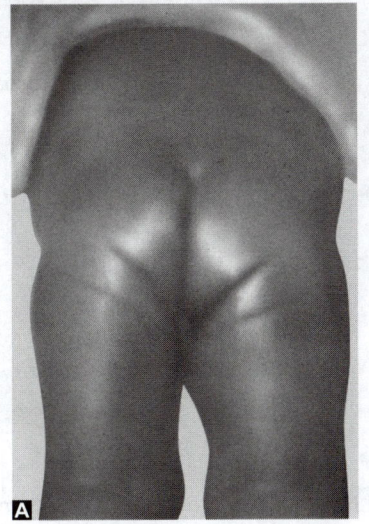
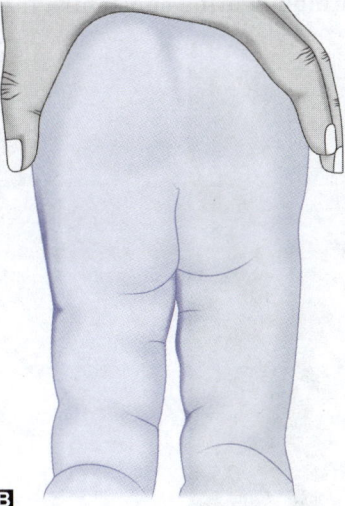

Figures 46.19A and B: Congenital hip dysplasia. (A) Normal gluteal and popliteal skin creases; (B) Abnormal skin creases in congenital dislocation of right hip.

buttock on the affected side is wider and flatter than normal. Radiographic examination should be used to confirm the diagnosis.

Early diagnosis is of vital importance in congenital hip dysplasia to prevent the development of persistent structural damage. Treatment is usually instituted as soon as the diagnosis is made. With early diagnosis, the sole therapy generally required is maintenance of the limb in a position of abduction and external rotation for 2–3 months. Application of double diapers help to keep the legs abducted. A splint or harness such as Pavlik harness may be applied to keep the legs in flexed and abducted position. Parents will require additional support in learning how to handle and care for their baby. Particular attention should be paid to skin care and checking for signs of chafing, and excoriation.

Streeter's Dysplasia (Fig. 46.20)

Streeter's dysplasia is a rather infrequent condition in which constricting bands (Streeter's bands) encircle one or more extremities. The constrictions are of varying depth and may appear on the digits, feet, hands or any part of the legs, or arms. Somewhat more common on the legs than on the arms, their causation is unknown, although hereditary factors have been thought responsible in some instances. The bands vary considerably in depth, sometimes being deep enough to cause congenital amputation and sometimes being so superficial that no treatment is required. Between these extremes, bands deep enough to interfere with circulation of lymphatic drainage call for surgical correction.

ABNORMALITIES OF THE GENITOURINARY SYSTEM

At birth, the first indication that there is an abnormality of the renal tract may be finding a single umbilical artery in the umbilical cord or alternatively recognizing the abnormal facies associated with Potter's syndrome (discussed later). Attention should be paid at the time of delivery to see if the baby passes urine. If no urine is passed within 24 hours or the baby is noted to be dribbling urine constantly, the pediatrician should be informed. Dribbling of urine is a sign of neural damage, which occurs with neural tube defects.

Hypospadias and Epispadias (Fig. 46.21)

In *hypospadias*, the urethral meatus opens on to the undersurface of the penis. It can be at any point along the length of the penis and in some cases will open on to the perineum. This abnormality often coincides with another condition named *chordee* in which the penis is short and bent. Some of these babies may require surgical intervention in the neonatal period to release the chordee and enlarge the urethral meatus. In *epispadias*, the urethral meatus opens on the upper (ventral) surface of the penis.

Cryptorchidism (Fig. 46.22)

If on examination of the baby after delivery, the scrotum is empty, the undescended testes may be found in the inguinal pouch. Sometimes, the testis in this position can be manipulated into the scrotal pouch. Testes that are found too high in the inguinal canal to manipulate into the scrotum may be malformed. Cryptorchidism may be unilateral or bilateral. Parents should be encouraged to have their baby examined at regular intervals. If descend of the testes do not occur by the time, the child has to go to school, orchidopexy will be required.

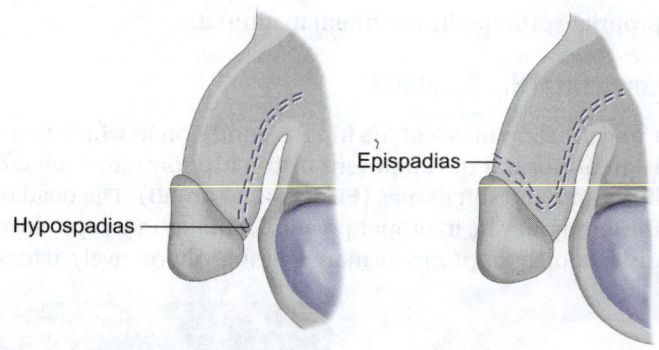

Figure 46.21: Hypospadias and epispadias.

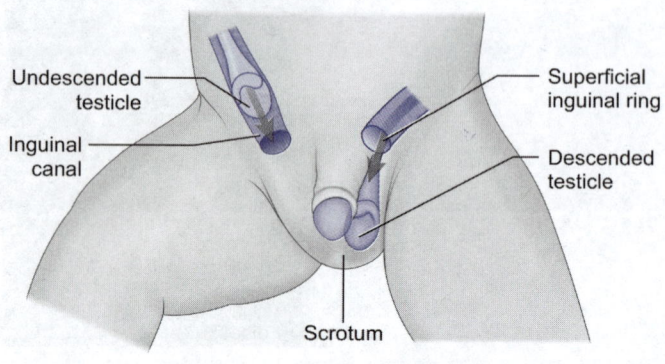

Figure 46.22: Cryptorchidism.

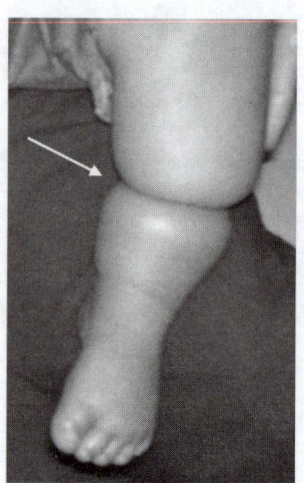

Figure 46.20: Streeter's dysplasia.

Ambiguous Genitalia (Figs. 46.23A to D)

On some occasions, the genitalia of a baby is such that it is difficult to determine the sex in order to give a definitive answer. Examination of the baby may reveal any of the following conditions such as a small hypoplastic penis, chordee, bifid scrotum, undescended testes or enlarged clitoris and incompletely separated, or poorly differentiated labia. Most of these babies are found to be females.

One of the reasons for ambiguous genitalia is an autosomal recessive condition called *adrenal hyperplasia*. The adrenal gland is stimulated to overproduce androgens because of a deficiency of an enzyme called 21-hydroxylase. If aldosterone production is reduced, these babies will rapidly loose salt. Urea and electrolyte levels should be measured and appropriate fluid replacements given. Baby girls with this condition may require later cosmetic surgery. The condition is not always recognized in boys in the neonatal period.

Intersex

In intersex condition, the internal reproductive organs are at variance with the external appearance of the genitalia.

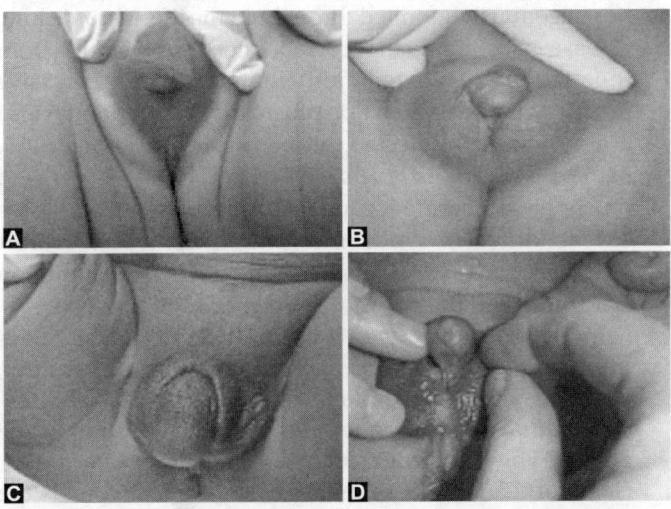

Figures 46.23A to D: Ambiguous genitalia.

Ultrasound examination will help identify the nature of internal reproductive organs. True *hermaphroditism* is extremely rare. Following chromosomal studies to determine the genetic makeup, hormone assays and consideration of the potential for cosmetic surgery and the decision of sex attribution is made. The difficulties of parents in accepting the condition and naming the baby are to be tackled with understanding. It is more common for a child of truly ambiguous gender to be raised as a girl.

GENETIC DISORDERS

The majority traits in the human body are controlled by several genes working together to produce the final effect or polygenic traits. For example, the distribution of height or the distribution of various body shapes of individuals.

Gene disorders may be single gene disorder or multiple gene (polygenic) disorders. Several pathologic conditions are polygenic and multifactorial. There is genetic disposition to conditions such as diabetes mellitus, hypertension, obesity and common psychiatric illnesses such as bipolar disorder and schizophrenia along with influence of environmental factors, such as lifestyle, dietary habits and stressful events.

Autosomal Dominant Gene Disorders

Autosomal disorders are single gene disorders involving the autosomes, which include both dominant gene disorders and recessive gene disorders.

An alteration in a single gene may cause multiple, physical and mental derangements without changing the gross structure of a chromosome or altering the total chromosome number of an individual. Therefore, the disorders may be classified under gene disorders (**Fig. 46.24**) and chromosome abnormalities.

- *Achondroplasia:* It is the most common form of dwarfism (adult stature is 122–127 cm), that is characterized by shortened limbs and a normal length torso. Common features include lordosis, prominent forehead with flattened nasal bridge and short hands with stubby fingers. Lifespan and intelligence quotient (IQ) are within normal limits among heterozygotes.

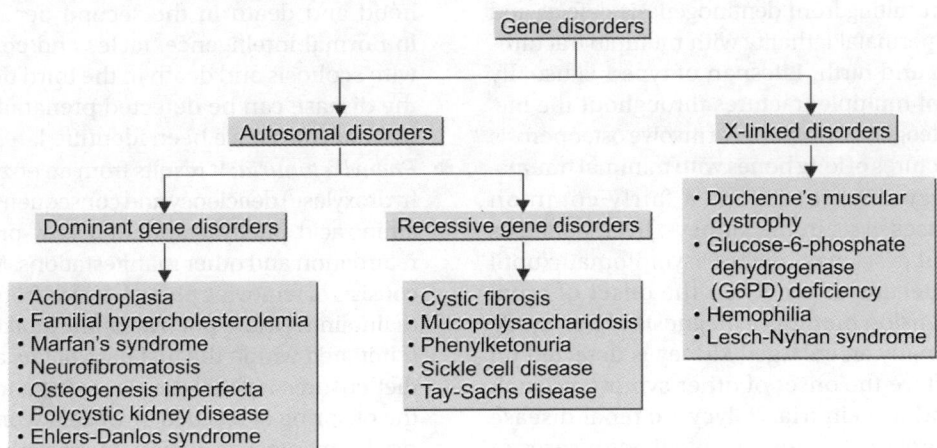

Figure 46.24: Types of gene disorders.

Gynecologic problems include premature menarche, enlarged breasts and premature menopause. Pregnancy results in several difficulties due to skeletal malformations. Increased paternal age is seen as a factor in producing achondroplasia.

- *Familial hypercholesterolemia:* Also known as hyperlipoproteinemia, familial hypercholesterolemia is one of the most common single gene disorders in which the manifestations are sensitive to dietary variations. Individuals who are homozygous for this gene tend to develop severe and life-threatening atherosclerotic disease that affects the coronary artery and cerebral and peripheral circulation.
- *Marfan's syndrome:* It is another disorder of connective tissue involving a triad of ocular, skeletal and cardiovascular alterations. The most common ocular abnormality is a partial dislocation of the lens. Common skeletal findings include tall stature, arachnodactylic (spider-like) hands and feet and scoliosis. The major life-threatening risk, however, is the frequent occurrence of aortic fusiform or dissecting aneurysms. About 50% of aortic aneurysms in affected women under age 40 occur during pregnancy with rupture most likely to occur in the third trimester. Aortic valve abnormalities found in Marfan's syndrome also contribute to an increased mortality rate during pregnancy. Average lifespan with the syndrome is 40–50 years.
- *Neurofibromatosis:* The condition also referred to as von Recklinghausen's disease is the multiple development of soft tumors of peripheral nerves or neurofibromas and abnormal skin pigmentation. In early childhood, the disease presents with multiple brown spots, usually on the torso and then progresses from adolescence onwards in the form of neurofibromas. About 75% of individuals go through life without developing some of the complications of this disease. Some individuals develop scoliosis, moderate to severe mental retardation, learning difficulties, hypertension, seizures, spinal cord compression, optic gliomas, pheochromocytomas and malignant changes in the neurofibromas.
- *Osteogenesis imperfecta:* Type I osteogenesis imperfecta is characterized by blue sclera, conductive deafness and discolored teeth resulting from dentinogenesis defects and type II results in perinatal lethality with multiple fractures during gestation and birth. Lifespan of type I is usually normal in spite of multiple fractures throughout the life. Other forms of osteogenesis imperfecta involve osteoporosis and recurrent fractures of long bones with minimal trauma.
- *Polycystic kidney disease:* This is a fairly common disorder that causes cysts in the kidneys, liver, pancreas and spleen. Renal cysts may remain asymptomatic until third or fourth decade of life when the onset of renal failure or hypertension prompts a diagnosis of polycystic disease. Occasionally an enlarged kidney is detected on X-ray studies before the onset of other symptoms such as hematuria and proteinuria. Polycystic renal disease accounts for approximately for 10% of all adult cases of chronic renal failure.
- *Ehlers-Danlos syndrome:* This genetic disease includes a group of disorders of connective tissue that result in hyperplasticity of skin, hyperflexible joints, vascular fragility and poor wound healing. Common complications include a tendency for bruising, hernias and varicose veins all of which increase during pregnancy. Poor wound healing and a predisposition to hemorrhage is risk factors during and after delivery (e.g. episiotomy healing may be delayed or complicated by these factors). The lifespan may be limited by vascular events such as aneurysms and rupture of large vessels.

Autosomal Recessive Disorders

The most common autosomal recessive disorders include cystic fibrosis, mucopolysaccharidosis, phenylketonuria (PKC), sickle cell disease and Tay-Sachs disease (TSD).

- *Cystic fibrosis:* It is a lethal genetic disease more common in Caucasians. Clinical manifestations include abnormal exocrine gland function with pancreatic insufficiency and malabsorption, chronic pulmonary disease and excessive salt in sweat. The pancreatic insufficiency results in pancreatic juice that lacks trypsin, an enzyme that must be exogenously supplied throughout the life. Chronic lung disease is secondary to recurrent infections resulting from the inability of ciliated epithelium to secrete excessive mucus. Pulmonary function progressively deteriorates and a large number of affected children die before the age of 10.
- *Mucopolysaccharidosis:* This diverse group of mucopolysaccharide accumulation disorders encompasses several different syndromes, which are type I, Hurler syndrome; type II, Hunter syndrome; type III, Sanfilippo syndrome and type IV, Morquio syndrome.

  Individuals with type I disease exhibit coarse facies in infancy, short stature, skeletal and joint deformities, deafness, corneal clouding, umbilical hernia, progressive mental retardation and death in the second decade of life. Type II is similar to type I, except for later onset, clear cornea and death in the third decade. Type I is the most common type with normal facies, stature and corneas, progressive mental retardation in the early childhood and death in the second decade. Type IV results in normal intelligence, facies and corneas; short stature with scoliosis and death in the third decade. Some type of the disease can be detected prenatally since their defective enzymes have been identified.
- *Phenylketonuria:* It results from an enzyme (phenylalanine hydroxylase) deficiency and consequent accumulation of the amino acid, phenylalanine and its by-products cause mental retardation and other manifestations. Management of PKU consists of removing phenylalanine from newborn's diet and maintaining a low-phenylalanine intake throughout the life. If initiated within the first days of life, a low-phenylalanine diet ensures normal development and lifespan. However, the offspring of rescued or treated women with PKU are at risk for mental retardation, microcephaly, congenital heart disease and intrauterine growth retardation. The condition

develops as a result of intrauterine exposure to high levels of maternal phenylalanine and its metabolites.

- *Sickle cell disease:* It is a serious, chronic hemolytic anemia that results from homozygosity for a mutant allele (one of two or more alternative forms of gene) hemoglobin S (HbS) gene. As a result of this genetic imbalance, HbS, abnormal hemoglobin replaces the normal adult hemoglobin A. HbS has decreased oxygen-carrying capacity and red blood cells (RBCs) acquire a sickle-shaped appearance, a morphologic change that greatly contributes to obstruction of small vessels and further ischemia. Infarctions of the lungs, kidneys, spleen and bones are common. The result is a lifelong series of sickle cell crises with recurrent pneumococcal infections, painful ulcers, osteomyelitis, priapism and other symptoms. Renal failure is a common serious complication. The lifespan is seriously shortened even with aggressive management.
- *Tay-Sachs disease:* It is a lipid shortage disorder with accumulation of GM2 ganglioside in cells of the nervous system resulting in a progressive neurologic disorder. The genetic defect results in decreased production of the enzyme β-hexosaminidase A *(HEXA)*. During their short life, children with TSD experience a progressive and steady neurologic deterioration in a series of mental and motor deficits, which begin at approximately 6 months of age. Symptoms at various ages include loss of developmental milestones acquired before the onset of the disease along with deafness, blindness, seizure activity and death by age 3–5.

X-linked Disorders

Genetic disorders whose causative gene is located on the X chromosome include Duchenne's muscular dystrophy, glucose-6-phosphate dehydrogenase (G6PD) deficiency, hemophilia and Lesch-Nyhan syndrome.

Duchenne's Muscular Dystrophy

Duchenne's muscular dystrophy is one of two types of X-linked recessive muscular dystrophies (the other being Becker's muscular dystrophy). Duchenne's muscular dystrophy results in progressive muscular weakening, atrophy and contractures beginning in early childhood. In the majority of cases, the age of onset is 5 years and the disease is characterized by delayed walking. A pseudohypertrophy of the calf (in which the muscle is replaced by adipose tissue) may mask the disease.

Affected children are usually unable to run and 95% of affected children are using a wheelchair by age 12. Mild mental retardation occurs in about one of four cases. Death often from respiratory insufficiency that occurs in the second decade.

Glucose-6-phosphate Dehydrogenase Deficiency

The G6PD deficiency common self-limiting hemolytic anemia, is a disorder due to deficiency of G6PD and is usually asymptomatic until the affected male is exposed to one of many environmental triggers such as certain drugs (antimalarial agents, Aspirin, sulfonamides) or certain foods. The hemolytic episode may also be precipitated by infections. Carrier females remain asymptomatic even when exposed to a trigger agent. Pregnant women with G6PD deficiency suffer several complications. Hemolytic episodes are more frequent; urinary infections, which are common in pregnancy cannot be treated with sulfa-based drugs and exposure of fetus with G6PD deficiency to maternally ingested trigger substances may result in fetal hemolysis, hydrops fetalis and death. The incidence of anemia, hyperbilirubinemia and kernicterus is also increased among newborn's with G6PD deficiency.

Hemophilia A

Type A or classic hemophilia is a fairly common X-linked recessive disorder of coagulation resulting from deficiency or defect in clotting factor VIIIC. In 10% of clients, the factor VIIIC level is normal, but activity is reduced. Variable degrees of deficiencies are probably caused by genetic heterogeneity (different mutations). In the presence of severe factor VIIIC deficiency, massive hemorrhages following trauma and surgical procedures (including dental procedures) can occur. 'Spontaneous bleeding' frequently occurs in areas subject to trauma such as joints resulting in hemarthrosis. Petechiae and ecchymoses are usually absent. Prenatal diagnosis by measurement of factor VIII is possible.

Lesch-Nyhan Syndrome

Lesch-Nyhan syndrome also known as hypoxanthine-guanine phosphoribosyltransferase (HGPRT), is a rare X-linked recessive disease characterized by a tendency toward self-mutilation, mental retardation, spasticity and hyperuricemia. Prenatal diagnosis is made by determination of fetal levels of HGPRT.

CHROMOSOMAL ABNORMALITIES

Chromosomal abnormalities may result from alteration in individual chromosomes (structural abnormalities) or from alterations in the total number of chromosomes (numerical abnormalities). Either situation may cause significant phenotype (observable characteristics of an individual) alterations and pathologic conditions.

Numerical Abnormalities of Autosomes

Numerical alterations of autosomes include some common trisomies found in humans such as trisomy 21 (Down syndrome), trisomy 18 (Edwards' syndrome), trisomy 13 (Patau syndrome) and Potter syndrome.

Trisomy 21 or Down Syndrome

Down syndrome is a common malformation due to a chromosomal defect. The defect is due to the inclusion of an additional chromosome, trisomy 21, i.e. 47 instead of 46 chromosomes. In a small percentage (5%), especially in young mothers, it occurs due to a translocation defect.

There is transfer of a segment of one chromosome to a different chromosome. The overall incidence is 1 in 600. The incidence rises with advancing age of the mother, reaching a peak of about 1 in 25 by the age of 45. The classic features of the syndrome were first described in 1866 by physician John Down. The commonly occurring features are as follows:

1. The head is round with flat occiput and a plump face, upward and outward slanting of the widely set eyes with epicanthic folds, short upper lip with small mouth and macroglossia.
2. The baby's face resembles that of the Mongolian race.
3. The hands are short and broad with a single palmar (simian) crease.
4. There is increased association of congenital heart disease [ventricular septal defect (VSD)], hypothyroidism, omphalocele, cataract and intestinal atresia.
5. The affected baby is often mentally retarded.

Expectation of life is reduced. An adult Mongol is likely to develop leukemia. Males are infertile. In females, puberty may be delayed and may be fertile. Diagnosis is established by chromosomal analysis (karyotyping) using bone marrow aspiration or leukocyte culture.

Parents who have a baby with Down syndrome should be offered genetic counseling to establish the risk of recurrence. Apart from emotional support, the mother may need help with feeding the baby as the baby may have generalized hypotonia.

Trisomy 18 or Edwards' Syndrome

Edwards' syndrome is found in about 1 in 5,000 births. An extra 18th chromosome is responsible for the characteristic features. The head is small with a flattened forehead, a receding chin and frequently a cleft palate. The ears are low set and maldeveloped. The sternum tends to be short, the fingers often overlap each other and the feet have a characteristic rocker-bottom appearance. Malformations of the cardiovascular and gastrointestinal systems are common. The lifespan of these babies is short and the majority dies during their 1st year.

Trisomy 13 or Patau Syndrome

An extra copy of the 13th chromosome leads to multiple abnormalities. The affected infants are small and are microcephalic. Midline facial abnormalities are common and limb abnormalities are frequently seen. Brain, cardiac and renal abnormalities may coexist with this trisomy. These babies have a short life. Only 5% live beyond 3 years.

Potter Syndrome

The baby's face will have a flattened appearance, low-set ears, antimongoloid slant to the eyes with deep epicanthic folds and a beaked nose. The babies are usually severely asphyxiated at birth because they have lung hypoplasia. They also have renal agenesis. It is a syndrome incompatible with sustained life.

Numerical Abnormalities of the Sex Chromosomes

Numerical abnormalities are caused by alterations in the total number of chromosomes. Some of the most common genetic disorders caused by sex chromosome aneuploidies (having an abnormal number of chromosomes) are Klinefelter's, Jacobs and Turner's and triple X female syndromes.

47,XXY (Klinefelter's Syndrome)

Klinefelter's syndrome is characterized by multiple X chromosomes and one Y chromosome. Physical abnormalities include elements of decreased masculinization such as gynecomastia, hypogonadism and increased pubis-to-sole length reflecting elongated lower limbs. Mental development is normal in most cases; mental retardation, if it occurs, is in the intelligence quotient (IQ) range of 50–85. Delayed language skills, however, are common.

47,XYY (Jacob's Syndrome)

Individuals with an extra Y chromosome are of tall stature (more than 183 cm) and suffer skin disorders such as adult acne. Children of XYY fathers often have normal chromosomal constitution.

45,XO (Turner's Syndrome)

Clinical manifestations of Turner's syndrome include low birth weight and short adult stature (135–140 cm); low posterior hairline and webbing of the neck, shield-shaped chest with divergent nipples, short metacarpals, cubitus valgus, coarctation of the aorta, urinary tract abnormalities, lymph edema of hands and feet in the newborn and fetal cystic hygroma and hydrops. Intellectual development is normal with verbal IQ exceeding performance IQ. Due to decreased secondary sex characteristics, administration of female hormones at puberty is a common practice.

47,XXX (Triple X Females)

Triple X females is a common condition (1:1,000 female live births) and display a normal phenotype with perhaps a slight decrease in mental capacity when compared to their euploid sisters. Gynecologic problems include delayed menarche and premature menopause. As with XXY males, the offspring of XXX females are largely normal.

Structural Chromosomal Abnormalities

Structural abnormalities include a variety of chromosome defects (e.g. deletions and translocations) that do not alter the total chromosome number. These are alterations in a single gene.

46,XX or XYB (5p- or Cri-du-chat/Cat's Cry Syndrome)

Cri-du-chat syndrome is a rare (1:50,000 live births) chromosome deletion syndrome resulting from loss of the small arm of chromosome B (5). In early infancy, this syndrome presents with a typical, but non-distinctive facial appearance often 'moon-shaped' face with wide-spaced eyes. As the child grows, this feature diminishes and by age 2, the child is undistinguishable from age-matched children. Profound mental retardation persists throughout a short life; most affected children die in infancy from multiple genetic imbalances. Typical of this disease is a crying pattern that is abnormal and cat-like. At times, it sounds like an angry cat and other times like a soft mewling sound. This is a result of laryngeal atrophy, which improves with age. By age 3, the crying pattern is still abnormal, but it acquires a normal pitch and loses its cat-like quality.

Fragile X Syndrome

Fragile X syndrome acquired its name from the fact that in vitro conditions, the X chromosome frequently displays breaks and gaps in its terminal portions. However, this is an X-linked dominant condition with increased prevalence among males. Clinical features include mental retardation and a typical facial appearance including an elongated face and long elf-like ears.

Chromosome Instability Syndrome

Chromosome instability syndrome is a heterogeneous group of genetic disorders characterized by a high frequency of chromosome breakage that is observed in vitro. They include ataxia-telangiectasia (or Louis-Bar syndrome), Fanconi anemia and xeroderma pigmentosum. These syndromes are associated with decreased immune function and an increased incidence of cancer mostly lymphomas and leukemia.

GENETIC SCREENING

Genetic screening is the process by which individuals or populations can be assessed for various genetic disorders to detect the presence of a gene before it expresses a genetic disease or to identify the carrier of a recessive state. Treatment for genetic disorders is rarely successful because of the complexity and magnitude of genetic damage. The primary weapon against increase in the prevalence of genetic disease is an aggressive program of genetic screening and counseling. The requirement of any such intervention must include voluntary participation, equal access to all and confidentiality (both in conducting the tests and in handling records and results). In addition, education and counseling about tests and procedures must be an integral part of any screening program.

Purposes

1. To provide early recognition of a disease for which effective intervention and therapy exist before symptoms occur, e.g. PKU.
2. To provide identification of carriers of genetic disease for the purpose of maximizing parenthood planning options, e.g. Tay-Sachs disease.
3. To obtain population data on frequency, spectrum and natural history of genetic disease, e.g. chromosomal abnormalities in newborns.

Timings of Genetic Disorders

Screening of genetic disorders can be performed during various times in a person's life:
1. Screening of selected populations for heterogeneous carriers, e.g. sickle cell disease.
2. Screening of relatives of a known carrier or affected individuals within a family for the purpose of reproductive decision-making.
3. Preconception screening for carriers, e.g. screening for Tay-Sachs disease among couples contemplating parenthood.
4. Postconception (prenatal) testing, e.g. screening for Tay-Sachs disease in the product of conception by two heterozygous carriers.
5. Newborn testing, e.g. testing for PKU in all newborns as mandated by law in some countries.

Among prenatal benefits of screening for carriers is the removal/reduction of anxiety and restoration of self-esteem, when the results do not reveal carrier status. It also facilitates genetic counseling and reproductive planning. Testing newborns for genetic defects provides for early detection and treatment initiation, maximizing quality of life.

Risks incurred in genetic screening include the potential stigmatization of those identified as carriers or affected individuals and for the development of feelings of inadequacy and guilt often seen in conjunction with genetic disease. A positive test result for one family member may result in the disclosure of genetic risks to other family members, who did not seek or want to know the outcome of the tests.

Candidates for Genetic Screening

- Women over 35 years
- Family history of neural tube defects
- Previous baby born with neural tube defect
- One or both parents, carriers of sex-linked autosomal traits
- A mentally retarded child with or without congenital anomaly
- Previous child with chromosomal anomaly
- History of recurrent abortion

Detection Tests

Improved prenatal screening and diagnostic techniques are now available for detection of abnormalities in early pregnancy, which include:
- Maternal serum alpha-fetoprotein (MSAFP)
- Triple test: MSAFP, unconjugated estriol (uE3) and human chorionic gonadotropin (hCG)
- Amniocentesis
- Chorionic villus biopsy (CVS)
- High-resolution ultrasonography
- Fetoscopy
- Embryo biopsy.

Termination of pregnancy is considered following early detection of certain genetic disorders, chromosomal abnormalities and structural abnormalities.

Management of 'At Risk' Couples

Preconceptional counseling is an important step in the management so that the couple has adequate information beforehand. Option of termination of pregnancy is offered if the fetus is affected with serious genetic, chromosomal or structural abnormality.

GENETIC COUNSELING

Genetic counseling consists of one or more encounters with the probands and their families with the objective of providing information about their genetic disease. A proband is a clinically identified individual, who displays the characteristics or features of the disease in question. The information includes risk figures and options, and provides a framework for a course of action to be taken by the individual or family.

It also includes an assessment of psychosocial family dynamics, which are an integral part of a genetic disease and exploration of feelings and perceptions often elicited by the newly obtained knowledge. Genetic counseling in its broader definition refers to a series of procedures that include processing the initial referral, assessing the needs, deciding on the appropriate tests, interpreting the results and finally communicating these findings to the proband, and family. The counseling process can be considered as a form of family counseling. However, two factors make genetic counseling a unique process:

1. Counselors must work with the grief and anticipatory grief issues. Even with the knowledge of a potentially negative outcome, a certain amount of hope and denial usually prevails until the birth of the affected child brings the family back to the reality.
2. The parent's knowledge that they are biologically responsible for their child's condition is a burden, often too heavy to carry without emotional damage. The physical contact with the individual, sometimes for a lifetime is a constant reminder of what may be perceived as reproductive failure. Emotional support can be provided by family members, counselors, social workers or even through question-answer column in newspaper, television and internet.

Many genetic disorders are not treatable with conventional techniques. In many instances, the prevention of a genetic disease is only possible though genetic counseling of persons at risk.

Stages of Counseling Interview

1. In the first interview, the counselor gathers pertinent information from family members. Once a detailed pedigree chart is generated, the counselor identifies the mode of inheritance and confirms the initial diagnosis. Testing of other family members, if recommended, is initiated at this time. The family members are made to feel at ease and ample time allotted for answering all questions.
2. In the second interview with all the previous information processed, the counselor discusses with the family all the implications of the findings, present options and clarifies possible outcomes, e.g. possibility of therapeutic abortion or sterilization. It is of topmost importance that genetic counseling remains a non-directive process with the counselor remaining supportive, but neutral about decisions that must be made. It must be remembered that the family members are the ones, who will have to live with their decision and therefore their decision, once made must be respected and supported by all health team members.

Prenatal Diagnosis for Genetic Counseling

One of the tools for genetic counseling is prenatal diagnosis of genetic disorder. These include a trisomy profile test, an ultrasound-assisted nuchal translucency test, a midtrimester amniocentesis and chorionic villi sampling (CVS).

Trisomy Profile Test

Trisomy profile test involves testing of MSAFP, hCG levels and uE3. The MSAFP levels are found lower in pregnancies affected by Down syndrome. Serum levels of hCG are found twice as high in Down syndrome pregnancy. This test presently includes maternal age, MSAFP, hCG and uE3, and has high rate of identification of common chromosome disorders.

Nuchal Translucency on Intravaginal Ultrasonography

Nuchal translucency high-resolution ultrasonography is used to detect increased nuchal (backside of neck) translucency as an indicator of Down syndrome. An increased nuchal translucency or presence of cystic hygromas (septated fluid-filled sacs in the nuchal region) is a common feature of several aneuploidy conditions including the common trisomies such as 13, 18 and 21. The procedure can be performed earlier in pregnancy than serum screening and it may decrease the need for future CVS or amniocentesis.

Midtrimester Amniocentesis

Midtrimester amniocentesis procedure is commonly performed between 14th and 16th weeks of gestation under ultrasound guidance and consists of transabdominally withdrawing approximately 20 mL of amniotic fluid for analysis of cells sloughed off by the developing embryo. Chromosomal analysis and biochemical analysis of the fluid are also done to detect the defects.

Chorionic Villi Sampling

The CVS test can be performed at an earlier time than amniocentesis that is 9th to 12th week and yields results sooner. The test is accurate in about 99% of cases, provided true CV material is obtained. One major disadvantage of CVS is that α-fetoprotein determination for detection of neural tube defects cannot be obtained and must be attempted at a later date, when the concentration of this substance increases.

NURSING IMPLICATIONS

One of the most important advances in biomedical science is the mapping of the human genome. This has the potential to make dramatic changes in all health care and certainly will affect the care of women and infants.

The nurse is likely to interact with clients and their families in a number of ways related to genetics. The involvement can vary depending on the setting and level of education. The nurse should have a general knowledge of genetic terminology to answer client questions and direct them to resources.

There are major implications in supporting couples in reproductive decision-making and in coping with potential genetic risks. Nurses may also be in the position to provide education and support for risk management for clients, who have their own risk factors.

STUDY QUESTIONS

Short Notes

1. Omphalocele.
2. Gastroschisis.
3. Duodenal atresia.
4. Imperforate anus.
5. Cystic fibrosis.
6. Hirschsprung's disease.
7. Pyloric stenosis.
8. Microcephaly.
9. Syndactyly.
10. Polydactyly.

Short Answer Questions

1. Pierre Robin syndrome.
2. Diaphragmatic hernia.
3. Choanal atresia.
4. Laryngeal stridor.
5. Anencephaly.
6. Hydrocephalus.
7. Talipes equinovarus.
8. Trisomy 21 (Down syndrome).
9. Hypospadias and epispadias.
10. Cryptorchidism.

BIBLIOGRAPHY

1. Dutta DC. Textbook of obstetrics, 5th edition. Kolkata: New Central Book Company; 2001.
2. Halliday AC. Congenital abnormalities. In: Bennett RV, Linda KB (Eds). Myles textbook for midwives, 13th edition. Philadelphia: JB Lippincott; 1999. pp. 795-814.
3. Littleton LY, Engebretson JC. Maternity nursing care: Thomson Delmar Learning. Australia: 2005, First Indian reprint, Haryana: Sanat Printers; 2007. pp. 239-65.
4. May K, Mahlmeister L. Maternal and neonatal nursing, 3rd edition. Philadelphia: JB Lippincott; 1994.
5. Nixon H, O'Donnell B. Essentials of pediatric surgery, 4th edition. Oxford: Butterworth Heinemann; 1992.

CHAPTER 47

Jaundice and Infections in the Newborn

Learning Objectives

Upon completing this chapter, the learner will be able to:
- Describe the process of bilirubin conjugation and underlying etiology of jaundice.
- Describe the causes and management of physiological jaundice.
- Explain the causes and consequences of pathological jaundice.
- Explain the treatment of jaundice by phototherapy and exchange transfusion.
- Describe the infections that may be acquired by the neonate before, during or shortly after birth.
- Discuss the role of the midwife in the prevention, assessment, diagnosis and treatment of neonatal infections.

JAUNDICE

Jaundice is the yellow discoloration of the skin caused by accumulation of excess of bilirubin in the tissues and serum. Neonatal jaundice becomes apparent at serum bilirubin concentrations of 5–7 mg/dL. Jaundiced shoulders and trunk indicates a level of 8–10 mg/dL. Jaundice of the lower body appears at 10–12 mg/dL and jaundice of the entire body at 12–15 mg/dL.

FORMATION OF BILIRUBIN

Bilirubin is formed mainly from the non-iron fraction of heme of broken down hemoglobin. Red blood cells (RBCs) are removed from the circulation and broken down in the reticuloendothelial system. The hemoglobin in the RBCs breaks down into its byproducts of globin, iron and heme. Globin is reused by the body to make proteins and iron is stored or reused for making new RBCs. Heme is rapidly bound to serum albumin and form unconjugated bilirubin-albumin complex (indirect bilirubin). The complex so formed is carried to the liver cells for conjugation by enzyme glucuronyl transferase to form water soluble (direct bilirubin). It is nontoxic and is excreted either in urine or feces.

Unconjugated bilirubin is fat soluble, cannot be excreted easily either in bile or urine and can build-up in blood and be deposited in extravascular fatty and nerve tissues, e.g. under the skin and in the brain. Deposits under the skin lead to jaundice, while deposits in the brain can cause bilirubin toxicity or kernicterus.

EXCRETION OF BILIRUBIN

The conjugated or water-soluble bilirubin is excreted via the biliary system into the small intestine where it is converted into urobilinogen by intestinal bacteria. This urobilinogen is then oxidized to form orange-colored urobilin. Most of the conjugated bilirubin is excreted in the feces as stercobilinogen and a small amount is excreted in the urine.

COMPLICATIONS OF HYPERBILIRUBINEMIA

Kernicterus (Bilirubin Toxicity)

Kernicterus is the most important complication, which can be fatal if not detected promptly and treated effectively. It is an encephalopathy that is caused by deposits of unconjugated bilirubin in the basal nuclei of the brain. The critical level of hyperbilirubinemia causing kernicterus varies from 15 to 20 mg%, depending upon the maturity of the baby. Hypoxia, acidosis, hypoglycemia, hypothermia or sepsis enhances the pathogenesis so that the condition may develop even at a lower level of bilirubin. Excess level of conjugated bilirubin cannot produce kernicterus.

Clinical manifestations are lethargy, poor feeding, high-pitched cry and loss of Moro reflex. Gradually, severe illness is manifested by prostration, respiratory distress and finally opisthotonus, nystagmus, hyperpyrexia, convulsions, and enlarged liver and spleen. The jaundice is intense along with anemia.

Prevention includes regular and periodic estimation of blood bilirubin level in susceptible babies. Exchange transfusion and phototherapy are used to effectively treat the condition.

TYPES OF JAUNDICE

Physiological Jaundice/Icterus Neonatorum

More than 50% of full-term neonates and 80% of preterm neonates will have some physiological jaundice. There is regular rise of unconjugated bilirubin from 1.5 to 2.0 mg/dL in the cord blood serum to 5–7 mg/dL on the 3rd day of life. In a full-term well baby, physiological jaundice never appears before 24 hours of age, never exceeds 12–13 mg/dL and usually fades by 1 week of age **(Fig. 47.1)**.

Causes of Physiological Jaundice

- *Increased red cell breakdown:* The newborns' RBCs have a shorter life span (100 day in term infants and 60–80 day in preterm infants as opposed to 120 day in adults).
- *Decreased albumin binding capacity:* The ability of neonates to actively transport bilirubin to the liver for conjugation is reduced because of lower albumin concentration or decreased albumin-binding capacity. Levels of unbound (free), unconjugated, fat-soluble bilirubin in the blood rise as the binding sites on albumin are used up.
- *Enzyme deficiency:* Newborn infants have low levels of uridine diphosphate glucuronyltransferase (UDPGT) enzyme activity during the first 24 hours of life. It is the major enzyme involved in bilirubin conjugation. Normal adult levels are not reached for 6–14 days.
- *Increased enterohepatic reabsorption:* Enterohepatic reabsorption of bilirubin is increased in neonates as they lack the normal enteric bacteria that break down bilirubin to urobilinogen.

Management of Physiological Jaundice

No specific treatment is generally required:
1. Adequate feeding: Early, frequent feeding helps newborns deal with their increased bilirubin load. Demand feeding ensures adequate volume of colostrum and milk in the intestine. Effective feeding encourages bowel colonization with normal flora and increases bowel motility, which in turn helps in the production of enzymes needed for conjugation, and decreases enterohepatic reabsorption.
2. Careful observation of newborns will help to distinguish between healthy babies with normal, physiological response (needing no active treatment) and those for whom serum bilirubin testing is required.
3. In premature babies, rising bilirubin level to critical level require use of phototherapy or phenobarbitone administration.

Pathological Jaundice

Pathological jaundice usually appears within 24 hours of birth and is characterized by a rapid rise in serum bilirubin and prolonged jaundice.

Features of Pathological Jaundice

- Clinical jaundice appears within the first 24 hours of life
- Increase in bilirubin more than 5 mg/dL per day
- Total bilirubin more than 13 mg/dL
- Persistence of clinical jaundice for 7–10 days in full-term infants and 2 weeks in premature infants.

Causes of Pathological Jaundice

The underlying etiology of pathological jaundice is some interference with bilirubin production, conjugation, transport and excretion.

Increased production due to excessive red cell hemolysis
Conditions that can lead to increased hemolysis include:
- Hemolytic diseases of the newborn:
  - Fetomaternal blood group incompatibilities—Rh and ABO incompatibility
  - Increased red cell fragility—congenital spherocytosis
  - Deficient red cell enzyme—glucose-6-phosphate dehydrogenase (G6PD) deficiency.
- Neonatal sepsis, which can lead to increased hemoglobin breakdown
- Polycythemia, delayed cord clamping and infants of diabetic mothers
- Extravasated blood, such as in cephalohematoma and bruising.

Defective conjugation
- Diminished production of the enzyme glucuronyl transference:
  - Immature liver cells as in premature babies
  - Dehydration, starvation, hypoxia and sepsis because oxygen and glucose are required for conjugation
  - Metabolic disorders such as galactosemia.

Transport and excretion failure
- Hepatic obstruction caused by congenital anomalies such as biliary atresia, bile plugs or absence of common bile duct

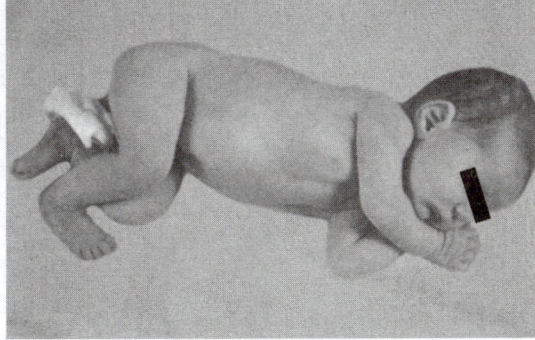

Figure 47.1: Physiological jaundice/icterus neonatorum *(For color version, see Plate 9).*

- Excess conjugated bilirubin caused by infection or idiopathic neonatal jaundice
- Umbilical cord sepsis leading to ascending thrombophlebitis, obstruction of biliary canaliculi and destruction of liver cells.

MANAGEMENT OF JAUNDICE

For the management of jaundice, it is important to differentiate between healthy babies whose jaundice is a normal physiological response and those with an underlying serious illness or liver disease. More than 50% of full-term infants and 80% of preterm babies will have some physiological jaundice. About 7 in 500 babies have some form of liver disease.

ASSESSMENT AND DIAGNOSIS

In evaluating neonatal jaundice, it is important to determine whether the jaundice results from the physiological breakdown of bilirubin or the presence of another underlying factor and whether the infant is at risk for kernicterus. Assessment includes observation of risk factors.

Risk Factors

- Birth trauma or evident bruising
- Prematurity
- Family history of jaundiced siblings or hemolytic disease
- Ethnic predisposition to jaundice or inherited disease (incidence of pathological jaundice is more in Asian, African and Mediterranean male infants)
- Delayed feeding or meconium passage
- Jaundice within the first 24 hours suggests hemolysis
- Prolonged jaundice may indicate serious disease such as hypothyroidism or obstructive jaundice
- Extent of changes in skin and scleral color
- Presence of lethargy, decreased eagerness to feed, vomiting, irritability, a high-pitched cry, dark urine or light stools
- Presence of dehydration, starvation, hypothermia, acidosis, hypoxia.

Laboratory Evaluation

- Serum bilirubin to determine if the bilirubin is unconjugated or conjugated
- Direct Coombs' test to detect the presence of maternal antibodies on fetal RBCs
- Indirect Coombs' test to detect the presence of maternal antibodies in serum
- Hemoglobin/Hematocrit estimation to assess any anemia
- Reticulocyte count (elevated with hemolysis when new RBCs are being formed)
- ABO blood group and Rh type for possible incompatibility
- Peripheral blood smear-red cell structure for abnormal cells
- White cell count to detect any infection
- Serum samples for specific immunoglobulins for the TORCH infections; TORCH stands for toxoplasmosis, other infections, rubella, cytomegalovirus (CMV), herpes simplex
- G6PD assay
- Urine for substances such as galactose.

TREATMENT

A number of treatment strategies are available to reduce bilirubin levels. These include phototherapy, exchange transfusion and possibly drug treatments.

Phototherapy (Fig. 47.2)

Phototherapy can be used to prevent the concentration of unconjugated bilirubin in the blood from reaching levels where neurotoxicity may occur. During phototherapy the neonate's skin surface is exposed to high-intensity light, which photochemically converts fat-soluble, unconjugated bilirubin into water-soluble bilirubin, which can be excreted in bile and urine.

Indications for Phototherapy

Phototherapy is started quickly, at lower bilirubin levels in infants:
- Who are smaller or preterm?
- Who are sick particularly with hemolysis?
- In whom jaundice appears within 12–24 hours?

Bilirubin levels indicating phototherapy are:
- For term infants who become jaundiced after 48 hours: 17–22 mg/dL (280–365 mmol)
- For preterm infants more than 1,500 g: 8–10 mg/dL (140–165 mmol)
- For preterm babies less than 1,500 g: 5–8 mg/dL (80–140 mmol).

The serum bilirubin level at which phototherapy is discontinued varies. Declining serum bilirubin levels below 13 mg/dL (215 mmol) are generally accepted as necessary for stopping phototherapy.

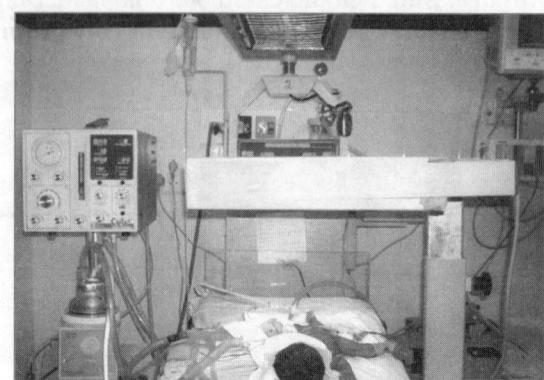

Figure 47.2: Baby undergoing phototherapy
(For color version, see Plate 9).

Types of Phototherapy

Conventional systems: Fluorescent lamps are used to deliver high-intensity light. The effectiveness depends on the wavelengths, the distance between the lights and the infant, and the amount of skin exposure. The infant usually is placed at a distance of about 45–60 cm from the phototherapy light with the skin exposed. The infants' testes/ovaries are covered with a nappy. Eyes are covered with eye shields or patches. Turning the neonate frequently ensures maximum skin exposure. Phototherapy treatment is generally continuous with interruption only for essential care, such as feeding or nappy changing. Intermittent therapy may be given for periods of 6 hours on and 6 hours off.

Fiberoptic light systems: Fiberoptic blankets or woven fiberoptic pads, which deliver high-intensity light with no ultraviolet or infrared radiation are wrapped around the infant under the clothing, thus ensuring that more skin is exposed to light. The pads can be used day and night with minimal supervision. They also reduce some of the side effects of phototherapy, e.g. increased insensible fluid loss. In addition, they eliminate the need for eye protection.

Fiberoptic phototherapy combined with the standard phototherapy is used to provide double phototherapy for optimum results. Fiberoptic mats were found more comfortable for infants and resulted in less restlessness.

Care of the Baby Undergoing Phototherapy

- *Observing any visible side effects:* These can include lethargy or irritability, decreased eagerness to feed, loose stools, hyperthermia, dehydration and fluid loss, skin rashes and skin burns, alterations in neurobehavioral organization, lack of usual sensory experiences including visual deprivation. Neonates may also experience hypocalcemia, low platelet counts, increased red cell osmotic fragility, bronze baby syndrome, riboflavin deficiency and DNA damage.
- *Eye care:* A potential side effect of phototherapy is the effect of the high-intensity light on the retina. The position of eye shields or patches is to be closely monitored to ensure that they are over the eyes, do not occlude the nose and that the headband is not tight. The infant is also observed for any eye discharge or weeping.
- *Estimation of bilirubin levels:* Bilirubin levels are usually estimated daily. The reduction in bilirubin levels appears to be greatest in the first 24 hours of phototherapy.
- *Skin care:* The skin is to be observed frequently for any rashes, dryness and excoriation, and cleaned with warm water when the midwife considers it necessary.
- *Temperature:* The infant is to be kept in a warm thermoneutral environment and observed for any hypo- or hyperthermia. If the infant is nursed in an incubator, servo control is usually used. Heat loss is to be minimized as far as possible.
- *Hydration:* Fluid intake and urine output are to be monitored (including the frequency, amount and color of urine and stool pattern). Good hydration is to be maintained with demand feeding, and if breastfeeding, the mother is to be encouraged to continue. Extra fluids may be required for severely ill or dehydrated infants. Intravenous fluids are not routinely required as they do not stimulate peristalsis or encourage meconium excretion.
- *Neurobehavioral status:* Infant's sleep and waking states, feeding behaviors, responsiveness, response to stress and interaction with parents and others are to be observed.
- *Sensory deprivation:* To reduce the effects of isolation when feeding, the eye patches are to be taken off and the infant is removed from the lights. Parents can be encouraged to hold, feed and care for their baby as much as possible.
- *Hypocalcemia:* Serum calcium level decreases in some babies and a level is less than 7 mg/dL is considered hypocalcemia in neonates. Symptoms include jitteriness, irritability, rash, loose stools, fever and dehydration and convulsions.
- *Needs of parents:* When the baby is undergoing phototherapy, parents will be in lot of distress due to anxiety about the baby's condition and the nature of treatment. The midwife has a particularly important role in providing information, support and reassurance. If the mother is breastfeeding, she may be encouraged to continue feeding as much as possible during her visit to the nursery.

Exchange Transfusion

Exchange transfusion is a life-saving procedure in severely affected hemolytic disease of the newborn. An exchange transfusion process removes bilirubin from the body and in cases of hemolytic disease, also replaces sensitized erythrocytes with blood that is compatible with the mother's and infant's serum.

Tan (1996) stated that phototherapy has largely replaced exchange transfusion when treating severe neonatal jaundice. Except in Rh incompatibility, exchange transfusion may now be seen as a second treatment of choice that is used only when phototherapy has failed. Exchange transfusion would certainly be considered when there is a risk of bilirubin toxicity or kernicterus.

Indications

Rh positive with direct Coombs' test positive babies having:
- Cord blood hemoglobin less than 15 g%
- Previous definite history of an affected baby due to hemolytic disease
- Birth weight less than 2,500 g
- Rapidly developing jaundice with unconjugated bilirubin above 5 mg%.

Objectives

The objectives of exchange transfusion are to:
- Correct the anemia by replacing the Rh-positive sensitized red cells (normal or hemolyzed) with compatible Rh-negative red cells

- Remove the circulating antibodies
- Eliminate the circulating bilirubin.

While about 80–90% of the fetal blood is exchanged during the procedure, transfusion of Rh-negative blood cannot alter the Rh factor of the baby's blood. The replacement temporarily helps to tide over the crisis from anemia and hyperbilirubinemia for about 2 weeks. Thereafter the baby produces its own Rh-positive blood.

Nature and Amount of Blood Transfused

1. Blood for exchange should be Rh negative, whole blood from unsensitized donors with the same ABO grouping to that of the baby or group 'O'. The blood should be cross-matched with the mother's serum (it does not cause any harm if Rh-negative blood is transfused to an Rh-positive individual).
2. The blood should be freshly collected.
3. The amount is about 170 mL/kg body weight of the baby.

A number of risks are associated with exchange transfusion. These include risks from the transfused blood and from the procedure itself, e.g. acquired immune deficiency syndrome and hepatitis B from the use of blood products. Exchange transfusion also increases the risk of necrotizing enterocolitis (Todd, 1995). Lack of experienced practitioners due to the infrequency of the procedure can also increase the morbidity and mortality.

Care of the Baby Undergoing Exchange Transfusion

The procedure is usually carried out in a neonatal intensive care unit with experienced neonatal nurses caring for the infant before, during and after the procedure. The transfusion is given by the umbilical vein. Removal of blood and replacement is conducted by removing approximately 10–15 mL at one time and replacing this with 10 mL, given slowly, taking at least 1 minute. This is usually continued until a total volume of 170 mL/kg of infant blood has been replaced.

For every 100 mL of blood transfused, one milliequivalent of sodium bicarbonate is given to combat metabolic acidosis and 1 mL of 10% calcium gluconate to prevent tetany due to transfusion of citrated blood. Bilirubin and hemoglobin levels are assessed prior to and after the exchange transfusion.

Following transfusion, the baby is placed under radiant warmer. The umbilicus is to be inspected frequently for any evidence of bleeding. Serum bilirubin is to be estimated 6 hours after transfusion and to be repeated as required. Blood glucose must be monitored four hourly to detect any hypoglycemia.

Complications of Exchange Transfusion

Immediate complications
- Cardiac failure due to raised venous pressure and overloading of the heart
- Air embolism
- Clotting and massive embolism
- Hyperkalemia
- Tetany
- Acidosis
- Sepsis
- Hypocalcemia
- Hypoglycemia
- Coagulopathies due to thrombocytopenia.

Delayed complications
- Necrotizing enterocolitis
- Extrahepatic portal hypertension due to thrombosis of portal vein.

Drug Therapy

Drugs are used as an adjuvant therapy:

1. *Phenobarbitone 2 mg/kg* body weight is administered thrice daily intramuscularly for babies undergoing phototherapy. Phenobarbitone increases the glucuronyl transferase enzyme activity in the fetal and neonatal liver to conjugate the bilirubin, which hastens its clearance.
2. *Antibiotics* are administered for 3–5 days.

HEMOLYTIC DISEASES OF THE NEWBORN

Hemolytic diseases of the newborn include:
- Fetomaternal blood group incompatibilities:
  - Rhesus incompatibility
  - ABO group incompatibility.
- Increased red cell fragility (congenital spherocytosis)
- Deficient red cell enzyme (G6PD).

Fetomaternal blood group incompatibilities are the most common cause of hemolysis in the newborn. Hemolysis occurs when the fetus possesses an antigen (Rh or ABO), which the mother does not have and becomes exposed to that antigen. The maternal antibodies so produced, i.e. an immunoglobulin G (IgG), crosses the placental barrier to the fetus to produce hemolysis of the RBCs by antigen-antibody reaction.

In spherocytosis the red cells are spherical instead of biconcave and are easily destroyed. In this case the abnormal gene is dominant and it may cause hemolytic jaundice in the neonate.

Glucose-6-phosphate dehydrogenase deficiency being an X-linked gene disorder is seen predominantly in male babies. G6PD is an enzyme necessary for the survival of the red cell. When it is deficient, red cells are destroyed. Jaundice occurs in newborns on the second or third day of life reaching a maximum by 6th day, subsiding by the end of 1st week.

RHESUS INCOMPATIBILITY

Rhesus or Rh (D) incompatibility can occur when a woman with Rh (D) negative blood type carries a baby with Rh (D) positive blood type. The antibodies produced in the maternal blood crosses the placenta and destroy the erythrocytes of the fetus. Usually sensitization occurs in the first pregnancy, and in subsequent pregnancies extensive destruction of fetal cells may occur.

Sensitization may also occur following such procedures as amniocentesis, abortion and external cephalic version or after antepartum hemorrhage. Antibodies once formed remain throughout life.

Effects on the Fetus

The effect on the fetus depends on the severity of the hemolysis:

- Congenital anemia—with lesser degrees of destruction
- Icterus gravis neonatorum—babies are born without evidences of jaundice at birth, but develop it within the first 24 hours of life
- Erythroblastosis fetalis—presence of increased number of immature RBCs
- Hydrops fetalis—infants are born with edema and ascites.

Management

When the bilirubin (unconjugated) level rises above 12 mg%, the condition is called *Hyperbilirubinemia of the newborn*. The palms and soles of the infant are usually stained yellow at this level and treatment is required. Treatment strategies to reduce bilirubin levels include phototherapy, exchange transfusion and drug treatments.

ABO INCOMPATIBILITY

ABO incompatibility occurs usually when the mother's blood group is O and the body contains both anti-A and anti-B antibodies. The antibodies are usually IgM class and are too large to cross the placenta. However, some women produce antibodies of IgG class, which are smaller than IgM and can cross the placenta. Once in the fetal circulation, the IgG anti-A and anti-B antibodies attach to fetal red cells and destroy them.

ABO sensitization can occur from blood transfusion and blood leakage due to pregnancy. Both first and subsequent babies are at risk. In subsequent pregnancies, the problem may become more severe because previous exposure of the fetus to type O antigens strengthens the anti-A response. The management of ABO immunization depends on the severity of the hemolysis. In most such cases where the mother's blood type is O and the baby's A or B, the hemolysis is mild.

NEONATAL INFECTIONS

Infection is one of the leading causes of neonatal death in the developing countries. The neonates are more susceptible to infection because they lack in natural immunity and take some time for the acquired immunity to develop. Full immunocompetence requires both natural (innate) and acquired immune mechanisms.

NATURAL OR INNATE IMMUNITY

Natural or innate immunity involves responses that do not require previous exposure to microorganisms. These include intact skin and mucous membranes and gastric acid and digestive enzymes that act as first line defense against infection in the neonate. Immediately after birth, the infant's bowel is not colonized with normal protective flora, and the skin is more easily irritated and damaged.

ACQUIRED IMMUNITY

Acquired or specific immune responses are the responses that develop and improve with ongoing exposure to a pathogen or organism. Although the infant has some immune protection from the mother, largely he must actively acquire this immune response. Immunoglobulins are deficient at birth. Antibody levels are limited (transfer of IgG across the placenta occurs after 32nd week of gestation). Breastfeeding increases the infant's immune protection through the transmission of secretary IgA in breast milk. During the early weeks of life, the infant also has deficiencies in both the quantity and quality of neutrophils.

Preterm infants are particularly vulnerable to infection. They have less well-developed defense mechanism and are more likely to be exposed to invasive procedures that increase the risk of infection.

MODES OF ACQUIRING INFECTION

Transplacental: Maternal infections that can affect the fetus through transplacental route are predominantly the viruses. They are rubella, CMV, herpes virus, human immunodeficiency virus (HIV), chickenpox and hepatitis B virus. Other infections are syphilis, toxoplasmosis and tuberculosis.

From amniotic fluid: Amnionitis following premature rupture of membranes can affect the baby following aspiration or ingestion of the infected amniotic fluid.

Intranatal:

1. Aspiration of infected liquor during labor in which early rupture of membranes and repeated internal examinations occur. This may lead to either congenital or neonatal pneumonia.
2. While the fetus is passing through the vagina, contamination of the eyes can occur with gonococci leading to ophthalmia neonatorum. Contamination with *Candida albicans* can lead to oral thrush.
3. Improper asepsis, while caring for the umbilical cord may lead to cord sepsis.

Postnatal:

1. Transmission of infection due to human contact as from infected mother, relatives or hospital staff.
2. Cross infection from an infected baby in the nursery or postnatal unit.
3. Infected utensils used for feeding or bathing—clothing or airborne.

ORGANISMS IN NEWBORN INFECTION

Soon after birth, the baby becomes colonized by bacteria derived from the mother, like *Staphylococcus* on the skin, *Streptococcus* in the respiratory tract and *Escherichia coli* in the gastrointestinal tract (GIT). This colonization takes place uneventfully in most newborns, but in some, particularly those who have been harassed during labor and delivered following distress in prolonged difficult labor, instrumental delivery or delayed emergency cesarean section, the same organisms turn virulent and produce severe infection.

The onset of infection is most often quiet and insidious. Except when the lesion is visible externally, the evidences of internal organ involvement are rarely detected. Minor changes in the baby's behavior should be identified as early detection and treatment gives good response and prognosis.

MANAGEMENT OF INFECTION IN THE BABY

The midwife's role in the management of fetal and neonatal infection includes prevention, assessment, diagnosis and treatment of infection.

Prevention

Midwives can play an important role in creating a safe environment that decreases the chances of infants acquiring infection after birth. They can do this by:
1. Encouraging and assisting the mother with breastfeeding, thus increasing the infant's immune protection.
2. Ensuring careful and frequent handwashing by all caregivers to prevent the spread of infection.
3. Having the infant rooming-in with his/her mother.
4. Adequately spacing the baby cots, when the infants are in the nursery with other infants.
5. Always using individual equipment for each infant.
6. Avoiding any irritation or trauma to the infant's skin and mucous membranes, as intact skin provides a barrier against infection.
7. Discouraging visitors, who have infections or who have been exposed to communicable disease, from visiting the baby.
8. Isolating infected babies when necessary.
9. Observing for and appropriately treating any infection in the mother prior to the infant's birth.
10. Ensuring the appropriate administration of immuno-globulin and antibiotics to mother or baby, if required.

Protection of midwives and other caregivers is also vital. The underlying assumption of universal precautions is that every patient is presumed to be a potential source of blood borne infections, e.g. hepatitis B, C and AIDS. Therefore, universal precautions must be used when dealing with any substance or article that may be contaminated with blood. General infection control measures must also be used with respect to any other body fluids that may be a potential source of other infections.

Assessment and Diagnosis

Prompt diagnosis and treatment of infection is critical in minimizing adverse or long-term effects for the neonate. Early signs of infection may be subtle and difficult to identify. Non-specific signs and symptoms can include temperature instability, lethargy, poor feeding, bradycardia or tachycardia and apnea. A maternal history of prolonged rupture of membranes, chorioamnionitis, pyrexia during birth, or offensive amniotic fluid increases the risk of infection for the baby. Laboratory evaluation may be dependent on the severity and type of signs and symptoms and may include:
- Complete blood cell count
- Testing of urine and stool for specific organisms
- Swabs from nose, throat and umbilicus
- Swabs from any skin rashes, pustules or vesicles
- Chest X-ray
- Lumbar puncture if central nervous system (CNS) signs are present
- Testing of cord blood, amniotic fluid and placental tissue for specific organisms.

Treatment of Infection

The objectives of treatment essentially are the prevention of septicemia and septic shock and a reduction in the short- and long-term effects of the infection:
1. The baby is to be nursed in a warm thermoneutral environment with the midwife observing for any temperature instability.
2. Maintenance of good hydration and the correction of electrolyte imbalance with demand of feeding and intravenous fluids, as required.
3. Systemic antibiotic or other drug therapy is always commenced as soon as possible as well as any local treatment of infection.
4. Monitoring of the infant's neurobehavioral status including sleep and wake states, feeding behaviors, responsiveness, response to stress and interaction with parents and other caregivers.
5. Any infant with septic shock is to be cared for in a neonatal intensive care unit as it is a life-threatening emergency.

The midwife has a particularly important role in providing information, support and reassurance to parents. Where possible, it is best to avoid separation of the mother and baby. If the baby requires, being in the nursery, parents could be encouraged to spend time with their baby. If the mother is breastfeeding she should be encouraged to continue or express the milk as appropriate and informed of the role of her milk in fighting infection.

INFECTIONS ACQUIRED BEFORE OR DURING BIRTH

Toxoplasmosis

Toxoplasmosis is a protozoal infection caused by *Toxoplasma gondii*. In adults infection is transmitted by encysted organism by eating infected raw or uncooked meat or through contact with infected cat and dog feces. It can also be acquired across the placenta. Transplacental infection to the fetus occurs during parasitemia.

Virulence of fetal infection is greatest, when maternal infection is acquired early in pregnancy. The affected baby may develop hydrocephalus, cerebral calcification, microcephaly and mental retardation. In less severe cases, infants may present with low birth weight, enlarged liver and spleen, jaundice, and anemia. Infants born asymptomatic at birth can later develop retinal disease and neurological abnormalities, usually by the age of 20. Maternal infection is rarely diagnosed clinically. On suspicion, serologic testing should be done for specific IgM antibody, which denotes acute infection. If current infection is confirmed amniocentesis and cordocentesis are done for detection of IgM antibody in the amniotic fluid and fetal blood. Ultrasonography is done at 20–22 weeks for ventricular dilatation.

If the fetus is infected and hydrocephalus is present, counseling for termination is done. If the fetus is infected, but is otherwise normal, drug treatment is given to the mother. Pyrimethamine, sulfadiazine, folic acid and spiramycin are given orally. If infection occurs late in pregnancy, only spiramycin is given.

Prevention includes advising women about proper handwashing and washing of kitchen surfaces following contact with uncooked meat. Uncooked meat, unpasteurized milk and contact with cat and dog litter to be avoided.

Rubella

Rubella or German measles virus causes mild and insignificant illness in the mother, but can have serious consequences for the fetus. The virus is transmitted by respiratory droplet exposure. Fetal affection is by transplacental route throughout pregnancy. Risk of major anomalies is about 80% if infection occurs in the first 12 weeks of pregnancy. Early infection may result in spontaneous abortion. The mother may also be advised termination of pregnancy.

Surviving infants can have cardiac defects, hearing problems, cataracts and very significant developmental delays. Infants born with congenital rubella are highly infectious and should be isolated from other infants and pregnant women for up to 1 year after birth.

Active immunity can be conferred in non-immune individuals by giving rubella vaccine (live, attenuated, rubella virus) preferably during adolescence to girls. It is not recommended in pregnant women. When given during childbearing period, pregnancy should be prevented for 3 months.

Cytomegalovirus Infection

Cytomegalovirus is the herpes class that is harbored in leukocytes and transmitted by saliva, semen, urine, cervical secretions and blood. Transmission may also occur by respiratory droplet or transplacental. Virus is excreted in urine and breast milk. Fetus is affected by transplacental route in about 30–40% of cases.

Infection in the mother may be primary or secondary. A primary infection in the mother during the first 20 weeks of pregnancy can result in spontaneous abortion, intrauterine growth retardation and premature birth of the infant. Infants with CMV may suffer from an enlarged liver and spleen, jaundice, developmental delay, blindness, epilepsy and hearing loss. Most congenitally infected babies are asymptomatic at birth with only 1% showing adverse clinical disease. However, they should be followed up for 5–7 years because of the possibility of long-term neurological problems. Infection can be confirmed by viral culture of urine and nasopharyngeal secretions. At this time, no specific antiviral treatment is effective against congenital CMV infection.

Herpes Simplex Virus

Infection with herpes simplex virus (HSV) is associated with genital herpes in the mother. Neonatal infection is more likely with a primary maternal infection during pregnancy and results in high morbidity and mortality. The infection may be acquired through the placenta or from an infected birth canal. The risk of intrapartum infection is about 50% when the mother has primary genital herpes lesions at the time of birth. Prolonged rupture of the membranes and the use of scalp electrodes both increase the risk of neonatal infection. Therefore, when active maternal infection is present, the baby should be delivered by cesarean section.

Signs of neonatal infection can be non-specific at birth. A herpetic rash (blisters and a papular vesicular rash) is usually, but not always, seen by the end of the 1st week of life. Multiple organs may be affected, in particular the brain, liver and adrenal glands. Mortality can be as high as 80%.

Untreated survivors can have long-term neurological damage, in particular microcephaly, blindness and severe developmental delay. Encephalitis occurs in a high proportion of children.

The virus is present in vesicles, urine and cerebrospinal fluid (CSF). An exposed infant should be isolated with the mother for care.

Acquired Immunodeficiency Syndrome

Acquired immunodeficiency syndrome (AIDS) is caused by HIV, which is a group of retrovirus, HIV-1 and HIV-2. The virus specifically reduces CD4 cells leading to immunodeficiency. As a result, the individual is susceptible to infections by opportunistic microorganisms and specific tumors. The incubation period is from 2 months to 4 years.

The main modes of transmission of HIV are sexual contact (homosexual or heterosexual), transplacental, exposure to infected blood or tissue fluids and through breast milk. Increased incidence of abortion, prematurity, intrauterine growth restriction (IUGR) and perinatal mortality are seen in HIV positive women.

The vertical transmission to neonates is about 30% in seropositive mothers. The baby may be affected in utero through transplacental transfer, during delivery by contaminated secretions and blood of the birth canal and through breast milk in neonatal period. Women with AIDS are discouraged to become pregnant.

Varicella Zoster Virus

Varicella zoster virus does cross the placenta and may cause congenital or neonatal chickenpox. Maternal mortality is high due to varicella pneumonia. In the neonate, infection can cause the milder symptoms associated with neonatal varicella or neonatal zoster. Maternal chickenpox from 4 months' gestation up to almost the time of birth usually results in these milder forms of the disease. However, at different stages of pregnancy more severe infections can also occur.

Varicella zoster immune globulin (VZIG) should be given to exposed non-immune mothers as it reduces the morbidity. VZIG should also be given to newborns exposed within 5 days of delivery. With maternal chickenpox during the first 20 weeks' gestation, up to 5% of infants will develop congenital varicella syndrome characterized by skin lesions, chorioretinitis and limb hypoplasia. About 24% will develop disseminated infection when the mother is infected from 5 days before to 2 days after delivery. This severe infection develops within days of birth and can result in disseminated skin lesions, viral pneumonia, liver problems, and death in 30% of cases.

Chlamydia Infection

Chlamydia infection may be acquired by the infant during birth from a mother with chlamydial cervicitis. Infected infants may develop ophthalmia neonatorum and a small number may develop pneumonia.

Hepatitis B Virus

The most common source of neonatal infection with hepatitis B virus (HBV) is maternal blood during birth. The virus can be detected in any body secretion including breast milk. About 90% of the infected infants will become carriers of the virus who are at risk of developing hepatocellular carcinoma in future. Infants with HBV positive mothers should be given hepatitis B immunoglobulin within 12 hours after birth. This is followed by administration of hepatitis vaccine during the 1st week, as part of an ongoing vaccination program. A booster dose is given at about 5 years of age.

Syphilis

Syphilis infection is caused by the spirochete *Treponema pallidum* and is transmitted by sexual contact or by maternofetal transmission. The infant may contract the disease through the placenta or from the birth canal. There are 50% chances of a mother with primary or secondary syphilis infecting her fetus during pregnancy. When active lesions are present in the birth canal, a cesarean birth is recommended.

Infants with congenital syphilis may be asymptomatic at birth or present with serious abnormalities. Symptoms may include maculopapular rash, enlarged liver and spleen, jaundice, skin lesions, deformed nails, alopecia, chorioretinitis and pseudoparalysis. Late congenital syphilis can also involve the CNS, bones, teeth and skin. Intravenous or intramuscular antibiotic treatment is recommended immediately on diagnosis with the infant isolated for the first 24 hours.

Gonococcal Infections

Neonatal gonococcal infection is acquired during the birth process. It can cause a variety of symptoms including ophthalmia neonatorum, scalp abscesses, vaginitis, proctitis, oropharyngeal infections and systemic infections. These systemic infections can include pneumonia, sepsis, arthritis or rarely meningitis. Diagnosis is difficult. Early and appropriate antibiotic treatment of both mother and baby is important.

Ophthalmia Neonatorum

Ophthalmia neonatorum is an inflammation of the conjunctiva during the first 3 days' life. The classical ophthalmia neonatorum caused by gonococcus is very rare these days. The most common cause for it is *Chlamydia trachomatis*. The other causes include—bacterial-staphylococcal, pseudomonal-pneumococcal, chemical silver nitrate and viral herpes simplex.

Infection occurs mostly during delivery by contaminated vaginal discharge. It is more likely in babies born by face and breech presentations. During neonatal period, there may be contamination from other sites of infection or by chemical. The clinical picture varies and the discharge may be watery, mucopurulent to frank purulent in one or both eyes. The eyelids may be sticky or markedly swollen. Cornea may be involved in severe cases.

The condition can be prevented by treating any suspicious vaginal discharge during the antenatal period and maintaining meticulous aseptic technique at birth. The newborn's closed eyelids should be thoroughly cleaned and dried. Sulfacetamide eyedrops or Soframycin eyedrops are instilled into each eye for few days.

The discharge from the eyes is taken for gram stain smear and culture and sensitivity tests. Treatment depends on the specific etiology. For gonococcal infections, eyes are irrigated with sterile isotonic saline every 1–2 hours and topical gentamicin eyedrops are instilled four times a day for 7 days. In severe cases, systemic benzylpenicillin 50,000 units/kg is given in two divided doses for 7 days or cefotaxime 100 mg/kg is given intravenously. For chlamydia, erythromycin suspension 40 mg/kg is given orally for 2–3 weeks with erythromycin eyedrops four times a day. For herpes simplex, systemic therapy with acyclovir 30 mg/kg for 2 weeks is given IV.

Candida Infections

Candida is a gram-positive yeast fungus. *Candida albicans* is responsible for most fungal infections including oral thrush in infants. Infection can affect the mouth (oral candidiasis), the skin (cutaneous candidiasis) and visceral organs (disseminated candidiasis).

Oral candidiasis or thrush presents as white patches on the gums, palate and tongue. It can also affect the skin around the mouth, perineum and anus. It can be acquired during birth or from caregiver's hands or feeding equipment. The fungus grows on the mucous membrane and produces milky white elevated patches resembling milk curd, which cannot be easily wiped off. Rarely, the infection may spread down to involve the gastrointestinal or respiratory tract. Removing the lesions is not recommended as this may leave raw areas. Nystatin (Mycostatin) oral suspension dropped under the tongue four times a day is effective to treat the infection. Application of boroglycerine is soothing.

Cutaneous candidiasis presents as a moist papular or vesicular rash, usually in the region of the axilla, neck, perineum or umbilicus. The area is kept as dry as possible and topical nystatin applied. Oral nystatin is also used to reduce the yeast population.

Disseminated candidiasis is usually found only in preterm and ill newborns. Complications can include meningitis, endocarditis, pyelonephritis, pneumonia and osteomyelitis.

INFECTIONS ACQUIRED AFTER BIRTH

Skin Infections

Most neonatal skin infections are caused by *Staphylococcus aureus (S. aureus)*. In newborn babies, the most likely skin lesions are septic spots or pustules, which may be either found as a solitary lesion or clustered in the umbilical and buttock areas. In a well neonate with limited lesions, regular cleansing with an antiseptic solution may be all that is required. Lesions that are more extensive require antibiotic treatment.

Pemphigus neonatorum is a serious form of skin infection in the newborn caused by *S. aureus*. It can cause septicemia or pyemia. Superficial ulcers appear on any part of the skin; become pustules and then burst. They tend to appear in crops and are usually associated with systemic illness.

The baby is to be isolated. The blisters are pricked with a sterile needle and after removal of the dead skin; the area is to be smeared with antibiotic ointment. Systemic administration of gentamicin or cloxacillin is required in severe infections. *Pemphigus* may also be due to syphilis when the blisters appear on the palms, soles or trunk. Other features of syphilis are present. Antisyphilitic treatment is to be instituted.

Omphalitis

Omphalitis (infection of the umbilicus) can include localized infection and an offensive discharge. Treatment includes regular cleansing, administration of an antibiotic powder and appropriate antibiotic therapy. Untreated infection can spread to the liver via the umbilical vein and cause hepatitis and septicemia.

Respiratory Infections

Nasopharyngitis and Rhinitis

These conditions though not severe, may be distressing for the infant. Babies with nasal pharyngitis may be isolated with their mothers to prevent the spread of the infection. Symptomatic treatment and antibiotics may be required.

Neonatal Pneumonia

Pneumonia is the most serious of neonatal respiratory infections. It may be acquired before, during or after birth. In newborns, pneumonia is life-threatening and early diagnosis is essential. Symptoms of general infection may be accompanied by nasal flaring, grunting, substernal and intercostal retraction and cyanosis. Blood evaluation and chest X-ray are done to diagnose pneumonia. Appropriate antibiotic therapy must be instituted promptly.

Gastrointestinal Infections

Gastroenteritis

Causative organisms include *Salmonella, Shigella* and a pathogenic strain of *Escherichia coli*. Rotavirus is the most important cause of viral gastroenteritis in the newborn. Treatment depends upon the severity of symptoms. The correction of fluid and electrolyte imbalance is an urgent priority as vomiting and diarrhea can rapidly cause dehydration.

Infants with infective diarrhea are isolated and stool should be sent for culture and sensitivity prior to antibiotic therapy. Milk feeding is stopped and oral rehydration fluids are given in mild cases. In severe cases, parenteral therapy is required.

Necrotizing Enterocolitis

Necrotizing enterocolitis (NEC) is characterized by inflammation, ischemia and necrosis of the gastrointestinal tract (GIT). It is the most common and most lethal surgical abdominal emergency in the newborn.

Early symptoms can include temperature instability, lethargy, bradycardia, apnea, decreased appetite, vomiting, blood in the stool and abdominal distension. As the disease, progresses there may be severe abdominal distension and tenderness, grossly bloody stools and presence of hepatic portal venous gas. Diagnosis is confirmed by X-ray showing pneumatosis intestinalis (submucosal or subserosal cysts filled with a gaseous mixture). In the late stages, perforation of the gut, peritonitis, septic shock and death can occur.

Possible risk factors for developing NEC include prematurity, low birth weight, enteral feeding, asphyxia, patent ductus arteriosus and bacterial infection. Treatment depends on the stage and severity of the disease. Nonsurgical treatment includes the prevention of shock, the correction of electrolyte imbalance and the administration of broad spectrum antibiotics. When surgical treatment is needed, the necrotic tissue is resected with the objective of preserving as much bowel as possible.

Urinary Tract Infections

Urinary tract infections can occur because of bacterial invasion or congenital anomaly that obstructs urine flow. The causative organisms include *E. coli*, group B *Streptococcus* and other organisms. The signs and symptoms are usually those of an early non-specific infection. Diagnosis is usually confirmed through laboratory evaluation of a urine sample. Specific treatment according to the organisms identified is instituted.

Meningitis

Meningitis is inflammation of the membranes lining the brain and spinal column. The most common organisms causing neonatal meningitis are *E. coli*, group B streptococci and *Listeria monocytogenes*. Other types found include candidal meningitis and herpes meningitis.

Maternal infections and pyrexia at birth are often identified as the associated factor. In the early stages, the infant may have non-specific signs of generalized infection. Specific signs of meningeal irritation may also be present, including irritability, raised intracranial pressure demonstrated by a bulging fontanel, increasing lethargy, crying, tremors and twitching, severe vomiting, alterations in consciousness and diminished muscle tone. Infants may also present with hemiparesis, decreased pupillary reaction of the eye, decreased retinal reflex and an abnormal Moro reflex.

Diagnosis is usually confirmed by lumbar puncture and examination of CSF. Very ill babies will require intensive nursing care including intravenous fluids and antibiotic therapy. Early diagnosis and treatment offers better prognosis. About 30–50% of surviving infants suffer long-term neurological complications such as feeding problems and minimal brain damage.

STUDY QUESTIONS

Short Notes

1. ABO incompatibility.
2. Rhesus incompatibility.
3. Natural immunity.
4. Kernicterus.
5. Omphalitis.
6. Pathological jaundice.

Short Answer Questions

1. Candida infection in newborn.
2. Ophthalmia neonatorum.
3. Types of phototherapy treatment.
4. Care of the baby undergoing phototherapy.
5. Acquired immunity.

Essay Questions

1. Explain physiological jaundice, its causes, diagnostic measures and management.
2. Explain pathological jaundice, its causes, diagnostic measures and management.

BIBLIOGRAPHY

1. Adhikari M, Coovadia YM, Singh D. A 4-year study of neonatal meningitis: clinical and microbiological findings. Journal of Tropical Pediatrics. 1995;41(2):81-5.
2. Blackburn S. Hyperbilirubinemia and neonatal jaundice. Neonatal Network. 1995;14(7):15-25.
3. Brown LP, Arnold L, Allison D, et al. Incidence and pattern of jaundice in healthy breast-fed infants during the first month of life. Nursing Research. 1993;42(2):106-10.
4. Costello SA, Nyikal J, Yu VY, et al. Biliblanket phototherapy system versus conventional phototherapy: a randomized controlled trial in preterm infants. Journal of Paediatric and Child Health. 1995;31(1):11-3.
5. Dutta DC. Textbook of obstetrics, 5th edition. kolkata: New Central Book Company; 2001. pp. 511-4.
6. Lott JW, Kenner C. Assessment and management of immunologic dysfunction. In: Kenner CA (Ed). Comprehensive Neonatal Nursing. A Physiologic Perspective. Philadelphia: WB Saunders; 1994.
7. McFadden EA. The Wallaby Phototherapy System: a new approach to phototherapy. Journal of Pediatric Nursing. 1991;6(3):206-8.
8. Percival P. Jaundice and infection. In: Bennett RV, Linda KB (Eds). Myles Textbook for Midwives, 13th edition. Edinburgh: Churchill Livingstone; 1999. pp. 814-42.
9. Rubaltelli FF, Griffith PF. Management of neonatal hyperbilirubinaemia and prevention of kernicterus. Drugs 1992;43(6):864-72.
10. Sater K. Color me yellow: caring for the new infant with hyperbilirubinemia and prevention of kernicterus. Journal of Intravenous Nursing. 1995;18(6):317-25.
11. Stephenson K. Neonatal jaundice. Physician Assistant. 1996;20(4):19-38.
12. Tan KL. Phototherapy for neonatal jaundice. Acta Paediatrics. 1996;85(3):277-9.
13. Todd NA. Isovolemic exchange transfusion of the neonate. Neonatal Network. 1995;14(6):75-7.

CHAPTER 48

Metabolic and Endocrine Disorders in the Newborn

Learning Objectives

Upon completion of this chapter, the learner will be able to:
- Review the common disorders of metabolic and endocrine disorders.
- Outline the screening methods available for the early detection of disorders.
- Discuss the features, causes and management of diarrhea and vomiting in newborn.
- Discuss the identification and management of babies with drugs or substance withdrawal.

INBORN ERRORS OF METABOLISM

Transient disorders of glucose and electrolyte balance are common in preterm and stressed neonates. Permanent disorders such as those caused by inborn errors of metabolism (IEM), may also present in the neonatal period. These disorders have the potential to cause brain damage, poor growth and development or even death. However, the occurrence of individual conditions is rare. As a group, IEM contribute significantly to neonatal morbidity and mortality.

Common Features of IEM

Most IEM are autosomal recessive inherited conditions. Certain conditions are more rare in different populations. In IEM, normal metabolism is disrupted by the absence or deficiency of an enzyme. Metabolites can then accumulate, which are toxic to the body tissues, including the brain. In utero, the fetus is usually not affected as the placenta removes toxins. It is mostly after birth, the neonate will start to show signs of IEM. Many of these signs can be nonspecific and could be attributed to other neonatal problems such as sepsis. The signs may become apparent within hours, days or weeks.

Possible Indicators of IEM

1. History of previous unexplained neonatal death in the family or parental consanguinity.
2. Failure of a sick neonate to respond to usual management.
3. History of a period of apparent health after birth, followed by adverse signs after the introduction of milk feeding.
4. Severe metabolic acidosis.
5. Diarrhea, vomiting and failure to thrive.
6. Apnea or respiratory distress secondary to neurological depression and/or severe metabolic acidosis.
7. Unusual odor from the baby's skin or urine, discoloration of urine, abnormally colored or offensive stool.
8. Prolonged or early jaundice.

Diagnosis of IEM

Antenatal diagnosis can be made by DNA analysis of fetal cells obtained at amniocentesis or chorionic villus biopsy. After birth, screening procedures done for neonates in developed countries ensures early diagnosis and prompt initiation of treatment.

One of the most common screening procedures used is the Guthrie test in which blood dropped onto an absorbent filter paper is examined using microbiological techniques. Antibiotics may interfere with the microbiological methods used in this test. If the baby is on antibiotic therapy or is breastfeed and the mother is taking antibiotics, the information is included in the Guthrie test card. Conditions screened will vary in different conditions. However, in most developed countries, all newborn babies are screened for phenylketonuria (PKU) and hypothyroidism.

Common investigations for IEM involve general tests such as:
- Blood glucose
- Blood gases
- Urine for ketones or reducing substances
- Metabolic tests for blood and urine
- Enzyme analysis of blood and urine.

PHENYLKETONURIA

Phenylketonuria is an autosomal recessive condition with an incidence of about 1 in 10,000. It is due to the deficiency of enzyme phenylalanine hydroxylase, which converts phenylalanine (an amino acid) to tyrosine in the liver. Because of the failure of conversion, phenylalanine levels rise and although some will be excreted in the urine, most will be converted to phenylpyruvic acid. The raised level of phenylalanine in the blood is found within a few days of birth, after the baby has been subjected to dietary protein. The build-up of phenylpyruvic acid takes longer. It is toxic to the developing brain and without treatment mental retardation results.

Clinical Features

At birth, the baby looks and behaves normally. Signs usually appear after 3 months. These include vomiting, feeding difficulties, eczema, fair skin and hair, blue eyes and 'musty' (stale) smelling urine due to presence of phenylacetic acid.

Diagnosis

1. Positive result on Guthrie test done on capillary blood drawn between 6th and 8th postnatal day.
2. Assessment of phenylalanine level in blood.

Management

Low phenylalanine diet is prescribed. Milk substitutes with iron supplements are usually given. After puberty, the child will be able to tolerate normal diet. Continued follow-up will be required. In females, a return to low phenylalanine diet is essential prior to conception and during pregnancy.

GALACTOSEMIA

Galactosemia is the most common disorder of carbohydrate metabolism, which appears in the neonatal period. It is an autosomal recessive condition and can be screened during the antenatal period and in the newborn period. The enzyme, which aids the conversion of galactose to glucose, is absent. Galactose and glucose are the component sugars present in the disaccharide lactose.

Clinical signs include vomiting, diarrhea, failure to gain weight, jaundice, lethargy and hypotonia. An affected baby may also present with septicemia secondary to damage to intestinal mucosa by high levels of galactose in the intestines. The diagnosis is confirmed by urine and blood enzyme assessment. Affected babies need to be fed lactose-free milk.

G6PD DEFICIENCY

Glucose-6-phosphate dehydrogenase (G6PD) is an inherited disorder of red blood cell metabolism. Hemolysis occurs resulting in jaundice and anemia in the neonate. This condition is more prevalent in Asian, Middle Eastern and Mediterranean populations. Management includes treating the jaundice, correcting anemia and reducing the baby's exposure to oxidants, which can damage fragile red blood cells. Vitamin E is prescribed for its antioxidant properties.

CYSTIC FIBROSIS

Cystic fibrosis is an autosomal recessive condition, which causes dysfunction of secretary glands. Mucus secretions are thick and may block glands and ducts. The condition is more common in Northern European population. It may be present in the neonatal period as meconium ileus. Delayed passage of meconium is usually present. Other signs are failure to thrive, prolonged jaundice, bulky pale stools and respiratory tract infections, which are easily affected. Diagnosis in the newborn period is by measuring the serum immunoreactive trypsin. Treatment is aimed at preventing complications and optimizing growth and development. Parents will need genetic counseling and antenatal screening for future pregnancies.

ENDOCRINE DISORDERS

Endocrine disorders are rare in the newborn period. They are usually treatable and if untreated, may lead to significant morbidity. The most common disorders involve the thyroid gland, adrenal cortex and developing sexual organs.

THYROID PROBLEMS

Congenital Hypothyroidism

The incidence of congenital hypothyroidism is approximately 1 in 3,500. Often there is a strong family history of hypothyroidism. Some rare forms of hypothyroidism are autosomal recessive conditions. Hypothyroidism in the neonate can also be caused by the mother taking antithyroid drugs or treatment with radioactive iodides in pregnancy. Low circulating levels of thyroid hormones cause impaired intellectual and motor function.

Clinical Presentation

Depending on the amount of thyroid hormone produced, there are different degrees of hypothyroidism. Severe hypothyroidism has the following manifestations:
- Coarse facial expression with a low hairline
- Wrinkled forehead and flat nasal bridge

- Short and thick neck
- Prolonged jaundice
- Constipation
- Lethargy
- Poor feeding
- Hypothermia.

Diagnosis and Treatment

Routine neonatal screening for hypothyroidism is done in many countries at the same time as the PKU screening. With this type of screening, diagnosis is often made before the baby shows signs and symptoms. A positive screening test will be followed up by radioimmunoassays of the thyroid hormone thyroxine (T_4) or the thyroid-stimulating hormone (TSH) before starting treatment with T_4 replacement.

Prognosis is good if treatment is instituted quickly, but infants with complete absence of thyroid tissue will have a less favorable outcome. Genetic counseling should be offered to parents.

ACQUIRED METABOLIC DISORDERS

Hypoglycemia

Hypoglycemia is the most common acquired metabolic disorder. The management of the neonate is important as any prolonged or recurrent hypoglycemia can result in mental retardation and permanent neurological damage.

In term infants, hypoglycemia occurs when blood glucose is 40 mg/dL, within the first 3 days of life. After the first 3 days of life 45 mg/dL signifies hypoglycemia. The fetus stores glucose as glycogen in the liver and muscles, and in subcutaneous and body fat, and this occurs largely in the third trimester. After birth, the baby must make metabolic adjustments to maintain a normal blood sugar. To meet the baby's energy needs during the initial hours after birth, hepatic glycogen is released. After the first few hours, the neonate is able to use fatty acids as an alternative energy source.

Normal term babies who have not been stressed have adequate stores of glycogen to meet their energy requirements, if they are kept warm and are able to feed.

Etiology

- Decreased stores:
  - Prematurity
  - Intrauterine growth retardation
  - Starvation.
- Hyperinsulinism:
  - Infant of diabetic mother
  - Erythroblastosis (Rhesus hemolytic disease)
  - Islet cell hyperplasia or hyperfunction
  - Beckwith-Wiedemann syndrome
  - Insulin-producing tumors
  - Inborn errors of metabolism
  - Maternal tocolytic therapy with β-sympathomimetic agents.
- Other causes:
  - Sepsis, shock
  - Asphyxia
  - Hypothermia
  - Glycogen storage disease
  - Galactosemia
  - Adrenal insufficiency
  - Abrupt stoppage of glucose 10% given intravenously (IV)
  - Hemorrhage of central nervous system (CNS).
- Iatrogenic causes:
  - Cessation of the hypertonic glucose infusions
  - Exchange transfusions.

Clinical Signs of Hypoglycemia

Many infants are asymptomatic, particularly the preterm. Common signs described are:
- Tremors and jittery movements
- Hypotonia
- Lethargy
- Poor feeding and refusal to suck
- Apnea and cyanosis
- Seizures
- Weak- or high-pitched cry.

Management of Hypoglycemia

It is important for the midwife to have the knowledge to identify the infants who are at risk. Effective management of the baby's feeding and temperature control will help to prevent hypoglycemia. Blood glucose screening, using whole blood obtained by capillary heel stab, must be done.

Early oral or gavage feeding with 10% glucose water every 2 hours until blood glucose levels are stable and then wean to breast or formula.

Minimize calorie expenditure by minimizing stress and keeping the baby warm. The prognosis is good unless the hypoglycemia has been severe or has been prolonged over days.

Hyperglycemia

Blood glucose levels greater than 130 mg/dL in newborn is considered as hyperglycemia. It is found most commonly in preterm infants. It is thought to be the result of immature infant's inability to handle glucose. It can occur also as a response to infection, dehydration, intravenous glucose, stress and steroids used to treat bronchopulmonary dysplasia. Treatment is to reduce the concentration of administered dextrose infusions and give a continuous insulin infusion if necessary. Neonatal diabetes mellitus is a rare occurrence. The cause is thought to be immaturity of the pancreatic islets with a resultant insulin insufficiency. Treatment with insulin until the condition resolves, when the pancreas matures.

Electrolyte Imbalance

Electrolyte levels will become imbalanced in the neonate when the normal hydration is not maintained. The midwife should be aware of the factors that can cause fluid and electrolyte imbalance, which include:
1. Fluid loss through the skin, which is increased under radiant warmer and in phototherapy.
2. Dehydration from inadequate feeding.

Sick and premature infants are more at risk of electrolyte and fluid imbalance.

Hypernatremia

Hypernatremia is the condition in which the serum sodium level is greater than 148 mEq/L. It may be due to an excessive intake of sodium, from incorrectly made feeds or a consequence of intravenous therapy, and the administration of sodium bicarbonate. Excessive water loss due to increased insensible water loss can also cause hypernatremia. The baby is usually dehydrated and may present with signs of cerebral irritation, which, if left untreated, can lead to intraventricular hemorrhage.

Management is to restore fluid and electrolyte balance and treat the underlying cause. It is important that the midwife ensures the baby under phototherapy receives sufficient fluid to prevent dehydration.

Hyponatremia

Hyponatremia occurs when the serum sodium is less than 133 mEq/L. It is the result of water retention or excessive sodium loss. Preterm babies are more at risk because of the immaturity of their kidneys, which allow a high sodium loss in the urine. The baby may be asymptomatic or present with signs of edema. If the sodium loss is acute, the baby may present with convulsions.

Management is to replace sodium either orally or intravenously and correct the imbalance.

Hypocalcemia

Hypocalcemia is a condition where the serum calcium is less than 8.0 mg/dL. It occurs most commonly in low-birth-weight babies, infants of diabetic mothers, babies who have acquired exchange transfusion or in very sick babies. Other causes are deficiency of maternal and fetal vitamin D, renal failure and hypoparathyroidism in the infant.

Signs of hypocalcemia are irritability, rapid jerky limb movements or even convulsions. Management is to supplement the baby with either oral or intravenous calcium.

Hypercalcemia

Neonatal hypercalcemia is diagnosed when the serum calcium is over 11.0 mg/dL. This is rare in newborn babies. High calcium levels can lead to renal damage and pathological changes in the heart. It may be the result of over treatment with calcium infusion or occur when there is insufficient phosphate in the baby's diet. It can also occur when the baby has abnormal vitamin D metabolism. Treatment will depend on the underlying cause.

Diarrhea in Newborn

Diarrhea is one of the serious problems in newborn. However, frequent passage of stool occurs in newborns, which should be differentiated from infective diarrhea or gastroenteritis.

Causes

Specific and non-specific organisms such as *Escherichia coli*, *Staphylococcus* or virus are usually responsible.

Clinical Features

True diarrhea of gastroenteritis is manifested by:
❖ Frequent watery stools
❖ Green stools due to unchanged bile
❖ Containing mucus and blood.

It is common in artificially fed babies because of problems in the quality of milk and maintaining asepsis of the utensils used. Associated features include:
❖ Colic and crying
❖ Evidences of dehydration are:
  – Dry, inelastic skin
  – Sunken eyes
  – Depressed anterior fontanel
  – Loss of weight
  – Ultimately circulatory collapse.

Dietetic Causes of Diarrhea (Noninfective)

Overfeeding: Increased amount and/or frequent feeds lead to undue irritation of the gut and intestinal hurry causing diarrhea. The stool is bulky without any mucus. Maintenance of regularity and adjusting the amount of feeds cure the condition.

Underfeeding: It is called hunger diarrhea. There is frequent passage of small green stools. Increasing the quantity of the feeds by test feeding solves the problem.

Excessive carbohydrate: It produces flatulence, frequent frothy stools with excoriation of the buttocks. The reaction of the stool is acidic.

Excessive fat (addition of cream): This may lead to vomiting and diarrhea with pale stool.

Protein diarrhea: This is associated with colic, vomiting and frequent bloody stools.

Treatment of Infective Diarrhea

The baby should be isolated and the stool should be sent for culture and sensitivity test prior starting the antibiotic therapy.

Mild diarrhea is managed as follows:
1. Milk feeding is stopped.
2. Oral rehydration solutions (ORS) is started. The WHO recommended ORS packet containing:
   - Glucose 20 g
   - Sodium chloride 3.5 g
   - Sodium citrate 2.9 g
   - Potassium chloride 1.5 g.

   The contents of a packet should be dissolved in 1 liter of drinking (potable) water and used within 24 hours.
3. The total fluids should be at least 200 mL/kg body weight per day and should be given at 2–3 hourly intervals. If the baby fails to take the necessary amount by mouth, parenteral therapy is started.
4. After diarrhea is controlled, breastfeeding is resumed. Alternatively, half-strength skimmed milk is given before the usual milk feeds are restored.
5. Antibiotics: If there is systemic infection with gastrointestinal manifestations, oral or parenteral antibiotics (colistin sulfate, ampicillin, amikacin or cefotaxime) are given.

Severe diarrhea with dehydration
Dehydration should be corrected with intravenous fluids. About 5% dextrose in one-fifth saline or half-strength Hartmann's solution or Ringer lactate is administered. Once urine output is adequate, oral rehydration is started. Other treatment measures are same as for mild diarrhea.

Vomiting in Newborn

Vomiting is one of the common manifestations in the neonates. Vomiting in neonates may either be trivial or manifestation of some graver pathology. Mucus vomiting tinged with blood is quite common soon after birth. It is due to irritation of the gastric mucosa by the swallowed materials during birth.

Causes of Vomiting

Obstructive: Vomiting may be a manifestation of congenital gastrointestinal tract obstruction. The conditions include esophageal atresia, cardiospasm, chalasia (continuous relaxation of esophageal-gastric sphincter), pyloric stenosis, duodenal atresia, diaphragmatic hernia or hiatus hernia, meconium ileus and imperforate anus.

Intracranial injuries: Raised intracranial tension due to hemorrhage or depressed skull bone fracture.

Dietetic: Overfeeding or qualitative change in the food constituents or excessive air swallowing.

Milk allergy: Allergy to cow's milk is manifested with mucus and blood in the vomitus. Recurrence of diarrhea after reintroducing cow's milk is very much suggestive.

Infective: Gastroenteritis, meningitis or septicemia.

Treatment

1. Early diagnosis and correction of fluid imbalance.
2. Medical or surgical therapy as appropriate for the underlying pathology.

Drug or Substance Withdrawal

Drugs and substances that have been prescribed or abused in pregnancy can cause neonatal withdrawal symptoms. Among these are narcotics, alcohol, amphetamines, barbiturates, codeine, benzodiazepines, pentazocine, cocaine, lithium and tricyclic antidepressants. The drugs and substances abused vary according to current trends, availability and geographical location. Drug and substance abuse is associated with increased fetal and neonatal deaths, prematurity and intrauterine growth restriction. Pregnant users often have accompanying social, economic and housing problems. This group of women is also at more risk for sexually transmitted diseases such as chlamydia, gonorrhea, human immunodeficiency virus (HIV) and hepatitis B infection.

Neonatal Abstinence Syndrome or Withdrawal Signs

Neonatal abstinence syndrome (NAS) or withdrawal signs are nonspecific and should be observed by the midwife when the mother presents with history of drug or substances use. The signs are:
- Tremor
- High-pitched cry
- Irritability
- Hyperactivity
- Sweating
- Pyrexia
- Sneezing
- Vomiting
- Disorganized suck
- Diarrhea
- Convulsions
- Respiratory distress.

In opiate misuse, the symptoms of withdrawal will generally appear within the first 24–48 hours of life. Barbiturate abstinence signs may not appear for 2 weeks and may go on for a period of several weeks or months.

Care of a baby undergoing withdrawal includes the following aspects:
1. Provision of a quiet environment with reduced light and noise stimulus.
2. Swaddling the baby to make him/her feel secure.
3. Small frequent feeds for comfort and adequate nutrition.
4. Administration of phenobarbitone to control convulsions.
5. If oral feeding is not tolerated administer IV fluids.

Treatment

Treatment will vary according to the drug of misuse and the severity of presenting signs. Narcotics such as morphine may be used until observable signs are controlled. Chlorpromazine is also used until presenting symptoms are controlled.

Midwife's management of the baby and mother must include providing opportunities for parents to participate in the care of the baby and adequate explanation of the baby's behavior. Adequate follow-up arrangements, including community health and social services, must be ensured when planning discharge from the hospital.

Fetal Alcohol Syndrome

Fetal alcohol syndrome (FAS) is characterized by intrauterine growth restriction, failure to thrive, developmental delay and dysmorphic (deformed) facial features. It is thought that ethanol (a component of alcohol) disrupts cell differentiation and growth in the fetus and impairs normal placental function.

Characteristics of Babies with FAS

1. Small eyes with exaggerated epicanthic folds.
2. Poorly formed nasal bridge.
3. Fretfulness and difficulty to feed.
4. Associated abnormalities of the heart and musculoskeletal system, intestinal atresias, skin lesions and cleft palate.
5. The baby will also have delay in mental and motor development, and may have learning and behavioral problems in later life.

Management

The midwife has an important role in the prevention and management of FAS by identifying women at risk and in giving effective antenatal education. In managing the baby suspected of having FAS, the midwife will need to monitor the signs of alcohol withdrawal. Follow-up care including community health and social services must be arranged prior to discharge from the hospital.

STUDY QUESTIONS

Short Answer Questions

1. Phenylketonuria (PKU) in newborn.
2. Galactosemia.
3. Congenital hypothyroidism.
4. Hypocalcemia.
5. Fetal alcohol syndrome.
6. Neonatal abstinence syndrome.

Essay Questions

1. Describe hypoglycemia of newborn, its causes, clinical manifestations and management.
2. Explain diarrhea in newborn, its causes, clinical features and management.

BIBLIOGRAPHY

1. Aynsley-Green A, Soltesz G. Metabolic and endocrine disorders. In: Roberton N (Ed). Textbook of Neonatology, 2nd edition. London: Churchill Livingstone; 1992.
2. Brown J, Philips CA, Hussain S. Glucose testing in the neonate. Journal of Neonatal Nursing. 1997;3(3):22-3.
3. Dutta DC. Textbook of obstetrics, 5th edition. Kolkata: New Central Book Company; 2001.
4. Jones KL. Fetal alcohol syndrome. Pediatric Review. 1986;8(4):122.
5. Livingston A. Metabolic and endocrine disorders and drug withdrawal. In: Bennett RV, Brown KL (Eds). Myles Textbook for Midwives, 13th edition. Edinburgh: Churchill Livingstone; 1999. pp. 843-85.
6. Roberton NRC. A Manual of neonatal intensive care, 3rd edition. London: Edward Arnold; 1993.

CHAPTER 49

Neonatal Intensive Care Unit

> **Learning Objectives**
>
> Upon completing this chapter, the learner will be able to:
> - Discuss the concept and goals of neonatal intensive care.
> - Enumerate the levels of NICU and the various health professionals involved in the care ill and preterm neonates in such a unit.
> - Explain the need for control of infection in NICU and the measures to be implemented for hand-washing, housekeeping and waste segregation prior to disposal.
> - Describe the importance of "baby care records" and nurses' responsibilities for maintenance and care of records.
> - List the types of reports in NICU, its purpose and nurses' role related to writing and safe-guarding the reports.

INTRODUCTION

A neonatal intensive care unit (NICU), also known as Intensive Care Nursery is a unit specializing in the care of ill and premature newborn infants. NICU has healthcare providers who have special training, and equipment to give best possible care to neonates. Neonates in NICU receive care in safe, controlled environment. The NICU combines advanced technology and skilled healthcare professionals to provide specialized care for babies.

BABIES WHO NEED SPECIAL CARE IN NICU

Most babies admitted to NICU are premature (born before 37 weeks of pregnancy), have low birth weight (less than 2,500 g) or have medical conditions that require special care. Twins and other multiples often are admitted to the NICU, as they tend to be born earlier and are smaller than single birth babies.

High-risk factors that can place the babies as high-risk and needing admission in NICU:
- Maternal factors:
  - Age younger than 16 or older than 40 years
  - Drug or alcohol abuse
  - Diabetes
  - Hypertension
  - Bleeding
  - Sexually transmitted diseases
  - Multiple pregnancy
- Delivery factors:
  - Fetal distress/birth asphyxia
  - Breech delivery
  - Meconium-stained amniotic fluid
  - Nuchal cord
  - Forceps/cesarean delivery
- Baby factors:
  - Pre or post-term deliveries (less than 37 weeks or more than 42 weeks)
  - Birth weight less than 2,500 g or over 4,000 g.
  - Resuscitation in the delivery room
  - Birth defects
  - Respiratory distress such as grunting or apnea
  - Infections such as herpes, group B streptococci, chlamydia
  - Seizures
  - Hypoglycemia
  - Hypoxia
  - Needing blood transfusion.

LEVELS OF NICU

- *Level-1:* Nurseries that care for healthy, full term babies. They are able to stabilize faster and be ready for transfer to special care nurseries.
- *Level-2 or specialty care nurseries:* Nurseries that have infants who are moderately ill with problems that are expected to resolve rapidly and are recovering from serious illnesses.
- *Level-3:* NICU capable of caring for very small or very sick newborn babies. Nursery is staffed with a variety of staff on site including neonatologists, neonatal nurses, and respiratory therapists who are available for 24 hours a day.

Baby's care-givers in NICU include:
- Doctors: Neonatologists, Pediatricians
- Nurses: Staff nurses, Nurse in-charge
- Other healthcare professionals such as pharmacist, and group of developmental team (paramedical staff).

GOALS OF NICU CARE

- To improve the condition of the critically ill neonate, keeping in mind the survival of the neonate so as to reduce the neonatal morbidity and mortality.
- To provide continuing in-service training to medical and nursing personnel in the care of newborn.
- To maintain the functions of the pulmonary, cardio-vascular, renal and nervous systems.
- To monitor the heart rate, body temperature and central venous pressure by non-invasive techniques.
- To ensure the oxygen concentration of the blood by oxygen analyzers.
- To check/observe the alarm system signals to find out the changes beyond certain fixed limits set on the monitors.
- To administer precise amounts of fluids and minute quantities of drugs through IV infusion pumps.

PREPARATION OF NICU (FIGS. 49.1 AND 49.2)

- Warm (33–36°C) incubators
- Adequate light source
- Resuscitation and treatment trolley stocked
- All required patient records.
- Oxygen, air and suction apparatus available
- Oxygen line connected to oxygen and air flow meter
- Complete suction unit tubing and various sizes of suction catheter, ventilation bag and mask of appropriate sizes
- Vital signs monitors
- Specific equipment as indicated by diagnoses.

HISTORY AND EXAMINATION

- All babies admitted to the neonatal intensive care units should have the following data taken carefully within 24 hours of admission.

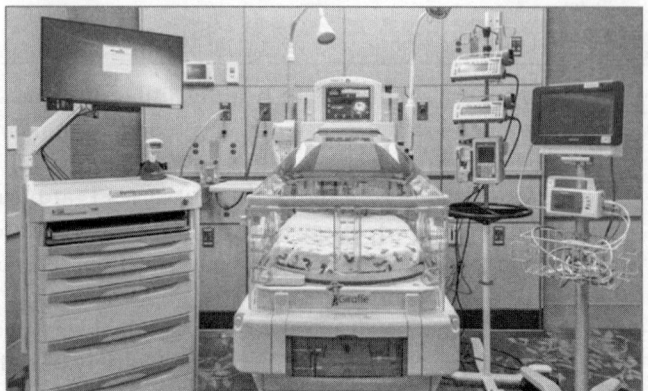

Figure 49.1: View of newborn care area in NICU.

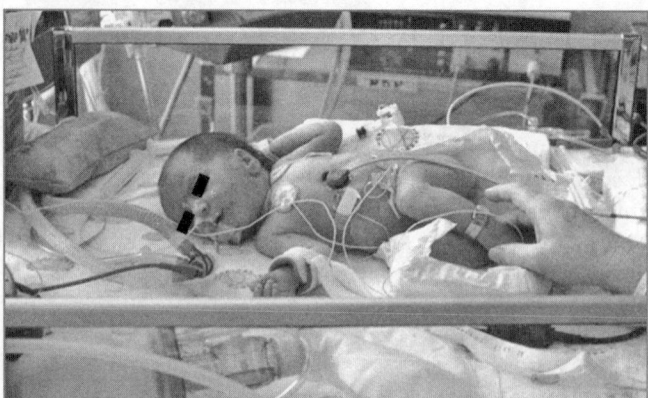

Figure 49.2: An ill baby in NICU incubator.

- History: Maternal health history, paternal health history, previous obstetric history, details of present pregnancy, labor, delivery, APGAR score.

On Admission

- Notify the doctor and nurse-in-charge
- Resuscitate infant as necessary and maintain warmth
- Check the infants' identification bands
- Quickly examine the infant from head to toe for obvious abnormality, if condition permits
- Record weight, length and head circumference as soon as possible
- Transfer to warm environment as soon as possible

Most common observations are:
- Temperature, heart rate, respirations, color and activity.
- Health status in appropriate medical records of the infant and reports in ICU

INFECTION CONTROL IN NEONATAL INTENSIVE CARE UNITS

Most babies admitted to NICU are preterm (born before 37 weeks of gestation) or have health conditions that require special care. Neonates in NICU must receive care in a safe, controlled environment. An incubator helps provide the baby with constant body temperature. These babies are given high-calorie nutrition, intravenous hydration and other therapies based on their specific condition. Babies with mild respiratory distress syndrome (RDS) are treated with oxygen therapy as well as placed in a ventilator. Hypoglycemia in babies born to diabetic mothers and those with any infection are treated appropriately in NICU. Twins, triplets and other multiples are often admitted in NICU. A difficult birth can cause decreased supply of oxygen and blood and such babies are managed in NICU. Sepsis is more likely in babies born earlier than full term. Protocols for care and maintenance of the unit are detailed below.

Newborn care is one of the important areas of concern and need special attention in all respects of the units design, layout, staffing, policies and practice. Newborn babies especially premature infants are susceptible to blood-borne infections. Babies in NICU often have immature immune system. They are exposed to many different care-givers and may have multiple blood tests. The approach towards prevention of neonatal sepsis is multidisciplinary, comprising of neonatologists, hospital administrators, nursing staff and engineers. Microbes enter the NICU via visitors and health-care workers (HCWs) and proliferate in susceptible sites. They spread in the neonates via contaminated articles and contaminated hands of HCWs. Once the babies are colonized, the organisms then enter through the umbilical cord, and skin during procedures, such as venous access, parenteral fluids, feeds, intubation and suctioning of endotracheal tubes.

Infection Control Measures in NICU

In order to reduce or minimize morbidity and mortality in NICU babies, several measures are recommended by the Center for Disease Control (CDC).

- ❖ *Prevent entry of microbes into NICU.*
  - Clean the immediate environment.
  - Organisms from labor room, resuscitation room environment and maternal vaginal flora can colonize the newborn skin. This can be prevented by the following clean measures:
    » Clean the mother's perineum
    » Clean the delivery surface
    » Clean the cord and cutting instruments
    » Ensure clean cord care
    » Ensure that nothing unclean is introduced into mother's vagina
    Equipment for resuscitation in the 'baby receiving' area should be regularly cleaned and articles autoclaved.
- ❖ *Standardize the NICU design:* Location of NICU should have a controlled access. Each infant space has to be a minimum of 120 sq. ft. clear floor space excluding the hand washing area and corridor. There should be a minimum of 4 ft. between two infant beds.
- ❖ *Airborne infection in isolation room:* An airborne infection isolation room should be available with the following facilities.
  - A hands-free hand washing station for hand hygiene.
  - An area for gowning and storage of clean materials near the entrance to the NICU.
  - According to the American Institute of Architecture (AIA) guidelines, the NICU and isolation room using an exhaust to the exterior should have a minimum of six air exchanges per hour (AEH).
- ❖ *Hand washing station:* Every infant bed should be within 20 ft. of a hands-free hand washing station. Hand washing sink should be large enough to control splashing. Pictorial hand washing instructions should be provided. There should be space for soap and towel dispensers. Non-absorbent wall material should be used around the sink to prevent the growth of mold.
  - Hand hygiene: The Center for Disease Control (CDC) recommends hand washing before and after contact with every infant for 30 seconds, and 40–60 seconds of hand washing before entering the NICU. CDC recommended hand washing steps for infection control which must be followed are:
    » No wrist watch, no bracelet and no rings on fingers.
    » Turn on water wet hands, and apply antimicrobial soap
    » Wash palms of hands
    » Wash between fingers at back of hands
    » Wash between fingers palm to palm
    » Wash palm area
    » Pay particular attention to thumb area and thumb joint
    » Wash fingertips paying particular attention to thumb area and thumb joint
    » Wash fingertips paying particular attention to finger nails
    » Rinse under running water
    » Turn off water without contamination
    » Wipe from fingertips to wrist
    » Discard paper towel in garbage bin
    Each of the action or step should take 5 seconds, taking a total of 30 seconds **(Fig. 49.3)**.
  - Use of alcohol-based hand rubs (ABHR): Alcohol-based hand rubs can be used as hand hygiene agents if hands are not visibly dirty or contaminated. Alcohol rubs may be used in between patient examination. At least 2–3 mL. of hand rubs should be applied over surface of palms and fingers. ABHRs are not useful after touching an infected patient or when the hands are soiled.
  - Visitors policy: Usually microbes enter into NICU through personnel who enter into NICU and hence restriction of entry is a must. People with active infection (respiratory, mucocutaneous, and gastrointestinal) and children should not be allowed inside NICU. Infected

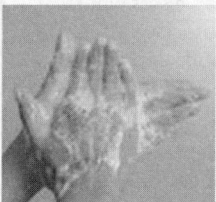 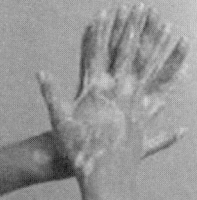 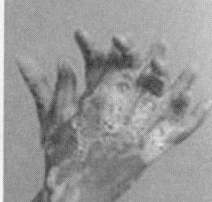

1. Soap palms, rub together for a minimum of 20 seconds
2. Rub back of each hand with the other palm
3. Interface fingers and rub together

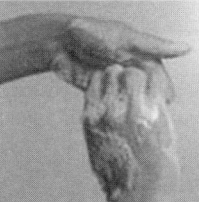 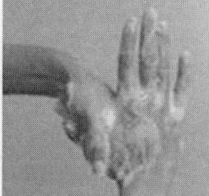 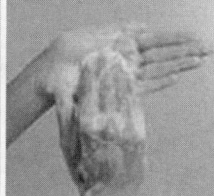

4. Curl the backs of the fingers into one palm then the other
5. Hold thumb and rotate, repeat with both hands
6. Hold fingers and rotate, repeat with both hands

Figure 49.3: Hand washing steps.

BOX 49.1: Housekeeping measures recommended for NICU.

Daily cleaning:

Incubators, warmers, infusion pumps, phototherapy units, mattresses, pulse-oximeter, monitors, oxygen hoods, ventilators, CPAP machines and telephones	Dry dusting followed by cleaning using a moist wipe
Suction bottles, humidifier chambers of CPAP	Change and fill with distilled water
Bag and mask	Immerse in 2% bacillocid for 6–8 hours after dismantling and cleaning with running water
Incubator, radiant warmers	Clean with 2% bacillocid if not occupied by an infant
Laryngoscopes, masks, stethoscopes, measuring tapes, thermometers, BP cuff, temperature and SpO_2 probes, flash lights	Wipe with alcohol after each use
Walls, floors, wash basins	Clean with phenol or lysol or 2% bacillocid or 0.5% chlorine (for walls only) in each shift
Dustbins, buckets for waste	Empty in each shift and clean with soap and water

Weekly cleaning:

Ventilators and CPAP circuits	Change with a new circuit
Window air conditioners	Surfaces and filters with soap and water
Procedure sets	Use disposable sets where possible. Autoclave after every use and keep ready the sets
Refrigerators	Sorted and cleaned once a week. Use separate fridge for milk and laboratory samples

■ **TABLE 49.1:** Color-coded bins for segregation of waste.

Black drums/bins	Needles without syringes, blades, sharps and all metal articles
Yellow drums/bins (disposal by incineration)	Infectious waste, bandages, gauze, cotton or any other things in contact with body fluids human body parts placenta
Blue drums/bins	All types of glass bottles and articles, outdated and discarded medicines
Red drums/bins Made non-infectious by autoclaving and disposed by shredding	Plastic waste, such as catheters, infected syringes, tubings, IV bottles

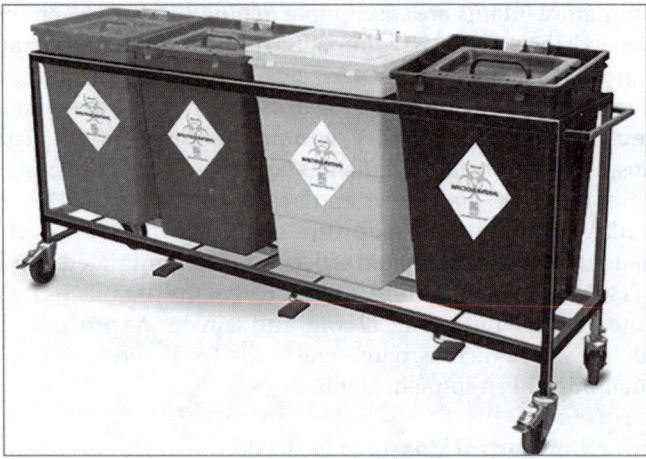

Figure 49.4: Colored bins for segregation of waste (For color version, see Plate 10).

and out-born infants should be managed in the isolation room. NICU should be a 'cell phone-free' zone.
- Growing to reduce nosocomial infection: Studies have shown no reduction of infection during gowning period as compared to no gowning. The focus should be more on adequate hand washing by all hospital personnel and visitors before handling neonates.
- Jewelry and finger-nails policy: Health-care workers should not wear artificial finger nails or extenders while having contact with neonates, and natural nails should be kept short.
- Measures to prevent proliferation of microbes in NICU: In order to prevent proliferation of microbes, in the NICU good housekeeping measures are to be followed: Avoid wet areas inside the NICU. A dry and clean NICU is unlikely to harbor microbes. Details of housekeeping routines and waste disposal are described in **Box 49.1**.
- Feeding utensils such as feeding paladai/katori should be cleaned and boiled for 15 minutes after each feeding.
- Waste segregation protocol adopted in India (**Table 49.1 and Fig. 49.4**).
- Prevention of cross contamination: In order to prevent spread of infection from proliferation sites to baby and from one baby to another, the following steps are important:
  » Nurse-to-patient ratio: All neonatal intensive and high dependency care units should have appropriate number of neonatal nurses. Recommended ratio is 1:1, if baby has multidrug resistant microbes, 1:2 if babies have similar organisms or susceptible organisms, 1:3, if babies are already on adequate antibiotics cover.
  » Use of disposables: Ample disposables are needed for each baby. A baby kit containing a stethoscope, measuring tape, thermometer and a flash light in a sterile container should be available at each bed. All articles used for the baby such as syringes, suction catheter, gloves and antibiotic vials should be disposable. Do not keep articles such as files, X-ray films and pens on the baby cot.

- » Measures to prevent entry of microbes into the infant through umbilical cord, skin and into the circulation.
- » Cord care
  - Careful application of adhesive tapes and take precautions during removal of adhesive.
  - Use skin friendly Duropore instead of Dynaplast and micropore.
  - Bath should be avoided in hospitals, instead sponging may be done.
- » Precautions during procedures
  - Aseptic precautions should be taken during procedures
  - Hand scrub to be done prior to each procedure
  - Skin area should be cleaned with alcohol, betadine and then again with alcohol
  - Cannulation sites should be monitored daily for signs of thrombophlebitis.
  - Catheters should be removed as soon as the baby's condition is stabilized.
- » Feeding of breast milk/breastfeeding/formula feeding
  - Encourage use of colostrum and expressed breast milk
  - Mother's entry into NICU and pumping of milk to ensure adequate breast milk for the infant to be encouraged
  - If the infant needs formula feed, reconstituted formula at right temperature is recommended.

Infection Control Protocols

Prevention of nosocomial infections is the prime responsibility of all individuals. Therefore, infection control protocols should be in place in all departments and patient care units. Every hospital should have an infection control committee in place with the goals to review and approve promptly.

- ❖ Programs of activity for surveillance and prevention
- ❖ Epidemiological surveillance data and identify areas for interventions.
- ❖ Ensure appropriate staff training in infection control and safety
- ❖ Provide input into investigation of epidemics.

The morbidity and mortality of neonates can be significantly reduced by instituting strict infection control strategies. Prevention of entry of microbes to NICU can be achieved by clean environment, hand hygiene and conducive infrastructure. Curtailing proliferation of microbes in NICU can be successful by daily and weekly maintenance of equipment like incubators, warmers, syringes, pumps, ventilator filters, circuits and bag and mask. Efficient biomedical waste disposal is important. Early breastfeeding, use of colostrum and early discharge plan are important in prevention of neonatal morbidity. The role of hospital management and an efficient infection control committee play an important role in prevention of infection, related to neonatal morbidity and mortality.

RECORDS AND REPORTS IN NEONATAL INTENSIVE CARE UNIT

NICU is a very specialized unit where critically ill neonates are treated and cared to reduce the neonatal morbidity and mortality. All professional persons need to be accountable for the performance of their duties and nursing being a profession, nurses need to record their work in completion. Every ICU keeps several records and reports. Records are administrative tools used to classify and prevent duplication of the information. Reports are administrative tools used to classify and prevent duplication of the information. Reports are document forms which include conclusions or findings based on facts or recommendations concerning the patient. The ICU nurse has to be highly-skilled today due to technological advances and complex care of the critically ill patients or neonates. Documentation and care required are complex and time consuming activities.

Purpose of Documentation in ICU

Documentation in the ICU is carried out for a number of reasons. It ensures continuity of care and provides up-to-date patient status. It fulfills hospital policies which furnish the legal aspects of 'duty of care'.

Principles of Record Keeping

- ❖ Since the clinical records is a legal document, it is essential that they should be written clearly, accurately, appropriately and legibly.
- ❖ All entries should be signed by the individual who writes them.
- ❖ Care to be taken not to make any errors in the records. If anything is crossed out, it should be dated and initialed.
- ❖ All records should be written with black ink or typed for better legibility.
- ❖ Records should be written in chronological order as to date and time. When recording medications and treatments, enter exact time and date when they are carried out.
- ❖ Records should be written continuously with no blank spaces. If any space is left out, it should be crossed out, dated and signed.
- ❖ Lengthy corrections of records are to be written as amendments.
- ❖ Each page of the record should be properly identified with the patient's name, age, IP no., OP no., date, etc.
- ❖ Use only standard abbreviations.

Importance of Records

The records form a permanent account of a patient's illness. Their clarity and accuracy is paramount for effective communication between healthcare professionals and patients. Maintenance of good records ensures that a patient's or neonate's assessed needs are met comprehensively.

- ❖ Records should be truthful, brief and complete. It should include all the services carried out or care given to the

patient from day-to-day and results of treatment or nursing activity.
- Records are to be factual, consistent and accurate.
- Provide current information of the care given and condition of the infant.
- Document clearly in such a way that the text cannot be erased.

Types of NICU Records

Every ICU maintains complete patient record. This will contain the biodata of the patient/neonate, diagnosis, mothers health and obstetric history, type of delivery, findings of neonatal assessment (APGAR score), resuscitation information if done, treatments and medications given, progress notes and summary made at the time of discharge or transfer to NICU.
- *Nurses' notes:*
  - Large parts of patient's records are filled by the nurse.
  - Nurses' notes are a record of treatments and nursing measures carried out by the nurse, their effects and observations made on the patient. Avoid bulky reports containing unnecessary and irrelevant materials.
  - Observation of the baby is continuous and it is impossible for the nurse to record all the observations. Observations should be specific and objective as possible.
- *Doctors' order sheet:* The doctors' orders (prescriptions) regarding medications, investigations and nutrition supply.
- *Graphic charts of TPR:*
  - On this, the neonate's temperature, heart rate and respirations are written in a graphic form so that any slight deviation from the normal can be noted at a glance.
  - Other information such as heart rate, respirations, number of bowel movements, body weight, name and date of any surgery performed, etc., are recorded in the chart according to the hospital policy.
- *Intake output chart:* Babies on intravenous fluids, enteric feeds, vomiting, diarrhea etc., should have intake-output maintained.
- *Registers:* To maintain the statistics, every NICU maintains certain registers in order to register admissions, discharges, and operations, census, etc. It is the nurses' responsibility to maintain those registers up-to-date. Other registers include:
  - Register with entries of laboratory examinations, biochemistry, hematology reports, etc.
  - Diet sheet entries.
  - Consent forms of parents for anesthesia and operations.

Nurses' Responsibility for Care of Patient Records

- Records are kept under the safe custody of the nurse in each unit or department.
- No individual sheet is separated from the complete record.
- Records are to be kept in a place not accessible to patients or visitors.
- No stranger is ever permitted to read patient records.
- Patients' records are not to be handed over to legal advisors without the written permission of the administration.
- All hospital personnel are legally and ethically obliged to keep in confidence all the information provided in the records.
- All records are to be handled carefully to avoid damage.
- All records are filed according to the hospital policy, so that they can be traced easily. It may be arranged alphabetically or numerically with index cards.
- All records are identified with the biodata of the patient such as name, age, unit, bed number, IP no., OP no., diagnosis, etc.

REPORTS

A report is a document that presents information in an organized format for a specific audience and purpose. Although summaries of reports may be delivered orally, complete reports are almost always in the form of written documents.

Reports in Patient Care Units

1. Incident Reports

An ancient is an unfavorable event that affects patient or staff safety. Typical healthcare incidents are related to physical injuries medical error, equipment failure or patient care; anything that endangers a patient's or staff's safety is called an incident in the medical system.

The principle regarding errors is that "to err is human, to cover up is unforgivable, and to fail to learn is inexcusable". The process of collecting incident data and presenting it properly is known as "incident reporting in healthcare system with incident reporting, an emerging problem is highlighted in a non-blaming way to provide a catalyst for changing the factors contributing to the error. Designated staff with authority to file a report or staff who has witnessed an incident firsthand, usually file the incident. Usually, nurses or other hospital staff who has witnessed an incident report within 24 to 48 hours after the incident occurred.

A situation for incident reporting
While injecting an IV pain medication, the nurse misread the label and administered a heavier dosage than prescribed, which increased the patient's blood pressure level. In this situation, it is necessary to fill in the incident report, simply because an unexpected event occurred and led to harm. It does not matter how severe or minor the incident is, it is essential to report all such incidents.

Purpose of incident reports
Incident reports provide valuable information to hospital administration. They capture data required to highlight necessary measures to improve the overall safety and quality of services of the hospital. An accurate incident report serves multiple purposes such as:

- Root cause identification
- Policy and process improvements
- Clinical risk management
- Continuous quality improvement
- Better training and continuous learning

Types of incident reports
- *Clinical incidents:* Unpleasant and unplanned event that causes or can causes physical harm to a patient.
  Example:
  – A patient falls out of bed while sleeping.
  – A patient brutally scratched a nursed while she was taking his temperature.
  – Nurse mislabeled the medicine box while storing it.
- *Near miss incidents:* An error or unsafe condition is caught before it reaches the patient.
  Example: A patient attempts to leave the hospital facility before discharge, but the security guard stopped him and brought him back to the ward.
- *Work place incidents:*
  Example: Patient or next of kin abuses a care provider verbally or physically leading to unsafe work conditions.

Most hospitals have incident reporting forms available in all units and departments in which details can be entered and forwarded to administration through proper channel.

Day and Night Reports

In hospitals, nurses provide patient care around-the-clock and prepare bedside shift reports. These are written reports, tape recorded report or verbal face-to-face report conducted in a private setting, and face-to-face beside patients (hand-over time report). These reports are verbal or written communication of data regarding the clients' health status needs, treatments, outcomes and responses. Advantages of reporting are that it facilitates clinical decision making, continuity of care and coordination among health team members, particularly nursing personnel. Day and night reports are used at change of duty shifts.

Transfer Report

Patients will be frequently transferred from one unit to another to receive different levels of care. When giving transfer request the nurse should include the following information:
- Client's name, age, primary doctor and medical diagnosis.
- Summary of medical progress up to the time of transfer.
- Current health status—physical and psychosocial.
- Current nursing diagnosis or problems and care plans.
- Any critical assessment or "interventions" to be completed shortly.
- Needs of any special equipment.

CONCLUSION

Admission to the neonatal intensive care unit often happens when a baby is in critical condition and needs the care in an incubator. Mostly neonates go to NICU from labor rooms, operation theater or referred and transferred from another hospital. Premature and critically ill babies are placed in NICU. Information in NICU records include ICU treatment, medications, visitation by specialists, daily health status and progress made. NICU records of the neonate provide the nurse a basis for analyzing the needs of the baby in terms of what has been done, what is being done and what needs to done. Nursing records of the neonate must be maintained correctly and accurately and safeguarded carefully according to the agency policies as well as in accordance with the legal and ethical standards. Reports are oral or written exchange of information shared between care givers or health personnel in a number of ways.

Different kinds of reports are prepared to meet specific purpose in the unit. An organized account of an event, unit activities or requirements in the unit for patient care are prepared for oral presentation or written and submitted to personnel in authority.

BIBLIOGRAPHY

1. Halliday HL. Handbook of Neonatal Intensive Care. London. Balliere Tindal; 1989.
2. Kattiwinkel J. University of Virginia. 1995; Newborn assessment and resuscitation. Virginia. www.vital.com.
3. Robertson NRC. Disorders of respiratory tract. A Manual .of Neonatal Intensive Care. 3rd edition: Edward Arnold; 1993.
4. The newborn intensive care unit. https://www.stanford-childrens.org
5. The newborn intensive care unit (NICU)-March of Dimes. https://www.marchofdimes.com
6. Neonatal Intensive Care Unit (NICU) https:/www.cimarindia.com.

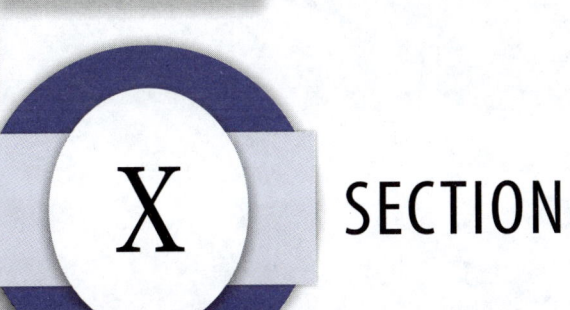

SECTION X

COMMUNITY MIDWIFERY

Section Outline

50. Preventive Obstetrics and Domiciliary Care in Maternity Nursing
51. Primary Helath care and Maternal/Child Health Services in India

SECTION 5

COMMUNITY MIDWIFERY

CHAPTER 50

Preventive Obstetrics and Domiciliary Care in Maternity Nursing

Learning Objectives

Upon completing this chapter, the learner will be able to:
- Describe the concept of community midwifery.
- Describe the role of the midwife and the scope of her practice during the antenatal, intrapartum and postpartum periods.
- Review the skills a midwife requires for home birth.

The concept of home care combines obstetrical concerns with the concepts of primary health care. Such midwifery care takes into account the woman's and her family's personal, and social circumstances, which influence the health and well-being of her and her baby.

Community midwifery is one of the functions of community health care. It aims to promote the well-being of mothers and babies, and to support sound parenting and stable families. It is a component of the maternal and child health (MCH) program in India, which has its specific objectives for reduction of maternal, perinatal, infant and childhood mortality and morbidity and promotion of reproductive health.

ANTENATAL CARE

The aim of antenatal care is to achieve at the end of a pregnancy—a healthy mother and a healthy baby. Ideally, this care should begin soon after conception and continue throughout pregnancy.

Objectives

1. Promote, protect and maintain the health of the mother during pregnancy.
2. Detect 'high-risk' pregnancies and give the mother's special attention.
3. Foresee complications and prevent them.
4. Remove anxiety and fear associated with delivery.
5. Reduce maternal and infant mortality and morbidity.
6. Teach mother, elements of childcare, nutrition, personal hygiene and environmental sanitation.
7. Sensitize the mother to the need for family planning.

Antenatal Visits

Ideally, the care should begin soon after conception and continue throughout pregnancy. A schedule to follow for the mother is to attend the antenatal clinic once a month during the first 7 months, twice a month during the next 2 months, and thereafter once a week if everything is normal. In India a large proportion of mothers are of low-socioeconomic group for whom attendance at the antenatal clinic may mean loss of daily wages and hence a minimum of three visits are encouraged as below:
- First visit, as soon as the pregnancy is known or at 20th week
- Second visit, at 32nd week
- Third visit, at 36th week.

Further visits may be made if justified by the condition of the mother. At least one visit should be paid in the home of the mother.

PRENATAL CARE

Preventive Services for Mothers in the Prenatal Period

The first visit irrespective of when it occurs should include:
- Health history
- Physical examination
- Laboratory examination:
  - Complete urine analysis
  - Stool examination
  - Complete blood count including Hb estimation
  - Serological examination
  - Blood grouping and rhesus (Rh) determination
  - Chest X-ray, if needed
  - Gonorrhea test, if needed.

On subsequent visits:
- Physical examination including weight and blood pressure
- Laboratory tests including urine examination and hemoglobin estimation
- Iron and folic acid supplementation and medications as needed
- Immunization against tetanus
- Group or individual teaching on nutrition, self-care, family planning, delivery and parenthood
- Home visiting by a female health worker or trained dai (trained traditional birth attendant)
- Referral services, when necessary.

Risk Approach

While continuing to provide appropriate care for all mothers, 'high risk' cases must be identified as early as possible and arrangements to be made for skilled care. These cases comprise the following:

1. Elderly primigravida (30 year and above).
2. Short-statured primigravida.
3. Malpresentations, e.g. breech, transverse lie, etc.
4. Antepartum hemorrhage, threatened abortion.
5. Preeclampsia and eclampsia.
6. Anemia.
7. Twins, hydramnios.
8. Previous stillbirth, intrauterine death, manual removal of placenta.
9. Elderly grand multipara.
10. Prolonged pregnancy (14 day beyond expected date of delivery).
11. Previous cesarean or instrumental delivery.
12. Pregnancy associated with medical conditions, e.g. cardiovascular disease, kidney disease, diabetes, tuberculosis, liver disease, etc.

The purpose of risk approach is to provide maximum services to all pregnant women with attention to those who need them most. Maximum utilization of all resources, including human resources is involved in such care. Services of traditional birth attendants, community health workers and women's groups are utilized. The risk strategy is expected to lead to improvements in both the quality and coverage of health care at all levels, particularly at primary healthcare level.

Home Visits

Home visits are paid by the female health worker or public health nurse. If the delivery is planned at home, several visits are required. The home visit will provide opportunities to study the environmental and social conditions at home, and to provide prenatal advice. In the home environment, the woman will have more confidence to make an informed decision about home birth.

Prenatal Advice

A major component of antenatal care is prenatal advice or education. The mother is more receptive to advice concerning herself and her baby at this time than any other time. The topics should cover not only the specific problems of pregnancy and childbirth but must also include family and child health care.

Diet

A balanced and adequate diet is of utmost importance during pregnancy and lactation to meet the increased needs of the mother, and to prevent nutritional stress. On an average a pregnant woman, gains about 12.5 kg of weight during pregnancy. Studies have indicated that Indian women of low-income group gain an average weight of 6.5 kg during pregnancy. Thus, pregnancy induces the need for calorie and nutritional requirements. If maternal stores of iron are poor as may happen after repeated pregnancies and if adequate iron is not available to the mother during pregnancy, it is possible that the fetus will lay down insufficient iron stores. Such a baby may show normal hemoglobin at birth, but will lack the stores of iron necessary for rapid growth, and increase in blood volume and muscle mass in the 1st year of life.

Personal Hygiene

Advice regarding personal hygiene is equally important. The need to bathe every day and to wear clean clothes should be explained. About 8 hours of sleep and at least 2 hours rest after midday meals should be advised. Constipation should be avoided by regular intake of green leafy vegetables, fruits and extra fluid. Purgatives such as castor oil to relieve constipation should be avoided. Light household work should be encouraged, but manual physical labor during pregnancy may adversely affect the fetus.

Smoking should be cut down to a minimum, as heavy smoking by the mother can result in babies much smaller than average size due to placental insufficiency. The perinatal mortality amongst babies whose mothers smoked during pregnancy is between 10% and 40% higher than in nonsmokers. Mothers who are moderate to heavy drinkers (alcohol) become pregnant, have greater risk of pregnancy loss and if they do not abort, their babies may have various physical and mental problems. Heavy drinking has been associated with fetal alcohol syndrome (FAS), which includes intrauterine growth retardation and developmental delay. Advice should also be given about dental care and sexual behavior during pregnancy. Sexual intercourse should be restricted during the last trimester of pregnancy.

Drugs

The use of drugs that are not absolutely essential should be discouraged as certain drugs taken by the mother during pregnancy may affect the fetus adversely and cause fetal malformations. Some of the drugs known to cause damage include streptomycin that may cause eighth nerve damage and deafness in the fetus, iodide-containing drugs that may cause congenital goiter, corticosteroids that may impair fetal growth, sex hormones that produce virilism and tetracyclines that affect the growth of bones and enamel formation of teeth. A great deal of caution is required in the drug intake by pregnant women.

Radiation

Exposure to radiation is a positive danger to the developing fetus. The most common source of radiation is abdominal X-ray during pregnancy. Studies have shown that mortality rates from leukemia and other neoplasms were significantly greater among children exposed to intrauterine X-ray. Congenital malformations such as microcephaly are known to occur due to radiation. Hence, X-ray examination in pregnancy should be carried out only for definite indications.

Warning Signs

The mother should be given instructions that she should report immediately, any of the following warning signals such as swelling of the feet, convulsions, headache, blurring of the vision, bleeding or discharge per vagina and any other unusual symptoms.

Childcare

Mothers attending antenatal clinics must be given mother craft education that consists of nutrition education, hygiene and childrearing, childbirth preparation and family planning information.

Specific Health Protection

Specific protection for pregnant women's health is an essential aspect of prenatal care. This is because 50%–60% of women, belonging to low-socioeconomic groups, are anemic in the last trimester of pregnancy. The major causative factors are iron and folic acid deficiencies. Anemia is known to be associated with high incidence of premature births, postpartum hemorrhage, puerperal sepsis and thromboembolic phenomena in the mother. The Government of India has initiated a program in which 60 mg of elemental iron and 500 µg of folic acid are being distributed daily to pregnant women through antenatal clinics, primary health centers and their subcenters.

Other Nutritional Deficiencies

Protection is required against other nutritional deficiencies that may occur during pregnancy such as protein, vitamin and mineral deficiencies. In some MCH centers, fresh milk is supplied free of cost to all expectant and lactating mothers; where this is not possible skimmed milk is given. Vitamin A and D capsules are also supplied free of cost.

Tetanus Protection

If the mother was not immunized earlier, two doses of tetanus toxoid should be given, the first dose at 16th–20th week and the second dose at 20th–24th week of pregnancy. For a woman who has been immunized earlier, one booster dose will be sufficient. When such a booster dose is given, it will provide necessary cover for subsequent pregnancies for the next 5 years.

Syphilis

Syphilitic infection in the woman is transmissible to the fetus, especially when she is suffering from primary or secondary stages after the 6th month of pregnancy. Neurological damage with mental retardation is one of the most serious complications. Blood should be tested for syphilis [Venereal Disease Research Laboratory (VDRL)] at the first visit and late in pregnancy. 10 daily injections of procaine penicillin (600,000 units) are usually adequate to treat the infection.

German Measles

Rubella infection contracted during the first 16 weeks of pregnancy can cause major defects such as cataract, deafness and congenital heart diseases. Vaccination of all women of childbearing age, who are seronegative, is desirable. Before vaccinating, it is desirable that pregnancy is ruled out and effective contraception be maintained for 8 weeks after vaccination because of possible risk to the fetus from the virus, should the mother become pregnant.

Rh Status

Rh status is a routine procedure in antenatal clinics to test the blood for Rh type in early pregnancy. If the woman is Rh negative and the husband is Rh positive, she is kept under surveillance for determination of Rh-antibody levels during antenatal period. The blood is further examined at 28th week and 34th–36th week of gestation for antibodies. Rh (anti-D) immunoglobulin should be given at 28th week of gestation so that sensitization during the first pregnancy can be prevented. If the baby is Rh positive, the Rh (anti-D) immunoglobulin is given again within 72 hours of delivery. It should also be given after abortion. Postmaturity should be avoided. Whenever there is evidence of hemolytic process in fetus in utero, the mother should be shifted to an equipped center specialized to deal with Rh problems. The incidence of hemolytic disease due to Rh factor in India is estimated to be approximately one for every 400–500 live births.

Infections of HIV

Human immunodeficiency virus (HIV) may pass from an infected mother to her fetus through the placenta or to her infant during delivery or by breastfeeding. About one-third of the children of HIV-positive mothers become infected through this route. The risk of transmission is higher if the mother is newly infected or if she has already developed acquired immunodeficiency syndrome (AIDS). Prenatal testing for HIV infection should be done as early in pregnancy as possible for pregnant women, who are at risk (if they or their partners have multiple sexual partners, have sexually transmitted disease or use illicit injectable drugs). Universal confidential voluntary screening of pregnant women in high-prevalence areas may allow infected women to choose therapeutic abortion, make an informed decision on breastfeeding or receive appropriate care.

Prenatal Genetic Screening

Screening for genetic abnormalities and for direct evidence of structural anomalies is performed in pregnancy in order to make the option of therapeutic abortion available, when severe defects are detected. Typical examples are—screening for trisomy 21 and severe neural tube defects. Women aged 35 years and above, and those who already have an afflicted child are at high risk.

Mental Preparation

Mental preparation is as important as physical or material preparation. Sufficient time and opportunity must be given to expectant mothers to have free and frank talk on all aspects of pregnancy and delivery. The 'mother craft' classes at the MCH centers help a great deal in removing their fears and in gaining confidence.

Family Planning

Family planning is related to every phase of the maternity cycle. Educational and motivational efforts must be initiated during the antenatal period. If the mother has had two or more children, she should be motivated for puerperal sterilization. The All India Postpartum Services (AIPS) are available to all expectant mothers in India.

INTRANATAL CARE

The need for effective intranatal care is paramount, even if the delivery is expected to be a normal one. Complications such as septicemia and tetanus neonatorum can occur from the use of improperly sterilized instruments. There must be emphasis on cleanliness, which includes clean hands and fingernails, a clean surface for delivery, clean cutting and care of the cord, and keeping birth canal clean by avoiding harmful practices. Hospitals and health centers should be equipped with midwifery kits, a regular supply of sterile gloves and drapes, towels, cleaning materials, soap and antiseptic solution as well as equipment for sterilizing instruments and supplies. Delivery kits [United Nations Children's Fund (UNICEF)] are available with the items needed for basic hygiene for delivery at home.

Objectives

The objectives of good intranatal care are to achieve:
1. Thorough asepsis.
2. Delivery with minimum injury to the newborn and mother.
3. Readiness to deal with complications such as prolonged labor, hemorrhage, convulsions, malpresentations, prolapse of the cord, etc.
4. Care of the baby at delivery—resuscitation, care of the cord, care of the eyes, etc.

Domiciliary Care

Mothers with normal obstetric history may be advised to have their delivery in their own homes, provided the home conditions are satisfactory. In such cases, the delivery may be conducted by the Female Health Worker or Assistant Nurse Midwife or trained dai (trained traditional birth attendants). This is known as *domiciliary midwifery service.*

Domiciliary midwifery service continues to be a necessary mode of practice in India as a large portion of the population (74%) is in the rural areas where there may be no more than one physician per 20,000–30,000 populations. Domiciliary outreach is a major component of intrapartum care.

Advantages of the Domiciliary Midwifery Service

1. The mother delivers in the familiar surroundings of her home, which may remove her fear associated with delivery in a hospital.
2. The chances of cross-infection are generally fewer than in the hospital/nursery.
3. The mother is able to keep an eye upon her children and domestic affairs.
4. The fear associated with hospitals is eliminated, which may tend to ease her mental tension.
5. The financial strain on the family is reduced, which would otherwise be a burden.
6. The load on hospital/health center facilities is reduced, so that other clients in greater need for urgent medical care can be adequately treated.

Disadvantages

1. The mother may have less medical and nursing supervision than in the hospital.
2. The mother may have less rest as she may resume domestic duties too soon.
3. Her diet and medications may be neglected.
4. Many homes in India are unsuitable for even a normal delivery.
5. Even though childbirth is a natural event, which should take place at home, not everything may be normal every time and hence extreme caution is essential in domiciliary midwifery.

A home delivery is contraindicated in certain home situations and when the mother and/or fetus present with *risk factors.* These include the following:
1. Home:
   - Overcrowding
   - Presence of infectious disease
   - Poor (unsanitary) environmental conditions.
2. Maternal factors:
   - Cephalopelvic disproportion
   - Pregnancy-induced hypertension
   - Eclampsia
   - Multiple pregnancy
   - Hydramnios
   - Antepartum hemorrhage

- Rh isoimmunization
- Elderly primigravida
- Grand multipara
- Previous cesarean section, forceps delivery, postpartum hemorrhage
- Associated medical disorders.

3. Fetal factors:
   - History of previous stillbirths or neonatal deaths
   - Malpresentation
   - Prematurity
   - Intrauterine growth retardation.

Preparation for Home Delivery

The midwife/female health worker should assess the home conditions and provide necessary instructions. The mother must be told what she should prepare and provide for the event to take place at home.

All pregnant women must be instructed to make necessary preparations for delivery. They should be provided with a disposable delivery kit (DDK) from the health center. In case the DDK is not available, they should be advised to buy a new razor blade, and some thread themselves and keep them ready. The thread should be boiled for 20 minutes and sun dried before delivery. They should be advised to keep ready cotton cloth for themselves and for the newborn. It is important that these are clean to prevent infection. Clothes should be washed with soap and sun dried and kept away from dust.

All women, who are pregnant, must be informed about the nearest hospital, so that they can be taken there immediately, if there is an emergency.

Room

In the week prior to delivery, the ceiling and walls should be dusted and the floor scrubbed. The mattresses should be beaten and exposed to sunlight for a day or two. The bed sheets should be washed and dried. Dirty surfaces should be wiped with a cloth wrung out of an antiseptic solution. The bed should be conveniently placed to have adequate light and access for health workers from both sides.

As the woman goes into labor, and the female health worker's arrival is awaited, the family should prepare the following:

- Boil two pots of water, one of which to be set to cool
- Bed linen and baby clothes to be kept ready
- A plastic sheet to be placed over the mattress to protect it from fluid and blood
- Arrangement to burn or deep bury the placenta.

Instruments, syringes and needles will have to be sterilized and brought from the hospital/health center along with the delivery kit. The management of labor and delivery is as in the hospital.

The female health worker or community health nurse, who is the pivot of domiciliary care, should be adequately prepared to recognize the 'danger signals' during labor and seek immediate help in transferring the mother to the nearest Primary Health Center or hospital, should the need arises.

Danger signals

- Sluggish contractions or no contractions after rupture of membranes
- Good contractions for an hour after rupture of membranes, but no progress
- Prolapse of cord or hand
- Meconium-stained liquor or a slow irregular or excessively fast fetal heart rate
- Excessive show or bleeding during labor
- A placenta, which is not separated within half an hour after delivery of the baby
- Postpartum hemorrhage or collapse
- A temperature of 38°C or over, during labor.

There should be close liaison between domiciliary and institutional delivery service.

Equipments for Conducting Home Delivery

From home for mother

- Clean newspapers
- A large pot to boil articles
- Two shallow mud pots to use as bedpan and placenta receiver
- Clean sheets and linen
- A clean mat to spread on the floor or cot
- Clean rags.

For baby

- Clothes for baby (old pieces washed with soap, dried by hanging in the sun and ironed with hot iron)
- A mild soap
- Small pieces of rags or cotton
- A cradle with firm bottom.

From the bag and midwifery kit (as suggested by UNICEF)

- Plastic apron
- Plastic sheet
- Two kidney trays
- Two bowls for lotion
- Two artery forceps
- Two thumb forceps
- Scissors
- Two to three packets of sterile gloves
- Syringe and needles
- Enema set
- Urethral catheter
- Mucus extractor (bulb syringe)
- Spring balance
- Thermometers (oral and rectal)
- Sterile cotton swabs and 4 × 4 gauze pieces
- Cord tie/Cord clamp
- Dettol or any antiseptic solution
- Alcohol
- Eyedrops/Ointment for the baby
- Injection vitamin K for the baby
- Methergine (injection and tablets)
- Fetoscope

- Measuring tape
- Episiotomy scissors
- Suture items.

Other items from the health center
- Prenatal record/card of the woman
- Notebook and pen.

Upon receiving the call for a home delivery, the midwife needs to:
1. Collect information regarding the time of onset of labor and the intensity of contractions.
2. Take out the woman's antenatal card or record.
3. Check the midwifery kit and public health bag and add any articles needed.
4. Leave information in the call register including name and address of the woman and the time of leaving.

Upon arrival in the home, further information regarding the onset of labor and other relevant data must be obtained. Monitoring the progress of labor, health of the mother and fetus, and conducting the delivery are same as in a clinic or hospital setting.

About 1% of deliveries tend to be abnormal and 4% 'difficult', requiring the services of a physician. Institutional care may be sought for all difficult cases.

The health status of the mother and baby must be stable before the midwife leaves the home. She must ensure that the woman's:
1. Vagina and perineum are intact, and does not have lacerations that require suturing in the health center.
2. Uterus is firm and contracted and bleeding is minimal.
3. Vital signs are stable and desirous of feeding and bonding with the baby.

An *initial assessment of the newborn* must be done to ensure that:
1. The cord is tied or clamped securely.
2. The neonate's temperature and breathing are stable.
3. The neonate is able to feed from the mother's breasts.
4. There are no visible/identifiable congenital anomalies.
5. Injection vitamin K and prophylactic eye medication are administered.

Instructions regarding the continued care, and observations of the mother and baby must be reviewed with the family. In the mother's antenatal card/record, the information about the management of labor and delivery are recorded including the medications used.

Articles used for the conduct of delivery must be cleaned and wrapped for transport to the health center for sterilization. Materials to be destroyed by burning must be sorted and the family instructed about it. Before leaving the home, the midwife must leave with the family clear instructions as to where she can be contacted if any need arises.

POSTNATAL CARE

Care of the mother and the newborn after delivery is known as postnatal or postpartal care. The objectives of postpartal care are to:
- Prevent complications of the postpartal period
- Promote rapid restoration of the mother's health to optimum level
- Check the adequacy of breastfeeding
- Provide family planning instructions and services
- Provide basic health education to mother/family.

Following delivery, the mother and baby are visited daily for 10 days. During each of these visits the midwife/FHW checks temperature, pulse and respirations of the mother, examines her breasts, checks the progress of normal involution of uterus, examines lochia for any abnormality, checks urine and bowels and advices on perineal toileting. The immediate postnatal complications such as puerperal sepsis, thrombophlebitis and secondary hemorrhage must be kept in mind. At the end of 6th week, the woman needs an examination by the physician in the health center to check up involution of the uterus, which should be complete by then. Further visits should be done once a month during the first 6 months and thereafter once in 2–3 months until the end of 1 year. In rural areas, where only limited care is possible, efforts should be made by the FHW to give at least 3–6 postnatal visits. The common conditions found during the late postnatal period are subinvolution of uterus, prolapse of uterus and cervicitis. Postnatal examination offers an opportunity to detect and correct these defects. Anemia if present needs to be treated. Health education regarding affordable nutritious diet and postnatal exercises to restore the stretched abdominal and pelvic muscles must be provided to enable the mother have a normal postpartum period.

The psychological aspect of postnatal care needs to be addressed based on a needs assessment. New mothers may have timidity and fears due to ignorance and insecurity regarding the care of the baby. In order to endure the emotional stress of childbirth, she requires the support and companionship of her husband as well as encouragement and assistance of family. Fear and insecurity may be eliminated by proper prenatal instructions, postnatal enforcing and supportive care.

Breastfeeding

Postnatal care includes helping the mother to establish successful breastfeeding. For many babies, breast milk provides the main source of nourishment in the 1st year of life. When the standard of environmental sanitation is poor and education is low, the content of feeding bottle is likely to be as nutritionally poor as it is bacteriologically dangerous. It is therefore very important to advise mothers to provide exclusive breastfeeding in the initial months. At the age of 4–5 months, breast milk should be supplemented by additional foods rich in protein and other nutrients (e.g. animal milk, soft-cooked mashed vegetables, fruits, etc.). These supplementary foods should be introduced very gradually and in small amounts.

Family Planning

Every attempt should be made to motivate mothers when they attend postnatal clinics or during postnatal contacts to adopt a suitable method for spacing the next birth or for limiting the family size as appropriate. Postpartum tubal ligation is generally recommended on the 2nd day after delivery. Contraceptives that will not affect lactation may be prescribed immediately following delivery after a physical examination.

Health Education

Health education during the postnatal period should cover the following areas:
- Hygiene—personal and environmental
- Feeding of infant
- Care of the umbilical cord/umbilical stump
- Bathing the baby
- Nutritious diet for the mother
- Pregnancy spacing
- Health check-up for mother and baby
- Birth registration.

STUDY QUESTIONS

Short Answer Question

1. Risk approach in antenatal care.

Essay Questions

1. Explain domiciliary care and list the advantages and disadvantages of domiciliary midwifery service.
2. Describe how you would prepare a client for home delivery. Explain the preparation of materials and physical environment of her house.

BIBLIOGRAPHY

1. Government of India, Annual report 1999–2000. Ministry of Health and Family Welfare. New Delhi; 2000.
2. Government of India, MCH division. National child survival safe motherhood programme. New Delhi; 1971.
3. Government of India, Ministry of Health and Family Welfare. Manual of orientation for midwives and supervisors. New Delhi; 1996.
4. Government of India, Ministry of Health, Department of Family Planning. Plan of operation for hospitals postpartum family planning programme. New Delhi; 1971.
5. Park K. Park's Textbook of Preventive and Social Medicine, 21st edition. Jabalpur: M/s Banarsidas Bhanot Publishers; 2011. pp. 408-526.
6. Parulekar SV. Textbook for Midwives, 2nd edition. Mumbai: Vora Medical Publications; 1998. pp. 585-602.

Primary Health Care and Maternal/Child Health Services in India

Learning Objectives

Upon completing this chapter, the learner will be able to:
- Describe the levels of health care in the country.
- Describe the objectives and evolution of maternal and child health (MCH) services program in India.
- Explain the plan of care for prenatal, intranatal and postnatal mothers.
- Describe the plans for neonatal care in MCH program.
- Explain the roles of female health worker (FHW), health assistant and trained birth assistant (TBA)/trained dai in implementing the MCH program.

The system of healthcare practiced in India presently includes treatment of illness, promotion of health and prevention of illness. Community participation is recognized as a major component. The stress is on the provision of these services to the people representing a shift from medical care to health care and from urban population to rural population.

HEALTH CARE

In India, the complex of primary health centers and their subcenters through the agency of multipurpose health workers, village health guides/TBA provide primary health care. Since India has opted for 'Health for All by 2000 AD', the primary healthcare system has been recognized and strengthened to make the primary healthcare delivery system more effective.

Levels of Health Care

The healthcare service is organized at three levels, i.e. primary, secondary and tertiary. These levels represent different types of care involving varying degrees of complexity.

Primary Care Level

The first level of contact of individuals, families and community with the national health system, where primary health care (essential health care) is provided. As a level of care, it is close to the people, where most of their health problems can be dealt with and resolved. At this level, the health care will be most effective within the context of the needs and limitations of the area.

Secondary Care Level

The next higher level of care is the secondary (intermediate) healthcare level. At this level, problems that are more complex are dealt with. In India, this kind of care is generally provided in district hospitals and community health centers, which also serve as the first referral level facility.

Tertiary Care Level

The tertiary level is a more specialized level than secondary care level and requires specific facilities, and attention of highly specialized health workers. This care is provided by the regional or central level institutions, e.g. medical college hospitals, All India Institutes, regional hospitals and specialized hospitals.

A fundamental and necessary function of the healthcare system is to provide a sound referral system. It must be a two-way exchange of information and returning patients to those who referred them for follow-up care. This will ensure continuity of care and inspire confidence of the consumer in the system.

Health Care at the Village Level

The Government of India evolved a national health policy based on primary health approach in 1983. Steps for implementing the national health policy were implemented during the sixth (1980–1985) and seventh (1986–1991) Five-year Plans. One of schemes adopted to implement the policy was the training of local dais in the country to improve their knowledge in the elementary concepts of maternal and child health and sterilization (asepsis) besides obstetric skills. The dais were trained for 30 working days at the primary health center (PHC), subcenters or MCH centers. During the training, the dais were to conduct two home deliveries under the guidance and supervision of the female health worker (FHW) or assistant nurse midwife (ANM). The emphasis during training was on asepsis so that home deliveries are conducted under safe hygienic conditions thereby reducing the maternal and infant mortality.

After successful completion of training, each dai was provided with a delivery kit and a certificate. These TBAs were also expected to play a vital role in propagating small family norm, since they were more acceptable to the community. The national target was to train one local dai in each village.

Health Care at the Subcenter Level

The subcenters are the peripheral outposts of the health delivery system in rural areas. These were established on the basis of one subcenter for every 5,000 population in general and one for every 3,000 population in the hilly, tribal and backward areas. Each subcenter is manned by a male and a female multipurpose health worker. The functions of subcenters are limited to MCH care, family planning and immunization and implementation of some aspects of national health programs such as Malaria Eradication Program.

Primary Health Center Level

The primary health centers and its subcenters provide the infrastructure to provide health services to the rural population. The National Health Plan of 1983 proposed reorganization of primary health centers on the basis of one PHC for every 30,000–50,000 population in the plains and one PHC for every 20,000 population in hilly, backward and tribal areas for effective coverage. In every community development block, there are one or more PHCs, each of which covers a rural population of 30,000 with a 15 member staff.

Community Health Center Level

Community health centers were established by upgrading the primary health centers (established earlier). Each community health centers covering a population of 80,000–125,000 (one in each community development block), with 30 beds and specialists in surgery, medicine, obstetrics and gynecology, and pediatrics with X-ray and laboratory facilities. A community health officer has been included in the 25 member staff in order to strengthen the preventive and promotive aspects of health care.

MATERNAL AND CHILD HEALTH SERVICES

Maternal and child health services are a method of delivering health care to special groups in the population, which are especially vulnerable to disease, disability or death. These groups include children under the age of 5 years and women in the reproductive age group of 15–44 years, which comprise 32.4% of the population in India. The MCH services encompass the curative, preventive and social aspects of obstetrics, pediatrics, family welfare, nutrition, child development and health education.

Objectives

The objectives of MCH services are:
- Re-education of morbidity and mortality rates for mothers and children
- Promotion of reproductive health
- Promotion of the physical and psychological development of the child and family.

Evaluation of Maternal and Child Health Programs in India

The MCH program has undergone several changes and inclusions in the services over the years, based on the assessment of health status and measurements of mortality, morbidity, growth and development:
- 1952: Family planning program adopted by Government of India
- 1971: Medical Termination of Pregnancy Act
- 1977: Renamed Family planning as Family Welfare Planning
- 1978: Expanded Program of Immunization (EPI)
- 1985: Universal Immunization Program (UIP) and Oral Rehydration Therapy (ORT) Program
- 1992: Child Survival and Safe Motherhood (CSSM) Program
- 1996: Target-Free Approach
- 1997: Reproductive and Child Health Program-1 (RCH-1)
- 2005: Reproductive and Child Health Program-2 (RCH-2), and National Rural Health Mission (NRHM).

Several healthcare services are included in the program to achieve positive health for mothers and children.

ANTENATAL CARE

Antenatal care is the care of the woman during pregnancy. The primary goal of antenatal care is to achieve at the end of a pregnancy a healthy mother and a healthy baby. Ideally this care should begin soon after conception and continue throughout pregnancy.

Objectives

- To promote, protect and maintain the health of the mother during pregnancy
- To detect 'high-risk' cases and give special attention
- To foresee complications and prevent them
- To alleviate anxiety and dread associated with delivery
- To reduce maternal and infant mortality and morbidity

- To teach the mother elements of child care, nutrition, personal hygiene and environmental sanitation
- To sensitize the mother to the need for family planning including advice to seek medical termination of pregnancy in deserving cases
- To attend to the under-fives accompanying the mother.

Antenatal Visits

Antenatal visits should ideally be encouraged to occur once a month during the first 7 months; twice a month during the next month and thereafter once a week if everything is normal. For women from low socioeconomic group who may find it difficult to attend the antenatal clinic so often (owing to loss of wages), a minimum of three visits covering the entire period of pregnancy as first visit at 20 weeks or as soon as the pregnancy is known, second visit at 32 weeks and third visit at 36 weeks may be considered.

Preventive Services

Services offered to prenatal mothers should include:
- Health history
- Physical examination
- Laboratory examinations:
  - Urine analysis
  - Stool examination
  - Complete blood count including hemoglobin estimation
  - Serological examination
  - Blood grouping and Rh determination
  - Chest X-ray, if needed
  - Venereal disease tests.

Risk Approach

The purpose of this approach is to identify 'high-risk' mothers as early as possible and arrange for them skilled care. These high-risk cases comprise the following:
- Elderly primigravida (35 years or over)
- Short statured primigravida (140 cm and below)
- Malpresentation (breech, transverse lie, etc.)
- Antepartum hemorrhage, threatened abortion
- Anemia
- Multiple pregnancy, hydramnios
- Previous stillbirth, intrauterine death, manual removal of placenta
- Elderly grand multipara
- Prolonged pregnancy [14 days after expected date of delivery (EDD)]
- History of previous cesarean or instrumental delivery
- Pregnancy associated with medical conditions such as cardiovascular diseases, kidney diseases, diabetes, tuberculosis, liver disease, etc.

The risk approach aims to provide better services for all, but with special attention to those who need them most. Inherent in this approach is maximum utilization of all resources such as TBA, community health workers and women's groups.

Maintenance of Records

The antenatal card is prepared at first visit to the clinic. The card contains a registration number, identifying data, previous health history and main health events. The record is kept in the maternal and child health/family planning (MCH/FP) center, a link is maintained between the antenatal card, postnatal card and under-fives card. Maintenance of records is essential for evaluation and further improvement of services.

Home Visits

All expectant mothers attending antenatal clinics must be paid at least one home visit by the FHW or public health nurse. More visits are required if the delivery is planned at home. The mother generally is relaxed at home. The home visit will also provide an opportunity for the health worker to observe the environmental and social conditions at home and also an opportunity to give prenatal advice.

Prenatal Advice

A major component of antenatal care is antenatal or prenatal advice. The mother is more receptive to advice concerning herself and her baby at this time. The topic for teaching should cover not only the specific problems of pregnancy and childbirth but also overflow into family and child health care.
- *Diet:* A balanced and adequate diet is of utmost importance during pregnancy and lactation, to meet the increased needs of the mother and to prevent 'nutritional stress'.
- *Personal hygiene:* Advice regarding this must include personal cleanliness, rest and sleep, exercise during pregnancy, smoking and alcohol drinking, dental care and sexual intercourse.
- *Use of drugs:* The use of drugs that are not absolutely essential should be discouraged. Certain drugs taken by mother during pregnancy may affect the fetus adversely and cause fetal malformations.
- *Warning signs:* The mother should be given clear-cut instructions that she should report immediately in the case of warning signals such as swelling of the feet, fits, headache, blurring of vision, bleeding or discharge from vagina and any other unusual symptoms.
- *Child care:* Mothers attending antenatal clinics are taught mother—craft lessons, which consist of nutrition education, advice on hygiene, child rearing, family planning and family budgeting.

Specific Health Protection

Surveys in different parts of India indicate that women belonging to low socioeconomic group have several health risks and require measures to prevent problems for mother and baby.
- *Anemia:* Iron and folic acid deficiencies cause high incidence of premature births, postpartum hemorrhage, puerperal

sepsis and thromboembolic phenomena in the mother. The Government of India has initiated a program in which 100 mg of elemental iron and 500 µg of folic acid are being distributed daily to pregnant women through antenatal clinics, primary health centers and their subcenters.

- *Other nutritional deficiencies:* In order to protect mothers against other deficiencies such as protein, vitamins and minerals such as vitamin A and iodine deficiency, milk and vitamin A and D capsules are supplied free of cost in selected areas.
- *Tetanus:* If the mother was not immunized earlier, two doses of tetanus toxoid are given —the first dose at 16–20 weeks and the second dose at 20–24 weeks of pregnancy. For women who have been immunized earlier, one booster dose will be sufficient and that provides necessary cover for subsequent pregnancies during the next 5 years.
- *Syphilis:* Mother's blood is tested for syphilis both early and late in pregnancy (at first visit and at 6th month of pregnancy) as the infection is transferable to the fetus. Injections of procaine penicillin are given daily for 10 days to infected mothers.
- *German measles:* Infection with Rubella virus during pregnancy should be prevented by preventing and controlling the disease in the general population. Community control of the infection can be achieved by vaccination of all women of childbearing age who are seronegative. Before vaccinating, it is advisable that pregnancy is ruled out and effective contraception be maintained for 8 weeks after vaccination because of the possible risk to the fetus from the virus.
- *Rhesus status:* It is a routine procedure in antenatal clinics to test blood for Rh type in early pregnancy. If the woman is Rh negative and the husband is Rh positive, she is kept under surveillance for determination of Rh-antibody levels during antenatal period. The blood should be further examined at 28 weeks and 34–36 weeks of gestation for antibodies. Rh (anti-D) immunoglobulin should be given at 28 weeks of gestation, so that sensitization during the first pregnancy can be prevented. If the baby is Rh positive, Rh (anti-D) immunoglobulin is given again within 72 hours of delivery. It should also be given after abortion. Whenever there is evidence of hemolytic process in fetus in uterus, the mother should be sent to an equipped center specialized to deal with Rh problems.
- *Human immunodeficiency virus (HIV) infection:* It may pass from an infected mother to her fetus through the placenta or to her infant during delivery or by breastfeeding. The risk of transmission is higher, if the mother is newly infected or if she has already developed acquired immunodeficiency syndrome (AIDS). Voluntary prenatal testing for HIV infection should be done as early in pregnancy as possible for pregnant women who are at great risk (if they or their partner has a number of sexual partners; has a sexually transmitted disease; uses illicit injectable drugs, etc.). Universal confidential voluntary screening of pregnant women in high-prevalence areas may allow infected women to choose therapeutic abortion, make an informed decision on breastfeeding or receive appropriate care.
- *Prenatal genetic screening:* It includes screening for chromosomal abnormalities associated with serious birth defects, screening for direct evidence of congenital structural anomalies, and screening for hemoglobinopathies and other inherited conditions detectable by biochemical assay. Screening for chromosomal abnormalities and for direct evidence of structural anomalies is performed in pregnancy in order to make the option of therapeutic abortion available when severe defects are detected. Typical examples are screening for trisomy 21 (Down syndrome) and severe neural defects. Women over 35 years and above and those, who already have an afflicted child are at higher risk.

Mental Preparation

Mental preparation is as important as physical or material preparation. Sufficient time and opportunity must be given to the expectant mothers to have a free and frank talk on all aspects of pregnancy and delivery. This will go a long way in removing her fears about confinement. 'Mothercraft' classes at the MCH centers help a great deal in achieving the objective.

Family Planning

Family planning is related to every phase of the maternity cycle. The mother in prenatal period is more receptive to advice on family planning than at other times. Educational and motivational efforts must be initiated during the antenatal period. If the mother has had two or more children, she should be motivated for puerperal sterilization.

Pediatric Component

Pediatric component is suggested that a pediatrician should be in attendance at all antenatal clinics to pay attention to the under-fives accompanying the mothers.

INTRANATAL CARE

Childbirth is a normal physiological process, but complications may occur. Septicemia may result from unskilled and septic manipulations, and neonatal infections from the use of unsterilized instruments. The need of effective intranatal care is therefore indispensable. It entails clean hands, clean surface for delivery, clean practices of cutting and care of cord and keeping birth canal clean. Hospitals and health centers should be equipped for delivery with midwifery kits, regular supply of sterile gloves and drapes, towels, cleaning materials, soap and antiseptic solution.

Objectives

The aims of good intranatal care are:
- Thorough asepsis
- Delivery with minimum injury to the newborn and mother

- Readiness to deal with complications such as prolonged labor, antepartum hemorrhage, malpresentations, convulsions and prolapse of the cord
- Care of the baby at delivery—resuscitation, care of the cord, care of the eyes, etc.

Domiciliary Care

Mothers with normal obstetric history may be advised to have their confinement in their homes, provided the home conditions are satisfactory. The delivery may be conducted by a FHW or TBA. This is known as 'domiciliary midwifery service'.

Advantages

- The mother delivers in the familiar surroundings of home, which may remove fears associated with hospital delivery
- The chances of cross-infection are generally fewer at home than in the hospital
- The mother is able to keep an eye upon her other children and domestic affairs.

Disadvantages

- The mother may have less medical and nursing supervision
- The mother may get less rest
- She may resume her domestic duties too soon
- Her diet may be neglected.

Many homes in India are unsuitable for safe normal delivery. The FHW, who is a pivot of domiciliary care, should be adequately trained to recognize the 'danger signals' during labor and seek immediate help in transferring the mother to the nearest primary health center or hospital. The danger signals are:

- Sluggish uterine contractions or no contractions after rupture of membranes
- Good contractions after rupture of membranes, but no progress
- Prolapse of the cord or hand
- Meconium-stained liquor, or slow, irregular or fast fetal heart tones
- Excessive show or bleeding during labor
- Maternal collapse during labor
- A placenta not separated within half-an-hour of delivery
- Postpartum hemorrhage
- A temperature of 38°C or over during labor.

There should be a close liaison between domiciliary and institutional delivery services.

Institutional Care

Institutional care is recommended for all 'high-risk' cases and where home conditions are unsuitable. About 1% of deliveries tend to be abnormal and 4% difficult. The mother is allowed to rest in bed on the 1st day after delivery. From the next day, she is allowed to be up and about. The woman may be discharged after 3–4 days following a normal delivery.

Rooming-in

Keeping the baby's crib by the side of the mother's bed is called 'rooming-in'. This arrangement gives an opportunity for the mother to know her baby. Mothers interested in breastfeeding usually find there is a better chance for success, with rooming-in. Having the baby's presence throughout, builds up her self-confidence.

POSTNATAL CARE

Care of the mother and newborn after delivery is known as postnatal care or postpartal care. This involves care of the mother, which is primarily the responsibility of the obstetrician and care of the newborn, which is the combined responsibility of the obstetrician and pediatrician. The combined responsibility is also known as perinatology.

Objectives

The objectives of postpartal care are:
- To prevent complications of the postpartal period
- To provide care for the rapid restoration of the mother to optimum health
- To check adequacy of breastfeeding
- To provide family planning services
- To provide basic health education to mother/family.

Complications

Certain complications may arise during the postpartal period, which should be recognized early and dealt with promptly. These are as follows:

1. *Puerperal sepsis:* Infection of the genital tract within 3 weeks after delivery. This is accompanied by rise in temperature and pulse rate, foul-smelling lochia, pain and tenderness in lower abdomen.
2. *Thrombophlebitis:* An infection of the veins of the legs frequently associated with varicose veins. The leg may become tender, pale and swollen.
3. *Secondary hemorrhage:* Bleeding from vagina any time from 6 hours after delivery to the end of the puerperium (6 weeks).
4. *Other infections:* Urinary tract infection and mastitis are common in postpartum period. It is important to look for these complications and prevent or treat them promptly.

Restoration of Mother's Health

In order to recuperate physically and emotionally from her experience of delivery, the care falls into three divisions—physical aspects, psychological aspects and social aspects.

Physical Aspects

- *Postnatal examination:* The health checkup must be frequent soon after delivery, i.e. twice a day during the first 3 days and subsequently once a day till she leaves the hospital and, if following home delivery, for a week. At each of these visits the FHW checks her vital signs temperature, pulse, respiration (TPR); examines the breasts, and progress of involution of uterus, examines lochia for any abnormality, checks urine and bowel pattern, and advises on care of stitches if any, perineal toileting and care of the newborn. At the end of 6 weeks, an examination to check involution of uterus is necessary (involution should be complete by them). Further visits should be done once a month during the first 6 months and then once in 2–3 months till the end of 1 year. In rural areas, efforts must be made by FHW to give at least three to six postnatal visits.

- *Anemia:* Hemoglobin estimation should be done during postnatal visits, and when anemia is detected it should be treated. It may be necessary to continue treatment for a year or more in some cases.
- *Nutrition:* The nutritional needs must be met adequately. When the family budget is limited, the mother should be instructed about how she can eat better with less money.
- *Postnatal exercises:* They are necessary to bring the stretched abdominal and pelvic muscles back to normal as quickly as possible. Gradual resumption of normal house-hold duties may be sufficient to restore one's figure.

Psychological Factors

Psychological factors peculiar to the recently delivered woman need special consideration. Some of the commonly seen problems are fear due to ignorance and insecurity regarding the baby. The woman requires the support and companionship of her husband to endure the stresses of childbirth. In rare cases, there may be postpartum blues, postpartum depression or postpartum psychosis. Such conditions must be detected promptly and treated appropriately.

Social Factors

This aspect of postpartal care emphasizes the importance of providing for the mother to nurture and raise the child in a wholesome family atmosphere. She must be helped to develop with her husband, their own methods for such a family life.

Breastfeeding

For many children, breast milk provides the main source of nourishment in the 1st year of life. It is important to instruct mothers to feed only breast milk for 6 months and to avoid feeding bottles. When the standard of environmental sanitation is poor and education low, the content of the feeding is likely to be nutritionally poor, as it is bacteriologically dangerous. At the age of 6 months, breast milk should be supplemented by additional foods rich in protein and other nutrients such as animal milk; soft, cooked and mashed vegetables; and fruits. These are called supplementary foods, which should be introduced very gradually in small quantities.

Family Planning

Family planning is related to every phase of maternity cycle. Every attempt should be made to motivate mothers during postnatal contacts and when they attend postnatal clinics to adopt suitable method for spacing the next birth or for limiting the family size as the case may be. Postpartum sterilization is generally recommended on the 2nd day after delivery. Contraceptives have to be supplied immediately postpartum. Contraceptives that will not affect lactation in the early postpartum period such as intrauterine contraceptive device (IUCD) and non-hormonal methods are the choices in the first 6 months following delivery.

Basic Health Education

Health education during the postnatal period should cover the following broad areas:
- Hygiene—personal and environmental
- Feeding for mother and infant
- Pregnancy spacing
- Importance of health checkup
- Birth registration.

NEONATAL CARE

The 1st week of life is the most critical period in the life of an infant. In India 61.3% of all infant deaths occur within the 1st month of life. Of these more than half may die during the 1st week of birth. This is because the newborn has to adapt itself rapidly and successfully to an alien external environment. The risk of death is greatest during the first 24–48 hours after birth. The problem is more acute in rural areas where expert obstetric care is scarce and the home environmental conditions where the baby is born are usually unsatisfactory.

Objectives

The objective of early neonatal care is to assist the newborn in the process of adaptation to an alien environment, which involves:
- Establishment and maintenance of cardiorespiratory functions
- Maintenance of body temperature
- Avoidance of infection
- Establishment of satisfactory feeding regimen
- Early detection and treatment of congenital and acquired disorders, especially infections.

Immediate Care

Clearing the Airway

Establishment and maintenance of cardiorespiratory functions (respiration) is the most important thing at the moment the baby is born. To help establish breathing, the airway should be cleared of mucus and other secretions. Positioning the baby with low head may help in the drainage of secretions. This process can be helped by gentle suction to remove mucus and amniotic fluid. Resuscitation becomes necessary, if natural breathing fails to establish within 1 minute; as in the case of babies who have already been subject to hypoxia during labor. In these cases, resuscitation may require more active measures such as suction, application of oxygen mask, intubation and assisted respiration. All delivery rooms should be equipped with resuscitation equipment including oxygen.

Apgar Scoring

The Apgar score is taken at 1 minute and again at 5 minutes after birth. It requires immediate and careful observation of the heart rate, respiration, muscle tone, reflex response and color of the infant. Each sign is given a score of 0, 1 or 2. The score provides an immediate estimate of the physical condition of the baby. A perfect score is 9 or 10; 0-3 indicates that the baby is severely depressed and 4-6 moderately depressed. A score below 5 needs prompt action. Infant with low Apgar score at 5 minutes of age are subject to high risk of complications and death during the neonatal period [*refer* **Table 39.1** (Chapter 39) for Apgar score chart].

Care of the Cord

In the case of the normal infant, the umbilical cord should be cut and tied when it has stopped pulsating. The body receives about 10 mL of extra blood if the cord is cut after pulsation ceases. Care must be taken to use sterilized instruments and cord ties as well as use antiseptic preparation on the cord stump and the skin around the base to prevent infection. The cord should be kept as dry as possible. It dries and shrivels up and separates by aseptic necrosis in 5-8 days.

Care of the Eyes

Before the eyes are open, the lid margins should be cleaned with sterile wet swabs, one for each eye from inner to outer canthus. A drop of freshly prepared silver nitrate 1% or tetracycline 1% ointment is placed in the eyes to prevent ophthalmia neonatorum.

Care of the Skin

When the baby is a few hours old and in stable condition, the first bath is given with warm water and soap to remove vernix, meconium and blood stains. The first bath is given by the nursing staff/midwife. Thereafter no further bath is given until the day of discharge.

Maintenance of Body Temperature

The normal body temperature of a newborn is 36.5-37.50°C. A newborn baby leaves the warm environment of the womb of the mother into an environment, which may be 10-20°C cooler especially in the winter months in India. A newborn has little thermal control and can lose body heat quickly. Immediately after birth, most of the heat loss occurs through evaporation of the amniotic fluid from the body of the wet baby. As much as 75% of the heat loss can occur from the head. It is therefore important that immediately after birth the baby is quickly dried (head and body) with a clean cloth and wrapped in a warm cloth or baby blanket, and given to mother for skin-to-skin contact and breastfeeding.

Breastfeeding

Breastfeeding should be initiated within an hour of birth. Although there is little milk at that time, it helps to establish feeding and a close mother-baby relationship known as bonding. The first milk, which is called 'colostrum', is the most suitable food for the body during this early period because it contains a high concentration of protein and other nutrients, the baby needs. It is also rich in anti-infective factors, which protect the baby against respiratory infections and diarrheal diseases. The regular milk comes on the 3rd-6th day after birth. The baby should be allowed to breastfeed whenever it wants. Feeding the baby on demand helps the baby to gain weight. It is very important to advise mother to avoid feeding bottles.

Neonatal Examinations

First Examination

The first examination is done soon after birth. This is to ascertain that the baby has not suffered injuries during the birth process, to detect malformations that require immediate treatment and to assess maturity. Abnormalities found on examination that require immediate alternation are:
- Cyanosis of the lips and skin
- Difficulty in breathing
- Imperforate anus
- Signs of cerebral irritation such as twitching, convulsions, neck rigidity and bulging of anterior fontanel
- Temperature instability.

Second Examination

The second examination is done by a pediatrician within 24 hours after birth. It is a detailed systematic examination from head to foot, conducted in good light. The following protocol is usually followed:
- Body size, which include body weight, crown-heel length, head and thoracic circumferences
- Body temperature
- Skin for cyanosis, jaundice, pallor, generalized erythema, vesicular and bullous lesions
- Cardiorespiratory activities such as cardiac murmur, central cyanosis, thoracic cage retraction on inspiration and respiratory rate over 60 per minute
- Neurobehavioral activity—neck retraction, frog-like posture, hyperextension of all limbs, asymmetrical posture, reflexes and cry
- Head and face—hydrocephalus, abnormalities of eyes, ears and mouth
- Abdomen—distension, abnormal masses imperforate anus

- Limbs and joints—joint deformities, congenital dislocation of hips and extra digits
- Spine—neural tube defects
- External genitalia—hypospadias, epispadias, undescended testes and hydrocele in male, fused labia and enlarged clitoris in female.

Measuring the Baby

Measurements of birth weight, length and head circumference are done to evaluate the health and maturity of the baby:
1. *Birth weight:* The birth weight should be taken within the 1st hour of life, before significant postnatal weight loss has occurred. Weight is taken by placing the naked baby on a clean towel on the scale pan. In home delivery, weight is taken by placing the baby in a sling bag using a salter weighing scale.
2. *Length:* It can be taken with a measuring board (infantometer) with a fixed head piece on which the infant is placed supine with legs fully extended and feet flexed at right angles to the lower legs. The sliding board is moved firmly against the feet by a second person and the reading is taken.
3. *Head circumference:* This measurement is taken with a tape measure at the maximum circumference of the head in the occipitofrontal diameter. The purposes of taking these measurements are as follows:
   a. To assess the baby's size against known standards for the population.
   b. To compare the size with estimated period of gestation.
   c. To provide a baseline against which subsequent progress can be measured.

Neonatal Screening

The objective of screening newborns is to detect babies with treatable genetic developmental and other abnormalities, and to provide their parents with genetic counseling. 10–15 mL of cord blood should be collected at birth for typing, Coombs' testing and other tests, if indicated. The most common disorders for which newborns are screened are the following:
1. Phenylketonuria (PKU), a rare disorder of amino acid metabolism. This is an autosomal recessive trait in babies who are homozygous with a deficiency in the enzyme phenylalanine hydroxylase, which converts phenylalanine to tyrosine. The deficiency causes raised serum phenylalanine concentration causing mental retardation and tendency to seizures, if the child does not receive low phenylalanine diet. Screening for this and other metabolic errors namely galactosemia, and maple syrup urine disease are tested on all babies in many countries by taking 4–5 drops of blood of baby by heel prick and placing on thick absorbent filter paper before discharge from the hospital.
2. Congenital hypothyroidism is a condition if present, leads to serious sequelae, including severe mental retardation. By measuring the levels of thyroxine (T_4) and thyroid-stimulating hormone (TSH), the condition can be identified and treatment started within the first 1–2 months of life.
3. Coombs' test is done on infants of all Rh-negative mothers.
4. Tests for hemoglobinopathies such as sickle cell disease, thalassemia and glucose-6-phosphate dehydrogenase (G6PD) deficiency.

Identification of 'At Risk' Infants

Identifying the babies 'at risk' and providing intensive care are important to reduce perinatal, neonatal and infant mortality. The basic criteria for identifying these babies include:
- Birth weight—less than 2.5 kg
- Twins
- Birth order—5 and more
- Artificial feeding
- Second and third degree malnutrition (weight below 70% of the expected weight)
- Failure to gain weight during 3 successive months
- Children with protein-energy malnutrition (PEM) and diarrhea.

Low-birth-weight Babies

The birth weight of infants is the single most important determinant of their chances of survival, healthy growth and development. Low-birth-weight (LBW) babies are of two groups; those born prematurely (short gestation) and those with fetal growth retardation.

Low-birth-weight babies have a high risk of dying not only during the neonatal period but also during their infancy, thus significantly raising the rate of perinatal and infant mortality, and contribute greatly to immediate and long-term health problems. Most of them become victims of malnutrition and infection.

There is strong and significant correlation between the maternal nutritional status and the length of pregnancy and birth weight. A high percentage of LBW therefore points to deficient health status of pregnant women, inadequate prenatal care and need for improved care of newborn. Direct interventional measures to reduce the incidence of LBW are to identify pregnant women with risk factors early in pregnancy and taking steps to reduce the risk. The risk factors are malnutrition, heavy work load, diseases, infections and high blood pressure. Added to malnutrition are too many and too frequent pregnancies, which contribute to continued depletion of her body. The interventions that can be taken for correction and prevention are:
1. *Increasing food intake:* Dietary improvement in the malnourished pregnant mother, even during the last trimester can result in a significant improvement in the birth weight of the newborn. Measures such as supplementary feeding, distribution of iron and folic acid tablets, and fortification and enrichment of foods.

2. *Controlling infections:* Maternal infections should be diagnosed and treated. Malaria, urinary tract infections, infections due to cytomegalovirus, toxoplasmosis, rubella and syphilitic infection are the common conditions seen in pregnant women, which can affect fetal growth. Indirect interventions include family planning, avoidance of excessive smoking, improved sanitation measures and measures aimed at improving the health and nutrition of young girls. These measures can be expected to be more effective and to have lasting effects only, if at the same time there are improvements in the socioeconomic and environmental conditions and in the distribution of health and social services especially in the underserved areas.

Management of LBW babies

For the purpose of management, the LBW babies can be divided into two groups:

1. Those under 2 kg.
2. Those between 2 and 2.5 kg.

Babies under 2 kg need care in an intensive care unit (ICU) until the weight reaches above 2 kg. Babies between 2 and 2.5 kg may be with mother for kangaroo care after 2 days of care in the ICU. LBW babies given to mothers for kangaroo care must be instructed to follow specific instructions, which include:

- Skin-to-skin positioning of the baby on the mother's chest
- Adequate nutrition through breastfeeding
- Ambulatory care as a result of early discharge from hospital
- Support for the mother and her family in caring for the baby.

Intensive care in the hospital consists of:

- Incubatory care, i.e. adjustment of temperature, humidity and oxygen supply
- Feeding by nasal catheter of breast milk, if available
- Prevention of infection.

In the care of LBW babies, all precautions must be taken to prevent the leading causes of death, such as atelectasis, pulmonary hemorrhage, intracranial bleeding secondary to anoxia or birth trauma and pneumonia and other infections.

SYSTEM OF DELIVERING MCH SERVICES IN THE COUNTRY

Maternal and child health services encompasses all the activities, which promote health and prevent or solve health problems of mother and children, irrespective of whether they are curative, diagnostic, preventive or rehabilitative, and whether they are carried out in health centers or in the home by primary healthcare workers, TBA or highly trained specialists.

Recent Trends in MCH Care

The emergence of certain new concepts is now changing the organization and management of MCH care in several countries. The concepts are as given below.

Integrated Care

The integrated approach is based on the fact that it is inconvenient for the mother to go to one place to receive care for herself, to another for care of her children and yet another for family planning services.

An integrated approach implies that all those involved in maternity care from the obstetrician down to the local dai or TBA, must work as a team. Obstetric and pediatric units should be closely linked so that there can be regular contact between obstetricians, pediatricians, community physicians, health and social workers so that services for the care of the mother and the child in the hospital and community be planned and reviewed including teaching and research. This approach helps to promote continuity of care as well as improves efficiency and effectiveness of MCH care.

Risk Approach

Risk approach is a means of improving the coverage and efficiency of MCH care and family planning. It is also a managerial tool for better use of scarce resources. It is based on the early detection of mothers and children with high-risk factors. All mothers and children with high-risk factors are given additional and more skilled care including hospitalization, while at the same time essential care is provided for the rest of the mothers and children so that everyone gets care appropriate to their need.

It is also possible to assess the 'degrees' of risk of each factor, by scoring according to the following:

- Magnitude, i.e. extent and severity
- Treatability—responsiveness to treatment and control
- Cost effect—in terms of alleviating suffering
- Community attitude—social concern.

Such an approach when applied on a community-wide basis enables the determination of priority activities, within the MCH program based on the 'degrees' of risk. Application of this approach is a departure from the past or traditional practices to promote the health of mothers and children.

Manpower Changes

The special category of 'maternal and child health workers' (e.g. auxiliary nurse-midwives and health visitors) at the peripheral level is gradually being phased out. A wide range of workers are now considered necessary for maternal and child health services. They include as following:

1. *Professionals:* Specialists.
2. *Fieldworkers:* Multipurpose workers, health guides, TBA, Balsevikas, Anganwadi workers, extension workers, accredited social health activists (ASHA), etc.
3. *Voluntary workers:* Members of women's organizations—in India, where 70% of population lives in rural areas, there are not enough obstetricians to attend to all deliveries. Therefore, a trained dai or midwife is essential in every village. The same thing is true about pediatricians. It is now recognized that obstetric and pediatric services can only be improved by cooperation and liaison with these practitioners.

Primary Health Care

Primary health care is now recognized as a way of making essential health care available to all. It has all the elements necessary to make a positive impact on MCH care, i.e. care of mothers and children, family planning, control of infections, education about health problems and how to prevent them, and measures to ensure nutritional food. Primary health care emphasizes family-oriented care and support, and community self-reliance in health matters.

The infrastructure in rural areas is based on the complex of community health centers, primary health centers and their subcenters. They provide preventive and promotive healthcare services. Since deliveries by trained dais or other healthcare workers are crucial in reducing maternal and infant mortality in rural areas, the Government of India undertook a scheme to train local dais to conduct safe deliveries. The dais or TBA is now available in most villages.

The Integrated Child Development Services (ICDS) are functioning all over the country providing a package of basic health services (e.g. supplementary nutrition, immunization, health checkup, referral, nutrition and health education, non-formal education) to mothers and children. In urban areas, the general trend is toward institutional delivery. In some of the larger cities, almost 90% of deliveries take place in maternity hospitals and maternity homes. Some of the institutions are under the auspices of the municipal corporations and voluntary organizations. The services of obstetricians are available at district hospitals. For specialized care of children, pediatric units have been established in several district hospitals.

ASSESSING MATERNAL AND CHILD HEALTH CARE

Maternal and child health status is assessed through measurements of mortality, morbidity and growth, and development. The commonly used mortality indicators of MCH care are:
- Maternal mortality rate
- Mortality of infant and child.

MATERNAL MORTALITY

Maternal deaths occur due to complications of pregnancy or childbirth and also deaths beyond the 6 weeks of postpartum period.

Maternal mortality rate (MMR) is the number of maternal deaths in a given period per 100,000 women of reproductive age during the same time period.

Maternal mortality ratio is the number of maternal deaths during a given time period per 100,000 live births during the same time period.

Maternal mortality ratio strongly reflect the overall effectiveness of health systems, which in many developing countries suffer from weak administrative, technical and logistical capacity, adequate financial investment and lack of skilled health personnel.

Measures to reduce the MMR are increasing the number of births attended by skilled health personnel, providing access to emergency obstetric care when necessary and providing postnatal care for mothers and babies. These measures could reduce both maternal and neonatal deaths. Enhancing women's access to family planning, adequate nutrition, improved water and sanitation facilities, and affordable basic health care. Protection from abuse, violence, and discrimination, empowerment of women and greater involvement of men in maternal and child care will further lower mortality rates.

Causes of Maternal Deaths

Causes of maternal deaths worldwide are obstetric hemorrhage puerperal infections, hypertensive disorders of pregnancy, prolonged or obstructed labor and other direct causes such as ectopic pregnancies, embolism, and deaths due to indirect causes such as anemia, cardiovascular diseases and infections such as tuberculosis and HIV/AIDS.

The life time chances of maternal death in the world as a whole is about 1 in 92. It varies from region to region and country to country. In the least developed countries, the chances are 1 in 24 and in the developing countries 1 in 76. In the sub-Saharan region, the chances are very high about 1 in 26 pregnancies.

India is among those countries, which have very high maternal mortality rate. It was 407 per 100,000 live births in 1997. It declined to 301 per 100,000 live-births in 2003 (24% reduction) and to 254 per 100,000 by 2006 (16% reduction). Major causes of maternal mortality in India according to 2001–2003 survey are; hemorrhage 38%, sepsis 11%, hypertensive disorders 5%, obstructed labor 5%, abortion 8%, anemia 19% and other conditions 34%.

Newer approaches taken in the recent years such as 'risk approach' and 'primary health care' are steps in the right direction to reduce maternal mortality and mobility. Essential obstetric care and first referral units (FRU) for emergency obstetric care are therefore a high priority under the safe motherhood component of reproductive and child health (RCH) program. Equally important is the improvement of sociocultural factors such as female literacy, level of nutrition, environmental sanitation, etc.

Preventive Measures

Any attempt to lowering MMR must consider the following measures:
- Early registration of pregnancy
- At least three antenatal checkups
- Dietary supplementation including correction of anemia
- Prevention of complications, e.g. eclampsia, malpresentations and ruptured uterus
- Prevention of infection and hemorrhage in puerperium
- Treatment of medical conditions such as hypertension, diabetes and tuberculosis
- Antimalarial and tetanus prophylaxis
- Clean delivery practice
- Delivery by trained personnel, e.g. FHW or TBAs
- Institutional deliveries for women with bad obstetric history and risk factors

- Promotion of family planning
- Identification of the cause of every maternal death
- Safe abortion services.

MORTALITY IN INFANCY AND CHILDHOOD

Mortality rates are good indicators to measure the level of health and health care in different countries. They also help in assessing the overall socioeconomic development of a country. Mortality is considered in and around infancy in a number of time periods as:
- Perinatal period
- Early neonatal period
- Neonatal period
- Late neonatal period
- Postneonatal period.

Perinatal Mortality

The WHO definition of perinatal mortality is as follows.

Perinatal mortality rate (PMR) is the number of late fetal deaths (28 weeks gestation and more) plus early neonatal deaths (1st week) in a given year per 1,000 live births in the same year.

$$\text{Perinatal mortality rate} = \frac{\text{Late fetal deaths (28 weeks gestation and more) + Early neonatal deaths (1st week) in 1 year}}{\text{Live births + Late fetal deaths in the same year}} \times 1,000$$

Perinatal mortality is a problem of serious dimension in all countries as it accounts for 90% of all fetal and infant mortality in the developed countries. The estimates of perinatal mortality rate in India for the year 2007 was about 37 per 1,000 live births and stillbirths with 41 for rural areas and 24 for the urban areas.

Causes of Perinatal Mortality

A number of social, biological and medical factors are known to be associated with perinatal mortality. Many of these factors endanger the life of the mother, causing high maternal mortality. The overall risk is increased in the following categories:

1. Prenatal causes:
   - Advanced maternal age (35 years and more)
   - Low maternal age (under 16 years)
   - High parity (fifth and subsequent pregnancies)
   - Maternal height (short stature)
   - Heavy smoking (10 or more cigarettes daily)
   - Poor past obstetric history (one or more past stillbirths and neonatal deaths)
   - Malnutrition and severe anemia
   - Multiple pregnancies
   - Maternal diseases: Hypertension, cardiovascular diseases, diabetes and tuberculosis
   - Uterine anomalies and pelvic diseases
   - Endocrine imbalances
   - Antepartum hemorrhage.
2. Intranatal causes:
   - Birth injuries
   - Asphyxia
   - Prolonged effort
   - Obstetric complications.
3. Postnatal causes:
   - Prematurity
   - Respiratory distress syndrome
   - Respiratory and alimentary infections
   - Congenital anomalies.

In some cases, the causes are unknown and clinically not ascertainable.

Prevention

Measures to reduce perinatal mortality rate are essential to accelerate the declining trend in neonatal and infant mortality rates. These include preventive and timely corrective measures for the causes identified in the prenatal, intranatal and postnatal period and improvement of socioeconomic status of mothers and families.

Neonatal Mortality

Neonatal deaths are deaths occurring during the neonatal period. Commencing at birth and ending 28 completed days after birth. Neonatal mortality rate is the number of neonatal deaths in a given year per 1,000 live births in that year.

$$\text{Neonatal mortality rate} = \frac{\text{Number of deaths of children under 28 days of age in a year}}{\text{Total live births in the same year}} \times 1,000$$

Causes of Neonatal Mortality

The causes of neonatal mortality are multifactorial:
- LBW
- Birth asphyxia and atelectasis
- Birth injuries
- Congenital malformations
- Infections
- Preterm birth.

The neonatal mortality is directly related to the birth weight and gestational age. Prematurity and congenital anomalies account for one third of newborn deaths and these often occur in the 1st week of life. The main causes of neonatal mortality are intrinsically linked to the health of the mother and the care she receives before, during and immediately after giving birth. Asphyxia and birth injuries usually result from poorly managed labor and delivery, and lack of access to obstetric services. Inadequate calorie or micronutrient intake also results in poor pregnancy outcomes. Many neonatal infections such as tetanus and congenital syphilis can be prevented by care during pregnancy and delivery. However, the endogenous factors, which are not sensitive to improvement in environmental conditions, are the difficult part of neonatal mortality to alter.

In India, the estimate for the year 2007 was about 29 per 1,000 live births in early neonatal period (0–7 day) with about 32 for rural areas and 16 for urban areas.

Prevention

Measures to reduce neonatal mortality rates and to improve newborn health are enumerated below:

1. During pregnancy:
   - Well-timed, well-spaced and wanted pregnancies
   - Well-nourished and healthy mother
   - Pregnancy free of drug abuse, and use of tobacco and alcohol
   - Tetanus and rubella immunization
   - Prevention of mother-to-child transmission of HIV
   - Early contact with healthcare system for prevention, detection and treatment of associated problems
   - Good diet.
2. During and soon after delivery:
   - Safe and clean delivery by trained attendant
   - Early detection and management of fetal complications
   - Emergency obstetric care for maternal and fetal complications
   - Newborn resuscitation
   - Newborn cord, skin and eye care
   - Early initiation of exclusive breastfeeding
   - Early detection and treatment for neonatal complications
   - Prevention and control of infections
   - Information and counseling on home care, danger signs and timely care seeking.
3. During the 1st month of life (neonatal period):
   - Protection, promotion and support of exclusive breastfeeding
   - Prompt detection and management of diseases in the neonate
   - Immunization
   - Protection of girl baby.

Studies show that neonatal mortality is dominated by endogenous factors and postneonatal neonatal mortality by exogenous factors (e.g. social and environmental). Diarrhea and respiratory infections are the main causes of death during the postneonatal period. Malnutrition is an additional factor reinforcing the adverse effects of the infections. In the developing countries, the main cause of postneonatal mortality is congenital anomalies. Postneonatal mortality increases steadily with birth order that infants born into already large families run a higher risk of death from infectious diseases.

Infant Mortality Rate

Infant mortality rate (IMR) is defined as the ratio of infant deaths registered in a given year to the total number of live births registered in the same year; usually expressed as a rate per 1,000 live births. It is given by the formula:

$$\text{Infant mortality rate} = \frac{\text{Number of deaths of children less than 1 year of age in a year}}{\text{Number of live births in the same year}} \times 1{,}000$$

The IMR is universally regarded not only as the most important indicator of the health status of a community but also the level of living of the people in general and the effectiveness of MCH services in particular. There are wide variations between countries in the levels of infant mortality. The IMR varies from 5 per 1,000 live births in the developed countries to 82 per 1,000 live births in the least developed countries according to estimates done in 2003. The decline in IMR has been attributed to:

- Improved obstetric and perinatal care
- Improvement in the quality of life that is economic and social progress
- Better control of communicable diseases
- Advances in chemotherapy, antibiotics and insecticides
- Better nutrition and emphasis on breastfeeding
- Family planning, e.g. birth spacing.

Infant Mortality in India

India is still among high IMR countries, though it has declined from 129 in 1970, 114 in 1980 to 53 in 2008. Despite significant decline the rates are very high as compared to developed countries.

India is a vast country with widely differing populations. An examination of state wise IMR shows a vast regional variation with Madhya Pradesh having IMR of 70 and Kerala as low as 12 per 1,000 live births during the year 2008. A critical IMR runs through Odisha, Madhya Pradesh, Assam, Uttar Pradesh and Rajasthan; all these states have IMR above the national average of 53.

The state of Kerala has managed to surpass all the Indian states in certain important measures of social development. It has the lowest IMR, the lowest birth rate and highest literacy rate.

Causes of Infant Mortality

The principal causes of infant mortality in India are LBW, respiratory infections, diarrheal diseases, congenital malformations and birth injuries. In developing countries the high IMR is due to LBW and the combined effects of infection such as diarrhea and respiratory infections, whereas in developed countries, it is mainly due to congenital anomalies, anoxia and hypoxia.

Factors Affecting Infant Mortality

Infant mortality is due to the interaction of several factors in combination. This may be classified as biological, economic and social factors:

1. *Biological:*
   a. Birth weight: Babies of LBW (under 2.5 kg) and high birth weight (over 4 kg) are at special risk.

b. **Age of the mother:** Infant mortality rates are greater, when the mother is either very young (below the age of 19 years) or relatively older (over 30 years).
c. **Birth order:** The highest mortality is found among first born and the lowest among those born second. The risk of mortality escalates after the third birth. Infant mortality from nutritional deficiencies is three to four times higher for infants born with fifth or higher birth order compared to the first three.
d. **Birth spacing:** Repeated and closer pregnancies cause malnutrition and anemia in the mother, and predispose to LBW resulting in higher infant deaths. Babies weaned prematurely due to births of younger babies are more prone to develop protein-energy malnutrition (PEM) and diarrhea both of which increase mortality in infants.
e. **Multiple births:** Infants born in multiple births face a greater risk of death than do those in single births due to the greater frequency of LBW among the former.
f. **Family size:** Frequency of disease and duration of illness were found more in families with three or more children. Deprivation of maternal care is also found in larger families. Fewer children would mean better maternal care, a better share of family resources, less morbidity and greatly decreased infant mortality.
g. **High fertility:** High fertility goes with high infant mortality.

2. *Economic factors:* One of the most important variables affecting infant mortality rates both directly and indirectly is socioeconomic status. Mortality rates are highest in the slums and lowest in the richer residential localities. The availability and quality of health care and the nature of child's environment are closely related to socioeconomic status. Major improvements in health status and a decrease in infant normality require continuing socioeconomic development including provision of health care.

3. *Cultural and social factors:*
   a. Infant health is related to breastfeeding because of the nutritional content and immunizing agents contained in breast milk. Early weaning and bottle-fed infants living in poor hygienic conditions are more prone to die than breastfed infants living in similar conditions.
   b. **Early marriages:** The baby of teenage mother has the highest risk for neonatal and postneonatal mortality.
   c. **Sex of the baby:** In most parts of India, female infants receive for less attention than male infants. In many families, birth of a female baby is unwelcome. Statistics show that female infant mortality is higher than the male infant mortality. However, the neonatal death rate is seen higher for male infants though postneonatal death rate is higher for female infants.
   d. **Quality of mothering:** Even in conditions of extreme poverty, child could reasonably survive if they had an efficient mother. It is the 'quality of mothering' that helps to reduce infant mortality.
   e. **Maternal education:** Mother's education level, even within the same economic class is a key determinant of their children's health. Maternal education plays a major role in the reduction of infant and child mortality because of their health behavior, care and access to use of health services. Women with schooling tend to marry later, delay childbearing and are more likely to practice family planning.
   f. **Quality of health care:** In India, inadequate prenatal care and infrequent attendance at delivery are factors affecting infant mortality. The percentage of deliveries attended by untrained personnel or relatives is still high in rural India. Shortage of trained personnel like TBAs, midwives and health visitors contributes to high infant mortality.
   g. **Broken families:** Infant mortality tends to be high where the mother or father has died or separated.
   h. **Illegitimacy:** A child born out-of-wedlock is generally unwanted both by the mother as well as the society. Consequently, such a child does not receive the care in terms of nutrition and medical care that it needs.
   i. **Brutal habits and customs:** Certain age-old customs and beliefs greatly influence infant mortality rate. These include depriving the baby of colostrum, frequent purgation, branding the skin, applying cow dung to the cut end of the umbilical cord, faulty feeding practices and early weaning.
   j. **Delivery by indigenous dai:** The untrained dai, who is an illiterate person lacks knowledge of rules of hygiene. Her unhygienic delivery practice is an important cause of high infant mortality.
   k. **Bad environmental sanitation:** Lack of safe water supply, poor housing conditions, bad drainage, overcrowding and insect breeding, all increase the risk of infant mortality as infants are highly susceptible to infections.

Preventive and Social Measures

As the etiology of infant and perinatal mortality is multifactorial, a multipronged approach will be needed to reduce the mortality:

1. *Prenatal nutrition:* The risk of death begins even before birth, if the mother in malnourished. Therefore, the very first need is to improve the state of maternal nutrition. Food supplementation to mother's basic diet would improve the birth weight of babies. The ICDS programs in India are a step in this direction.
2. *Prevention of infection:* Many of the infections causing death in children are preventable by immunization. Tetanus toxoid to pregnant mothers and Universal Immunization Program aim at providing protection against vaccine preventable diseases, and thereby ensures greater child survival.
3. *Breastfeeding:* The most effective measure for lowering infant mortality is to promote breastfeeding, which is a safeguard against gastrointestinal and respiratory infections and PEM.
4. *Family planning:* Family limitation and spacing of births contribute substantially to lowering of infant mortality

rate. Smaller number of children and longer spacing between pregnancies are associated with improved infant and child survival.
5. *Growth monitoring:* All infants should be weighed periodically (at least once a month) and maintained their growth charts. These charts help to identify children at risk for malnutrition early.
6. *Sanitation:* For infants and young children, the risk of dying is very closely related to the environment in which they live. Exposure to infection through contaminated food and polluted water, lack of elementary hygiene, insects and poor housing are hazards, which the young children cannot escape.
7. *Provision of primary health care:*
   a. Prenatal care must improve with a view to detecting mothers with 'high-risk factors' and those with prenatal conditions associated with high risk for hospitalization and treatment.
   b. Special baby care units must be provided for all babies weighing less than 2 kg.
   c. Proper referral services must be available.
   d. All those involved in maternity care from the obstetrician to the local dai should collaborate and work together as a team.
8. *Socioeconomic development:* This must include spread of education especially female literacy, improvement of nutritional standards, provision of safe water and basic sanitation, improvement of housing conditions and growth of agriculture and industry. This implies an all-round health and social development of the community.

Child Mortality Rate (1–4 Years)

Child death rate is the number of deaths of children aged 1–4 years per 1,000 children in the same age group in a given year. This is computed by the formula:

$$\text{Child death rate} = \frac{\text{Number of deaths of children aged 1-4 years during a year}}{\text{Total number of children aged 1-4 years at the middle of the year}} \times 1{,}000$$

Child mortality rate is a more refined indicator of the social situation in a country than IMR. Mortality in this group no longer depends on perinatal hazards and other endogenous factors, which often cause loss of life during the 1st year of life. It reflects the adverse environmental health hazards (e.g. malnutrition, poor hygiene, infections and accidents) including economic, educational and cultural characteristics of the family.

In the age group 1–4 years, the 2nd year is the period, when the young child runs the highest risk of dying. After the 2nd year, death rates decline progressively. The infectious diseases of childhood such as measles, whooping cough, diphtheria, diarrhea and acute respiratory infections affect mostly this age group.

Mortality rate at ages 1–4 years is about 30 in some developing countries, whereas it is less than one in developed countries. In India, for the year 2007, child mortality was estimated as 4.2% of total deaths. Like infant mortality, child mortality also shows wide state-wise variations. The states reporting rates higher than national average are Madhya Pradesh 5.8%, Uttar Pradesh 6.3%, Bihar 8.7 and Rajasthan with 5.3% of total deaths. Kerala recorded the lowest with 0.5% followed by Tamil Nadu 1.1%.

Leading Causes of Death

The leading causes in the 1–4 years age group are the following:
- Diarrheal diseases
- Respiratory infections
- Malnutrition
- Infectious diseases such as measles, whooping cough
- Other febrile diseases
- Home accidents and injuries.

In developed countries deaths from infectious diseases are quite rare, while accidents are the leading causes of death from the age of 1 year. Four groups of home accidents have been identified such as:
1. Falls from unprotected stairs and balconies.
2. Poisoning.
3. Burns and scalds. Almost all accidents are preventable.

Causes, such as congenital anomalies and neoplasms are not easy to prevent or care. These conditions also affect children in developing countries, but their relative importance is overshadowed by infections.

Preventive Measures

The current trend in India as in many other countries is to provide integrated MCH and family planning services as compact family welfare service. This implies a close relationship of maternity health to child health, maternal and child health to the health of the family, and family health to the general health of the community. In providing these services, specialists in obstetrics and child health (pediatrics) have joined hands, and are now looking beyond the four walls of hospitals into the community to meet the health needs of mothers and children aimed at positive health.

JOB FUNCTIONS OF HEALTH WORKERS FOR IMPLEMENTING MCH SERVICES

Female Health Worker

Under the multipurpose health worker scheme, a FHW in the subcenter has the following functions.

Registration

1. Registration of all pregnant women, married women in the reproductive period and children through systematic home visits and at clinics.

2. Maintenance of maternity records, register of antenatal cases, eligible couples register and children register.
3. Categorize the eligible couples according to the number of children and age of mothers.

Care at Home

During home visits, she will:
1. Provide care to pregnant women especially, registered mothers, throughout the period of pregnancy.
2. Give advice on nutrition to expectant and nursing mothers.
3. Distribute iron and folic acid tablets to pregnant and nursing mothers, children and family planning adopters and vitamin A solution to children.
4. Immunize pregnant mothers with tetanus toxoid.
5. Refer women with abnormal pregnancies and medical or gynecological problems.
6. Conduct about 50% of total deliveries.
7. Supervise deliveries conducted by TBAs whenever called in.
8. Refer cases of difficult labor and newborns with abnormalities and help them to get institutional care and provide follow-up care to patients referred to or discharged from the hospital.
9. Provide at least three postdelivery visits for each delivery case and render advice regarding feeding of the newborn as well as diet and hygiene.
10. Spread the message of family planning to the couples; motivate them for family planning individually and in groups.
11. Distribute conventional contraceptives to the couples, provide facilities and help to prospective adopters in getting family planning services, if necessary by accompanying them or arranging TBA (dai) to accompany them to hospital.
12. Provide follow-up services to family planning adopters, identify those who develop side effects and minor complaints and refer those cases that need attention by physicians, to the PHC/hospital.
13. Assess the growth and development of the infant and take necessary action.
14. Administer diphtheria, tetanus and pertussis (DPT), polio, Bacille Calmette-Guérin (BCG) and measles vaccination to all the infants in her area, where facilities for these are available.
15. Provide treatments for minor ailments, first aid in case of emergencies and refer cases beyond her competence to PHC or nearest hospital.
16. Notify all the notifiable diseases, which she comes across during her visits.
17. Record and report all the births and deaths occurring in her area to the local birth and death registrar and to her supervisor.
18. Test urine for albumin and glucose during her home visits.
19. Identify clients who require help for medical termination of pregnancy, provide information on the availability of services and refer them to the nearest approved institution.
20. Provide health education on all health matters and healthful living.

At the Health Center

1. Arrange and help the Medical Officer and the female health assistant in conducting MCH and family planning (FP) clinics at the subcenters.
2. Conduct urine examination and estimate hemoglobin percentage.
3. Educate mothers individually and in groups in better family health including MCH and FP, nutrition, immunization, hygiene and minor ailments.

In the Community

1. Identify women leaders, help the female health assistant and participate in the training of women leaders.
2. Set up women depot-holders for condom distribution and help the health assistant in training them.
3. Participate in Mahila Mandal meetings and utilize such gatherings for educating women in family welfare programs.
4. Utilize satisfied customers, village leaders, dais and others for promoting family welfare program.

Other Responsibilities

1. Maintain the cleanliness of the centers.
2. Attend staff meetings at PHC and community development block.
3. List dais in her area and involve them in promoting family welfare work.
4. Help the female health assistant in the training program for dais.
5. Coordinate activities with health workers particularly male health workers.
6. Prepare and maintain all registers, records, maps and charts for her area in the subcenters and submit the prescribed periodical reports in time to the health assistants as per standing orders and instructions (Park, 2001).

Female Health Assistant

The female health assistant will:
1. Carry out supervisory house visiting.
2. Guide the FHW in establishing women depot holders for distribution of conventional contraceptives.
3. Conduct MCH and family planning clinics, and carry out educational activities.
4. Organize and conduct training for dais and women leaders with the help of women health workers.
5. Visit each of the four subcenters at least once a week.

6. Respond to urgent calls from the health workers and trained dais and render necessary help.
7. Organize and utilize Mahila Mandals (women's groups), teachers, etc. in the family welfare programs.
8. Personally, motivate resistant cases for family planning.
9. Provide information on availability of services for medical termination of pregnancy and refer suitable cases to the approved institutions.
10. Supervise the immunization of all pregnant women and children 0–5 years.

Selection of ASHA

For job functions of Accredited Social Health Activist, *refer* Chapter 60, Page 596.

STUDY QUESTIONS

Short Notes

1. Primary level health care.
2. Tertiary level health care.
3. Objectives of maternal and child health (MCH) services.
4. Rooming-in practice.

Short Answer Questions

1. Objectives of antenatal care in MCH service.
2. Risk approach in MCH service.
3. Breastfeeding policies.
4. Immediate care of newborn.
5. Apgar scoring.

Essay Questions

1. Describe the advantages and disadvantages of domiciliary midwifery. Explain how you will prepare a prenatal client for home delivery.
2. Describe the initial and second examinations of a neonate.
3. Enumerate the recent trends in MCH care.

BIBLIOGRAPHY

1. Ministry of Health and Family Welfare. Manual for orientation for Auxiliary Nurse Midwives and Supervisors, Reproductive and Child Health Approach. New Delhi; August 1996.
2. National Institute of Health and Family Welfare, Reproductive and Child health, Module for Staff Nurses' (PHC/CHC), Integrated skill Development Training, NIHEW Munirka. New Delhi; July 2001.
3. Park K. Park's Textbook of Preventive and Social Medicine, 16th edition. Jabalpur: M/s Banarsidas Bhanot Publishers; 2000.
4. Park K. Park's Textbook of Preventive and Social Medicine, 21st edition. Jabalpur: M/s Banarsidas Bhanot Publishers; 2011.
5. WHO/UNICEF. Report of joint committee of health policy. Geneva: World Health Organization; 1987.
6. World Health Organization Chronicle 32, 33. Geneva: World Health Organization; 1977.
7. World Health Organization. Report of training courses on organization of MCH field practice programmes. SEA/MCH, New Delhi; 1969.

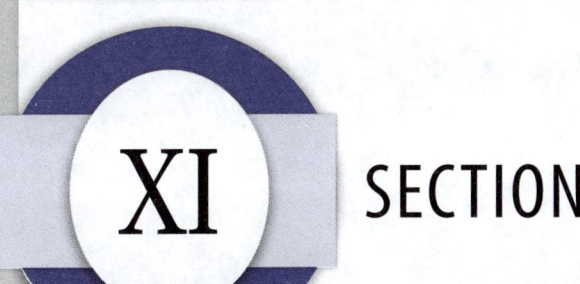

SPECIAL TOPICS

Section Outline

52. Pain Relief and Comfort in Labor
53. Childbirth Education and Preparation
54. Special Exercises for Pregnancy, Labor and Puerperium
55. Drugs Used in Obstetrics
56. Vital Statistics in Obstetrics
57. Perinatal Loss and Grief
58. Radiology and Ultrasonics in Obstetrics
59. Legal and Ethical Aspects of Nursing
60. National Population Policy and Family Welfare Programs
61. Obstetric and Gynecological Instruments
62. Quality Assurance and Audit in Maternity Nursing

CHAPTER 52

Pain Relief and Comfort in Labor

Learning Objectives

Upon completing this chapter, the learner will be able to:
- Identify the factors affecting perception of pain and individual reactions to it.
- Identify the causes of pain during labor and delivery.
- Discuss the effects of various pain relief methods on the well-being of the fetus.
- Describe the advantages and disadvantages of the various methods of analgesia and anesthesia for use during labor and delivery.
- Identify the nonpharmaceutical methods of pain relief that are effective for laboring women.

Most women expect and experience pain in labor and childbirth. Pain is a subjective experience and it is whatever the woman says it is for her. Labor pain is often described as the most intense ever experienced and in many cases, it is the aspect of childbirth most feared by the expectant mother. Physical, psychological and cultural factors play an important role in the woman's response to childbirth, although the intensity of pain experienced varies a great deal from one woman to another.

Pain is managed in various ways according to the following indicators; the frequency, duration and intensity of uterine contractions; the character of labor, the woman's emotional behavior, her response to pain; the dilatation of cervix, the condition of mother and fetus, the skill, attitude and experience of healthcare team, and the preferences of the woman and her family. Pain relief ranges from none or very mild sedation to regional anesthesia to heavy sedation and/or anesthetic medication. When considering any form of analgesia or anesthesia, the safety of the mother and fetus are paramount. Pain relief in labor presents unique problems. Sedatives and anesthesia cross the placenta and can cause respiratory distress in the fetus. Unlike its use in surgery, which is brief, obstetrical analgesia may be needed for as long as 12 hours. In addition, since labor begins without warning, the woman invariably has not had sufficient time to empty her gastric contents, leading to the threat of aspiration of vomitus. Therefore, the risks versus benefits of pain relief in labor must be carefully weighed prior to its administration. 'Comfort' in labor is not merely an emotional or physical relieving of malaise and pain. It is a complex process in which the midwife combines research-based knowledge and skills, with warmth, empathy and sensitivity in order to provide a birth environment, which is safe, caring and conducive to a satisfying birth experience.

PERCEPTION OF PAIN

The way in which an individual perceives and reacts to pain is affected by many different factors.
- *Fear and anxiety:* This will heighten the individual's response to pain. Fear of the unknown, fear of being left alone to cope with an experience such as labor and fear of failing to cope well will increase anxiety. A previous bad experience will also increase anxiety.
- *Personality:* The woman who is naturally tense and anxious will cope less well with stress than one who is relaxed and confident.
- *Fatigue:* The woman who is already fatigued by several hours of labor, perhaps preceded by a period when sleep was disturbed by the discomforts of late pregnancy, will be less able to tolerate pain.
- *Cultural and social factors:* Some cultures expect fortitude in suffering, while others encourage expression of feeling. The perception of pain may be altered if the woman has experienced pain and hardship previously.
- *Expectations:* The woman who is realistic in her expectations of labor and about her likely response to it is probably the best equipped, as long as she feels confident that she will receive the help and support she needs, and is assured that she will receive appropriate analgesia.

CAUSES OF PAIN

During the first stage of labor, pain occurs due to dilatation of the cervix, hypoxia of the uterine cells during contractions, stretching of the lower uterine segment and pressure on adjacent structures. Initially contractions are felt in the lower back and then progress to the lower torso in the back and abdomen.

In the second stage of labor, pain is due to hypoxia of the contracting uterine muscle cells, distension of the vagina and perineum, and pressure on adjacent structures.

During delivery, there is often a decrease in pain, although many women describe the sensations of stretching, splitting or burning. Most third-stage pain results from contractions and cervical dilatation as the placenta is expelled. After the third stage, anesthesia is needed primarily for episiotomy repair.

ANALGESICS

In the recent years, with the family involvement in childbearing, the use of anesthesia and analgesia has diminished to some extent. Approaches to labor and delivery have been shifting from 'always medicate' to 'rarely medicate' in the western world. The practice of obstetrics now takes a middle of the road approach and the value of anesthesia and analgesia is in the process of re-evaluation.

Analgesics and their Fetal/Maternal Side Effects

When cervical dilatation and uterine contractions cause discomfort, a narcotic such as Demerol (meperidine) and a tranquilizer such as promethazine, usually are indicated. Administration is either by intramuscular (IM) or intravenous (IV) route. The advantage of the IM or subcutaneous injection is that this is the fastest route in regard to midwife time and observation. The disadvantages include the length of time it takes for the drug to cause relief of pain, the danger of the drug's crossing the placental barrier and affecting the fetus, and unequal absorption of the drug. The advantage of the IV route is prompt pain relief with predicable results and that small amounts can be given in equally divided doses. The disadvantage of IV administration is the possibility of a bolus, but if given in the correct manner this is not of concern.

Commonly Used Narcotic Analgesics

- *Meperidine hydrochloride (Demerol):* It is typically administered IV in 12.5–25 mg doses (with 50 mg maximum) and IM in 75 mg doses (with 100 mg maximum). Pain relief usually occurs within 10 minutes after IV administration. Maternal side effects include central nervous system depression, especially respiratory, nausea, vomiting and/or dry mouth, drowsiness, dizziness, flushing, transient hypotension, tachycardia, palpitation and convulsions. Fetal/newborn side effects include neonatal hypotonia and lethargy, interference of thermoregulatory response for up to 72 hours after delivery, neonatal respiratory depression, neurologic and behavioral alterations for up to 72 hours postdelivery and depressed attention and social responsiveness for the first 6 weeks of life.
- *Meptazinol:* It has similar analgesic and sedative property as that of pethidine. It causes less respiratory depression of the newborn.
- *Pentazocine (Fortwin):* It is given intramuscularly in a dose of 30–40 mg. Its duration of action is shorter and causes some respiratory depression. It also causes some drug dependence.
- *Butorphanol (Stadol):* It is a synthetic narcotic agonist-antagonist analgesic. The typical dose is 2 mg IM every 3–4 hours. When given IV, lower doses are used. Its effects compare favorably to 40–60 mg of pethidine. Since it can cause respiratory depression, it is contraindicated in women with respiratory disease. Other side effects include sedation, nausea, dizziness, a clammy, sweaty sensation and a tendency to elevate cerebrospinal fluid pressure. Fetal side effects can include respiratory depression in the fetus. It must be used with great caution if premature delivery is expected. Nubain and Stadol must be used with extreme caution in women who are addicted to drugs, since narcotic antagonists can induce acute withdrawal symptoms in mother and fetus if the mother is addicted to heroin.

Patient-controlled Analgesia

Narcotics can be administered by the mother herself from a pump at an intermittent demand rate through intravenous route. This offers better pain control than high doses given at long intervals by the midwife. Client satisfaction is high with this method. Drugs commonly used are Demerol (meperidine) and fentanyl.

Assessment and Intervention

Nursing intervention in pain relief should start with nonpharmaceutical methods, which will be discussed later in this chapter. For some women however, those methods will not bring adequate relief and increasing discomfort will interfere with their ability to perform breathing techniques and maintain a sense of control.

Under these circumstances, pharmacological analgesics may be used to decrease discomfort, increase the woman's ability to relax, and reestablish her sense of control. However, since analgesics will affect the mother, the fetus and the contraction pattern, the midwife must first assess the woman's vital signs to determine that they are stable and must establish that the woman is willing to receive analgesia after being advised about its effects. She should understand the type of medication being administered, its route of administration, its expected effects, its implications for the fetus/neonate and the safety measures required for its use. The fetus must also be assessed to determine that the fetal heart rate (FHR) is between 120 and 160 beats per minute with no late or variable decelerations present; normal accelerations are present with fetal movement, the fetus is at term and there is no meconium staining.

Labor assessment includes a well-established contraction pattern, cervical dilation of 4-5 cm in nulliparas and 3-4 cm in multiparas, engagement of the fetal presenting part and progressive descend of the fetal presenting part with no complications existing.

When administering analgesic drugs, careful and continuous observation of maternal respirations and FHR are mandatory with baseline FHR and maternal vital signs recorded on the monitor strip (if on continuous monitoring) both before and after administration. The physician's written order is checked and the drug is prepared and signed out on the narcotic sheet. The woman's arm band is checked/the woman correctly identified and she is again asked if she is allergic to any drug. The drug is administered by the route ordered and the medication, time, dosage and site of administration are charted on the nurse's notes. Safety precautions include side rails and continuous observation for nausea and vomiting to prevent aspiration. While receiving analgesia, the woman should preferably be in an individual birthing or labor room, with the environment free from sensory stimuli. She should be encouraged to empty her bladder before drug administration and she should not be left alone.

ANESTHESIA

Regional Anesthesia

Regional anesthesia is the injection of local anesthetic agents that block the transmission of painful stimuli from the uterus, cervix, vagina and perineum to the thalamic pain centers in the brain. The methods most often used in labor are the pudendal block, the paracervical block, the peridural (lumbar, epidural and caudal) block, subarachnoid or saddle block (spinal for cesarean birth, low spinal for vaginal delivery) and local infiltration. These blocks are accomplished by means of a single injection or continuously by means of an indwelling plastic catheter. Paracervical and peridural blocks are used in the first stage of labor. During the second stage pudendal, peridural or subarachnoid blocks are used.

Pudendal Block

Pudendal block consists of a local anesthetic agent injected around the pudendal nerve, which causes perineal analgesia. Used late in second stage, just before spontaneous or low forceps delivery of the infant, it provides anesthesia for birth and for repair of the episiotomies. It does not alter maternal or fetal respirations or other body functions, and does not affect uterine contractions. However, it may affect the woman's bearing down reflex and may cause broad ligament hematoma.

Paracervical Block

Paracervical block is accomplished by injecting a local anesthetic transvaginally, adjacent to the outer rim of the cervix. It may be administered during the active phase of labor, achieving rapid and complete relief of uterine pain during cervical dilatation. It does not anesthetize the lower vagina or the perineum and it does not interfere with the bearing-down reflex. However, it has several maternal disadvantages including systemic toxic reaction and uterine vessel damage leading to severe hematoma. Fetal risks include bradycardia, acidosis and death. Because of these risks, electronic fetal monitoring is indicated. Paracervical blocks are used infrequently.

Peridural (Epidural) Anesthesia

Peridural (epidural) anesthesia, which can be used during the first or second stages of labor, consists of injecting an anesthetic agent into the extradural space. It does not penetrate the dura or the spinal cord, and may be administered into the caudal space within the sacrum or into the epidural space at the second, third or fourth lumbar interspace. It may be given by a single injection or by continuous injection over several hours. A small amount relieves the discomfort of uterine contractions, while a larger dose extends anesthesia to the vagina. An additional dose may be given to provide perineal anesthesia.

Its advantages are that it can be given during active labor, providing effective pain relief during uterine contractions and cervical dilatation. It also enhances the woman's rest, relaxation and ability to cope. However, it has several disadvantages; if given too early, it may slow labor and may result in maternal hypotension and decrease in placental blood flow. The second stage of labor may be lengthened, since the mother does not feel the bearing down sensation, thus possibly requiring a forceps delivery. It may interfere with the woman's ability to void and it may cause infection. In addition, the dura mater may be punctured, resulting in inadvertent spinal anesthesia. Epidural anesthesia is contraindicated when maternal hemorrhage is present or likely to occur, in the presence of local infection at the injection site and when the woman has cardiac, pulmonary or central nervous system disease.

Spinal Anesthesia (Subarachnoid)

Spinal anesthesia (subarachnoid) involves the injection of a local anesthetic directly into the spinal fluid, providing anesthesia for vaginal or cesarean delivery. For vaginal delivery, it is given late in the second stage, when the fetal head is on the perineum. It has no effect on maternal or fetal respirations, but may cause temporary hypotension and a postspinal maternal headache. A spinal block eliminates the bearing-down reflex, but proper patient preparation will usually allow for spontaneous delivery. If not, forceps are easily applied due to perineal relaxation. Its advantages are simplicity, rapidity of action, high success rate and a low incidence of maternal and fetal side effects.

Contraindications: Include severe hypovolemia, central nervous system disease, infection at the puncture site, severe hypotension or hypertension, cephalopelvic disproportion and fear of the procedure.

Actions Specific to Blocks

1. *Paracervical:* Assess maternal blood pressure, pulse and FHR, assure continuous FHR tracing, assess maternal bladder.
2. *Epidural:* Initially assess maternal blood pressure and pulse, and the FHR for baseline. An electronic fetal monitor must be used for continual tracing. Maternal blood pressure and pulse are assessed every 2 minutes during the first 15 minutes after the injection and every 10–15 minutes until stable. Assess bladder at frequent intervals for distention after delivery. Delay ambulation until all motor control has returned. Assess for orthostatic hypotension.
3. *Spinal:* Assess maternal vital signs and FHR for baseline. Assist with positioning during administration. Assess for uterine contractions and inform anesthesiologist. Place a wedge under patient's right hip to tip the uterus off the vena cava. Assess maternal blood pressure and pulse every 2–5 minutes until stable and continue to monitor contractions. Provide safety and prevent injury when moving the patient. Provide bedrest for 6–12 hours following delivery.
4. *Pudendal:* Provide support and assess for development of hematoma.
5. *Local infiltration:* Provide support and assess for perineal trauma, such as swelling or bruising.

Advantages and Disadvantages of Regional Anesthesia

Regional anesthesia has become increasingly popular due to its compatibility with the goals of psychoprophylactic preparation for childbirth. Its many advantages include the following.

The area blocked is completely relieved from pain, depression of maternal vital signs is rare and aspiration of gastric contents is eliminated when no additional sedative is given, administration does not alter the course of labor and the woman remains alert and able to participate in the birth.

The *disadvantages* of regional anesthesia include the high degree of skill required for its administration, the possibility of failure to adequately block pain, the side effects of some agents and the possibility of systemic toxic reactions, which can range from mild symptoms to cardiovascular collapse. Mild reactions include palpitations, vertigo, tinnitus, apprehension, confusion, headache and a metallic taste in the mouth. Moderate reactions include more intense degree of the above mentioned mild symptoms plus nausea; vomiting hypotension and muscle twitching that can lead to convulsions and loss of consciousness, coma, severe hypotension, bradycardia, respiratory depression and cardiac arrest. Because of the possibility of adverse reactions, regional anesthetics should always be used with an intravenous line in place.

Nursing Considerations

Nursing considerations during the administration of regional anesthesia include the following:

1. Support for the laboring woman, encouraging her participation in decision-making.
2. Continuous monitoring of vital signs and fetal status.
3. Adequate knowledge of medications, their proper dosages, possible complications, early signs and symptoms of complications and actions to initiate in the event of untoward reaction until the arrival of appropriate medical personnel.

General Anesthesia

General anesthesia is inhalation anesthesia, which provides pain relief through the administration of a gaseous agent mixed with oxygen and inhaled until the client becomes unconscious. Its advantages are that it produces overall relaxation, which is useful in difficult forceps deliveries, breech and cesarean sections. The likelihood of convulsions in preeclamptic or eclamptic women is reduced when general anesthesia is administered and perhaps its greatest advantage is that it can be administered rapidly in emergencies when delivery must be immediate and pain relief is essential. However, its disadvantage is that delivery must occur within 5–7 minutes after administration, because inhalation anesthesia crosses the placenta quickly and can cause hypoxia and respiratory depression in the fetus. There is always risk of maternal aspiration of gastric contents, which can result in pulmonary complications and immediate postpartum recovery is more complicated due to the risks of nausea, vomiting, uterine atony and postpartum hemorrhage. With this type of anesthesia, the bearing-down reflex is stopped and the mother cannot participate in the birth nor can she interact with the baby immediately following birth.

General anesthesia is used today because of previous complications or high-risk problems due to pregnancy. Women, whose regional anesthesia is ineffective, those with pregnancy-induced hypertension, prolapsed cord; severe bleeding or fetal distress with a second twin may be candidates.

Contraindications for general anesthesia are fetal prematurity or distress, maternal upper respiratory infection, multiple births and if the woman who has eaten before administration.

The patient receiving general anesthesia requires preoxygenation, IV fluid loading and tracheal protection with cricoid pressure to prevent aspiration and a pelvic tilt for maximum uterine circulation to the fetus. The midwife attending the patient under general anesthesia must observe the FHR constantly, while monitoring maternal vital signs and checking for uterine bleeding. Although it may slow down uterine contractions, general anesthesia can also relax perineal musculature and cause rapid expulsion of the fetus for which the midwife must be alert.

Types of General Anesthesia

Nitrous oxide (Entonox): The anesthetic, which is 40% nitrous oxide and 60% oxygen is administered by facemask or inhaler. Its induction is fast and pleasant and it is nonirritating, nonexplosive, and less disruptive of physiological functions than any other general anesthetic. Its main use is in the second stage of labor as an induction agent or as a supplement to more potent general anesthesia.

Halothane (Fluothane): Not used as frequently as nitrous oxide, halothane nevertheless bears mention for obstetrical anesthesia. Its induction is rapid, predictable and safe, since it causes little or no nausea or vomiting. It provides moderate to good uterine relaxation, although it may cause respiratory depression as well as irritability of cardiac tissue, which can result in arrhythmia. It may also cause increased uterine contraction along with the risk of postpartum hemorrhage.

Methoxyflurane (Penthrane): Administered by inhaler for analgesia or in combination with other agents for anesthesia, methoxyflurane induction is pleasant, but slower than with gas agents. Uterine contraction may result from its use and administration is restricted to low doses for short periods, because of the risk of postpartum bleeding.

Thiopental sodium (Pentothal): This ultrashort-acting barbiturate is given intravenously and it produces narcosis within 30 seconds. Induction and emergence are smooth and pleasant, with little nausea or vomiting. It is most frequently used for induction or as an adjuvant to more potent anesthetics.

Recovery

The recovery period from general anesthesia requires particular vigilance from the midwife. If the woman is conscious, her physiological and psychological well-being demands that she be with her baby and significant other. At the same time, the midwife must monitor temperature, blood pressure, pulse and respiration, while watching for bleeding, checking uterine tone and observing bladder filling. Vital signs and observations of the uterus, bladder and episiotomies or abdominal incision must be recorded every 15 minutes. The recovery period is generally of 2 hours.

Balanced Anesthesia

Today's trend is toward 'balanced anesthesia' for both vaginal and cesarean births. This is achieved by giving several different agents by different routes, which increases effectiveness and safety. Because of the combined effect, smaller doses can be given of each agent than if given separately. For example, IV thiopental sodium may be given for sedation and induction, followed by halothane by facemask for analgesia and anesthesia.

NONPHARMACEUTICAL METHODS OF PAIN RELIEF

Gate Control Theory

According to the gate control theory, pain is the result of interactions between several specialized neural systems. This theory postulates that a mechanism in the dorsal horn of the spinal column serves as a valve (or gate) that can increase or decrease the flow of nerve impulses from the periphery to the central nervous system. The gate mechanism is influenced by the size of the fibers that transmit impulses and by the impulses that descend from the brain. Pain perception and response may activate the gate system and influence psychological processes including experiences, attention and emotion. Therefore, according to the theory, the gates can either be opened or closed by central nervous system activities such as anxiety, excitement or through selective localized activity.

The gate control theory as it applies to obstetrics has vast implications. It suggests that pain can be controlled by tactile stimulation and can be modified by activities controlled by the central nervous system. These include back rub, sacral pressure, suggestion, distraction and conditioning. Abdominal effleurage, a specific type of cutaneous stimulation is used before the transitional phase of labor. It consists of light abdominal stroking. It is used in the Lamaze method of childbirth preparation. It is particularly effective in relieving mild-to-moderate pain, but is ineffectual for intense pain. The application of deep pressure over the sacrum is more effective for relieving back pain.

Other nonpharmaceutical methods of pain relief include acupuncture, acupressure, therapeutic touch, transcutaneous electrical nerve stimulation (TENS), bathing or showering, warmth and positioning.

Acupuncture

Acupuncture has been widely used in the Orient for many years and there is increasing evidence that it may be an effective tool during labor. In some cultures, women have pressed combs into the palms of their hands to reduce the pain of contractions. Similarly, acupuncture involves the insertion and rotation of needles on specific points of the body, which is thought to produce analgesia and sedation through the release of β-endorphin. However, acupuncture is an invasive technique that may cause infection.

Acupressure

Acupressure is also used in the Orient and is thought to activate the release of endorphins in the body. It is defined as finger pressure or massage over 'pain prevention (or acupressure) points' and is another form of touch therapy. Proponents of the gate control theory speculate that the acupressure's pain relieving qualities are based on blocking the gate at the level of the spinal cord.

This technique is now taught in many childbirth education classes in the developed countries.

Acupressure may be used to alleviate some of the common discomforts of pregnancy such as dizziness, faintness, headache or sciatic nerve pain and leg cramps. In labor, acupressure is used as a part of pain control routine that includes relaxation, concentration and rhythmic breathing.

Contraindications to this technique include any site where there is red, swollen, broken or infected skin and selected points that should not be used during pregnancy, because of the potential to induce labor.

Yoga and Meditation

Yoga and meditation are claimed to have calming effect, assist the mother in becoming attuned to her body and give a focus for distraction from pain and tension.

Therapeutic Touch

Throughout history, people have used touch (the ancient art of laying on of hands) as a means of calming a person. Now, according to researchers, there is evidence of an actual transfer of energy taking place in some forms of touching, as evidenced in muscular relaxation. Therapeutic touch offers several advantages. No devices are required, no physician's order is needed, the technique is non-invasive and it incurs no cost since the technique is incorporated into nursing care. Indeed, there has been extensive research by nurses into the background and application of therapeutic touch, which was originally described by a nurse—Dolores Krieger. The technique has no religious base and requires only the conscious intent of the healer.

Therapeutic touch may offer a powerful means of enhancing relaxation, reducing anxiety and controlling pain. It can be of help to couples to increase their communication and alleviate the discomforts of pregnancy. During labor and birth, it is used along with breathing and other relaxation strategies; and in the early months of parenting, it is frequently used as a means of calming a crying baby, relaxing a distraught parent or helping a woman through 'postpartum blues'. Therapeutic touch can benefit not only the client but also the healer through enhancing her sense of inner harmony, well-being and relaxation, enabling her to cope, while healing. Touch is a means of making coping skills more powerful and effective.

Transcutaneous Electrical Nerve Stimulation

Transcutaneous electrical nerve stimulation method of alleviating pain by electrical nerve stimulation generally requires the services of a physiologist or other professional. Although TENS is widely used outside obstetrics, its use in labor is questionable. It may interfere with continuous electronic fetal monitoring, since it must be applied constantly to gain relief. Moreover, it is most effective only if introduced before crisis.

Bathing, Showering, and Warmth

During the early stage of labor, bathing or showering may afford a measure of pain relief for the woman. No physician's order is needed for showering. Whichever method is employed, the midwife should remain in close attendance to avoid the possibility of accidents and hyperthermia. The midwife must also be alert to the mother's need for bodily warmth in cold climates and should provide blankets as needed or keep the room temperature at a comfortable level as appropriate.

POSITIONING

The midwife should encourage the laboring woman to assume whatever position she finds most comfortable. However, any position used during labor and delivery should facilitate the alignment of the presenting part to the axis of the pelvis, and should encourage the mother's effort toward accomplishing delivery.

Women may require help to find positions, which are comfortable for them. Leaning forward with the arms resting on a convenient windowsill, table or shelf during a contraction may help the woman cope with backache. A rocking chair provides a soothing, rhythmic distraction during contractions, the motion probably encourages release of endogenous opioids and most rocking chairs give good support to the back. A reclining chair also gives good support, but a recumbent position should be avoided because of the risk of aortocaval occlusion. Birthing beds and chairs are designed specifically for women in labor and most are very versatile. Ideally, they are used for delivery only and the woman is encouraged to walk about and use alternative positions during the first stage of labor.

An alternative position may be described as any position other than recumbent, semi-recumbent or sitting on the bed; the woman follows her natural instincts and finds a position and movements, such as pelvic rocking, which feel right for her, making use of gravity to assist descend of the presenting part. An upright or kneeling position also allows maximum 'give' of the pelvic girdle, whereas sitting causes pressure over the sacrum and coccyx. Any woman in normal labor may benefit from freedom of mobility.

During delivery, the upright position was considered normal in most societies until recent times and only within the past two centuries has the recumbent (lithotomy) position been used, mainly for the convenience of the physician or midwife. Now some countries have accepted alternative positions based on the comfort of the laboring woman. These include sitting in a birthing chair, semi-Fowler's position and left lateral Sims' position, squatting and sitting in a birthing bed.

In active birth, the woman participates fully in her labor, is very aware of all that is going on in her body and aims to respond to these events naturally. She will have to prepare herself during her pregnancy by exercising. She will not wish to have any form of medical intervention if this can be avoided.

HYGIENE AND COMFORT

The woman in labor will become very hot and will perspire profusely. If she is able, she will prefer a bath or shower. If the woman is not able to get up, she will appreciate frequent sponging, particularly of her face and neck with cold water. A clean, cool gown will be appreciated and a fan is comforting. Her mouth will feel much fresher if she can clean her mouth or have a mouthwash.

Care of the bladder and bowels is an important aspect of the mother's comfort. In helping the laboring woman to achieve pain relief, the midwife should focus on the body's natural resources and should emphasize supportive pain management techniques for labor and childbirth. The midwife must respect the woman's right to her feelings about pain medication and other aspects of labor and delivery. She must attempt to convey a realistic picture of the childbirth pain experience, assist the woman in her efforts to manage pain and bolster her confidence, so that she can cope with the experience of childbirth.

STUDY QUESTIONS

Short Notes
1. Pudendal block anesthesia.
2. Paracervical block anesthesia.

Short Answer Questions
1. Factors that affect pain perception.
2. Epidural anesthesia in labor.

Essay Question
1. Describe the nursing management of a client in labor, who is receiving regional anesthetic.

BIBLIOGRAPHY

1. Bevis R. Pain relief and comfort in labor. In: Bennett RV, Linda KB (Eds). Myles textbook for midwives, 13th edition. Edinburgh: Churchill Livingstone; 1999. pp. 429-40.
2. Cunningham FG, MacDonald PC. Grant NF. Williams Obstetrics, 18th edition. London: Prentice Hall International; 1989.
3. Fairs PJ. Relieving pain and discomfort in labor. The role of the midwife. Nursing Times. 1966;62(18):599-600.
4. Field Peggy A. Relief of pain in labor. Canadian Nurse. 1974;70(12):17-23.
5. Karpen M, Conrad L, Chitwood L, et al. Essentials of maternal-child nursing, 2nd edition. Western Schools Press; 1995. pp. 99-110.
6. Kemp S. The dignity of labor. Nursing Times. 1970;66(45):1436.
7. Ladewig PW, London ML, Olds SB. Essentials of maternal-newborn nursing, 1st edition. New York: Addison-Wesley; 1990.
8. Martin E. Intrapartum management modules. Baltimore: Williams & Wilkins; 1990.
9. Moore S. Physiology of pain. In: Moore S (Ed). Understanding pain and its relief in labor. Edinburgh: Churchill Livingstone; 1997.
10. Neeson JD. Clinical manual of maternity nursing. Philadelphia: JB Lippincott; 1987.
11. Page L. Putting principles into practice. In: Page L (Ed). Effective Group Practice in Midwifery. Oxford: Blackwell Science; 1995.
12. Schott J, Henley A. Culture, religion and childbearing in a multiracial society. Oxford: Butterworth-Heinemann;1999.
13. Simkin P. Stress, pain and catecholamines in labor: Part 2. Stress associated with childbirth events: a pilot survey of new mothers. Birth. 1986;13(4):234-40.
14. Thornton JA. The relief of pain in labor. Nursing Times. 1961;16:1128-30.

CHAPTER 53

Childbirth Education and Preparation

> **Learning Objectives**
>
> Upon completing this chapter, the learner will be able to:
> * State the goals of childbirth education and preparation.
> * Describe the different philosophical approaches to childbirth education.
> * Identify the role of the 'coach' or support person.
> * Specify the responsibilities of the childbirth educator (midwife) in providing effective prenatal and parenting education.

Childbirth is one of the greatest events in every woman's life. Having had fantasies about pregnancy and motherhood, when confronted with the reality, many of them have doubt in their ability to cope with this great event in their lives. Influenced by family, friends and relatives, they get prepared in different ways as they approach the experience of childbirth. This preparation may be positive or negative, realistic or inaccurate.

At this time, the mother needs a lot of help for the realization and acceptance of childbirth as a normal physiological phenomenon. She needs to develop a healthy attitude toward pregnancy so that she might have a safe and emotionally satisfying experience of labor and a rapid recovery both mentally and physically in the puerperium. Realization of this need by the obstetricians led to the development of psychosomatic methods of preparation for childbirth.

NATURAL CHILDBIRTH APPROACH

The natural childbirth movement was originated by Dr Grantly Dick-Read. He developed the method in 1933 in England. The basis of the program was the realization that childbirth was a normal physiological occurrence and as such should not be painful. He believed that the pain of labor and delivery was mental in origin. He attributed the cause of pain to culturally induced fear and anxiety. "The belief was that fear of labor and delivery was a learned response and fear created tension, which was responsible for the pain that occurred".

The physical exercise component of the Read's method was largely due to the work of Helen Heardman, a physiotherapist in England, who strongly supported Read's contentions. She believed in the necessity of a healthy positive mental attitude in the prospective mother. She advocated a vigorous program of physical education in preparation for parturition. Thus, through the combined efforts of Grantly Dick-Read and Helen Heardman—education, psychological training and physical exercise to enhance relaxation comprised the original natural childbirth program.

CHILDBIRTH PREPARATION PROGRAM

Childbirth education classes were developed for meeting women's pain-reduction needs during labor and delivery. Early contributors, such as Grantly Dick-Read and Lamaze, formed the basis of today's childbirth education classes, which in addition to pain management is designed to help women cope with childbirth through active participation and increased decision-making. Childbirth education emphasizes making childbirth a more rewarding experience for the mother, her mate and her entire family.

Goals of Educational Programs

Antepartal education programs vary in content, leadership techniques and teaching methods. The ideal childbirth education program should help the woman/couple to cooperate through the 'problem' of labor in a satisfactory manner to both. It should provide them with coping skills and impetus to practice what they have learned and it should encourage mutual participation. As the couple works toward assuming an active and independent role in the childbirth experience, they will learn to become more flexible and their potential for working together in future situations will be enhanced. Therefore, the objectives of childbirth education should include the following:

- Providing a supportive milieu
- Reducing anxiety
- Providing factual information
- Maintaining a focus on current concerns.

Methods of Childbirth Preparation

Read Method

Read method is a method of psychophysical preparation for childbirth designed by Grantly Dick-Read. It was the 'natural childbirth' program, a term coined by Read. Read held the view that childbirth is a normal, physiologic process and that the pain of labor and delivery is of psychogenic origin; the fear-tension-pain syndrome (fear causes tension, which in turn causes pain). He countered women's fears with education about the physiologic process, encouraged a positive, welcoming attitude, corrected false information and led tours of the hospital before birth. In order to decrease tension, he developed a series of breathing exercises for use during the various stages of labor. To foster relaxation and optimal physical function in labor, and in recovery after delivery, he incorporated a series of physical exercises to be performed regularly in classes, and to practice at home during pregnancy. The woman is helped to manage labor and delivery using the Read method in the following ways.

- *During the early and mid-first stage of labor:* Before cervical dilatation has reached 7 cm, contractions are 2–5 minutes apart and last for 30–40 seconds, the mother lies on her back with the knees bent. Abdominal breathing is used during contractions. Her hands are placed over her lower abdomen, fingers touching. She breaths slowly and deeply—in through the nose and out through the mouth. The abdominal wall rises with each inhalation, which she can feel with her hands. The rate of breathing is no more than 6 breaths in 30 seconds or 12–18 in one contraction.
- *During the late part of the first stage of labor:* After 7 cm of cervical dilatation, the contractions are 1½–2 minutes apart and last for 40–60 seconds. Costal or diaphragmatic breathing is used during contractions. Her hands are placed on her sides over the ribs. She breaths in more shallowly feeling her ribs move sideways against the hands. Each breath is drawn in through her nose and exhaled through the mouth. The abdominal wall does not rise and fall with this kind of breathing. The rate of breathing is no more than 6 breaths in 30 seconds or 12–18 in one contraction.
- *At the end of the first stage of labor:* Near full dilatation, contractions may be very strong occurring every 1½–2 minutes and lasting 60–90 seconds. The mother lies on her back with her knees bent. Panting respirations are used during contractions. The mother holds one of her hands on the sternum, which rises and falls as she pants lightly and rapidly through her mouth. Panting continues through the end of the first stage to full dilatation as the urge to push grows. Panting helps the woman to avoid pushing.
- *During the second expulsive stage of labor:* After full dilatation of the cervix, the contractions occur every 1½–2 minutes, last for 60–90 seconds and are accompanied with an urge to bear down and push. The woman lies back with head and shoulders supported in a semisitting position. She is helped to draw the legs up, holding them with her hands behind the lower thighs, thighs on her abdomen and legs apart.
- *As each contraction begins:* She raises her head, takes a deep breath, tucks her chin on her chest, blocks the escape of air from her lungs and bears down. During each contraction, she may need to blow the air out, refill her lungs and push again two or three times.
- *Throughout labor:* The woman is helped to understand what is occurring to participate and accept the experience in anticipation of the birth of the baby. Currently, many authorities that advocate the use of other aspects of the Read method strongly recommend that a woman in labor not lie on her back. Supine hypotension is frequently the result of this position, because the uterus can fall back occluding the vena cava and decreasing the volume of blood returned to the heart, thus reducing the volume of cardiac output. Maternal hypotension follows, resulting in decreased placental perfusion and an inadequate supply of oxygen to the fetus. Today, the woman using the Read method spends much of her labor lying on her side or in a semisitting position with her knees, back and head well-supported.

Lamaze Method (Psychoprophylaxis)

A method of psychophysical preparation for childbirth was developed in the 1950s by a French obstetrician, Fernand Lamaze. It uses Pavlov's stimulus-response theory to decondition women in labor. His method of 'painless childbirth' became popular in the 1960s and now it is one of the most frequently used methods of childbirth education in several countries. The classes consist of two components:

1. Education to dispel fears, coupled with training to achieve relaxation of body musculature.
2. Conditioning for labor, which is achieved through the development of consciously controlled activities displace the pain sensations of contractions in the brain. Relaxation is achieved by means of breathing techniques for each stage of labor and by massage, and counter pressure. Positioning is used as a means to assist in increasing maternal comfort and exercises to strengthen pelvic musculature are taught.

It requires classes, practice at home and coaching during labor and delivery, often by a trained coach called 'monitrice'. The classes given during pregnancy teach the:

- Physiology of pregnancy and childbirth
- Exercises to develop strength in the abdominal muscles and control of isolated muscles of the vagina and perineum
- Techniques of breathing and relaxation to promote control and relaxation during labor.

The woman is conditioned by repetition and practice to dissociate herself from the source of a stimulus by concentration on a focal point, by consciously relaxing all muscles and by breathing in a special manner at a particular rate, thereby training herself not to pay attention to the stimuli associated with labor.

Kind and Rate of Breathing Change with Advancing Stages of Labor

- *During the early part of the first stage of labor:* When the cervix is dilated less than 5 cm and the contractions occur every 2–4 minutes lasting 40–60 seconds and are of mild to moderate strength, the mother does slow chest breathing during contractions. The abdominal wall does not move with respiration. She may perform an effleurage or rhythmic fingertip massage of her lower abdomen during the contractions. The rate of respiration is 10 or fewer breaths per minute increasing to 12 per minute as labor intensifies. A deep cleansing breath is taken before and after each contraction.

- *During the active part of the first stage of labor:* The transition occurs up to the second stage, the cervical dilatation is from 5 cm to nearly full dilation, the interval between contractions is 2–3 minutes and the duration of contraction is from 45 to 90 seconds. During this phase, the mother breathes quietly and slowly in her chest. The rate of her breathing varies with the strength of the contractions, increasing during a contraction to as fast as once a second at the peak slowing to once every 6 seconds as the uterus relaxes. She is coached to concentrate on the focal point and has selected to perform the effleurage of her abdomen to relax her perineal and vaginal muscles and to take a cleansing breath at the beginning and end of each contraction.

- *At the end of the first stage of labor:* When the cervix is almost completely dilated and the contractions are strong, occurring every 1½–2 minutes and lasting 60–90 seconds, the mother begins to feel the urge to bear down and push during contractions. She avoids pushing before full dilatation by combining several light, shallow breaths in the chest with short puffing exhalations as the urge increases during contractions.

- *During the second stage of labor:* The cervix is fully dilated and contractions are strong, frequent and expulsive. The mother's head and shoulders are supported on pillows. During contractions, she is helped to draw her legs back flexing the thighs against the abdomen, holding them behind the lower thigh with her hands. Her chin is tucked on her chest, the air is blocked from escaping from her lungs, her perineum is relaxed and she bears down forcibly.

Depending on the strength of contraction, several pushes of 10–15 or more seconds may be possible during a contraction. As the head of the baby crowns, she is asked to pant lightly so that the head maybe delivered slowly.

The advantages of the method include the need for little or no analgesia for pain relief and participation in the labor by the mother giving her a great sense of satisfaction at delivery. The father of the baby also benefits by participating in the birth of his baby.

Modified Lamaze Method

Childbirth educators have enhanced the Lamaze method by adding information on prenatal nutrition, infant feeding, cesarean birth and variations from the usual labor, discussions on sexuality, parenting and coping skills for the postpartum period (**Box 53.1**). The original Lamaze theory specified the presence of a female monitor (monitrice), but now a father-husband coach is encouraged along with a medical attendant. The exercises have been modified to enhance comfort in pregnancy and birth. However, perhaps the most important modification involves a change in philosophy concerning the goals of expectant parents. The original Lamaze theory virtually demanded that in order to have a successful childbirth experience, the delivery was to be painless and without anesthetic. In many cases, the parturient that was unable to fulfill this goal was left with a feeling of inadequacy. Today childbirth educators encourage the couple to set their own goals, supplying them with the tools for accepting these goals while providing reassurance and information about other options for those who cannot achieve a pain free and anesthetic-free delivery.

Bradley Method

A method of psychophysical preparation for childbirth developed by Dr Robert Bradley, involves education about physiology of childbirth, exercise, nutrition during pregnancy, techniques of breathing and relaxation for control and comfort during labor and delivery. The father is extensively involved in the classes and acts as the mother's 'coach' during labor. Among the advantages of the method are its simplicity, the involvement of the father and the realistic approach to the efforts and discomforts of labor. This is also called the husband-coached childbirth.

Teaching Content

Childbirth preparation classes are designed to help the couple make informed decisions during the childbearing period and should contain information regarding changes in the woman and the development of the fetus. They are best conducted in chronological sequence, with both parents taught breathing and relaxation techniques, infant care and coping strategies.

First trimester classes

The content of the first trimester classes included the following—early gestational changes, self-care during pregnancy, fetal development and environmental dangers for the fetus, sexuality in pregnancy, birth settings, nutrition, rest and exercises; relief measures for common discomforts of pregnancy and psychological changes in pregnancy. These

> **BOX 53.1:** Content outline for Lamaze prepared childbirth classes.
>
> 1. Theory of the Lamaze method.
> 2. Anatomy and physiology as they relate to:
>   - Pregnancy
>   - Labor and birth
>   - The postpartum period (mother)
>   - The newborn.
> 3. Emotional responses of expectant parents to:
>   - Pregnancy experience
>   - Childbirth experience
>   - Early parenting experience (includes role changes).
> 4. Physical conditioning for childbirth:
>   - Prenatal exercises
>   - Posture/body mechanics
>   - Guidelines for exercises.
> 5. Stages and phases of labor:
>   - Overview
>   - First stage:
>   – Latent phase
>   – Active phase
>   – Transition phase.
>   - Second stage
>   - Third stage
>   - Woman's physical responses
>   - Woman's emotional responses
>   - Coach's role.
> 6. Nonpharmacological analgesia:
>   - Progressive relaxation
>   - Touch relaxation
>   - Imagery
>   - Focusing techniques
>   - Effleurage
>   - Massage
>   - Comfort measures (back rub, positioning, etc.)
>   - Support (role of the coach, hospital staff, physician or midwife).
> 7. Pharmacological analgesia and anesthesia:
>   - Types used (describe and explain)
>   - How and when administered?
>   - Effects on mother and baby.
> 8. Breathing techniques:
>   - Respiratory theory and principles
>   - Respiratory techniques:
>   – Slow paced
>   – Modified paced
>   – Patterned paced.
>   - Second stage expulsion:
>   – Physiologic techniques
>   – Modified valsalva technique.
> 9. Birthing process:
>   - Vaginal birth
>   - Cesarean birth:
>   – Indications
>   – Procedure
>   – Use of prepared childbirth techniques
>   – Coach's role.
>
> *Contd...*
>
> 10. Variations in labor and birth:
>   - Amniotomy
>   - Fetal monitoring:
>   – External
>   – Internal.
>   - Induction and augmentation
>   - Forceps and vacuum extraction
>   - Episiotomies.
> 11. Hospital procedures:
>   - Admission
>   - Labor and birth
>   - Postpartum care (mother and baby)
>   - Parent-infant interaction.
> 12. Other content:
>   - Nutrition
>   - Infant feeding (breast or bottle)
>   - Signs of premature labor (prevention of prematurity)
>   - Grieving and loss of unexpected outcome
>   - Postpartum 'blues'
>   - Family planning (contraception).

(*Source:* Karpen, Conrad and Chitwood, 1995).

classes should also highlight factors that place the woman at risk for preterm labor and discuss its signs and symptoms. The pros and cons of breastfeeding and bottle feeding should be covered, since many women make their decisions regarding feeding before the third trimester.

Second and third trimester classes

Later classes should focus on preparation for labor, birth and early parenthood, stressing and allowing time for body conditioning, relaxation, breathing techniques and other measures that promote comfort and participation during the birth experience. Postpartum self-care should be taught, as well as early adjustment to parenthood and infant care including feeding, family nutrition, child health and safety, growth and development, infant stimulation, and family development. A discussion of the car seat is important where applicable for child safety.

Refresher Courses

Refresher courses may be given for experienced mothers who have previously taken a course in prepared childbirth and who want to update their skills and knowledge. These classes may review the process of labor and delivery as well as methods of promoting comfort and participation during childbirth. They most often include a segment on sibling adjustment.

Cesarean Birth Preparation

With the increase in the proportion of cesarean deliveries, preparation for the possibility should be included in every childbirth education class. To help the couple avoid the feelings of anger, loss and grief that can occur with cesarean birth, it should be approached as a normal event, with the instructor stressing the similarities between it and vaginal birth. Information should be provided that will help a couple make personal choices and participate in the experience. The content should cover the details of a cesarean delivery and describe what the mother and father will feel as well as what they can do.

For the couple who know ahead of time that cesarean birth is planned (for instance, the handicapped woman or the woman with pelvic insufficiency) should receive more detailed cesarean preparation classes. The classes will also benefit those couples that anticipate a repeat cesarean birth. The instructor should stress that subsequent cesarean deliveries are often less painful than the first and for the woman whose first cesarean was preceded by a long or strenuous labor, there will be much less fatigue the second time around.

Prenatal Exercise Classes

A well-conditioned body will perform better and more reliably under the stresses of labor than a body in poor physical condition. However, because of the body's changes during pregnancy, the pregnant woman must learn how to exercise safely and effectively to condition her body with minimum risk to herself and the fetus. The goal of these exercises is to strengthen muscle tone in preparation for delivery and promote faster restoration of muscle tone after delivery.

The exercises taught include the pelvic tilt, abdominal exercises (tightening abdominal muscles in synchronization with respiration, partial sit-ups, inner thigh exercises (done cross-legged in tailor position) and Kegel's exercises to strengthen the perineal muscles. An exercise prescription from the physician is encouraged (for details on exercises, *refer* Chapter 54).

Effectiveness of prenatal education

Prenatal education serves many purposes on many different levels. Although prepared childbirth does not preclude the use of medication when necessary, it allows for a decreased use of analgesics and anesthetics during labor, thereby lowering the probability of drug-related side effects to mother and baby. It also intensifies the mother-father-child relationship by allowing for full participation in the birth process. It reduces fear, anxiety and pain by providing knowledge and understanding, helping to make the experience of parenthood one of joy. In sharing experience with other couples, lateral supports are strengthened, reducing the couples' feelings of isolation. The understanding gained concerning changes in the woman's body during pregnancy, labor and postpartum period provides a feeling of preparedness and calm. Added to this are the benefits of increased circulation and respiratory exchange, a reduced perception of contractions as painful and increased confidence in the couple's ability to cope with the discomforts of labor.

As a counselor, teacher, professional and friend, the childbirth educator helps parents evaluate their feelings. Since pregnancy and childbirth are 'normal crises of life', the educator helps parents gain internal as well as external resources for handling crises situations, which aids them in achieving a satisfactory and healthy adjustment. In the open and permissive classroom atmosphere, the educator encourages parents to examine their feelings and discuss how and why they react the way they do to situations. Through discussions and role playing, the responsibility of learning to adjust is placed on the parents and the educator guides them through process of exploring their reactions and trying new ones. With the proper guidance, it becomes easier to choose appropriate responses in labor and cope with the stresses of the postpartum period.

ROLE OF COACH OR SUPPORT PERSON

Providing a supportive milieu is one of the most important functions of childbirth preparation programs. The childbirth coach, an integral member of the support team, goes to classes with the expectant mother, asks questions regarding issues of concern and uses the discipline of repetitive practice with the expectant mother to begin the process of conditioning. The coach's role is to help the mother use the techniques she has learned. During labor, the coach comforts and supports the woman with care-taking activities, such as soothing conversations, touching, staying close by giving back rubs, applying cool clothes to the face and forehead and maintaining eye contact. Using verbal clues, the couple practices together, the coach reinforces learned responses while encouraging and working with the laboring mother to achieve a satisfying birth experience. The coach is particularly important in helping the woman time her contractions, identifying the beginning of each one and breathing through it with her or encouraging and supporting her as she breathes.

ROLE OF THE CHILDBIRTH EDUCATOR

The childbirth educator has three responsibilities—assessment of parents, intervention and fulfillment of their educational needs.

Assessment includes determining the accuracy and completeness of the parents' information regarding parenting, determining their misconceptions (if any) about the maternity role, determining their ability to understand information and instructions, assessing their motivation to learn and becoming familiar with any personal or cultural values that may influence their acceptance of information, and their compliance with instructions.

Intervention may include conducting parents' classes, dispensing of literature (if any) appropriate to their level of understanding and educational level and individual counseling and teaching. Effectiveness of teaching is enhanced by:

1. Choosing the time of optimum readiness for motivation to learn (for example, not teaching labor and delivery during the first trimester).
2. Limiting the amount of new information given at one time.
3. Summarizing and writing down points.
4. Providing feedback mechanism to assess learning, such as asking clients to repeat the information, asking if they understand the material and verifying their understanding by non-verbal clues, and providing an atmosphere where questions can be asked freely.

Educational Needs

- Anatomical and physiological changes in pregnancy
- The labor and delivery process
- Signs of labor, nutrition and signs of complications in pregnancy
- The rationale for early and regular prenatal care
- Safety precautions
- Hospital admission and daily routine procedures, hospital policies affecting mother-child interaction
- Planning and purchasing baby clothes and other materials
- Preparation for natural childbirth—exercises, hygiene and fetal development
- General health care and newborn care.

STUDY QUESTIONS

Short Note

1. Goals of childbirth education (preparation for childbirth).

Short Answer Question

1. Role of a coach or support person with the laboring woman.

Essay Question

1. Describe the effectiveness of prenatal preparation and education.

BIBLIOGRAPHY

1. Chertock J. Psychosomatic methods of preparation for childbirth. American Journal of Obstetrics and Gynecology. 1967;98(5):698-707.
2. Davis CD, Morrone FA. An objective evaluation of a prenatal childbirth program. American Journal of Obstetrics and Gynecology. 1962;84: 1196-206.
3. De Santo P, Hassid P. Evaluating exercises, childbirth educator, american baby; 1983.
4. Dick-Read G. Revelation of childbirth: The principles and practice of natural childbirth, 2nd edition. London: William Heinemann; 1943.
5. Elizabeth B. Six practical lessons for an easier childbirth, 1st edition. New York: Bantam Books; 1967.
6. Grantly Dick-Read. Childbirth without fear. New York: Harper and Row Publishers; 1972.
7. Karpen M, Conrad L, Chitwood L. Essentials of maternal-child nursing, 2nd edition. Western Schools Press, 1995. pp. 47-57.
8. Ladewig PW, London ML, Olds SB. Essentials of maternal newborn nursing, 1st edition. New York: Addison-Wesley; 1990.
9. Margo E. Ego states and stroking in childbirth experience. The Transactional Analysis Journal. 1971;3-6.
10. Raff B, Friesner A. Quick reference to maternity nursing. 1st edition. Aspen Publishers: Rockville; 1989.
11. Sclare AB. Psychoprophylaxis in obstetrics. Nursing Times. 1965;61(41):1373-4.
12. Yahia, Clement and Ulin. The theory and technique of psychoprophylactic preparation for childbirth. American Journal of Obstetrics and Gynecology. 1968;93:942-8.

CHAPTER 54

Special Exercises for Pregnancy, Labor and Puerperium

Learning Objectives

Upon completing this chapter, the learner will be able to:
- Develop an insight into the postural and circulatory changes that may occur during pregnancy, which may lead to discomforts.
- Discuss the measures for relaxation and relief of discomforts during pregnancy and labor.
- Describe the posture for comfort in different positions in the prenatal period.
- Describe the exercises that can be practiced during pregnancy.
- Describe the exercises for relieving aches and pains following vaginal delivery and cesarean section.

Preparation for parenthood outlined in Chapter 53 'Childbirth Education and Preparation' includes information about physiology of pregnancy and childbirth as well as breathing and relaxation techniques, which the prospective parents can learn from a professional in a relaxed atmosphere. In such an atmosphere, prospective parents develop confidence to cope with pregnancy, labor and delivery. In this chapter, information related to postural and lifestyle changes and exercises for relief of discomforts during antenatal period, labor and postpartum period are explained.

POSTURAL CHANGES IN PREGNANCY

Accompanying the gradual weight gain in pregnancy and its centralizing distribution is the hormonal effect on ligamentous structures. These factors alter the posture of the pregnant women. The body's center of gravity moves forwards and when this is combined with stretching of weak abdominal muscles, it often leads to a subsequent hollowing of the lumbar spine with a rounding of the shoulders and poking chin. There is a tendency for back muscles to shorten and abdominal muscles to stretch, extra strain is placed on the ligaments and the result is backache, usually of sacroiliac or lumbar origin. Postural re-education, including correction of the 'pelvic tilt' should be taught. Advice relating to comfortable positions in sitting, standing, lying and general mobility, and how to lift correctly must be given to avoid back pain.

POSTURE FOR COMFORT IN DIFFERENT POSITIONS

Sitting

The pregnant woman should choose a comfortable chair, which supports both back and thighs **(Figs. 54.1A and B)**. She should sit well back and if necessary, place a small cushion or folded towel behind the lumbar spine for additional comfort. The seat height should allow the feet to rest on the floor, or a small stool. If relaxing in an easy chair, the head can be supported and the legs elevated on stool.

Standing

The posture should be as tall as possible with both the abdomen and buttocks tucked in. Weight must be evenly distributed on both legs, to prevent undue strain on the pelvic ligaments and spread between the heels and the balls of the feet. A medium or low-heeled shoe, which gives support, should be used; high heels should be avoided, as it will throw the balance of the pregnant woman too far forwards. Shoulders are to be down and relaxed to prevent thoracic aches.

Lying

Equal pressure on all parts of the body will lead to a good posture in lying with no undue strain on any one area. Lying flat on the back should be avoided as far as possible because of the danger of supine hypotension. Lying with two to three pillows to raise the head and shoulders, will avoid the risk. It may be more comfortable with an additional pillow under the thighs to reduce the tension behind the knees **(Fig. 54.2A)**.

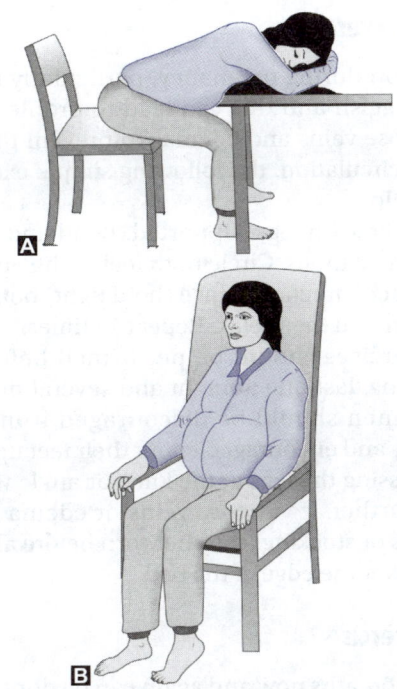

Figures 54.1A and B: Relaxation in sitting position.

Side lying with pillows under the top arm and knee is usually a comfortable position in pregnancy (**Fig. 54.2B**).

Getting up from lying can be done by bending the knees, rolling on to one side, and then using the arms to push up into a sitting or kneeling position. This would avoid strain on both back and the abdominal muscles.

Household Activities

Household tasks may be performed in a sitting position as much as possible. When activities are done in standing position, the working surface should be at the correct height to avoid the need to stoop and subsequent backache. For jobs at the floor level, kneeling position prevents lumbar strain.

Lifting heavy objects should be avoided during pregnancy, if possible. If lifting is unavoidable, then the object must be held close to the body with the knees bent and the back kept straight (**Fig. 54.3**). This way the strain is taken by the thigh muscles and not those of the back. Twisting movements, while lifting are dangerous and must not be performed.

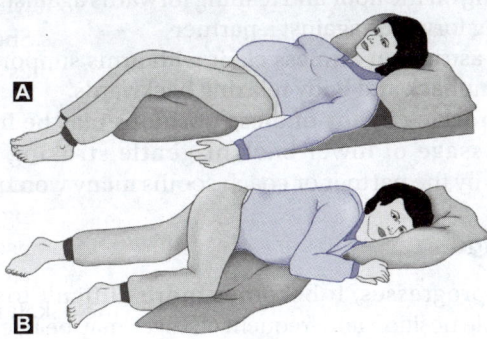

Figures 54.2A and B: Relaxation in lying position.

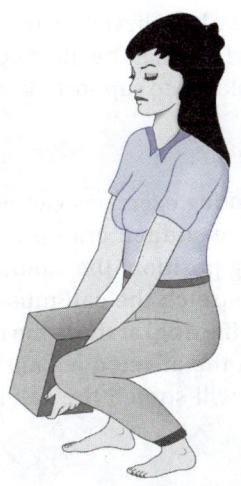

Figure 54.3: Proper position for lifting.

EXERCISES DURING PREGNANCY

Moderate exercises during pregnancy stimulates circulation, helps to keep joints flexible, creates good muscle tone and promotes a general scene of well-being. It has also been observed that women who exercise regularly during pregnancy have an improved course of pregnancy and compared to those who lead a sedentary lifestyle.

Walking

Walking in the fresh air remains one of the most natural and simplest forms of exercise and should be encouraged.

Cycling

Cycling is a good form of exercise, which allows for good mobility of the lower limbs with the body weight supported. Cycling when done should only be short distances and care must be taken to avoid steep areas. It is also advisable to stop before feeling tired.

Swimming

Swimming is another excellent exercise, as water relieves the effects of gravity on the body and muscles can be strengthened and flexibility of joints retained without undue fatigue. Light swimming with gentle supporting arm movements is often most comfortable. Strenuous strokes and diving should be avoided.

POSTURE FOR RELIEF OF ACHES AND PAINS

Back and Pelvic Pain

A good number of women experience backache at some stage of their pregnancy. Women who suffer from backache can be helped by encouraging good posture and the practice of pelvic tilting exercise in standing, sitting and lying position.

Sciatic-like pain may be relieved by lying on the side away from the discomfort, so that the affected leg is uppermost. Pillows should be placed to support the whole limb.

Cramp

Practicing foot and leg exercises can achieve prevention of cramp. To relieve sudden cramp in the calf muscles, whilst in the sitting position, the woman should hold the knee straight and stretch the calf muscles by pulling the foot upwards (dorsiflexing) at the same time. Alternatively, standing firmly on the affected leg and striding forwards with the other leg will stretch the calf muscles and solve the problem.

Rib Discomfort

Discomfort around the rib cage can often be relieved by adopting a good posture or by specifically stretching one or both arms upwards, depending on which side the pain is present.

ANTENATAL EXERCISES

Muscles of good tone are more elastic and will regain their former length more efficiently and more quickly after being stretched than muscles of poor tone. Exercising the abdominal muscles antenatally will ensure a speedy return to normal postnatally, effective pushing in and the lessening of backache in pregnancy. The overstretched ligaments and weakened abdominal muscles during pregnancy can lead to chronic skeletal problems postnatally as well as backache antenatally. In order to prevent this and to maintain good abdominal tone, abdominal tightening and pelvic tilting exercises are to be taught.

Abdominal Tightening

The woman has to sit comfortably or kneel on all fours. Breathe in and out, and then pull the lower part of the abdomen below the umbilicus, while continuing to breathe normally. Hold up to 10 seconds and repeat up to 10 times.

This exercise strengthens the deep transverse abdominal muscles, which are the main postural support of the spine and will help to prevent backache in the future. When the woman masters this exercise, it can be practiced in any position whilst doing other activities.

Pelvic Floor Exercise (Kegel Exercise)

Sit, stand or half-lie with legs slightly apart. Close and draw up around the anal passage as though preventing a bowel action, then repeat front passages (vagina and urethra) as if to stop the flow of urine in midstream. Hold for as long as possible up to 10 seconds, breathing normally, then relax. Repeat up to 10 times. All pregnant women should practice this exercise very regularly antenatally, particularly after emptying the bladder.

Foot and Leg Exercises

The circulation during pregnancy, particularly the venous return, is sluggish and this can lead to problems such as cramp, varicose veins and edema. To prevent these and to improve the circulation, the following simple exercises and advice will help.

Sit or half-lie with legs supported. Bend and stretch the ankles at least 12 times. Circle both feet at the ankle at least 20 times in each direction. Brace (hold tight) both knees for a count of four and then relax. Repeat 12 times.

These exercises should be performed before getting up from resting, last one at night and several times during the day. Women should be discouraged from standing unnecessarily and encouraged to put their feet up whenever possible. Crossing the legs at the knee or ankle will impede circulation further. If varicose veins or edema is present, support tights or stockings may be worn before allowing the legs to drop over the edge of the bed.

Breathing Exercise

A few deeper breaths now and again can be done every day. This will help the venous return and aid the oxygen supply to both pregnant woman and her fetus. Only three or four breaths are to be taken at a time. More deep breaths at one time can lead to hyperventilation.

POSITIONS FOR COMFORT DURING LABOR

First Stage of Labor

Early Stage

A woman in labor should be encouraged to keep mobile and active, if there are no complications. She should be encouraged to try alternative positions of ease as alteration of position leads to productive uterine contractions. When discomfort increases during contractions, the woman should be encouraged to stay relaxed and concentrate on rhythmical, easy breathing.

The following positions of ease may help during the early stages of labor and can be practiced in the antenatal period:
- Sitting against a table and relaxing forwards so that shoulders, arms and head are supported
- Standing, leaning backwards against the wall of the room
- Kneeling on the floor and leaning forwards against a chair
- Leaning forwards against a partner
- Sitting astride on armless chair with arms supported on the chair back and body relaxing backwards.

Pelvic rocking in any of these positions may be helpful. Deep massage of lower back or gentle stroking of the abdomen by the partner or coach sooths many women.

Later Stage

As labor progresses, it becomes more difficult to find a comfortable position and frequent changes may be necessary. Some prepared women are content to sit back against pillows on the bed and concentrate on breathing and relaxation at this stage. If there is an urge to push, they must be encouraged to use an interrupted outward breath pattern that is two shorter breaths followed by a longer breath (pant-pant-blow). This prevents the increase in intra-abdominal pressure. An alteration in position, such as the side lying, may take away some of the urge to push.

Second Stage of Labor

Position for second stage of labor will depend largely on the obstetric practice in the institution. In most places, women are delivered in supine position. However, alternative positions are possible, depending on the method of pain relief and obstetric factors. The positions that may be used include:
- Side lying
- Squatting on the bed
- Supported squatting with partner supporting from behind
- Sitting fairly upright against the back rest with knees bent and feet resting on the bed
- Kneeling on all fours.

As the contraction starts, the mother is reminded to breathe in and out gently. When the urge to push becomes overwhelming, she will tuck in her chin and bear down, keeping the pelvic floor relaxed. Breath holding should not be encouraged because of the danger of fetal hypoxia in an already compromised baby. To prevent pushing whilst the head is delivered, deep panting may be useful.

POSTNATAL EXERCISES

Postnatal exercise should be started as soon as possible after delivery in order to improve circulation, strengthen pelvic floor and abdominal muscles and prevent transient and long-term problems.

Circulatory Exercises

Foot and leg exercises must be performed very frequently in the immediate postpartal period to improve circulation, reduce edema and prevent deep vein thrombosis. If edema is present, the foot of the bed may be raised slightly.

Pelvic Floor Exercises (Kegel Exercise)

The pelvic floor muscles have been under strain during pregnancy and stretched during delivery, and it may be both difficult and painful to contract these muscles postnatally. Mothers should be encouraged to do the exercise as often as possible, in order to regain full bladder control, prevent uterine prolapse and ensure normal sexual satisfaction in future. The contraction should be held for 10 seconds (to a count of 6) and repeated up to 10 times at any one session, breathing normally throughout.

The mother should continue to do this exercise for 2–3 months. After 3 months, if the mother is able to cough deeply with a full bladder without leaking urine (stress incontinence), she may stop the exercise. If leaking occurs, she may continue the exercise for the rest of her life.

Abdominal Exercises

Abdominal muscles need to regain tone as soon as possible after delivery in order to protect the spine, prevent back problems and help the mother to regain her former physical fitness. These include abdominal breathing, head and shoulder raising, leg raising, pelvic tilt, knee rolling, hip hitching and sit-ups.

Abdominal Breathing

The mother is taught deep abdominal breathing to strengthen the diaphragm. This may be started on the first postpartum day. She is taught to take a deep breath, raising her abdominal wall and exhale slowly. To ensure that the exercise is being done correctly, place one hand on the chest and another on the abdomen. When inhaling, the hand on the abdomen should be raised and the hand on the chest should remain stationary. Repeat the exercise five times **(Fig. 54.4)**.

Head and Shoulder Raising

On the 2nd postpartum day, lie flat without pillow and raise head until the chin is touching the chest. On the 3rd postpartum day raise both head and shoulders off of the bed and lower them slowly. Increase gradually until able to do 10 times **(Fig. 54.5)**.

Leg Raising

Leg raising exercise may be begun on the 7th postpartum day. Lying down on the floor with no pillows under the head,

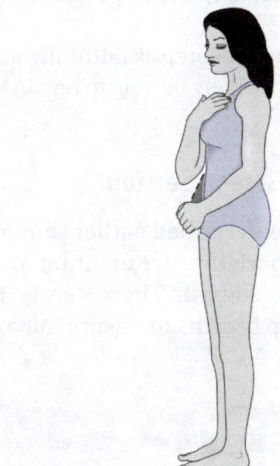

Figure 54.4: Abdominal breathing.

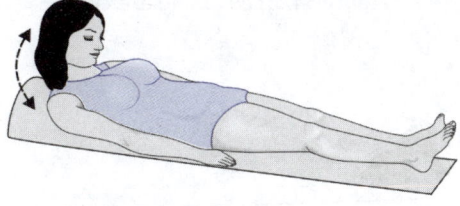

Figure 54.5: Head and shoulder raising exercise.

point toe and slowly raise one leg keeping the knee straight. Lower the leg slowly and gradually increase to 10 times each leg **(Fig. 54.6)**.

Pelvic Tilting or Rocking

Lie flat on the floor with knees bent and feet flat. Inhale and while exhaling, flatten the back hard against the floor so that there is no space between the back and the floor. While doing this, tighten abdominal muscles and the muscles of the buttocks, and then tilt pelvis towards ceiling and inhale normally, hold breath for up to 10 seconds, and then relax. Repeat up to 10 times **(Fig. 54.7)**.

Knee Rolling

Knee rolling exercise will strengthen the oblique abdominal muscles and may be done only if there is no undue separation of the rectus muscles (diastasis of the rectus muscle). In back lying with knees bent, pull in the abdomen and roll both knees to one side as far as comfortable, keeping shoulders flat. Return knees to and upright position and relax the abdomen. Pull in again and roll both knees to the other side. This exercise can be performed up to 10 times.

Hip Hitching

Hip hitching or leg shortening is performed in back lying with one knee bent and the other knee straight. Slide the heel of the straight leg downwards thus lengthening the leg. Shorten the same leg by drawing the hip up toward the ribs on the same side. Repeat up to 10 times, keeping the abdomen pulled in. Change to the opposite side and repeat **(Figs. 54.8A and B)**.

If the mother does these exercises faithfully and follows a sensible diet, she will most likely be able to regain her physical fitness quickly.

Exercises Following Cesarean Section

Foot and leg exercises as described earlier should be started as soon as possible, especially after epidural anesthesia, as distal circulation will be sluggish. These may be followed by not more than four deep breaths to ensure full expansion of

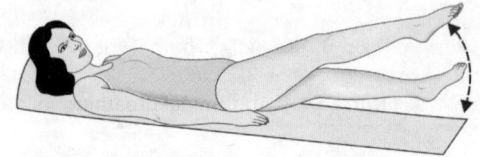

Figure 54.6: Leg raising exercise.

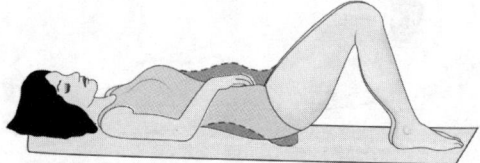

Figure 54.7: Pelvic tilt exercises.

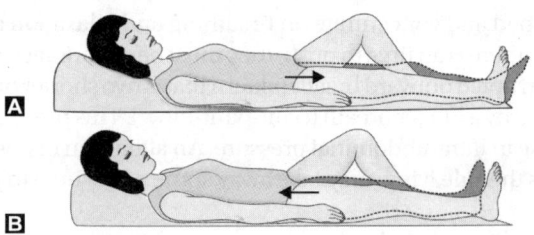

Figures 54.8A and B: Hip hitching (up drawing) exercise.

the lungs and pumping action on the inferior vena cava. If a general anesthetic has been given, the mother may have extra secretions and needs to be taught how to clear them by coughing in a sitting position with the sutures supported by both hands and a pillow. Deep breathing and coughing will help to loosen the secretions.

To ease backache and flatulence the *abdominal tightening*, *pelvic tilting* and *knee rolling* exercises can be practiced gently after 24 hours.

Mothers will progress to the pelvic floor exercises, head raising and hip hitching when they feel more comfortable, usually after 4–5 days if there is no undue separation of the rectus muscles. Pelvic floor exercises are still important following cesarean section even though the women in this group are less likely to suffer stress incontinence.

Adequate rest is essential postnatally to allow the tissues to regain their normal function. After a cesarean section, the woman has not only given birth but also has undergone major surgery, yet she has to cope with her baby. The midwife must take every opportunity to remind relatives of the need to help with chores and the organization of rest periods for the mother.

Care of the Back Postnatally

It may take up to 6 months for the ligaments to completely resume their normal functions. Therefore, it is vital that mothers receive advice on back care in relation to everyday activities during this period.

When feeding the baby, she should sit back in a chair, well-supported with the baby raised up on pillows to prevent a slouched forward position. Diaper changing and bathing of the baby are best carried out at waist level or with the mother kneeling at a coffee table height **(Figs. 54.9A and B)**.

Lifting should be avoided, if at all possible and the object should be as light as possible and kept close to the body. While lifting, the knees must be bent and back kept straight.

IMMEDIATE POSTNATAL PHYSICAL PROBLEMS

Diastasis Symphysis

Diastasis symphysis condition may be present in late pregnancy, occur during labor or appear after delivery. If the pain is severe, indicating complete separation of the pubic joint, complete bedrest with some support around the pubis is advised. The woman must be instructed to press her knees together when moving in bed. She should be encouraged to

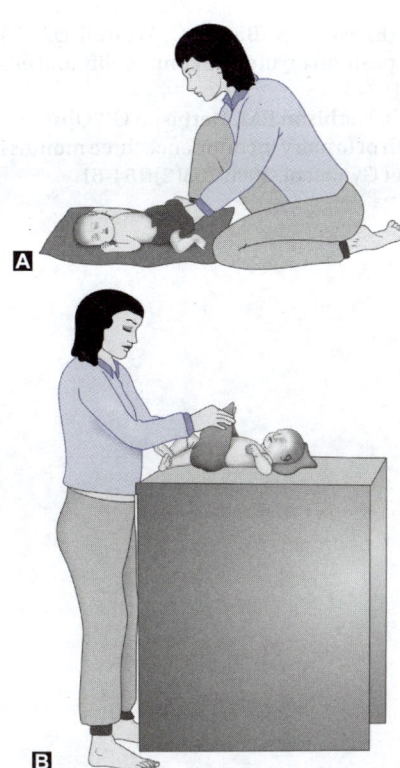

Figures 54.9A and B: Positions for changing baby's diaper. (A) Changing diaper in sitting position; (B) Changing diaper in standing position.

perform the abdominal tightening and pelvic tilting exercises plus circulatory exercises, while she is resting. Mobilization of the woman may be allowed only when the acute pain has subsided. Therapeutic ultrasound, transcutaneous nerve stimulation or ice applications may be prescribed to relieve local pain.

Diastasis Recti

If the woman's rectus muscles are found more than two fingers width apart, the only exercises, which should be permitted are abdominal tightening, pelvic tilting and head lifting. While performing head lifting, the woman should keep her hands crossed over the abdomen to support the muscles and draw them towards the midline.

Painful Perineum

Painful perineum is a common problem and advice on positioning should be given with analgesia and local pain-relieving measures, such as ice application. To avoid the possibility of local skin injury, ice should not be in direct contact with the skin. It may be crushed and placed inside a polythene bag or gauze and positioned against the painful area for no longer than 5–10 minutes. The woman will be most comfortable in side lying position and should be reminded not to sit on the ice pack, as the pressure would impede circulation. Alternatively, the perineum may be massaged for 5–10 minutes at a time by an ice cube, held in a disposable cloth or clean plastic bag. When the pain is less, pelvic floor exercises should be encouraged with the aim of increasing the local circulation.

Incontinence

Stress incontinence occurs in some women following delivery. Pelvic floor exercises will help to rehabilitate the pelvic floor, but the woman will usually require specific obstetric exercises prescribed by her physician.

Backache

Early postnatal backache is usually postural and can be relieved by warmth and pelvic tilting exercises. Persistent and severe back pain if present, the woman will need physiotherapy.

Coccydynia

An acutely painful coccyx occasionally presents, which may be incapacitating for a new mother. Placing pillow strategically may give some relief and alternative positions in feeding may be given. Specific physiotherapy or manipulation may be required for a displaced coccyx.

During pregnancy, labor and the puerperium, mothers should be influenced to incorporate a sensible approach to exercise. Relaxation, walking, cycling and other forms of exercises can be encouraged as part of a general lifestyle. Specific exercises for strengthening pelvic floor and abdominal muscles or relieving aches and pains such as cramps or backache will be useful even beyond the months of childbearing.

▌STUDY QUESTIONS

Short Notes

1. Kegel exercise.
2. Hip hitching exercise.
3. Diastasis recti.
4. Coccydynia.
5. Knee rolling exercise.

▌BIBLIOGRAPHY

1. Brayshaw EM. Special exercises for pregnancy, labour and the puerperium. In: Bennett RV, Linda KB (Eds). Myles Textbook for Midwives, 13th edition. Edinburgh: Churchill Livingstone; 1979. pp. 873-89.
2. Caldeyro Barcia R. The influence of maternal position on labor and the influence of maternal bearing-down efforts in the second stage of labor on fetal well-being. In: Simkin PR (Ed). Kaleidoscope of Childbearing Preparation, Birth and Nurturing. Seattle: Penny Press; 1978.
3. Clapp J. The courses of labor after endurance exercise during pregnancy. Am J Obstet Gynecol. 1992;163(6):1799-805.
4. Clausen JP. Maternity Nursing Today. New York: McGraw Hill Publishing Company; 1973.

5. Fry D. Diastasis symphysis pubis. Journal of the Association of Chartered Physiotherapists in Obstetrics and Gynecology. 1992;71:10-3.
6. Jacobson B, Smith A. The Nation's Health: A Strategy for the 1990s, London: Kings Fund; 1991.
7. Polden M, Mantle J. Physiotherapy in Obstetrics and Gynecology. London: Butterworth-Heinemann; 1990.
8. Roberts JE, Mendez-Bauer C, Wodell DA. The effects of maternal position on uterine contractility and efficiency. Birth. 1983;10(4):243-9.
9. Wilson PD, Herbison RM, Herbison GP. Obstetric practice and prevention of urinary incontinence three months after delivery. Br J Obstet Gynaecol. 1996;103(2):154-61.

CHAPTER 55

Drugs Used in Obstetrics

Learning Objectives

Upon completing this chapter, the learner will be able to:
- Describe the use of oxytocic drugs and the nursing considerations related to each.
- Describe the use of antihypertensive drugs for maternity clients.
- Describe the use and nursing considerations for tocolytic agents.
- Discuss the effects of maternal medications on fetus and breastfeeding infants.

Drugs commonly used for maternity clients are described in this chapter. The midwife should have thorough knowledge of the indications, actions and side effects of these drugs as well as the nursing considerations related to each of them in order to plan and implement effective nursing process.

OXYTOCICS

Oxytocics are the drugs that have the power to excite contractions of the uterine muscles. Among a large number of drugs belonging to this group, the ones that are important and extensively used are oxytocin, ergot derivatives and prostaglandins.

Oxytocin

Oxytocin is an octapeptide synthesized in the hypothalamus and stored in the posterior pituitary.

Preparations

Synthetic oxytocin available for parenteral use includes:
- *Syntocinon:* 5 unit/mL in ampules of 1 mL
- *Pitocin:* 10 unit/mL in ampules of 0.5 mL
- *Syntometrine:* A combination of syntocinon 5 units and ergometrine 0.5 mg
- Oxytocin nasal solution 40 unit/mL.

Actions

Acts directly on myofibrils producing uterine contraction and stimulates milk ejection by the breasts.

Indications for Use

1. Pregnancy:
   - To induce abortion (inevitable, missed)
   - To expedite expulsion of hydatidiform mole
   - For oxytocin challenge test
   - To stop bleeding following evacuation
   - To induce labor.
2. Labor:
   - To augment labor
   - In uterine inertia
   - To prevent and treat postpartum hemorrhage.
3. Postpartum:
   - To initiate milk let-down in breast engorgement.

Contraindications

1. In late pregnancy:
   - Grand multipara
   - Contracted pelvis
   - History of cesarean section or hysterotomy
   - Malpresentation.
2. During labor:
   - All contraindications mentioned in pregnancy
   - Obstructed labor
   - Incoordinate uterine action.
3. Anytime:
   - Hypovolemic state
   - Cardiac disease.

Adverse Effects

- Hypertonic uterine activity
- Fetal distress and fetal death
- Uterine rupture
- Hypotension
- Neonatal jaundice
- Water retention and water intoxication.

Dosage and Routes of Administration

- Controlled intravenous (IV) infusion (10 units of oxytocin in 1 L of Ringer's lactate or 5% dextrose in water)
- Nasal spray for milk let-down.

Nursing Considerations

1. Assess:
   - Intake and output ratio
   - Uterine contractions and fetal heart rate (FHR)
   - Blood pressure (BP), pulse and respiration.
2. Administer:
   - By IV infusion
   - After having crash cart (emergency trolley) available in the ward.
3. Evaluate:
   - Length and duration of contractions
   - Notify physician of contractions lasting over 1 minute or absence of contractions.
4. Teach client/family:
   - To report increased blood loss, abdominal cramps or increased temperature.

Ergot Derivatives

Ergot alkaloids are either natural or semisynthetic.

Preparations

- Ergometrine (ergonovine): 0.25 mg or 0.5 mg ampules and 0.5–1 mg tablets
- Methergine (methylergonovine): 0.2 mg ampules and 0.5–1 mg tablets
- Syntometrine with ergometrine: 0.5 mg + Syntocinon 5.0 units ampules.

Ergometrine and Methergine can be used parenterally or orally. As the drug produces titanic uterine contractions, it should only be used after delivery of the anterior shoulder or following delivery of the baby. It should not be used in induction of labor or abortion. Syntometrine should always be administered intramuscularly.

Mode of Action

Ergometrine acts directly on the myometrium. It stimulates uterine contractions and decreases bleeding.

Indications

1. *Therapeutic:* To stop the atonic uterine bleeding following delivery, abortion or expulsion of hydatidiform mole.
2. *Prophylactic:* As a prophylaxis against excessive hemorrhage; it may be administered after the delivery of the anterior shoulder (active management of third stage) with crowning or following delivery of the baby.

Contraindications

1. *Suspected plural pregnancy:* If given accidentally with the delivery of the first baby, the second twin is likely to be compromised by the titanic contractions of the uterus.
2. *Organic cardiac disease:* It may cause sudden squeezing of blood out of the uterine circulation into the general circulation causing overloading of the right heart and precipitating failure.
3. *Severe preeclampsia and eclampsia:* There may be sudden rise of blood pressure.
4. *Rhesus (Rh)-negative mother:* There is more chance of fetomaternal microtransfusion.

Note: For women with heart diseases or hypertension, oxytocin is a better substitute.

Adverse Effects/Side Effects

- A rise of blood pressure is precipitated because of its vasoconstrictive action
- Prolonged use in puerperium may interfere with lactation by decreasing the concentration of prolactin
- Prolonged use may lead to gangrene of the toes due to its vasoconstrictive effect.

Nursing Considerations

1. Assess:
   - Blood pressure, pulse and respiration
   - Watch for signs of hemorrhage.
2. Administer:
   - Orally or intramuscular (IM) in deep muscle mass
   - Have emergency cart readily available.
3. Evaluate:
   - Therapeutic effect: Decreased blood loss.
4. Teach client/family:
   - To report increased blood loss, abdominal cramps, headache, sweating, nausea and vomiting or dyspnea.

Prostaglandins

Prostaglandins (PGs) are synthesized from one of the essential fatty acids, arachidonic acid, which is widely distributed throughout the body. In the female, these are identified in the menstrual fluid, endometrium, decidua and amniotic membrane.

Preparations

- PGE$_2$—Prostin E$_2$ (dinoprostone)
- PGF$_{2\alpha}$—Prostin F$_{2\alpha}$ (dinoprost tromethamine)
- PGE$_1$—misoprostol.

Actions

Both PGE$_2$ and PGF$_{2\alpha}$ have an oxytocic effect on the pregnant uterus. They also sensitize the myometrium to oxytocin. PGF$_{2\alpha}$ acts predominantly on the myometrium, while PGE$_2$ acts mainly on the cervix.

Indications

- For induction of abortion during second trimester and expulsion of hydatidiform mole
- For induction of labor in intrauterine death of fetus
- In augmentation or acceleration of labor
- To stop bleeding from the open uterine sinuses as in refractory cases of atonic PPH
- Cervical priming.

Contraindications

Hypersensitivity, uterine fibrosis, cervical stenosis, pelvic surgery, pelvic inflammatory disease, respiratory disease.

Side Effects/Adverse Reactions

Headache, dizziness, hypotension, leg cramps, joint swelling, blurred vision.

Dosage and Routes of Administration

- *Tablets:* Containing 0.5 mg Prostin E$_2$
- *Vaginal suppository:* Containing 20 mg PGE$_2$ or 50 mg PGF$_{2\alpha}$
- *Vaginal pessary:* Containing 3 mg PGE$_2$
- Injectable ampules or vials of Prostin E$_2$, 1 mg/mL Prostin F$_{2\alpha}$, 5 mg/mL
- Misoprostol (PGE$_1$) 50 mg, given 4 hourly by oral, vaginal or rectal route for induction of labor.

Nursing Considerations

1. Assess:
   - Respiratory rate, rhythm and depth
   - Vaginal discharge, itching or irritation indicative of infection.
2. Administer:
   - Antiemetic or antidiarrheal preparations prior to giving this drug
   - High in vagina (if vaginal preparations are used)
   - After warming the suppository by running warm water over package.
3. Evaluate:
   - For length and duration of contractions, notify physician of contractions lasting over 1 minute or absence of contractions
   - Fever and chills.
4. Teach client/family:
   - To remain supine for 10–15 minutes after vaginal insertion.

ANTIHYPERTENSIVE DRUGS

Antihypertensive drugs are used in hypertensive disorders of pregnancy. The commonly used drugs are:

- *Adrenergic inhibitors:* Methyldopa
- *Adrenergic blocking agents:* Labetalol, propranolol
- *Vasodilators:* Hydralazine, Diazoxide, sodium nitroprusside
- *Calcium channel blockers:* Nifedipine.

Methyldopa

Preparations

Aldomet, Dopamet.

Action

Stimulates central α-adrenergic receptors or acts as false transmitter resulting in reduction of arterial pressure.

Indication

Hypertension.

Contraindications

Active hepatic disease, congestive cardiac failure, blood dyscrasias, psychiatric disorders.

Side Effects/Adverse Reactions

- Nausea, vomiting, diarrhea, constipation
- Bradycardia, orthostatic hypotension, angina, weight gain
- Drowsiness, dizziness, headache, depression
- Leukopenia, thrombocytopenia, Coombs' test may be positive.

Dosage and Route of Administration

- Orally: 250 mg twice a day (bid) to 1 g three times a day (tid)
- Intravenous infusion: 250–500 mg.

Nursing Considerations

1. Assess:
   - Blood values: Neutrophils, platelets
   - Renal studies: Protein, blood urea nitrogen (BUN), creatinine

- Liver function tests
- Blood pressure before beginning treatment and periodically thereafter.
2. Perform/Provide:
   - Storage of tablets in tight containers.
3. Evaluate:
   - Decrease in blood pressure (therapeutic response)
   - Allergic reaction: Rash, fever, pruritus, urticaria
   - Symptoms of congestive heart failure (edema, dyspnea, wet rales)
   - Renal symptoms: Polyuria, oliguria, frequency.
4. Teach client/family:
   - To avoid hazardous activities
   - Administer 1 hour before meals
   - Not to discontinue drug abruptly or withdrawal symptoms may occur
   - Not to use over the counter (OTC) medications (nonprescription) for cough, cold or allergy, unless directed by physician
   - Compliance with dosage schedule even if feeling better
   - To rise slowly to sitting or standing position to minimize orthostatic hypotension
   - Not to skip or stop drug unless directed by physician
   - Notify physician of untoward signs and symptoms.

Labetalol

Preparations
Trandate, Normodyne.

Action
Non-selective beta blocker.

Indication
Hypertension.

Contraindications
Hepatic disorders, sinus bradycardia, bronchial asthma.

Side Effects/Adverse Reactions
Orthostatic hypotension, bradycardia, chest pain, ventricular dysrhythmias, drowsiness, headache, nightmares, lethargy, agranulocytosis, thrombocytopenia, sore throat, dry burning eyes.

Dosage and Routes of Administration
- Orally: 100 mg tid up to 800 mg daily
- The IV infusion (hypertensive crisis): 1–2 mg/min until desired effect.

Nursing Considerations
1. Assess:
   - Intake, output and weight daily
   - Blood pressure and pulse check every 4 hours (q4h)
   - Apical or radial pulse before administration.
2. Administer:
   - Per os (po), before food and at bedtime (hs)
   - Intravenous (IV) keep client recumbent for 3 hours.
3. Perform/Provide:
   - Storage in dry area at room temperature.
4. Evaluate:
   - Therapeutic response: Decreased BP after 1–2 weeks
   - Edema in feet, legs daily
   - Skin turgor and dryness of mucous membranes for hydration status.
5. Teach client/family:
   - Not to discontinue drug abruptly, taper over 2 weeks
   - Not to use over the counter medications containing α-adrenergic stimulants such as nasal decongestants and cold medications, unless directed by physician
   - To report bradycardia, dizziness, confusion or depression
   - To avoid alcohol, smoking and excess sodium intake
   - Take medication at bedtime to prevent the effect of orthostatic hypotension
   - Wear support hose to minimize effects of orthostatic hypotension.

Propranolol (Inderal)

Action
β-adrenergic blocker: Decreases preload, afterload, which is responsible for decreasing left ventricular end-diastolic pressure and systemic vascular resistance.

Indications
Hypertension, prophylaxis of angina pain.

Contraindications
Bronchial asthma, renal insufficiency, diabetes mellitus, cardiac failure.

Side Effects/Adverse Reactions
1. Maternal:
   - Severe hypotension, sodium retention, bradycardia, bronchospasm, cardiac failure.
2. Fetal:
   - Bradycardia and impaired fetal responses to hypoxia, intrauterine growth restriction (IUGR) with prolonged therapy, neonatal hypoglycemia.

Dosage and Routes of Administration
Orally: 80–240 mg in divided doses.

Nursing Considerations
1. Assess:
   - Pulse, BP and respirations during therapy
   - Weight daily and report excess weight gain
   - Intake and output ratio.

2. Administer:
   - Administer with 240 mL of water on empty stomach.
3. Evaluate:
   - Tolerance, if taken for long period
   - Headache, lightheadedness, decreased BP.
4. Teach client/family:
   - There may be stinging sensation when the drug comes in contact with mucous membranes
   - The drug may be taken before stressful activity exercise
   - Client compliance with treatment regimen
   - To make position changes slowly to prevent fainting.

Hydralazine

Preparations

Apresoline, Hydralyn, Rolazine.

Actions

Vasodilates arteriolar smooth muscles by direct relaxation, reduction in BP with reflex increase in cardiac function.

Indication

Essential hypertension.

Contraindications

Coronary artery disease, mitral *valvular*, rheumatic heart disease.

Adverse Effects

Maternal: Hypotension, tachycardia, arrhythmia, palpitation, acute rheumatoid state, muscle cramps, headache, dizziness, depression, anorexia, diarrhea, pruritus.

Dosage and Routes of Administration

- Orally: 100 mg/day in 4 divided doses
- Intravenous/Intramuscular bolus 20–40 mg q4–6 h.

Nursing Considerations

1. Assess:
   - Every 15 minutes BP initially for 2 hours then every hour for 2 hours and then q4h, pulse q4h
   - Blood studies: Electrolytes, complete blood count (CBC) and serum glucose
   - Intake, output and weight daily.
2. Administer:
   - To patient in recumbent position, keep in that position for 1 hour after administration.
3. Evaluate:
   - Edema in feet and legs daily
   - Skin and mucous membrane for hydration
   - Rales, dyspnea, orthopnea
   - Joint pain, tachycardia, palpitation, headache and nausea.

4. Teach client/family:
   - To take with food to increase bioavailability
   - To notify physician if chest pain, severe fatigue, muscle or joint pain occurs.

Nifedipine

Preparations

Adalat, Procardia.

Actions

- Calcium channel blocker
- Produces direct arteriolar vasodilatation by inhibition of inward calcium channels in vascular smooth muscles.

Indications

Hypertension, angina pectoris.

Contraindications

- Simultaneous use of magnesium sulfate could be hazardous due to synergistic effect
- Second or third degree heart block.

Side Effects/Adverse Reactions

Flushing, hypotension, palpitations, bradycardia, inhibition of labor, headache, fatigue and drowsiness, nausea, and vomiting.

Dosage and Routes of Administration

Orally: 5–10 mg tid.

Nursing Considerations

1. Assess:
   - Blood levels of the drug, therapeutic levels 0.025–0.1 µg/mL.
2. Administer:
   - Before meals and hs.
3. Evaluate:
   - Therapeutic response, cardiac status, BP, pulse, respiration and electrocardiogram (ECG).
4. Teach client/family:
   - To limit caffeine consumption
   - To avoid over-the-counter (OTC) drugs unless directed by the physician
   - Stress patient compliance to all aspects of drug use.

Diazoxide

Preparation

Hyperstat.

Action
Vasodilator.

Indication
Hypertensive crisis when urgent decrease of diastolic pressure is required.

Contraindications
- Diabetes, heart disease
- Diuretics should be used simultaneously.

Side Effects
1. Maternal:
   - Fluid and sodium retention
   - Inhibition of uterine contraction
   - Hyperglycemia
   - Severe hypotension
   - Palpitations.
2. Fetal:
   - Hypoxia.

Dosage and Routes of Administration
Intravenous—30–50 mg may be repeated every 10–15 minutes or continuous infusion.

Nursing Considerations
1. Assess:
   - Blood pressure q5 min for 2 hours, then q1h for 2 hours and then q4h
   - Pulse, jugular venous distention q4h
   - Serum electrolytes, CBC, serum glucose
   - Weight daily, intake and output.
2. Administer:
   - To patient in recumbent position, keep in that position for 1 hour after administration.
3. Perform/Provide:
   - Protection from light.
4. Evaluate:
   - Therapeutic response: Primarily decreased diastolic pressure
   - Edema in feet and legs
   - Hydration status
   - Dyspnea and orthopnea
   - Postural hypotension: Take BP sitting and standing.
5. Teach patient/family:
   - To limit caffeine consumption
   - To report side effects, if present
   - To comply with the regimen.

Sodium Nitroprusside

Preparations
Nipride, Nitropress.

Actions
Peripheral vasodilator, directly relaxes arteriolar, venous smooth muscle, resulting in reduction of cardiac preload and afterload.

Indications
- Hypertensive crisis
- To decrease bleeding by creating hypotension during pregnancy.

Contraindications
- Should be used in critical care unit for short time
- Compensatory hypertension is possible.

Side Effects/Adverse Reactions
1. Maternal:
   - Nausea, vomiting, severe hypotension
   - Restlessness, decreased reflexes, loss of consciousness.
2. Fetal:
   - Toxicity due to metabolites: Cyanide and thiocyanate.

Dosage and Route of Administration
Intravenous infusion—0.5–10 mg/kg/min.

Nursing Considerations
1. Assess:
   - Serum electrolytes, BUN and creatinine
   - Hepatic function [aminotransferase (AST), alkaline phosphatase (ALP) and alkaline transaminase (ALT)]
   - Blood pressure and ECG
   - Weight, intake and output.
2. Administer:
   - Using an infusion pump only
   - Wrap bottle with aluminum foil to protect from light.
3. Evaluate:
   - Therapeutic response: Decreased BP, absence of bleeding
   - Edema: Feet and legs
   - Hydration status.

DIURETICS

Diuretics are used in the following conditions during pregnancy:
- Pregnancy-induced hypertension with massive edema
- Eclampsia with pulmonary edema
- Severe anemia in pregnancy with heart failure
- Prior to blood transfusion in severe anemia
- As an adjunct to certain antihypertensive drugs, such as hydralazine or diazoxide.

Furosemide (Lasix)

Action

A loop diuretic: Acts on loop of Henle by increasing excretion of sodium and chloride.

Dosage

Tablet 40 mg, daily following breakfast for 5 days a week. In acute conditions, the drug is administered parenterally in doses of 40–120 mg daily.

Side Effects

1. Maternal:
   - Side effects include weakness, fatigue, muscle cramps, hypokalemia, hyponatremia, hypocalcemia, hypochloremic alkalosis and postural hypotension.
2. Fetal:
   - May occur due to decreased placental perfusion leading to fetal compromise. Thrombocytopenia and hyponatremia are other hazards.

Contraindications

Hypersensitivity to sulfonamides, hypovolemia.

Interactions/Incompatibilities

- Increased toxicity—lithium, skeletal muscle relaxants and digitalis
- Decreased effects of antidiabetics
- Increased anticoagulant activity
- Increased action anticoagulants.

Nursing Considerations

1. Assess:
   - Weight, intake and output daily to determine fluid loss
   - Respiration: Rate, depth and rhythm
   - Blood pressure: Lying and standing
   - Electrolytes: Sodium, chloride, potassium, BUN, blood sugar, CBC, serum creatinine, blood pH and arterial blood gases (ABGs)
   - Glucose in urine, if patient is diabetic.
2. Administer:
   - In morning to avoid interference with sleep
   - Potassium replacement, if serum potassium is less than 3.0 mEq/L
   - With food, if nausea occurs, absorption may be decreased slightly.
3. Evaluate:
   - Improvement in edema of feet, legs and sacral area
   - Signs of metabolic acidosis: Drowsiness, restlessness
   - Signs of hypocalcemia, postural hypotension, malaise, fatigue, tachycardia and leg cramps
   - Rashes and temperature elevation.
4. Teach patient/family:
   - To increase fluid intake 2–3 L/day unless contraindicated
   - To rise slowly from lying or sitting position
   - To report adverse reactions such as muscle cramps, nausea, weakness or dizziness
   - To take with food or milk
   - To take early in day to prevent nocturia.

Hydrochlorothiazide

Preparations

Esidrex, Hydrodiuril, Hydrozide.

Actions

- Sulfonamide derivative
- Acts on distal tubule by increasing excretion of water, sodium, chloride and potassium.

Uses

Edema, hypertension.

Dosage and Route

Per os, 25–100 mg/day.

Side Effects/Adverse Reactions

- Polyuria, glycosuria, frequency
- Nausea, vomiting, anorexia
- Rash, urticaria, fever
- Increased creatinine, decreased electrolytes.

Contraindications

Hypersensitivity to thiazides or sulfonamides.

Nursing Considerations

1. Assess:
   - Weight, intake and output to determine fluid loss
   - Rate, depth and rhythm of respiration
   - Blood pressure: Lying and standing
   - Electrolytes: Potassium, sodium and chloride
   - Blood sugar, BUN, CBC, serum creatinine, blood pH and ABGs
   - Glucose in urine, if patient is diabetic.
2. Administer:
   - In morning to avoid interference with sleep
   - Potassium replacement, if serum potassium is less than 3.0 mEq/L
   - With food, if nausea occurs.
3. Evaluate:
   - Improvement in edema
   - Improvement in central venous pressure (CVP)
   - Signs of metabolic acidosis, drowsiness and restlessness

- Signs of hypokalemia, postural hypotension, malaise, fatigue, tachycardia, leg cramps and weakness
- Rashes and temperature elevation.
4. Teach patient/family:
   - To increase fluid intake to 2-3 L/day unless contraindicated
   - To notify physician of muscle weakness, cramps, nausea and dizziness
   - Drug may be taken with food or milk
   - To take early in day to avoid nocturia.

Spironolactone (Aldactone)

Mode of Action

The drug antagonizes aldosterone by competitive inhibition in the distal tubules, thereby preventing the potassium excretion and decreasing the sodium reabsorption.

Dose

Initially 25 mg po may be increased to 100 mg in divided doses.

Advantages

There is no potassium loss. It has some hypotensive action.

Nursing Considerations

1. Assess:
   - Weight, intake and output daily to determine fluid loss
   - Blood pressure: Lying and standing as postural hypotension may occur
   - Serum electrolytes (sodium, potassium, chloride), BUN, blood glucose, serum creatinine and CBC.
2. Administer:
   - In morning to avoid interference with sleep
   - Potassium replacement, if serum potassium is less than 3.0 mEq/L
   - With food, if nausea occurs.
3. Evaluate:
   - Improvement in edema: Feet, legs and sacral area daily
   - Signs of metabolic acidosis—drowsiness, restlessness
   - Signs of hypokalemia: Postural hypotension, fatigue, tachycardia, leg cramps and weakness.
4. Teach client/family:
   - To increase fluid intake
   - To rise slowly from lying or sitting position
   - To take with food or milk for gastrointestinal (GI) symptoms
   - To take early in day to prevent nocturia.

TOCOLYTIC AGENTS

Tocolytic drugs can inhibit uterine contractions and used to prolong the pregnancy. In women who develop premature uterine contractions in addition to putting them to absolute bedrest and sedating, tocolytic drugs are administered in an attempt to inhibit uterine contractions.

The commonly used drugs are isoxsuprine (Duvadilan), ritodrine hydrochloride (Yutopar) and magnesium sulfate.

Isoxsuprine (Duvadilan)

Actions

Acts directly on vascular smooth muscle, causes cardiac stimulation and uterine relaxation.

Dosage and Routes

1. Initial:
   - Intravenous drip 100 mg in 5% dextrose. Rate 0.2 µg/min. To continue for at least 2 hours after the contractions cease.
2. Maintenance:
   - Intramuscular 10 mg 6 hourly for 24 hours, tablet 10 mg 6-8 hourly.

Side Effects

Hypotension, tachycardia, nausea, vomiting, pulmonary edema, cardiac arrhythmias, adult respiratory distress syndrome, hyperglycemia, hypokalemia, lactic acidosis.

Contraindications

Hypersensitivity, postpartum.

Nursing Considerations

1. Assess:
   - Pulse and BP during treatment
   - Take BP, lying and standing—orthostatic hypotension is common
   - Intensity and length of uterine contractions
   - Fetal heart tones (FHT).
2. Administer:
   - With meals to reduce GI upset.
3. Perform/Provide:
   - Storage at room temperature.
4. Evaluate:
   - Therapeutic response
   - Reduced uterine contractions
   - Absence of preterm labor
   - Increased pulse volume.
5. Teach patient/family
   - To avoid hazardous activities until stabilized on medication, dizziness may occur
   - To make position changes slowly or fainting may occur
   - To notify physician if rash, palpitations or severe flushing develops.

Ritodrine Hydrochloride (Yutopar)

Action

Uterine relaxant: Acts directly on vascular smooth muscle causes cardiac stimulation and uterine relaxation.

Dosage and Routes

1. Initial:
   a. Intravenous drip 100 mg in 5% dextrose. Rate, 0.1 mg/min gradually increased by 0.05 mg/min q10min until desired response. To continue for at least 2 hours after the contractions cease.
2. Maintenance:
   a. Tablet 10 mg 6–8 hourly.
   b. Per os 10 mg given half an hour before termination of IV, then 10 mg q2h × 24 hours, then 10–20 mg q4h not to exceed 120 mg/day.

Side Effects/Adverse Reactions

- Hyperglycemia, headache, restlessness, sweating, chills and drowsiness
- Nausea, vomiting, anorexia and malaise
- Altered maternal and FHT and palpitations.

Contraindications

Hypersensitivity, eclampsia, hypertension and dysrhythmias.

Nursing Considerations

1. Assess:
   - Maternal and FHT during infusion
   - Intensity and length of uterine contractions
   - Fluid intake to prevent fluid overload, discontinue if this occurs.
2. Administer:
   - Only clear solutions
   - After dilution 150 mg in 500 mL 5% dextrose in water (D5W) or normal saline (NS), give at 0.3 mg/mL
   - Using infusion pumps or monitor carefully.
3. Perform/Provide:
   - Positioning of patient in left lateral recumbent position to decrease hypotension and increase renal blood flow.
4. Evaluate:
   - Therapeutic response
   - Decreased intensity
   - Length of contraction
   - Absence of preterm labor
   - Decreased BP.
5. Teach patient/family:
   - To remain in bed during infusion.

ANTICONVULSANTS

The commonly used anticonvulsant is magnesium sulfate. Diazepam, phenytoin and phenobarbitone are also used.

Magnesium Sulfate

Actions

Decreases acetylcholine in motor nerve terminals, which is responsible for anticonvulsant properties thereby reduces neuromuscular irritability. It also decreases intracranial edema and helps in diuresis. Its peripheral vasodilatation effect improves the uterine blood supply and has depressant action on the uterine muscle and CNS.

Uses

It is a valuable drug lowering seizure threshold in women with pregnancy-induced hypertension. The drug is used in preterm labor to decrease uterine activity.

Dosage and Route

1. For control of seizures, 20 mL of 20% solution IV slowly in 3–4 minutes; to be followed immediately by 10 mL of 50% solution IM, and continued 4 hourly till 24 hours postpartum. Repeat injections are given only if the knee jerks are present, urine output exceeds 100 mL in previous 4 hours and the respirations are more than 10 minutes. The therapeutic level of serum magnesium is 4–7 mEq/L.
2. 4 g intravenous slowly over 10 minutes, followed by 2 g/h and then 1 g/h in drip of 5% dextrose for tocolytic effect.

Side Effects

1. Maternal: Severe CNS depression (respiratory depression and circulatory collapse), evidence of muscular paresis (diminished knee jerks).
2. Fetal: Tachycardia, hypoglycemia.

Antidote

Injection calcium gluconate 10% 10 mL IV.

Nursing Considerations

1. Assess:
   - Vital signs q15min after IV dose. Do not exceed 150 mg/min
   - Monitor magnesium levels
   - If using during labor, time contractions, determine intensity
   - Urine output should remain 30 mL/h or more, if less notify physician
   - Uterine contractions when used as tocolytic agent
   - Reflexes—knee jerk, patellar reflex.

2. Administer:
   - Only after calcium gluconate is available for treating magnesium toxicity
   - Using infusion pump or monitor carefully; IV at less than 150 mg/min circulatory collapse may occur
   - Only dilutions.
3. Perform/Provide:
   - Seizure precautions: Place client in single room with decreased stimuli, padded side rails
   - Positioning of client in left lateral recumbent position to decrease hypotension and increase renal blood flow.
4. Evaluate:
   - Mental status, sensorium, memory
   - Respiratory status: Respiratory depression, rate and rhythm, hold drug if respirations are less than 12 minutes
   - Hypermagnesemia: Depressed patellar reflex, flushing, confusion, weakness, flaccid paralysis, dyspnea
   - Respiratory rate, rhythm and reflexes of newborn if drug was given within 24-hours prior to delivery
   - Reflexes: Knee jerk and patellar reflex decrease with magnesium toxicity
   - Discontinue infusion if respiration are below 12 minutes, reflexes severely hypotonic, urine output below 30 mL/h or in the event of mental confusion or lethargy, or fetal distress.
5. Teach client/family:
   - On all aspects of the drug: Action, side effects and symptoms of hypermagnesemia
   - To remain in bed during infusion.

Diazepam (Valium)

Actions

Depresses subcortical levels of CNS, anticonvulsant and antianxiety.

Dosage and Route of Administration

- Per os, 2–10 mg tid–qid
- Intravenous, 5–20 mg (bolus), 2 mg/min, may repeat q5–10 minutes, not to exceed 60 mg, may repeat in 30 minutes, if seizures reappear.

Side Effects

- Mother: Hypotension, dizziness, drowsiness, headache
- Fetus: Respiratory depressant effect, which may last for even 3 weeks after birth, hypotonea and thermoregulatory problems in newborn.

Nursing Considerations

1. Assess:
   - Blood pressure in lying and standing positions; if systolic pressure falls 20 mm Hg, hold drug and inform physician
   - Blood studies: CBC
   - Hepatic studies.
2. Administer:
   - Intravenous into large vein to decrease chances of extravasation
   - Per os with milk or food to avoid GI symptoms.
3. Provide:
   - Assistance with ambulation during beginning therapy since drowsiness and dizziness may occur
   - Safety measures include side rails.
4. Evaluate:
   - Therapeutic response
   - Mental status, sensorium, sleeping pattern
   - Physical dependence, headache, nausea, vomiting.
5. Teach patient/family:
   - Drug may be taken with food
   - To avoid alcohol ingestion
   - Not to discontinue medication abruptly
   - To rise slowly as fainting may occur.

Phenytoin (Dilantin)

Action

Inhibits spread of seizure activity in motor cortex.

Dosage and Route of Administration

- Eclampsia: 10 mg/kg IV at the rate not more than 50 mg/min, followed 2 hours later by 5 mg/kg
- Epilepsy: 300–400 mg daily orally in divided doses.

Side Effects

1. Maternal:
   - Hypotension, cardiac arrhythmias and phlebitis at injection site.
2. Fetal:
   - Prolonged use by epileptic patients may cause craniofacial abnormalities, mental retardation, microcephaly and growth deficiency.

Nursing Considerations

1. Assess:
   - Blood studies: CBC, platelets every 2 weeks until stabilized
   - Discontinue drug if neutrophils are less than 1,600/mm^2.
2. Administer:
   - After diluting with normal saline, never water.
3. Evaluate:
   - Mental status, sensorium, affect memory
   - Respiratory depression
   - Blood dyscrasias: Sore throat, bruising.
4. Teach patient/family:
   - All aspects of drug administration, when to notify physician.

Phenobarbital (Luminal)

Actions

Decreases impulse transmission and increases seizure thresholds at cerebral cortex level.

Dose and Route of Administration

About 120–240 mg/day in divided doses.

Side Effects

1. Maternal:
   – Sedation, drowsiness, hangover, headache, hallucinations.
2. Fetal:
   – Withdrawal syndrome.

Nursing Considerations

1. Assess:
   – Blood studies, liver function tests during long-term treatment
   – Therapeutic level 15–40 mg/mL.
2. Evaluate:
   – Mental status, mood, sensorium, affect and memory
   – Respiratory depression
   – Blood dyscrasias: Fever, sore throat bruising, rash.
3. Teach patient/family:
   – All aspects of drug administration and when to notify physician.

ANTICOAGULANTS

Heparin Sodium

Action

Prevents conversion of fibrinogen to fibrin.

Indications

Deep vein thrombosis, thromboembolism, disseminated intravascular coagulation, patients with prosthetic valves in the heart.

Dosage and Routes

Administered parenterally; only 5,000–7,000 IU to be administered initially as IV push, followed by 2,500 units subcutaneously every 24 hours.

Side Effects

Leukopenia, thrombocytopenia, osteoporosis, hemorrhage, alopecia.

Nursing Considerations

1. Assess:
   – Blood studies: Hematocrit, platelets, occult blood in feces
   – Partial prothrombin time
   – Blood pressure: Signs of hypertension.
2. Administer:
   – At same time, each day to maintain steady blood levels
   – Avoid all IM injections that may cause bleeding.
3. Evaluate:
   – Therapeutic response: Decrease of deep vein thrombosis
   – Bleeding gums, petechiae, ecchymosis, black tarry feces, hematuria
   – Fever, skin rash, urticaria.
4. Teach patient/family:
   – To avoid use of drugs unless prescribed by physician
   – To use soft-bristled toothbrush to avoid bleeding gums
   – To comply with instructions
   – To recognize and to sign of bleeding—gums, under skin, urine, feces.

Warfarin Sodium (Coumadin)

Action

Interferes with blood clotting by indirect means—depresses hepatic synthesis of vitamin K-dependent coagulation factors (II, VII, IX and X).

Indications

Deep vein thrombosis, pulmonary embo-lism.

Dosage and Route

Orally 10–15 mg daily for 2 days followed by 2–10 mg at the same time each day depending upon the prothrombin time.

Side Effects

1. Maternal:
   – Hemorrhage.
2. Fetal:
   – Skeletal and facial deformities, optic atrophy, microcephaly.

Nursing Considerations

1. Assess:
   – Blood studies: Hematocrit, platelets, occult blood in feces
   – Prothrombin time
   – Blood pressure: Watch for signs of hypertension.
2. Administer:
   – At same time each day to maintain steady blood levels
   – Alone—do not give with food
   – Avoid all IM injections that may cause bleeding.
3. Perform/Provide:
   – Storage in tight container.
4. Evaluate:
   – Therapeutic response: Decrease of deep vein thrombosis

- Bleeding gums, petechiae, ecchymosis, black tarry feces, hematuria
- Fever, skin rash, urticaria.
5. Teach patient/family:
   - To avoid OTC preparations unless prescribed by physician
   - Drug may be held during menstruation
   - To use soft-bristled toothbrush
   - Stress client compliance
   - To report any sign of bleeding.

ANALGESICS

Pethidine (Meperidine)

Pethidine is synthetic narcotic analgesic agent, well-absorbed by all routes of administration.

Actions

Inhibits ascending pain pathways in CNS, increases pain threshold and alters pain perception.

Indications

Moderate to severe pain in labor, postoperative pain, abruptio placentae, pulmonary edema.

Dosage and Route of Administration

Injectable preparation contains 50 mg/mL, can be administered subcutaneous (SC), IM, IV. Its dose is 50–100 mg IM combined with promethazine 25 mg.

Contraindication

Pethidine should not be used intravenously within 2 hours and intramuscularly within 3 hours of the expected time of delivery of the baby for fear of birth asphyxia. It should not be used in cases of preterm labor and when the respiratory reserve of the mother is reduced.

Side Effects/Adverse Reactions

1. Mother:
   - Drowsiness, dizziness, confusion, headache, sedation, euphoria, nausea and vomiting.
2. Fetus:
   - Respiratory depression, asphyxia.

Nursing Considerations

1. Assess:
   - Urinary output: May cause urinary retention.
2. Administer:
   - With antiemetic (promethazine) to prevent nausea and vomiting
   - When pain is beginning to return—determine dosage interval by patient response.
3. Perform/Provide:
   - Storage in light-resistant container at room temperature
   - Assistance with ambulation
   - Safety measures: Side rails, night light, call bell within easy reach.
4. Evaluate:
   - Therapeutic response: Decrease in pain
   - Changes in CNS: Dizziness, drowsiness, euphoria
   - Allergic reactions: Rash, urticaria
   - Respiratory depression, notify physician if respirations are less than 12 minutes.
5. Teach patient/family:
   - To report symptoms of CNS changes, allergic reactions.

Fentanyl

Fentanyl is a synthetic narcotic analgesic agent.

Actions

Inhibits ascending pain pathways in CNS, increases pain threshold and alters pain perception.

Indications

Moderate to severe pain in labor, postoperative pain and as adjunct to general anesthetic.

Dosage and Routes

Intramuscular: 0.05–0.1 mg q 1–2 hours as needed (prn), available in injectable form, 0.05 mg/mL.

Contraindications

Hypersensitivity to opiates.

Side Effects/Adverse Reactions

Dizziness, delirium, euphoria, nausea, vomiting, muscle rigidity, blurred vision.

Nursing Considerations

1. Assess:
   - Vital signs
   - Note muscle rigidity.
2. Administer:
   - By injection (IM or IV), give slowly to prevent rigidity
   - Only with resuscitative equipment available.
3. Perform/Provide:
   - Storage in light-resistant container at room temperature
   - Coughing, turning and deep breathing for postoperative patients
   - Safety measures: Side rails, night light, call bell within reach.

4. Evaluate:
   - Changes in CNS: Dizziness, drowsiness, hallucination, euphoria, level of consciousness (LOC), pupil reaction
   - Allergic reaction: Rash, urticaria
   - Respiratory dysfunction, respiratory depression: Notify physician if respirations are more than 12 minutes.
5. Teach patient/family:
   - To report any symptoms of CNS changes, allergic reactions.

Promethazine (Phenergan)

Promethazine is an antihistamine, H_1-receptor antagonist belonging to the phenothiazine group.

Actions

Decreases allergic response by blocking histamine, sedative and antiemetic.

Indications

- Treatment of vomiting in pregnancy
- Sedation during labor
- Pregnancy-induced hypertension
- Combined with pethidine to prevent vomiting
- In Rh isoimmunization to decrease the production of antibodies
- Allergic reactions.

Dosage and Route of Administration

Available for oral use as 12.5 mg, 24 mg and 50 mg tablets and for parenteral use as 25–50 mg/mL solutions. The dose is 25 mg, 8 hourly orally and 25 mg intramuscularly to be repeated as necessary.

Contraindications

- Acute asthma attack
- Lower respiratory tract disease.

Side Effects/Adverse Reactions

Drowsiness, dizziness, poor coordination, fatigue, anxiety, confusion, neuritis, paresthesia.

Nursing Considerations

1. Assess:
   - Urinary output: Be alert for urinary retention, frequency, dysuria; drug should be discontinued if these occur.
2. Administer:
   - Coffee, tea and cola (caffeine) to decrease drowsiness
   - With meals if GI symptoms occur when given orally
   - Deep IM in large muscle; rotate site.
3. Perform/Provide:
   - Hard candy or gum, frequent rinsing of mouth for dryness
   - Storage in light-resistant container.
4. Evaluate:
   - Therapeutic response
   - Respiratory status: Wheezing, chest tightness
   - Cardiac status: Palpitation, hypotension, increased pulse.
5. Teach patient/family:
   - Drug may cause photosensitivity, to avoid prolonged sunlight
   - To notify physician if confusion or hypotension occurs
   - To avoid concurrent use of alcohol or other CNS depressants
   - To avoid drinking or other hazardous activity, if drowsiness occurs.

EFFECTS OF MATERNAL MEDICATIONS ON FETUS AND BREASTFEEDING INFANTS

During early embryogenesis, the drugs taken by the mother reach the conceptus through the tubal or uterine secretions by diffusion. The harmful effect on the blastocyst is usually death. In case of survival, there is chance of congenital anomalies.

From 2nd to 12th weeks (period of organogenesis), drugs taken by the mother can cause serious damages. Gross congenital malformations and even death of the fetus may result depending on the route, length of time and dose of exposure.

From the second trimester onwards, transfer of drugs takes place through the uteroplacental circulation. The drug transfer across the placenta is increased due to the lowered serum albumin concentration, which results from hemodilution. As the albumin-binding capacity of the drugs is decreased, more free drug is available for placental transfer. In addition, the metabolism of the drugs may be hampered by the increase in plasma steroids. Increased uteroplacental blood flow, increased placental surface area and decreased thickness of the placental membrane are the additional causes for increased drug transfer.

Fetotoxic or teratogenic drugs are prescribed only when the benefits outweigh the potential risks. Prior counseling is mandatory and minimum therapeutic dosage is used for shortest possible duration.

Maternal Medications with Established Teratogenic Properties and their Effects

1. *Cytotoxic drugs:* Multiple fetal malformations and abortion.
2. *Androgenic steroids, hydroxyprogesterone:* Masculinization of the female offspring.
3. *Lithium:* Increased congenital malformations when used in the first trimester, neonatal goiter, hypotonia and cyanosis.
4. *Diethylstilbestrol:* Vaginal stenosis, cervical hoods and uterine hypoplasia in female fetuses.

Possible Teratogens

1. *Antithyroid drugs:* Goiter, mental retar-dation.
2. *Oral antidiabetic drugs:* Abnormalities in the eyes, central nervous system, skeletal system and neonatal hypoglycemia.
3. *Vitamin D:* Cardiopathies, hypercalcemia and mental retardation.
4. *Lysergic acid diethylamide (LSD):* Chromosomal abnormality and stunted growth.
5. *Anticonvulsants (phenytoin, valproate):* Mental retardation, cardiac abnormalities, limb defects, neonatal bleeding, epilepsy.

Fetotoxic Drugs

1. *Aspirin:* High doses in the last few weeks can cause premature closure of ductus arteriosus, persistent pulmonary hypertension and kernicterus in the newborn.
2. *Corticosteroids (prednisolone):* Doses above 10 mg daily may produce fetal and neonatal adrenal suppression.
3. *Aminoglycosides (antibiotics, e.g. amikacin, streptomycin):* Auditory or vestibular damage.
4. *Chloramphenicol:* Peripheral vascular collapse (gray baby syndrome).
5. *Tetracycline:* Dental discoloration (yellowish) and deformity, inhibition of bony growth.
6. *Long-acting sulfonamides:* Neonatal hemolysis, jaundice and kernicterus.
7. *Nitrofurantoin (furadantin):* Hemolysis in newborn with glucose-6-phosphate dehydrogenase (G6PD) deficiency, if used at term.
8. *Vitamin K (large doses):* Hyperbilirubinemia and kernicterus.
9. *Alcohol and smoking:* Intrauterine growth retardation, preterm labor, mental retardation.
10. *Narcotics:* Depression of CNS, apnea, bradycardia and hypothermia.
11. *Anesthetic agents:* Convulsion, bradycardia, acidosis, hypoxia, hypertonia.
12. *Antihistamines:* Tachycardia, vomiting, diarrhea.
13. *Anticoagulants:* Optic atrophy, microcephaly, chondrodysplasia punctata.
14. *Diuretics:* Fetal compromise due to diminished placental perfusion.
15. *Beta blockers (antihypertensive drugs):* IUGR, fetal bradycardia and impaired fetal responses to hypoxia.

Maternal Drug Intake and Breastfeeding

Maternal drug intake of nursing mothers has adverse effects on lactation and also on the baby as it may be present in the breast milk.

Milk concentration of some drugs such as iodides may even exceed those in the maternal plasma so that therapeutic doses in the mother may cause toxicity to the infant. Certain drugs in breast milk may cause hypersensitivity in the infant when used in therapeutic doses. Transfer of drugs through breast milk depends on the following factors:

- Chemical properties
- Molecular weight
- Degree of protein binding
- Ionic dissociation
- Lipid solubility
- Tissue pH
- Drug concentration
- Exposure time.

Drugs that are nonionized, of low molecular weight and lipid soluble compounds are usually excreted through breast milk. Drugs identified as having effects on lactation and the neonates are listed below:

1. *Bromides:* Rash, drowsiness and poor feeding.
2. *Iodides:* Neonatal hypothyroidism.
3. *Chloramphenicol:* Bone marrow toxicity.
4. *Oral pill (combined preparations):* Suppression of lactation.
5. *Bromocriptine (Parlodel):* Suppression of lactation.
6. *Ergot:* Suppression of lactation.
7. *Metronidazole (Flagyl):* Anorexia, blood dyscrasias, irritability, weakness, neurotoxic disorders.
8. *Anticoagulants:* Hemorrhagic tendency (warfarin appears safe in therapeutic doses).
9. *Isoniazid:* Anti-deoxyribonucleic acid (DNA) activity and hepatotoxicity.
10. *Antithyroid drugs and radioactive iodine:* Hypothyroid-ism and goiter, agranulocytosis.
11. *Antimetabolites (methotrexate):* Anti-DNA activity, immunosuppression.
12. *Diazepam, opiates, phenobarbitone:* Sedation effect with poor sucking reflex.

Breastfeeding is discouraged for mothers on medications that are harmful for the infant **(Table 55.1)**.

TABLE 55.1: Maternal medications with established teratogenic properties and their use.

Medication	Effect on fetus	Use in therapy
Alcohol	Growth retardation, congenital defects	Avoided
Amphetamines	Congenital heart defects	Avoided
Antimetabolites	Eye abnormalities	Avoided
Anesthetics	Depressed fetal vital centers	Avoided
Antithyroid drugs	Causes goiter	Avoided
Anticonvulsants	Cleft lips/palate, congenital heart defects, abnormalities of fingers and toes	Avoided
Chloroquine	Affects ears (hearing)	Avoided
Chlorpromide	Intrauterine death	Avoided
Chloramphenicol	Neonatal gray baby	Avoided
Chlorthiazide	Decreased blood count	Avoided

Contd...

Contd...

Medication	Effect on fetus	Use in therapy
Caffeine	Abortion, growth retardation, stillbirth	Avoided
Carbamazepine	Neural tube defects	Avoided
Cocaine	Growth retardation, uterine rupture and placental insufficiency	Avoided
Glucocorticoids	Intrauterine growth retardation	Avoided
Lithium	Heart defects	Avoided
Lysergic acid diethylamide (LSD)	Chromosome abnormalities	Avoided
Metronidazole	Embriotoxic	Avoided
Estrogen	Vaginal carcinoma	Avoided
Progestogens	Masculinization of female fetus	Avoided
Phenobarbitone	Fetal bleeding is a rare complication	Used with vitamin K
Prednisolone	Cleft palate, fetal death	Used with care
Phenytoin	Fetal congenital anomalies	Avoided
Streptomycin	Fetal congenital anomalies	Avoided
Sulphonilamide	Neonatal jaundice	Avoided at term
Steroids	Congenital deformities	Used with care
Tetracycline	Effects on bones and teeth	Avoided
Trimethoprim	Antifolate action	Avoided
Thalidomide	Limb deformities	Avoided
Tolbutamide	Multiple deformities	Avoided
Valporic acid	Neural tube defects	Avoided
Warfarin	Skeletal and limb defects, low birth weight	Avoided

STUDY QUESTIONS

Short Answer Questions

1. Use of isoxsuprine (Duvadilan).
2. Use of magnesium sulfate.
3. Use of pethidine (meperidine).
4. Heparin sodium.

Essay Questions

1. Describe the use of oxytocics in obstetrics.
2. Describe the use of prostaglandins in obstetrics.

BIBLIOGRAPHY

1. Clark JB, Queener SF, Karb VB. Pharmacological Basis of Nursing Practice, 4th edition. St Louis: Mosby Year Book; 1994.
2. Dutta DC. Textbook of Obstetrics, 5th edition. Kolkata: New Central Book Company; 2001.
3. Goodman A. Goodman and Gilman's, The Pharmacological Basis of Therapeutics, 9th edition. New York: Pergamon Press; 1994.
4. Linda S. Mosby's Nursing Drug Reference. St Louis: CV Mosby; 1996.
5. McKenry LM, Salerno E. Mosby's Pharmacology in Nursing, 18th edition. St Louis: Mosby Year Book; 1992.
6. Nima B. Midwifery and Obstetrical Nursing, 2nd edition. Bangalore: EMMES Medical Publishers; 2015.
7. Parulekar VS. Textbook for Midwives, 2nd edition. Kolkata: New Central Book Company; 2001.

Vital Statistics in Obstetrics

Learning Objectives

Upon completing this chapter, the learner will be able to:
- Explain the vital events' registration system in the country and the place of it in health care.
- Describe the maternal vital statistics, the magnitude of the problem and the measures to reduce the mortality and morbidity.
- Describe the perinatal and neonatal mortality, the prevailing causes and the preventive measures for a faster decline of the rates.
- Enumerate the role of midwives for record keeping.

Many of the advances in health services have come because of public health interventions. The ability to intervene the health of population is dependent on the development of appropriate tools for measuring health, illness and interventions. Only by standardizing communication on such issues, as infant and maternal mortality, the health managers hope to target high-risk populations with effective interventions.

REGISTRATION OF VITAL EVENTS

Much importance is given for the registration of vital events (e.g. births, deaths) in all countries, as it is the precursor of health statistics. If registration of vital events is complete and accurate, it can serve as reliable source of health information.

The United Nation defines vital events registration system as including 'legal registration, statistical recording and reporting of the occurrence of, and collection, compilation, presentation, analysis and distribution of statistics pertaining to vital events, i.e. live births, deaths, fetal deaths, marriages, divorces, adoptions, legitimations, recognitions, annulments and legal separations'.

India had Births, Deaths and Marriage Registration Act since 1873, but the act provided only for voluntary registration. However, the registration system tended to be very unreliable, the data being grossly deficient in regard to accuracy, timeliness, completeness and coverage. The extent of under-registration was high in several states because of illiteracy, ignorance, lack of concern and motivation. Reasons such as lack of uniformity in the collection, compilation and transmission of data and the working of multiple registration agencies contributed to the lack of adequacy and accuracy of the data.

In an effort to improve the civil registration system, the Government of India promulgated the Central Births and Deaths Registration Act in 1969. The Act came into force in 1970. The Act provides compulsory registration of births and deaths throughout the country, and compilation of vital statistics in the states to ensure uniformity and comparability of data. The Act fixes the responsibility for reporting births and deaths, while citizens (e.g. parents and relatives) should report events occurring in their households, the heads of hospitals, nursing homes, hotels, jails or dharamshalas are to report events occurring in such institutions to the concerning Registrar. The time limit for registering the event of birth is 14 days and that of death is 7 days. In case of default, a fine up to ₹50.00 can be imposed.

MATERNAL VITAL STATISTICS

The quality of healthcare delivery system of a country is reflected by its maternal and perinatal mortality rates (PMR). During the last 50 years, there has been marked reduction in the maternal and perinatal death rates in the developed countries and to some extent in the developing countries. Maintenance of accurate vital statistics, their critical analysis and formulation of the preventive measures contributed to the reduction of death in advanced countries. Unregulated fertility, inadequate prenatal care and lack of trained birth attendants are mainly recognized as the factors responsible for high maternal and perinatal deaths in the developing countries.

MATERNAL MORTALITY

Maternal death is defined as death of a woman who is pregnant or within 42 days of the termination of pregnancy irrespective of the duration and the site of pregnancy from any cause related to or aggravated by the pregnancy or its management, but not from accidental or incidental causes.

Maternal Mortality Rate

Maternal mortality rate (MMR) measures the risk of women dying from 'puerperal causes' and is defined as:

$$\frac{\text{Total number of female deaths due to complications of pregnancy, childbirth or within 42 days of delivery from puerperal causes in an area during a given year}}{\text{Total number of live births in the same area and year}} \times 1{,}000$$

Ideally, the denominator should include all deliveries and abortions. However, the rate is expressed as a rate per 1,000 live births. In developed countries, MMR has declined significantly and because of this decline; they use the multiplying factor 100,000 instead of 1,000 to avoid fractions in calculating MMR.

In a study carried out jointly by WHO and UNICEF, it is estimated that globally some 585,000 maternal deaths occur every year from pregnancy-related causes. About 99% of these deaths occur in developing countries. For the year 1997, MMR for India was estimated as 408 per 100,000 live births. The trend has not changed much in the last 5 years. The MMR in developed countries such as the USA, the UK and Europe ranges from 5 to 8 per 100,000. The causes for high maternal mortality in India are attributed to large number of deliveries conducted at home by untrained persons, in addition, lack of adequate referral facilities to provide emergency obstetric care for complicated cases also contribute to high maternal morbidity and mortality.

Classification of Maternal Deaths

Direct Maternal Deaths (75%)

Direct maternal deaths are defined as deaths from complications of pregnancy, delivery or puerperium. Such conditions are abortion, ectopic pregnancy, preeclampsia, eclampsia, hemorrhage, chorioamnionitis and puerperal sepsis, and include any complications arising from their treatment, omissions, incorrect treatment or events resulting from any of the above.

Indirect Maternal Deaths (25%)

Indirect deaths often represent underlying medical conditions aggravated, but not caused by pregnancy. This would include conditions present before or developed during pregnancy. These are anemia, cardiac disease, diabetes, thyroid disease and connective tissue disease of which anemia is the most important single cause in the developing countries. Viral hepatitis when endemic, contributes significantly to maternal deaths.

Virtually all the direct maternal deaths demand intense scrutiny because most deaths shown to have been preventable under optimal circumstances. Indirect maternal deaths, however, may reflect the remarkable advances in medical care that allow these women to achieve reproductive age and in some cases to voluntarily undertake pregnancy in the face of enormous disadvantages.

Nonobstetric or Unrelated Deaths

Nonobstetric or unrelated deaths rate measures death of pregnant or postpartum women, which were neither caused by nor aggravated by pregnancy and include those due to motor vehicle accidents, homicides and infectious diseases such as malaria and typhoid.

Reproductive Mortality

The term reproductive mortality is used currently to include direct maternal deaths and mortality resulting from the use of contraceptives.

Magnitude of the Problem

Maternal mortality statistics reveal an alarming picture in the developing countries. Out of an estimated 585,000 annual maternal deaths in the globe, 99% are distributed in the developing countries. There are more maternal deaths in India in the space of a week than there are in Europe in a whole year. In India, 148,000 women die every year because of pregnancy and childbirth, which is about one maternal death every 4 minutes. It is further estimated that for one maternal death, at least 15 more suffer from severe morbidities.

Factors Associated with Maternal Mortality

Age

The optimum reproductive efficiency appears to be between 20 and 25 years. In the young adolescent, pregnancy carries a higher risk due to preeclampsia, cephalopelvic disproportion and uterine inertia. In women aged 35 years or over, the risk is three to four times higher.

Parity

The risk is slightly higher in primigravida and it is three times greater in para 5 or above due to postpartum hemorrhage (PPH), malpresentations and rupture of uterus. The risk is lowest in the second pregnancy.

Socioeconomic Strata

Mortality rates are higher in women of low socioeconomic level as these women are likely to be less privileged in the areas of nutrition, education, housing and prenatal care.

Antenatal Care

Availability and acceptance of antenatal care is low among women of lower socioeconomic status and those who live in rural areas of the country.

Social Factors

Presence of social evils such as illiteracy, ignorance, prejudice, inadequate maternity services and underutilization of existing facilities are responsible for increased number of avoidable maternal deaths.

Causes of Maternal Death

Hemorrhage

Hemorrhage is accounted for 20-25% of maternal deaths and is mostly due to PPH, antepartum hemorrhage (APH), abortion and ectopic gestation.

Sepsis

Deaths due to infections associated with labor and puerperium, and unsafe abortions contribute to 20-25% of deaths.

Hypertensive Disorders in Pregnancy

About 5-15% of maternal deaths are attributed to preeclampsia and eclampsia, and are mostly due to lack of antenatal care.

Anemia

About 40% of obstetric clients in the developing countries suffer from anemia and if it is severe, they may die from congestive cardiac failure during pregnancy or labor. Deaths among anemic women account for 15-20%.

Infective Hepatitis

Infective hepatitis, when present in an epidemic form, results in a mortality rate of up to 20-25% in India. This risk of death is most in the last trimester with hepatic coma and coagulation failure leading to hemorrhage.

Thromboembolism

Thromboembolism accounts for about 2-5% of deaths in India. Deaths due to thrombophlebitis are higher (15-20%) in western countries.

Lack of Assistance of Trained Personnel

A large number of deliveries take place at home without the services of trained midwifery personnel. The risk of maternal death is higher for such women and is estimated to be 1 in 41.

Preventive Measures

High maternal mortality reflects not only an inadequacy of healthcare services for mothers but also a low standard of living and socioeconomic status of the community. An attempt to lower MMR must take the following measures into consideration:

1. Early registration of pregnancy.
2. At least three antenatal checkups.
3. Improvement of nutritional status including correction of anemia.
4. Identification of high-risk cases and their referrals to appropriate referral hospitals.
5. Prevention of complications such as eclampsia, malpresentations and ruptured uterus.
6. Treatment of medical conditions such as hypertension, diabetes and tuberculosis.
7. Antimalarial and tetanus prophylaxis.
8. Integration of domiciliary, rural and institutional deliveries with efficient referral system.
9. Institutional deliveries for women with bad obstetric history and risk factors.
10. Promotion of family planning to control the number of children to not more than two and spacing of births.
11. Identification of every maternal death and searching for its causes through regular maternal mortality review conferences.
12. To provide safe delivery services to all mothers by training the traditional birth attendants (TBA), upgrading the health centers, making government vehicles available in emergencies and increasing the number of healthcare providers such as midwives, multipurpose health workers, health assistants and other ancillary personnel.
13. Frequent joint consultation amongst specialists in the management of medical disorders of pregnancy such as anemia, diabetes, hypertension and heart disease.
14. Periodic refresher courses for continuing education of all levels of health workers to highlight the preventive measures.

MATERNAL MORBIDITY

Maternal morbidity originates from any cause related to pregnancy or its management, at any time during antepartum, intrapartum and postpartum period usually up to 42 days after delivery. The parameters of maternal morbidity are:

- Temperature more than 100.4°F (38°C) and continuing for more than 24 hours
- Blood pressure more than 140/90 mm Hg
- Recurrent vaginal bleeding
- Hemoglobin less than 10.5 g% irrespective of gestational period
- Asymptomatic bacteriuria of pregnancy.

Classification

Direct Obstetric Morbidity

Direct obstetric morbidity include temporary conditions such as APH, PPH, eclampsia, obstructed labor, rupture of uterus, sepsis, ectopic pregnancy and molar pregnancy. Chronic or permanent causes of morbidity include vesicovaginal fistula (VVF), rectovaginal fistula (RVF), uterine prolapse, secondary infertility and Sheehan's syndrome.

Indirect Morbidity

Indirect conditions of morbidity are exaggerated previously existing diseases like malaria, hepatitis, tuberculosis, anemia, etc. by changes in the various systems during pregnancy.

Reproductive Morbidity

Reproductive morbidity is term the used to include obstetric morbidity, gynecological morbidity and contraceptive morbidity.

PERINATAL MORTALITY

Perinatal mortality is defined as death among fetuses weighing over 1,000 g at birth, which die before or during delivery or within the first 7 days of delivery (late fetal and early neonatal deaths). The PMR is expressed in terms of such deaths per 1,000 total births.

$$PMR = \frac{\text{Late fetal deaths (28 weeks of gestation and more) + Early neonatal deaths (1st week) in 1 year}}{\text{Live births in the same year}} \times 1,000$$

The PMR includes stillbirths and deaths within the 1st week of life. In India, stillbirths are seldom registered. Consequently, most studies on perinatal mortality in this country are hospital based. The PMR in India is reported to be 49.1 per 1,000 live births in rural areas and 32.7 per 1,000 live births in urban areas. Both rural and urban areas combined, the figure was 46.0 per 1,000 live births in 1991. In developed countries, the level has declined in the past decade for about 15–20 per 1,000 total births due to improved obstetric and perinatal technologies.

Causes of Perinatal Mortality

About two-third of all perinatal deaths occur among infants with 2,500 g weight. The causes involve one or more complications in the mother during pregnancy or labor, in the placenta, fetus or neonate.

The main causes of death are intrauterine and birth asphyxia, low birth weight, birth trauma and intrauterine or neonatal infections. The various causes of perinatal mortality may be grouped as follows:

Antenatal Causes

- *Maternal diseases:* Hypertension, cardiovascular diseases, diabetes, tuberculosis and anemia
- *Pelvic diseases:* Uterine myomas, endometriosis and ovarian tumors
- *Anatomical defects:* Uterine anomalies and incompetent cervix
- *Endocrine imbalance:* Inadequate uterine preparation
- Blood incompatibilities
- Malnutrition
- Toxemias of pregnancy
- Antepartum hemorrhage
- Congenital defects
- Advanced maternal age
- Preterm labor and preterm rupture of membranes.

Intranatal Causes

- Birth injuries
- Asphyxia
- Prolonged labor
- *Obstetric complications:* Dystocia, abnormal uterine action and malpresentation.

Postnatal Causes

- Prematurity
- Respiratory distress syndrome
- Respiratory and alimentary infections
- Congenital anomalies.

Measures for Reduction of Perinatal Mortality

Measures to reduce PMR are essential to accelerate the declining trend in neonatal and infant mortality rates (IMR). These are:

- Advice to women with medical problems to avoid pregnancy until health improves
- Birth spacing
- Tetanus toxoid immunization
- Iron and folic acid supplements for anemia control
- Early treatment of maternal complications
- Institutional delivery for women at high risk
- Immediate referral and appropriate care of emergency obstetric complications
- Safe and clean delivery practices
- Essential newborn care
- Resuscitation of newborns without spontaneous cry at birth.

Preventive Measures

Many of the perinatal deaths are preventable with proper care and good organizational set-up. The following measures may help greatly in reducing the perinatal mortality:

1. Prepregnancy health care and counseling.
2. Genetic counseling to detect genetic, chromosomal or structural abnormalities.
3. Regular antenatal care, with advice regarding health, diet and rest.

4. Improvement of maternal nutrition.
 5. Screening of high-risk mothers: Those of poor socioeconomic status, high parity, very young and those with multiple pregnancies for hospital delivery.
 6. Careful monitoring during labor and avoidance of traumatic vaginal delivery.
 7. Efficient neonatal service for preterm babies.
 8. Health education to mothers about care of newborn.
 9. Autopsy studies of perinatal deaths.
 10. Continued study of perinatal mortality problems.

Stillbirths

A stillbirth is a birth of newborn after 28 completed weeks (weighing 1,000 g or more) and the baby does not breathe or show any sign of life after delivery. Such deaths include antepartum deaths (macerated) and intrapartum deaths (fresh stillbirths).

Stillbirth rate is the number of such deaths per 1,000 total births (live and still).

Causes

Antepartum deaths

1. Pregnancy complications such as preeclampsia and APH.
2. Pre-existing medical diseases and acute illnesses during pregnancy such as chronic hypertension, diabetes, chronic nephritis, syphilis, hyperpyrexia (malaria), severe anemia and infections.
3. Fetal causes such as congenital malformations, Rh-incompatibility and postmaturity.
4. Iatrogenic as due to administration of quinine group of drugs and external version.
5. Placental insufficiency.

Intrapartum deaths

The common causes are:
- Acute fetal distress
- Traumatic vaginal delivery leading to asphyxia or intracranial hemorrhage
- Asphyxia especially in premature babies
- Congenital malformations of the fetus.

NEONATAL MORTALITY

Neonatal deaths are deaths occurring during the neonatal period, commencing at birth and ending at 28 completed days after birth. Neonatal mortality rate (NMR) is the number of neonatal deaths in a given year per 1,000 live births in that year. It is tabulated as:

$$\text{NMR} = \frac{\text{Number of deaths of babies under 28 days of age in a year}}{\text{Total live births in the same year}} \times 1{,}000$$

Causes of Neonatal Deaths

About two-third of the neonatal deaths are related to prematurity and majority of the deaths occur within 48 hours of birth:

- Low birth weight
- Birth injury due to difficult labor
- Congenital anomalies
- Hemolytic disease of the newborn
- Conditions of placenta and cord
- Acute respiratory infections
- Tetanus
- Diarrheal diseases.

As the high concentration of neonatal deaths occur in the early neonatal period, there is need to improve the antenatal and postnatal services to mothers. Neonatal mortality is seen greater in boy babies throughout the world, because newborn boys biologically are more fragile.

Neonatal mortality varies from 53 per 1,000 live births for the least developed countries to about 5 per 1,000 live births for the developed countries. In India, about 50–60% of infant death occurs within the neonatal period (first 28 days). Of these, more than half may die during the 1st week of birth, first 24 hours being the time of greatest risk. The NMR for the year 1995 was 50 per 1,000 live births.

INFANT MORTALITY RATE

Infant mortality rate is defined as the ratio of infant deaths registered in a given year to the number of live births registered in the same year; usually expressed as a rate per 1,000 live births. It is given by the formula:

$$\text{IMR} = \frac{\text{Number of deaths of children less than 1 year of age in a year}}{\text{Number of live births in the same year}} \times 1{,}000$$

During the past decades, there have been steady decline in IMR throughout the world and more so in the developed countries. By 1980s, most developed countries achieved rates below 10 per 1,000 live births. India had the goal of reducing the IMR of 72 in 1998 to 60 per 1,000 live births by the year 2000.

The decline in infant mortality has been attributed to:
1. Improved obstetric and perinatal care, e.g. availability of oxygen, fetal monitoring during labor, improved techniques for induction of labor.
2. Improvement in the quality of life, i.e. economic and social progress.
3. Better control of communicable diseases, e.g. immunization and oral rehydration.
4. Advances in chemotherapy, antibiotics and insecticides.
5. Better nutrition especially emphasis on breastfeeding.
6. Family planning, e.g. birth spacing.

In India, the states, those have higher female literacy and improved primary health care have achieved lower IMR.

RECORD KEEPING

Records of activities and events related to vital statistics that occur in healthcare facilities, such as in hospitals and primary health centers must be maintained as accurate and complete as possible. Standard forms and acceptable formats are often available in the workplace. Midwives functioning in different settings are required to keep detailed records, which must be made as contemporaneously as is reasonable.

Records commonly maintained by midwives include:
1. Antenatal record for individual clients in which details of the pregnancy and treatments prescribed is entered.
2. Antenatal register with record of all women attending the clinic.
3. Birth register with details of childbirth, including mode of delivery, sex of the baby, birth weight, weight of placenta, Apgar score, etc.
4. Postnatal record contains details of childbirth, condition of the newborn, condition of the mother, etc.
5. Under-five record/card: A card for each baby with information such as serial weight and height, immunization, weaning and vitamin supplements given. These are entered until the child becomes 5 year old.
6. Eligible couples register: Record of all couples in the reproductive age group and the mode of contraceptives used is maintained in the health centers.
7. Register for recording contraceptives: Condom distribution, oral pill register, register for intrauterine device (IUD), and sterilization register for males and females.
8. Morbidity registers for different categories of clients.
9. Admission and discharge register.
10. Outpatient treatment register: Name, diagnoses and treatments given to patients.
11. Referral register.
12. Stock register.
13. Contraceptive follow-up register.
14. Death register: Record of all deaths of mothers and babies including details such as full name, age address, age at the time of death and cause of death.

General Guidelines for Maintaining Records

1. All information must be entered in the proper place/particular column in the appropriate register or record.
2. Information must be entered as soon as possible to avoid incompleteness and inaccuracies.
3. All information to be written clearly and legibly for use by supervisors and others for statistical and related purposes.
4. All records must be arranged in order and safeguarded.
5. Records should be treated as confidential material and away from handling by unauthorized persons.
6. All records should be kept safely for prescribed period of time, minimum period of 5 years in government institutions.

All the records written must be legible, accurate and complete with all the required details for effective tabulation and communication. The information may be used currently as well as retrospectively and hence, all records and reports must be preserved.

STUDY QUESTIONS

Short Notes
1. Maternal mortality.
2. Stillbirth.

Short Answer Questions
1. Factors associated with maternal mortality.
2. Causes of neonatal mortality in India.
3. Causes of infant mortality in India.

Essay Questions
1. Explain the causes of maternal deaths in India and preventive measures being taken.
2. Explain perinatal mortality, its causes and measures for reduction and prevention.

BIBLIOGRAPHY

1. Dutta DC. Textbook of Obstetrics, 5th edition. Kolkata: New Central Book Company; 2001. pp. 642-50.
2. Government of India, MCH Division. National Child Survival and Safe Motherhood Program; 1994.
3. Hogarth J. Glossary of Health Care Terminology. Copenhagen: WHO; 1978.
4. National Institute of Health and Family Welfare. Reproductive and Child Health Module for Staff Nurses' Integrated Skill Development Training. Munirka, New Delhi: NIHF; 2000.
5. Park K. Park's Textbook of Preventive and Social Medicine, 16th edition. Jabalpur: Banarsidas Bhanot Publishers; 2000. pp. 305-50.
6. WHO. Health for All Series, No. 4; 1981.

CHAPTER 57

Perinatal Loss and Grief

Learning Objectives

Upon completing this chapter, the learner will be able to:
- Describe the grief situations in perinatal period.
- Describe the nature of perinatal grieving/mourning.
- Explain the phases of mourning.
- Explain the help to be given to grieving parents.
- Explain the care needed by caregivers.

All expectant parents expect a healthy baby as the outcome of pregnancy. For most parents and families, healthy pregnancy, normal childbirth and healthy baby are realities, but for a few others the reality is loss, grief and mourning. The grieving parents experience the death of their infant, along with the end of their hopes and dreams for the infant. When an unexpected death or loss occurs, there is disappointment and loss of what could have been. A person's response to the loss results from a combination of factors such as life experience, education, culture, tradition and beliefs. The feeling of being in crisis and the need for support can depend on the type of loss experienced, and on the background and beliefs of the person. Caring for mothers who confront perinatal or neonatal loss are occasional yet important grief situations a midwife has to deal with. Providing assistance to cope with the loss through healthy grieving process is important for resumption of balance or homeostasis in the life of the bereaved person.

LOSS, GRIEF AND MOURNING

Loss

Loss is defined as the anticipated or actual removal of something or someone of value to a person. Perinatal loss includes those which involve loss of the baby to abortion, miscarriage, stillbirth or having a baby, but with loss of expectations of perfect baby image, such as prematurity or congenital abnormalities.

Grief

Grief is an intense and personal experience, manifested as emotional reactions in response to a significant loss. When it is related to perinatal loss, it is termed perinatal grief. Grief as a response of sadness to a death has common characteristics although the process is very individual. A person's response to a death or loss depends on culture, traditions, reaction to past losses, circumstances surrounding the death and the perceived available support networks.

Mourning

Mourning is the expression of sorrow with outward signs of grief, which include crying, fatigue, feeling of emptiness and a depressed mood. The process of mourning involves accepting the loss and experiencing the pain in response to the loss and redirecting the energy from grieving to reconstruction of one's life.

REPRODUCTIVE LOSS

Reproductive loss includes those which involve loss of the baby to abortion, miscarriage, stillbirth or having a baby, but with loss of expectations of perfect baby image such as prematurity or congenital abnormalities, neonatal death or relinquishment (a mother's decision to give up her right to parent her child).

Perinatal loss triggers many obvious signs of grieving process. Feelings of guilt and anger are more common. Delivery of an infant with congenital anomaly or an infant who is relinquished is considered incomplete losses and may lead to a chronic grief state. Expectations and dreams of the infant are never fulfilled.

Loss of the Perfect Baby

Once the pregnancy test result is positive, a woman begins to make plans. She knows the possible due date and begins to fantasize about her child's future. Her hopes and dreams that may extend into the child's adult years can be halted abruptly by the birth of an infant who does not meet the parents' expectations or by the death of the infant. Parents will grieve the loss of their expectations, which may be a full-term healthy baby boy or girl with certain features. They also grieve the loss of the idealized infant before they will be able to adapt and attach to the real child. Parents of premature infants and infants who have anomalies or deformities will ask themselves how a thing such as this could have happened.

As the parents attempt to attach, they also have concerns that the baby may not survive. The roller coaster of emotions may be overwhelming. The degree of their grief reaction may not be equal to the level of severity or critical state of the child. It is the personal meaning of the anomaly or the reaction to shock of not having the baby they imagined that will give form to the grief. It is frightening to see one's infant for the first time attached to equipment and wires. The death of an infant will have a lifelong effect on the family. The care provided to them in the hospital and the follow-up care during the first 18 months after the death will shape their future.

Grief Situations in the Perinatal Period

Feeling of loss and the need to grieve may occur at any time in the childbearing period:
- Grieving related to infertility occurs in those who have difficulty to conceive.
- Spontaneous and induced abortions, termination of pregnancy for fetal abnormalities and ectopic pregnancies are losses in the first and early second trimester.
- Intrauterine fetal deaths, induced abortions and premature births are losses in the late second and third trimesters.
- Stillbirths, neonatal deaths and birth of infants with congenital anomalies are losses in the immediate period before and after childbirth.
- Birth of a baby of a sex different from that expected by the parents is a grief situation for some.
- Mothers who choose elective termination of pregnancy also mourn their infants.
- Death of an infant in the neonatal nursery following the immediate period after birth is also included as perinatal loss.
- The baby with a handicap, which may or may not be expected.

Nature of Perinatal Loss and Grief

Perinatal loss and grief are different from other types of grief in several respects.

Intense Feelings

For parents who experience an outcome of pregnancy different from their expectation and from the experience of most people they know, the feelings are intense. To them a traumatic event has substituted for what was expected to be a joyful event.

Anticipatory Grief

When an intrauterine fetal anomaly or death is diagnosed before the onset of labor, there may be few hours or days of anticipatory grief.

Emotional and Physical Stress

In some instances, perinatal loss follows a period of maternal illness. This leaves parents emotionally and physically stressed.

Mourning

Mourning in the absence of a visible object or baby. For losses in the first trimester, parents mourn the absence of a visible object or baby.

Guilt and Anger

With abortions or miscarriages, they experience the loss of both the baby and the pregnancy, and feel guilt if they engaged or failed to engage in activates, they think were related to the experience. When a seemingly perfect baby is stillborn or extremely premature, there is also aggravated guilt and anger, wondering if they failed to do something.

Loss of Relationship

A mother develops a unique and special relationship with her fetus during pregnancy that is different from her relationship to any other person. As a result, when the baby is lost either before birth or after birth, her experience of loss is also different from any other loss.

Limited Memories

When a baby is lost to miscarriage, to stillbirth or to loss in immediate period after birth, there are limited memories. For some it may be an ultrasound image, a single photograph or remembering the feel of a fetal kick.

Social Support

Family and friends may not recognize the significance of the loss to the parents and therefore, may not provide adequate support. The parents experiencing the loss may feel the need to be strong for each other. The loss often diminishes the ability of each to talk about the loss with the other.

SYMPTOMS OF NORMAL GRIEF

Upon perceiving the loss, the individual begins experiencing several distress symptoms in progressive manner:
- Acute distress—sensation of somatic distress occurring in waves and lasting 20–60 minutes
- Feeling of tightness in the throat
- Choking with shortness of breath
- Need for sighing (recovering oxygen level in the baby)
- Empty feeling in the stomach

- Lack of muscular power
- Intense subjective distress described as tension
- Frequent crying
- Slight sense of unreality
- Preoccupation with the image of the deceased
- Preoccupation with guilt ("I only.....")
- Irritability and anger
- Restlessness
- Lack of energy

PHASES OF GRIEVING/MOURNING

The stages grief through which a person is likely to have to work has been described by Kübler-Ross (1970). These stages are not negotiated in a consistent, sequential order and there will be individual variations. Often a person moves back and forth through them, eventually achieving resolution.

The stages of mourning include initial shock and disbelief, a phase of anxiety and searching, a phase of disorganization and a phase of resolution (reorganization). Each phase is characterized by physical symptoms, behaviors and feelings. Feelings such as anger or guilt may appear to be resolved, only to reappear at a later time. Feelings, behaviors and physical symptoms may intensify at certain times and worn out at other times.

Period of Shock and Denial (24 Hours to 3 Weeks)

Shock is always the initial response to loss. Responses associated with shock include disbelief, crying, wanting to escape and becoming numb or incoherent. The initial responses comprise a defense mechanism, which serves to protect the individual from the full impact of the loss in the period immediately after the loss. In this period, they may verbalize statements of denial and show apathy, inappropriate behavior, unexplained calm, impaired concentration, difficulty in decision-making and physical detachment. These feelings may last from several days to weeks. It is important for midwives to recognize that denial is a defense mechanism that serves a useful purpose of giving the person time to mobilize her coping recourses. As decision-making is difficult at this stage, they will need help.

Phase of Anxiety and Searching (3 Weeks to 7 Months)

Anxiety and searching is the second phase of mourning, which is commonly intense from the 2nd–4th or 5th month after a loss. Feelings of sorrow may be easily apparent. Some of the less acceptable emotions include guilt, anger and sorrow as well as compulsive searching and more worrying. Realization dawns in waves as the bereaved person tries various coping strategies to 'bargain' with herself to delay accepting the reality.

Phase of Disorganization (Intensity Reduces by 7 Months)

During this period, they find it difficult to accomplish their normal tasks. Physical symptoms such as body ache, restlessness, malaise and anorexia may be experienced. Feelings such as sadness, lowered self-esteem, social withdrawal and preoccupation with the lost baby are some of the characteristics of this period.

Resolution or Reorganization (18–24 Months)

In this stage, the restoration of the capacity to interact with others and to plan for the future takes place. This process may be slow and vary with setbacks in different individuals. Although, a mother is never likely to get over her loss, she will probably be able to eventually integrate it into her experience of life. This ultimate degree of resolution is recognizable in the person's ability to contemplate realistically the strengths and weaknesses of her lost relationship. Family relationships stabilize and the capacity to concentrate on activities and to interact with others is restored.

PATHOLOGICAL GRIEF

Pathological grief is a distortion of the normal bereavement process. Behaviors in the pathological grief are:
1. Over activity without a sense of loss.
2. Initial episodes or exacerbations of diseases known to be associated with stress or psychosomatic conditions such as ulcerative colitis, rheumatoid arthritis and asthma.
3. Alterations in relationship with friends and relatives owing to feelings of irritability and a marked desire to be left alone, which leads to progressive social isolation.
4. Furious hostility against a specific person, particular professionals such as physicians and nurses.
5. Lasting loss of social interaction patterns that also include lack of decision-making and lack of initiative to participate in social activities without the intervention of another individual.
6. Activities detrimental to personal, economic and social existence including spending large sums of money or engaging in activities such as excessive drinking.
7. Agitated depression including tension, insomnia and feeling of restlessness, bitter self-accusation and suicidal tendencies.

Caring for a Bereaved Family

Many of the behaviors that began in the initial crisis period will continue through the continuum of care. Nursing interventions to assist parents who face stillbirth or neonatal death goes through the mourning process requires several support strategies.

Immediate Support

Immediate support includes calling a support person such as a close friend, family or clergy and ensuring that the mother is not left alone.

Attitude and Empathy

The attitude and empathy of the staff are important in terms of how the process is remembered and perhaps resolved.

Conveying an understanding that each fetus or infant is special and significant to the mother is important.

Validating the Loss

This includes understanding and accepting the family's feelings about their loss and encouraging the acceptance of the baby's existence:
1. Be sensitive to the family's cultural values related to disposing the infant's body.
2. Encourage the father to share the grief of the mother and participate in her care.
3. Avoid rationalizing that she would have another baby and not to worry.
4. Provide opportunity to grieve and encourage verbalizing their feelings.
5. Hold or touch the mother when she cries, to convey a feeling of caring.
6. Give some mementos for the mother to keep such as a card with information of the baby, a lock of hair or certificate of life or death.

Making the Loss Real

1. Prepare parents for what they will see, if they choose to see and hold the dead baby. Give them some description like body temperature, color, size, bruises and deformities.
2. Stay with them unless they request time alone, allow the parents to see and hold the dead baby if they wish.
3. Wrap the baby in a clean and warm blanket or sheet; the care taken with the baby demonstrates respect.
4. Refer to the baby by name; if a name has been given; if no name, refer to the baby by the correct sex.
5. If the parents wish, take a photograph of the baby.
6. Encourage parents to have a burial or funeral for the baby.
7. Discuss medical findings and autopsy results (if done) in a frank and sensitive manner.

For Mothers Who Grieve the Loss through Miscarriage

1. Convey an understanding that they mourn their fantasized baby.
2. Empathize the intense grieving they go through.
3. Provide privacy and support as they go through the process.

Death of an Infant in the Nursery

When a baby dies after surviving the immediate period of days or weeks, parents need special help:
1. During the period between birth and death, encourage parents to spend as much time as possible with their baby.
2. Provide opportunities to hold and touch the baby or care for the baby as appropriate.
3. Provide opportunity to be with the baby in the final period before death.
4. Immediately after death, be with the family or be available for support and family should not be left to feel alone or abandoned.

RIGHTS OF PARENTS WHEN AN INFANT DIES

When an infant dies, parents need special attention and care, and their rights to such care must be respected. Their rights to be respected include:
1. To be given the opportunity to see, hold and touch their baby any time before or after death within reason and to be alone with their baby.
2. To have photographs taken of their baby and to make them available when they wish to see them.
3. To be given as many mementos as possible, i.e. the crib card, identification bands, ultrasound pictures, a lock of hair, footprints and a record of the baby's weight and length.
4. To name their baby and to bond with the baby.
5. To be cared for by an empathetic staff, who respects their feelings, thoughts, beliefs and individual requests.
6. To be with each other as much as possible throughout hospitalization.
7. To be informed of the grieving process.
8. To have information presented in terminology understandable to the parents regarding their baby's status and cause of death, pathology reports and medical records.
9. To plan a farewell ritual, burial or cremation in accordance with their personal beliefs or cultural traditions.
10. To be provided with information about support resources that assist in the healing process.

CARING FOR THE CAREGIVER

The sense of loss and grief that accompanies perinatal loss is not limited to parents and family members. Nurses and other professionals grieve as well. Before nurses can be helpful to parents and families, they must recognize their own potential for grief. It is difficult for most nurses not to identify with young parents who grieve. Many nurses are in their own childbearing years and some may have experienced a perinatal loss themselves or may fear such a loss in the future. Shock and disbelief may be experienced for loses which occur suddenly. The inability to prevent the death may be perceived as a threat to self-esteem. They may try to cope with their anxiety by remaining detached. There may be feelings of anger at the baby, parents or other team members. Nurses need opportunities to express their feelings and ask questions. They need acceptance of colleagues. An effective counseling service and team spirit will prevent staff burnout.

RECORD KEEPING

Records regarding fetal demise, infant death or miscarriage are essential for accurate vital statistics of the country and for taking measure for preventing such occurrences in future when possible. Details of events and management must therefore be entered in all the relevant records and registers.

CONTINUED CARE

Ongoing support of the grieving mother/parents will need to be provided by community health nurses or other health workers. The suppression of lactation may require particular attention during this period. If follow-up at home cannot be arranged, clear and detailed instructions will have to be given before the parents leave the hospital. For a mother to go through a healthy grieving process and to come to terms with her loss, the care and attention given to her must be of the highest standard, empathetic and individualized.

NURSING PROCESS FOR THE CLIENT EXPERIENCING A LOSS

Nursing process provides a structure to make certain that all steps in caring for a family experiencing loss are addressed.

Assessment

1. History of pregnancy including any medications and complications for the mother.
2. Whether pregnancy was wanted or unwanted.
3. Whether parents had other pregnancy losses.
4. Physical and emotional health during pregnancy.
5. Support of friends and family.
6. Grief behaviors such as sleep disturbances, dependence, withdrawal, anger or guilt.

Nursing Diagnoses

1. Fear related to the initial diagnosis of pregnancy loss or infant death as evidenced by increased tension and expression of dread.
2. Ineffective coping related to inadequate social support as evidenced by lack of goal-directed behavior, poor coordination or fatigue.
3. Spiritual distress related to perinatal loss as evidenced by energy consuming anxiety, physical and psychological stress.
4. Health-seeking behaviors related to effective managing of adaptive tasks by family as evidenced by the family moving in the right direction of health-promoting lifestyle that promotes maturation process.

Expected Outcomes

1. Mother and father will be able to work through the bereavement process, each at their own pace with understanding and support for each other.
2. Parents will go through mourning process making healthy adaptations and seeking necessary support.
3. At 1 or 2 years after the loss, the parents will be able to identify positive growth for them from the experience.

Nursing Interventions

Physical Care

1. After delivery, the mother has same needs for physical care, as does a mother whose baby was born alive. For example, nutrition, perineal care, postpartum exercise, postpartum recovery of genital organs.
2. Implement measures for milk suppression and reduction of discomfort of engorged breasts, because there is no infant to empty the breasts.

Psychological and Emotional Care

1. Keep parents and family informed of the situation.
2. Support seeing and holding the infant, and create memories including photographs and mementos.
3. Support decision-making regarding paper work and disposition of infant's body.
4. Listen to stories and concerns.
5. Encourage choices and increased sense of control.

Educational Care (Health Education)

1. Provide instructions for self-care and related pamphlets or leaflets.
2. Discuss bereavement process.
3. Encourage questions and concerns.
4. Address issues such as burial arrangements, funeral and informing other children (siblings), friends and others who know the mother was pregnant.
5. Identify available resources such as support groups, reading materials and websites.
6. Follow-up visits by health workers in the home and/or clinic or hospital in the community.

Evaluation

1. Ongoing evaluation of the bereavement process.
2. Referral to social services if appropriate.

STUDY QUESTIONS

Short Notes

1. Perinatal loss.
2. Perinatal grief.
3. Perinatal mourning.

Short Answer Questions

1. Grief situations in perinatal period.
2. Phases of perinatal mourning.

Essay Question

1. A mother who gave birth to a full term, stillborn baby is assigned to you as one of four postpartum mothers.

Describe your nursing care to the mother in assisting her go through the mourning process.

BIBLIOGRAPHY

1. Glen D. Undertaking Mourning. Minneapolis, MN: Augsburg Publishing House; 1984.
2. Iles S. The loss of early pregnancy. In: Oats MR (Ed). Psychological Aspects of Obstetrics and Gynecology. London: Bailliere Tindall; 1989.
3. Kowalski K. Perinatal loss and bereavement. In: Sonstegard L, Kowalski K, Jennings B (Eds). Women's Health: Crisis and Illness in Childbearing. Orlando: Grune & Straffon; 1987.
4. Kübler-Ross E. On Death and Dying. London: Tavistock Publications; 1970.
5. Lewis E, Bourne S. Perinatal death. In: Oates M (Ed). Psychological Aspects of Obstetrics and Gynecology. London: Bailliere Tindall; 1989.
6. Littleton LV, Engebretson JC. Maternity Nursing Care. Haryana: Thomson Delmar Learning, Sanat Printers; 2007. pp. 343-96.
7. Littlewood J. Aspects of Grief: Bereavement in Adult Life. London: Tavistock Publications, Rutledge; 1992.
8. Ma Caffery M. Nursing Management of the Patient with Pain. Philadelphia: Lippincott; 1979.
9. Nicholas FN, Zwelling E. Maternal Newborn Nursing: Theory and Practice. Philadelphia: WB Saunders Co; 1997.
10. Nima B. Midwifery and Obstetrical Nursing, 2nd edition. EMMES Medical Publishers; 2015.
11. O'Hare T, Creed F. Life events and miscarriage. Br J Psychiatry. 1995;167(6):799-805.
12. Rådestad I, Steineck G, Nordin C, et al. Psychological complications after stillbirth-influence of memories and immediate management: population based study. BMJ. 1996;312(7045):1505-8.

CHAPTER 58

Radiology and Ultrasonics in Obstetrics

Learning Objectives

Upon completing this chapter, the learner will be able to:
- Describe the use of radiology in obstetrics and list the hazards of radiation.
- Enumerate the use of ultrasound in the present day obstetric practice.
- Describe how ultrasound works and the different methods available for diagnostic purposes.
- Explain the responsibilities of midwives regarding prenatal ultrasound screening.

RADIOLOGY IN OBSTETRICS

Radiology in obstetrics is used mainly to supplement and confirm findings, which have been made on clinical examination during pregnancy. Until recently, radiological examinations have been used extensively in obstetric clients. With the advent of ultrasonography and magnetic resonance imaging (MRI), the use of radiology is declining. Currently, radiological examinations are done on pregnant women only if the following principles are met:
- The benefits of radiation must outweigh the risks of the procedure
- Minimum radiation dose to be used
- Appropriate fetal shielding to be done
- First trimester should preferably be avoided
- Benefits and safety of ultrasonography must be considered as an alternative.

Indications

- *Diagnosis of pregnancy:* The fetal skeletal shadow is visible at 16th week of pregnancy.
- *Diagnosis of hydatidiform mole:* Negative fetal shadow beyond 16th to 18th week.
- *Multiple pregnancies:* To confirm the diagnosis, to note the lie of the fetus and to exclude malformations.
- *Hydramnios:* To exclude multiple preg-nancies and to diagnose congenital bone malformations such as open spina bifida or anencephaly.
- *Intrauterine death of the fetus:* Overlapping of skull bones and hyperflexion of the spine may be present.
- Diagnosis of congenital anomalies such as the extent of imperforate anus, intestinal obstruction, diaphragmatic hernia.
- *Diagnosis of limb defects* such as amelia (absence of limb), ectromelia (absence of a part of a limb), phocomelia (absence of proximal part of a limb) and mermaid (single lower limb).
- *Fetal maturity:* Evidenced by overall fetal shadow, thickness and density of ossification centers of the upper end of the tibia and lower end of the femur (usually after 38 week).
- Placental localization.
- Pelvimetry in cases suspected to have pelvic contraction.
- Secondary abdominal pregnancy.
- Hydrops fetalis.
- *Amniography:* Abnormalities such as atresia of gastrointestinal tract could be revealed.
- Patients having cardiopulmonary disease may require X-ray during pregnancy.

Radiation Hazards

The risk is primarily based on the estimated dose of radiation and period of gestation:
1. *Teratogenic effects:* Irradiation of less than 5 rad is not associated with any defects. Higher doses can cause microcephaly, mental retardation, cataracts, retinal degeneration, cleft palate, hypoplasia of genitalia, etc.
2. *Oncogenicity:* Fetal exposure in the first trimester is associated with an increased risk of malignancy.

Measures that Help to Reduce Radiation

- Avoiding as far as possible any radiological examination during pregnancy
- Use of minimum essential plates
- Use of high frequency X-rays
- Use of short exposure times
- Use of fast films
- Use of filters
- Use of screens when possible, e.g. shielding of the abdomen during chest radiography.

ULTRASONICS IN OBSTETRICS

The ultrasound is a sound wave beyond the audible range of frequency greater than 2 MHz (cycles per second). The commonly used frequency range in obstetrics is 3.5–5 MHz. SONAR stands for 'sound, navigation and ranging'. In clinical practice, two main varieties of ultrasound (sound that is produced at a very high pitch) are used depending upon whether the reflected waves give audible or visual signals:

1. The apparatus, which interprets the audible signals—doptone and sonicaid are easy to carry and simple to use even with batteries. It can detect fetal heartbeats as early as 10th week of gestation.
2. The apparatus for interpretation of visible signals—the sonar system, which is a much more sophisticated and bulky apparatus, is used in three forms:
   a. The A-scan, that gives a one-dimensional picture.
   b. The B-scan, that gives a composite two-dimensional picture.
   c. The real-time scanner that depicts movements to display cardiac and breathing activity.

How does Ultrasound Work?

Scanners are used to produce static pictures. The picture is built up as a single crystal transducer (a thin disk to which a wire is attached), which is moved backwards and forwards across the area scanned. When the transducer is placed on the body and as it encounters a structure, a fraction of that sound is reflected back. The echo is detected electronically and transmitted on to the screen as dots. The amount of sound from each organ varies according to the type of tissue encountered:

- Strong echoes give bright dots, e.g. bone
- Weaker echoes give various shades of gray according to their strength
- Fluid-filled areas cause no reflexion and give rise to a black image.

Real-time scanners are so called because it produces a moving picture on the screen as opposed to scanners that give static picture. The real-time scanner can have several types of transducers attached to it, which are interchangeable and are used according to the type of image needed and the part of the anatomy to be examined. Types of transducers in common use include—the linear array; the curved linear array; the sector and the vaginal probe. Instead of a single crystal, all these types of transducers have many crystals that fire off electrical energy and collect the echoes very rapidly, thus producing the moving picture.

Use of Ultrasound in Obstetrics

Sonography is a non-invasive procedure and has been proved safe to the conceptus, even with repeated exposures at any stage of pregnancy. Routine sonography in early months is used for:

1. *Diagnosis of pregnancy:* Detects gestational ring at 5th week, fetal poles and gestational sac at 6th week, cardiac pulsation at 7th week and embryonic movements at 8th week of gestation.
2. Detection of abnormal conceptus prior to clinical manifestations and fetal malformations.
3. Accurate determination of gestational age is possible, which is helpful later in pregnancy when intrauterine growth restriction (IUGR) is suspected. For this, crown-rump length (CRL) at 10–11 weeks gives the best predictive value.
4. Diagnosis of twins can be made early in pregnancy for effective management.
5. To diagnose unsuspected placenta previa: Because of the possibility of placental migration to the upper segment, repeat scanning should be performed later at around 34th week **(Figs. 58.1 and 58.2)**.

Selective Sonography

Selective sonography is done when indicated at any time during pregnancy for the following reasons:

1. To determine the maturity of the fetus: Biparietal diameter (BDP), CRL and femur length (FL) are the measurements of choice for assessment of gestational age. Determination of the maturity is important in cases of:
   - Uncertain gestational age
   - Discrepancy between amenorrhea and uterine size
   - Prior to elective induction for postmaturity or elective cesarean section.
2. Suspicion of fetal and/or placental abnormalities such as:
   - Suspected ectopic pregnancy
   - Blighted ovum (empty sac)
   - Incomplete abortion
   - Hydatidiform mole
   - Localization of placenta as in placenta previa
   - Abruptio placentae
   - Intrauterine growth retardation
   - Intrauterine death
   - Malpresentations such as breech, transverse or face
   - Structural defects such as neural tube defects, absent or abnormal limbs
   - Defects of gastrointestinal and urinary system, and heart defects.

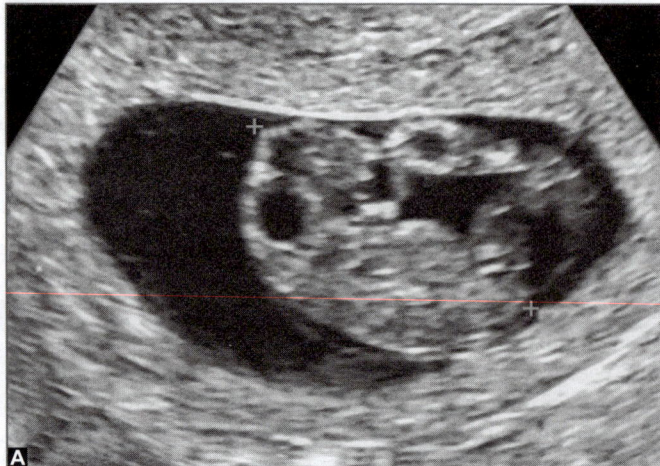

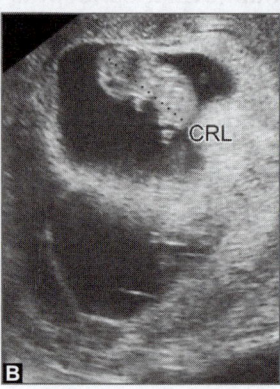

Figures 58.1A and B: Ultrasound images of fetus. (A) Fetus at 8 weeks; (B) Fetus at 6 weeks (CRL: crown-rump length).

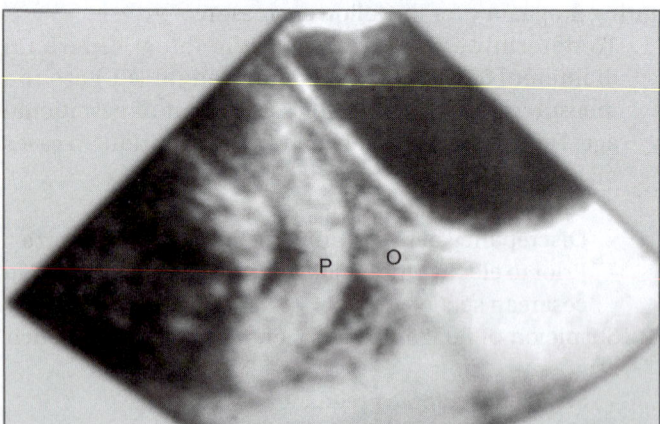

Figure 58.2: Placenta previa: Longitudinal scan shows the placenta (P) lying just above the cervical os (O).

3. Prior to invasive procedures such as chorionic villus biopsy, amniocentesis, cordocentesis, fetoscopy and intrauterine fetal therapy.
4. As a part of antepartum or intrapartum fetal surveillance: Biophysical profile.
5. Integrity of a previous cesarean scar—a weak scar or placental implantation over the scar can be detected.
6. Postpartum period:
   – Secondary postpartum hemorrhage (PPH)
   – Retained placental bits
   – Subinvolution due to fibromyoma.
7. Neonatal head screening to diagnose:
   – Intraventricular hemorrhage
   – Hydrocephalus.

Transvaginal Ultrasonography

Transvaginal ultrasonography is usually done during the first trimester of pregnancy. As the transducer is closer to the object, the images are of enhanced quality. A full bladder is not required. Transvaginal sonography is superior to transabdominal sonography in diagnosing placenta previa.

Doppler Ultrasound (Audible Signal)

Ultrasound transmitted into the body in a narrow beam is transferred back at the same frequency when the object is still. When moving, there is a change in frequency known as the Doppler shift. The frequency increases or decreases according to whether the movement is toward or away from the source of energy.

It is used for monitoring the fetal heart rate, which can be picked up as early as 10th week of gestation. Uterine and fetal blood flow can be assessed and the fetus at risk of compromise could be identified. Leg vein thrombosis can be diagnosed by noting the absence of hissing sound of blood flow through the veins.

MIDWIFE'S RESPONSIBILITY REGARDING PRENATAL SCREENING

Midwives take care of pregnant women in different stages of their pregnancy. They often need to involve themselves in preparing and counseling women through the process. When giving information about the screening tests available or prescribed, it is important to include information regarding:
- Why the test is offered?
- What the test involves?
- When and how the results will be given?

In order to advise women regarding the tests that are available, the midwife needs to keep up-to-date with current technological advances.

Information given to women should also include how the woman needs to prepare herself, e.g. by attending with a full bladder for a scan.

The midwife needs to be available for women, when ambiguous or screen positive results plunge them and their spouses into a period of anxiety as they try to make decisions regarding further tests and/or termination of the pregnancy.

STUDY QUESTIONS

Short Notes

1. Doppler ultrasound examination.
2. Transvaginal ultrasonography.

Short Answer Questions

1. Use of ultrasound in obstetrics.
2. Indications for ultrasound examination in pregnancy.

BIBLIOGRAPHY

1. Chudleigh P, Pearce MJ. Obstetric ultrasound. Edinburgh: Churchill Livingstone; 1983.
2. Dutta DC. Textbook of obstetrics, 5th edition. Kolkata: New Central Book Company; 2001. pp. 683-93.
3. Lockwood C, Benacerraf B, Krinsky A, et al. A sonographic screening method for Down syndrome. Am J Obstet Gynecol. 1987;157:803-8.
4. Luck CA. Value of routine ultrasound scanning at 19 weeks: a four year study of 8849 deliveries. BMJ. 1992;304(6840):1474-8.
5. Proud J. Specialized antenatal investigations. In: Bennett RV, Linda KB (Eds). Myles textbook for midwives, 13th edition. Edinburgh: Churchill Livingstone; 1999.

CHAPTER 59

Legal and Ethical Aspects of Nursing

Learning Objectives

Upon completion of this chapter, the learner will be able to:
- Identify the legal and ethical standards in the practice of maternal-newborn nursing.
- Discuss the legal regulations of nursing practice and legal roles of nurses.
- Discuss the laws related to nursing practice and areas of potential liability.
- Outline the practice guidelines for legal protection.
- Enumerate the ethical principles that assist nurses in making decisions during difficult situations.
- Discuss the special ethical issues and ethical principles that guide nursing practice.

INTRODUCTION

The practice of professional nursing is governed by legal concepts and ethical standards. A nurse is accountable for her professional judgments and actions. Knowledge of laws that affect nursing practice is essential to ensure that her decisions and actions are consistent with established legal principles and that she will have protection from legal liability. A law is a standard rule of human conduct established by authority and enforced by government. Laws are intended chiefly to protect the rights of people and to regulate the action of all persons.

Nurses deal with intimate and sensitive life events such as birth, death and suffering. They experience dilemmas and conflicts as a result of their unique nurse-patient relationships in their professional practice. Advances in medical and reproductive technology, client's rights, special and legal changes and use of technical resources are among the things that have contributed to an increase in ethical concerns. Standards of conduct for nurses are set forth in codes of ethics developed by international, national and state nursing councils. Nurses need to be able to apply ethical principles in decision making and consider their own values, and beliefs of clients, of the profession and of all concerned parties. Ethics is the branch of philosophy which is concerned with human character and conducts a system of morals or rules of behavior. While ethical and legal considerations are a component of all areas and specialties of nursing, some unique issues exist in maternal-newborn nursing. Many of these issues occur because two parties, tightly linked are involved—the mother and fetus/newborn. Adequate knowledge of legal concepts and standards of care for practicing within legal boundaries is essential for all practitioners of nursing in general and midwifery in particular.

FUNCTIONS OF THE LAW IN NURSING

The law serves following functions in nursing.
- Provides a framework for establishing which nursing actions in the care of clients are legal.
- Differentiates the nurse's responsibilities from those of other health professionals.
- Helps establish the boundaries of independent nursing actions.
- Assists in maintaining a standard of nursing practice by making nurses accountable under the law.

MECHANISMS OF REGULATION OF NURSING PRACTICE

The regulation of nursing practice is a function of state laws. State legislatures pass statues that define and regulate nursing. The regulations are nurse practice acts which are in line with the constitutional or national laws.

Licensing (nurse registration) requirements of State Nursing Councils serve as legal controls for the scope of nursing practice in India. These include nurse registration, approval of basic nursing education programs, standards of care, and contracts.

Nurse Registration

Registration in the State Nursing Council, a government agency grants to individual nurse the permission to engage in the practice of the profession and to use a particular title. Nursing registration is mandatory in all states and union territories of India. The State Nursing Council has the right to revoke the registration for just causes such as incompetent nursing practice or professional misconduct. The legal controls, licensing (registration) requirements and standards of care are meant to protect the public.

Approval of Basic Nursing Education Programs

One of the functions of the National Council of Nurses (Indian Nursing Council) and the State Nursing Councils is to ensure that schools and colleges preparing nurses maintain minimum standards of education. All educational institutions in India require approval from State Nursing Councils and Indian Nursing Council (INC) as legal requirements.

Standards of Care

Standards of care are the skills and learning (theoretical knowledge) possessed by members of the nursing profession. The purpose of standards of care is to protect the consumer (clients). They are also used to evaluate the quality of care nurses provide and therefore become legal guidelines for nursing practice. Standards of care include the nurse's educational level, expertise, job description, institutional policies and procedures, and standards of the professional organization.

Contracts

A contract is an agreement between two or more competent persons on sufficient consideration (remuneration) to do or not to do some lawful acts. It is the basis of the relationship between a nurse and her employer. A contract may be written or oral. The terms of an oral contract may however, be difficult to prove in a court of law. A contract is considered to be expressed when the two parties discuss and agree orally or in writing to terms and conditions during the creation of the contracts. For example, a nurse will work at a hospital for a stated length of time and under stated conditions.

A written contract cannot be changed legally by an oral agreement. If two people wish to change some aspect of a written contract, the change must be written into the contract, because one party cannot hold the other to an oral agreement that differs from the written one.

LEGAL ROLES OF NURSES

Nurses have three different legal roles, each with rights and associated responsibilities. These are as provider of service, employee or contractor for service, and citizen.

Provider of Service

The nurse is expected to provide safe and competent care. She has legal responsibility or liability for her actions as a nurse. For example, a nurse has an obligation to practice and direct the practice of others under her supervision so that harm or injury to the client is prevented and standards of care are maintained. The nurse has the responsibility to document all the care provided to patient accurately and maintain her clinical competency. Even when a nurse carries out treatments ordered by the physician, the responsibility for the nursing activity belongs to the nurse. When a nurse is asked to carry out an activity that the nurse believes to be injurious to the client, the nurse's responsibility is to refuse to carry out the order and to report this to the nurse's supervisor.

Employee or Contractor for Service

A nurse, who is employed by an agency or hospital, works as a representative of the agency and her contract with the client is an implied one. However, if the nurse is employed directly by a client, for example, a private duty nurse may have a written contract with that client in which the nurse agrees to provide professional services for a definite fee, where the contractual relationship is an individual one. When the nurse functions as a hospital employee she represents and acts for the hospital and therefore must function within the policies of the employing agency. This type of relationship creates the legal doctrine known as *respondent superior* (let the master answer). In other words the employer (master) assumes responsibility for the conduct of the employee (servant) and also be held responsible for mal practice by the employee. By virtue of the employee role, therefore, the nurse's conduct is the hospital's responsibility.

This doctrine will not prevail if the nurse's actions are extraordinarily inappropriate, that is beyond those expected or foreseen by the employer. For example, if the nurse hits a client, the employer could disclaim responsibility, because this behavior is beyond the expected behavior.

The nurse in the role of an employee or contractor for service has obligations to the employer, the client and other personnel. She must practice according to the nurse-practice act, and policies and procedures of the organization. The nurse is expected to respect the rights and responsibilities of other health professionals.

Citizen

The rights and responsibilities of a nurse in the role of a citizen are same as those of any individual under the legal system. As a citizen, she has the right to respect by others and right to physical safety. She has responsibility to protect the rights of recipients of care.

LAWS RELATED TO NURSING PRACTICE

Nurses need to understand the laws that regulate and affect nursing practice, in order to ensure that their actions are consistent with legal principles and to protect them from liability. Laws govern the relationship of private individuals with government and with each other.

Criminal Law

Criminal law deals with crimes. A crime is an act committed in violation of criminal law, and is punishable by a fine or imprisonment. An action does not have to be intended for it to be a crime. For example, a nurse may accidentally give a client an additional or lethal dose of a narcotic to relieve pain. Crimes are classified as either felonies or misdemeanors.

- A *felony* is a crime of serious nature such as murder, punishable by a term in prison. *Manslaughter* is a second degree murder. A nurse who accidentally gives an additional and lethal dose of narcotic can be accused of manslaughter.
- A *misdemeanor* is an offense of less serious nature and is usually punishable by a fine or short-term jail or both. A nurse who slaps a client on his face could be charged with a misdemeanor.

Civil Law

Civil law refers to the body of law that deals with the relationship between individuals and the governmental agencies. Two types of civil laws that are most relevant to practice of nursing profession are contract law and civil law.

Contract law involves the enforcement of agreements among private individuals or the payment of compensation for failure to fulfill the agreements.

Tort law defines and enforces duties and rights among private individuals that are not based on contractual agreements. Examples of tort laws applicable to nurses are negligence and malpractice, invasion of privacy, and assault and battery.

Nursing liability is usually involved with tort law. Liability is an obligation, one incurred or might incur through any act or failure to act. However, it is important for nurses to know the difference between crimes and torts.

A tort is a civil wrong committed against a person or a person's property. The person or persons claimed to be responsible for the tort are sued for damages. A tort liability is based on the fault which is something that was done incorrectly (unreasonable act of commission) or something that should have been done was not done (act of omission). Torts may be unintentional or intentional.

Unintentional Torts

- *Negligence (breach of duty):* It is the failure of an individual to provide care that is expected of an ordinary, reasonable and prudent person. Such conduct places another person at risk for harm. Both nonmedical and professional persons can be liable for negligent acts.

  Gross negligence involves extreme lack of knowledge, skill or decision-making that the person clearly should have known would put others at risk for harm.
- *Malpractice:* This is "professional negligence" that is negligence that occurred while the person was performing as a professional. This includes wrongful conduct, improper discharge of professional duties, or failure to meet the standards of acceptable care which result in harm to another person. Malpractice applies to physicians, dentists, lawyers and generally includes nurses.

For a case of nursing malpractice, the following six elements are to be present.
  1. *Duty:* The nurse must have had a relationship with the client that involves providing care and following an accepted standard of care. For example, a nurse assigned to the care of a patient in the home or hospital.
  2. *Breach of duty:* There must be a standard of care that is expected in the specific situation, but that the nurse did not observe. That is, something was done that should not have been done or nothing was done when it should have been done. This is failure to act as a reasonable, prudent nurse, under the circumstances.
  3. *Foreseeability:* A link must exist between the nurse's act and the injury suffered.
  4. *Causation:* It must be proved that the harm occurred as a direct result of the nurse's failure to follow the standard of care and the nurse should have known that failure to follow the standard of care could result in such harm.
  5. *Harm or injury:* The client or plaintiff must demonstrate some type of harm or injury (physical, financial or emotional) as a result of the breach of duty owned by the client.
  6. *Damages:* The nurse or accused is held liable for damages that may be compensated financially.

Intentional Torts

These are torts carried out with intent, i.e. the defendant executed the act on purpose. No harm needs to be caused by intentional torts for liability to exist. Also, since no standard is involved, no expert witnesses are needed. The intentional torts related to nursing are listed below.

- *Assault:* It is described as an attempt or threat to touch another person in an offensive, insulting or intimidating manner. It is an act that caused the person to believe a battery is about to occur (often an assault proceeds a battery). A person who threatens another with a club or closed fist is guilty of assault. A nurse who threatens a client with an injection after the client refuses to take the medication orally, would be committing assault.
- *Battery:* It is the willful touching of a person (or a person's clothes or even something the person is carrying) that may or may not cause harm. To be actionable at law, the touching must be wrong in some way; for example, touching done without permission that is embarrassing or that causes injury.

If the nurse followed through the threat (mentioned as example for assault) and gave the injection without the client's consent, the nurse would be committing battery. Liability applies even though the physician ordered the medication or the procedure and even if the client benefits from the nurse's action. Consent is required before procedures are performed. Battery exists when there is no consent. Unless there is implied consent, a procedure performed in an unconscious patient is considered battery. If the nurse is uncertain whether a client refusing a treatment is competent (elderly, with mental disorder, or those on particular medications), the supervisor and the physician should be consulted so that another ethical treatment that does not constitute battery can be provided.

- *False imprisonment:* This is the unjustifiable detention of a person without legal warrant to confine the person. Legally, restraining can be used only when it is needed to treat a patient's medical symptom. False imprisonment accompanied by forceful restraint or threat of restraint is battery. Although the nurse may suggest under certain circumstances that a client remain in the hospital room or in bed, the client must not be detained against his will. The client has the right to insist on leaving even though it may be detrimental to his health. In this instance the client may leave by signing an AMA (against medical advice) form.
- *Invasion of privacy:* It is a direct wrong of personal nature. It injures the feelings of a person and does not take into account the effect of revealed information on the standing of the person in the community. The right to privacy is the right of individuals to withhold themselves and their lives from public scrutiny. It is also described as the right to be left alone. Liability can result if the nurse breaches confidentiality by passing along confidential client information to others or intrudes into the client's private domain. Nurses must hold each patient's care in complete confidentiality; information can only be shared with other members of the patient's healthcare team.
- *Defamation:* This is communication that is false or made with careless disregard for truth and results in injury to the reputation of another.
- *Libel:* Libel is defamation by print, writing or pictures. Writing in nurse's notes that a physician is incompetent because he did not respond immediately to a call is an example of libel.
- *Slander:* It is defamation by spoken word or a false word by which one's reputation is damaged. An example of slander would be for the nurse to tell a client that another nurse is incompetent.

CONSUMER PROTECTION ACT (CPA)

Medical profession has been brought under the Section 2(1)(o) of CPA, which underlines that a medical professional can be held responsible in case he/she fails exercise rational caution and capability during diagnosis and treatment of a patient in accordance with the prevailing standards in force at that point of time.

The Judicial Process

The judicial process functions to settle disputes peacefully and in accordance with the law. A law suit has strict procedural rules. There are generally five steps.

1. A *document*, called a complaint is filed by a person referred to as *plaintiff*, who claims that his or her legal rights have been infringed on by one or more persons referred to as defendants.
2. *A written response*, called answer, made by the defendant.
3. *Discovery:* Both parties engage in pretrial activities referred to as discovery in an effort to obtain all the facts of the situation.
4. *Trial:* In the trial of the case, all the relevant facts are presented to a jury or a judge.
5. *Decision or verdict:* The judge renders the verdict. If the outcome is not acceptable to any one party, an appeal can be made for another trial.

During a trial, a plaintiff must offer evidence of the defendant's wrong doing. This duty of proving a wrong doing is called the *burden of proof.*

AREAS OF POTENTIAL LIABILITY IN NURSING

Nursing liability is usually involved with tort law. Negligence and malpractice which are unintentional torts usually occur when errors in basic nursing care are made.

Errors generally occur in the following areas:

1. *Patient assessment*
   Failing to:
   - Assess whether a patient is steady on his feet prior to ambulation
   - Recognize the significance of certain data e.g. laboratory values, vital signs
   - Monitor patients who are using medical equipment.
2. *Planning nursing care*
   Failing to:
   - Know the patient's medications in order to take preventive measures against adverse effects.
   - Bring questionable orders or protocols to the attention of the physician and nursing supervisor.
   - Give adequate explanation and discharge instructions that the patient understands.
3. *Implementation and evaluation of nursing care.*
   Failing to:
   - Document clearly all nursing interventions
   - Understand the medications being administered
   - Monitor the client as the condition warrants and as ordered
   - Document frequency of monitoring and client status
   - Promptly bring distressing, symptoms and changes in patient's status to the physician
   - Document the time and content of all telephone conversations about the patient with the physician.

Selected Activities and Procedures that Carry Higher Legal Implications for Nurses

Informed consent: This is an agreement by a client to accept a procedure or a course of treatment after being provided complete information, including the benefits and risks of the treatment, alternatives to the treatment and prognosis if not treated by a health care provider. Usually, the patient signs a form provided by the hospital. The signed form is a record of informed consent. The major elements of informed consent are that it must be given voluntarily by the client or individual with the capacity and competence to understand and that he must be given sufficient information to be the ultimate decision maker.

Expressed consent: For procedures that are invasive and/or with greater potential for risk to the client, *express consent* in written form is needed. Generally the physician who performs the procedure explains the procedure to the client and obtains consent and nurses witness the consent. By entering the witness signature in the consent form, the nurse confirms that the client gave the consent voluntarily, his signature is authentic and that he appeared competent to give consent. The nurse could be liable for giving incorrect information or interfering with client-provider relationship.

Implied consent: For routine nursing procedures non-verbal or oral consent is obtained after adequate explanation. This type of consent is called *implied* consent. Implied consent exists when the individual's non-verbal behavior indicates agreement. For example, clients who position their bodies for an injection or co-operate with taking of vital signs infer implied consent. Consent is also implied in a medical emergency when the individual cannot provide express consent because of physical condition.

LAWS CONCERNING MEDICAL AND NURSING PRACTICE

Abortions: Abortion laws provide specific guidelines for nurses about what is really permissible under the medical termination of Pregnancy Act (MTP Act, 1971).

Prenatal detection of sex: The Pre-Natal Diagnostic Technique (PNDT) Act and Rules is a federal legislation enacted by the Parliament of India to stop female feticides and arrest the declining sex ratio in India. The Act has banned prenatal sex determination.

Transplantation of human organs: The Transplantation of Human Organs Act 1994 provides for the regulation of removal, storage and transplantation of human organs for therapeutic purposes and for the prevention of commercial dealings in human organs and for matters connected therewith. Nurses assisting for organ transplantations need to be aware of the regulations given in this act.

Biomedical waste management: Biomedical waste (management and handling) rules 1998 deals with the generation/handling/treatment/disposal of biomedical waste. These rules apply to all persons who generate, collect, receive, store, transport, treat, dispose or handle biomedical waste in any form. Nurses are closely associated with generation and handling of biomedical waste and hence they need to be aware of these regulations.

Care of mentally ill: Mental Health Act, 1987 is an act to consolidate and amend the law relating to the treatment and care of mentally ill persons, to make better provision for care of mentally-ill persons.

Narcotic and psychotropic medicines: Under Narcotic Drugs and Psychotropic Substances Act and Rules 1985 (NDPS Act), it is illegal for a person to produce/manufacture/cultivate, possess, sell, purchase, transport, store, and/or consume any narcotic drug or psychotropic substance. Nurses are responsible for ensuring appropriate storage and usage of narcotic and psychotropic medications for medical purposes in hospital.

Medications: Administering wrong medications, wrong doses, wrong routes or timing resulting in harm can be considered an act of malpractice.

Death and related issues: Legal issues associated with death include advance directives, euthanasia; do not resuscitate orders, certification of death, autopsy and organ donation.

LEGAL ISSUES IN MIDWIFERY PRACTICE

As in the practice of nursing in any medical especially or health care facility, nurses practicing maternal-newborn care nursing and gynecology nursing need also to be knowledgeable of the legal issues that may occur.

1. *Professional negligence:* Medical negligence is the legal error committed by medical personnel. In legal terms this error is a tort. A tort is a civil wrong that injures a person. If a tort is international, it becomes a crime of assault or battery. Negligence is an intentional tort—a form of malpractice. In order to prove that a negligent act or tort has occurred, four elements must be present.
    i. A duty must exist between the injured party and the professional accused of wrong doing.
    ii. A breach of duty must have occurred, i.e. the midwife must have practiced outside the standard of care of her profession.
    iii. The breach of duty must be proximate to cause of the claimed injury.
    iv. There must be damage or injury to the claimant that are recognized by law and compensational.
2. *Medication error:* Nurses are to administer medications correctly to patients. Administering wrong medications, wrong doses, and wrong routes or timing resulting in harm may be considered an act of malpractice.
3. *Failure of monitoring:* A nurse is responsible to monitor clients admitted with obstetric or gynecologic problems. Monitoring during intrapartum and postpartum periods requires great care.
4. *Informed consent:* Based on client's right to self-determination, informed consent demands that information regarding treatment procedures be given to clients and their consent obtained by concerned physician, and nurses witness the patient's signing in the form. If he/she finds that a valid consent is missing, it must be reported on time.
5. *Nursing care of newborn:* Newborns require professional and specialized care. Failure of the neonatal nurse to meet

her obligations can result in liability in employment or even a civil suit.

6. *Failure in assessing:* Failure in assessing and reporting changes in a client's condition for timely action can be considered a malpractice.
7. *Abortion:* Nurses assist in the performance of abortions under the act of "medical termination of pregnancy" (MTP) and take care of patients following the procedure. They have the right to refuse to assist in the procedure if the abortion is illegal.

Although most nurses assume that they will never be named in a law suit, it is true that a few are. Nurses these days take up employment in institutions of different levels in several countries of the world. Increasing awareness of health care and patients' rights in communities makes it imperative for health professionals to be more alert in delivering quality care that is ethically and morally right, and to exercise adequate care not to give chance for legal issues.

PRACTICE GUIDELINES FOR LEGAL PROTECTION

1. Function within the scope of your education, job description and practice guidelines.
2. Follow the procedures and policies of the employing agency.
3. Develop and maintain good rapport with clients.
4. Always check the identity of a client prior to any procedure.
5. Apply nursing process for providing safe and effective care.
6. Assess and monitor the client accurately. Communicate and record significant changes in the client's condition to the physician.
7. Document accurately and promptly all assessments and care given as well as response to management and care.
8. Perform procedures correctly and appropriately.
9. Make sure the correct medications are given in the correct dose, by the right route at the scheduled time and to the right client.
10. When delegating responsibilities, make sure that the person who is delegated a task understands what to do and that the person has the required knowledge and skill.
11. Always anticipate sources of client- injury and educate clients about hazards and implement measures to prevent injury.
12. Report promptly all incidents involving clients.
13. Always check any order that a patient questions or you find questionable.
14. Ask for assistance and supervision in situations for which you feel inadequately prepared.
15. Maintain your clinical competence through continued study and updating clinical knowledge and skills. For nursing students study and practice are essential before caring for clients.

LEGAL RESPONSIBILITIES OF NURSING STUDENTS

Nursing students are responsible for their own actions and liable for their own acts of negligence committed during the course of their clinical practice. When students perform nursing procedures that are within the scope of professional nursing such as administering, medications, they are legally held to the same standard of skill and competence as a registered professional nurse. Lower standards are not applied to the actions of nursing students.

In cases of negligent actions involving students, the hospital and the educational institution will be held potentially liable under the doctrine of *respondent superior*.

Nursing students in clinical posting must be assigned learning experiences within their capabilities and be given reasonable guidance and supervision. Nursing, instructors with them in the clinical area are responsible for assigning students to the care of clients and providing adequate guidance. Failure to provide reasonable assignment of a client or supervision to a student who is not prepared and competent can be a basis for liability.

In order to fulfill the responsibilities to clients and to minimize chances of liability, nursing students need to do the following:
- Make sure they are prepared to carry out the necessary care for assigned clients
- Ask for additional help or supervision in situations for which they are inadequately prepared
- Comply with the policies of the agency in which they obtain their clinical experience
- Comply with the policies and guidelines given by the educational institutions (school/college of nursing).

ETHICAL PRINCIPLES RELATED TO NURSING PRACTICE

Ethics is the science of morals and that branch of philosophy which is concerned with human character and conduct. It is a system of morals or rules of behavior that relates to professional standards of conduct which are in accord with approved with moral behavior.

The study of ethics has led to the identification of basic concepts or principles including rights, autonomy, beneficence, nonmaleficence, justice, fidelity, and selflessness. Character and confidentiality form the basis of ethical management of patient care. Understanding these principles assists nurses in making decisions during difficult situations.

Rights

Webster defines *right as* "something to which one has a just claim or the power or privilege to which is justly entitled". "A patient's bill of rights" was initially developed by the American Hospital Association in 1973 and revised in 1992. In the United States, all hospitals are now required by law to inform patients of these rights upon admission to the hospital. In India, it is not mandated by law to inform patients of their rights, however all patients are entitled to same rights.

Autonomy

The term *autonomy* comes from the Latin words '*auto*' meaning "*self*" and '*nomy*' which means "control". Individuals must be given the right to assist in their own decision making. This ethical concept has led to the need for *informed consent*. Sometimes patient's religious or cultural beliefs lead them to make decisions regarding their own care that may seem controversial or even dangerous. However, the concept of autonomy gives them the right to make those decisions unless they are mentally impaired.

Beneficence and Nonmaleficence

Beneficence means 'do good' and not harm to other people. Nonmaleficence is the concept of preventing intentional harm. Both these ethical concepts relate directly to patient care. Nurses are often faced with making decisions about extending life with technology which might not be in the best interest of the patient. Often the concept of weighing potential benefit against potential harm is used in making those difficult decisions along with the patient's own stated wishes.

Justice

The term justice is closely tied with the legal system. However, the word refers to the obligation to be fair to all the people. Economic decisions about healthcare resources have to be made on the number of patients who would benefit. The need to make health care available to the frail elderly poor and disabled is sure to be addressed in all societies.

Fidelity

Fidelity refers to the concept of keeping a commitment. Although the word is more closely used to describe a marital relationship, fidelity is the concept of accountability. Privacy and confidentiality are concepts that are considered under the concept of fidelity in health care.

Selflessness

Within the paradigms of hospital jobs, a nurse is expected to go beyond the call of duty and walk that extra mile to provide the necessary medical assistance.

Healthcare has placed many demands on the profession and so have patients. Selflessness is a virtue without which the profession lacks substance. A nurse should ideally be able to stay vigilant and be aware of each patient in her charge and be there whenever required. Treating every patient as an extension of self is a very important aspect of nursing ethics.

Character and Integrity

The 'Professional Codes of Nursing' do spell out essentials applicable on job. But ethics in the nursing profession comes from the deepest recesses of human psyche and experience. It hardly matters what remuneration a nurse is drawing or at what level in the hierarchy he or she features. The person's show of character and solidarity is what makes him or her special. A nurse is expected to be a person of immense character; one who can shoulder the weight of neglect that a patient might feel or the suffering of a little child while delivering dedicated care. A nurse is expected to deliver patient-care with respect and attend to life and death situations in the most caring and professional manner. The ethics need to be lived rather than read and developed forcefully. Nursing is a profession that is, not to be opted for 'by chance' instead it is a calling "by choice".

Honesty and Confidentiality

A nurse is expected to adhere to strict honesty and confidentiality. The need for this arises out of the fact that many patients confide in a nurse in tender and sensitive moments. The patients do move on, so do the nurses, but what happens with the information shared is what really matters. Becoming a nurse involves giving up on many negative vices like lying and squealing. The very objective of the nursing ethics is delivering the best medical and moral support to the patients at hand.

ETHICS IN CLINICAL NURSING PRACTICE

The Standards of Clinical Nursing Practice prepared by the American Nurses Association (ANA) has standard V, on ethics and states that "the nurse's decisions and actions on behalf of patients are determined in an ethical manner".

The measurement criteria stated or the ethical standards are:
- The nurse's practice is guided by the *code of ethics for nurses*
- The nurse maintains patient confidentiality within legal and regulatory parameters
- The nurse acts as a patient-advocate and assists patients in developing skills so they can advocate for themselves
- The nurse delivers care in a nonjudgmental and nondiscriminatory manner that is sensitive to patient diversity
- The nurse delivers care in a manner that preserves patient autonomy, dignity and rights
- The nurse seeks available resources in formulating ethical decisions.

NURSING CODES OF ETHICS

A code of ethics is a formal statement of a group's ideals and values. It is a set of ethical principles that is shared by members of the group and reflects their moral judgments. A code serves as a standard for their professional actions. *Ethical codes are systematic guidelines for shaping ethical behaviors that answer the normative questions of what beliefs and values should be normally accepted.* An ethical code is adopted by an organization in an attempt to assist those in the organization called upon to make decisions understand the difference between right and wrong and to apply this understanding to their decisions. A code of ethics contains specific set of professional behaviors and values the professional practitioner must know and abide by including confidentiality, accuracy, privacy and integrity.

Types of Ethics

The code of ethics links to and gives rise to a code of conduct for employees: (1) Employee ethics and (2) Professional ethics.

Employee Ethics

A code of conduct is a document designed to influence the behavior of employees. They set out the procedures to be used in specific ethical situations. The effectiveness of such codes of ethics depends on the extent to which the management supports them with rewards and sanctions. Violations of a code of conduct may subject the violator to organizational remedies which can under particular circumstances result in the termination of employment.

Professional Ethics

A code of practice adopted by a profession or by a governmental or nongovernmental organization to regulate that profession. A code of practice may be styled as a code of professional responsibility, which will discuss difficult issues, difficult decisions that often need to be made, and provide a clear account of what behavior is considered "ethical" or "correct" or "right" in the circumstances.

The code of ethics for nurses gives the professionals various guidelines that tell how they should behave with each other, with the public and with governments. These are guidelines which the professional should follow when they are dealing with their clients. Ethics also tell the public what they can expect from a professional and tells the professionals what the public expects from them.

Nursing ethics refers to ethical issues that occur in nursing practice. Nursing is a profession that provides a healing touch to patients along with care for their health problems (diseases) and maintenance of their health. Adherence to the code of ethics leads to credibility of the profession and esteem of that profession rises automatically. In India, the Indian Nursing Council (INC) has laid down code of ethics and code of professional conduct.

Professional conduct

The code of professional conduct for nurses is critical for building professionalism and accountability. Ethical considerations are vital in any area that deals with human beings because they represent values, rights and relationships. The nurse must have professional competence, responsibility and accountability with moral obligations. The nurse is obliged to provide services even if it is in conflict with her/his personal beliefs and values.

International and National Nursing Associations have established codes of ethics. The International Council of Nurses (ICN) first adopted a code in 1953 and the most recent revision was in 2000. National nurses associations such as The American Nurses Association (ANA), The Canadian Nurses Association (CAN), The British Nurses Association, The Australian Nurses Association and The Indian Nursing Council have formulated codes of ethics for nurses to follow. Most of the codes are similar and several National Associations including the one of India use the codes of INC.

Purposes of the Codes of Ethics

- To inform the public about the minimum standard of the profession and professional nursing conduct.
- To provide a sign of the profession's commitment to the public it serves.
- To outline the major ethical considerations of the profession.
- To provide ethical standards for professional behavior.
- To guide the profession in self-regulation.
- To remind nurses of the special responsibility they assume when caring for the sick.

Uses of the Codes of Ethics

- Acknowledges the rightful place of individuals in health care delivery system.
- Contributes towards empowerment of individuals to become responsible for their health and well-being.
- Contributes to quality care.
- Identifies obligations in practice, research and relationships.
- Informs individuals, families, community and other professionals about expectations of a nurse.

THE INTERNATIONAL COUNCIL OF NURSES CODE OF ETHICS (2000)

Preamble

Nurses have four fundamental responsibilities which are; to promote health, to prevent illness, to restore health and to alleviate suffering. The need for nursing is universal.

Inherent in nursing is respect for human rights, including right to life, to dignity, and to be treated with dignity. Nursing care is unrestricted by consideration of age, color, creed, culture, disability or illness, gender, nationality, politics, race or social status. Nurses render health services to the individual, the family and the community and coordinate their services with those of related groups.

The Code

The *ICN code of ethics* for Nurses has four principal elements that outline the standards of ethical conduct.
1. *Nurse and people:*
   - The nurse's primary responsibility is to people requiring nursing care

- In providing care, the nurse promotes an environment in which the human rights, values, customs and spiritual beliefs of the individual, family and community are respected
- The nurse ensures that the individual receives sufficient information on which to base consent for care and related treatment
- The nurse holds in confidence personal information and uses judgment in sharing this information
- The nurse shares with society the responsibility for initiating and supporting actions to meet the health and social needs of the public, in particular those of vulnerable populations
- The nurse shares responsibility to sustain and protect the natural environment from depletion, pollution, degradation and destruction.

2. *Nurse and practice:*
   - The nurse carries personal responsibility and accountability for nursing practice, and for maintaining competency by continual learning
   - The nurse maintains a standard of personal health such that the ability to provide care is not compromised
   - The nurse uses judgment regarding individual competence when accepting and delegating responsibility
   - The nurse at all times maintains standards of personal conduct that reflect well on the profession and enhance public confidence
   - The nurse in providing care ensures that use of technology and scientific advances are compatible with the safety, dignity and rights of people.

3. *Nurse and profession:*
   - The nurse assumes the major role in determining and implementing acceptable standards of clinical practice management, research and education
   - The nurse is active in developing a core of research-based professional knowledge
   - The nurse acting through the professional organization participates in creating and maintaining equitable social and economic working conditions in nursing.

4. *Nurse and coworkers:*
   - The nurse sustains a cooperative relationship with coworkers in nursing and other fields.
   - The nurse takes appropriate actions to safeguard individuals when their care is endangered by a coworker or any other person.

INDIAN NURSING COUNCIL CODE OF ETHICS

1. The nurse respects the uniqueness of individuals in provision of care.
   - Provides care for individuals without consideration of caste, creed, religion, culture, ethnicity, gender, socioeconomic and political status, personal attributes, or any other grounds.
   - Individualizes the care considering the beliefs, values and cultural sensitivities.
   - Appreciates the place of the individual in the family and community and facilitates participation of significant others in the care.
   - Develops and promotes trustful relationship with individuals.
   - Recognizes the uniqueness of responses of individuals to interventions and adapts accordingly.

2. The nurse respects the rights of individuals as partner in care and helps in making informed choices.
   - Appreciates individual's rights to make decisions about their care and therefore gives adequate and accurate information for enabling to make informed choices
   - Respects the decisions made by individuals regarding their care
   - Protects public from misinformation and misinterpretations
   - Advocates special provisions to protect vulnerable individuals/groups

3. The nurse respects individual's right to privacy, maintains confidentiality, and shares information judiciously.
   - Respects the individual's right to privacy of their personal information
   - Maintains confidentiality of privileged information except in life-threatening situations and uses discretion in sharing information.

4. The nurse maintains competence in order to render quality nursing care.
   - Nursing care must be provided only by registered nurse.
   - Nurse strives to maintain quality nursing care and upholds the standards of care.
   - Nurse values research as a means of development of nursing profession and participate in research adhering to ethical principles.

5. The nurse is obliged to practice within the framework of ethical, professional and legal boundaries.
   - Adheres to code of ethics and code of professional conduct for nurses in India developed by the Indian Nursing Council.
   - Familiarizes with relevant laws and practices in accordance with the law of the state.

6. The nurse is obliged to work harmoniously with members of the health team.
   - Appreciates the team efforts in rendering care.
   - Cooperates, coordinates and collaborates with members of the health team to meet the needs of people.

7. The nurse commits to reciprocate the trust invested in nursing profession by society.
   - Demonstrates personal etiquettes in all dealings.
   - Demonstrates professional attributes in all dealings.

INC Code of Professional Conduct for Nurses

1. *Professional responsibility and accountability:*
   - Appreciates sense of self-worth and nurtures it
   - Maintains standards of personal conduct reflecting credit upon the profession

- Carries out responsibilities within the framework of professional boundaries
- Is accountable for maintaining practice standards set by the Indian Nursing Council
- Is accountable for own decisions and actions
- Is compassionate
- Is responsible for continuous improvement of current practices
- Provides adequate information to individuals that enable them make informed choices
- Practices healthful behavior.

2. *Nursing practice:*
   - Provides care in accordance with set standards of practice
   - Treats all individuals and families with human dignity in providing physical, psychological, emotional, social and spiritual aspects of care
   - Respects individuals and families in the context of traditional and cultural practices and discourages harmful practices
   - Presents realistic picture truthfully in all situations for facilitating autonomous decision making by individuals and families
   - Promotes participation of individuals and significant others in the care of clients
   - Ensures safe practice
   - Consults, coordinates, collaborates and follows up appropriately when individuals' care needs exceeds the nurse's competence.

3. *Communication and interpersonal relationship.*
   - Establishes and maintains effective interpersonal relationship with individuals, families and communities
   - Upholds the dignity of team members and maintain effective interpersonal relationship with them
   - Appreciates and nurtures professional role of team members
   - Cooperates with other professionals to meet the needs of individuals, families and communities.

4. *Valuing human being*
   - Takes appropriate action to protect individuals from harmful unethical practice
   - Consider relevant facts while taking conscientious decisions in the best interest of individuals
   - Encourage and support individuals in their right to speak for themselves on issues affecting their health and welfare
   - Respects and supports choices made by individuals.

5. *Management:*
   - Ensures appropriate allocation and utilization of available resources
   - Participates in supervision and education of students and other formal care providers
   - Uses judgment In relation to individual competence while accepting and delegating responsibility
   - Facilitates conductive work culture in order to achieve institutional objectives
   - Communicates effectively following appropriate channels of communication
   - Participates in performance appraisals
   - Participates in evaluation of nursing ervices
   - Participates in policy decisions, following the principal of equity and accessibility of services
   - Works with individuals to identify their needs and sensitizes policy makers and funding agencies for resource allocation.

6. *Professional advancement:*
   - Ensures protection of human rights while pursuing advancement of knowledge
   - Contributes to the development of the profession
   - Participates in determining and implementing quality care
   - Takes responsibility for updating own knowledge and competencies
   - Contributes to the core of professional knowledge by conducting and participating in research.

(*Source:* Rajamani S. Ethics in Nursing Practice, Presentation transcript, 12/10/2012) www.indiannursingcouncil.org

Making Ethical Decisions and Strategies that Enhance Ethical Practice

Because of their unique position in the health care system, nurses experience conflicts among their loyalties and obligations to clients, families, physicians, employing institutions and licensing bodies. Client needs may conflict with institutional policies, physician preferences and needs of the client's family. According to the code of ethics, the nurse's first loyalty is to the client. However, it is not always easy to determine which action best serves the client's needs.

Responsible ethical reasoning is rational and systematic. Decision making should be based on ethical principles and codes rather than on emotions, fixed policies or precedent occurrences. In making ethical decisions, the nurse needs to apply the following obligations.

❖ Maximize the client's well-beings.
❖ Balance the client's need for autonomy with family members' responsibilities for the client's well-being.
❖ Support each family member and enhance the family support system.
❖ Carry out hospital policies.
❖ Protect other client's well-being.
❖ Protect the nurse's own standards of care.

A good decision is one that is in the client's best interest and at the same time preserves the integrity of all involved. Nurses have ethical obligations to their clients, to the institution that employs them, and to physicians. Therefore nurses must weigh all competing factors when making ethical decisions. Several people are usually involved in making ethical decisions. Therefore collaboration, communication and compromise are important skills for health professionals. When nurses do not have the autonomy to act on their moral or ethical choices, compromise becomes essential.

Strategies that Enhance Ethical Practice of Nursing

- Be aware of your own values and ethical aspects of nursing
- Be familiar with nursing code of ethics
- Respect the values, opinions and responsibilities of other healthcare professionals
- Strive for collaborative practice, in which Nurses function effectively in cooperation with other health care professionals
- Participate in ethical rounds and discussions that focus on the ethical dimensions of client care rather than the client's clinical diagnosis.

Special Ethical Issues

Some of the ethical problems nurses encounter most frequently include issues in the care of HIV/AIDS clients, abortions, organ transplantation, end-of-life decisions, cost-containment issues that jeopardize client welfare and access to health care and breaches of client confidentiality.

Some of the most frequent and disturbing ethical problems for nurses involve issues that arise around death and dying. These include euthanasia, assisted suicide, termination of life-sustaining treatment and withdrawing or withholding of food and fluids.

Many problems involving end of life procedures can be resolved if clients complete *advance directives*. Advance directives direct caregivers as to the client's wishes about treatments, providing ongoing voice for clients when they have lost capacity to make or communicate their decisions.

Euthanasia is popularly known as "mercy killing". *Active euthanasia* involves actions to directly bring about the client's death; with or without client consent. An example of this would be the administration of a lethal medication to end the client's suffering. Regardless of the caregiver's intent, active euthanasia is forbidden by law and can result in criminal charge of murder.

Active euthanasia includes *assisted suicide* or giving clients the means to kill themselves if they request it (e.g. providing pills or a weapon). This also is forbidden by law and is in violation of the code of ethics for nurses.

Passive euthanasia involves the withdrawal of extraordinary means of life support, such as removing a ventilator or withholding special attempts to revive a client (e.g. giving the client "no code" status).

Termination of Life-sustaining Treatment

Clients may specify that they wish to have life-sustaining measures withdrawn; they may have advance directive on this matter or may appoint a surrogate decision maker. However, nurses must understand that a decision to withdraw treatment is not a decision to withdraw care. As the primary caregivers nurses must ensure that sensitive care and support measures are given as the client's illness progresses.

Withholding or Withdrawing Food and Fluids

A nurse is morally obligated to withhold food and fluids (or any other treatment) if it is determined to be more harmful to administer them than to withhold them. The nurse must also honor competent patient's refusal to food and fluids.

Nonclinical Behaviors Viewed as Unethical for Nurses

- Deliberately providing misinformation to public about the profession
- Improper use of the internet; personal, or commercial
- Intercepting private e-mail
- Taking secretly (stealing) copyrighted material and credit for intellectual property
- Misusing research material.

A Patient's Bill of Rights

A patient's Bill of Rights was first adopted by the American Hospital Association in 1973 and later revised in 1992. The rights can be exercised on patient's behalf by a designated surrogate or proxy decision maker if the patient lacks decision-making capacity, legally incompetent or is a minor.

1. The patient has the right to considerate and respectful care.
2. The patient has the right to and is encouraged to obtain from physician and other caregivers relevant, current and understandable information concerning diagnosis, treatment and prognosis.
3. The patient has the right to make decisions about the plan of care, prior to and during the course of treatment and to refuse a recommended treatment or plan of care to the extent permitted by law and hospital policy and to be informed of the medical consequences of this action.
4. The patient has the right to have an advance directive (such as a living will, health care proxy or durable power of attorney for health care) concerning treatment or designating a surrogate decision maker (An advance directive specifies what life-saving treatments he or she does or does not wish to have).
5. The patient has the right to every consideration of privacy. Case discussions, consultation, examination and treatment should be conducted so as to protect each patient's privacy.
6. The patient has the right to expect that all communications and records pertaining to his/her care will be treated as confidential by the hospital, except in cases such as suspected abuse and public health hazards when reporting is permitted or required by law.
7. The patient has the right to review the records pertaining to his/her medical care and to have the information explained or interpreted as necessary, except when restricted by law.
8. The patient has the right to expect that within its capacity and policies, a hospital will make reasonable response to the request of a patient for appropriate and medically indicated care and services.
9. The patient has the right to ask and be informed of the existence of business relationships among the hospital, educational institutions, other health care providers or payers that may influence the patients' treatment and care.

10. The patient has the right to consent to or decline to participate in proposed research studies or human experimentation affecting care and treatment or requiring direct patient involvement and to have those studies fully explained prior to consent.
11. The patient has the right to expect reasonable continuity care when appropriate and to be informed by physicians and other caregivers of available and realistic patient care options when hospital care is no longer appropriate.
12. The patient has the right to be informed of hospital policies and practices that relate to patient care, treatment and responsibilities.

A patient's Bill of Rights was presented with the expectation that it will contribute to more effective patient care. The collaborative nature of health care requires that patients or their families/surrogates participate in their care. The effectiveness of care and patient satisfaction depend, in part, on the patient fulfilling certain responsibilities.

Patient's Responsibilities

- Be responsible for providing information about past illnesses, hospitalizations, medications and other matters related to health status
- Take responsibility for requesting additional information or clarification about their health status or treatment when they do not fully understand information and instructions
- Ensure that the hospital has a copy of the written advance directive if they have one
- Inform their physicians and other caregivers if they anticipate problems in following prescribed treatment
- Make reasonable accommodations to the needs of the hospital, other patients, medical staff and hospital employees
- Provide necessary information for insurance claims and for working with the hospital to make payment arrangements, when necessary.

Most of the responsibilities of nurses and professional nursing ethics are not spelt on paper because he or she is expected to emulate the best under any circumstance. The nursing profession is considered noble and beyond a "pricing". The nurse is expected to be the embodiment of high values and tolerance. She is supposed to stand for undaunted faith in the treatment being extended and accordingly help the patients towards a speedy recovery.

There are many statements of ethics and values, but more important is the realization and understanding that nursing goes beyond the administering of medicines or prescribed list of therapies when the doctor is not around. Nursing is for the brave hearts—those driven beyond time and quantity to deliver medical/nursing care in attending to the sick and dying. The profession should ideally be the calling of those who understand the evolution of nursing ethics and feel intensely about social service.

SUMMARY

Nursing codes of ethics are formal statements of the profession's ideals and values that serve as standard for professional actions and inform the public of its commitment. Ethical problems are created as a result of changes in society, advances in technology, conflicts within the nursing role itself, and nurses' conflicting loyalties and obligations to clients, families, employees, physicians and other nurses. Nurses' ethical decisions are influenced by their role perceptions, moral theories and principles, nursing codes of ethics, level of cognitive development, and personal and professional values. The goal of ethical reasoning, in the context of nursing, is to reach a mutual, peaceful agreement that is in the best interest of client; reaching an agreement may require compromise. The focus of client advocacy is to respect client's decisions and enhance client autonomy. Its goal is to protect the rights of clients.

STUDY QUESTIONS

Short Notes

1. Respect for autonomy.
2. Nonmaleficence.
3. Beneficence.
4. Justice.

Essay Questions

1. Explain the legal issues that can occur in the practice of midwifery and measures of safeguard that can be adopted.
2. Explain the areas of potential liability in nursing.
3. List the ethical principles related to nursing practice.

BIBLIOGRAPHY

1. Beauchamp T, Childress J. Principles of biomedical ethics, 5th edition. New York: Oxford University Press: 2001.
2. Fry ST. The ethics of caring: can it survive in nursing? Nursing Outlook. 1983; (1):48.
3. Hall K. Nursing ethics and law. Philadelphia: WB Saunders; 1996.
4. Jacob A, Rekha R, Jadhav S. Clinical nursing procedures, the Art of nursing. 3rd edition. New Delhi: Jaypee Brothers Medical Publishers (P) Ltd: 2015. pp. 656-671.
5. Kozier B, Erb G, Bergman A, et al. Fundamentals of nursing. 7th edition. India Dorling Kindersley Pvt Ltd; 2007.pp. 84-104.
6. Kumari N, Shama S, Gupta P. Midwifery and gynecological nursing. Jalandar City: S Vikas & Company; 2010.
7. Littleton L, Engebretson J. Maternity nursing care. India: Thompson Delmar Learning; 2007. pp. 77-102.
8. Tschudin V. Ethics in nursing. 3rd edition. Philadelphia, USA: WB Saunders; 2003.

CHAPTER 60

National Population Policy and Family Welfare Programs

Learning Objectives

Upon completion of this chapter, the learner will be able to:
- Describe the present population status in India.
- List the measures adopted since 1950 and the demographic achievements after half a century.
- Describe the strategies and action plan of the National Population Policy (NPP).
- Describe the schemes under the National Family Welfare Programs (NFWPs) for maternal and child health.

India is currently the world's second largest country in population. India crossed the 1 billion mark in the year 2000; 1 year after the world population crossed the 6 billion thresholds. India is currently home to about 1.21 billion people representing a full 17% of the earth's population. India's 2011 census showed that the country's population had grown by 181 million people in the prior decade.

Demographers expect India's population to surpass the population of China, currently the most populous country of the world by 2030. At that time, India is expected to have a population of more than 1.53 billion, while China's population is forecast to be at its peak of 1.46 billion.

When India gained independence from the United Kingdom 64 years ago, the country's population was a mere 350 million. Since 1947, the population of India has more than triple. In 1950, India's total fertility rate (TFR) was approximately 6 children per women. Nonetheless since 1952, India has worked to control its population growth. In 1983, the country's National Health Policy (NHP) was to have a replacement value of TFR of 2.1 by the year 2000. That did not occur.

NATIONAL POPULATION POLICY 2000

In the year 2000, the country established a new National Population Policy (NPP), to stem the growth of the country's population. One of the primary goals of the policy was to reduce the TFR to 2.1 by 2010. One of the steps along the path toward the goal in 2010 was a TFR of 2.6 by 2012.

India's demographic achievements half a century after formulating the National Family Welfare Program (NFWP) are:
- Reduced crude birth rate (CBR) from 40.8 in 1951 to 26.4 in 1998
- Halved the infant mortality rate (IMR) from 146 per 1,000 live births in 1951 to 72 per 1,000 live births in 1998
- Quadrupled the couple protection rate (CPR) from 10.4% in 1971 to 44% in 1999
- Reduced crude death rate (CDR) from 25 in 1951 to 9 in 1998
- Added 25 years to life expectancy from 37 years to 62 years
- Achieved nearly universal awareness of the need for and methods of family planning
- Reduced TFR from 6 in 1951 to 3.3 in 1997.

Stabilizing population is an essential requirement for promoting sustainable development with more equitable distribution. However, it is as much a function of making reproductive healthcare accessible and affordable for all:
1. Increasing the provision and outreach of primary and secondary education.
2. Extending basic amenities including sanitation, safe drinking water and housing.
3. Empowering women and enhancing their employment opportunities and providing transport and communication facilities.

The National Population Policy 2000 (NPP 2000) affirms the commitment of government toward voluntary and informed choice and consent of citizens, while availing of reproductive health services, and continuing of 'target free' approach in administering family planning services. The NPP 2000 provides a policy framework for advancing goals and prioritizing strategies during the next decade to meet the reproductive and child health (RCH) needs of the people of India and to achieve net replacement levels by 2010.

Objectives of NPP

The objectives of the NPP 2000 were to address the unmet needs for contraception, healthcare infrastructure, and health personnel and to provide integrated service delivery for basic RCH care. The medium-term objective was to bring the TFR to replacement level by 2010, through vigorous implementation of intersectoral operational strategies. The long-term objective was to achieve a stable population by 2045, at a level consistent with the requirements of sustainable economic growth, social development and environmental protection.

In order to achieve these objectives, the following targets were set:

1. Address the unmet needs for basic RCH services, supplies and infrastructure.
2. Make school education up to age 14, free and mandatory and reduce drop outs at primary and secondary school levels to below 20% for boys and girls.
3. Reduce MR to below 30 per 1,000 live births.
4. Reduce maternal mortality ratio to below 100 per 100,000 child births.
5. Achieve universal immunization of children against all vaccine preventable diseases.
6. Promote delayed marriage for girls, not earlier than 18 and preferably after 20 years.
7. Achieve 80% institutional deliveries and 100% deliveries by trained persons.
8. Achieve universal access to information/counseling and services for fertility regulation, and contraception with a wide basket of choices.
9. Achieve 100% registration of births, deaths, marriages and pregnancies.
10. Contain spread of acquired immunodeficiency syndrome (AIDS) and promote greater integration between the management of reproductive tract infections (RTIs) and sexually transmitted infections (STIs) and National AIDS Control Organization.
11. Prevent and control communicable diseases. Integrate Indian Systems of Medicine (ISM) in the provision of RCH services and in reaching out to households.
12. Promote vigorously the small family norm to achieve the replacement levels of TFR.

Strategies of NPP 2000

- Decentralization of the plan and program implementation
- Convergence in services at delivery points
- Strengthening measures for child survival
- Meeting the unmet needs for family welfare
- Special services to slum dwellers
- Attending to adolescents
- Increasing male participation.

Promotional Measures

- Providing fertility regulating information and services
- Furnishing family life/sex information
- Improving the status of women
- Improving the health and nutrition status
- Providing incentives and disincentives
- Improving research and evaluation
- Carrying out specific legal reforms to influence internal and international migration.

Legislation

As a motivational measure, in order to enable state governments to fearlessly and effectively pursue the agenda for population stabilization contained in the NPP 2000, legislation was considered necessary. It was recommended that the 42nd constitutional amendment that freezes till 2001, the number of seats to the Lok Sabha and Rajya Sabha based on the 1971 census be extended up to 2016.

The NPP 2000 is to be implemented and managed at Panchayat and Nagar Palika levels in coordination with the concerned state/union territory administrations. This will require comprehensive and multisectoral coordination of planning, and implementation between health and family welfare on the one hand along with schemes for education, nutrition, women and child development, safe drinking water, sanitation, rural roads, communication, transportation, housing, forestry development, environmental protection, and urban development. Accordingly the following structures were recommended:

1. *National Commission on Population:* A National Commission on Population presided over by the Prime Minister will have the Chief Ministers of all states and union territories (UT) and the Central Minister-in-*Charge of the Department of Family Welfare* and other concerned central ministers and departments.
2. *State and UT commissions on population:* Each state and UT to have a state/UT Commission, presided over by the Chief Minister, on the analogy of the National Commission to oversee and review implementation of NPP 2000 in the state/UT.
3. Coordination cell in the planning commission.
4. *Technology mission in the department of family welfare:* This will be to provide technology support in respect of design and monitoring of projects and programs for RCH campaigns.

Action Plan of the NPP 2000

1. **Operational strategies:**
    a. Converge service delivery at village level.
    b. Utilize village self-help groups to organize and provide basic services for reproductive and child care, combined with the ongoing *Integrated Child Development Scheme* (ICDS).
    c. Implement at village levels a one-stop integrated and coordinated service delivery package for basic health care, family planning and maternal and child health-related services provided by the community for its members.
    d. At the village levels, the Anganwadi center may become the pivot of basic healthcare activities,

contraceptive counseling and supply, nutrition, education and supplementation as well as preschool activities.
   e. Providing maternity services. The Panchayat may appoint a competent and mature midwife, and volunteers to assist her. Trained birth attendants, traditional dais and auxiliary nurse midwives at subcenters are to monitor and respond to maternal morbidity/emergencies at village level.
2. **Empowering women for improved health and nutrition:**
   a. Create an enabling environment for women and children to benefit from products, and services disseminated under RCH program.
   b. Open more childcare centers in rural areas and in urban slums where a woman worker will have her children in responsible hands.
   c. Pursue drinking water schemes for increasing access to potable water.
   d. Give rewards and priority schemes for households who use energy saving devices such as solar cookers, making sanitation facilities or extending telephone facilities.
   e. Improve district, subdistrict and Panchayat level health management with coordination and collaboration between district health officer and Panchayat for planning and implementing healthcare activities:
      i. Encourage adequate transportation at village level, subcenter level, Zilla Parishads, primary health centers (PHCs) and at community health centers (CHCs), so that the women with complications can reach emergency care in time.
      ii. Strengthen the capacity of PHCs to provide basic emergency obstetric and neonatal health care.
      iii. Involve professional agencies in developing and disseminating training modules for standard procedures in the management of obstetric and neonatal health care.
      iv. Involve professional agencies in developing and disseminating training modules for standard procedures in the management of obstetric and neonatal health care.
      v. Improve supervision by developing guidance and supervision checklists.
   f. Monitor performance of maternal and child health services at each level by using various monitoring systems.
   g. Improve technical skills of maternal and child healthcare providers through in-service education and training.
   h. Develop and implement health package for adolescents.
   i. Expand the availability of safe abortion care.
   j. Develop maternity hospitals, district hospitals and CHCs to function as first referral units (FRUs) for complicated and life-threatening deliveries.
   k. Formulate and enforce standards of clinical services in the public, private and non-governmental organization (NGO) sectors.
   l. Focus on distribution of non-clinical methods of contraception such as condoms and oral pills.
3. **Improving child health and survival:**
   a. Support community activities from village level upwards to monitor early and adequate antenatal, natal and postnatal care. Focus attention on neonatal health care and nutrition.
   b. Promote compulsory registration of births in coordination with ICDS program.
   c. After birth of a child, provide counseling and advocacy about contraception to encourage adoption of a reversible or terminal method.
   d. Improve capacity of health centers in basic midwifery services and essential neonatal care including management of sick neonates.
   e. Sensitize and train health personnel in the integrated management of childhood illnesses.
   f. Strengthen critical interventions aimed at bringing about reductions in maternal malnutrition, morbidity and mortality by ensuring availability of supplies and equipment at village levels and subcenters.
   g. Pursue rigorously the pulse polio campaign to eradicate polio.
   h. Ensure 100% routine immunization for all vaccine preventable diseases.
   i. Expand ICDS to include children between 6 and 9 years of age, especially to promote and ensure 100% school enrolment.
4. **Meeting the unmet needs of family welfare services:**
   a. Address on priority, the different unmet needs in particular an increase in rural infrastructure, deployment of sanctioned and appropriately trained health personnel, and provisioning of essential equipment and drugs.
   b. Improve facilities for referral transportation at Panchayat, Zilla Parishad and PHC levels.
5. **Uplifting the underserved population:** Groups in urban slums, tribal communities, hill area population and displaced, and migrant populations:
   a. Integrate aggressive health education programs with health and medical care programs with emphasis an environmental health, personal hygiene and healthy habits, nutritional education and population education.
   b. Streamline the referral systems and linkage between the primary, secondary and tertiary levels of health care in urban areas.
   c. In tribal areas provide information and counseling in respect of infertility.
   d. Healthcare providers in tribal and hilly areas to adopt a 'burden of disease' approach to meet the special needs of such communities.
   e. Provide for adolescents the package of nutritional services under the ICDS program.

f. Enforce the Child Marriage Restraint Act, 1976, to reduce the incidence of teenage pregnancies.
g. Encourage increased participation of men in planned parenthood. Repopularize vasectomies, in particular the no-scalpel vasectomy as a safe, simple, painless procedure, more convenient and acceptable for men.

6. **Utilizing diverse healthcare providers:**
   a. At district and subdistrict levels, maintain block-wise database of private medical practitioners whose credentials may be certified by Indian Medical Association (IMA).
   b. Revive the earlier system of licensed medical practitioners who, after appropriate certification from IMA, may participate in the provision of clinical services.
   c. Involve nonmedical fraternity in counseling and advocacy.
   d. Modify the under/postgraduate medical, nursing and paramedical professional course syllabic and curricula in consultation with the relevant apex body [IMA, Indian Nursing Council (INC), etc.] in order to reflect the concepts and implementation strategies of the RCH program and the national population policy.
   e. Encourage the efficient functioning of the FRUs, i.e. 30-bed hospitals at block levels, which provide emergency obstetric and child health care to bring about reductions in maternal mortality rate (MMR) and infant mortality rate (IMR).

7. **Collaboration with and commitment from the non-government sector to augment advocacy, counseling and clinical services:**
   a. Collaboration between the voluntary sector and the NGOs will facilitate dissemination of efficient service delivery to village levels.
   b. Encourage voluntary sector to motivate village-level self-help groups to participate in community activities.
   c. Specific collaboration in social marketing of contraceptives to reach village levels.

8. **Mainstreaming of Indian Systems of Medicine and Homeopathy (ISMH):**
   a. Utilize the ISMH institutions, dispensaries and hospitals for health and population related programs.
   b. Utilize the ISM 'barefoot doctors' after appropriate training and orientation for providing advocacy, and counseling for disseminating supplies and equipment, such as depot holders at village levels.

9. **Promotion of research on contraceptive technology and RCH:**
   a. Promote and finance studies and research projects related to MCH services and contraceptive technology.

10. **Providing for older population.**

11. **Promoting information, education and communication:**
    a. Optimal use of folk media to successfully mobilize local population.
    b. Involve departments of rural development, social welfare, transport, co-operatives and education with special reference to schools to improve clarity and focus of the Indian Education Council (IEC) effort and to extend coverage and outreach. Health and population education must be included from the school level.
    c. Utilize radio and television as the most powerful media for disseminating relevant sociodemographic messages.
    d. Involve civil society for disseminating information, counseling and spreading education about small family norm, need for fewer, but healthy babies, higher female literacy and later marriages for women. Civil society could also be of assistance in monitoring the availability of contraceptives, vaccines and drugs in rural areas and in urban slums.

NATIONAL FAMILY WELFARE PROGRAM

India launched the National Family Welfare Program in 1951, with the objective of reducing the birth rate to the extent necessary to stabilize the population at a level consistent with the requirement of the national economy. The Family Welfare Program (FWP) in India is recognized as a priority area and is being implemented as a 100% centrally sponsored program.

Evaluation of the FWP

The approach under the program during the first and second Five Year Plan was mainly 'clinical' under which facilities for provision of services were created. However, on the basis of data brought out by the 1961 census, clinical approach adopted in the first two plans was replaced by 'extension and education approach', which envisaged expansion of service facilities along with spread of message on small family norm.

In the fourth plan (1961–1970) high priority was accorded to the program and it was proposed to reduce birth rate from 35 per 1,000 to 32 per 1,000 by the end of the plan. 16.5 million couples constituting about 16.5% of the couples in the reproductive age group were protected against conception by the end of fourth plan.

The objective of the fifth plan (1974–1979) was to bring down the birth rate to 30 per 1,000 by the end of 1978–1979 by increasing integration of family planning services with those of MCH and nutrition so that, the program become more, readily acceptable.

There was phenomenal increase recorded in the performance of sterilization in 1975–1977 periods. In view of the rigidity of enforcement of targets by field functionaries and an element of coercion in the implementation of the program in some areas the program received a set back during 1977–1978.

This led to a change in approach and the government made it clear that there was no place for force or coercion, or pressure of any sort and the program had to be implemented as an integral part of family welfare relying solely on mass education and motivation. The name of the program was changed to family welfare from family planning.

In the sixth plan (1980–1985), certain demographic goals of reaching net reproduction rate of unity were envisaged. These were to achieve the following by the year 2000:
- Reduction of average family size from 4.4 children in 1995 to 2.3 children
- Reduction of birth rate to 21 from the level of 33 in 1978 and death rate to 9 from 14, and infant mortality to 67 from 127
- Increasing the couple protection level from 22%–60%.

The FWP during the seventh Five Year Plan (1985–1990) was continued on a purely voluntary basis with emphasis on promoting spacing methods, securing maximum community participation and promoting MCH care. In order to provide facilities/services nearer to the door steps of population, the following initiatives were taken:
1. To have one subcenter for every 5,000 population in plain areas and for 3,000 population in hilly and tribal areas. At the end of seventh plan, i.e. 1990, 1.3 lakhs subcenters were established in the country.
2. To extend the postpartum program progressively to subdistrict level hospitals. At the end of seventh plan 1,012 subdistrict level hospitals and 870 health posts were established.
3. To extend the Universal Immunization Program (UIP) to cover all the districts in the country by 1990.
4. To improve primary health care in urban slums in the cities of Mumbai and Chennai with assistance from World Bank.
5. To implement area development projects in selected districts in 15 major states.

The achievements of the FWP at the end of seventh plan were:
- Reduction in crude birth rate from 41.7 (1951–1961) to 30.2 (1990)
- Reduction in TFR from 5.97 (1950–1955) to 3.8 (1990)
- Reduction in IMR from 146 (1970–1971) to 80 (1990)
- Increase in couple protection rate 10.4% (1970–1971) to 43.3% (1990)
- Setting up of a large network of service delivery infrastructure
- Over 118 million births were averted by the end of March 1990.

In the eighth Five Year Plan (1992–1997), several new initiatives were introduced to introduce new dynamism to the FWP. Ongoing schemes were revamped and new initiatives were introduced as under:
1. World Bank assisted area projects, which seek to upgrade infrastructure and development of trained manpower. Indian Population Project (IPP) eighth and ninth were initiated during the eighth plan. The IPP eighth project aims at improving health and family welfare services in urban slums of Delhi, Kolkata, Hyderabad and Bengaluru. IPP ninth will operate in the states of Rajasthan, Assam and Karnataka.
2. An United States Agency for International Development (USAID) assisted project named 'Innovations in Family Planning Services' was taken up in Uttar Pradesh with the specific objective of reducing TFR from 5.4 to 4 and increasing couple protection rate (CPR) from 35% to 50% over 10 years project period.
3. Realizing that government efforts alone in propagating and motivating the people for adoption of small family norm would not be sufficient, greater stress was laid on involvement of NGOs to supplement and complement the government efforts.

The UIP was launched in 1985 to provide universal coverage of infants and pregnant women with immunization against identified vaccine preventable diseases. From the year 1992–1993, the UIP has been strengthened and expanded into the Child Survival and Safe Motherhood (CSSM) project. It involves sustaining the high immunization coverage level under UIP, and augmenting activities under oral rehydration therapy (ORT), prophylaxis for control of blindness in children and control of acute respiratory infections. Under the safe motherhood component, training of traditional birth attendants (TBAs), provision of aseptic delivery kits and strengthening of FFUs to deal with high risk and obstetric emergencies were taken up.

The targets fixed for the eighth plan of national level birth rate of 26 was achieved by all states except the states of Assam, Bihar, Haryana, Madhya Pradesh, Orissa, Rajasthan and Uttar Pradesh.

In the ninth Five Year Plan (1997–2002), reduction in the population growth has been recognized as one of the priority objectives. The objectives were:
- To meet all the felt needs for contraception
- To reduce the infant and maternal morbidity and mortality so that, there is a reduction in the desired level of fertility.

The strategies during the plan would be:
- Assess the needs for RCH at PHC level and undertake area-specific micro planning
- To provide need-based demand-driven high quality, integrated RCH care.

The expected levels of achievement by the terminal year of 2002 were:
- Crude birth rate 23/1,000
- Infant mortality rate 50/1,000
- Total fertility rate 2.6
- Couple protection rate 60%
- Neonatal mortality rate 35/1,000
- Maternal mortality rate 3/1,000.

Vital Statistics 2011 (India)

Data from population and health statistics of India, based on census 2011, National Health Profile (NHP) 2011 and Sample Registration Bulletin (SRS Bull) December 2011.

Population

- *Population:* 1,210 million
- *Growth per year:* 18 million
- *Average annual growth rate:* 1.76%
- *Urban population:* 31%

- *Sex ratio:* 940 females for 1,000 males
- *0–4 years:* 10%
- *5–14 years:* 23%
- *15–44 years:* 48%
- *45–59 years:* 12%
- *60+ years:* 7%.

Vital Rates

- *Birth rate:* 22.1/1,000 population
- *Crude death rate:* 7.1/1,000 population
- *Infant mortality rate:* 47/1,000 population
- *Maternal mortality ratio:* 212/100,000 live births
- *Expectation of life at birth:* 64.2 years.

Fertility and Family Welfare

Couples using contraceptives (any method): 56.3%.

Implementation of the FWP

The following were the main components of FWP:
- Maternal health
- Child health
- Population control/Stabilization.

The following were the schemes and programs for implementation of National Family Welfare:
- Reproductive and Child Health Program
- Janani Suraksha Yojana (JSY)
- Vande Mataram Scheme
- Safe Abortion Services
- National Rural Health Mission (NRHM)
- Integrated Child Development Services.

REPRODUCTIVE AND CHILD HEALTH PROGRAM

Population growth and health of women and children had been a major problem in India despite implementation of several programs since 1951. MCH and CSSM programs were implemented through organized healthcare systems.

In 1994, during the International Conference on Population Development (ICPD), a new approach to tackle the problem was recommended. The Government of India adopted the Reproductive Health Approach and launched the RCH program in October 1997.

The objective of the RCH program was to provide quality, integrated and sustainable primary healthcare services to women in the reproductive age group, and children with special focus on family planning and immunization.

Essential Components of RCH Program

- Prevention and management of unwanted pregnancy
- Services for mothers during pregnancy, childbirth and postpartum period
- Child survival services for newborns and infants
- Management of RTIs and sexually transmitted diseases (STDs)
- Establishment of an effective referral system
- Reproductive services for adolescent health
- Health services including counseling on sexuality and family life.

Services Included in the Program for Mothers and Children

1. *Essential care for all mothers and children:*
   a. Registration by 12th–16th week of pregnancy.
   b. Antenatal check-up at least three times during pregnancy.
   c. Tetanus toxoid to all women as early as possible during pregnancy with two doses at 1 month interval.
   d. Iron and folic acid tablets daily for 100 days. Women with clinical signs of anemia to receive two tablets daily for 100 days.
   e. Deworming with mebendazole during second or third trimester in areas where hookworm infestation is common.
   f. Safe and clean delivery services.
   g. Preparation of women for exclusive breastfeeding and timely weaning.
   h. Postpartum care, including advises and services for limiting and spacing births.
2. *Early detection of complications:*
   a. Clinical examination to detect anemia.
   b. Referral and transportation to the nearest hospital of women with hemorrhage or complications.
   c. Referral of all women identified as having pregnancy-induced hypertension (BP >140/90 mm Hg and weight gain >3 kg/month).
   d. Referral of all women who develop signs of infection following delivery or abortion.
   e. Transfer of women in labor for more than 12 hours to the nearest hospital that has facilities for cesarean delivery.
3. *Emergency care to those who need it:*
   a. Early identification of obstetric emergencies.
   b. Initial management of emergencies and transfer to referral hospital without delay using the fastest available mode of transport.
4. *Care to women in the reproductive age group:*
   a. Counseling on:
      » Optimal timing and spacing of birth
      » Small family norm
      » Use and choice of contraceptives
      » Prevention of STDs and RTIs
      » Importance of girl child.
   b. Information on availability of:
      » Medical termination of pregnancy (MTP) services
      » Intrauterine contraceptive device (IUCD) and sterilization services.
   c. Family planning services:
      » Condom distribution
      » Oral contraceptive dispensing
      » Intrauterine contraceptive device services.

d. Recognition and referral of clients with STDs and RTIs.
5. *Provision of clean and safe delivery practices at the community level:*
   a. Creation of awareness about the need for clean and safe deliveries.
   b. Deliveries by trained personnel.
   c. Provision of disposable delivery kits for deliveries.
   d. Promotion of institutional deliveries.
   e. Early identification and referral of high-risk cases.
6. *Newborn care:*
   a. Weighing all newborns at birth. Normal weight 2,500–2,800 g. Referral of newborns weighing >2,000 g.
   b. Resuscitation of asphyxiated newborns using mucus sucker or breathing as required.
   c. Prevention of hypothermia.
   d. Breastfeeding within 1 hour of birth.
   e. Referral of newborns who show signs of illness.
   f. Education of mother on newborn care and feeding.
7. *Immunization:*
   Infants
   a. Bacille Calmette-Guérin (BCG) one dose at birth.
   b. Diphtheria, tetanus, pertussis (DPT): Three doses, beginning at 6th week at monthly interval.
   c. Polio: 'Zero' dose at birth for all institutional deliveries and three doses at 1 month interval.
   d. Measles: One dose at completion of 9 months.
   e. Vitamin A: First dose of 100,000 IU along with measles vaccination.
   Children 1 to 3 years
   a. Diphtheria, tetanus, pertussis.
   b. Oral polio vaccine (OPV) booster dose at 16th to 18th month.
   c. Vitamin A:
      » Second dose 200,000 IU at 16th to 18th month
      » Third to fifth doses 200,000 IU each at 6 monthly intervals.
   Children 3 to 5 years
   a. Iron and folic acid (smaller dose) for children with signs of anemia.
   b. Treatment for worm infestation with mebendazole.
8. *Prevention of deaths due to diarrheal diseases:*
   a. Correct management.
   b. Teaching mothers to increase body fluid with ORS and normal feeding.
9. *Prevention of deaths due to pneumonia:*
   a. Correct management of all cases of acute respiratory infections.
   b. Referral of children with severe pneumonia or severe illness.

Reproductive and child health phase II began in April 2005. The focus of the program was to reduce maternal and child morbidity and mortality with emphasis on rural health care.

Strategies

The major strategies of the second phase of RCH are:
- Essential obstetric care:
  - Institutional delivery
  - Skilled attendance at delivery
  - Policy decisions.
- Emergency obstetric care:
  - Operationalizing FRUs
  - Operationalizing PHCs and CHCs for round the clock delivery services.
- Strengthening the referral system.

Services Included

1. *Essential obstetric care:*
   a. Institutional delivery: In order to promote institutional deliveries, it is envisaged that 50% of the PHCs and all the CHCs would be made operational as 24-hour delivery centers in a phased manner by 2010. Basic emergency obstetric care essential newborn care and basic newborn resuscitation services will be provided in these centers round the clock.
   b. Skilled attendance at delivery: Guidelines for conducting normal delivery and management of obstetric complications at PHC and CHC for medical officers and for skilled attendance at birth for auxiliary nurse midwife (ANM) and lady health visitors (LHVs) have been formulated and disseminated to the states.
   c. Policy decisions regarding use of drugs and interventions: ANMs, LHVs and staff nurses (SNs) have now been permitted to use certain drugs in specific emergency situations to reduce maternal mortality. They have also been permitted to carry out certain emergency interventions when the life of the mother is at stake.
2. *Emergency obstetric care:*
   The FRUs will be made operational/functional with following services on a 24-hour basis:
   a. 24-hour delivery services including normal and assisted deliveries.
   b. Emergency obstetric care including surgical interventions like cesarean sections:
      » Newborn care
      » Emergency care of sick newborns
      » Full range of family planning services including laparoscopic services
      » Safe abortion services
      » Treatment for STIs and respiratory tract infections
      » Blood storage facility
      » Essential laboratory services
      » Referral (transport) services.
      In order to perform full range of FRU functions a health facility must have:
      » Minimum bed strength of 20–30
      » Fully functional operation theater
      » Fully functional labor room with well-equipped care area

» A functional laboratory and blood storage facility
» 24-hour water and electricity supply
» Arrangements for waste disposal
» Ambulance facility.

3. *Strengthening referral system:*
   In order to improve referral linkage practiced in RCH phase I, new initiatives were added:
   a. Training of MBBS doctors in life-saving anesthetic skills for emergency obstetric care.
   b. Setting up of blood storage centers at FRUs according to government of India guidelines.
   c. Janani Suraksha Yojana: The National Maternity Benefit Scheme (NMBS) has been modified into a new scheme called Janani Suraksha Yojana.

JANANI SURAKSHA YOJANA

Janani Suraksha Yojana program was launched on 12th April 2005. The objectives of the scheme are such as reducing maternal mortality and infant mortality through encouraging delivery at health institutions and focusing at institutional care among women below poverty line families.

Salient Features of the JSY

1. It is a 100% centrally sponsored scheme.
2. Benefit of cash assistance with institutional care during antenatal, delivery, and postpartum care to all women both rural and urban belonging to below poverty line households and aged 19 years or above, up to first two live births. In 10 low-performing states, the cash benefit will be extended up to the third child, if the mother chooses to undergo sterilization in the health facility where she delivered. The accredited social health activist (ASHA) will be responsible for making institutional care available. She would also be responsible for escorting the pregnant woman to the health center.

The cash assistance will be ₹1,400 to all mothers in rural areas of low-performing states and ₹1,200 to mothers in urban areas. All women including those from SC and ST families delivering in government institutions or accredited private institutions are eligible for cash assistance. Women from rural areas of high-performing states get ₹700, while those from urban areas get ₹600.

The Yojana gives cash assistance of ₹250 for transportation of women to the nearest health center for delivery. The women get a subsidy of ₹1,500 for cesarean deliveries and management of obstetric complications. According to the government report of 2008, in the years 2006–2008 about 28.11 lakhs pregnant women received benefits from this scheme, out which 18.72 lakhs had institutional deliveries.

VANDE MATARAM SCHEME

Vande Mataram Scheme is a voluntary scheme wherein any obstetric or gynecology specialist, maternity home or nursing home lady doctor or MBBS doctor can volunteer herself/himself for providing safe motherhood services. The enrolled doctor will display 'Vandemataram logo' at the clinic. Iron and folic acid tablets, oral pills, tetanus toxoid (TT) injections, etc. will be provided by the respective District Medical Officers (DMOs) to the 'Vande Mataram doctors or clinics' for distribution to beneficiaries. The cases needing special care and treatment can be referred to the government hospitals that have been advised to take due care of such patients coming with Vande Mataram cards.

SAFE ABORTION SERVICES

In India abortion is a major cause of maternal morbidity and mortality, and accounts for nearly 8.9% of maternal deaths. Majority of abortions take place outside authorized health services and/or by unauthorized and unskilled persons. Under RCH phase II, following facilities are provided:

1. *Medical method of abortion:* Termination of early pregnancy with drugs—mifepristone (RU-486) followed by misoprostol; currently, the use of these two drugs are recommended up to 7 weeks (49 days) of amenorrhea in a facility with provision for safe abortion services and blood transfusion. Termination of pregnancy using these two drugs is offered to women under the preview of the Medical Termination Pregnancy (MTP) Act 1971.
2. *Manual vacuum aspiration (MVA):* This is a safe and simple technique for termination of early pregnancy, and is feasible to be used in PHCs or comparable facilities, thereby increasing the access to safe abortion services.

All the below listed interventions included in RCH phase I will continue in the phase II implementation period:
   a. Appointing additional public health nurses, ANMs, anesthetists and safe motherhood consultants.
   b. Providing 24-hour delivery services at PHCs and CHCs.
   c. Providing referral transport and integrated financial package.
   d. Conducting RCH camps and training of Dais.
   e. Implementing interventions for newborn care and child health [immunization, control of acute respiratory injection (ARI) and diarrhea, vitamin A and iron supplementation, etc.].

NATIONAL RURAL HEALTH MISSION

The Government of India launched NRHM on 5th April 2005 for a period of 7 years (2005–2012) in order to improve the quality of life of its citizens. The mission seeks to improve the healthcare delivery system. It is operational in the whole country with special focus on North East states.

The main aim of NRHM is to provide accessible, accountable, effective and reliable primary health care and to bridge the gap in rural health care through creation of a cadre of ASHA, and strengthening the services of subcenters, PHCs and CHCs.

Goals to be Achieved by NRHM

At National Level

1. Reduction of IMR to 30/ 1,000 live births.
2. Reduction of MMR to 100/100,000.
3. Reduction of total fertility.
4. Reduction of mortality rates of malaria, filaria, dengue, kala-azar and Japanese encephalitis.
5. Reduction of prevalence rates of leprosy and tuberculosis.
6. Upgrading CHCs to Indian Public Health standards.
7. Increasing FRUs from less than 20% to 75%.
8. Engaging 250,000 female ASHA.

At Community Level

1. Availing trained community level workers at village level with a drug kit for general ailments.
2. Provision of immunization, antenatal and postnatal check-ups, and services related to health of mother and child including nutrition at Anganwadi level.
3. Availing of generic drugs for common ailments at subcenter level.
4. Providing good hospital care through assured availability of doctors, drugs and quality services at PHC and CHC level.
5. Improved access to universal immunization.
6. Improved facilities for institutional deliveries.
7. Availability of assured health care at reduced financial risk.
8. Improved outreach services through mobile medical units at district level.
9. Provision of household toilets.

Plan of Implementation of NRHM

Implementation of the NRHM program will be through ASHAs and ANMs.

Selection of ASHA

The ASHA must be a resident of the village—a woman (married/widowed/divorced) preferably in the age group of 25–45 with formal education up to eight class, having communication skills and leadership qualities. The general norm will be one ASHA for 1,000 populations. In tribal, hilly and desert areas, the norm could be relaxed to one ASHA per habitation. The selected ASHAs will be trained to carry out specific responsibilities.

Roles and Responsibilities of ASHA

The ASHA will function as a health activist in the community and carry out the following responsibilities:

1. Take steps to create awareness and provide information on health determinants such as nutrition, basic sanitation and hygienic practices, healthy living and the need for utilization of existing health and family welfare services.
2. Counsel women on birth preparedness, safe delivery, breastfeeding, complementary feeding, immunization, contraception and prevention of common infections including RTIs and STIs.
3. Mobilize community in accessing health-related services available at the Anganwadi, subcenter, and PHC such as immunization, antenatal check-up, postnatal check-up, supplementary nutrition, sanitation and other services being provided by the government.
4. Identify women in families below poverty line (BPL) as beneficiaries of the scheme (NRHM) and assist them to obtain BPL registration.
5. Ensure that the JSY card is filled up at least 16–20 weeks prior to delivery.
6. Work with the village health and sanitation committee of the Gram Panchayat to develop comprehensive village health plan.
7. Arrange escort/accompany pregnant women and children requiring treatment/admission to the nearest preidentified health facility (subcenter or PHC).
8. Provide primary medical care for minor ailments such as fever, diarrhea, and first aid for minor injuries.
9. Be a provider of 'directly observed treatment short-course' (DOTS) under national tuberculosis control program.
10. Will act as a direct depot holder for essential provisions like ORS, iron and folic acid tablets, chloroquine, disposable delivery kits, oral pills and condoms, and keep a medicine kit with Ayurveda, Yoga and Naturopathy, Unani, Siddha and Homoeopathy (AYUSH) and allopathic formulations recommended by the technical/expert advisory group of the government.
11. Ensure registration of births and deaths in her village, any unusual health problems or disease outbreaks in the community.
12. Promote construction of household toilets under total sanitation campaign.

Role and Integration with ANM

The ANM will guide ASHA in performing her functions through activities such as:

- Holding weekly/fortnightly meetings to discuss activities
- Acting as resource person for training of ASHA
- Guiding ASHA regarding arrangement for outreach programs
- Participating and guiding ASHA in organizing health days in Anganwadi center
- Utilizing ASHA to motivate pregnant women to go to the subcenter for checkups, take full course of iron and folic acid tablets and TT injections.

The ANMs will inform ASHA on date, time and place for initial and periodic training schedule, and also ensure that ASHA gets the compensation for performance and traveling allowance (TA)/daily allowance (DA) for attending training.

INTEGRATED CHILD DEVELOPMENT SERVICES

Integrated Child Development Service program adopts a multisectoral approach to child well-being incorporating health education and nutrition interventions, and is implemented through a network or Anganwadi centers at the community level. Malnutrition is fought through interventions targeted at unmarried adolescent girls, pregnant women, mothers and children up to 6 years.

The key services provided through ICDS are:
- Supplementary feeding
- Immunization
- Health and nutrition education
- Micronutrient supplementation
- Preschool education for 3–6 years old
- Nutrition, health awareness and skills development for adolescent girls
- Income generation schemes for women.

Supplementary nutrition service includes growth monitoring, prophylaxis against vitamin A deficiency and control of nutritional anemia. All families in the community are surveyed to identify children below the age of 6, pregnant and nursing mothers. They are given supplementary nutritional support for 300 days in a year. The program aims to bridge the caloric gap between the national recommended, and average intake of children and women in low income and disadvantaged groups.

Children below the age of 3 are weighed once a month and children below 3–6 are weighed quarterly. Growth rate and nutritional status are assessed, and malnourished children are given supplementary feeding and referred to medical centers.

Immunization of pregnant women against tetanus is undertaken toward reducing maternal and neonatal mortality. Vaccination of infants and children for six vaccine preventable diseases—poliomyelitis, diphtheria, pertussis, tetanus, tuberculosis and measles are also included.

Health check-ups are offered to children up to 6 years, and expectant and nursing mothers. The services are provided by Anganwadi workers and PHC staff and include weight checking, immunization, management of malnutrition, treatment of diarrhea, deworming and distribution of simple medicines. Through the 1.4 million Anganwadi centers, the education component of the ICDS program is implemented. The early learning provides foundation for cumulative, lifelong learning and development. This also contributes to universalization of primary education. Providing to children the necessary preparation for primary schooling, nutrition, and health education are key elements of the work of Anganwadi workers. Capacity building of women, especially in the age group of 15–45 years is a long-term goal to be achieved.

Integrated Child Development Service Team

The ICDS team comprises the Anganwadi workers, Anganwadi helper, supervisors, Child Development Project Officers (CDPOs) and District Program Officers (DPOs). Anganwadi workers are ladies selected from the local communities and as such community-based front line workers of the ICDS program. The health teams include medical officers, ANMs and ASHAs as functionaries of ICDS to provide different services.

STUDY QUESTIONS

Short Notes

1. Reproductive Child Health Program.
2. Accredited Social Health Activist (ASHA).

Short Answer Questions

1. Objectives of National Population Policy of India, 2000.
2. List the essential components of Reproductive and Child Health (RCH) program.
3. Essential obstetric care under RCH plan.
4. Emergency obstetric care under RCH plan.
5. Integrated Child Development Services (ICDS).

Essay Question

1. Describe the National Rural Health Mission (NRHM) plan made by Government of India for 2005–2012 including the goals and plan of implementation.

BIBLIOGRAPHY

1. Government of India, Ministry of Health and Family Welfare. Annual report 2005–2006; New Delhi: 2006.
2. Government of India, Rural Health Division. Bulletin for Rural Health Statistics in India; New Delhi: 2002.
3. Park K. Park's Textbook of Preventive and Social Medicine. 21st edition. Jabalpur: M/S Banarsidas Bhanot Publishers; 2011. pp. 408-526.
4. Sharma MP. (2012). Selected Health Statistics of India 2012. [online]. Available from www.ucms.ac.in
5. Sikdar SK. Government of India, Family Planning Division. Ministry of Health and Family Planning. [online]. Available from www.cami.health.org

CHAPTER 61

Obstetric and Gynecological Instruments

Learning Objectives

Upon completion of this chapter, the learner will be able to:
- Identify the instruments used in obstetrics and gynecology.
- Describe the features of different instruments.
- Enumerate the specifications and uses of specific instruments.

SPONGE HOLDING FORCEPS (FIG. 61.1)

Specifications and Uses

- A heavy metal instrument 23–75 cm in length
- Shafts are thin and blades are fenestrated
- Has a catch-lock, which gives firmness, while holding any material
- Has ring shaped tips, which may be serrated or smooth
- Used for cleaning the operative field
- Used for swabbing or packing body cavities like vagina
- Can be used to catch hold of soft organs like ovary and cervix in pregnancy

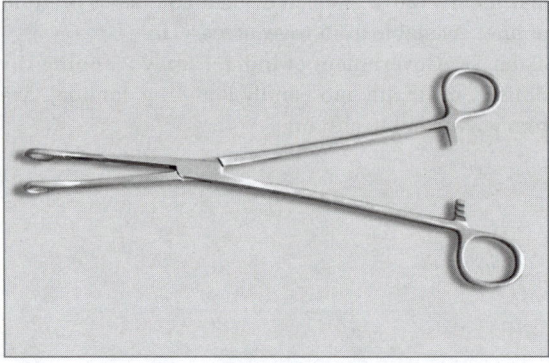

Figure 61.1: Sponge holding forceps.

- Can be substituted in the place of an ovum forceps
- Used for deep moping to clear the area during surgery.

KOCHER'S HEMOSTATIC FORCEPS (FIGS. 61.2A AND B)

Specifications and Uses

- A strong, straight metal instrument
- Has a catch-lock to bring the blades together for locking
- Inner surface of both blades are transversely serrated
- It may be straight or curved
- Single toothed at distal end
- Used to catch the edges of the incision, while suturing skin
- Used for artificial rupture membranes
- Used to clamp the umbilical cord.

HEMOSTATS (ARTERY FORCEPS) (FIGS. 61.3A AND B)

Specifications and Uses

- Artery forceps may be small or mosquito straight, or curved, strong metal instrument
- Medium or large in size
- Blades are tapering to the distal end, but blunt
- Has a catch-lock to bring the blades together and to lock it
- Inner surface of the blades are transversely serrated and when locked, the blades are well in apposition
- Blades are roughly half the size of the handle
- Used to stop bleeding by catching the blood vessel
- Used as a clamp for pedicles of internal organs like kidneys, spleen, ligaments of uterus, etc.
- Used to enlarge the opening of an abscess in the absence of a sinus forceps
- Can be used to substitute a needle holder
- Used to hold the incised edges of skin and fascia
- Used to hold the free ends of sutures at the beginning of suturing and to hold the cut ends of tension sutures before tying

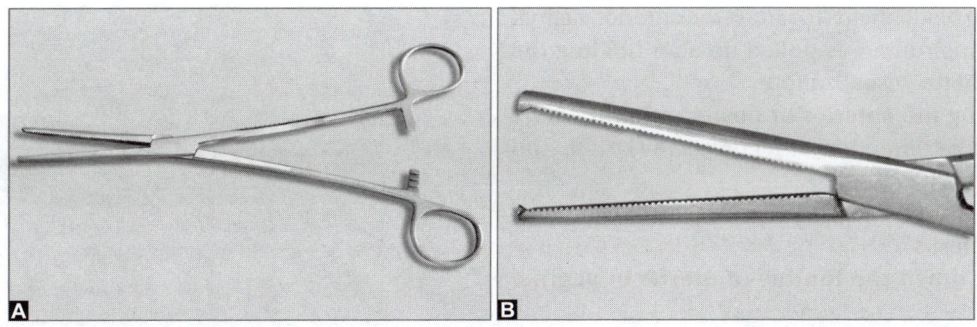

Figures 61.2A and B: Kocher's hemostatic forceps. (A) Kocher's forceps; (B) Toothed distal end.

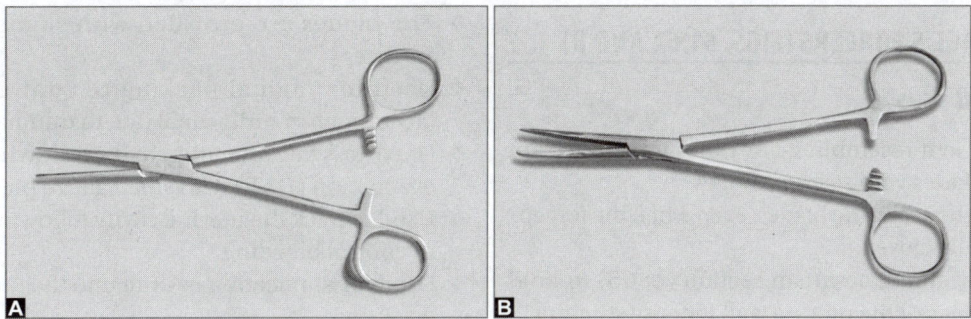

Figures 61.3A and B: Artery forceps. (A) Straight artery forceps; (B) Curved artery forceps.

- Used to hold the tape of abdominal pads or sponges during surgeries to prevent them missing in the cavity
- Mosquito forceps are used to hold the small bleeding points
- Used for blunt dissection by holding swabs.

OVUM FORCEPS (FIGS. 61.4A AND B)

Specifications and Uses

- A moderately heavy metal instrument having cupped blades with linear fenestrations
- The size and type of blades can hold a reasonable amount of tissues in between with good grip
- The length is about 30 cm
- Used for removing products of conception from the uterus in incomplete abortion
- Used to remove any foreign body from the uterine cavity, e.g. intrauterine device when threads are broken
- Used to remove any retained placental bits or membrane pieces from the uterus after delivery.

VULSELLUM FORCEPS (FIG. 61.5)

Specifications and Uses

- An average sized metal instrument resembling forceps at the distal end
- The proximal end has a lock for fixing and distal end has multiple sharp teeth for firm grip

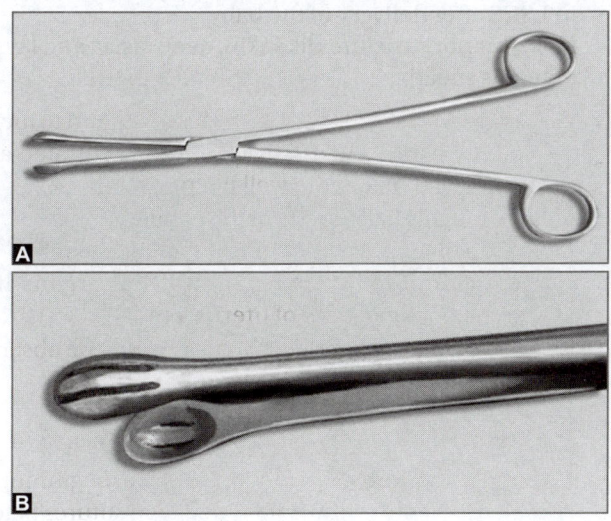

Figures 61.4A and B: Ovum forceps. (A) Ovum forceps with cupped blade; (B) Ovum holding tip of the forceps.

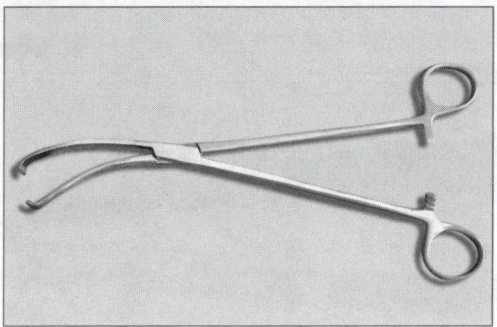

Figure 61.5: Vulsellum forceps.

- The curvature of blades helps to retract the anterior vaginal wall when the instrument is pulled up after holding the cervical lip for better visualization
- Used for holding the anterior or posterior lip of cervix in operations like dilatation and curettage (D&C), and cauterization of cervix
- Used to test the mobility of cervix and laxity of ligaments in prolapse of uterus
- Used to bring down the fundus of uterus in vaginal hysterectomy
- Used to hold the cervical lip for procedures like tubal insufflation or introduction of laminaria tent.

GREEN ARMYTAGE'S FORCEPS (FIGS. 61.6A AND B)

Specifications and Uses

- A metal instrument resembling any other forceps except for triangular blades with serrated edges
- Has small space between the blades, even when the forceps is locked and fully closed
- Used in lower segment cesarean section (LSCS) to hold the retracted edges of the uterine wall for easy stitching
- While holding the edges, it acts as a hemostat to decrease bleeding from the incision.

UTERINE PACKING FORCEPS/UTERINE DRESSING FORCEPS (FIG. 61.7)

Specifications and Uses

- A curved forceps about 35 cm in length, the curvature corresponding to axis of birth canal for easy packing
- Has blades, handles and finger bows

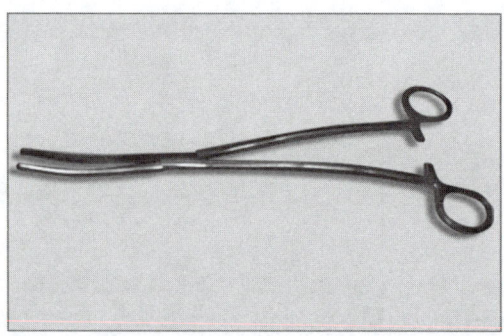

Figure 61.7: Uterine packing forceps.

- The blades are provided with slight groves on inner surfaces
- Used for vaginal packing to control bleeding from lacerations in birth canal due to trauma
- Used to swab uterine cavity following dilatation and evacuation (D&E) with small gauze pieces
- Used to pack the uterine cavity following D&C or delivery to control bleeding
- Used for application of drug into the uterine cavity.

ALLIS TISSUE FORCEPS (FIG. 61.8)

Specifications and Uses

- An instrument with straight blades and catch lock
- Have sharp teeth at the tip with interlock on closing
- The tips are slightly curved or angulated for better grip of tissues
- It is used to:
  - Catch hold of the anterior lip of the cervix during D&C operation
  - Hold the apex of the episiotomy wound during repair
  - Catch hold of the torn ends of the *sphincter ani prior* to suturing in repair of complete perineal tear
  - Catch hold of the margins and angles of the uterine flaps in LSCS after delivery of the baby
  - Hold thinner structures like skin, deep fascia and layers of rectus sheath.

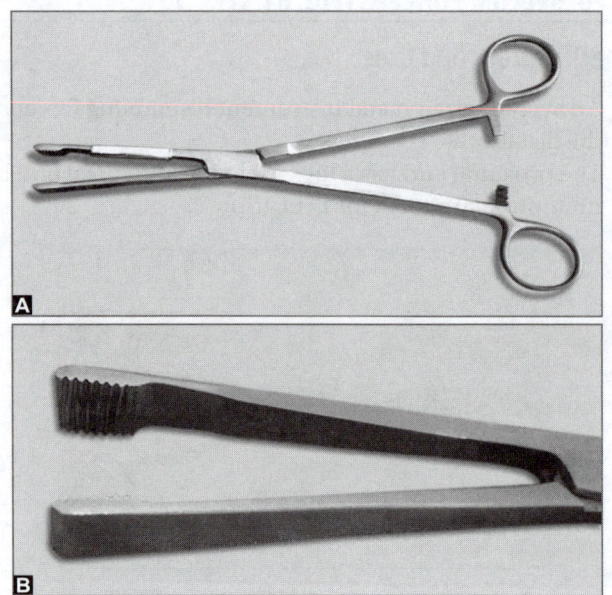

Figures 61.6A and B: Green Armytage's forceps.

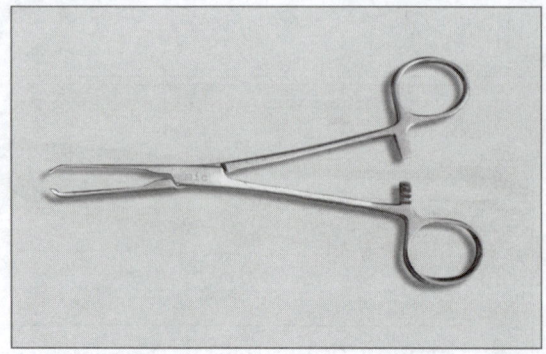

Figure 61.8: Allis tissue forceps.

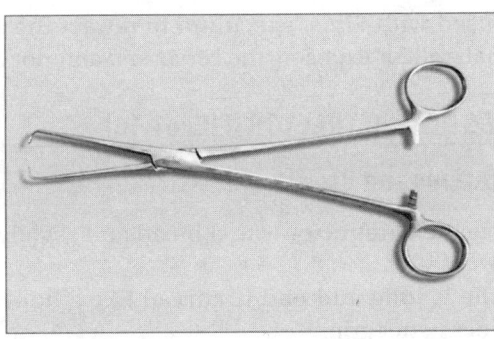

Figure 61.9: Tenaculum forceps.

TENACULUM FORCEPS (FIG. 61.9)

Specifications and Uses

- An instrument resembling vulsellum forceps except there is a single tooth at the distal end
- Used to hold the tissues at one point only, so as to minimize bleeding
- Used to hold the anterior lip of cervix transversely, while doing Rubin's test in order to fit the cannula airtight in the cervix.

LAMINARIA TENT INTRODUCING FORCEPS (FIG. 61.10)

Specifications and Uses

- A metal instrument with a handle and lock
- Almost similar to uterine dressing forceps
- Has a groove on either blade to catch the laminaria tent
- Used to hold and introduce the laminaria tent conveniently into the cervix.

LAMINARIA TENT (FIG. 61.11)

Specifications and Uses

- Laminaria tent is dehydrated, compressed, Chinese seaweed
- It is sterilized by keeping it immersed in absolute alcohol

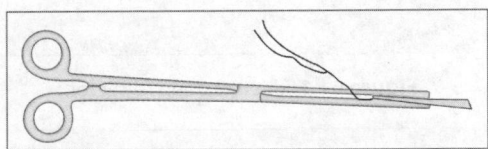

Figure 61.10: Laminaria tent introducing forceps.

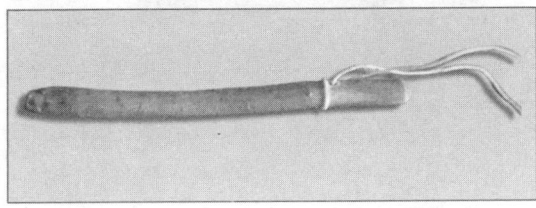

Figure 61.11: Laminaria tent.

- Tents are about 7–10 cm in length with an eye at one end and a thread hanging through the eye of each tent
- The thread attached to the tent facilitates easy removal
- Laminaria tents (more than one) are introduced into the cervical canal and kept for 12–24 hours
- The tent being hygroscopic swells up by absorbing fluid from cervix causing slow dilatation of cervical canal
- Used for dilating cervical canal in cases of spasmodic dysmenorrhea and for expulsion of products of conception in medically terminated pregnancy (MTP), incomplete abortion and hydatidiform mole.

DISSECTING FORCEPS (FIGS. 61.12A AND B)

Specifications and Uses

- It has two equal, flat shafts with a sharp curve at the middle and joined at the proximal end
- Toothed dissecting forceps have tooth in the inner surface of the distal end
- On pressing the shafts, the pointed tips are well-apposed, so that they do not slip against each other
- The outer surface of shafts is made rough and irregular to get a firm grip, while holding in the hand
- Plain dissecting forceps are used to hold delicate structures like peritoneum, vessels, bowel wall, etc. for suturing and to lift swabs, and gauze pieces for dressing
- Toothed dissecting forceps are used to hold tough structures like skin or fascia, while suturing
- It is used to lift the knots of sutures, while removing them after the wounds are healed. It is used to dissect soft, friable tissues.

DOYEN'S TOWEL CLIP (FIG. 61.13)

Specifications and Uses

- Doyen's towel clip is a light and strong metal instrument
- It has a catch lock to fix the grip of drapes
- The tips are sharply pointed for better grasping

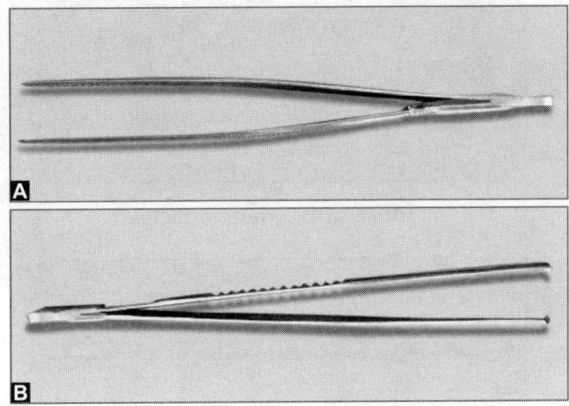

Figures 61.12A and B: Dissecting forceps. (A) Non-toothed dissecting forceps; (B) Toothed dissecting forceps.

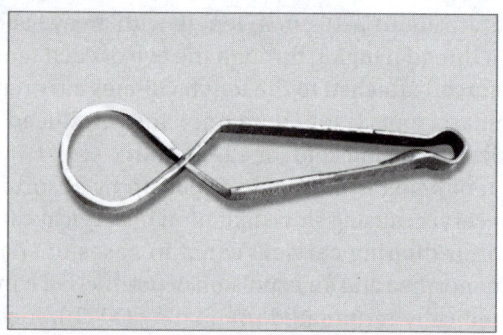

Figure 61.13: Doyen's towel clip.

- Used to fix drapes in order to expose only the required area
- Used to fix tubing such as suction tubes to drapes preventing displacement
- It can be used as tongue holding forceps in emergency situations, but it will perforate the tongue.

DOYEN'S RETRACTOR (FIG. 61.14)

Specifications and Uses

- Doyen's retractor is a metal instrument with flat solid blade on one end and a long handle
- Used to retract pelvic organs during cesarean section
- It is temporarily taken off, while delivering the baby and then reintroduced till toileting of peritoneal cavity is done.

ANTERIOR VAGINAL WALL RETRACTOR (FIG. 61.15)

Specifications and Uses

- A metal instrument with two oval shaped and fenestrated ends
- The fenestrated end has transverse serrations
- The oval shaped ends are connected at an angle of 45°C to both ends of the shaft

- It is used with Sims' speculum to retract the anterior vaginal wall for exposing the cervix and anterior fornix.

KELLY'S DEEP RETRACTOR (FIG. 61.16)

Specifications and Uses

- A large metal retractor with a broad and slightly curved blade
- Handle is long and end is curved like a hook, which provides better grip
- This type of retractor is available in various sizes
- It is used for retracting intra-abdominal viscera like liver and spleen during surgeries like cholecystectomy
- Smaller size retractor is used to retract the bladder walls in intravesical operations
- It is used to retract pelvic structures during surgery of appendix, cecum, etc. to prevent injury to pelvic organs.

SIMS' DOUBLE-BLADED VAGINAL SPECULUM (FIG. 61.17)

Specifications and Uses

- A moderately heavy metal instrument
- It has two thick blades of unequal breadths to facilitate introduction according to the size of vagina
- It is used to:
  - Toilet the vagina following delivery
  - Visualize any injured site on the cervix or vagina
  - Inspect the cervix to exclude any local lesion causing bleeding in suspected cases of abortion, ante- or post-partum hemorrhage (APH or PPH).

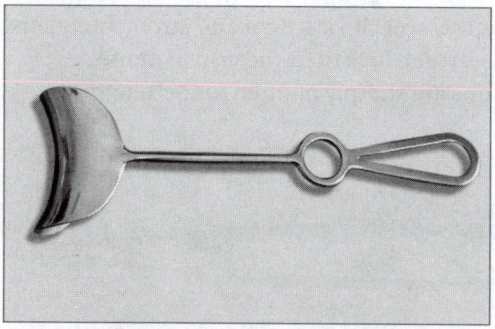

Figure 61.14: Doyen's retractor.

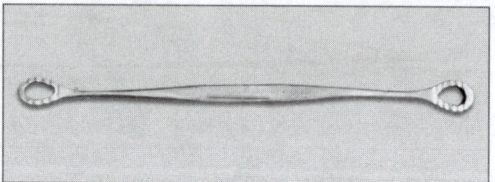

Figure 61.15: Anterior vaginal wall retractor.

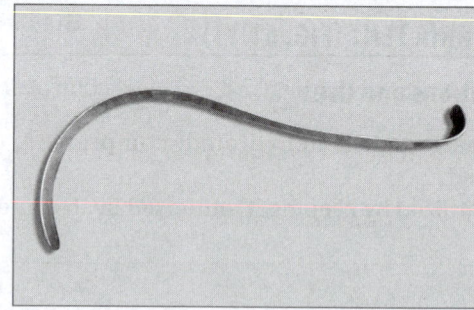

Figure 61.16: Kelly's deep retractor.

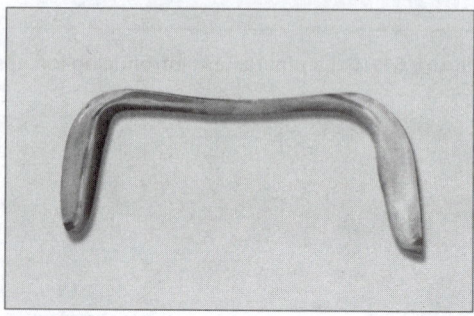

Figure 61.17: Sims' double-bladed vaginal speculum.

- Used in operations of the cervix and vagina in lithotomy position
- Used in D&C, and D&E surgery
- Used for taking biopsy from genital tract and for cauterization of erosions of cervix.

CUSCO'S BIVALVED SPECULUM (FIG. 61.18)

Specifications and Uses

- A self-retaining speculum with a special screw arrangement
- It has two blades, which can be opened laterally and adjusted at various angles by adjusting the screw after introducing in the vagina
- It is introduced into the vagina with its blades closed in vertical position and then made horizontal, opened and locked in position; it can be closed and rotated further, and opened again to see other sides of vagina after locking in required position
- Can be used without any assistance
- Used to visualize or inspect vagina and cervix
- Can be used without bringing the patient to the edge of bed
- Used in insertion of intrauterine contraceptive device (IUCD)
- Used to reach into the cervix to apply medications to take swabs for culture and sensitivity to get biopsy specimens, and to do electrocautery in the cervix.

AUVARD'S WEIGHTED VAGINAL SPECULUM (FIG. 61.19)

Specifications and Uses

- Auvard's weighted vaginal speculum is weighted vaginal speculum for retaining
- The weight is due to the metal weight attached to the handle
- There is a channel in the handle for collection of discharges and curette material
- It is used to retract the posterior vaginal wall in operations of the cervix and vagina in lithotomy position such as D&C, D&E or dilatation and insufflation.

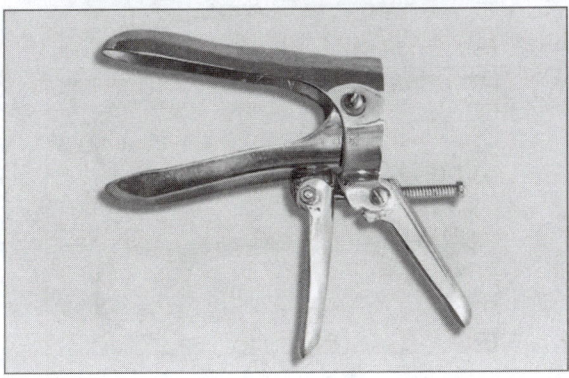

Figure 61.18: Cusco's bivalved speculum.

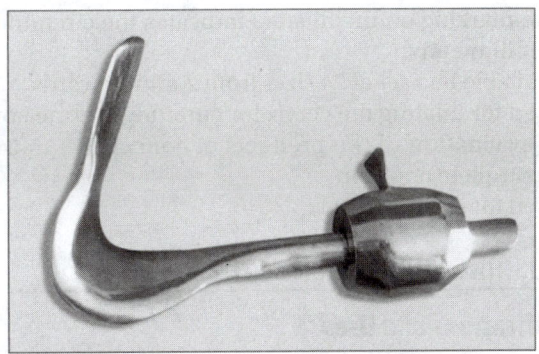

Figure 61.19: Auvard's weighted vaginal speculum.

SIMS' DOUBLE-ENDED UTERINE CURETTE (FIG. 61.20)

Specifications and Uses

- A flat metal instrument with small spoon-like arrangement for scarping
- Both ends are spoon shaped with fenestrations in the middle
- One end is blunt and the other end is sharp for curetting
- Used to take out the endometrium by curetting the uterine cavity for diagnostic or therapeutic purpose
- Used to empty the uterus by curetting the products of conception in incomplete or missed abortion.

DAS' CERVICAL DILATORS (FIG. 61.21)

Specifications and Uses

- Heavy metal instruments of gradually increasing sizes
- Has smooth, round body and tip having two different sizes in a single dilator

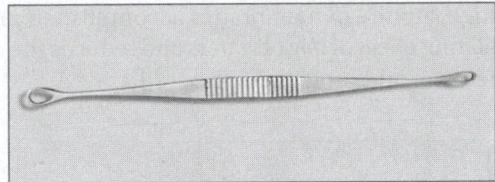

Figure 61.20: Uterine curette.

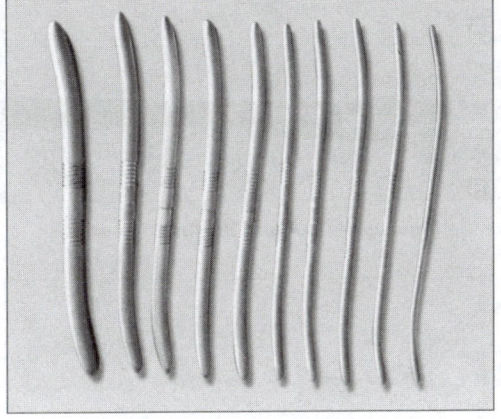

Figure 61.21: Das' cervical dilators.

- The marking on the dilators indicates the circumference in millimeters
- Available in a set of 24 sizes from 2 mm upwards
- Used for dilating the cervix for curetting uterine contents in evacuation of the products of conception in MTP or incomplete abortion
- Used for dilating cervix.

FLUSHING CURETTE (FIGS. 61.22A AND B)

Specifications and Uses

- A curette with small spoon-like arrangement at one end for scraping
- The stem of the curette is hollow for the passage of any fluid to the interior of the spoon-like end
- To the other end (proximal), rubber tubing can be attached from a reservoir to pass fluids through the hollow area to the curetting end, which is blunt
- Used to wash out the uterine cavity, usually with warm antiseptic solution.

DREW SMYTHE CATHETER MEMBRANE PERFORATOR (FIG. 61.23)

Specifications and Uses

- It is a S-shaped, double curved metal catheter with a blunt stilet
- It has two openings, one inlet and one outlet, and double tube; one inner tube and one outer tube
- It is used for high rupture of membranes
- It allows controlled escape of liquor amnii through it
- It can be passed between the membranes and uterus some length before puncturing
- The high rupture of membranes accomplished preserves the dilating effect of bag of waters and reduces the chances of infection, and prolapse of the cord.

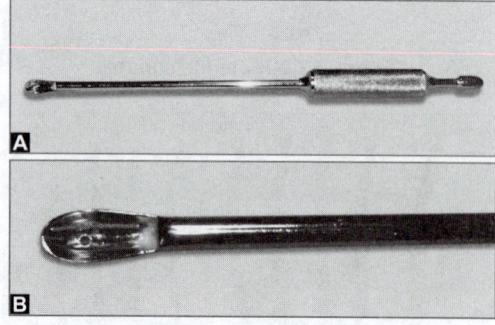

Figures 61.22A and B: Flushing curette.

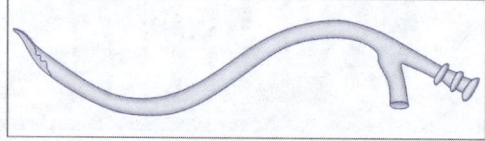

Figure 61.23: Drew Smythe catheter.

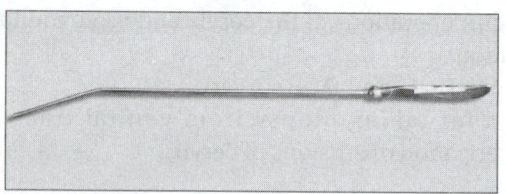

Figure 61.24: Uterine sound.

UTERINE SOUND (FIG. 61.24)

Specifications and Uses

- A slender, graduated, malleable metallic instrument
- It has an olive pointed tip and a broad handle
- The body is graduated and it can be used as a first dilator to dilate the cervix
- It is used to note the position of uterus and to measure the length of uterine cavity prior to D&E procedure
- It can be used to sound the uterine cavity to locate the IUCD with missing threads.

SCISSORS (FIGS. 61.25A TO C)

Specifications and Uses

- Scissors are used for blunt or sharp dissection
- Straight or curved Mayo scissors, which are very smooth at the ends, are used to cut the tissues and internal organs, so that adjacent tissues are protected, while using
- Episiotomy scissors are used for cutting the perineum to enlarge the vaginal opening to deliver the fetal head

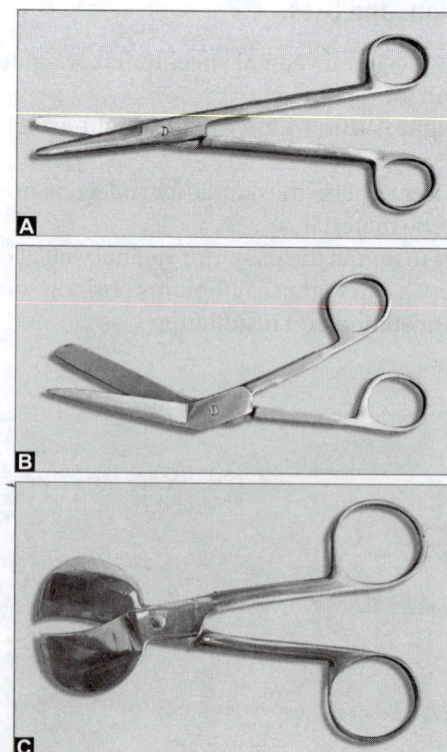

Figures 61.25A to C: Scissors. (A) Straight Mayo scissors; (B) Episiotomy scissors; (C) Umbilical cord cutting scissors.

- Umbilical cord cutting scissors with broad rounded end are used for cutting umbilical cord.

BULB SYRINGE (FIG. 61.26)

Specifications and Uses

- A rubber bulb with elongated tip
- Used to remove secretions from mouth and nostrils of neonates following delivery of head.

MUCUS SUCKER (FIG. 61.27)

Specifications and Uses

- A plastic device with graduated barrel and tubes
- Used to suck secretions from oropharynx and hypopharynx of neonates following birth, prior to the attempt of respiration.

CORD CLAMP (FIG. 61.28)

Specifications and Uses

- A plastic device fused to clamp the umbilical cord
- It is kept in place until the cord dries and falls off; the clamp falls off with the detached cord stump.

WRIGLEY'S OUTLET FORCEPS (FIG. 61.29)

Specifications and Uses

- A metal instrument in two pieces (halves) articulated by lock

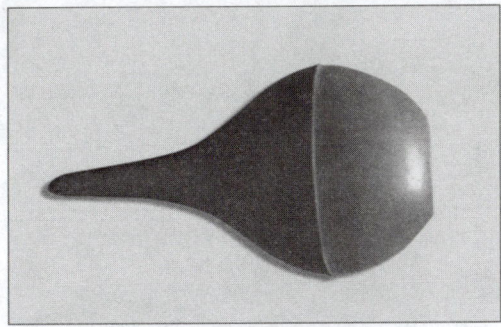

Figure 61.26: Bulb syringe.

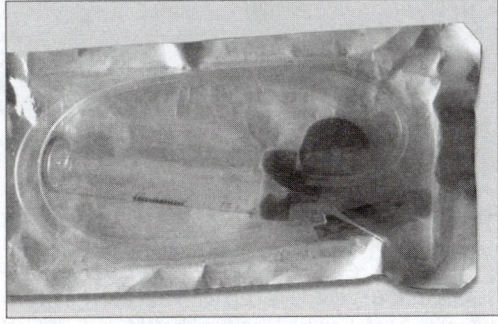

Figure 61.27: Mucus sucker.

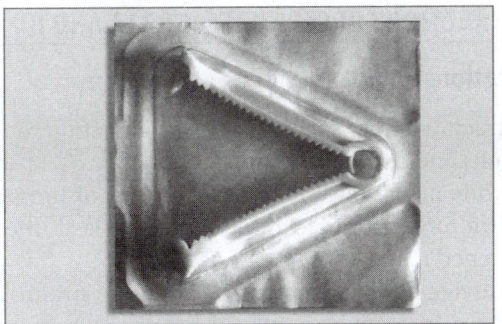

Figure 61.28: Disposable cord clamp.

- Each piece has a handle, lock, shaft and a fenestrated expanded blade
- The fenestrated portion of the blade allows good grip of the fetal head
- It is used to deliver the fetal head presenting at the pelvic outlet
- Delivery of the head is accomplished by extending it.

DAS' LONG CURVED OBSTETRIC FORCEPS (FIG. 61.30)

Specifications and Uses

- A heavy metal instrument about 37 cm (15 inch) long. Its parts are blade, shank, lock and handle
- The blades are named left or right in relation to maternal pelvis in which they lie when applied
- Each blade has a cephalic curve to grasp the fetal head without compression and a pelvic curve to fit the curve on the axis of pelvic canal (curve of Carus)
- In order to lock the two halves after application, the left blade needs to be inserted first
- It is used in low forceps operation.

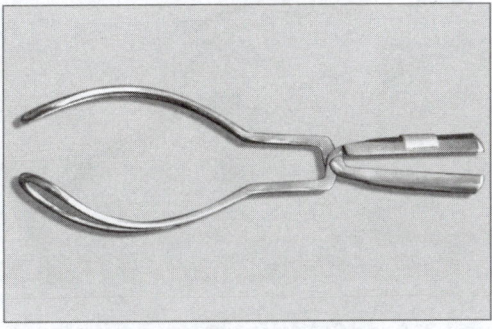

Figure 61.29: Wrigley's forceps.

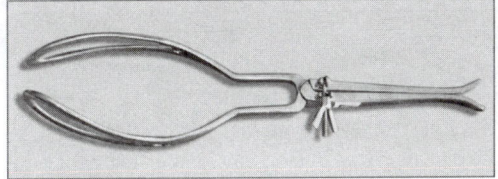

Figure 61.30: Long curved forceps.

AXIS TRACTION FORCEPS (FIGS. 61.31A AND B)

Specifications and Uses

- Axis traction forceps includes two axis traction rods (right and left) and a traction handle
- The rods are assembled in the blades of long curved obstetric forceps prior to introduction and lastly the handle is attached to the rods
- The devices are required (used) where much force is necessary for traction as in mid-forceps operation
- It provides traction in the correct axis of the pelvic curve and as such less force is necessary to deliver the head.

KIELLAND'S FORCEPS (FIG. 61.32)

Specifications and Uses

- Kielland's forceps is a long, almost straight (very slight pelvic curve) obstetric forceps with a sliding lock
- Usually used as rotation forceps in deep transverse arrest of occipitoposterior position of the head
- Facilitates grasping and correction of an asynclitic head because of its sliding lock.

VENTOUSE CUP WITH TRACTION DEVICE/ VACUUM EXTRACTOR (FIGS. 61.33A AND B)

Specifications and Uses

- An instrumental device designed to assist delivery by creating a vacuum between it and the fetal scalp
- The bell-shaped cups are of four sizes (30, 40, 50 and 60 mm)
- The cups have metallic plates at their apex; each cup has a traction tube (rubber tube through which the traction chain passes) and a traction bar
- The traction device is used with a vacuum pump
- It is used in the operation of vacuum extraction of the fetal head
- The cup is to be fitted to the scalp of the forthcoming head by producing a 'chignon' with the help of vacuum
- A manometer connects the traction bar and suction bottle
- It can be used with lesser force (10 kg) than required for forceps application to accomplish delivery of the head
- Silastic vacuum cups are softer, less traumatic and safer to use
- Vacuum extractor is used as an alternative to forceps
- It can be used on a fetal head at a higher station and not well-rotated.

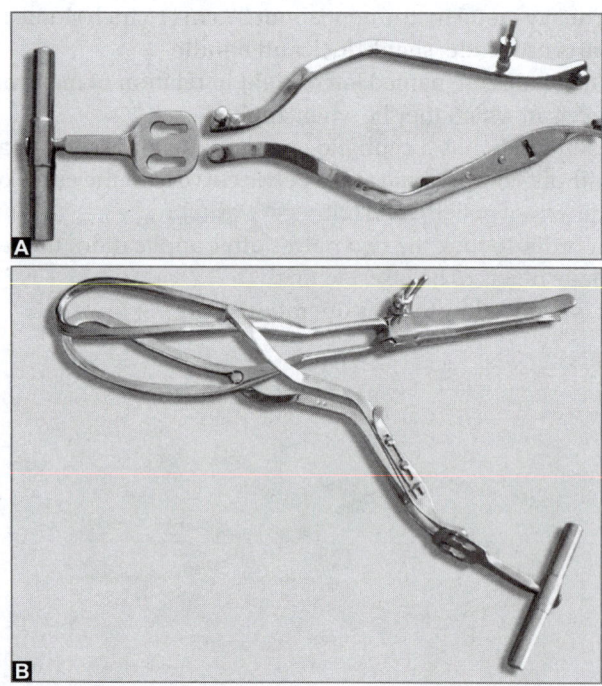

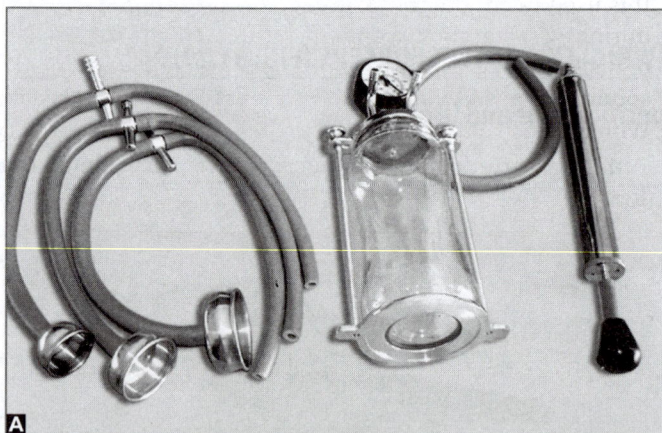

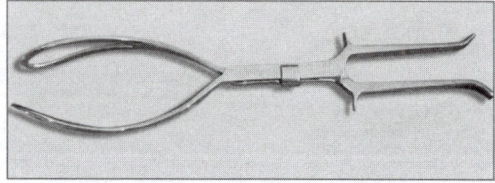

Figures 61.31A and B: Axis traction delivery forceps. (A) Axis traction devices; (B) Long curved forceps with axis traction device.

Figure 61.32: Kielland's forceps.

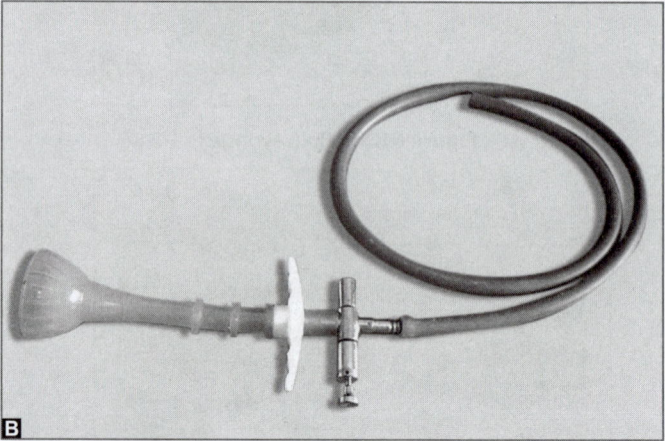

Figures 61.33A and B: Ventouse cup with traction device. (A) Metal suction cups with metal chain, vacuum bottle and vacuum pump and tube; (B) Silastic vacuum cup.

SIMPSON'S PERFORATOR (FIG. 61.34)

Specifications and Uses

- A heavy metal instrument with spear-shaped sharp blades and handles with ridges
- With the closed blades, it is introduced into the vagina and fetal skull is perforated using rotary movements
- It is used to churn the brain matter before withdrawal to facilitate evacuation of brain matter.

CRANIOCLAST (FIG. 61.35)

Specifications and Uses

- A heavy metal instrument with two blades, one blade is solid and the other fenestrated
- Used to compress the head following perforation
- The solid blade is introduced inside the cranium and the fenestrated blade outside for compression and extraction by traction.

EMBRYOTOMY SCISSORS (FIG. 61.36)

Specifications and Uses

- A heavy scissors used in destructive operation
- It is used to cut the thoracic cage or the abdominal wall during evisceration or to cut the remnant of the soft tissue of neck behind, during decapitation, or in cleidotomy or spondylotomy operation
- With this instrument, only the tissues of the baby are cut.

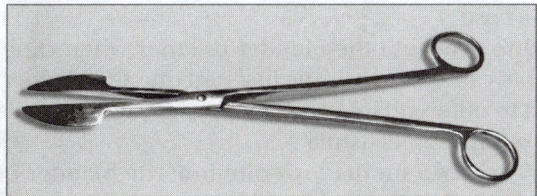

Figure 61.34: Simpson's perforator.

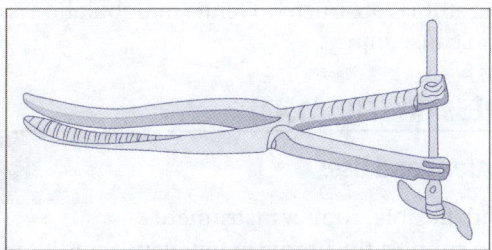

Figure 61.35: Cranioclast.

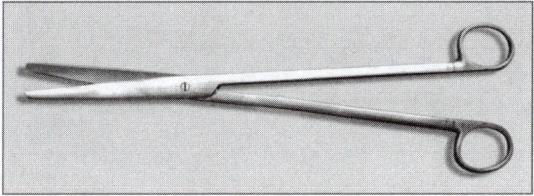

Figure 61.36: Embryotomy scissors.

BREECH HOOK AND CROCHET (FIG. 61.37)

Specifications and Uses

- A metal instrument, which has curves at both ends, one end is acutely curved (the crochet) and the other gradually bent (breech hook)
- The hook is used to give traction to groin of a dead baby when breech is impacted at the outlet
- The crochet is used to deliver the decapitated head by hooking the mandible through mouth or through a hole in the skull
- The middle portion is ridged to act as a handle and both ends may be used.

JARDINE'S DECAPITATION HOOK (FIG. 61.38)

Specifications and Uses

- Jardine's decapitation instrument has a handle and a head
- It is used in decapitation operation in neglected transverse lie or in impacted shoulder presentation where the fetal neck is accessible per vagina
- The hook with knife is used to severe both the vertebral column and soft tissue; in locked twins where disengagement is impossible, it is used to perform decapitation to save the second twin
- It is used in rare cases of double-headed fetus to facilitate extraction.

COMBINED CRANIOCLAST AND CEPHALOTRIBE (FIG. 61.39)

Specifications and Uses

- The instrument consists of three parts, which can be adjusted and locked by a screw
- The central piece is placed within the skull through the opening made by a perforator

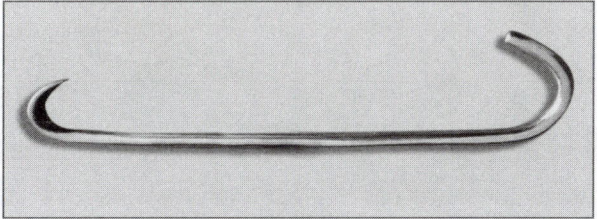

Figure 61.37: Breech hook and crochet.

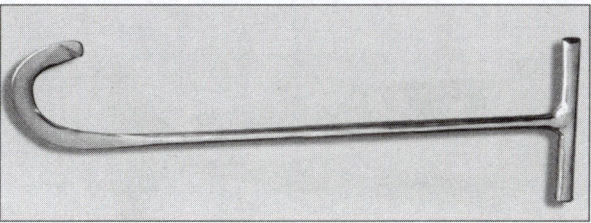

Figure 61.38: Decapitation hook.

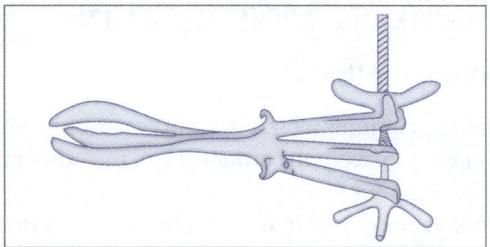

Figure 61.39: Cranioclast and cephalotribe.

- The other two blades are almost straight without any pelvic curve
- They are placed externally over the skull and brought together by a butterfly screw prior to extraction of a dead fetus.

EXTERNAL PELVIMETER (FIG. 61.40)

Specifications and Uses

- A metal instrument with a joint at one end and a graduated bar
- Used to determine the external pelvic measurements
- Used to measure fundal height from symphysis pubis.

PINARD'S STETHOSCOPE/FETOSCOPE (FIG. 61.41)

Specifications and Uses

- A light, aluminum instrument
- It has an open abdominal end and an aural end
- When used to listen to fetal heart tones, it should be held firmly at right angle to the point on abdominal wall
- While listening to the fetal heart tones, the fetoscope should not be touched by hand.

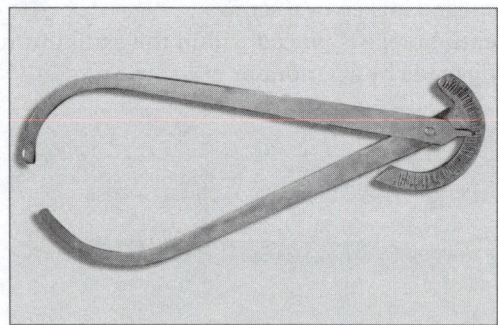

Figure 61.40: Pelvimeter.

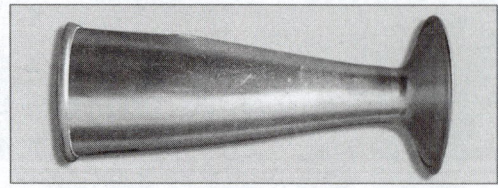

Figure 61.41: Fetoscope.

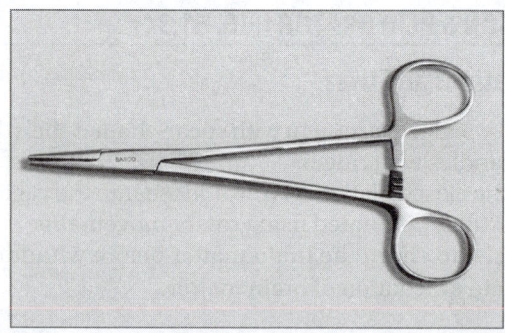

Figure 61.42: Needle holder.

NEEDLE HOLDER (FIG. 61.42)

Specifications and Uses

- The instrument has long handles and small blades and resembles an artery forceps
- The blades have cross serrations
- It has a groove for catching the needle on its inner surface
- It may be straight or curved
- Used to hold the needle for suturing
- Straight type is used for holding needles, while suturing a surface; curved type is used to work at depth or inside the cavity.

FEMALE METAL CATHETER (FIG. 61.43)

Specifications and Uses

- A hollow, metallic tube, which may be straight or curved, tapering at the tip with an opening in the side and a ring at the base
- Used to evacuate the bladder in labor when rubber or flexible catheter cannot be inserted into the bladder
- Used to differentiate between a vesicovaginal fistula and an urethrovaginal fistula
- Used to ascertain the lower limit of the bladder before operations for genital prolapse
- Used only when other softer catheters cannot be used or when urethra is obstructed. Gentle manipulation is needed as it can cause injury.

RING PESSARY (FIG. 61.44)

Specifications and Uses

- A round, flexible, rubber instrument
- Used to support the uterus in following conditions:
  - Prolapse in older age group

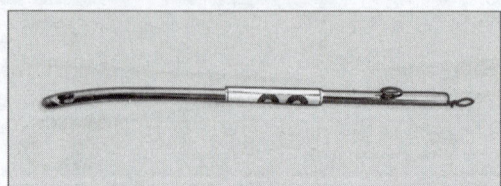

Figure 61.43: Female metal catheter.

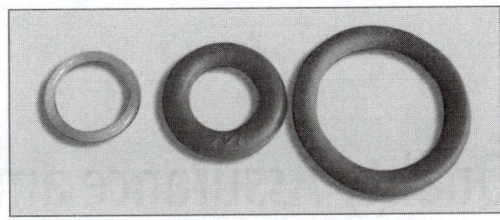

Figure 61.44: Ring pessary.

- Prolapse associated with pregnancy
- Puerperal prolapse or retroversion
- Prolapse when patient has a surgical risk or refuses to undergo surgery.
❖ Used as a temporary measure to support uterus
❖ The watch spring, inside the rubber ring of the instrument stretches the vaginal walls, which can thus act as a better support.

■ HODGE-SMITH PESSARY (FIG. 61.45)

Specifications and Uses

❖ A rubber or plastic device shaped as ring with one end broader
❖ Used to support uterus in the following conditions:
   - Symptom producing, mobile, uncomplicated retroverted uterus
   - Retroverted uterus in puerperal period
   - Retroverted gravid uterus up to 24th week of gestation.

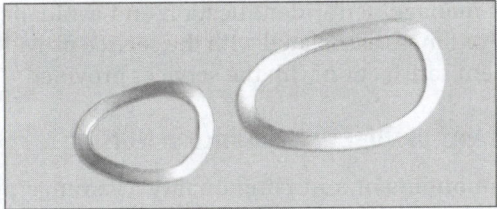

Figure 61.45: Hodge-Smith pessary.

■ BABCOCK'S TISSUE FORCEPS (FIG. 61.46)

Specifications and Uses

❖ A light and delicate instrument
❖ It is a non-traumatizing type of tissue forceps
❖ The blades are curved and fenestrated
❖ Tips of the blades are in the form of transverse bars with transverse serrations on its inner aspects
❖ It is used to hold soft and delicate tissues such as fallopian tubes, ureters, appendix and gut wall as in gastrostomy and colostomy
❖ It can be used as a hemostat when the bleeder is difficult to pinpoint. The whole chunk of tissue is held with Babcock's forceps to cause temporary hemostasis.

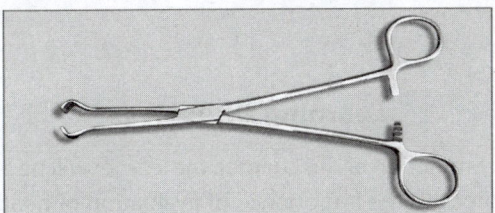

Figure 61.46: Babcock's tissue forceps.

■ BIBLIOGRAPHY

1. Adele P. Maternal and Child Health Nursing, 5th edition. Philadelphia: Lippincot Williams & Wilkins; 2007.
2. Arun Y, Arora VS. Synopsis of Medical Instruments and Procedures. New Delhi: Jaypee Brothers Medical Publishers (P) Ltd; 2003.
3. Bhowmik A, Chatterjee G. Medical Instruments, 3rd edition. New Delhi: BI Publications (P) Ltd; 2005.
4. Dutta DC. Textbook of Obstetrics. Kolkata; New Central Book Agency (P) Ltd; 2006.
5. Thresiamma CP. Operating Room Technique and Anesthesia for GNM Course, 2nd edition. New Delhi: Jaypee Brothers Medical Publishers (P) Ltd; 2003.

CHAPTER 62

Quality Assurance and Audit in Maternity Nursing

Learning Objectives

Upon completion of this chapter, the learner will be able to:
- Appreciate the importance of evaluation of healthcare practice.
- Describe the process of quality assurance in nursing.
- Enumerate the standards in midwifery care.
- Describe the importance and process of clinical audit.

INTRODUCTION

Quality assurance is an assessment of the effectiveness of healthcare provision, the efforts made to improve care as a result of assessment, combined with an assurance that quality care will be maintained.

Quality assurance in nursing is about assuring quality in nursing care by ensuring that practices are compliant with quality standards and that the desired health outcomes are consistent with current professional knowledge.

GOALS OF QUALITY ASSURANCE

Goals of an effective nursing quality assurance program as outlined by Maciorowski are:
- Evidence of nursing accountability for services rendered and compliance with standards of practice
- A defined mechanism to identify, measure and resolve clinical issues related to practice
- A defined mechanism for evaluating quality indicators, collecting data, developing corrective actions and assessing outcomes.

COMPONENTS OF QUALITY ASSURANCE PLAN

A quality assurance plan provides the foundation and framework of all quality control activities. A quality assurance plan should include the following components:

- Clearly stated goals
- Measurable objectives of how the goals will be achieved
- Designated accountability for written objectives
- Delineated methods of QA activities
- Outlined responsibilities for conducting QA activities
- Outlined mechanisms of reporting data
- Outlined mechanisms of corrective action
- Clear statements of confidentiality.

According to the principles of quality assurance given in WHO booklet (1983), there are four components that must be addressed in any quality assurance activity. These are:
1. Performance (technical quality).
2. Resources use (efficiency).
3. Risk management (identification and avoidance of injury or illness associated with the service provided).
4. Patient satisfaction with the services provided.

Components of Quality Assurance in Nursing

The components of a nursing quality assurance program were originally developed by Lang and adopted by the American Nurses Association as a model for quality assurance in nursing. The evaluation model is open and circular, indicating a cyclical process that can be entered at any point.

The American Nurses Association Model for Quality Assurance and Implementation of Standards

Identification of values emphasizes the need to clarify the social, institutional, professional and individual values, along with the advances in scientific knowledge which influences nursing practice.

The standards and criteria derived from the values describe the level of nursing care considered acceptable. These standards may range from minimal to achievable, excellent or comprehensive. Standards represent the agreed upon level of excellence, whereas criteria are specific and measurable statements which reflect the intent of the standards and can be compared to actual nursing practice.

The next component involves the measurement of current nursing practice against the established standards criteria.

- Here, process describes the nature and sequence of nursing activities which nurses do, how they do it and in what order
- Standards refer to the level of nursing care that is to be provided
- Criteria are the characteristics or behaviors used to measure the level of care
- Outcome standards and criteria reveal the end result of nursing care.

Quality circles: A quality control program, or quality circle (QC), is a group of people from the organizational area who meet regularly to solve problems they experience at work. Members are trained in solving problems, in applying statistical quality control and in working in groups. Usually a facilitator works with each group, which normally consists of six to twelve members. The QC group may meet about 4 hours a month. Although QC members may receive recognition, they usually do not receive monetary rewards.

Quality circles evolve from suggestion programs. In both approaches, workers participate in solving work related problems.

Factors Influencing Quality Management

- Good organization structure
- Good quality staff
- Continuing professional development
- Continuing functional performance evaluation
- Learning from failures and moving from low quality to high quality organization

Guidelines for Quality Control

Guidelines can be helpful for quality improvement:

- Quality improvement must be a long-term continuous effort. There are always opportunities for improvement.
- While top-management commitment is of vital importance, everyone in an organization from top to bottom must be committed to quality.
- Most quality problems require the cooperation and coordination of many functional departments such as production, design testing, engineering, manufacturing, marketing, etc.
- Ideas and suggestions for quality improvement can come from many, often unexpected sources.
- Quality control should be done at crucial steps in the operation process.
- A quality improvement plan is not sufficient. Provision for its implementation must be made.

Implementation of Quality Assurance in Nursing

Quality improvement is the commitment and approach used to continuously improve every process in every part of an organization, with the intent of meeting and exceeding customer expectations and outcomes. In order to implement an effective quality assurance program for nursing and midwifery care, competent and motivated nursing and midwifery personnel are essential. The organization must be committed to providing quality, equitable and accessible health services. Factors that are prerequisites for quality assurance in OBG nursing/professional nursing are:

1. Policy and planning
   - Involvement of nurses and midwives in health policy formulation and program planning
   - Strategic planning for nursing and midwifery workforce management as an integral part of human resource planning and health system development.
2. Education, training and development
   - Coordination between education and service
   - Standard recruitment
   - Competency-based education
   - Multidisciplinary learning
   - Lifelong learning culture
   - Continuing education system.
3. Deployment and utilization
   - Appropriate skill mix and competencies
   - Relevant nursing and midwifery infrastructure
   - Effective leadership and management
   - Good working conditions and efficiently organized work
   - Technical supervision systems
   - Career advancement opportunities
   - Incentive systems
   - Job satisfaction.
4. Regulations.
5. Evidence-based decision making.

STANDARDS IN MIDWIFERY PRACTICE

A nursing standard is a descriptive statement of desired quality against which to evaluate nursing care given to a patient. They reflect a desired and achievable level of performance against which actual performance can be compared. Their main purpose is to promote, guide and direct professional nursing practice [Registered Nurses Association of British Columbia (2003) and The College of Nurses Ontario (2002)].

Standards of nursing practice provide a guide to the knowledge, skills, judgement and attitudes that are needed to practice safely.

Purpose of Standards

- To give direction and provide guidelines for performance of nursing care
- To provide a baseline for evaluating quality of nursing care, ranging from excellent care to unsafe care
- To help to improve quality of nursing care, increase effectiveness of care and improve efficiency (quality assurance)
- To improve documentation of nursing care provided, i.e. maintain record of nursing care

- Help to determine the degree to which standards nursing care should be maintained and take necessary action on time
- To help supervisors to guide nursing staff to improve performance:
  - To help to improve the decision making and devise alternative system for delivering nursing care
  - It may help justify demands for resources for improvement
  - To help clarify nurses' area of accountability
  - To help nursing to define clearly different levels of care
  - To help decrease the costs of nursing tasks
  - To be used as a framework or basis for determining nursing negligence
  - To motivate nurses to achieve excellence.

Uses and Advantages of Standards

- They establish norms and allow community members and individuals to know what level of service to expect/demand. Because they are written down, they can be made public
- They demonstrate quality provision and act as bench mark to monitor quality performance
- They focus on the care and critical tasks that must be performed in the actual situation and can be tailored to meet specific and local situation
- They improve efficiency and lead to better utilization of resources
- They improve staff utilization and staff motivation
- They can be used to access the practical aspects of both basic and post-basic education and training.

Steps of Developing Standards

Step 1: Define and Agree

In this step, the goal is to define and agree on several areas and issues that will define the standards.
- Certify the consensus process both topic selection and approval
- Clarify the approval process for the standards.

Step 2: Select Who should be Involved

Identify at the outset of the process all those individuals or groups with a vested interest in the successful development of the standards.

Step 3: Gather Information

In this step, the working group gathers information about the topic under review and other resources that can help define the key elements that should be included in the standards. A flowchart may be developed to better understand the points in the current process, requiring the development of standards.

Step 4: Draft Standards

The components for drafting standards are:
- Decide the structure and format of the standards, depending on their purpose. After the format is decided, the working group drafts the standards
- Develop indicators to measure performance according to standards
- Prior to field testing, the draft standards should be evaluated internally

Step 5: Test the Standards

Once indicators are developed, the working group must decide whether a field test is needed.

Step 6: Communicate the Standards

Standards communication and implementation strategies are critical to achieving healthcare provider performance according to the standards. The impact of well-developed standards depend on healthcare providers using the standards.

Approaches for Implementing the Standards

Three possible approaches are possible:
1. *Centralized/national approach:* This relies on the center taking a lead, making all the decisions and initiating all the activities. For this approach to be effective, there should be an effective management system. A difficulty with this approach is that sometimes local level difficulties arise which cannot be foreseen at the national level/top level.
2. *Decentralized approach:* This approach is when the center takes lead in making the policy decisions to use midwifery standards, as major component of quality assurance. However, the planning of activities and adaptations of the midwifery standards are left to the local centers/lower level managers.
   Disadvantages
   - Lack of expertise in the local level
   - As each site may make their own adaptations at the local level, it is difficult to ensure the use of national norms and consistency.
3. *Combined approach:* The center at the national level remains responsible for the overall implementation of the midwifery standards, but uses local demonstration sites to try them out, to learn how they can be implemented elsewhere and what adaptations are required to make them specific to the national situation. The center must therefore work closely and take action with local demonstration sites at all stages, right from the initial decision making and planning stages to the evaluation stage.

Advantages
- The approach is flexible and allows for local differences, while at the same time ensuring consistence and uniformity in midwifery standards
- The approach is good for developing expertise within and across the country as each center is involved with all parts of the implementation process
- The approach lends itself to long-term sustainability.

Legal Significance of Standards

- Standards of care are guidelines by which nurses should practice
- Malpractice suit against nurses are based on the charge that the patient was injured as a consequence of the nurse's failure to meet the appropriate standards of care.

Implementation of Standards

Each employee of the institution should follow the standards developed by the organization.

Monitor Compliance on Structure Standards and Process Standards

Compliance monitoring is done by survey and auditing. Standards for nursing practice: The standards for nursing practice are interrelated and all are equally important.

- *Standard 1:* Accountability
  The registered nurse is accountable to the public for competent, safe and ethical nursing practice.
- *Standard 2:* Continuing competence
  The registered nurse attains and maintains competencies relevant to own scope of nursing practice.
- *Standard 3:* Application of knowledge, skill and judgment
  The registered nurse demonstrates competencies relevant to own scope of nursing practice.
- *Standard 4:* Professional relationship and advocacy
  The registered nurse establishes professional therapeutic relationships with the health care system.
- *Standard 5:* Professional leadership
  The registered nurse demonstrates professional leadership in the delivery of quality nursing and health care services to the public.
- *Standard 6:* Self-regulation
  The registered nurse assumes personal accountability to practice nursing competently and ethically.

Importance of Standards for Quality Maternity and Midwifery Care

A standard serves to establish norms and states what level of performance is required to obtain a specific desired outcome. In doing so it provides protection to the public by having criteria against which products and performance of practitioners can be assessed.

Standard statements are usually expressed in behavioral and measurable terms. They will say precisely what the workers will do and how they will carry out the task, e.g. correctly, accurately, gently. It is also important that standards of practice can help identify the actual competencies required by a midwifery trained personnel in routine normal practice. Such standards can be used as the basis for assessing current practice, organizing refresher and updating programs, as well as developing future criteria.

Format of Midwifery Standards

Each standard includes seven major components, i.e. *the aim, standard statement, outcome, prerequisites, process, audit, and action plan:*

1. The **aim** indicates the intended objectives of the standard
2. The **standard statement** described precisely what the midwifery trained personnel will do and to what level of competence
3. The **expected outcomes** are stated in measurable terms although some of the outcomes are long-term outcomes such as increased utilization of midwifery trained personnel
4. The **pre-requisites** include those elements that are to allow the health worker to perform the standards, e.g. training resources, knowledge, equipment, drugs and system
5. **Process** is the critical task to be followed for meeting the standard
6. **The audit** is an integral part of the standard. It includes a check list can be used to test or audit the standard. The action plan is the critical part of audit. It is intended to identify the areas which need strengthening or correcting and to assist the supervisors and managers in their routine supervisory visits. Without action following the audit, standards will be difficult to maintain and impossible to improve.
7. **Action plan** A check list can be used to test or audit the standard. The action plan which is the critical part of audit is intended to identify the areas which need strengthening or correcting, and to assist supervisors and managers in their routine supervisory visits. Without action plan following the audit, standards will be difficult to maintain and impossible to improve.

Example for an Antenatal Care Standard

Abdominal Palpation

Aim

To estimate gestational age, monitor fetal growth and accurately identify lie, presentation and position of the fetus.

Essential requirements
- Pregnant women must attend antenatal clinic
- Midwifery-trained personnel have been trained in the correct procedure for conduction of an abdominal palpation
- Essential equipment such as measuring tape and fetal

stethoscope are available and in good working condition
- A culturally appropriate place is available which allows privacy to conduct the abdominal palpation
- Prenatal records are available for use
- A fully operational referral system is in place for the pregnant woman identified as at risk or have complication to receive appropriate care and treatment.

Procedure

Midwifery trained personnel must:
- Carry out abdominal palpation at every antenatal visit
- Ask the pregnant woman prior to the palpation how she feels, if the baby is moving and when her last menstrual cycle occurred and the date she felt the first movement
- Ensure that the place for conducting palpation provides the woman adequate privacy
- Prior to an abdominal palpation ask the pregnant woman to empty her bladder
- Lay the pregnant woman on her back with upper part of her body supported with pillows
- Inspect the abdomen for scars, previous stretch marks, signs of over distension, signs of multiple pregnancy, and excessive or reduced amount of amniotic fluid. Record findings and refer for institutional delivery
- Estimate gestational age and assess fetal growth. After 24 weeks of pregnancy, the most effective way to estimate gestational age is to use a measuring tape
- Using measuring tape, measure from the upper border of the symphysis pubis to the top of the fundus. Record the measurement in centimeters. If measurement is different from calculated weeks by more than 3 cm or there is no growth or poor growth from the last examination, refer for further investigations
- Gently palpate the abdomen to assess the lie of the fetus
- Using two hands, palpate the abdomen and pelvic area to identify the presenting part
- After 37 weeks especially in primi gravida, assess if the fetal head is engaged. If the head will not go into the pelvis, refer to the first referral unit/hospital
- Identify where the fetal back is and listen to the fetal heart sounds
- Discuss the findings with the pregnant woman, her spouse/accompanying family members
- Record all findings accurately. Reveal all findings and if any deviations are found, refer to the first referral unit/hospital for more specialized investigation as appropriate.

AUDIT IN OBSTETRICS AND MIDWIFERY

Definition

Audit is defined as the systematic and critical analysis of the quality of obstetric/medical care.

Nursing Audit

This is the audit for which nurses themselves define the standards from their point of view and describe the actual practice of nursing.

Objective

Objective of carrying out an audit is to improve the quality of clinical care. It is done by changing and strengthening many aspects of practice and administration. Audit could be clinical, where scrutiny is done over the work done by all health professionals including the doctors.

Structuring an Audit

The important aspect to organize an obstetric audit is motivation of all doctors, midwives, and other health professionals. Proper documentation of facts and figures must be there. Audit should be kept confidential and is considered an educational tool.

When to Conduct an Audit?

The audit should be done six to twelve months after commencement of service and then:
- At regular intervals such as annually
- Immediately when major incident or problem occurs
- As soon as feasible when there is a complaint by the midwifery trained personnel that they are unable to fulfill the standard, or a complaint is raised by the community about the service quality
- When a new intervention related to the standard is implemented, such as the use of some new technology or treatment/drug. In this case, there should be an interval of a minimum of three months before the audit is conducted so that the full benefits/effects of the new treatment, equipment or drug can be seen.

How to Conduct an Audit?

Audit should be prearranged with the midwifery trained personnel. The auditor should go to the field/unit where the midwifery trained personnel is working, to observe the standard of practice in the local situation. This should be done over 2–3 days so that the auditor can observe the midwifery trained personnel in different situations.

Importance of Carrying Out an Audit

- A well-structured and efficient audit is based on scientific evidences with facts and figures
- It can replace the out of date clinical practice with the better one
- It can remove the disbelieving and agonistic attitudes between hospital management and professionals and also amongst professionals
- It improves awareness between health professionals and patients
- It is an effective educational tool.

Use of Audit Results

After conducting the audit and depending on the results, decisions will be made either to:

- Continue with the standard since it is working effectively. Take further specific action to strengthen the standard or correct deficiencies
- Revise the standard.

From the result of the audit check list, it will be possible to develop an action plan to further improve or strengthen the standard. It is important in action plan to set target dates for completion of each task. If the audit result shows that the standard is operating correctly, then a date should be set for re-audit of the standard annually or as national policy states. It may be necessary to re-audit earlier, if there is any major change or problem/incident or there is a complaint from either the midwifery trained personal that they cannot achieve the standard or from the community about the quality of care and performance.

Clinical Audit

Clinical audit is about improving practice and providing better service to consumers. Practitioners are expected to measure and demonstrate the effectiveness of the care they provide and one way of assessing practice is by clinical audit.

Clinical audit is a continuous process that involves—identifying an area to be examined, the collection of appropriate data and the introduction of changes in practice as a result of analysis of data. It is crucial that the effect of changes is monitored by repeating the audit and introducing further changes if indicated. Audit may influence aspects of service structure and process as well as the outcome of clinical care.

Process of Clinical Audit

When embarking on a process of clinical audit for the first time, it is better to concentrate on a small area of study and one that is amenable to change. It is extremely important to define objectives at the start of any process of audit and decide on how the results of the process might be used to influence practice. When an area of study has been chosen, it is vital to decide on a clinical consensus on what constitutes good care, that is, what should be the desired level of achievement—a standard.

Example of An Audit Checklist

Evaluation procedure: Bed bath
Date of evaluation:_____
Name of patient:_____
Hospital number:_____
Date of admission:_____
Condition of patient:_____
Name of nurse/student nurse:_____

Fundaments Steps of the Bed Bath Procedure (Table 62.1)

- Preparing the patient's unit
- Explanation to the patient
- Action of giving bed bath
- Comfortable position to the patient
- Care of articles used
- Recording and reporting.

Criteria for Evaluation

Poor   : 0–23
Fair   : 24–32
Good   : 33–41
Excellent : 42–48

Remarks

A performance rating that obtains a score of 40 or 41 is considered good. The performers (Midwifery trained personnel/students) are given necessary corrections and advised to practice correctly and regularly.

Unit Records

All records that are made by a midwife must be preserved for specified period of time/years according to the policy of the institution. The midwife's records are distinct from that of the doctors although they may contribute to the medical records especially during pregnancy. She must keep records of patient's medical and obstetric history and details of all antenatal examinations which she does. During labor, records of observations examinations and care are essential and it is particularly important to enter details promptly because events move on so rapidly. A register of controlled drugs is kept for the purpose of monitoring the issues and use of drugs. The midwife's register of births is usually kept communally by hospital midwives but individually by a community midwife.

Maternity units use a variety of records and notes including those which are designed to be entered into a computer and others which are appropriate to the midwifery process or to varying styles of individualized care.

All records that are made by a midwife and other health professionals must be preserved for a period of 25 years or according to the institution's policy. The reason for this, is that the records may be needed for any legal issues that may arise.

Norms and Policies

Norms are standards that guide, control and regulate individuals and groups. For planning nursing manpower, certain norms are followed. The nursing norms are recommended by various committees such as the Nursing Manpower Committee. Dr Bajaj Committee and the staff inspection committees of Indian Nursing Council (INC) and state Nurse Councils in each state. The norms have been recommended taking into account the workload projected in the wards (in-patient units) and other areas of the hospital.

TABLE 62.1: Observation checklist on admission procedure: Admission bath/bed bath.

Area of observation	Done (1)	Not done (0)	Remarks
Preparation of patient's unit: *Articles:* • Basin with warm water • Soap • Wash cloth/sponge cloth • Towel • Patients clothes			
Nursing actions of bed bath:			
1. Explain the procedure to the patient prior to starting			
2. Bring necessary articles to the bedside locker/table			
3. Close curtains/door			
4. Perform hand hygiene			
5. Loosen the patient's gown			
6. Keep the towel under head			
7. Fold the wash cloth like a mit on hand			
8. Wipe the face without soap • Wipe the eyes from inner canthus to outer canthus • Change side of wash cloth before wiping the other eye			
9. Clean the patient's face, neck and ears			
10. Expose the forearm of the patient and place the towel lengthwise under it			
11. Using firm strokes wash the arm and axilla			
12. Place a folded towel on the bed next to the patient' hand and place the basin on it			
13. Soak the patient's hand in basin, wash and rinse, and dry the hand			
14. Expose the near arm, of the patient and place the towel lengthwise under it			
15. Using firm strokes, wash the near arm and axilla			
16. Place the folded towel on the bed next to the patient's far hand and put the basin on it			
17. Soak the patient's far hand in the basin. Wash, rinse and dry the hand			
18. Spread the towel across the patient's chest			
19. Wash, rinse and dry the patient's chest			
20. Wash, rinse and dry the abdomen			
21. Place the towel under the far leg			
22. Using firm strokes, wash, rinse and dry the leg from ankle to knee and knee to groin			
23. Fold the towel near the foot area and place the basin on it			
24. Place the patient's feet in the basin, wash, rinse and dry paying special attention to toes			
25. Assist the patient to take prone position			
26. Wash, rinse and dry the patient's back and buttocks area			
27. Refill the basin with clean water			
28. Clean the perineal area			
29. Help the patient to put on clean clothes			
30. **Comfortable position to patient:** Provide comfortable position to patient			
31. Care of articles			
32. Discard the water in basin			
33. Wash the sponge cloth and basin			
34. Spread the sponge cloth for drying			
35. Recording and reporting Record the procedure and significant observations in patient's chart			
Total score			

Policies

Policies are general principles and directions. They are usually without the mandatory approach for addressing an issue, but might be considered mandatory in some national health services. Institutional policies are intended to guide and manage the services of different groups of employees for meeting the objectives of the institution such as a hospital or health center.

A policy is a general statement, which is in line with the organizational objectives and intents to provide guidelines for decision making. "Policies are plans in that they are general statements for an undertaking which guide or channel thinking and action in decision making. They limit an area within which a decision to be made and assure that the decision will be consistent with and contribute to the objectives" (Koonts and O'Donnel). This definition indicates that policies are standing plans that provide solutions to recurring problems by setting boundaries or limits for the decisions, telling people within the organization what can be done and what cannot be given answers in similar situations, which ensure uniformity in actions and thus make the decisions more predictable and transparent. Policies are generally written statements which guide setting up boundaries that explain the limits and directions in which management decisions and actions will take place. Policies on the basis of emergence are called originated, appealed, implied and imposed policies.

- Originated policies are formed at the initiative of top-level managers
- Appealed policies are formulated out of the appeal made by subordinates to their superior in relation to the actions to be taken on a given situation. Such decisions become the precedent for future actions
- Implied policies are stated neither in writing nor verbally expressed but believed to exist. They actually develop out of actions of superiors that people see about them and believe to exist as policies
- Imposed policies are policies that are externally imposed on an enterprise and must be followed. The government and professional organizations are examples of the external sources of imposed policies.

Characteristics of Good Policies

A good policy must have the following features:
- In order to help achieve the objectives, policies must be in line with organizational goals and for achieving the objectives and it must reflect the needs of those who will be affected by it
- It must be comprehensive enough to cover a wide range of actions and leave room for judgment and interpretation as required by the specific situation (not too rigid)
- In order to avoid ambiguity, every policy should be expressed in definite and precise words indicating as who is responsible for implementing it
- It should be formulated by using a participative approach to ensure compliance by employees
- It must be periodically reviewed in order to bring about necessary change or to abandon completely
- It must maintain reasonable balance between stability and flexibility, in other words policies must change with the change of conditions. However, some degree of stability must also prevail in order to give the sense of order and direction.

In order that a good standard of nursing care be maintained, nursing superintendent should develop written policies and procedures to serve as guides for nurses in various units of the hospital. Important topics that should be incorporated are as follows:
- Organization of the institution and its service departments
- Status and relationship to positions above and below
- Responsibilities of personnel
- Staffing pattern and shift pattern.
- Departmental functions.
- Requisitioning of supplies.
- Utilization, care and maintenance of equipment.
- Nursing procedures.
- Coordination with departments and domestic services.
- Handling of narcotics and dangerous drugs.
- Isolation techniques.
- Safety—hospital hazards, accidents, fire, etc.
- Public relations.
- Visiting hours and dealing with visitors and relatives.
- Records and reports.
- Admission, transfer and discharge of patients.
- Procedure for patients leaving against medical advice.
- Procedure following death of patients.

Protocols

A protocol is a written system for managing care that should include a plan for audit of that care. Most protocols are binding on employees as they usually relate to the management of consumers of care with urgent possibly life-threatening conditions. A protocol may exist for the care of the woman with antepartum hemorrhage, but not for the care of women in labor without complication.

A protocol is a multidisciplinary planned course of suggested actions in relation to specific situations. Protocols determine individual aspects of practice and should be studied using latest evidence.

In a hospital there may be prepared or written protocols to manage several possibly difficult and emergency, situations. Employees including nursing personnel must know the protocols for dealing with those situations. This may include communication with patients, relatives public who may be in a heightened/stressful emotional state. Several aspects related to the specific situation may have to be explained. Higher level staff may need to be consulted or the matter referred to them. Adequate documentation will be required. Some of the common examples of situations for which protocols are necessary are as follows:

1. Patient questions about the delay in examination by a physician in the out-patient unit:

- Listen and respond with empathy and concern
- Acknowledge and apologize for the delay
- Briefly explain the reason for delay, communicate a realistic and liberal time frame and do not blame other colleagues and departments for the delay
- Ensure that the patient gets attention and care
- Confirm the patient understands his or her plan of care
2. Patient verbalizes that he/she wants to leave against medical advice (AMA):
    - Immediately inform the charge nurse and the physician that the patient wishes to go against medical advice.
    - The physician will evaluate the situation and intervene with the patient as appropriate
    - Document in the patient's chart the intervention taken and the result
    - Complete the specific forms/documents.
3. Patient uses threats and profanity:
    - Tell the patient: "In order for me to help you, you need to stop profanity".
    - Immediately notify the charge nurse of the situation
    - Implement security management plan as required
    - Document the details in appropriate forms.

SUMMARY

Quality assurance in nursing is about assuring quality in nursing by ensuring that practices are compliant with quality standards. It looks for ways to improve procedures within a health facility. A standard is a descriptive statement of desired level of performance against which to evaluate the quality of service structure. All standards of practice provide a guide to the knowledge, skills, judgment and attitudes that are needed to practice safely. They reflect a desired and achievable level of performance against which actual performance can be compared. Protocols are specific written procedures that describes nursing actions in a given situation, e.g. protocol for ventilator weaning. A protocol may describe mandatory nursing assessments, behaviors and documentation for establishing and maintaining invasive appliances, method of administering specific drugs, special care modalities for patients with certain disorders, other components of patient care, and lines of authority or channels of communication under particular circumstances.

BIBLIOGRAPHY

1. Agarwal AK. Management of Hospitals in India. National Institute of Health and Family Welfare. New Delhi: 1989.
2. Alexander E. Nursing Administration in Hospital Health Care System. St. Louis: C V Mosby; 1972.
3. Anita F. Leadership and Management in Nursing. Dorling Kindersley Pvt. Ltd. New Delhi; 2009.
4. Nima B. Midwifery and Obstetrical Nursing. 2nd edition. Bangalore: EMMES Medical Publishers; 2015.
5. Vinita M. Quality Assurance in Nursing. F.Y. MSc Nursing, Mumbai. SNDT Women's University; 1915.

SECTION XII

GYNECOLOGICAL NURSING

Section Outline

63. Menstrual Cycle Disorders and Abnormal Bleeding
64. Displacement of Uterus
65. Infectious Conditions of Pelvic Organs
66. Benign Pelvic Conditions
67. Gynecological Examinations and Diagnostic Procedures
68. Congenital Malformations of Female Genital Organs
69. Genital Fistulae
70. Perioperative Care of Gynecological Patient
71. Infertility and Adoption
72. Genital Malignancies
73. Special Gynecological Conditions
74. Diagnostic Procedures in Gynecology

CHAPTER 63

Menstrual Cycle Disorders and Abnormal Bleeding

Learning Objectives

Upon completion of this chapter, the learner will be able to:
- Discuss the subjective and objective data, laboratory test results, and investigations for menstrual cycle disorders.
- Discuss the therapeutic interventions for menstrual cycle disorders.
- Discuss the nursing process appropriate for patients with menstrual disorders.

Abnormal conditions of the menstrual cycle are deviations from what is normal for an individual woman. The condition may occur in the frequency or length of the cycle, volume or length of menstrual follow or the total number of years of menstruation. Menstrual cycle conditions may be classified as amenorrhea, Mittelschmerz's, syndrome, dysmenorrhea, dysfunctional uterine bleeding, premenstrual syndrome, menorrhagia polymenorrhea, metrorrhagia, oligomenorrhea and hypomenorrhea.

AMENORRHEA

Amenorrhea is the absence or lack of menstruation during the reproductive years. Normal causes of amenorrhea include pregnancy, lactation and menopause. Other causes can be pathologic and may include stress, excessive exercise, eating disorders, weight loss, a low body mass index (BMI) or other potentially life-threatening disorders. It is of two types, primary and secondary.

Primary Amenorrhea

Primary amenorrhea is the absence of menarche until age 16 years or the absence of the development of secondary sex characteristics and menarche till age of 14 years.

Causes

Causes of primary amenorrhea include:
- Hypothalamic, pituitary or enzymatic problems
- Chromosomal abnormalities
- Genitourinary abnormalities
- Drugs.

Symptoms

- Failure to experience menarche when there has been development of secondary sex characteristics
- No menarche and absence of development of secondary sex characteristics as in Turner's syndrome.

Management

Therapeutic interventions depend on the cause of amenorrhea:
- Estrogen replacement therapy (ERT) to stimulate development of secondary sex characteristics and to prevent osteoporosis.

Secondary Amenorrhea

Secondary amenorrhea is the absence of menstruation for at least 6 months or for three cycles after menarche.

Causes

- Physiologic response to pregnancy, lactation or anovulation
- Hypothyroidism or hyperthyroidism
- Adrenal disease
- Chronic renal disease
- Polycystic ovary syndrome
- Chronic hepatic disease
- Anorexia nervosa
- Malnutrition
- Vigorous athletic training.

Investigations

- Thyroid function tests
- Blood glucose level
- Laparoscopy to check ovarian pathology
- Ultrasound to check polycystic ovary syndrome.

Management

- Cyclic progesterone therapy if the cause is anovulation
- Oral contraceptives for women who desire contraception
- Bromocriptine if there is hyperprolactinemia
- Gonadotropin-releasing hormone (GnRH), when the cause is hypothalamic failure
- Thyroid hormone replacement for hypothyroidism
- Calcium and estrogen to prevent development of osteoporosis.

DYSMENORRHEA

Dysmenorrhea is painful menstruation or cramping during menstruation. Typically dysmenorrhea begins up to 48 hours before onset of menstruation and resolves within 2–4 days of onset or by the end of menstrual period. Dysmenorrhea can be classified as primary (spasmodic) or secondary (congestive).

Primary Dysmenorrhea

Primary dysmenorrhea is one where there is no pelvic pathology. Usually occurs within 1–3 years of menarche.

Causes

Painful uterine contractions stimulated by prostaglandin produced by the endometrium during menstruation.

Symptoms

- Sharp, intermittent suprapubic pain radiating to the back or thighs
- Headache and backache
- Fatigue, dizziness and syncope
- Gastrointestinal (GI) symptoms: Nausea, vomiting and bloating.

Treatment

Women often experience reduction in dysmenorrhea after pregnancy. Therapeutic intervention includes:
- Nonsteroidal anti-inflammatory drugs (NSAIDs) started 1–3 days before the onset of menstruation (to decrease prostaglandin production)
- Oral contraceptives to decrease endometrial proliferation and production of prostaglandin.

Secondary Dysmenorrhea

Secondary dysmenorrhea is painful menstruation resulting from a pathologic process. The pain may be related to increasing tension in the pelvic tissues due to pelvic congestion or increased vascularity in the pelvic organs. Patients are usually in 30s and parous.

Causes

- Chronic pelvic infection
- Pelvic endometriosis
- Pelvic adhesions
- Uterine fibroids
- Endometrial polyp
- Intrauterine contraceptive device (IUCD) in utero.

Symptoms

- Dull pain situated in the back and front
- Pain starts 3–5 days prior to onset of menstruation and relieves with the start of bleeding
- Symptoms of associated pathology and no systemic discomfort.

Treatment

Treatment involves correction of the cause. The type of treatment depends on the severity, age and parity of the patient.

MITTELSCHMERZ'S SYNDROME (OVULAR PAIN)

Mittelschmerz's syndrome is a mid-menstrual pain that occurs around the time of ovulation in menstruating women. The pain is usually situated in the hypogastrium or one iliac fossa.

Characteristics

- The pain is usually located on one side and does not change according to which ovary is ovulating
- The pain usually lasts for about 12 hours
- It may be associated with slight vaginal bleeding or excessive mucoid vaginal discharge.

Probable Causes

- Increased tension of the Graafian follicle prior to rupture
- Peritoneal irritation by the follicular fluid following ovulation
- Contraction of the fallopian tubes and uterus.

Treatment

- Analgesics and reassurance
- Contraceptive pills to make the cycle anovular in obstinate cases.

DYSFUNCTIONAL UTERINE BLEEDING

Dysfunctional uterine bleeding (DUB) is abnormal uterine bleeding without any clinically detectable cause. It occurs more often in adolescents and perimenopausal women.

Causes
- Hormonal abnormalities such as anovulation
- Pelvic inflammatory disease (PID)
- Endometriosis
- Neoplasms.

Pathophysiology
Abnormal bleeding is probably due to local causes in the endometrium. There is disturbance of the endometrial blood vessels and capillaries, and coagulation of blood in and around these vessels. These are probably related to alteration in the ratio of endometrial prostaglandins, which are delicately balanced in homeostasis of menstruation.

Clinical Manifestations
1. *Polymenorrhea (frequent menstruation):* This occurs following childbirth and abortion, during adolescence and premenopausal period.
2. *Oligomenorrhea (light or infrequent menstruation):* This occurs in adolescence and preceding menopause.
3. *Menorrhagia:* Excessive and prolonged menstruation.

Investigations
1. History of the nature of menstrual abnormity.
2. Internal examination including speculum examination.
3. *Blood tests:* Hemoglobin, complete blood count (CBC), platelets, prothrombin time, bleeding time, partial thromboplastin and thyroid function tests.
4. *Ultrasound and color Doppler:* Transvaginal sonography and saline infusion sonography to detect abnormalities like fibroids and adenomyosis.
5. Endometrial biopsy through hysteroscopy to rule out endometrial cancer.
6. Laparoscopy to exclude pelvic pathology.

Management
1. *General:* Correction of anemia by diet, hematinics and blood transfusion if required.
2. Oral contraceptives for menstrual cycle regulation.
3. Cyclic progesterone for anovulatory bleeding.
4. Nonsteroidal anti-inflammatory drugs to reduce the amount of menstrual bleeding.
5. *Gonadotropin-releasing hormone agonists:* If the woman is infertile and wants pregnancy. In low doses, it reduces blood loss and produces hypoestrogenic features.
6. Endometrial ablation (separation) to decrease or eliminate tissue sloughing.
7. *Antiprogesterone:* Mifepristone (Ru486) to inhibit ovulation, induce amenorrhea and reduce myoma size.
8. Hysterectomy is done when abnormal uterine bleeding cannot be corrected by conservative treatment and the blood loss impairs the health of the patient.

PREMENSTRUAL SYNDROME
Premenstrual syndrome (PMS) is a cyclic cluster of behavioral, emotional and physical symptoms that occurs just prior to menstruation that is in the luteal phase of the menstrual cycle. There is a cyclic appearance of large number of symptoms during the last 7–10 days of the menstrual cycle. The symptoms must be sufficiently severe and fulfill the following criteria before the diagnosis can be made:
- Not related to any organic lesion
- Occurs regularly during the luteal phase of each ovulatory menstrual cycle
- Symptom-free period during the rest of the cycle.

Pathophysiology
The probable causes of the conditions are:
- Alteration in the level of estrogen and progesterone starting from the midluteal phase
- Neuroendocrine factors such as decreased synthesis of serotonin and withdrawal of endorphins (neurotransmitters) during the luteal phase
- Psychological and psychosocial factors producing behavioral changes.

Clinical Features
Related to Water Retention
- Abdominal bloating
- Breast tenderness
- Swelling of extremities
- Weight gain.

Neuroendocrine and Psychological Related
- Irritability, tearfulness
- Depression, anxiety
- Tension, mood swings
- Rejection sensitivity
- Insomnia/hypersomnia
- Decreased concentration
- Forgetfulness, confusion
- Restlessness
- Headache
- Increased appetite
- Change in libido.

Autonomic Symptoms
- Nausea, anorexia
- Diarrhea
- Palpitation
- Perspiration.

Behavioral Symptoms
- Fatigue, decreased motivation
- Tiredness, social isolation
- Clumsiness, paresthesia (numbness or tingling).

Treatment

Treatment is aimed aet alleviation of symptoms since PMS is not a disease. No single treatment may be effective. Drugs like tranquilizers, diuretics and antidepressants are used based on individual needs. Women are taught the following measures to reduce the intensity of symptoms:
- Modify diet
- Increase exercise
- Alleviate stress
- Change activities of daily living
- Reduce fatigue
- Enhance ability to sleep.

Menstrual Cycle Disorders

Nursing assessment for menstrual conditions involves careful medical and gynecologic history, assessment of symptoms, and assessment for specific suspected condition. The physical assessment focuses on collection of data regarding the suspected menstrual cycle abnormality including collection of data from laboratory tests and special investigations.

Applicable nursing diagnoses may include:
- Pain related to the specific menstrual condition
- Fear related to the medical diagnosis
- Anxiety related to unknown outcomes
- Deficient knowledge related to limited experience regarding specific menstrual cycle disorder.

Planning includes specific actions, the woman should complete to achieve the highest level of wellness. Plans prepared in collaboration with the client may include the following. The client will:
- Consume correct proportions of recommended food as evidenced by a 24-hour diet recall
- Exercise by walking 30 minutes each day
- Take prescribed medications according to instructions
- Return to the healthcare facility as scheduled for follow-up visits
- Contact the physician if symptoms do not improve
- Understand the health promotion counseling.

MENORRHAGIA

Definition

Menorrhagia is an abnormally heavy and prolonged menstrual period at regular intervals. Normal menstrual cycle is 25–35 days in duration with bleeding lasting an average of 5 days and a total blood flow between 25 and 80 mL. A blood loss greater than 80 mL or lasting longer than 7 days constitutes menorrhagia (also called *hypermenorrhea*).

Causes

Usually no causative abnormality can be identified and treatment is directed to the symptom rather than a specific mechanism. An overview of causes includes the following.

TABLE 63.1: Abnormal uterine bleeding.

Condition	Description
Oligomenorrhea	Light of infrequent menstruation
Hypomenorrhea	Scanty or infrequent menstruation. Menstrual periods occur less often than average 28 days cycle.
Menorrhagia	Heavy or prolonged vaginal bleeding with menstrual cycle (heavy or prolonged period)
Metrorrhagia	Uterine bleeding at irregular intervals, particularly between the expected menstrual periods
Menometrorrhagia	Prolonged or excessive uterine bleeding that occurs irregularly and more frequently than normal
Dysmenorrhea	Cramps and pelvic pain with menstruation
Amenorrhea	Absence of monthly menstrual periods
Mittelschmerz	One sided, lower abdominal pain associated with normal ovulation
Dysfunctional uterine bleeding (DUB)	Bleeding from the uterus that occurs in between periods, which may occur every few weeks and the flow may be heavier than usual.

Uterine
- Endometrial polyp
- Submucosal fibroid
- Endometrial hyperplasia
- Endometrial adenomyosis.

Ovarian
- Ovulatory DUB
- Anovulatory DUB
- Polycystic ovary syndrome
- Granulosa cell tumor of ovary.

Others
- Hematological causes
- von Willebrand's disease
- Hypothyroidism, hyperthyroidism
- Leukemia.

Diagnosis
- Pelvic and rectal examination
- Pap smear
- Pelvic ultrasound scan is the first line diagnostic study for identifying structural abnormalities
- Endometrial biopsy to exclude atypical hyperplasia or endometrial cancer
- Hysteroscopy.

Treatment

Where underlying cause can be identified, treatment may be directed at this. Clearly heavy periods at menarche and menopause may settle spontaneously.

Medications

- Iron supplements to counter anemia
- Nonsteroidal anti-inflammatory drugs to reduce blood loss
- Hormonal treatment for DUB:
  - Oral contraceptives, usually combined estrogen, progesterone pills for few months
  - Progesterone only pills or injection Depo-Provera
  - Progesterone releasing intrauterine system (IUS).
- Other options:
  - Antifibrinolytics: Gonadotropin-releasing hormone agonists.

Surgery

Surgical treatment is rarely resorted to:
- Endometrial ablation
- Dilation and curettage
- Hysteroscopic myomectomy to remove fibroids.

POLYMENORRHEA

Polymenorrhea or epimenorrhea is defined as cyclic bleeding where the cycle is reduced to an arbitrary limit of less than 21 days and remain constant at that rate. If the frequent cycle is associated with excessive and/or prolonged bleeding, it is called epimenorrhea.

Causes

- Dysfunctional uterine bleeding
- Common in adolescence, preceding menopause and following delivery, and abortion; hyperstimulation of ovaries by the pituitary hormone may be the causative factor
- Ovarian hyperemia
- Seen in PID or ovarian endometriosis.

Treatment

Hormone Therapy

Estrogen and progestogen are generally prescribed either separately or as combined oral pills. The preparations of progestogen used are norethisterone acetate and medroxyprogesterone acetate. Progestin alone therapy is highly effective in anovular DUB, while combined preparations of progestogen and estrogen are effective in ovular type. Norethisterone preparations (5 mg tablets) are used three times a day till bleeding stops, which is usually 3–7 days. Low-dose combined oral pills (estrogen and progestogen) used as cyclic therapy from 5th to 25th day for three cycles in ovular bleeding.

METRORRHAGIA

Metrorrhagia is defined as irregular, acyclic bleeding from the uterus. It is mostly related to surface lesions in the uterus. When the bleeding is so irregular and excessive that the menstruation (periods) cannot be identified, it is called *menometrorrhagia*.

Causes

Acyclic Bleeding

- Dysfunctional uterine bleeding (during adolescence, following childbirth or abortion and preceding menopause)
- Submucous fibroid
- Uterine polyp
- Endometrial or cervical cancer.

Contact Bleeding

- Carcinoma cervix
- Mucous polyp of cervix
- Infections: Chlamydial or tubercular cervicitis
- Cervical endometriosis.

Intermenstrual Bleeding

- Urethral caruncle
- Intrauterine contraceptive device in utero
- Breakthrough bleeding in pill users
- Ovular bleeding.

Treatment

Treatment is directed to the underlying pathology.

OLIGOMENORRHEA

Oligomenorrhea is defined as bleeding occurring more than 35 days apart and which remains constant at that frequency.

Causes

- *Age related:* During adolescence and preceding menopause
- Obesity
- Vigorous exercise
- *Endocrine disorders:* Polycystic ovary syndrome (PCOS), hypoprolactinemia, hyperthyroidism
- *Androgen producing tumors:* Ovarian, adrenal
- Tuberculous endometritis.

Treatment

Treatment according to the cause identified.

HYPOMENORRHEA

Hypomenorrhea is defined as menstrual bleeding that is unduly scanty and lasts for less than 2 days.

Causes

- Uterine synechiae
- Endometrial tuberculosis
- Use of oral contraceptives
- Thyroid dysfunction

- ❖ Malnutrition
- ❖ Premenopausal period.

Treatment

Treatment is directed to the specific cause.

STUDY QUESTIONS

Short Notes

1. Polymenorrhea (epimenorrhea).
2. Oligomenorrhea.
3. Hypomenorrhea.

Short Answer Questions

1. Metrorrhagia.
2. Menorrhagia.
3. Premenstrual syndrome.

Essay Questions

1. Describe amenorrhea; primary and secondary types, and causes, symptoms and treatment for each.
2. Describe dysmenorrhea; primary and secondary types and causes, symptoms and treatment for each.
3. Explain DUB. Describe the causes, clinical manifestations, diagnosis and management of DUB.

Displacement of Uterus

Learning Objectives

Upon completion of this chapter, the learner will be able to:
- Discuss the occurrences of uterine prolapse, retroversion and inversion.
- Describe the measures to be taken to prevent uterus displacement problems in gynecological and obstetrical patients.
- Describe the manifestations, diagnosis and management of the three gynecological problems.
- Discuss the nursing implications in the care of patients with specific gynecologic condition.

The uterus is not in a fixed position in pelvis. Minor variations in position occur with changes in posture with straining and with full bladder or rectum. When the uterus rests habitually in a position beyond the limit of normal variation, it is called displacement. The commonly occurring displaced positions are retroversion, prolapse and inversion of uterus.

RETROVERSION OF UTERUS (FIGS. 64.1A TO C)

Retroversion is the turning backward of the uterus with long axis of the corpus and cervix in line and the whole organ turns backwards in relation to the long axis of the birth canal. Retroflexion is a bending backwards of the corpus on the cervix at the level of the internal os. The two conditions are usually present together and are referred to as retroversion/retroflexion or retrodisplacement.

Degrees of Displacement

1. *First degree:* The fundus is vertical and pointing towards the sacral promontory.
2. *Second degree:* The fundus lies in the sacral hollow, but not below the internal os.
3. *Third degree:* The fundus lies below the level of internal os.

Causes

1. *Developmental defects:* The infantile position of the uterus is retained. There is lack of uterine muscle tone and the condition is associated with short vagina with shallow anterior vaginal fornix.
2. *Puerperal:* Due to stretched ligaments caused by childbirth.
3. Prolapse caused by traction following cystocele.
4. Fibroid tumor in the anterior or posterior wall of the uterus produces heaviness making it fall behind.
5. *Pelvic adhesions:* Adhesions either inflammatory, operative or due to endometriosis pull the uterus posteriorly.

Incidence

The condition is seen in about 15–20% of normal women.

Signs and Symptoms/Clinical Presentation

- Chronic premenstrual pelvic pain due to varicosities in broad ligament produced by the kinks
- Dyspareunia due to direct thrust by the penis against the retroflexed uterus or prolapsed ovaries lying in the pouch of Douglas
- Infertility as the external os is away from the seminal pool at the posterior fornix during coitus or it may be occluded by the anterior vaginal wall
- On bimanual examination, body of the uterus is felt in the posterior fornix and cervix directed upwards
- On speculum examination, the cervix is viewed easily and the external os points forwards.

Prevention

The following are guidelines to be followed during the weeks after childbirth or abortion to prevent retroversion:
- Empty the bladder regularly
- Increase the tone of the pelvic muscles by regular exercise

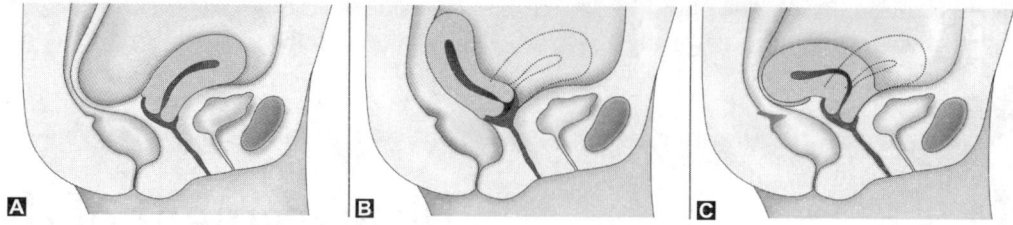

Figures 64.1A to C: Retroversion and retroflexion of the uterus. (A) The most common position; (B) Retroversion of uterus; (C) Retroversion and retroflexion of uterus.

❖ Encourage lying in prone position for 30–60 minutes twice daily in 2nd to 4th week postpartum.

Corrective Treatment

1. Hodge-Smith pessary is used for stretching the uterosacral ligaments, so as to pull the cervix backwards.
2. *Surgical correction:* Ventrosuspension of the uterus by plicating the round ligaments of both sides extraperitoneally to the under surface of the anterior rectal sheath. This will pull the uterus forwards and maintains it permanently.

UTERINE PROLAPSE (FIG. 64.2)

Definition

Prolapse of uterus refers to a collapse, descend or change in the position of the uterus in relation to surrounding structures in the pelvis.

Description

Uterine prolapse occurs when pelvic floor muscles and ligaments stretch and weaken providing inadequate support for the uterus. The uterus then descends into the vaginal canal. Uterine prolapse usually happens in women who have had one or more vaginal births. Congenital or nulliparous prolapse is a rare type of prolapse seen in young women.

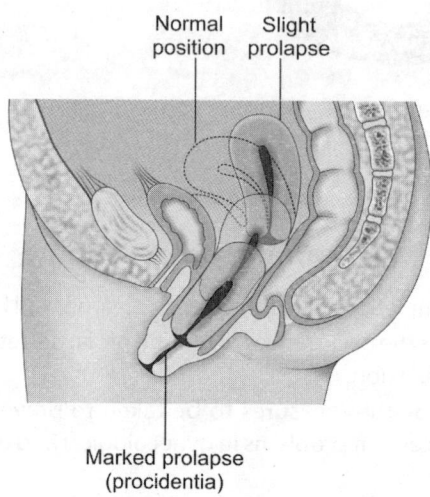

Figure 64.2: Degrees of uterine prolapse.

Associated Conditions

Other conditions associated with prolapsed uterus occur due to weakness of muscles that hold the uterus in place:

1. *Cystocele* **(Figs. 64.3A and B)***:* It is a herniation or bulging of the upper two-third of the anterior vaginal wall, where a part of the bladder bulges into the vagina. This leads to urinary frequency, urgency, retention and incontinence.

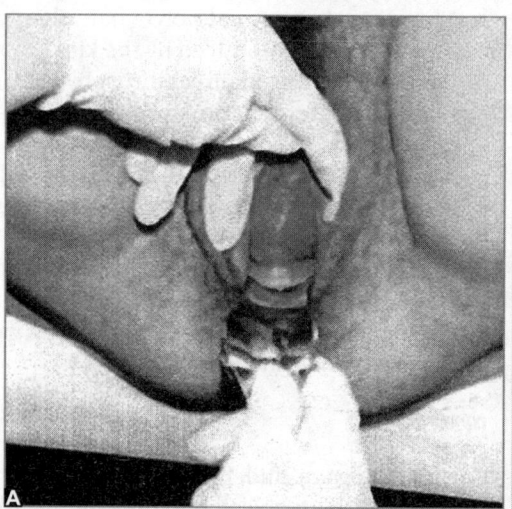 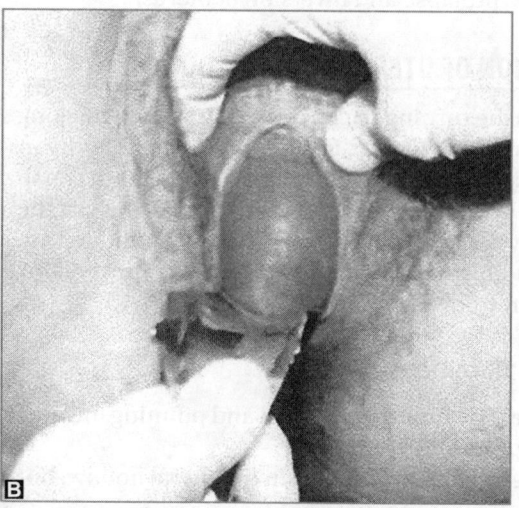

Figures 64.3A and B: Conditions associated with uterine prolapse. (A) Cystocele and uterovaginal prolapse; (B) Cystocele and enterocele with uterine prolapse *(For color version, see Plate 10).*

2. *Urethrocele:* There is herniation of the anterior vaginal wall. This may appear independently or along with cystocele and is called urethrocystocele.
3. *Enterocele:* There is herniation of the upper posterior vaginal wall, where a portion of small bowel bulges into the vagina. Standing leads to a pulling sensation and backache and this is relieved on lying down.
4. *Rectocele* **(Fig. 64.4)***:* There is herniation of the middle third of the posterior vaginal wall where the rectum bulges into the vagina. This makes bowel movements difficult to the point that the woman may need to push on the inside of vagina to empty the bowel.
5. *Relaxed perineum:* There is gaping of the introitus produced by torn perineal body with bulge of the lower part of the posterior vaginal wall.

DEGREES OF PROLAPSE (FIGS. 64.5A AND B)

Prolapse of the uterus may be one of three types, depending on severity:

1. *First degree:* The uterus sags downward from the normal anatomic position into the upper vagina. The external os remains inside the vagina.
2. *Second degree:* The cervix is at or outside the vaginal introitus, but the uterine body remains inside the vagina.
3. *Third degree:* This type is also referred to as complete prolapse or procidentia. The entire uterus descends to lie outside the introitus.

Causes

The uterus is held in position in the pelvis by muscles, special ligaments and other tissue. The uterus prolapses into the vaginal canal when these muscles and connective tissue weakens:

1. *Stretching of the pelvic support system:* Long and difficult childbirth or multiple childbirth causes the muscles and ligaments that normally hold the uterus in place to become stretched and slack.
2. *Pelvic relaxation that happens during pregnancy:* There is softening of the pelvic tissues and laxity of the supports during pregnancy as the weight of the gravid uterus continuously bears down upon the pelvic diaphragm.
3. Chronic increase in intra-abdominal pressure such as may be associated with obesity, abdominal or pelvic tumors, ascites or repetitive downward thrust of intra-abdominal pressure due to constipation or chronic cough.
4. Normal aging and lack of estrogen hormone after menopause.

Symptoms

1. A feeling of something coming down per vagina especially, while moving about. There may be variable discomfort on walking when the mass comes out of the introitus.
2. Backache or dragging pain in the pelvis, which may be relieved on lying down.

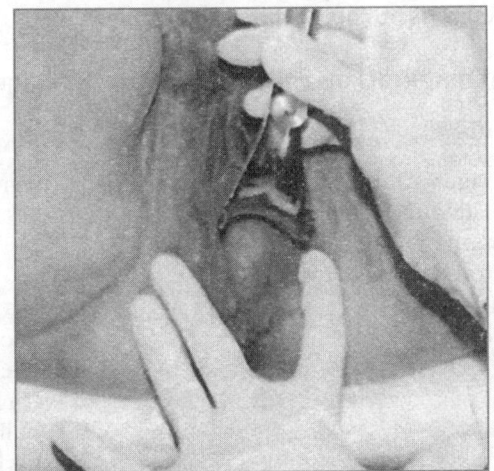

Figure 64.4: Rectocele *(For color version, see Plate 11).*

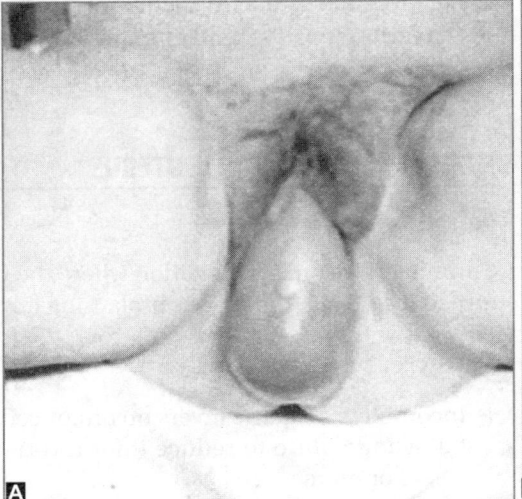
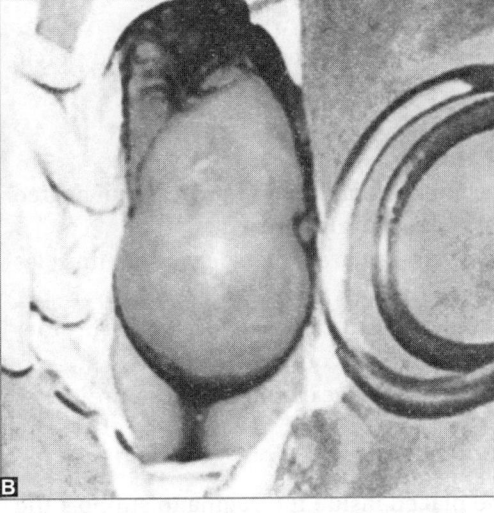

Figures 64.5A and B: Complete uterine prolapse in two different patients *(For color version, see Plate 11).*

3. Dyspareunia.
  4. *Urinary symptoms (in presence of cystocele):*
     - Difficulty in passing urine. Patient may have to elevate the anterior vaginal wall for emptying the bladder.
     - Incomplete emptying of the bladder, causing frequent desire to pass urine.
     - Urgency and frequency of micturition, which may also be due to cystitis.
     - Stress incontinence usually due to associated urethrocele.
     - Retention of urine may rarely occur.
  5. *Bowel symptoms (in presence of rectocele):*
     - Difficulty in passing stool. Patient may have to push back the posterior vaginal wall to complete the evacuation of feces. Fecal incontinence may be associated.
     - Excessive white or blood-stained discharge per vagina due to associated vaginitis or ulceration.

Examination and Diagnosis

1. Inspection and palpation: Vaginal, rectal and rectovaginal examination.
2. Pelvic examination in dorsal and standing positions. Patient may be asked to perform Valsalva's maneuver during examination.
3. Examination in squatting position, if reconfirmation is required.
4. Examination under anesthesia, if difficult to arrive at a conclusion.

Management of Uterine Prolapse

Preventive

1. *Adequate antenatal and intranatal care:* To avoid injury to the supporting structures during vaginal delivery either spontaneous or instrumental.
2. *Adequate postnatal care:* To encourage early ambulation and pelvic floor exercises (Kegel exercises) during puerperium.
3. *General measures:* To avoid strenuous activities, chronic cough, constipation and heavyweight lifting.
4. Limiting and spacing pregnancies help avoid pelvic relaxation.

Conservative

- Estrogen replacement therapy may improve minor degree prolapse in postmenopausal women
- In mild cases, exercises to strengthen pelvic floor muscles may help
- Obese patients may be instructed to reduce weight in order to reduce pressure on pelvic organs
- To avoid wearing constrictive clothing such as girdles.

Nonsurgical Management

A pessary may be placed inside the vagina to support the pelvic organs for patients who do not desire surgery. This serves to relieve the symptoms, but does not cure the condition. Pessary may also be used for patients waiting for surgery or unfit for surgery.

Surgical Management

Surgical management depends on the anatomical alteration of structures and the degree of prolapse. Patient's age, reproductive and sexual functions are also considered:

1. Anterior colporrhaphy for correction of cystocele and urethrocele.
2. Perineorrhaphy/colpoperineorrhaphy to repair the prolapse of posterior vaginal wall, which may include repair of *relaxed perineum, rectocele* and *enterocele.*
3. Fothergill's or Manchester operation: This is designed to correct uterine descend associated with cystocele and rectocele where preservation of uterus is desired. The operation combines repair of anterior and posterior vaginal walls with amputation of cervix and plication of Mackenrodt's ligaments in front of the cervix.
4. Vaginal hysterectomy with pelvic floor repair.
5. Cervicopexy or Purandare's operation for congenital or nulliparous prolapse without cystocele.

Possible Complications Following Surgical Management

Immediate

Hemorrhage within 24 hours following surgery (primary) or between 5th and 10th day (secondary):
- Retention of urine
- Infection leading to cystitis
- Wound sepsis
- Vault cellulitis.

Late

- Dyspareunia
- Recurrence of prolapse
- Vesicovaginal fistula (VVF) following bladder injury
- Rectovaginal fistula (RVF) following rectal injury
- Cervical stenosis—hematometra
- Infertility
- Cervical incompetency.

CHRONIC INVERSION OF UTERUS

Definition

Chronic inversion is a condition where the uterus becomes turned inside out, the fundus prolapsing through the cervix.

Causes

- Incomplete obstetric inversion unnoticed or left uncared following failure to reduce it for a variable period of 4 weeks or more
- Submucous myomatous polyp arising from the fundus causing traction effect

- Sarcomatous changes of fundal fibroma causing infiltration of malignancy into the myometrium leading to softening of the wall
- Senile inversion following high amputation of the cervix.

Types of Inversion

1. *Incomplete inversion:* The fundus protrudes through the cervix and lying inside the vagina.
2. *Complete inversion:* Whole of the uterus including the cervix is inverted. The vagina may also be involved.

Signs and Symptoms

1. Sensation of something coming down per vagina.
2. Irregular vaginal bleeding.
3. Offensive vaginal discharge.
4. On inspection, the protruding mass appears globular with no opening in the leading part. A tumor may be present at the bottom.
5. On vaginal examination, the cervical rim is either felt high up or not felt. A cup-shaped depression felt at the fundus or the uterus is not felt in position.
6. On rectoabdominal examination, displacement of uterus or fundal depression is felt.
7. Uterine sound test demonstrates shortness or absence of uterine cavity.
8. Examination under anesthesia (EUA) may be needed to confirm the diagnosis. When the inversion is secondary to a fibroid polyp or sarcoma and the inversion is incomplete, filling the vagina, diagnosis is more difficult.

Treatment

Rectification of inversion by surgery or removal of the uterus is determined by such factors as age, parity and associated complications.

Improvement of general condition by treating anemia and local sepsis is done, if required prior to surgery:
- Haultain's operation: Rectification per abdomen
- Spinelli's operation: Rectification per vagina
- Hysterectomy following rectification.

Nursing Implications

Nursing diagnoses are individualized to each client and her specific condition. Applicable diagnoses may include:
- Pain related to specific gynecologic condition
- Fear related to diagnostic and therapeutic procedures
- Anxiety related to treatment outcome
- Deficient knowledge regarding the pelvic condition, treatment and prognosis.

STUDY QUESTIONS

Short Answer Question

1. Clinical manifestations of inversion of uterus.

Essay Questions

1. Explain the degrees of uterine prolapse, causes, symptoms and management of a client admitted with third-degree prolapse.
2. Explain retroversion of uterus, causes, symptoms and corrective measures. List the preventive measures to be taken by women following childbirth and abortion.

CHAPTER 65

Infectious Conditions of Pelvic Organs

Learning Objectives

Upon completion of this chapter, the learner will be able to:
- List the common infections of pelvic organs.
- Describe the features of pelvic inflammatory disease.
- Discuss the common infections of vulva, vagina and cervix.
- Explain the nursing process for patients with pelvic infection.

Infection and inflammation affect upper genital tract organs together and individual organs of both upper and lower genital tracts. Depending on the causative organisms, pathological changes in the organs, nature and severity of the condition, medical and/or surgical management are required.

PELVIC INFLAMMATORY DISEASE

Pelvic inflammatory disease (PID) is a spectrum of infection and inflammation of the upper genital tract organs typically involving the endometrium, fallopian tubes, ovaries, pelvic peritoneum and surrounding structures.

Risk Factors

- Menstruating teenagers—ascending infections especially caused by *Escherichia coli* (*E. coli*), group B *Streptococcus* and *Staphylococcus*
- Previous history of acute PID
- Use of intrauterine contraceptive devices (IUCD)
- Multiple sex partners.

Types of Infections

- Uterus:
  - Acute endometritis
  - Chronic endometritis
  - Atrophic (senile) endometritis
  - Pyometra (collection of pus in the uterine cavity).
- Fallopian tubes:
  - Acute salpingitis
  - Chronic salpingitis.
- Ovaries: Oophoritis.

Causative Organisms

Acute PID is usually a polymicrobial infection caused by organisms ascending from the lower genital tract. The primary organisms are usually sexually transmitted and the secondary organisms are those normally found in the vagina:
- Sexually transmitted organisms:
  - *Gonococcus*
  - *Chlamydia trachomatis*
  - *Mycoplasma hominis*.
- Pyogenic infection causing organisms:
  - *Streptococcus*
  - *Staphylococcus*
  - *E. coli*
  - *Actinomyces* species
  - *Bacteroides* species, e.g. *B. fragilis* and *B. bivius*, *Peptostreptococcus* and *Peptococcus*.

Pathology

The pathological process is initiated in the endosalpinx with gross destruction of the epithelial cells, cilia and microvilli. In severe infection, it involves all the layers of the tube and produces acute inflammatory reaction; becomes edematous and hyperemic. The abdominal ostium is closed due to inflammatory adhesions. Depending upon the virulence, the exudate may be watery producing hydrosalpinx or purulent producing pyosalpinx.

On occasions, the exudate pours through the abdominal ostium to produce pelvic peritonitis and pelvic abscess or may affect the ovary producing ovarian abscess.

Clinical Features

Symptoms usually appear at and immediately following menses in acute infections:
- Bilateral lower abdominal and pelvic pain
- Fever—temperature > 38.3°C
- Tiredness and headache
- Irregular and excessive vaginal bleeding due to endometritis
- Increased vaginal discharge usually mucopurulent
- Nausea and vomiting
- Dyspareunia and dysuria
- Dysmenorrhea
- Postcoital spotting
- Cervical motion tenderness
- Hypoactive bowel sounds
- Adnexal fullness and tenderness
- Cervical friability
- Congested vulva, urethral meatus and openings of Bartholin's ducts
- Elevated erythrocyte sedimentation rate (ESR) and C-reactive protein
- Ultrasound evidence of fluid or pus collection.

Investigations

- Identification of organisms from the materials collected from the affected organ
- Blood tests for white blood cells (leukocytosis and elevated ESR)
- Sonography; dilated fluid-filled tubes, adnexal mass or fluid in the pouch of Douglas is suggestive of PID
- Laparoscopic examination in severe cases
- Culdocentesis and examination of the fluid.

Treatment

Patients with severe infection are hospitalized for management:
- Bedrest
- Restricted oral feeding
- Intravenous fluid to correct dehydration and acidosis
- Antibiotics intravenously; cefoxitin or gentamicin and metronidazole
- Draining of collected fluid or pus via laparotomy
- Nasogastric suction in the presence of ileus or abdominal distention.

Indications for Surgical Interventions

Need for surgical intervention is rare and indicated in:
- Generalized peritonitis
- Pelvic abscess
- Tubo-ovarian abscess, which does not respond to the antimicrobial therapy for 48–72 hours.

Complications

With chronic PID, which is diagnosed and treated late, there is increased risk of developing complications such as:
- Infertility
- Ectopic pregnancy
- Chronic pelvic pain.

Measures to Prevent Reinfection

Patients should be educated on following measures to prevent repeat infection:
- Avoid multiple sexual partners
- Use condom for sexual intercourse
- Get the sexual partner investigated and treated
- Have follow-up smears and culture tests until it becomes negative for infecting organisms. The tests are usually repeated following menstrual period until it becomes negative for three consecutive reports.

ENDOMETRITIS

Endometritis is an inflammation of the lining of the uterus—the endometrium.

Causes

Endometritis can stem from several underlying causes the most prevalent of which are bacterial infections:
1. Remnant tissues such as the placenta retained after a delivery or abortion is the most common cause of post-partum infection. Such infection may spread to the entire uterus, ovaries and pelvis.
2. Amniotic fluid can become infected from stool excreted by the fetus or from other sources of pathogenic bacteria during pregnancy.
3. Sexually transmitted diseases (STDs) such as gonorrhea and Chlamydia are often causes.
4. Pelvic inflammatory disease may also lead to endometritis.
5. Tuberculosis.
6. Normal vaginal bacteria can be a reason for endometritis.

Risk Factors

The risk of developing endometritis increases by number of factors:
1. A cesarean section significantly heightens the chances of postpartum infection.
2. Extended labor or premature rupture of fetal membranes.
3. Anemia may be a pre-existing condition or it may result from heavy bleeding during labor.
4. Steroid medications: Sometimes used to assist fetal lung development and functioning when premature birth is expected, are another risk factor.
5. The presence of an intrauterine device (IUD) can induce or exacerbate inflammation.
6. Use of special instruments or procedures such as hysteroscopy, dilatation and curettage (D&C) can induce inflammation.

Signs and Symptoms

The postpartum endometritis develop in 49-72 hours:
* Abdominal distention or swelling
* Abnormal vaginal bleeding
* Abnormal vaginal discharge often with a foul odor
* Lower abdominal or pelvic pain
* Fever with chills (temperature 100°F–104°F)
* Discomfort with bowel movement (constipation may occur)
* Malaise and general discomfort.

Tests and Investigations

* Abdominal palpation to discover tenderness or soreness
* Pelvic examination
* Blood tests; WBC, complete blood count (CBC), ESR
* Cultures from cervix for organisms
* Pap smear to detect the presence of abnormal cells
* Laparoscopy/Hysteroscopy and endometrial biopsy
* Computed tomography (CT) to assess the uterus and other internal organs.

Treatment

Patients with serious symptoms and postpartum infection need to be hospitalized and treated. Treatment measures include:
* Administration of intravenous antibiotics for 2-7 days
* Administration of oral or intravenous fluids to prevent dehydration
* Aspiration to drain pus from uterus
* Evacuation of remnant tissue from the uterus (placenta, membranes)
* Adequate rest
* A postpartum hysterectomy to remove a hopelessly damaged or infected uterus
* Analgesics for pain and fever, and isolation to avoid cross-infection are often instituted. Mild cases may be treated on an outpatient basis.

Prognosis

Most cases of endometritis clear up with antibiotics. Untreated endometritis can lead to more serious infection and complications with pelvic organs, reproduction and general health.

Possible Complications

* Infertility
* Pelvic peritonitis
* Pelvic or uterine abscess formation
* Septicemia
* Septic shock.

Prevention

Endometritis caused by sexually transmitted infections, can be prevented by:
* Early diagnosis and complete treatment of STDs
* Educating women on safe sex practices.

The risk of endometritis will be reduced by following sterile techniques by healthcare workers, while delivering a baby or performing an abortion, IUD placement or other gynecological procedures.

CERVICITIS

Cervicitis refers to infection of the endocervix including the glands and stroma. The infection may be acute or chronic and usually occurs following childbirth, abortion or any operation on the cervix. The infection may be acute or chronic.

Causative Organisms

Organisms causing cervicitis include *Streptococcus, Staphylococcus, E. coli, Gonococcus* and *Chlamydia trachomatis*. The organisms gain entry into the glands of the endocervix and produce acute inflammatory changes. The infection may be localized or spread upwards to involve the fallopian tubes and parametrium.

Clinical Features

* Spotting after sexual intercourse
* Yellowish white discharge
* Red, edematous, friable cervix
* Cervical motion tenderness
* Vaginal examination is painful.

Treatment

* Antibiotic therapy based on identified drug sensitivity (high vaginal and endocervical swabs are taken for bacteriological identification and drug sensitivity)
* In chronic cervicitis, the diseased tissue may be destroyed by electrosurgery, diathermy cauterization, laser or cryosurgery
* Any associated cervical tear, if present may be reconstructed
* Cervical scrape cytology must be done to exclude malignancy.

VULVAL AND VAGINAL INFECTIONS

Vulval and vaginal infections occur when the defense is lost following constant irritation by vaginal discharge or urine (incontinence), or following menopause when there will be atrophic changes.

Common Infectious Conditions

- Bartholinitis, Bartholin's abscess and Bartholin's cysts
- Vaginitis: Bacterial, viral, monilial and atrophic (postmenopausal)
- Vulvovaginitis.

Causative Organisms and Clinical Manifestations

1. Bacterial infections are caused by sexually transmitted organisms such as gonorrhea, *Chlamydia trachomatis* and syphilis:
   - Increased vaginal discharge
   - Musty or fleshy odor of discharge following sexual intercourse
   - Homogeneous, gray-white discharge
   - Bacterial infections are treated with local antiseptics and systemic antibiotics.
2. Monilial infections are caused by *Candida albicans*. Manifestations are:
   - Itching and burning
   - Thick curd-like discharge
   - Dyspareunia
   - Vulvar and/or vaginal erythema
   - Edematous cervix.

   Monilial infection is treated with local fungicidal preparations such as nystatin, clotrimazole, miconazole or econazole or fluconazole oral therapy.
3. Vulval infection is usually caused by varicella-zoster virus. It produces painful eruptions of groups of vesicles distributed over the skin. Vesicles may rupture or become dry with scab formation.

   It is treated with analgesics to relieve pain, antibiotics to prevent secondary infection and acyclovir as antiviral drug.
4. *Atrophic vulvovaginitis:* This type of infection is seen in postmenopausal women. There is atrophy of the vulvovaginal structures due to deficiency of estrogen. Vaginal mucosa is thin and more susceptible to trauma and infection.

Clinical Features

- Dryness and soreness
- Itching and burning
- Vulvar and vaginal atrophy
- Pale, thin, friable vaginal mucosa
- Sparse pubic hair
- Dyspareunia
- Yellowish or blood-stained discharge.

Treatment

- Intravaginal applications of estrogen cream
- Systemic estrogen, if there is no contraindication
- Treatment of local infection, if present.

NURSING PROCESS FOR CLIENTS WITH PELVIC INFECTIONS

Assessment

Nursing assessment for genital infections include assessment for risk, symptoms, medical history, gynecologic history and lifestyle behaviors. Physical assessment focuses on data from assessment and investigation findings to aid diagnosis of specific infection.

Nursing Diagnosis

Nursing diagnoses are formulated after diagnosis of infection. Applicable nursing diagnoses may include the following:
- Pain related to infection
- Fear related to the diagnosis
- Deficient knowledge related to the experience regarding the diagnosis.

Nursing care plans include specific actions the client completes to achieve the highest level of wellness possible. Sample goals for the client may include the following:
- Takes the prescribed medications correctly
- Returns to healthcare facility/physician as scheduled for follow-up assessment of infectious status
- Notifies physician of any failure of symptoms to improve as expected or adverse effects of prescribed medications
- Adopts recommended changes in lifestyle behaviors to prevent recurrent infection
- Learns measures for health promotion.

Nursing Interventions

Nursing interventions include teaching and counseling for prevention and explaining prescribed medications.

STUDY QUESTIONS

Short Answer Questions

1. Cervicitis.
2. Vulval and vaginal infections.
3. Prevention of pelvic inflammatory disease.

Essay Question

1. A client who developed endometritis following a difficult delivery is admitted. Describe the possible investigations, treatment and nursing management.

66: Benign Pelvic Conditions

Learning Objectives

Upon completion of this chapter, the learner will be able to:
- List the benign pelvic conditions that are structural and functional.
- Explain the common tumors of uterus and ovary.
- Describe polyps and cystic conditions of pelvic organs.
- Describe polycystic ovary disease and management of patients.
- Explain the nursing management of clients with benign pelvic conditions.

Benign pelvic conditions can be categorized as structural and functional growths. Common structural conditions include fibroid tumors, ovarian tumors, cysts and polyps. Common functional condition is polycystic ovary syndrome (PCOS).

FIBROID TUMORS

Fibroid tumors are benign tumors arising in the myometrium, which can protrude into the uterine cavity and bulge through the outer layer or grow within the myometrium.

Growth of Fibroids

1. Fibroids develop due to proliferation of smooth muscle cells. The tumors usually grow very slowly, about 1–2 cm per year.
2. Fibroids are estrogen dependent and thus grow rapidly during pregnancy. They do not occur before menarche and growth cessation occurs after menopause.

Incidence

The tumors are found most often during the fourth and fifth decades of life. The incidence of symptomatic fibroid is about 3% in Indian women. The incidence is higher in women in United States of America (USA) and United Kingdom (UK). Fibroids occur more often in nulliparous women or in those having secondary infertility. Higher incidence is seen in obese women and oral pill users.

Types of Fibroids (Fig. 66.1)

1. *Interstitial or intramural fibroids (75%):* These are fibroids that grow within the myometrium.
2. *Subserous or subperitoneal fibroids (15%):* These are intramural fibroids that are pushed outwards toward the peritoneal cavity. They are partially or completely covered by peritoneum. If the fibroid has a pedicle, it is called pedunculated submucosal fibroid.
3. *Submucosal fibroids (15%):* When the tumor protrudes into the uterine cavity and lies underneath the endometrium, it is called submucosal fibroid. This can make the uterine cavity irregular and distorted. Pedunculated submucosal fibroid may come out through the cervix.

Clinical Features

- Majority of fibroids (75%) remains asymptomatic and are detected during routine examination or at laparotomy, or laparoscopy

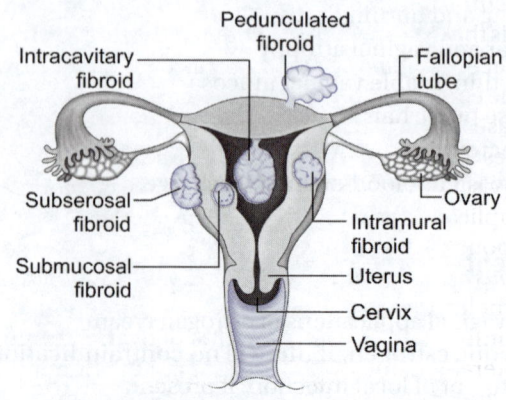

Figure 66.1: Uterine fibroids.

- The uterus reaches a 4–5 months gestation size without symptoms in most cases
- In symptomatic type, menorrhagia is the classic symptom
- Metrorrhagia or irregular bleeding is seen in some women
- Dysmenorrhea is a symptom when it is associated with pelvic congestion or endometriosis
- Infertility is seen in about 30% of women
- Recurrent pregnancy loss (miscarriage or preterm labor)
- Lower abdominal or pelvic pain.

Diagnosis

1. Majority of uterine fibroids can be diagnosed from history and pelvic examination.
2. Ultrasound and color Doppler are used to locate the fibroids accurately. Laparoscopy is useful, if the uterine size is less than 12 weeks and associated with pelvic pain and infertility.
3. Uterine curettage is done in the presence of irregular bleeding to detect any co-existing pathology and to study the endometrial pattern.

Management

Therapeutic intervention depends on the woman's desire for future pregnancy and the tumor size:

1. *Medical management:* Hormone therapy may be used as a short-term intervention to decrease the size of fibroid and to minimize blood loss. Drugs used are antifibrinolytics, antiprogesterone danazol, gonadotropin-releasing hormone (GnRH) analogs and prostaglandin synthetic inhibitors. Use of hormones for more than 6 months can increase the risk of osteoporosis.
2. *Surgical management:*
   - Myomectomy to remove submucosal fibroid for women, who desire future childbearing
   - Hysterectomy for women, who do not desire future pregnancies and with tumors, which are large.

BENIGN OVARIAN TUMORS

Benign ovarian neoplasms commonly seen are mucinous cystadenoma, serous cystadenoma, Brenner tumor and dermoid cyst:

1. *Mucinous cystadenoma:* It arises from the totipotent (cells that have ability to differentiate into any type of cells) surface epithelium of the ovary as a mucinous metaplasia of the epithelial cells. The tumors are bilateral in about 10% of cases. It may attain a huge size if left uncared for. It is the largest benign ovarian tumor. The content inside is thick and viscid mucin (a glycoprotein, which is colorless unless complicated by hemorrhage). The chance of malignancy is about 10%.
2. *Serous cystadenoma:* It arises from the totipotent surface epithelium of the ovary. This type of adenoma is quite common and accounts for 40% of ovarian tumors. It is bilateral in about 40%. The cyst appears smooth, shiny and grayish white. The content fluid is clear and rich in serum proteins—albumin and globulin.
3. *Brenner tumor:* This accounts for 1–2% of all ovarian tumors. About 8–10% is bilateral and is seen in women over the age of 40. Majority are solid, similar to that of fibroma and measure less than 2 cm in diameter. The cells look like coffee bean as the nuclei have longitudinal groves. Estrogen is secreted by the tumor and the women may present with abnormal vaginal bleeding.
4. *Dermoid cyst:* It arises from the germ cells arrested after first meiotic division. Its incidence is about 15–20% amongst ovarian tumors. The tumor is bilateral in about 15–20%. The cyst usually is of moderate size with tense, smooth capsule. The content is predominantly sebatious material with hair.

Clinical Features of Benign Tumors and Cysts of Ovary

1. Generally, manifests in the late childbearing period. Dermoid cyst is more common in pregnancy.
2. Often seen related with nulliparity.
3. Tumors are asymptomatic and usually detected during routine abdominal or pelvic examination, laparoscopy or laparotomy.
4. When the tumor becomes symptomatic, they present with:
   - Heaviness in the lower abdomen
   - Gradual growth of size of abdomen
   - Dull, aching pain in abdomen.
5. Gastrointestinal symptoms like nausea and indigestion in neglected cases, when the tumor becomes big enough to fill the whole abdomen.
6. With large mucinous cystadenoma, patient may be cachectic due to protein loss.
7. Pitting edema of legs when a huge tumors press on great veins.
8. On abdominal examination, the tumor is nontender, which can be moved from side to side.
9. On pelvic examination, the tumor mass is felt separated from the uterus and not movable, when the cervix is moved. Lower pole of the cyst can be felt through the fornix.

Special Investigations

- *Sonography:* Transvaginal sonography with color Doppler to note the tumor volume and vascularity
- Straight X-ray of the abdomen for evidence of teeth or bone tissue in dermoid cyst
- Computed tomography (CT) scan to identify presence of fat, calcification and teeth
- Laparoscopy, if there is pain and suspicion of ectopic pregnancy
- Cytology when the patient presents with ascites or pleural effusion.

Complications of Benign Ovarian Tumors

- Torsion of the pedicle
- Intracystic hemorrhage

- Infection
- Rupture
- Pseudomyxoma peritonei (peritoneal mass composed of mucus resembling myxoma)
- Malignancy.

Management

- Ovarian cystectomy, leaving behind the healthy ovarian tissue in young patients
- Salpingo-oophorectomy for a big tumor that has destroyed most of the ovarian tissues or for a gangrenous cyst
- Total hysterectomy with bilateral salpingo-oophorectomy for parous women above 40 years.

POLYPS

A polyp is a tumor attached by a pedicle. Two types of polyps are commonly seen; mucoid polyp and fibroid polyp.

Mucoid Polyp

Mucoid type of polyp arises from the body of uterus or from the cervix. The pedicle may at times be long enough to make the polyp protrude from the cervix or reach up to the vaginal introitus.

Clinical Features

1. There may not be any symptom. Polyps are usually discovered during speculum examination, hysteroscopy or hysterosalpingography.
2. Irregular uterine bleeding is seen either in pre or post-menopausal.
3. Contact bleeding, if the polyp is at or outside the cervix.
4. Excessive vaginal discharge, which may be offensive.
5. On speculum examination, the polyp looks reddish in color, attached usually by a slender pedicle. The size may be about 1–2 cm.

Fibroid Polyp

The fibroid polyp may arise from the body of the uterus or from the cervix. It is an extrusion of a submucosal fibroid from the uterine cavity. The polyp is usually single and of varying sizes. There may be infection, necrosis and hemorrhage at the tip.

Clinical Features

Patients are usually in reproductive period:
- Intermenstrual bleeding
- Colicky pain in lower abdomen
- Excessive vaginal discharge, which may be offensive
- Sensation of something coming down when the polyp becomes big distending the vulva
- Uterus may feel bulky
- Pale or hemorrhagic polyp can be visualized on speculum examination.

Management

- Small polyps such as mucus polyps are removed by twisting, after catching it with an Allis forceps or tissue forceps
- Polyps with thick pedicles are removed by placing a transfixation suture in the pedicle and then cutting it distal to the ligature
- Big fibroid polyp lying in the vagina is removed by morcellation (piecemeal).

POLYCYSTIC OVARY SYNDROME

Polycystic ovary syndrome (PCOS) is a complex endocrine disorder associated with long-term anovulation and an excess of androgen circulation in the blood. The syndrome is characterized by formation of cysts in the ovaries. PCOS is the leading cause of amenorrhea in young reproductive age group women (20–30%).

Clinical Features

- Increasing obesity, especially central obesity
- Menstrual abnormalities in the form of oligomenorrhea, amenorrhea or dysfunctional uterine bleeding
- Infertility
- Hirsutism and acne
- Acanthosis nigricans (thickened, pigmented skin) over nape of neck, inner thighs and axilla.

Causes

The disorder is characterized by excessive androgen production by the ovaries, which interfere with reproductive, endocrine and metabolic functions.

The syndrome begins with an imbalance of luteinizing hormone (LH) and follicle-stimulating hormone (FSH). LH is seen elevated and FSH low to normal.

The result of hormonal imbalance is continued follicular development, elevated estrogen levels, anovulation and multiple cysts. Diagnosis is based on the presence of any two of the following three criteria:
- Oligo and/or anovulation
- Hyperandrogenism
- Polycystic ovaries.

Investigations

1. *Sonography:* Transvaginal sonography will show enlarged ovaries with peripherally arranged cysts.
2. *Serum values:*
   - LH level is elevated, and LH:FSH ratio is elevated (> 3:1)
   - Raised level of estradiol and estrone
   - Reduced level of sex hormone-binding globulin (SHBG)
   - Raised serum testosterone (>150 ng/dL)
   - Raised fasting insulin levels (>25 µIU/mL)
   - Raised level of prolactin.
3. *Laparoscopy:* Bilateral polycystic ovaries.

Possible Late Sequelae

- Risk of developing diabetes mellitus due to insulin resistance (15%)
- Risk of developing endometrial carcinoma due to persistently elevated level of estrogens
- Risk of hypertension and cardiovascular disease due to abnormal lipid profile (dyslipidemia)
- Postmenopausal breast cancer.

Management

Management of PCOS needs to be individualized. It depends on her presenting symptoms like menstrual disorder, infertility, obesity and hirsutism or combined symptoms.

Medical Management

- Correction of biochemical abnormalities with combination oral pills, GnRH agonists and medroxy-progesterone (Provera)
- For patients wanting pregnancy, ovulation induction is done by giving clomiphene citrate with or without dexamethasone or bromocriptine
- For patients with hyperinsulinemia, metformin is given with clomiphene.

Surgical Management

Surgical treatment is indicated for those resistant to medical therapy. Endoscopic cauterization or carbon dioxide (CO_2) laser vaporization of multiple cysts is usually done.

Nursing Process

Nursing Assessment

Nursing assessment for pelvic conditions involves assessing risk factors, presenting symptoms and medical and gynecological history. Data from physical assessment, laboratory tests and diagnostic procedures are considered.

Nursing Diagnosis

Nursing diagnosis are formulated based on assessment data and findings. Applicable nursing diagnosis may include:

- Pain related to pelvic condition
- Fear related to procedures and treatment
- Anxiety related to effects of condition or treatment
- Anxiety related to future childbearing
- Deficient knowledge regarding specific pelvic condition.

Nursing Care Plans

Nursing care plans include specific actions, the client will complete to achieve the highest level of wellness. Goals for the client may be that she will:

- Develop strategies for coping with pain
- Reduce stress and promote wellness by following exercise regimens
- Consume recommended food to control obesity and maintain optimum body weight
- Return to physician for follow-up care
- Notify physician of response to therapy and improvement or lack of it
- Be informed about the choices of medical management and expected outcomes of therapy.

Nursing Interventions

Nursing interventions include education about the condition, specific procedures, expected outcomes of therapy and providing emotional support.

STUDY QUESTIONS

Short Notes

1. Types of fibroid tumors.
2. Fibroid polyp.

Essay Question

1. Explain polycystic ovary syndrome (PCOS), diagnostic measures and medical management of the condition. Prepare a nursing care plan for a young, newly married client, who is anxious to become pregnant and newly diagnosed as having PCOS.

CHAPTER 67

Gynecological Examinations and Diagnostic Procedures

Learning Objectives

Upon completion of this chapter, the learner will be able to:
- Gather patient information and relevant history from gynecological patients for identifying health problems.
- Describe the gynecological examinations that are performed for clients with various problems.
- Discuss the tests and procedures in gynecology for diagnostic and therapeutic purposes.

Examination of a gynecological patient includes history taking as well as general, abdominal and internal examinations. A detailed and composite history using different formats can be obtained.

HISTORY TAKING (BOX 67.1)

Past medical history: Information regarding relevant medical disorders such as systemic illness, metabolic or endocrine disorder and infection.

Past surgical history: General, obstetrical or gynecological surgeries, postoperative recovery and any special information related to investigations are included.

Personal history: Data related to occupation, marital status, sexual life, contraceptive practices, any infertility problems and if not married status of genitourinary functions are included. History of medications taken in the past and currently and any allergies are also entered.

Family history: Information on diseases in family that can have some value such as malignancies of genital organs, colon, tubercular infections, etc. is taken.

BOX 67.1: History taking.

Demographic data	Menstrual history
Name:	Age of menarche:
Age:	Regularity of cycle:
Marital status:	Duration of period:
Education:	Length of cycle:
Occupation:	Amount of bleeding:
Income:	Menstrual discomfort:
Religion:	Amenorrhea:
Address:	Last menstrual period:

Obstetrical history

Sl. No.	Date of delivery	Duration of pregnancy	Abnormalities in pregnancy	Delivery (vaginal/cesarean)	Puerperium, baby (alive/stillborn)

EXAMINATION

Examination of a gynecologic patient includes general, systemic examination and gynecological examination.

General and Systemic Examination

Aspects included in this examination are:
- General body built (obese/thin)
- Development of social characteristics
- Appearance—inspection (head to foot)
- Systems examination—gastrointestinal, cardiovascular and respiratory
- Vital signs.

Gynecological Examination

Breast examination is done especially for women above 30 years with special attention to the presence of any lump or pathology.

Abdominal Examination

Using different methods such as *inspection, palpation, percussion and auscultation*, abdominal and pelvic organs and their functions are assessed. Some of the important observations include presence of old scar, striae, prominent veins, hernia and abnormal distention of abdomen.

Palpation can reveal muscle tension, rigidity or guarding. Any tumor or growth if felt may be further tested for consistency, mobility and location.

Percussion may be useful to study the details of any tumor or fluid collection palpated. *Auscultation* method is used to identify intestinal sounds, uterine soufflé over a vascular fibroid or pregnant uterus and fetal heart rate (FHR) over a pregnant uterus.

Pelvic Examination

Internal examination for gynecological patients includes:
- Inspection of vulva
- Vaginal examination
- Rectal examination
- Rectovaginal and bimanual examination.

Inspection of Vulva

Vulvar inspection is done to note any anatomical abnormality, visible pathological changes, discharges, enital prolapse, stress incontinence and hemorrhoids.

Vaginal Examination

Examination is done for inspection of vagina and cervix. A speculum examination followed by a bimanual examination is done by the physician to evaluate the structures. Cervical scrape cytology and endocervical sampling for cytological testing are done in all or selected gynecological patients. Digital examination of the vagina using a gloved index finger lubricated with sterile ubricant is done to palpate any swelling in the labia or adjacent structures. In virgins with intact hymen, this examination is done only under anesthesia.

The vaginal cervix is examined for following features:
- *Direction:* Anteverted or retroverted
- *Station:* External os at the level of ischial spines or not
- *Texture:* Firm-like tip of nose or soft
- *Shape:* Conical or cylindrical
- *External os:* Round or dilated
- *Movement:* Painful or not.

Tendency to bleed on touch—present or not

Integrity and tone of the perineal body are checked by flexing the internal finger posteriorly and palpating it with the thumb placed externally. A bimanual examination will be done to palpate the uterus, uterine appendages and pouch of Douglas.

Vaginal or cervical discharge and scraping
- Microscopic examination
- Culture examination.

Cervical smear for cytological and hormonal study
Cervical mucus for bacteriological study, hormonal status and infertility investigation.

Rectal Examination

Rectal examination is done in isolation or as an adjunct to vaginal examination. It is indicated in:
- Children or adult virgins
- Painful vaginal examination
- Carcinoma cervix
- Vaginal atresia
- Rectocele or enterocele.

Rectovaginal and Bimanual Examination

Rectovaginal or bimanual examinations may also be performed when indicated, e.g. adnexal mass.

Blood Investigations

Commonly included blood tests are:
- Hemoglobin estimation
- White blood cells (WBCs) counts
- Erythrocyte sedimentation rate
- Venereal disease research laboratory (VDRL) test
- Platelet count
- Bleeding and coagulation time.

Urine Examination

- Routine examination
- Culture and drug sensitivity.

DIAGNOSTIC PROCEDURES

Colposcopy

Colposcopy is examination of the cervix and vagina using an instrument called colposcope and colpomicroscope.

Patient Selection

- Women with abnormal smear report
- Women with history of contact bleeding despite negative smear.

Procedure

1. Patient is placed in lithotomy position after ensuring that her urinary bladder is empty.
2. Cusco's speculum is placed to visualize the cervix.
3. Colposcope is inserted and cervix and vagina examined using low-power magnification.
4. During examination, cervix is wiped with normal saline and 3% acetic acid for better assessment. Findings include normalcy of epithelium and changes due to condyloma or papilloma.

X-ray Examination

Plain X-ray of pelvis is used to locate an intrauterine contraceptive device (IUCD) or shadows of teeth or bone in a cystic teratoma. Special X-rays used for gynecologic patients are:

- Hysterosalpingography to note tubal patency
- Lymphangiography to locate the lymph glands involved in pelvic malignancy.

Ultrasound Examinations

Ultrasonographic examinations are common diagnostic modalities in gynecology:

1. *Transabdominal sonography (TAS)* is used in conditions, where patient has large masses like fibroid or ovarian tumor.
2. *Transvaginal sonography (TVS):* This is done with a probe, which is placed close to the target organ. Detailed evaluation of pelvic organs (within 10 cm of the field) is possible with TVS. This method is not suitable for use in women with narrow vagina as in virgins, postmenopausal women or postradiation vaginal stenosis.
3. *Transvaginal color Doppler sonography:* This examination provides additional information of blood flow to, from or within an organ (uterus or adnexal). This flow can be measured by analysis of the waveform using the pulsatility index.

Use of Ultrasound Examinations

1. *Infertility work-up:* Monitoring of follicular maturation and ovulation for induction of ovulation, artificial insemination and ovum retrieval in cases of in vitro fertilization (IVF) and gamete intrafallopian transfer (GIFT).
2. Detection of ectopic pregnancy as a 'tubal ring' separate from ovary in a patient with empty uterine cavity.
3. Detection of pelvic mass such as uterine fibroid, ovarian mass, endometriomas, tubo-ovarian mass, etc. with regard to its location and consistency [transvaginal color Doppler sonography (TV-CDS)] can assess the vascularity of the mass that raises suspicion of malignant tumor.
4. Detection of submucosal fibroids and polyps using sonohysterographic studies, which involve instillation of saline in the uterine cavity and aspiration of material from cysts and masses.

Computed Tomography

Computed tomography (CT) scan provides high resolution, two-dimensional images. CT differentiates tissue densities and these gray-scale pictures can be read on X-ray film or a television monitor. Pelvic organs can be differentiated from gastrointestinal and urinary systems using contrast media given orally, intravenous (IV) or rectally.

The CT scan is most useful in the diagnosis of lymph node metastasis, depth of myometrial invasion in endometrial cancer, ovarian mass and myomas. CT scan also facilitates the percutaneous needle biopsy of suspicious lymph nodes. CT scan is also useful in assessing tumor extent and detecting metastases. It is useful in staging of ovarian cancer and deposits of cancer cells in other organs such as the liver.

Magnetic Resonance Imaging

Magnetic resonance imaging (MRI) creates cross-sectional images of body using a combination of radiowaves (nonionizing radiation) and magnetic fields.

In gynecology, MRI is found superior to CT scan in the delineation of pelvic organs in multiple planes.

Uses of Magnetic Resonance Imaging

1. To measure the depth of myometrial penetration of endometrial cancer preoperatively MRI is used.
2. It can detect accurately the parametrial invasion of cervical cancer and distinguish post-treatment fibrosis and recurrence.
3. Tumor volume can be measured with 3D imaging system. MRI is thus useful in determining the invasion of bladder, rectum, parametrium and uterine body.
4. Leiomyomas are better diagnosed with MRI.
5. The MRI is useful in the diagnosis of endometriosis as it can measure the depth of penetration, which is responsible for pelvic pain.
6. The MRI is useful and even superior in the evaluation of metastatic lymph nodes or recurrent pelvic tumor.

Positron Emission Tomography

Position emission tomography (PET) is based on the tissue uptake of 18-fluoro-2 deoxyglucose. Fluorodeoxyglucose

(FDG) PET can measure the difference between the normal tissue and cancerous tissue. The glucose analog is given IV, scan is then done and images are interpreted.

The scan is more sensitive for detection of metastatic diseases and recurrence of ovarian malignancy. It is also useful to assess the response following tumor therapy.

Surgical Methods

1. *Endometrial sampling:* It is one of the diagnostic tests done in the clinical work-up of women with infertility or abnormal uterine bleeding, or for periodic screening during hormone replacement therapy. A uterine sampler, which has a thin plastic cannula and plunger, is used to obtain a sample of endometrium. Endometrial sample obtained by suction from the fundus and upper part of the body is used for the test.
2. *Endometrial biopsy:* This is the method of obtaining endometrium by curettage after dilatation of the cervix. It is usually performed under general anesthesia.
3. *Cervical biopsy:* It is done to confirm the clinical diagnosis of cervical pathology. Biopsy can be taken in the outpatient unit, if the pathology is detectable, but for wider tissue excision as in cone biopsy, it is done as an inpatient procedure.
4. *Culdocentesis:* It is the transvaginal aspiration of peritoneal fluid from the cul-de-sac or pouch of Douglas. The procedure is done in suspected ectopic pregnancy or other conditions producing hemoperitoneum and pelvic abscess.
5. *Laparoscopy:* It is a technique of visualization of peritoneal cavity by means of a fiber optic endoscope introduced through the abdominal wall. Prior to introducing the endoscope pneumoperitoneum is achieved by introduction of carbon dioxide or air. Either local or general anesthesia may be used for performing the procedure.
6. *Hysteroscopy:* This is an operative procedure for visualizing the endometrial cavity with the aid of fiber optic telescope. Uterine distension is achieved by carbon dioxide, normal saline or glycine. The instrument is passed transcervically after paracervical block or general anesthesia. Hysteroscopy is done for the following indications:
   – Unresponsive irregular uterine bleeding
   – Recurrent abortion
   – Missing threads of IUCD
   – Intrauterine adhesions (uterine synechiae)
   – To visualize transformation zone with microcolpohysteroscopy, when colposcopic finding is unsatisfactory.
7. *Salpingoscopy:* In this, a firm telescope is inserted through the abdominal ostium of the fallopian tube, so that the tubal mucosa can be visualized by distending the lumen with saline infusion. The telescope is introduced through laparoscope. This is used to study the anatomy and physiology of the tubal epithelium for selecting patients for IVF.
8. *Cystoscopy:* The use of cystoscopy in gynecology is
   – to evaluate cervical cancer prior to staging and to
   – investigate the urinary symptoms including hematuria, incontinence and fistula.
9. *Culdoscopy:* It is the procedure of visualizing the pelvic structures through an incision in the pouch of Douglas. Use of culdoscope is limited as compared to laparoscope.
10. *Proctoscopy:* It is done following a digital examination of the rectum in cases of rectal involvement of genital malignancy.
11. *Examination under anesthesia (EUA):* It is indicated where bimanual examination cannot be conducted properly either because of extreme tenderness or inadequate relaxation of abdominopelvic muscles, or non-cooperative patient. It is also done in cases of uterine malignancy for clinical staging and also to examine virgins and children with gynecological problems.
12. *Laser (light amplification by stimulated emission of radiation):* Laser is used in gynecology for the purpose of tissue cutting, coagulation or vaporization. It is used widely in genital tract surgeries and with endoscopic surgeries.

■ STUDY QUESTIONS

Short Notes

1. Endometrial sampling.
2. Cervical sampling.
3. Culdocentesis.
4. Hysteroscopy.
5. Salpingoscopy.

Short Answer Questions

1. Explain ultrasound examination in gynecological patients.
2. Discuss the use of magnetic resonance imaging in gynecology.

CHAPTER 68

Congenital Malformations of Female Genital Organs

Learning Objectives

Upon completion of this chapter, the learner will be able to:
* List the common congenital malformations of female genital organs.
* Describe the manifestations of malformations of different organs.
* Describe the management of different congenital problems.
* Describe the nursing managements of clients and families facing problems related to congenital malformations of genital organs.

Congenital malformations are anomalies, which may be either hereditary or occurring during gestation and evident at the time of birth. Development of the female genital tract is a complex process dependent upon a series of events involving cellular differentiation, migration, fusion and canalization. Failure of any one of these processes results in a congenital anomaly.

The development of female genital tract begins at 3 weeks of gestation and continues into the second trimester of pregnancy.

While, major abnormalities escape attention, the moderate and severe ones produce gynecologic and obstetric problems. Female genital abnormalities often do not present until or well after puberty. Although genital abnormalities may be isolated, careful assessment for possible underlying disorders particularly chromosomal or metabolic is essential.

CONGENITAL UTERINE ANOMALIES/ABNORMALITIES

Definition

Congenital anomalies of the uterus are defects of uterine development and shape that occur during intrauterine life.

Development of Uterine Anomalies

Congenital anomalies, also called Müllerian duct anomalies are malformations that develop during embryonic life. During fetal development period, it actually starts as two small uteri which migrate down separately and ultimately fuses to form a single uterus. Normally, the wall where the two uteri join, reabsorbs completely from the bottom to the top resulting in a triangular shaped uterine cavity. Any alteration to this developmental process of cellular differentiation, migration, fusion and canalization leads to what is called congenital uterine anomaly.

Types of Uterine Anomalies (Figs. 68.1 to 68.6)

Uterus Didelphys

Didelphys uterus also called double uterus is a rare uterine abnormality in which the two halves of the uterus develop completely separate. There will be two separate uteri each one with a cervix. A uterus with double cervix is named a bicollis and that with a single cervix is unicollis. These may have double vagina or single vagina as shown in **Figure 68.1**. Women with this type of uterus often have successful pregnancies, however, they are at higher risk of preterm delivery or miscarriage. This is seen in 7.5% of women.

Arcuate Uterus (Fig. 68.2)

Here the uterus looks normal, but the internal surface of the single endometrial cavity shows a shallow groove of 1 cm or less which forms a short septum. This is seen in 7% of women.

Unicornuate Uterus (Fig. 68.3)

This abnormality of the uterus is also called single-horned uterus and happens when the tissues that form the uterus do not develop properly. Only one half of the uterus develops from a single Müllerian duct. The unicornuate uterus has only one fallopian tube. Seen in 15% of women.

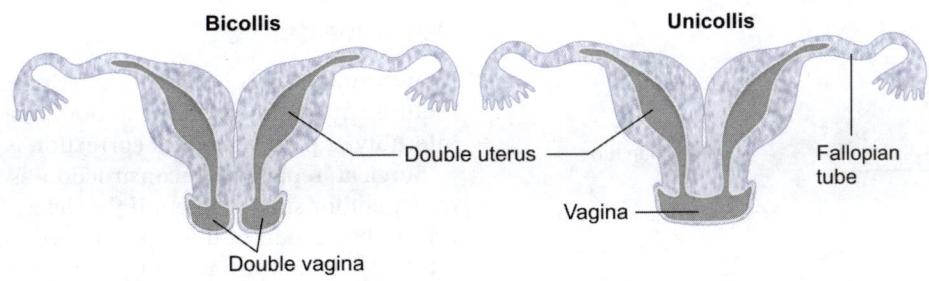

Figure 68.1: Uterus didelphys.

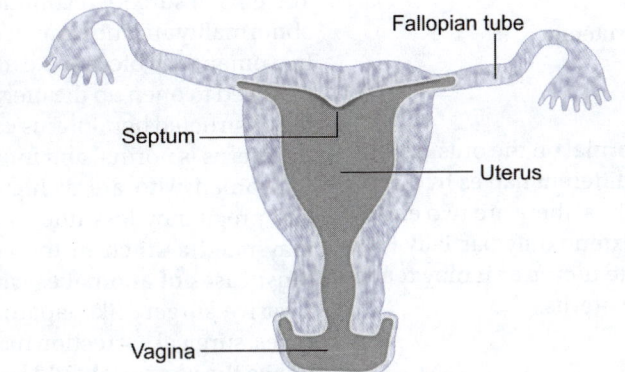

Figure 68.2: Arcuate uterus.

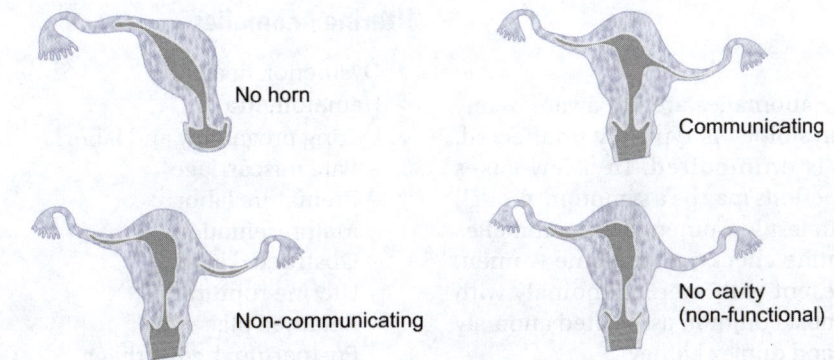

Figure 68.3: Unicornuate uterus.

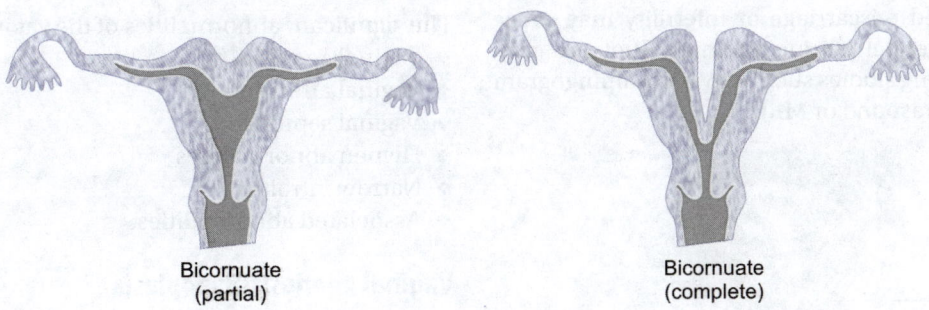

Figure 68.4: Bicornuate uterus.

Bicornuate Uterus (Fig. 68.4)

In this type, the uterus has an external indentation or groove marking its division internally into two endometrial cavities. The two halves of the uterus may appear almost completely separated except at the lower part. When pregnancy occurs, the baby has less space to grow in the uterine cavity. This makes up about 25% of such anomalies.

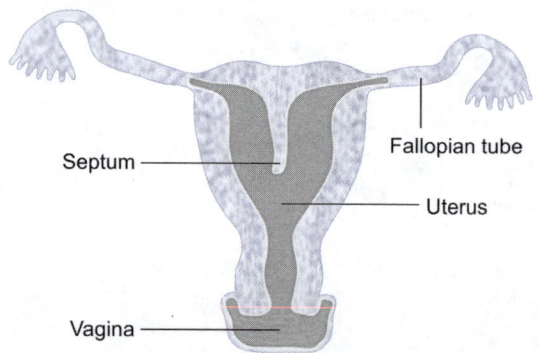

Figure 68.5: Septate uterus.

Septate Uterus (Fig. 68.5)

Here the uterus looks completely normal on the outside, but is separated on the inside into two different halves by a septum of varying size and thickness. Thus, there are two endometrial cavities. The septum may extend only partially into the uterus resulting in partial septate uterus or it may reach up to the cervix as complete septate uterus.

Uterine Agenesis (Fig. 68.6)

The uterus fails to form at all in about 10% of women with uterine anomalies.

Clinical Features

Most women with uterine anomalies are not aware of any defect as their female physiology is typically unaffected. In most cases, fertility is unimpaired. In a few cases dysmenorrhea or painful periods may be a symptom, though this is very nonspecific. In fertile women, these anomalies are picked up during routine check-up. In some women, renal defects are also present with uterine anomaly with renal agenesis being the most common associated anomaly followed by renal ectopic and duplex kidney.

Diagnosis

A history of repeated miscarriage or infertility may cause a suspicion of congenital uterine anomaly. They are confirmed only by imaging studies such as hysterosalpingogram or scanning with ultrasound or MRI.

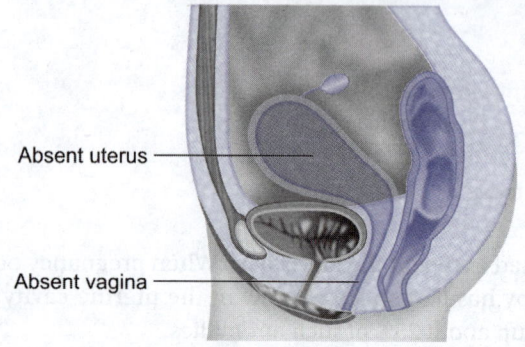

Figure 68.6: Uterine agenesis.

Management

Many women with congenital uterine abnormality do not require any treatment. If the anomaly causes a miscarriage, infertility or pain, a surgical correction is required.

Surgical repair or reconstruction is the only form of treatment for such women. If the defect is severe enough to cause obstruction of the reproductive tract, associated with infertility or miscarriage surgery is recommended. Septate uteri are most commonly repaired to improve the chances of having a baby, but the other types are generally left alone. The type of surgery recommended depends upon the type of abnormality and the woman's reproductive history and health. In women with bicornuate uterus, the dividing septum can be removed to open up the uterus. In case of unicornuate uterus, the obstructed hemiuterus can be removed if the other part of the uterus is normal and functional.

Women who are at higher risk for preterm delivery or late pregnancy loss due to congenital uterine abnormality may need a stitch in the cervix (called cervical cerclage). Most cases of anomalies can be corrected using a minimal invasive surgery like laparoscopy or hysteroscopy. In some cases, surgical correction may not result in improvement and hence the women should be told what to expect beforehand.

Possible Complications Associated with Uterine Anomalies

- Dysmenorrhea
- Hematometra
- During pregnancy and labor:
  - Late miscarriage
  - Premature labor
  - Malpresentation
  - Obstructed labor
  - Uterine rupture
  - Retained placenta
  - Postpartum hemorrhage.

VAGINAL MALFORMATIONS

The significant abnormalities of the vagina are:
- Vaginal agenesis
- Vaginal atresia
- Vaginal septum
- Hymen abnormalities
- Narrow introitus
- Associated abnormalities.

Vaginal Agenesis/Hypoplasia

Vaginal agenesis occurs in approximately 1 in 5,000–7,000 female births. It results from a problem during the early development of the reproductive system of a fetus. The condition is also known as Rokitansky's syndrome. It is often associated with hypoplasia, which is less development than usual. There is absence of vagina, fallopian tubes, cervix and uterus.

Some women have incompletely developed uterine remnants or horns. The ovaries and external genitalia are normal and the chromosome makeup is normal. The syndrome (complete agenesis) is known as Mayer-Rokitansky-Küster-Hauser (MRKH) syndrome.

Diagnosis

Diagnosis of vaginal agenesis or hypoplasia is commonly made between the ages of 15 and 18 years, when women present themselves with concerns that they have not started menstruating.

As they have normal functioning ovaries, they would have gone through puberty and have normal breasts and pubic hair. Careful physical examination, hormonal and genetic tests, imaging studies such as ultrasound, MRI and intravenous pyelography (IVP) are done to confirm the diagnosis.

Treatment

- Reconstructive operation (vaginoplasty) is done if the patient wishes to marry
- Pressure dilatation—expanding and enlarging the tissue already present at the vaginal entrance by applying pressure over an extended period of time.

Vaginal Atresia

The lower portion of the vagina consists of fibrous tissue. Some methods of correction as for vaginal hypoplasia can be done for this abnormality also.

Vaginal Septum

Transverse vaginal septa can be present as single or multiple in the upper or lower segments and may be complete or patent. Septum located in the lower vagina is often complete and can be the cause of hematometra or other fluid collections. Septum located in the upper vagina is often perforated. Longitudinal septum of vagina may be present when the distal parts of the Müllerian ducts fail to fuse. It may be associated with double uterus and double cervix. This may cause dyspareunia or may obstruct delivery. Management depends on the type of septum. Incision or excision of the septum is done for relief of symptoms.

Hymen Abnormalities

Imperforate hymen is the common abnormality. It is due to failure of disintegration of the central cells of the Müllerian eminence that projects into the urogenital sinus. This may first present with obstruction of menstrual flow after puberty. The menstrual blood collects behind the hymen (cryptomenorrhea). The accumulated blood first distends the vagina (hematocolpos). The uterine cavity gets filled after that (hematometra). In late and neglected cases, the tubes may also get distended after the fimbrial ends become closed by adhesions (hematosalpinx).

Clinical Features

Girls aged about 14–16, present with:
- Periodic lower abdominal pain
- Primary amenorrhea
- Urinary frequency, dysuria or retention
- Suprapubic swelling
- On vaginal examination, the bulging bluish membranes, which may be the transverse vaginal septum close to the inner aspect of hymen, are detected.

Ultrasonography can be used to make the diagnosis of the condition. Treatment is draining the collected blood through a cruciate incision in the hymen. Antibiotic therapy and treatment of any residual pathology are generally required.

Narrow Introitus

The existence of narrow introitus is revealed after marriage, when the woman complains of dyspareunia or during investigation for infertility. Treatment is manual stretching under general anesthesia or surgical enlargement (perineoplasty).

Associated Abnormalities

Abnormalities associated with congenital malformations of vagina are vesicovaginal fistula, rectovaginal fistula and persistent urogenital sinus.

Vesicovaginal fistula is formed, when the Müllerian eminence ruptures into the vesicoureteral part of the cloaca instead of the pelvic part of the urogenital sinus.

Rectovaginal fistula forms, when the Müllerian eminence opens in the dorsal segment of the endodermal cloaca. Persistent urogenital sinus presents with various irregularities of urethral and vaginal orifices.

ABNORMALITIES OF EXTERNAL GENITALIA

Labia Minora Abnormalities

Labia minora abnormalities can have *labial fusion* or *hypertrophy* in otherwise normal females. Hypertrophy can be unilateral or bilateral and may occasionally require surgical correction.

Labia Majora Abnormalities

Labia majora abnormalities can be hypoplastic or hypertrophic. Abnormal fusion is usually associated with *ambiguous genitalia* of female and *pseudohermaphroditism* due to congenital adrenal hyperplasia.

Clitoral Abnormalities

Clitoral abnormalities are generally rare and are double clitoris or bifid clitoris. Hypertrophy can be associated with a number of *intersex disorders*.

ANOMALIES OF THE OVARIES

Ovarian Agenesis/Dysgenesis

1. Ovarian agenesis/dysgenesis includes *Turner's syndrome* and a wide range of chromosomal anomalies.
2. The anomaly results in the production of *streak ovaries* and is associated with a number of other somatic abnormalities.
3. Neonates with streak ovaries often have edema of the hands and feet; many present in adolescence with short stature.
4. Girls with Turner's syndrome have genital infantilism, webbing of the neck, cubitus valgus and retarded growth.
5. Girls with streak (indistinct) ovaries have shield chest, obesity, high palate, micrognathia, epicanthal folds, low-set ears, hypoplasia of nails, osteoporosis, pigmented moles, hypertension, lymph edema, coarctation of aorta, deafness and mental retardation.
6. There are also patients of normal height without those abnormalities, but with gonadal streaks in which there are two cell types—one with two normal sex chromosomes and another with only a single X chromosome.
7. Follicle-stimulating hormone (FSH) and luteinizing hormone (LH) are raised, estrogens are low and non-gonadal endocrine functions are normal.
8. Treatment is with estrogen for development of secondary sex characteristics, growth hormone to increase height and surgical removal of gonadal streaks to prevent malignant degeneration.

True Hermaphroditism

True hermaphroditism is characterized by the presence of both ovarian and testicular tissue in a single patient. The testes will develop in the presence of a single Y chromosome even with more than a single X chromosome. No single clinical feature can distinguish the condition from other forms of intersexuality. Diagnosis is possible after hormone assay and ultrasonography.

Often patients are reared as males because of appearance of external genitalia. However, with early diagnosis and treatment with hormones, most can be reared as females. Many menstruate and some, who had testicular tissue removed, have become pregnant. Treatment is to remove contradictory organs and reconstruct external genitalia corresponding to the sex of rearing.

Female Hermaphroditism due to Congenital Adrenal Hyperplasia

Usually, this condition is due to a genetic defect in the synthesis of the enzyme required for the synthesis of cortisol. Adrenal glands secrete abnormally large amounts of virilizing steroids, even in the fetus. The baby is born with scrotolabial folds fused and a greatly enlarged clitoris that can easily be mistaken for a penis. No testes are palpable. Normally, only a single urinary meatus at the base of the phallus is seen with the vagina entering a urogenital sinus.

Babies exhibit rapid growth in infancy, but this stops early creating short structure. Pubic hair can appear as early as 2 years, but generally later than this followed by the appearance of pubic and facial hair and acne. Puberty does not occur and there is no breast development. Diagnosis is by pelvic ultrasound in the newborn in the presence of ambiguous external genitalia, assay of urinary *17-ketosteroid* and serum *17-hydroxyprogesterone*. Treatment is with hydrocortisone and surgical correction of external genitalia.

Accessory Ovary and Supernumerary Ovaries

Accessory ovary occurs due to division of the original ovary into two. This is seen very rarely. Supernumerary ovaries may be found in the broad ligament or elsewhere. This can explain a rare event where menstruation continues even after removal of two ovaries.

STUDY QUESTIONS

Short Notes

1. Bicornuate uterus.
2. Unicornuate uterus.
3. Didelphic uterus (double uterus).
4. Septate uterus.
5. Uterine agenesis.
6. Arcuate uterus.
7. True hermaphroditism.

CHAPTER 69

Genital Fistulae

Learning Objectives

Upon completion of this chapter, the learner will be able to:
- Define the different types of fistulae of the genital tract.
- Describe the obstetrical and gynecological causes of fistulae formation.
- List the preventive measures for different fistulae.
- Describe the diagnosis of fistulae and management of clients following fistulae repair.

GENITOURINARY FISTULA

Definition

Genitourinary fistula is an abnormal communication between the urinary and genital tract either acquired or congenital with involuntary escape of urine into the vagina.

Types (Fig. 69.1)

The communication may occur between the bladder, urethra or ureter and genital tract.

Bladder

- Vesicovaginal (most common)
- Vesicourethrovaginal
- Vesicouterine
- Vesicocervical.

Urethra

- Urethrovaginal

Ureter

- Ureterovaginal
- Ureterouterine
- Ureterocervical.

Rectum

- Rectovaginal

VESICOVAGINAL FISTULA

There is communication between the bladder and the vagina, and urine escapes into the vagina causing true incontinence. Vesicovaginal fistula (VVF) is the most common type of genitourinary fistula.

Causes

1. *Obstetrical*: The most common cause is obstetrical and constitutes 80–90% of cases in developing countries as against 5–15% in developed countries. The fistula may occur due to ischemia or following trauma:
   - *Ischemic*: The fistula results from prolonged compression effect on the bladder base between the fetal head and symphysis pubis in obstructed labor. The compression causes ischemic necrosis, infection, sloughing and fistula in 3–5 days following delivery.
   - *Traumatic*: This may be caused by:
     » Instrumental vaginal delivery such as destructive operations or forceps, especially with Kielland's forceps

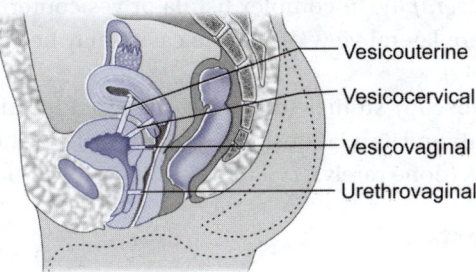

Figure 69.1: Types of genitourinary fistula.

» Abdominal operations such as hysterectomy for rupture uterus or cesarean hysterectomy; traumatic fistula usually follows soon after delivery.
2. *Gynecological*: Fistulae due to gynecological causes are rare in the developing countries and is the most common in the developing countries. The common gynecological cases are:
   – *Operative injury*: During operations like anterior colporrhaphy, abdominal hysterectomy or removal of Gartner's cyst.
   – *Traumatic*: Injury to anterior vaginal wall and the bladder wall following fall on a pointed object, use of a stick for criminal abortion, following fracture to pelvic bone or due to retained pessary.
   – *Malignancy*: Advanced carcinoma of the cervix, vagina and bladder may produce fistula by direct spread.
   – *Radiation*: Ischemic necrosis may occur when carcinoma cervix is treated by radiation in 1–2 years.
   – *Infective*: Chronic granulomatous lesions such as vaginal tuberculosis, lymphogranuloma venereum and actinomycosis may produce fistula.

Sites

1. *Juxtacervical (close to the cervix)*: The communication is between the supratrigonal region of the bladder and the vagina.
2. *Midvaginal*: The communication is between the base (trigone) of the bladder and vagina.
3. *Juxtaurethral*: The communication is between the neck of the bladder and vagina (may involve the upper urethra as well).

Clinical Features

1. *Patient profile:* The patients are usually young primiparous with history of difficult labor or instrumental delivery in recent past. In others it is related with relevant events.
2. Continuous escape of urine per vagina is the classic symptom. The patient has no urge to pass urine. If the fistula is small, the escape of urine occurs in certain positions and the patient can also pass urine normally.
3. Pruritus vulva.
4. Escape of watery discharge per vagina of ammoniacal smell.
5. Excoriation of the vaginal skin.
6. Varying degrees of perineal tear may be present.
7. On speculum examination; the bladder mucosa may be seen prolapsed through a big fistula. Puckered area of vaginal mucosa is evidenced in tiny fistula.

Diagnosis of Fistula

1. Examination under anesthesia (EUA).
2. *Examination in Sims' or knee-chest position:* Bubbles of air are seen through the tiny fistula when the woman coughs.

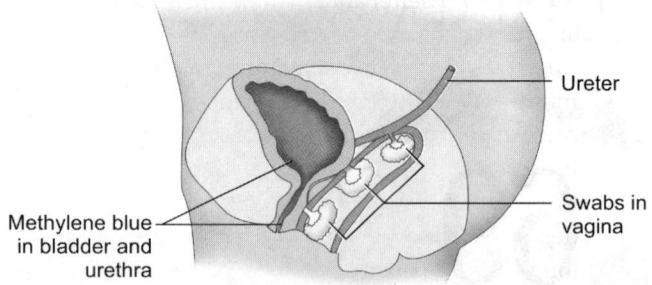

Figure 69.2: Three swab test using methylene blue.

TABLE 69.1: Three swab test.

Observation	Inference
Upper most swab socked with urine, but unstained with dye; the lower two swabs remain dry	Ureterovaginal fistula
Upper and lower swabs remain dry, but the middle swab stained with dye	Vesicovaginal fistula
The upper two swabs remain dry, but the lower swab stained with dye	Ureterovaginal fistula

3. *Dye test:* A speculum is introduced and the anterior vaginal wall is swabbed dry. When the methylene blue solution is introduced into the bladder by a catheter, the dye will be seen coming out through the opening.
4. *Catheter test:* A metal catheter passed through the external urethral meatus, when passes out through the fistula, VVF is confirmed.
5. *Three swab test* (**Fig. 69.2 and Table 69.1**): Three cotton swabs are placed in the vagina, one at the vault, one at the middle and one just above the introitus. Methylene blue is instilled into the bladder through a rubber catheter and the patient is asked to walk about for 5 minutes. She is then asked to lie down and the swabs are removed for inspection.

Investigations

1. *Intravenous urography:* For the diagnosis of ureterovaginal fistula.
2. *Retrograde pyelography:* For the diagnosis of exact site of ureterovaginal fistula.
3. *Cystography:* In complex fistula or vesicouterine fistula where lateral view of uterine cavity may be seen (done rarely).
4. Endoscopy studies to identify the exact location of the fistula and its relationship to ureteric orifices and bladder neck (done rarely).

Treatment

1. *Prevention:* Obstetric fistula is prevented with safe motherhood initiative. Gynecologic fistula can be

prevented with better anticipation and improved surgical skill. The measures to be taken are:
- Adequate antenatal screening to identify 'at risk' mothers likely to develop obstructed labor.
- Anticipation, early detection and ideal approach in the method of delivery in relieving the obstruction.
- Continuous bladder drainage for 5–7 days following delivery either vaginally or abdominally in a case of long-standing obstructed labor.
- Care to avoid injury to the bladder during pelvic surgery—obstetrical or gynecological.

2. *Immediate management:* Once the diagnosis is made, catheterization and continuous bladder drainage for 6–8 weeks is maintained. This may cause spontaneous closure of the fistula tract that is small, with minimal tissue damage.
3. *Operative management:* Local repair of the fistula is the surgery of choice:
   - Preoperative assessment includes identifying the site, size, number and status of the margins of the fistula, and urethral involvement.
   - Improvement of general condition is essential as most patients may be of poor socioeconomic status:
     » Local infection in the vulvar region if present, should be treated with local application of bland ointments or glycerine
     » Urinary infection if any, should be treated
     » Psychological preparation of the patient and family with adequate explanation of the expected management and recovery.

The ideal time for surgery is after 3 months following delivery in case of old VVF. Surgical fistula recognized within 24 hours may be repaired immediately provided it is small.

Repair is done by flap splitting method or by using tissue graft depending on the site and size of the fistula.

Postoperative Care

Special Care Following VVF Repair

1. Urinary antiseptic either at random or appropriate to the sensitivity report.
2. Continuous bladder drainage for about 10–14 days.
3. Advise to pass urine 2 hourly following removal of catheter. The interval to be increased gradually.

Instructions during Discharge from Hospital

- To pass urine more frequently
- To avoid intercourse for at least 3 months
- To differ pregnancy for at least 1 year
- If conception occurs to report to the physician and must have mandatory antenatal checkup and hospital delivery.

URETHROVAGINAL FISTULA

Causes

The causes are the same as those of VVF. Part or whole of the urethra is involved along with the bladder.

Small isolated urethrovaginal fistula is caused by:
- Injury inflicted during anterior colporrhaphy, urethroplasty or sling operation for stress incontinence
- Residual fistula left behind following repair of vesicourethrovaginal fistula.

Diagnosis

1. The patient has urge to pass urine, but urine dribbles out into the vagina during the act of micturition.
2. A sound or a metal catheter passed through the external urethral meatus comes out through the communicating urethrovaginal opening.
3. 'Three swab test' may be employed to confirm the diagnosis.

Treatment

- Surgical repair in two layers followed by continuous bladder drainage as outlined for VVF is done
- Prior suprapubic or vaginal cystostomy ensures better success
- In cases of complete destruction of the urethra, reconstruction of urethra is performed
- Stress incontinence may occur in 10–15% of cases following repair.

URETEROVAGINAL FISTULA

Causes

1. *Congenital:* The aberrant ureter may open into the vault of vagina, uterus or into urethra.
2. *Acquired:* This is the most common type and usually follows trauma during pelvic surgery. It is commonly associated with difficult surgery like abdominal hysterectomy in cervical fibroid, broad ligament fibroid, endometriosis, ovarian malignancy or radical hysterectomy.

Diagnosis

Signs and symptoms are subtle and often overlooked. Patient may develop fever, flank pain, hematuria, abdominal distension, urine leakage through vagina, peritonitis and retroperitoneal urinoma.

Investigations

1. Three swab test.
2. *Intravenous Indigo Carmine test:* Indigo Carmine is injected intravenously. If urine in the vagina becomes blue in 4–5 minutes, the diagnosis of ureterovaginal fistula is established.

3. *Cystoscopy:* To determine the side of ureterovaginal fistula.
4. *Excretory urography/intravenous urography (IVU)* confirms the side, site and tract of ureterovaginal fistula.
5. Renal ultrasound.
6. Computed tomography (CT).

Management

When injury is recognized during operation:
1. *Ureteral sheath denudation:* No intervention and rarely ureteral stenting, if a long segment is involved.
2. *Ureteral kinking (due to closely placed sutures):* Immediate removal of suture.
3. *Ureteral ligation:* Immediate delegation—assessment of viability by blood flow and ureteral peristalsis. Stenting may be needed, if any doubt.
4. Extraperitoneal drainage.
5. Ureteric implantation into the bladder, if the length of ureter is sufficient.
6. Bladder flap procedure when the ureter is short or injury is at the level of pelvic brim.

Complications Following Repair of Ureteric Injury

- Stricture
- Infection
- Ureteric obstruction
- Reflux of urine
- Stent or flap complications.

RECTOVAGINAL FISTULA

Causes

Abnormal communication between the rectum and vagina with involuntary escape of flatus and/or feces into the vagina is called rectovaginal fistula.

Acquired

Obstetrical
- Incomplete healing or unrepaired recent complete perineal tear (CPT)
- Obstructed labor causing pressure necrosis, which leads to infection, sloughing and fistula
- Instrumental injury inflicted during destructive operation.

Gynecological
- Following incomplete healing of repair of old CPT (most common).
- Trauma inflicted inadvertently and remains unrecognized in pelvic operations like perineorrhaphy, repair of enterocele, vaginal tubectomy, posterior colpotomy, reconstruction of vagina, etc.
- Fall on sharp pointed object.
- Malignancy of the vagina, cervix or bowel.
- Radiation.
- Lymphogranuloma venereum or tuberculosis of vagina.
- Diverticulitis of the sigmoid colon, when the abscess bursts into the vagina.
- Crohn's disease involving the anal canal or lower rectum.

Congenital

The anal canal may open into the vestibule or into the vagina.

Diagnosis

- Involuntary escape of flatus and/or feces into the vagina
- Rectovaginal examination reveals the size and site of fistula
- *Dye test:* Methyl ene blue introduced into the rectum, is seen escaping through the fistula into the vagina
- *Probe test:* Passing a probe through the vagina into the rectum
- Examination under anesthesia.

Investigations

- Barium enema
- Barium meal and follow through to confirm the site of intestinal fistula
- Sigmoidoscopy and proctoscopy in case of inflammatory bowel disease for taking biopsy of fistula edge.

Treatment

Preventive
- Good antenatal care
- Identification of complete perineal tear and effective repair
- Care to prevent injury during gynecologic surgeries.

Definitive
- Extension to CPT and repair if the defect is situated low down
- Repair by flap method for injury situated in the middle third
- For defect situated high-up, preliminary colostomy for local repair after 3 weeks and closure of colostomy after 3 weeks.

STUDY QUESTIONS

Short Notes

1. Sites of vesicovaginal fistula (VVF).
2. Diagnostic tests used for VVF.

Essay Questions

1. Describe vesicovaginal fistula, causes for the condition, clinical features and treatment.
2. Describe the obstetrical causes of rectovaginal fistula, its diagnosis and management.

CHAPTER 70

Perioperative Care of Gynecological Patient

Learning Objectives

Upon completion of this chapter, the learner will be able to:
- Describe the phases of perioperative period.
- Discuss various types of surgery according to degree of urgency, risk and purpose.
- Identify essential aspects of perioperative assessment of gynecological patient.
- Identify nursing responsibilities in planning perioperative nursing care.
- Describe essential preoperative preparation including teaching.
- Identify essential nursing assessments and interventions for the postoperative patient.

Surgery is a unique experience of planned physical alteration encompassing three phases.

Preoperative, intraoperative and *postoperative are* three phases and together referred to as the perioperative period.

- The preoperative phase begins when the decision to have surgery is made and ends when the patient is transferred to the operating table. Nursing activities associated with this phase include assessing the patient, identifying potential or actual health problems, planning specific care based on the individual's needs and providing preoperative teaching for the patient and family.
- The intraoperative phase begins when the patient is transferred to the operating table and ends when the patient is transferred to the recovery or postanesthetic room. Nursing activities related to this phase include a variety of special procedures to maintain the health status of the patient.
- The postoperative phase begins with the admission of the patient in the postoperative unit or ward and ends when the healing is complete. Nursing activities during this period include assessing the patient's response (physiologic and psychologic) to surgery, performing interventions to facilitate healing and preventing complications, teaching and providing support and planning for home care.

Some gynecological operations are performed in an outpatient setting. In such situations, the three phases of perioperative period are shortened and the postoperative period continues at home. With such patients, the nurses' role in assessing, teaching and following up is vital to successful outcome for the patient.

TYPES OF SURGERY

Surgical procedures are commonly grouped according to purpose, degree of urgency and degree of risk.

Purposes of Surgical Procedure

1. *Diagnostic:* Confirms or establishes diagnosis, e.g. biopsy of a mass or growth.
2. *Palliative:* Relieves or reduces pain or symptoms of a disease, but does not cure, e.g. draining a hematoma.
3. *Ablative:* Removes a diseased body part, e.g., removal of breast (mastectomy).
4. *Constructive:* Restores function or appearance that has been lost or reduced, e.g. perineoplasty.

Degrees of Urgency

Surgery is classified by its urgency and necessity to preserve the patient's life, body part or function:
1. Emergency surgery is performed immediately, e.g. rupture of an ectopic pregnancy.
2. Elective surgery is performed when surgical intervention is the preferred treatment for a condition that is not immediately life-threatening. An example is hysterectomy for fibroids in the uterus.

Degree of Risk

Surgery is classified as major or minor, according to the degree of risk to the patient. The degree of risk involved in a surgical procedure is affected by the patient's age, general health, nutritional status, use of medications for conditions unrelated to the indication for surgery and the mental status (disorders that affect cognitive function). Some surgeries are thus referred to as high-risk surgeries.

MANAGEMENT IN PREOPERATIVE PHASE

The overall goal of nursing care during the preoperative phase is to prepare the patient mentally and physically for surgery.

Preoperative Evaluation

Preoperative evaluation of a patient includes a detailed history (general, medical and surgical), a complete physical examination and laboratory investigations.

History

- *Age:* Very young and older patients are greater surgical risks than children and adults.
- *General health:* Surgery is least risky when the client's general health is good. Any infection or pathophysiology increases the risk.
- *Nutritional status:* Adequate nutrition is required for normal tissue repair. Surgery increases the body's need for nutrients for the needed tissue healing and prevention of infection during the postoperative period. Obesity contributes to postoperative complications such as pneumonia and wound infection. A malnourished client also is at risk for delayed wound healing. If the surgery cannot be delayed, parenteral or enteral nutrition may be initiated.
- *Medications:* Regular use of certain medications can increase surgical risk. Examples are anticoagulants, tranquillizers, corticosteroids and diuretics. Information related to the use of such medications can help the surgeon plan relevant management.
- *Allergies:* Allergies to drugs, food, latex, antiseptics, etc. can alert the hospital staff in using medications and procedures.
- *Previous surgeries:* Previous surgical experiences may influence the client's physical and psychological responses to surgery.
- *Mental status:* Clients mental status and ability to understand and respond appropriately can affect the entire perioperative experience.
- *Smoking:* Smokers may have more difficulty clearing respiratory secretions after surgery; increasing the risk of postoperative pneumonia and atelectasis.
- *Alcohol and other mind-altering substances:* Use of these can affect the central nervous system, liver and other body systems.
- *Family and social resources:* Availability of family, caregivers and social support are important for recovery.
- *Coping:* Patients with healthy self-concept and coping mechanisms deal better with stressors of surgery.

Physical Examination

Assessment of physiological status is done by review of body systems such as respiratory system, circulatory system, gastrointestinal system, neurological system, etc.

Routine Investigations

Routine investigations are:
1. *Blood—hemoglobin and hematocrit:*
   - Total and differential leukocyte count and platelet count
   - Blood group and crossmatching
   - *For older patients*, liver function, renal function, serum electrolytes and blood glucose.
2. *Urine:* Routine and microscopic analysis, which includes tests for protein, glucose, casts and pus cells.
3. Chest X-ray and electrocardiogram for patients over 40 years. If there is history of any systemic disease, relevant investigations such echocardiography, blood coagulation profile, etc. will be required.
4. Special investigations, which are appropriate for certain lesions such as vesicovaginal fistula (VVF) or malignancy may be included.
5. Screening for human immunodeficiency virus (HIV) antibodies and hepatitis B virus may be included for patients in high-risk group.

Preoperative Consent

Prior to any surgical procedure, the patient must sign a consent form, which is generally, supplied by the hospital or healthcare facility.

Although the surgeon maintains legal responsibility for ensuring that the client gives informed consent, the nurse may witness the client's signature on the consent form. A preoperative informed consent form should include the following information:

- Nature and intention of the surgery
- Name and qualification of the surgeon
- Risks including tissue damage, disfigurement or even death
- Chances of success
- Possible alternative measures
- The right of the client to refuse consent or later withdraw consent.

Preoperative Teaching

Preoperative teaching should include information about the specific gynecologic condition of the patient, for which she needs surgery, role of the client throughout the perioperative period, expected discomforts and training for the postoperative period and psychological support.

Teaching for postoperative period should include moving, leg exercises and coughing and deep breathing exercises to prevent postoperative complications.

Physical Preparation

Physical preparation for the surgical patient will include special attention to meet their needs of nutrition and fluids, elimination, hygiene, rest, medications and surgical skin preparation:

1. Light diet in the previous evening and nothing in the morning of operation. Nothing by mouth for at least 8 hours to keep the stomach empty at the time of anesthesia.
2. A cleansing enema in the evening before surgery. If bowel involvement is suspected, additional bowel preparation with osmotic oral purgative may be prescribed.
3. Skin preparation (local preparation) by shaving of the operative area or clipping of hair is done to reduce the chance of wound infection. Cleansing with soap, water and povidone iodine will be done in the ward and in the operating room.

Preoperative Checklist

A preoperative checklist is completed before the patient goes to operating room. This is a guide to the adequacy of patient preparation and documentation.

Presurgery Medications

- Tranquilizer or sedative medication in the night before surgery
- Tranquilizer and preanesthetic medication 2 hours before surgery
- Prophylactic antibiotics.

MANAGEMENT IN INTRAOPERATIVE PHASE

The overall goal of nursing care during the intraoperative phase is maintaining the patient's safety. Anesthesia may be general or regional. Regional anesthesia includes topical, local, nerve block, spinal anesthesia (subarachnoid block) and epidural anesthesia. Preparations include:

1. A surgical skin preparation should be carried out as close to the time of surgery as possible. Intravenous line will be established if not already done.
2. Positioning of patient: Dorsal or lithotomy position is chosen according to type of operation.
3. Draping is done using sterile linen and towel clips as required for the specific surgery.
4. The surgeon then makes an appropriate incision and performs the intended procedure (surgery) and closure of the incision.
5. In the case of minor or 'day care' surgery, patients are admitted, operated and discharged on the same day. Common 'day care' gynecological operations are:
   - Dilatation and curettage (D&C)
   - Dilatation and evacuation (D&E)
   - Biopsy procedures
   - Examination under anesthesia (EUA)
   - Endoscopic procedures.

Immediate postanesthetic care focuses on assessment and monitoring parameters to prevent complications from anesthesia or surgery.

MANAGEMENT IN POSTOPERATIVE PHASE

The overall goals of nursing care during the postoperative period are to promote comfort and healing, restore the highest possible wellness and prevent associated risks such as infection or respiratory and cardiovascular complications.

Initial and ongoing assessment of the postoperative patient includes:
- Level of consciousness
- Vital signs
- Oxygen saturation
- Skin color and temperature
- Comfort
- Fluid balance
- Dressings and drains.

Ongoing postoperative nursing interventions include:
- Managing pain
- Appropriate positioning
- Encouraging deep breathing and coughing exercises
- Promoting leg exercises and ambulation
- Maintaining adequate hydration and nutrition status
- Promoting urinary elimination
- Providing wound care.

Surgical aseptic technique (sterile technique) is used when changing dressing on surgical wounds to promote healing and to reduce risk of infection.

Sutures or clips used to approximate skin and underlying tissue after surgery are generally, removed 7–10 days after surgery. Instructions for home care and follow-up are reviewed with the patient and family prior to discharge from the hospital.

STUDY QUESTIONS

Short Answer Questions

1. List the preoperative investigations routinely done prior to any gynecological surgery.
2. Postoperative nursing management of a client following a gynecological surgery.

71. Infertility and Adoption

Learning Objectives

Upon completion of this chapter, the learner will be able to:
- Explain the factors related to male and female infertility.
- Enumerate the investigations for infertile couples.
- Discuss the regimens to treat infertility of male and female partners.
- Explain the procedures of assisted reproductive technology.
- Describe briefly the process of adoption, its reasons and causes.
- Explain the types of adoptions, its advantages and disadvantages to the adoptive and birth parents and children.
- Explain the process and steps of legal adoptions in India.

INFERTILITY

Definitions

Infertility is defined as a failure to conceive within one or more years of regular unprotected intercourse.

Subfertility refers to a state in which a couple has tried unsuccessfully to have a child for a year or more. The term subfertile means less fertile than a regular couple.

Primary infertility denotes couples who have never been able to conceive.

Secondary infertility indicates difficulty conceiving after already having conceived (either carried the pregnancy to term or had a miscarriage).

Incidence

Generally, worldwide it is estimated that one in seven couples have problems conceiving. Nearly 80% of couples achieve conception, if they so desire within 1 year of having regular intercourse with adequate frequency (four to five times a week). Another 10% will achieve the objective by the end of 2nd year. About 10% remain infertile by the end of 3rd year.

Factors Required for Fertility (Male and Female)

- Healthy spermatozoa should be deposited high in the vagina at or near the cervix
- *Capacitation and acrosome reaction:* Spermatozoa should undergo changes and acquire motility in cervical canal
- *Motility:* Spermatozoa should ascend through the cervix into the uterine cavity and fallopian tube
- *Ovulation:* Ovum should reach the fimbriated end of the tube
- *Patent fallopian tube:* Fertilization should occur at the ampulla of the tube
- Transportation of fertilized ovum to uterine cavity in 3–4 days, the fertilized ovum should reach the uterine cavity for nidation.

Causes of Infertility

Conception depends on the fertility potential of both male and female partner. For infertility, male factor contribution is about 30–40%, female factor 40–55% and combined factor about 10–15%. In about 10% of the couple, the cause is unexplained. About 4 out of 10 in the unexplained group conceive within 3 years without any specific treatment.

Male Factors that Cause Infertility

1. *Defective spermatogenesis:* Spermatogenesis and sperm maturation need a high androgenic environment. Spermatogenesis is predominantly controlled by the genes on the 'Y' chromosome. The process of spermatogenesis takes approximately 74 days for completion. Additional 12–20 days are needed for spermatozoa to travel the epididymis. The causes of defective spermatogenesis are:

a. *Congenital:* Undescended testes are a congenital condition in which spermatogenesis is depressed. Vas deferens is absent bilaterally in 1–2% of such men
b. Hypospadias causes failure to deposit sperm high in the vagina. In Kartagener's syndrome (autosomal disease), there is loss of ciliary function and sperm motility
c. *Thermal factor:* The scrotal temperature has to be 1°F–2°F less than the body temperature. It is raised in conditions such as varicocele, big hydrocele or filariasis. Other causes are using tight undergarment or working in hot atmosphere
d. *Infection:* Mumps orchitis after puberty may permanently damage spermatogenesis. In chronic systemic illnesses like bronchiectasis, the quality of sperm is adversely affected. Infection of the seminal vesicle or prostate depresses sperm count
e. *Gonadotropin suppression:* This happens in chronic debilitating diseases, malnutrition, heavy smoking and with high alcoholic consumption
f. *Endocrine factors:* Follicle-stimulating hormone (FSH) level is seen raised in idiopathic testicular failure. Hypoprolactinemia is associated with impotence
g. Loss of sperm motility (asthenozoospermia and abnormal sperm morphology are seen in some males)
h. *Genetic:* Common chromosomal abnormality in azoospermic male is Klinefelter's syndrome (47, XXY)
i. *Iatrogenic:* Radiation, cytotoxic drugs, nitrofurantoin, cimetidine, beta (β)-blockers, antihypertensives, anticonvulsants and antidepressant drugs are likely to hinder spermatogenesis
j. *Immunological factor:* Antibodies against spermatozoa surface antigens may cause infertility. This causes clumping of spermatozoa after ejaculation.

2. *Obstruction of the efferent ducts:* The efferent ducts may be obstructed by gonococcal or tubercular infections. Surgical trauma during vasectomy or herniorrhaphy may lead to obstruction.
3. *Failure to deposit sperm high in the vagina (coital problems):*
   a. Erectile dysfunction
   b. Ejaculatory defects such as premature, retrograde or absence of ejaculation
   c. Hypospadias
4. *Errors in seminal fluid:*
   a. Unusually high or low volume of ejaculate (normal volume is 2 mL or more)
   b. Low-fructose content
   c. High-prostaglandin content
   d. Undue viscosity

Normal semen values as determined by World Health Organization (WHO) are given in **Table 71.1**.

TABLE 71.1: Normal semen values as given by World Health Organization (2002).

Semen parameters	Reference value
Volume	20 mL or more
pH	7.2–7.8
Sperm concentration	20 million per mL or more
Motility	50% or more with progressive forward motility
Morphology	15% or more in normal form
Viability	75% or more living
Leukocytes	Less than one million per mL
Sperm agglutination	<2

Causes of Female Infertility

Ovarian factors

1. *Anovulation or oligo-ovulation:* Ovarian activity depends on gonadotropins, which are related to the release of gonadotropin-releasing hormone (GnRH) from hypothalamus (hypothalamic-pituitary-ovarian axis).

   Disturbance of these may result in anovulation, oligomenorrhea or even amenorrhea. In these conditions, there is inadequate growth and function of the corpus luteum.
2. *Tubal and peritoneal factors:* Tubal and peritoneal factors are responsible for about 30–40% of cases of female infertility. These include:
   – Peritubal adhesions
   – Endosalpingeal damage
   – Previous tubal surgery or sterilization
   – Salpingitis
   – Tubal or peritoneal endometriosis
   – Polyps within the lumen
   – Tubal spasm.

Uterine factors

Uterine factors include interfere with reception and nidation of fertilized ovum (unfavorable endometrium).

Common conditions

- Uterine hyperplasia
- Inadequate secretary endometrium
- Fibroids
- Endometritis
- Uterine synechiae
- Congenital malformations.

Cervical factors

Ineffective sperm penetration due to following factors:
- Chronic cervicitis
- Presence of antisperm antibodies
- Congenital elongation of cervix
- Second-degree uterine prolapse
- Acute retroversion of uterus

- Occlusion of cervical canal with polyp
- Pinhole os
- Scanty vaginal mucus
- Abnormal constituents in the mucus (excessive, viscous or purulent).

Vaginal factors (implicated)
- Atresia (partial or complete)
- Septum
- Narrow introitus.

Combined factors
It include presence of factors both in female and male causing infertility:
- Age of wife beyond 35 years and advancing age in men
- Infrequent intercourse (less than 4–5 per week) during fertile period (around ovulation)
- Apareunia (failure of emission of semen/ejaculation) and dyspareunia
- Anxiety and apprehension
- Use of lubricants during intercourse, which may be spermicidal
- Immunological factors (antisperm antibodies).

Investigations of Female

History

1. *History:* Age, duration of marriage, history of previous marriage with proven infertility, if any.
2. *Medical history:* Tuberculosis, sexually transmitted disease (STD), pelvic inflammatory disease and diabetes.
3. *Surgical history:* Abdominal or pelvic surgery that can cause peritubal adhesions.
4. *Menstrual history:* Hypomenorrhea or oligomenorrhea that is associated with hypothalamic-pituitary-ovarian axis which may be either primary or secondary to adrenal, or thyroid dysfunction.
5. *Previous obstetric history:* In the case of secondary infertility, history of previous pregnancies, interval, premature rupture of membranes or puerperal sepsis are taken.
6. *Contraceptive practice:* Use of intrauterine contraceptive device (IUCD) that have chance to produce pelvic inflammatory disease (PID).
7. *Sexual problems:* Dyspareunia and loss of libido.

Examinations

1. *General examination:* Obesity or marked reduction in weight, abnormal distribution of hair and underdevelopment of secondary sex characteristics.
2. *Systemic examination:* Hypertension, organic heart disease, chronic renal lesion or endocrinopathies.
3. *Gynecologic examination:* To look for adequacy of hymenal opening, evidence of vaginal infection, undue elongation of cervix, uterine size, position and mobility, and presence of adnexal mass and nodules in the pouch of Douglas.
4. *Speculum examination:* For presence of cervical discharge, which if present needs to be tested for infection.

Diagnostic Evaluation

In the presence of major fault in male partner such as azoospermia or intersex, there is very little scope in investigating the female partner. However, considering the scope of assisted reproductive technology (ART), investigations may be done if the couple so desire. Similarly, if a major defect is identified in female partner such as Müllerian agenesis or intersex, further investigations may be suspended. Any correctable abnormality found should be rectified prior to investigations, e.g. narrow vaginal introitus, hypothyroidism or diabetes mellitus. Noninvasive and minimal invasive methods are to be carried out prior to major invasive ones:

1. *Menstrual history:* Look for evidences of ovulation such as:
   a. Regular, normal menstrual loss between the ages of 20 and 35.
   b. Mid-menstrual bleeding (spotting) or pain, or excessive mucoid vaginal discharge suggestive of mittelschmerz syndrome.
   c. Features of primary dysmenorrhea or premenstrual syndrome (PMS).
2. *Basal body temperature (BBT):* Patient is instructed to take and record body temperature daily on waking in the morning, before rising out of bed. The body temperature maintaining throughout the first half of the cycle, drops about 0.5°F about middle of cycles then is raised to 0.5°F–1°F (0.2°C–0.3°C) following ovulation. The rise is sustained throughout the second half of the cycle and falls about 2 days prior to the next period. The drop in temperature of 0.5°F before the rise coincides with either luteinizing hormone (LH) surge or ovulation. Maintenance of BBT chart helps in determining ovulation and timing of postcoital test, endometrial biopsy, cervical mucus or vaginal cytology test for ovulation. It also helps the couple to determine the most fertile period, if the cycle is regular.
3. *Cervical mucus study:* Alteration of the physiochemical properties of the cervical mucus occurs due to the effect of estrogen and progesterone. Disappearance of fern pattern of the mucus beyond 22nd day of cycle, progesterone causes dissolution of sodium crystals. Following ovulation, there is loss of stretchability or elasticity, which was present in the midcycle. This loss of elasticity is an evidence of ovulation. Fern test during the cycle aids in determining ovulation.
4. *Hormone estimation:*
   a. Serum progesterone: Estimation on day 8 and 21 of cycle. An increase in value from 1 mg/mL to greater than 6 mg/mL suggests ovulation.
   b. Serum LH: Daily estimation of serum LH at midcycle can detect LH surge. Ovulation occurs about 34–36 hours after beginning of LH surge and coincides about 10–12 hours after the LH peak.

c. *Serum estradiol:* This hormone attains peak rise approximately 24–36 hours prior to ovulation (these tests are used for in vitro fertilization).
d. *Urinary LH:* Ovulation usually occurs within 14–26 hours of detection of urine LH surge and almost always within 48 hours (the test should be done on a daily basis, starting 2–3 days before the day of expected surge).

5. *Endometrial biopsy:* Biopsy is done on 21st to 23rd day of the cycle (if the cycle is irregular, it is done within 24 hours of the period). Evidence of secretory activity of the endometrial glands in the second half of the cycle gives the diagnosis of ovulation. The secretary changes are due to the action of progesterone on the estrogen-primed endometrium.

6. *Sonography:* Serial sonography during midcycle can precisely measure the Graafian follicle just prior to ovulation (18–20 mm). The features of recent ovulation are collapsed follicle and fluid in the pouch of Douglas.

7. *Laparoscopy:* Laparoscopic visualization of recent corpus luteum or detection of the ovum from the aspirated peritoneal fluid to the pouch of Douglas is the direct evidence of ovulation.

8. *Insufflation test (Rubin's test):* It is done to see the patency of fallopian tubes. It is done by pushing air or carbon dioxide under pressure through the cervical canal. If the tubes are patent, air reaches the peritoneal cavity. It is done in the postmenstrual period at least 2 days after stoppage of menstrual bleeding. Positive findings include:
   a. Fall in the pressure when raised beyond 120 mm Hg.
   b. Hissing sound heard on auscultation on either iliac fossa.
   c. Shoulder pain experienced by the patient due to irritation of diaphragm by air.

   The procedure should not be done in the presence of pelvic infection. In about one-third of cases, the test gives false-negative findings and hence not very reliable. This test is not commonly alone these days.

9. *Hysterosalpingography (HSG):* In this test, instead of air or carbon dioxide, dye is introduced transcervically. The test is done in the postmenstrual phase, 2 days after the stoppage of menstruation. It is avoided if the woman has pelvic infection. HSG has definite advantages over insufflation test. It can precisely detect the site of block in the tube. It can reveal any abnormality in the uterus such as fibroid or synechiae. Disadvantage of HSG is radiation risk.

10. *Laparoscopic chromotubation:* This is an invasive investigation and hence performed only after male factors and ovulation functions have been found normal or corrected. It involves checking for tubal patency laparoscopically by injecting methylene blue through the cervix into the fallopian tubes to confirm spillage of the dye into the pelvic cavity. It also helps in the detection of PID, endometriosis and pelvic adhesions along with tubal patency. Chromotubation is a diagnostic and therapeutic procedure as it can allow for release of peritubal adhesions and fimbrial block. Appropriate surgery for infertility can be planned based on the findings.

11. *Sonosalpingography:* This test involves a slow injection of physiological saline into the uterine cavity using a pediatric Foley's catheter. The catheter balloon is inflated at the level of the cervix to prevent fluid leak. Ultrasonography of the uterus and fallopian tubes is then done. Ultrasound can follow the fluid through the tube up to the peritoneal cavity and in the pouch of Douglas.

Management of Infertility

Management of infertility or subfertility would depend upon the cause identified, duration and age of the couple, especially the female.

General Instructions

When minor defects are detected in both the husband and wife, each of which alone could not cause infertility, but in combination they decrease the fertility potential, the faults should be treated simultaneously:

1. *Body weight:* Overweight or underweight of any partner should be adequately dealt with to obtain an optimal body weight.
2. *Smoking and alcohol:* Excess smoking or alcohol consumption to be avoided.
3. *Ideal coital frequency:* Intercourse on multiple days during the fertile window period, which includes the five preceding and the day of anticipated ovulation should be reviewed with the couple.
4. Use of at home 'fertility monitor' and checking of vaginal mucus discharge to determine the optimal timing of intercourse may be most helpful.
5. *Use of LH surge kit:* Use of the kit can detect LH surge in urine by getting a deep blue color of dipstick. The test performed between 12th and 16th day of regular cycle and timed intercourse over 24–36 hours after the color change reasonably succeeds to conception.
6. Avoidance of lubricants and douches to be stressed.
7. The use of fertility impairing medications should be avoided by both partners if possible, e.g. hormones.
8. Psychological support should be offered as the couple may face significant stress and sadness as the investigations and consultations progress.

Management of Male Infertility

The treatment of male partner is indicated in *extreme oligospermia, azoospermia, low-volume ejaculate* and *impotency*. Measures to improve spermatogenesis are advised:

1. General care:
   a. Improvement of general health:
      » Reduction of weight in obese
      » Avoidance of alcohol and heavy smoking
      » Avoidance of tight and warm undergarments
      » Avoidance of occupation that may elevate testicular temperature.

b. Avoiding medications that interfere with spermatogenesis such as:
      » Cytotoxic drugs, nitrofurantoin, cimetidine, anticonvulsants, antidepressants and beta blockers.
2. Medications to treat specific causes:
   a. Human chorionic gonadotropin (hCG) and human menopausal gonadotropin (hMG) for hypogonadism.
   b. Dopamine agonist (cabergoline) for hyperprolactinemia and altered testosterone level and to improve libido, potency and fertility.
   c. The GnRH therapy for hypogonadism.
   d. Clomiphene citrate to increase serum levels of FSH, LH and testosterone.
   e. Antibiotics for genital tract infections.
3. Special treatments for causes identified such as:
   a. Intrauterine insemination (IUI).
   b. In vitro fertilization (IVF).
   c. Intracytoplasmic sperm injection (ICSI).
   d. Artificial insemination with donor (AID) sperm.
4. Surgical treatment:
   a. In men, whose testicular biopsy shows normal spermatogenesis and obstruction is suspected, vasoepididymostomy or vasovasostomy may help.
   b. Correction of hydrocele.

Management of Female Infertility

Treatment for females is also according to the disorders identified:
1. For ovulatory dysfunction:
   a. Induction of ovulation using drugs such as clomiphene citrate, letrozole, FSH, hCG and GnRH.
   b. Correction of biochemical abnormality: Metformin for hyperinsulinemia, dexamethasone for androgen excess, bromocriptine for prolactin excess.
   c. Substitution therapy: Thyroxin for hypothyroidism, antidiabetic drugs for diabetes mellitus.
2. Surgery:
   a. Laparoscopic ovarian drilling (LOD) or laser vaporization for polycystic ovarian syndrome (PCOS).
   b. Surgical removal of virilizing or functioning ovarian, or adrenal tumor.
   c. Tubotubal anastomosis for adhesion in tube.
   d. Cannulation and balloon tuboplasty for block in tube.
   e. Fimbrioplasty for fimbrial adhesion.
   f. Adhesiolysis for separation or division of adhesion.
   g. Salpingostomy to create an opening in tube in a completely occluded tube.

Management of Unexplained Infertility

Unexplained or persistent infertility refers to those couples who have undergone complete basic infertility workup and in whom no abnormality has been detected and still remains infertile. The reported evidence is about 10–20%. About 60–80% of those couples become pregnant within 3 years without any treatment.

The recommended treatment for unexplained infertility is induction of ovulation, IUI and superovulation combined with IUI.

ASSISTED REPRODUCTIVE TECHNOLOGY

Assisted reproductive technology encompasses all methods used to achieve pregnancy by artificial or partially artificial means. It involves manipulation of gametes and embryos outside the body for the treatment of infertility. In ART, the process of intercourse is bypassed either by IUI or fertilization of the oocytes in the laboratory environment as in IVF.

Different Techniques of ART

- Intrauterine insemination
- In vitro fertilization and embryo transfer (IVF-ET)
- Gamete intrafallopian transfer (GIFT)
- Zygote intrafallopian transfer (ZIFT)
- Intracytoplasmic sperm injection.

Intrauterine Insemination

Intrauterine insemination involves placing increased concentration of motile sperms close to the fallopian tubes bypassing the endocervical canal which is abnormal. IUI may be *artificial insemination husband (AIH), AID or insemination with donor egg.*

Indications
- Hostile cervical mucus
- Cervical stenosis
- Oligospermia or athenospermia
- Immune factor (male or female)
- Male factor impotency or anatomical defect, but normal ejaculate can be obtained, e.g. hypospadias (AIH)
- Unexplained infertility.

Technique
About 3 mL of washed and concentrated sperms are injected through a flexible polyethylene catheter within the uterine cavity around the time of ovulation. The processed sperms for insemination should at least be 1 million. Fertilizing capacity of spermatozoa is 24–48 hours. The procedure may be repeated two to three times over a period of 2–3 days. Generally, four to six cycles of insemination with or without superovulation are advised.

When large volumes of washed and processed sperms are placed within the uterine cavity around the time of ovulation, it causes perfusion of the fallopian tubes with spermatozoa. Hence, this method is known as *fallopian tube sperm perfusion*.

In conjunction with ovulation induction, pregnancy rate is 25–30% per cycle.

Artificial insemination donor
When the semen of a donor is used for insemination, it is called *artificial insemination* donor.

Indications
- Untreatable azoospermia or athenospermia of husband
- Genetic disease affecting spermatogenesis in husband
- Rh-sensitization of the woman.

Technique

The donor should be healthy and serologically and bacteriologically free from venereal disease, human immunodeficiency virus (HIV) and hepatitis. The recipient and donor must be matched for blood group and Rh typing, either fresh or frozen semen is used.

About three to six cycles may be used for success. Insemination when combined with superovulation enhances success rate. Two inseminations 18–42 hours after hCG administration (for ovulation) give higher result when compared to single insemination after 36 hours.

Artificial insemination husband

An AIH is done for four cycles. The results are better, if combined with ovulation induction for multiple ovulations.

Indications
- Oligospermia
- Impotency
- Premature ejaculation or retrograde ejaculation
- Hypospadias
- Antisperm antibodies in cervical mucus
- Unexplained infertility
- X-Y fractionation of sperms for sex selection in genetic and chromosomal abnormalities.

Technique

Semen collection, washing, centrifugation and swim-up methods are done. Washed and concentrated sperm is then placed in uterine cavity as in AID technique.

In Vitro Fertilization and Embryo Transfer

Fertilization of an ovum outside the body is a technique used when a woman has blocked fallopian tubes or some other impediment to the union of sperm and ovum in the reproductive tract. The woman is given hormone therapy causing a number of ova to mature at the same time (superovulation). Several of them are then removed from the ovary through a laparoscope.

The ova are mixed with spermatozoa from her spouse and incubated in a culture medium until a blastocyst is formed. The blastocyst is then implanted in the mother's uterus and the pregnancy allowed to continue normally.

Indications
1. Tubal disease or block.
2. Endometriosis.
3. Cervical hostility.
4. Unexplained infertility.
5. Ovarian failure (donor oocyte IVF).

Donor oocyte IVF is done for women with no eggs due to surgery, chemotherapy, genetic causes or poor egg quality.

Patient selection
1. Age of women (egg donor) less than 35 years.
2. Presence of at least one functioning ovary.
3. Normal seminogram for husband.
4. Couple negative for HIV and hepatitis.

Technique/Procedure steps
1. Induction of superovulation using drugs clomiphene citrate and GnRH.
2. *Monitoring of follicular growth:* This is done by cervical mucus study, sonographic measurement of the follicle and serum estriol estimation.
3. *Ovum retrieval:* This is done either laparoscopically or vaginally. If vaginal route is used, a small needle is inserted through the back of the vagina and guided via ultrasound into the ovarian follicle to collect the fluid that contains the ova about 36 hours after hCG administration, but before ovulation occurs.
4. *Fertilization (in vitro):* The sperm for insemination in vitro is prepared by the wash and swim technique. Approximately 50,000–100,000 sperms are placed into the culture media containing the oocyte within 4–6 hours of retrieval. The semen is collected just prior to ovum retrieval. Sperm density and motility are most important criteria for successful IVF.
5. *Embryo transfer:* The fertilized ova at the four to eight cell stages are placed into the uterine cavity close to the fundus about 48–72 hours later though a fine flexible tube transcervically. Not more than three embryos are transferred per cycle to minimize multiple pregnancies.

Gamete Intrafallopian Transfer

In this procedure, both the sperm and the unfertilized oocyte are transferred into the fallopian tubes using laparoscopy following transvaginal ovum retrieval. Fertilization is then achieved in vivo.

The prerequisite for GIFT procedure is to have normal fallopian tubes. The result is poor in male factor abnormality. Superovulation is done as in IVF. About 2 hours prior to ovum retrieval, semen specimen is obtained. The semen is washed by 'swim-up' technique and the most fertile fraction of the sperm is obtained and used for transfer.

Zygote Intrafallopian Transfer

In ZIFT, egg cells are removed from the woman's ovaries and fertilized in the laboratory. The resulting zygote is then placed in the fallopian tube following one day in vitro fertilization through laparoscope or through a uterine opening under ultrasonic guidance.

The technique is a suitable alternative of GIFT. GIFT procedures are avoided when tubal factors of infertility are present.

Intracytoplasmic Sperm Injection

Intracytoplasmic sperm injection method is beneficial in the case of male factor infertility where the sperm counts are very low or failed fertilization with previous IVF attempts. The ICSI procedure involves a single sperm carefully injected into the center of an egg using a microneedle. Sperm is retrieved from the ejaculate or by testicular sperm extraction (TESE) or by microsurgical epididymal sperm aspiration (MESA). Indications are azoospermia, severe oligospermia, sperm antibodies and obstruction of afferent duct system and failure of IVF.

Prognosis of Artificial Reproductive Methods

The pregnancy rate within 2 years after the start of investigations ranges from 30% to 40%. The rate is higher, if AID cases are included. However, if pregnancy occurs, there is two-fold increased chance of abortion, five times ectopic pregnancy and the perinatal mortality doubles.

ROLE OF NURSES IN MANAGEMENT OF INFERTILITY

Nurses meet couples seeking help for treatment of infertility in special centers or clinics, where such services are available. Those working in infertility centers usually are the first contact persons who coordinate various activities for the couple's treatment. Their role with such couples includes assessing, educating and counseling in addition to therapeutic assistance as they undergo tests and procedures.

When a couple presents with concerns about infertility, it is important for the nurse to understand that men and women are very concerned and possibly emotionally fragile. Entering a medical facility for evaluation is in itself for some an admission of failure.

Before or even beginning, the medical aspects of care is important to understand and assist the couple to understand their motivation for pregnancy and to offer support. The couple should understand and accept that the evaluation and treatment for infertility will be stressful and will involve both partners throughout the process. It is important to meet the couple together.

An important step in evaluation for infertility is taking a detailed medical and family history from each partner. Treatment may be individualized for each partner. Nursing interventions include assisting in reducing stress in the relationship, encouraging cooperation, protecting privacy and fostering understanding. Because infertility evaluations and treatments are expensive, time consuming, invasive, stressful and not always successful, couples need great support in working together to deal with the process. During the period of therapy, couples need to avoid smoking, continue good diet, exercise, maintain health and take folic acid supplements, if prescribed.

ADOPTION

Description

Adoption is the legal procedure that allows someone to become the parent of a child even though the child and parent are not related by blood. But in every way adoptive parents are the child's parents with all the rights, privileges and responsibilities that are attached to a biological child.

Fundamental Principles Governing Child Adoption

- The child's best interest shall be the paramount consideration, while processing any adoption placement.
- Preference shall be given to place the child in adoption with Indian citizens and with regard to the principle of placement of the child in his own sociocultural environment as far as possible.
- All adoptions shall be registered on 'Child Adoption Resource Information and Guidance System' and the confidentiality of the same shall be maintained by the authority.

Adoption Laws in India

1. The Indian Adoption and Maintenance Act 1956.
2. The Juvenile Justice (JJ) Act (Care and Protection of Children) 2000.
   The main strength of the JJ Act are:
   - Any Indian citizen can adopt a child who is legally free for adoption.
   - The adoptee gets the same rights that a biological child might.
   - The religion of the adoptive parent is not relevant.
   - Single person can adopt.
   - The adoption is irrevocable.
     Some, time limits have been set to ensure that children are considered legally free for adoption.
   - The trust is on the best interest of the child.

Stakeholders in Adoption Process

1. Central Adoption Resource Authority (CARA) ensures smooth functioning of the adoption process from time to time, issues adoption guidelines laying down procedures and processes to be followed by different stakeholders of adoption programme.
2. State Adoption Resource Agency (SARA) acts as a nodal body within the state to promote and monitor adoption and non-institutional care in coordination with CARA.
3. Specialized Adoption Agency (SAA) is recognized by the state Governments under subsection 4 of section 41 of the act for the purpose of placing children in adoption.
4. Authorized Foreign Adoption Agency (AFAA) is recognized as a foreign social or child welfare agency that is authorized by the CARA on the recommendation of concerned central authority as CARA or Government department of that country for coordinating all matters relating to adoption of Indian child by a citizen of that country.
5. District Child Protection Unit (DCPU) means a unit set-up by the state Government at district level under section 61A of the Act. It identifies orphaned, abandoned and surrendered children in the district and get them, declared legally free for adoption by child Welfare Committee.

Eligibility Criteria for Prospective Adoptive Parents

- The prospective adoptive parents should be physically, mentally and emotionally stable; financially capable, motivated to adopt a child and should not have any life-threatening medical condition.
- Any prospective adoptive parent, irrespective of his marital status and whether or not he has his own biological son or daughter, can adopt a child.
- Single female is eligible to adopt a child of any gender.
- Single male person shall not be eligible to adopt a girl child.
- In case of a couple, the consent of both spouses shall be required.
- No child shall be given in adoption to a couple unless they have at least two years of stable marital relationship.
- The age of the prospective adoptive parents as on the date of registration shall be counted for deciding the eligibility of the PAA, to apply for children of different age groups shall be as under.

Age of child	Maximum composite age of prospective adoptive parents (couple)	Maximum age of single prospective adoptive parent
Up to 4 years	90 years	45 years
Above 4 and up to 8 years	100 years	50 years
Above 8 and up to 18 years	110 years	55 years

- In case of a couple, the composite age of prospective adoptive parents shall be counted.
- The minimum age difference between the child and either of the prospective adoptive parent should not be less than 25 years.
- The age of eligibility will be as on date of registration of the prospective parents.
- The age criteria of PAP shall not be applicable in case of relative adoption by step parents.
- Couples with three or more children shall not be considered for adoption except in cases of special need children as defined in subregulation (21) of regulation (2), and hard to place children as mentioned in regulation 50, and as in case of relative adoption and adoption by step parent.

Adoption Procedure

One can adopt a child through submission of an online application available at *www.cara.nic.in*, and following the procedure steps provided in the "Adoption Regulation 2017". For further details, one can visit the website *www.cara.nic.in*. It is now mandatory to register online. The applicant can then approach the District Child Protection Officer (DCPO) of the applicant's district.

Steps to Adopt a Child in India

In-country adoption

1. Parents register online on CARINGS (*www.cara.nic.in*).
2. Select preferred adoption agency for Home Study Report (HSR) and state user ID and password are generated.
3. Upload documents within 30 days of registration.
4. Register number is generated.
5. The Specialized Adoption Agency (SAA) prepare the home study report (HSR) of the prospective adoptive parents (PAPs) and upholds it on CARINGS within 30 days from the date of submission of required documents on CARINGS.
6. Suitability of PAPs is determined and if not found suitable, PAPs are informed with reasons for rejection.
7. PAPs reserve one child as per their preference from up to 6 children.
8. PAPs visit the adoption agency within 15 days from the date of reservation and finalize the child.
9. If the child is not finalized within the stipulated time, the PAPs come down in the seniority list.
10. On acceptance of the child by PAPs, the SAA completes the referral and adoption process (on CARINGS).
11. PAPs take the child (bring the child home) under a pre-adoption foster care agreement and SAA files a petition in the court to get the adoption formally approved by a judge. When the judge approves the adoption, the child becomes the adoptive parents' son/daughter.
12. Adoption court order is then issued.
13. The adoption agency will receive the court's formal order, based on which they will procure the birth certificate and mail to parents.

The child becomes officially the child of adoptive parents.

STUDY QUESTIONS

Short Answer Questions

1. List the causes of female infertility.
2. Assisted reproductive technology (ART).
3. Intrauterine insemination (IUI).
4. Artificial insemination donor (AID).
5. In vitro fertilization and embryo transfer (IVF-ET).
6. Gamete intrafallopian transfer (GIFT).
7. Zygote intrafallopian transfer (ZIFT).

Essay Questions

1. Explain the diagnostic evaluation methods for infertility.
2. Explain the measures of infertility management in females and males.
3. Describe the legal adoption in india.

BIBLIOGRAPHY

1. Adoption Process Overview .https: https://www.adoptionnetwork.com
2. Baram DA. Sexuality and sexual function. Novak's Gynecology, 13th edition. Baltimore: Williams & Wilkens; 1998.
3. Bhaskar Nima. Midwifery and Obstetrical Nursing, 2nd edition. Bangalore: EMMES Medical Publishers; 2015.
4. CARA Central Adoption Resource Authority. https://cara.nic.in
5. Cheryl R, Marina E, Cassandsra M, Catherine W. Normal family processes: growing diversity and complexity. 3rd edition. Newyork: Guilford Press; 2003.
6. Freudnlich Madelyn. Adoption and Assisted Reproduction. Child Welfare League of America. Washington D. C; 2001.
8. Harold GD, Nora D, Kohler JL, Lash Esau Amy. Handbook of adoption: implications for researchers, practitioners, and families. Thousand Oaks, CAGE Publications; 2007.
9. Introduction to adoption-Child Welfare Information Gateway. https://www.childwelfare.gov
10. James CA. The nursing role in assisted reproductive technologies. NAACOGS Clinical Issues Perinatal Women Health Nursing. 1992;3(2):328-44.
11. Jirka J, Schuett S, Foxall MJ. Loneliness and social support in infertile couples. Journal of Obstetric. Gynecologic and Neonatal Nursing. 1996;25(1):55-60.
12. Kaplan CR. Workup of infertility diagnosis and treatment of anovulation. The Female Patient. 1966;21(3):35-42.
13. Madelyn F. Adoption and assisted reproduction. Child Welfare League of America. Washington D. C; 2001.
14. Nima B. Midwifery and obstetrical nursing, 2nd edition. Bangalore: EMMES Medical Publishers; 2015.
15. Adoption Laws in India. https://www.legalserviceindia.com
16. Child Adoption in India-Laws and Rules/Eligibility/Procedure. https://www.restthecase.com
17. Overview of Child Adoption Process in India https://www.vikaspedia

Genital Malignancies

Learning Objectives

Upon completion of this chapter, the learner will be able to:
- Identify the factors that have been found to cause genital organ malignancies.
- Describe the significance of health education and preventive care in decreasing the incidence of cancer of pelvic organs.
- Describe the roles of surgery, radiation therapy, chemotherapy and other therapies in treating cancer.
- Describe the special nursing needs of patients receiving treatment for cancer.
- Describe the common nursing diagnoses for patients with malignancies of generative organs.

Cancer is a disease in which cells of the body grow out of control. The new growth is termed neoplasm and that with locally invasive, destructive and metastatic properties is termed as malignancy. A malignant growth or cancer is always named for the part of the body where it starts even if it spreads to other parts later. Genital cancers develop in the ovaries, uterus, cervix, vulva, vagina and fallopian tubes.

OVARIAN CANCER

Ovarian cancer is a term that includes a variety of malignant growths that originate in the ovary. There are about 20 microscopically distinct types. They can be classified into three large groups; *epithelial cancers, germ-cell tumors and specialized stromal cell cancers*. There are three such groups because the ovary contains collections of cells with three distinct origins and functions.

Incidence

Ovarian malignancy constitutes about 15–20% of genital malignancy. It is more prevalent in the United States of America (USA) and Scandinavian countries, but much less in Oriental or Latin American and Asian countries including Japan and India.

Epidemiology

Nulligravida carry a higher risk for ovarian malignancy. Repeated ovulatory trauma to the ovarian epithelial lining is seen as a promoting factor for carcinogenesis. There is a significant reduction in the risk with increasing parity. Combined oral contraceptive pills reduce the risk significantly as also repeated pregnancies.

The use of coffee, tobacco, alcohol and dietary fat has also been associated with reduction in the risk.

Origin

During embryonic development, when the fetus is about 8 weeks postconception, the organ systems begin to form. There is, on each side of the abdominal cavity, an area that is destined to become ovary. Into this area, special cells migrate from the yolk sac, which are destined to become ova. These cells are called **germ cells**. Also in these two areas cells are specialized for manufacture of steroid hormones. Covering all these are the mesothelium, which becomes the peritoneum—the lining of abdominal cavity that contains all of the intestines, liver and in women, the uterus and ovaries. From puberty and through adult life, the ovary will function as a producer of ova and steroid hormones such as estrogen and progesterone.

During each menstrual cycle, a germ cell will mature into an ova or egg contained in a follicle or cyst. While maturing the ova, the ovary produces estrogen. The follicle cyst is covered with the epithelium that once was the mesothelium. At ovulation the follicle breaks and releases the ova. The remnant of the follicle cyst called corpus luteum produces progesterone.

The epithelial covering gives rise to **epithelial ovarian cancers**, the germ cells to the **germ cell tumors** and the steroid producing cells to the **specialized stromal cells cancers**.

About 80% of ovarian cancers are epithelial, 10–20% are of germ cell origin and very little are of stromal cell origin, 3–5%.

Genetics and Ovarian Malignancy

Hereditary ovarian cancer occurs in two forms:
1. *Hereditary breast ovarian cancer (HBOC) syndrome:* When gene mutation occurs to chromosome 17q, it is called *BRCA1*. When gene mutation happens in chromosome 13q, it is *BRCA2*. These produce serous carcinoma in early age.
2. *Hereditary non-polyposis colorectal cancer (HNPCC) or Lynch syndrome:* This is an autosomal dominant transmission. Women with HNPCC have lifetime risk of about 50% for endometrial cancer and 12% for ovarian cancer. However, majority of epithelial ovarian cancers are not familial or hereditary. They are less than 10% of all ovarian cancers.

Classification of Ovarian Cancers

Epithelial Ovarian Cancers

- Serous
- Endometrioid
- Clear cell
- Papillary serous
- Brenner cell
- Undifferentiated adenocarcinoma and sarcoma.

Stromal Cell Cancers

- Immature teratoma
- Mature teratoma
- Carcinoid tumor
- Dysgerminoma
- Embryonal cell carcinoma
- Endodermal sinus tumor
- Primary choriocarcinoma
- Gonadoblastoma.

Specialized Stromal Cell Cancers

- Granulosa cell tumor
- Theca cell tumor
- Sertoli-Leydig cell tumor
- Hilar cell tumor.

In addition, there are others that are very rare. These rare tumors are not discussed in this chapter. The ovary is also a site for metastasis from other cancers, especially the intestinal cancer and breast cancer. Cancers metastatic to the ovaries are termed as **Krukenberg tumors**.

Features of Specific Types of Tumors

Epithelial Cancers

1. Malignant epithelial tumors are both cystic and solid types, with the cystic type more common.
2. These are bilateral in about 50%.
3. These may arise de novo as malignant or more commonly result from malignant changes of benign cystic tumors.
4. In 20%, it is seen associated with endometrial carcinoma and in 10% with ovarian endometriosis. In less than 5%, it may arise from an endometrial cyst.

Germ Cell Tumors

1. Germ cell tumors commonly occur in young women: 50% are women younger than 21 years of age.
2. These are very aggressive and virulent cancers.
3. The teratomas have the potential to form complete adult type tissues.
4. The mature teratoma is called 'dermoid' and can contain hair, teeth, bone, and brain tissue; often they are full of skin.
5. They are generally not malignant, but very rarely can have a secondary malignancy such as melanoma or squamous cell cancer of skin.
6. Some contain thyroid tissue and can cause hyperthyroidism.
7. If the tissues remain immature or fetal in appearance, then they are malignant.

Specialized Stromal Cell Tumors

1. Granulosa and theca cell tumors are often mixed and can produce estrogen.
2. If it occurs in a young girl, it can produce premature sexual development, which will also stop the bones from growing, causing short stature.
3. Sertoli-Leydig cell tumors produce male hormones and will cause defeminization, then masculinization with male pattern baldness, deep voice, excessive hair growth and enlargement of clitoris.
4. The specialized stromal cell cancers are not aggressive cancers and usually involve only one ovary.

Risk Factors for Ovarian Cancer

Majority of ovarian cancers are epithelial cell type cancers characteristics are:
1. Epithelial ovarian cancers tend to be a cancer of affluent societies where expected life spans are long. Most ovarian cancers occur in women over age 50.
2. An increased risk factor other than age is nulliparity or delayed childbearing.
3. Use of fertility drugs that induce ovulation.
4. Familial cancers includes breast, endometrial, ovarian, colorectal.
5. History of removal of benign ovarian tumor or breast carcinoma.
6. Postmenopausal palpable ovary (volume > 8 cm^2).
7. Women workers in asbestos related industries.
8. A decreased risk is seen with multiparity and with prolonged use of birth control pill. The mechanism for this protective effect may be that the number of ovulations is reduced. Each ovulation requires the breakage of the

ovarian follicle and the repair of the ovarian surface. A repair process means increased cell divisions or mitosis. Each mitotic division is a time of risk for mutation to occur.

Clinical Features

Ovarian cancer is very difficult to detect in its early stages because at first there are often no obvious symptoms. A cyst can break and bleed and can cause enough symptoms to cause the woman to seek help. Otherwise the cancer is usually far advanced before it is diagnosed. When symptoms do appear, they may include:

- An ongoing feeling of abdominal discomfort or pain, which the patient may express as gas, indigestion, bloating, swelling or cramps
- Nausea, diarrhea, constipation
- Loss of appetite
- Feeling full even after a light meal
- Sudden loss of weight
- Urinary frequency or incontinence
- Abnormal vaginal bleeding
- Pelvic pain, back pain
- Fatigue and pallor
- Edema leg or vulva
- Respiratory distress due to ascites or pleural effusion.

Special Investigations

Investigations are aimed at identifying the extent of lesion to detect the primary site and to confirm malignancy prior to surgery, which includes:

1. Cytology examination of fluid collected from abdominal paracentesis or cul-de-sac aspiration.
2. Blood test for carcinoma antigen 125 (CA 125)—tumor maker. Level above > 35 U/mL with a pelvic mass may be suggestive of epithelial ovarian cancer.
3. Chest X-ray to exclude pleural effusion and chest metastasis.
4. Barium enema to detect any lower bowel malignancy.
5. Sonography to detect involvement of the omentum or contralateral ovary.
6. Computed tomography (CT) for retroperitoneal lymph node assessment and to detect metastasis in liver or omentum.
7. Magnetic resonance imaging (MRI) to detect involvement of lymph nodes relapse following initial treatment.
8. Positron emission tomography (PET) is a more sensitive test than MRI or CT to differentiate normal tissues from cancer tissues.
9. Intravenous pyelography.
10. Diagnostic and dilatation and curettage (D&C).

In all, but the earliest cancers, there is often some cancer remaining after surgery. This is because it spreads throughout the abdomen in little nodules, some are only barely visible and others are too small to see.

The surgical goal is not to leave any nodule larger than 1 cm. If the residual is smaller, debulking or cryoreduction may be done. If small nodules are detected on the intestine, then removal of a piece of intestine and even a colostomy may be necessary to achieve the goal.

In addition to stage (size and extent of spread) the grade (microscopic appearance) is also important. Grade '0' refers to an epithelial carcinoma of low malignant potential, which is borderline cancer.

Grade 1 adenocarcinoma is easily identified as being from a glandular origin. Grade 3 cancers are difficult to identify as glandular and are poorly differentiated and expected to behave the worst. Grade 2 cancers are intermediate in appearance.

Preventive Management

Primary Prevention

1. Genetic screening for BRCA for women who are at high risk for breast and ovarian cancer.
2. Annual mammographic screening for women with strong family history of breast cancer.
3. Periodic screening for other malignancies. For example, colonoscopy and endometrial biopsy for women with Lynch II syndrome.
4. Combined contraceptive pills for women belonging to HNPCC families.
5. Prophylactic oophorectomy with hysterectomy in high-risk women such as:
   - Nulliparous women aged above > 45 years
   - Women with history of ovarian, endometrial or colonic cancer in the first degree relative (mother, sister)
   - Grossly abnormal ovary in premenopausal women (ovarian volume > 20 cm^2)
   - Women who had one ovary removed for neoplasm
   - Previous history of breast carcinoma
   - Any woman with radiation induced menopause.
6. Careful follow-up of any ovarian enlargement of about 8 cm or more during childbearing period.
7. In postmenopausal women any ovarian enlargement should be assessed by CA 125 and transvaginal sonography.
8. Follow-up of women who had ovarian cyst with ultrasound and serum CA 125 at an interval of 4 months.
9. Laparotomy for any enlargement of ovary beyond 8 cm and symptomatic ovarian tumor, while the woman is under observation.

Secondary Prevention

Screening as secondary preventive measure aims at detecting early ovarian malignancy in asymptomatic women:

1. Tumor marker: Test for specific antigen CA 125. Values more than 35 U/mL are suggestive of epithelial ovarian cancer.

2. Transvaginal ultrasonography and study of vascular parameters.

Treatment

Surgery

Surgery is the key treatment for ovarian malignancy. Surgery chemotherapy, radiotherapy and combination therapy are used according to the stage and degree of the malignancy **(Table 72.1)**.

Borderline ovarian cancer: This category of epithelial ovarian cancers is of low malignant potential and slow growing. Recurrence after surgery may not develop for 15–20 years or may not recur at all. Most are stage I, but can be stage III when diagnosed. These are usually treated only by surgery.

Epithelial ovarian cancer: For this type of cancer, the initial treatment is surgery, which is removal of uterus, tubes and ovaries as well as any large nodules of cancer. Removal of only one ovary is done in the following situations:
- The patient has strong desire for further childbearing
- The cancer is stage IA grade '0' or stage II epithelial cancer
- The cancer is stage I germ cell or a specialized stromal cell type.

When unilateral oophorectomy is done, the woman is advised to have the remaining ovary removed when childbearing is completed. All ovarian cancer patients will receive a maximal surgical effort, so that the residual is small and there is a better chance for complete response to chemotherapy. In advanced stage, a segment of intestine may be removed with a colostomy.

TABLE 72.1: Surgical stages of ovarian cancer (FIGO).

Stages	Features
Stage I	Limited to the ovaries
Stage IA	One ovary involved
Stage IB	Both ovaries involved
Stage IC	One or both ovaries involved, but with cancer on the surface of an ovary, rupture of an ovarian cyst, malignant ascites or positive abdominal washings
Stage II	Spread to adjacent pelvic structures
Stage IIA	Spread to uterus or fallopian tubes
Stage IIB	Spread to pelvic peritoneum
Stage IIC	Confined to the pelvis, but with malignant ascites or positive abdominal washings
Stage III	Spread to the upper abdomen
Stage IIIA	Microscopic spread to the upper abdomen
Stage IIIB	Cancer nodules less than 2 cm
Stage IIIC	Nodules more than 2 cm or positive pelvic or aortic lymph nodes
Stage IV	Distant spread beyond the abdomen, liver, lung, etc.

(FIGO: International Federation of Gynecology and Obstetrics).

Chemotherapy

Chemotherapy is accomplished by giving chemotherapeutic drugs soon after surgery. The drugs are repeated every 3–4 weeks and usually six courses are given. Single agent drugs commonly used are melphalan, cisplatin, carboplatin and paclitaxel. For combination therapy the drugs used are cyclophosphamide, adriamycin and cisplatin.

Radiation

Radioactive isotope of phosphorus called ^{32}P is instilled in the abdominal cavity. This is used when microscopic amount of cancer only is present. With a one-time instillation, the entire abdominal contents receive a dose of several thousand rads to a depth of several millimeters.

The unit used to measure the amount of ionizing radiation absorbed by human tissues is 'rad' or 'cGy' (centigray). 100 rads (cGy) is equal to 1 Gy (gray), which is the amount of energy absorbed by one kilogram of human tissue. Currently, the term centigray is used (one cGy is equivalent to one rad). Primary tumors should receive high dose as instillation therapy (peritoneal or pleural cavity).

External beam therapy is usually fractionated and is given once daily for 5 days a week for 4 weeks (for example, a dose of 40 Gy in 20 fractions given five times weekly for 4 weeks gives 2 Gy per fraction). A planning computer is used to calculate the dose and field size from different angles of the treatment machine.

Immunotherapy

Use of cytokines, interferon- or interleukin- 2 has shown improvement in response rate.

Prognosis

1. Stage IA and IB grade 1 cancers require no further treatment after surgery. The 5-year survival rate is 95%.
2. All stage IC and all stage III cancers receive treatment either with chemotherapy or ^{32}P. The prognosis is usually good with cure rate of 65–80%.
3. All stage II and stage III cancers with minimal or microscopic residual receive chemotherapy. The 5 year survival is 30–35%.
4. For those with stage III and IV cancers with bulky residual, the short-term response is good, but the long-term outlook is poor.

UTERINE CANCER

Uterine cancer also called endometrial cancer and uterine adenocarcinoma involves a malignant growth that originates in the lining of the uterus—the endometrium. Endometrial cancer is the most common cancer of the female reproductive system. Cancer of the uterus mainly affects postmenopausal women between the ages of 50 and 60, and is uncommon below 40 years.

Incidence

The incidence is higher amongst the white population of USA and lowest in India and Japan. The high incidence within a few decades of menopause is associated with excessive exposure to estrogen.

Etiology

The following are found to be related to carcinoma body of the uterus:
1. *Estrogen:* Persistent stimulation of endometrium with unopposed estrogen is the single most important factor for the development of endometrial cancer.
2. *Age:* About 75% postmenopausal cancers are diagnosed at median age of 60. About 10% of women with postmenopausal bleeding have endometrial cancer.
3. *Parity:* It is more common in unmarried and nulliparous women (about 30%).
4. *Late menopause:* The chance of carcinoma increases if menopause fails to occur beyond 52 years.
5. *Corpus cancer syndrome:* Encompasses obesity, hypertension and diabetes.
6. *Obesity:* Leads to high level of free estradiol as the sex hormone binding globulin level is low.
7. *Unopposed* estrogen stimulation that occurs in conditions such as functioning ovarian tumor, polycystic ovarian disease (PCOD), and estrogen replacement therapy in postmenopausal women is associated with endometrial cancer.
8. Tamoxifen used for treatment of breast cancer is noted as contributing to endometrial cancer due to its weak estrogenic effect.
9. Family history or personal history of colon, ovarian or breast cancer increases the risk of endometrial cancer.
10. Fibroid is associated in 30% of cases.

Classification

Carcinoma

Most endometrial cancers are **carcinomas** usually **adenocarcinomas** meaning that they originate from the single layer of epithelial cells that line the endometrium and form the endometrial glands. The microscopic type of endometrial carcinoma include the:
- Endometrioid type
- Papillary serous carcinoma
- Clear cell endometrial carcinoma.

Sarcoma

Endometrial stromal sarcomas are cancers that originate in the non-glandular connective tissue of the endometrium.

Carcinosarcoma

Carcinosarcoma is a rare uterine cancer that contains cancerous cells of both glandular and sarcomatous appearance. In this case, the cell of origin is unknown.

Signs and Symptoms

- Vaginal bleeding and/or spotting in postmenopausal women
- Abnormal uterine bleeding and abnormal menstrual periods
- Bleeding between normal periods in premenopausal women; extremely long, heavy or frequent episodes of bleeding may indicate premalignant changes
- Anemia caused by chronic loss of blood
- Lower abdominal pain or cramping
- Thin white or clear vaginal discharge in postmenopausal women
- Abdominal mass
- Pain during sexual intercourse.

Risk Factors

- High level of estrogen
- Endometrial hyperplasia
- Obesity, diabetes, hypertension
- Polycystic ovary syndrome
- Nulliparity and infertility
- Early menarche
- Late menopause
- Endometrial polyps or other benign growths of uterine lining
- History of irregular and excessive premenopausal bleeding
- Use of tamoxifen for breast cancer treatment
- High intake of animal fat
- Pelvic radiation therapy
- Ovarian cancer
- Anovulatory cycles.

Diagnosis

- History and clinical examination
- Pap smear may be either normal or show abnormal cellular changes
- Endometrial biopsy using a Sharman curette or aspiration using a soft, flexible plastic suction cannula
- Transvaginal ultrasound and color Doppler to evaluate the endometrial thickness in women with postmenopausal bleeding
- Hysteroscopy and direct visualization of the uterine cavity to take biopsy
- Fractional curettage to detect the extent of growth.

Preoperative Evaluation

- Complete medical history, physical examination and pelvic examination
- Blood examination—hemoglobin, complete blood count (CBC), blood glucose, urea, creatinine and electrolytes
- Urine examination—routine examination for protein, sugar and pus cells
- Chest X-ray and electrocardiogram (ECG)

- Pelvic ultrasonography
- Liver and renal function tests
- Serum tumor marker such as AC 125.

Treatment

Choice of treatment is based on the surgical staging (Table 72.2). The primary treatment is surgery:

1. Surgical treatment consists of:
   - Cytologic sampling of the peritoneal fluid
   - Abdominal exploration
   - Palpation and biopsy of suspicious lymph nodes
   - Abdominal hysterectomy
   - Bilateral salpingo-oophorectomy and lymphadenectomy (pelvic and para-aortic lymph nodes), if the tumor has high-risk features or extension to the cervix or adnexa.
2. Surgery in combination with radiotherapy for women with stage I disease that are at risk for recurrence and for those with stage II cancer.
3. Chemotherapy for those with stage III and IV disease.
4. Hormonal therapy with progestins and antiestrogens for treatment of endometrial and stromal sarcomas.

Complications of Treatment

1. Uterine perforation may occur during a D&C or an endometrial biopsy.
2. Asherman's syndrome: Intrauterine adhesions may occur from D&C, resulting in infertility and an increased risk of future obstetric complications.

Prognosis

1. Prognosis is poor for tumors that are poorly differentiated with greater degree of myometrial penetration, lymphovascular space invasion and advanced stages.
2. Aneuploid tumors are prognostically worse.

TABLE 72.2: Staging of endometrial carcinoma FIGO, 2010.

Stages	Features
Stage IA	Tumor confined to the endometrium
Stage IB	Invasion of less than half the endometrium
Stage IC	Invasion of more than half the endometrium
Stage IIA	Endocervical glandular involvement only
Stage IIB	Cervical stromal invasion
Stage IIIA	Tumor invades serosa or adnexa
Stage IIIB	Vaginal and/or parametrial involvement
Stage IIIC1	Pelvic node involvement
Stage IIIC2	Para-aortic lymph node involvement with or without pelvic node involvement
Stage IVA	Tumor invasion to bladder and/or bowel mucosa
Stage IVB	Distant metastasis including abdominal metastasis and/or inguinal lymph nodes

(FIGO: International Federation of Gynecology and Obstetrics)

GESTATIONAL TROPHOBLASTIC DISEASE

Gestational trophoblastic disease (GTD)/neoplasia is a generic name for a group of pregnancy related disorders that arise from trophoblasts (primitive cells, which are placental stem cells). When there is persistence of GTD beyond pregnancy, the condition is referred to as **gestational trophoblastic neoplasia** (GTN).

Types

Gestational trophoblastic disease is the common name for five closely related tumors, most of which are malignant; benign—hydatidiform mole.

The malignant types are:
- Invasive mole
- Choriocarcinoma
- Placental site trophoblastic tumor
- Persistent trophoblastic disease.

The tumors arise from trophoblastic cells. Trophoblast is the membrane that forms the wall of the blastocyst in the early development of the fetus. In a normal pregnancy, trophoblastic cells aid the implantation of the fertilized egg into the uterine wall. But in GTD, they develop into tumor cells.

Invasive Mole

Invasive mole (choriocarcinoma destruens) consists of 15% of all gestational trophoblastic neoplasms. Features of invasive mole are:
- Abnormal penetration through the muscle layers of the uterus
- Perforation of the uterine wall at multiple areas showing purple fungating growth
- Intraperitoneal hemorrhage
- Metastasis to vagina or distant sites as in choriocarcinoma.

Diagnosis
1. On laparotomy:
   - Perforation of the uterus through which purple fungating growth is visible
   - Hemoperitoneum.
2. On histological examination, hyperplasic, trophoblastic cells, which still retain villus structure are seen.
3. Persistent high level of urinary and serum hCG.

Choriocarcinoma

Choriocarcinoma is a highly malignant and aggressive cancer arising from the chorionic epithelium. The abnormal cells start in the tissue that would normally become placenta. About 3–5% of all patients with molar pregnancy develop choriocarcinoma. Choriocarcinoma of the placenta is preceded by hydatidiform mole in 50% of cases, spontaneous abortion in 20% of cases, ectopic pregnancy in 20% of cases and normal term pregnancy in 20–30% cases.

Pathology

Characteristic feature is the identification of intimately related syncytiotrophoblasts and cytotrophoblasts without formation of definite placenta type villi.

Placental Site Trophoblastic Tumor

The tumor arises from the trophoblasts of the placental bed. Incidence is about 1% of all patients with GTN. 15–20% of these patients develop metastasis. Intermediate trophoblast cells are predominant. α-hCG secretion is low, but human placental lactogen (HPL) is secreted and this is monitored during follow-up. Hysterectomy is the preferred treatment. This neoplasm is not responsive to chemotherapy.

Persistent Trophoblastic Disease

The term persistent trophoblastic disease (PTD) is used when after treatment of a molar pregnancy, some molar tissue is left behind which again starts growing into a tumor. Patient presents with irregular vaginal bleeding, subinvolution of uterus, persistence of theca lutein cysts and elevation of hCG (after molar evacuation serum β-hCG becomes normal in about 7–9 week). Majority of these patients need treatment with chemotherapy (90%). About 10% of patients can be treated successfully with a second curettage.

Spread of GTN

Apart from the local spread, vascular erosion takes place early and hence metastases occur rapidly. The common sites of metastases are lungs, anterior vaginal wall, brain and liver.

Clinical Features of GTN

Clinical features depend on the location of the primary growth and on its secondary deposits:
1. History of molar pregnancy in the recent past. It is rarely related to a term pregnancy, abortion or ectopic pregnancy. GTN after a molar pregnancy is always a choriocarcinoma.
2. Persistent ill health.
3. Hyperemesis.
4. Irregular vaginal bleeding, at times brisk.
5. Uneven swelling of the uterus.
6. Cough breathlessness and hemoptysis with lung involvement.
7. Headache, convulsion and paralysis with cerebral involvement.
8. Epigastric pain and jaundice with liver involvement.
9. Pallor of varying degree.
10. On bimanual examination—subinvolution of uterus is seen; there may be a purplish red nodule in the lower third of the anterior vaginal wall; unilateral or bilateral enlarged ovaries palpable through lateral fornices.
11. On chest X-ray, multiple infiltrates of various shapes in both lungs giving a 'snowstorm' appearance and pleural effusion may be present.
12. Raised level of serum hCG and urine hCG.
13. Pelvic sonography helps to localize the lesion.
The anatomical staging is described in **Table 72.3**.

TABLE 72.3: FIGO anatomical staging of gestational trophoblastic tumor (GTT).

Stages	Features
Stage I	The lesion is confined to the uterus
Stage II	The lesion spreads outside the uterus, but is confined to the genital organs
Stage III	The lesion metastasizes to the lungs
Stage IV	The lesion metastasizes to sites such as brain, liver or gastrointestinal tract

(FIGO: International Federation of Gynecology and Obstetrics)

Management of GTN

Preventive

1. Prophylactic chemotherapy following evacuation of molar pregnancy to 'at risk' women who are:
   a. Age over 35 years.
   b. Initial serum hCG ≥100,000 U/mL.
   c. Level of hCG level fails to become normal in 7–9 weeks or there is an elevation.
   d. Previous history of molar pregnancy.
   e. Unable for follow-up.
2. Meticulous follow-up following evacuation of hydatidiform mole for at least 6 months, to detect early evidence of GTN.
3. Selective hysterectomy in hydatidiform mole, i.e. women over 35 years.
4. Diagnostic uterine curettage in unexplained abnormal bleeding 8 weeks following term delivery or abortion.

Curative

1. *Chemotherapy:*
   a. Single drug regimen in low-risk cases (stage I) using methotrexate or folinic acid.
   b. Combination therapy for stages II, III and IV based on individualized assessment. Drugs include methotrexate, folinic acid, actinomycin D, cyclophosphamide and vincristine.
2. *Surgery:*
   a. Hysterectomy for lesions confined to the uterus in women above 35 years, with intractable hemorrhage or in whom accidental perforation occurred during uterine curettage.
   b. Lung resection in pulmonary metastasis, in drug resistant cases.
   c. Craniotomy for control of bleeding.
3. *Radiation:*
   a. Whole brain radiation for patients with brain metastasis.
   b. Whole liver radiation along with chemotherapy in hepatic metastasis.

Prognosis

Most women whose cancer has not spread can be cured and will maintain reproductive function. Complete cure is harder if:
- The disease has spread to liver or brain
- Level of hCG level is more than 40,000 m U/L when treatment begins
- Cancer recurred after chemotherapy
- Carcinoma occurred after a pregnancy that resulted in the birth of a baby (GTD coexisting with a normal fetus).

Prevention of Recurrence and Follow-up

For prevention of recurrence, additional chemotherapy following normalization of hCG level is recommended as follows:
- *Non-metastatic disease*: One cycle
- *Metastatic disease*: Two to three cycles based on the assessment of prognosis.

Follow-up is mandatory for all patients at least for 2 years. Serum hCG levels are to be monitored weekly for 3 months, monthly for 6 months and 6 monthly for life. Future conception is recommended after 1 year of completion of treatment with instruction for regular checkups.

CANCER OF CERVIX

Cancer cervix is the most common cancer in women of the developing countries where screening facilities are inadequate. It is a preventable disease as the different screening, diagnostic and therapeutic procedures are effective. Incidence of cervical cancer is steadily decreasing in the developed world.

The incidence in India according to the 2004 Indian Council of Medical Research (ICMR) report was between 14% and 24% of all female cancers. Major factors affecting the prevalence of carcinoma cervix in a population are economic factor, sexual behavior and degree of effective screening.

Epidemiology

Worldwide, cervical cancer is 12th most common and fifth most deadly cancer in women. It affects about 16 per 100,000 women per year and kills about 9 per 100,000 each year. Approximately 80% of cervical cancers occur in developing countries.

Causes

Human papilloma virus (HPV) infection is a necessary factor in the development of all cases of cervical cancer.

Other cofactors and risk factors provided by the American Cancer Society include:
1. Human immunodeficiency virus (HIV) infection, chlamydia infection, hormonal contraception, exposure to the hormonal drug diethylstilbestrol (DES) and family history of cervical cancer.
2. Early age at first intercourse and first pregnancy are also considered risk factors.

Signs and Symptoms

Patients are usually multiparous, in premenopausal age group. The early stages of cervical cancer may be completely asymptomatic. They may have previous history of postcoital or intermenstrual bleeding, which they ignored. Other symptoms are:
1. Vaginal bleeding: Irregular or continued and contact bleeding.
2. Offensive vaginal discharge.
3. Pelvic pain of varying degree due to involvement of uterosacral ligament or sacral plexus.
4. Leg edema due to progressive obstruction of lymphatics and/or iliofemoral veins by the tumor.
5. Back pain and leg pain.
6. Bladder symptoms such as frequency of micturition, dysuria, hematuria or true incontinence due to fistula formation.
7. Rectal involvement symptoms such as diarrhea, rectal pain, bleeding per rectum or even rectovaginal fistula.
8. Frequent attacks of pyelonephritis due to ureteric obstruction.
9. In late stages, patient may be cachectic and anemic with edema of legs.
10. Uremia in advanced stage.

Diagnosis

1. Pap smear is an effective screening test.
2. Speculum examination reveals the nature of the growth—ulcerative or fungating or bleeds on touch.
3. Bimanual examination reveals the induration and extent of growth to the vagina and to the sides.
4. Rectal examination to note the involvement of parametrium and extent to the lateral pelvic wall.
5. Biopsy for confirmation of diagnosis. Wedge biopsy is done for small lesion, which includes a portion of the healthy tissue as well. If the lesion is big and infected, a bit of tissue from the non-infected area is taken.
6. Ancillary aids for staging are cystoscopy, chest X-ray, intravenous pyelography and proctoscopy.
7. Scanning such as MRI and PET scanning are used to detect parametrial extension, and to define the tumor volume.

Diagnosis of Precancerous Lesions

Cervical intraepithelial neoplasia (CIN), the potential precursor to cervical cancer is often diagnosed on examination of biopsies. For premalignant dysplastic changes, the CIN grading is used. It classifies mild dysplasia as CIN1, moderate dysplasia as CIN2 and severe dysplasia as CIN3 in a pathology report. Histologic subtypes of invasive carcinoma of cervix are the following:
- Squamous cell carcinoma
- Adenocarcinoma

- Adenosquamous carcinoma
- Small cell carcinoma
- Neuroendocrine carcinoma.

Staging

Cervical cancer is staged by the International Federation of Gynecology and Obstetrics (FIGO) based on clinical examination **(Table 72.4)**. Diagnostic tests used in determining the stages are colposcopy, proctoscopy, endometrial curettage, hysteroscopy, cystoscopy, intravenous urography, X-ray of lungs and, skeleton and cervical conization.

Complications

The following complications may occur sooner or later as the lesion progresses:
- Hemorrhage
- Frequent attacks of ureteric pain due to pyometra especially with endocervical variety
- Vesicovaginal fistula
- Rectovaginal fistula, which is a comparatively rare complication
- Cystitis pyelonephritis and bladder dysfunction.

TABLE 72.4: Staging of cervical cancer FIGO.

Stages	Features
Stage 0	Full thickness involvement of the epithelium without invasion into the stroma (cancer in situ)
Stage I	Limited to the cervix
Stage IA	Diagnosed only by microscopy; no visible lesions
Stage IA1	Stromal invasion less than 3 mm in depth and 7 mm or less in horizontal spread
Stage IB	Visible lesion or a microscopic lesion with more than 5 mm of depth or horizontal spread of more than 7 mm
Stage IB1	Visible lesion 4 cm or less in greater dimension
Stage IB2	Visible lesion more than 4 cm
Stage II	Invades beyond cervix
Stage IIA	Without parametrial invasion, but involve upper two-third of vagina
Stage IIB	With parametrial invasion
Stage III	Extends to pelvic wall or lower third of vagina
Stage IIIA	Involves lower third of vagina
Stage IIIB	Extends to pelvic wall and/or causes hydronephrosis or non-functioning kidney
Stage IV	Extends outside the vagina
Stage IVA	Invades mucosa of bladder or rectum
Stage IVB	Distant metastasis

(FIGO: International Federation of Gynecology and Obstetrics).

Management

Primary Prevention

- Identifying high-risk women:
    - History of early sexual intercourse
    - History of age of first pregnancy
    - History of too many or too frequent birth
    - Low socioeconomic status
    - Poor maintenance of local hygiene
    - Sexually transmitted oncogenes [HPV and herpes simplex virus (HSV) type 2].
- Identifying high-risk men (spouses):
    - Multiple sex partners
    - Previous wife died of cancer.
- Employing positive measures:
    - Use of condom during early intercourse
    - Raise the age of marriage and first childbirth
    - Limitation of family size
    - Maintenance of local hygiene
    - Effective treatment of sexually transmitted disease (STD).

Secondary Prevention

Screening

The widespread introduction of screening for cervical cancer using papanicolaou test (Pap smear) has been found to reduce the incidence and mortality of cervical cancer in developed countries. It is recommended to start testing 3 or more years after first sex.

Treatment

The types of treatment employed for the invasive cancer are:
- Primary surgery
- Primary radiotherapy
- Chemotherapy
- Combination therapy.
  Treatment measures based on stages are:
1. Stage IA (microinvasive cancer) is usually treated by hysterectomy (removal of the whole uterus including part of the vagina).
2. Stage IA2: In addition to hysterectomy, the lymph nodes are also removed. For patients who desire to remain fertile, a local surgical procedure called '*loop electrical excision procedure*' (LEEP) or cone biopsy is done; another surgical option for patients who want to preserve fertility is *trachelectomy.*
3. For stages IB1 and IIA less than 4 cm can be treated with *radical hysterectomy* with removal of lymph nodes and radiation therapy. Radiation therapy with or without chemotherapy is given for patients who show high-risk features on pathologic examination. Tumors more than 4 cm can be treated with radiation therapy and cisplatin-based chemotherapy followed by hysterectomy.

Prognosis

Prognosis depends on the stage of cancer. With treatment, the 5-year relative survival rate for the earliest stage of invasive cancer is 92% and overall (all stages combined) 5-year survival rate is 72%.

According to the FIGO, survival improves when radiotherapy is combined with cisplatin-based chemotherapy.

As the cancer metastasizes to other parts of the body, prognosis drops drastically because treatment of local lesions is generally more effective than the whole body treatment such as chemotherapy.

CANCER OF THE VULVA

Vulval cancer is an abnormal growth of malignant cells (neoplasm, tumor) in the vulva. The vulva is defined as the female external genitalia and includes the labia majora, labia minora, clitoris and vestibule.

Incidence

The lesion is rare, about 1.7/100,000. About 70% of vulval cancers involve the labia majora, 15–20% involves the clitoris and another 15–20% involves the perineum. In about 5% of cases, the cancer is present at more than one site.

Etiology

The etiology remains unclear, but the following factors are seen related:

- Usually seen in postmenopausal women with median age of 60 years
- More common among white people
- Increased association with obesity, diabetes, hypertension and nulliparity
- Associated with local lesions such as chronic vulval dystrophy of atypical type
- Human papillomavirus
- Condyloma accuminata, herpes simplex, syphilis and lymphogranuloma venereum
- Chronic pruritus and poor hygiene
- Malignancies in other sites of genital tract.

Types of Vulval Cancer

- *Squamous cell carcinoma:* The vast majority (90%) of vulval cancers are squamous cell carcinomas, which originate from the epidermis of the vulval tissue. Carcinoma in situ is a precursor stage of squamous cell cancer prior to invading through the basement membrane. Most lesions originate in the labia majora. Other areas affected are the clitoris, fourchette and the local glands. Squamous cell lesions tend to grow with local extension and spread via local lymph system. The tumor may also invade adjacent organs such as the vagina, urethra and rectum and spread via their lymphatics.
- *Melanoma:* About 5% of vulval malignancy is caused by melanoma of the vulva. Such melanomas behave like melanomas in other locations and may affect a much younger population. Melanomas have a risk of metastasis unlike squamous cell carcinomas.
- *Basal cell carcinoma:* Basal cell carcinoma constitute about 1–2% of vulval cancer. It is a slowly growing lesion and affects the elderly. It behaves similar to basal cell carcinoma in other locations, i.e. it spreads to grow locally with low potential of deep invasion or metastasis.
- *Other lesions:* Vulvar lesion can be caused by other lesions such as adenocarcinoma or sarcoma.

Clinical Features

- The lesion is present in the form of a lump or ulceration, often associated with itching, irritation and sometimes local bleeding and discharge
- Dysuria, dyspareunia and pain in the vulvar region
- Melanomas have a typical dark discoloration
- Adenocarcinomas may arise from the Bartholin's gland and appear as a painful lump
- Inguinal lymph glands of one or both sides may be enlarged and palpable if there is associated infection
- Vulval ulceration, which bleeds on touching
- Edematous, indurated tissue surrounding the lesion.

Diagnosis

- Examination of the vulva
- Biopsy from the margin
- Supplemental evaluation including chest X-ray, intravenous pyelogram (IVP), cystoscopy and proctoscopy.

Staging

The clinical staging as outlined by FIGO is tabulated in **Table 72.5**.

Treatment

- Adequate treatment for persistent pruritus vulva in postmenopausal women
- Simple vulvectomy for advanced cancers where the disease has spread to adjacent organs such as urethra, vagina and rectum
- Radiation therapy and chemotherapy are usually not a primary choice of therapy, but may be used in selected cases of advanced cancer
- Chemotherapy followed by surgery, radiotherapy or both.

Prognosis

With negative groin nodes, the 5 year survival rate is about 75% of course it depends on factors such as stage and type of lesion, age and general health. Survival rate of 5 years is about 20% when pelvic lymph nodes are involved.

TABLE 72.5: Staging of vulval carcinoma (FIGO, 1995).

Stages	Features
Stage 0	Carcinoma-in situ: Vulval intraepithelial neoplasia (VIN-3)
Stage I	Tumor confined to the vulva and/or perineum is 2 cm or less in greatest dimension, nodes are not palpable
Stage IA	Stromal invasion no greater than 1 mm
Stage IB	Stromal invasion greater than 1 mm
Stage II	Tumor confined to the vulva and/or perineum is more than 2 mm in greatest dimension; nodes are not palpable
Stage III	Tumor of any size with: 1. Adjacent spread to the lower urethra and/or vagina, or the anus 2. Unilateral regional node metastasis
Stage IV	1. Tumor invades any of the following: Upper urethra, bladder mucosa, rectal mucosa, pelvic bone and/or bilateral regional node metastasis 2. Any distant metastasis including pelvic lymph nodes

(FIGO: International Federation of Gynecology and Obstetrics).

BARTHOLIN'S GLAND CANCER

A distinct mass or lump on either side of the opening to the vagina can be the sign of Bartholin's gland carcinoma. A lump in this area may sometimes be a Bartholin's gland cyst, which is more common. Treatment is surgery like that of squamous cell carcinoma of the vulva.

VAGINAL CANCER

Types

There are two main types of primary vaginal cancers and they are named after the cells from which they develop:
1. *Squamous cell carcinoma:* This is the most common type of vaginal cancer and found in the upper part of the vagina. It affects women between the ages of 50 and 70. Exact etiology is unknown. Following factors are often related:
   – Human papillomavirus
   – Progression from vulval intraepithelial neoplasia (VIN)
   – Previous irradiation therapy to the vagina or immunosuppression
   – Prolonged use of pessary.
2. *Clear cell carcinoma:* This type of carcinoma is found in adolescent girls who have had history of intrauterine exposure to diethylstilbestrol in first trimester.

The risk of developing clear cell adenocarcinoma of the vagina following DES exposure is 1 in 1,000 or less. These patients are more likely to develop adenomyosis and rarely adenocarcinoma. The lesion usually involves the upper third of the anterior vaginal wall.

Treatment is radical hysterectomy and vaginectomy with pelvic lymphadenectomy. Radiotherapy is reserved for advanced cases.

Signs and Symptoms of Primary Vaginal Cancer

The mean age of the patient is 55 years. The cancer may be asymptomatic, being accidentally discovered during routine screening procedure.

The most common symptoms are:
- Blood-stained vaginal discharge
- Postcoital vaginal bleeding and pain
- Urinary frequency, nocturia and hematuria
- Foul smelling vaginal discharge
- Rectal pain
- On vaginal examination ulcerative, nodular or exophytic growth.

Diagnosis

- Smear test for cytology
- Colposcopic examination and biopsy
- Biopsy from clinically suspected lesion
- Computed tomography scan
- Magnetic resonance image scan.

Staging

The clinical staging as outlined by FIGO is tabulated in **Table 72.6**.

Treatment

The treatment for vaginal cancer depends on a number of factors including age, general health, stage (size and extent of spread) grade (microscopic appearance) and the type of cancer. Radiotherapy, surgery and chemotherapy are used separately or in combination.

Surgery

1. *For growth limited to upper third:* Radical hysterectomy, partial vaginectomy, bilateral vaginal lymphadenectomy.

TABLE 72.6: Staging of vaginal carcinoma (FIGO, 1995).

Stages	Features
Stage 0	Carcinoma in situ
Stage I	Carcinoma is limited to the vaginal wall
Stage II	Carcinoma has involved subvaginal tissue, but has not extended to the pelvic wall
Stage IV	Carcinoma has extended beyond the true pelvis or has involved the mucosa of bladder or rectum
Stage IVA	Adjacent organs such as bladder, rectum involved
Stage IVB	Distant organs are involved

(FIGO: International Federation of Gynecology and Obstetrics)

2. *For growth limited to the lower third:* Radical vulvectomy with removal of bilateral inguinofemoral lymph nodes along with partial vaginectomy.
3. *For growth limited to middle third:* Radiation by external beam therapy with intracavitary or interstitial radiation. Care to be taken to prevent bladder or rectal injury.
4. In cases of failure with radiation therapy, pelvic exenteration operation (very extensive surgery) can be done.

Radiotherapy

For many patients with vagina cancer, radiotherapy is the most suitable treatment. In younger women, radiotherapy may be combined with chemotherapy, which is known as chemoradiation.

Teletherapy, a method of external radiation is administered on the pelvis encompassing the vagina. Additional radiation is delivered locally in the form of interstitial therapy or brachytherapy with iridium.

External radiation reduces the tumor volume and sterilizes the regional lymph nodes. Complications of radiotherapy include vaginal stenosis and bladder, and rectal fistulae.

Prognosis

The overall 5 year survival rate ranges from 80% for stage I disease to 10% for stage IV disease.

CANCER OF FALLOPIAN TUBE

Primary Fallopian Tube Cancer

Primary fallopian tube cancer is the rarest of all gynecologic cancers representing less than 1%. It is an abnormal growth of malignant cells in one or both of a woman's fallopian tubes.

Fallopian tube cancers are found in women between 60 and 64 years of age, but can also manifest in women in their mid 80s.

Pathology

The site is usually the ampullary part and the mucosa. Fimbrial end usually gets blocked resulting in hydrosalpinx. It is unilateral in 80% and mostly adenocarcinoma. In most cases, cancer that affects the fallopian tubes originates from some other part of the uterus like the cervix or endometrium. The cancer cells metastasize and then spread to the tubes.

Clinical Manifestations

- Patients are usually postmenopausal and nulliparous
- History of infertility and pelvic infection
- Vaginal bleeding after menopause
- Colicky pain in lower abdomen
- Intermittent vaginal discharge that is white, clear, watery or pink in color
- On bimanual examination, unilateral mass, which may be tender.

Diagnosis

- Many cases of fallopian tube cancer are accidentally discovered on laparotomy and histologic examination of the excised tube
- Clinical features as mentioned above
- CA 125 test, which measures the level of blood protein that is linked to certain gynecological cancers
- A CT scan and ultrasound examination of the pelvic region and uterus
- Laparoscopy in case of persistent postmenopausal bleeding with a negative cervical and endometrial pathology
- Ultrasound can help in the preoperative diagnosis.

Treatment

- Total hysterectomy with bilateral salpingo-oophorectomy along with omentectomy
- External pelvic radiation following surgery
- Chemotherapy after surgery to destroy residual tumor cells.

Prognosis

The prognosis is mostly unfavorable due to late diagnosis. Survival rate of 5 years ranges between 25% and 40%.

Secondary Fallopian Tube Cancer

Secondary fallopian tube cancers are more common (90%) than the primary. The common primary sites are ovary, uterus, breast and gastrointestinal tract. The mode of spread from the ovary or uterus is probably by lymphatics rather than direct spread. Diagnosis and treatment are same as for primary fallopian tube cancer.

BREAST CANCER

Breast cancer is a malignant tumor that starts in the cells of the breast. A malignant tumor is a group of cancer cells that can grow (invade) into surrounding tissues or spread (metastasize) to a distant area of the body. The disease occurs mostly in women, but men can also get it. Breast cancer is the second most prevalent cancer in women. The chance of developing breast cancer for an average 40-year-old woman is 1 in 1,000. The risk increases as women gets older. There is an increase of new cases in the recent years, which were attributed in part to the earlier detection of breast cancer through increased use of breast self-examination, clinical breast examination and diagnostic screenings, including mammography. Statistical evidence indicates that over an entire life time, a woman's risk for developing breast cancer is one in eight. When broken by age, the risk by age 39 is 1 in 209 and it increases to 1 in 24 by age 59. Approximately 80% of breast cancers are diagnosed after 50 years of age.

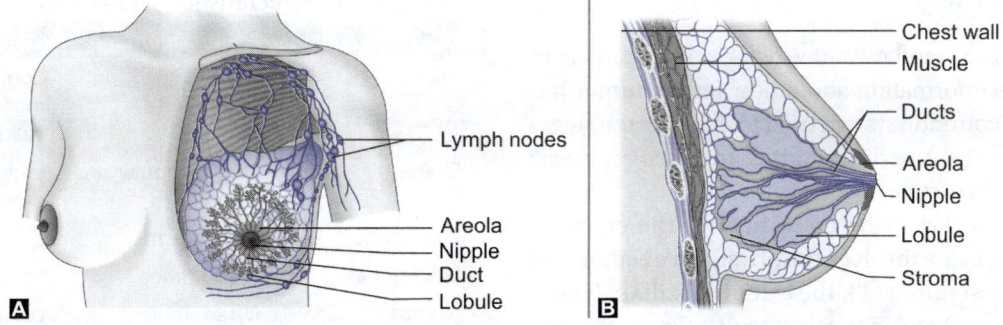

Figures 72.1A and B: Normal breast tissue. (A) Anteroposterior view; (B) Lateral view.

Normal Breast (Figs. 72.1A and B)

The female breast is made up mainly of lobules, which are milk producing glands; ducts, which are tiny tubes that carry the milk from the lobules to the nipple; and stroma, which contain fatty tissue and connective tissue surrounding the ducts and lobules as well as blood vessels and lymphatic vessels.

Lymphatic System of Breast (Fig. 72.2)

The lymph system is one way through which breast cancers can spread. This system has several parts. Lymph nodes are small bean-shaped collections of immune system cells (cells that are important in fighting infections) that are connected by lymphatic vessels. Lymphatic vessels carry clear fluid called lymph away from the breast. Breast cancer cells can enter lymphatic vessels and begin to grow in lymph nodes. Most lymphatic vessels are connect to lymph nodes under the arm (axillary lymph nodes) and those above or below the collar bones (supraclavicular or infraclavicular) near the nodes.

Risk Factors of Breast Cancer

The risk of breast cancer rises as women ages, mostly notable after age 40. Risk factors for breast cancer include:
- Family history of breast cancer (first-degree relative, i.e. mother, sister, daughter)
- Biopsy confirmed atypical hyperplasia
- Early menarche (before age 12)
- Late menopause (after age 55)
- Recent use of contraceptives or postmenopausal use of estrogen therapy
- Never having children or having the first child after age 30
- High socioeconomic status and high level of education
- Alcohol consumption of more than 2–5 drinks per day
- Presence of *BRCA1* or *BRCA2* (genes on chromosome-17) is responsible for majority of inherited breast cancers
- Obesity and high fat intake (controversial)
- Exposure to chemical carcinogens
- Poor diet and lack of exercise (lifestyle changes).

Malignant Breast Conditions

Localized Breast Cancer

Localized breast cancer, is one in which the cancer has not metastasized (spread), is usually less than 2 cm in size, is considered as noninvasive beyond the breast and has potential for the best client outcome. The lower the stage of breast cancer at the time of diagnosis, the better the outcome will be. According to the size of tumor, nodal involvement and metastasis the tumor size, node involvement, metastasis (TNM) method of staging cancer is used.

Management of localized breast cancer in which the cancer is confined to one area, can include lumpectomy (removal of the tumor and a small amount of surrounding tissue) and radiation therapy. Adjacent lymph nodes may also be removed.

Invasive Breast Cancer

Invasive breast cancer is that which has extended beyond the local epithelium and has the potential to spread from the breast to other areas of the body. Invasive cancer meets TNM criteria for stage 2 and 3.

Metastatic Breast Cancer

Metastatic breast cancer is the breast cancer that has spread to other parts of the body. It meets the criterion for TNM stage 4, which is a metastasized tumor of any size. Once metastasis occurs, there is no cure and life expectancy is short. Thus, therapeutic intervention is primarily supportive in nature.

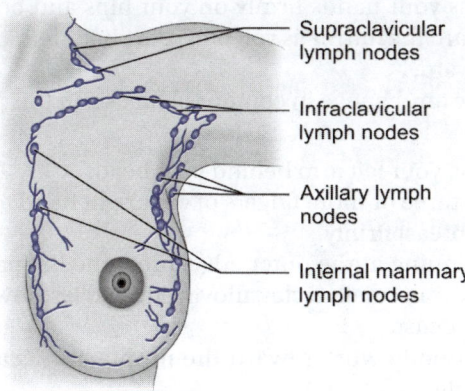

Figure 72.2: Lymph nodes in relation to the breast.

Staging of Breast Cancer

A staging system is a standardized way for cancer care team to summarize the information about how far the tumor has spread. The most common system used to describe the stages of breast cancer is the American Joint Committee on Breast Cancer (AJCC) TNM system.

Staging involves classifying the cancer by the extent of disease. Clinical staging involves the physician's estimate of the size of the breast tumor (T), the extent of axillary lymph node involvement (N) and metastasis to distant organs (M). The staging is determined by physical examination and imaging studies.

Stage 0: A precancer state of the breast; ductal carcinoma in situ (DCIS) and Paget's disease of the nipple with no invasion are precancer states of the breast.

Stage 1A: The tumor is 2 cm or less and has not spread to lymph nodes or to distant sites.

Stage 1B: The tumor is 2 cm or less with micrometastasis in 1–3 axillary lymph nodes.

Stage 2A: The tumor is 2 cm or less. Has spread to 1–3 axillary lymph nodes with the tumor in lymph nodes larger than 2 cm or less (sentinel, axillary or mammary lymph nodes).

Stage 2B: The tumor is larger than 2 cm, but less than 5 cm. It has spread to 1–3 axillary lymph nodes.

Stage 3A: The tumor is not more than 5 cm. It has spread to 4–9 axillary lymph nodes and no spread to distant sites.

Stage 3B: The tumor has grown into the chest wall or skin. It has spread to 1–3 axillary lymph nodes or it has enlarged the internal mammary glands.

Stage 3C: The tumor is of any size with spread to 10 or more axillary lymph nodes.

Stage 4: The cancer is of any size. It has spread to distant organs or to lymph nodes far from the breast. The most common sites are bone, liver, lung and brain.

Clinical Manifestations (Table 72.7)

Breast cancers can occur anywhere in the breast, but are usually found in the upper outer quadrant, where the most breast tissue is located. Generally, the lesions are nontender, fixed rather than mobile and hard with irregular borders. With the increased use of mammography, more women are seeking treatment at earlier stages of illness. These women often have no signs or symptoms other than a mammography abnormality. Women who ignore symptoms in early stages show up with signs of dimpling, nipple retraction or skin ulceration. Nipple thickening, pain and discharge are seen in patients with Paget's disease.

Diagnosis of Breast Cancer

Breast Self-examination

By regularly examining her own breasts, a woman is likely to notice any changes that occur. The best time for breast self-examination (BSE) is about a week after periods, when the breasts are not tender or swollen. If the periods are not regular, BSE is best done on the same day every month. It may be done either in standing position, in front of a mirror or in lying down (supine) position.

TABLE 72.7: Characteristics of breast masses.

	Fibroadenoma	Malignancy
• Age	Puberty to menopause	Common after menopause, 40 to 80 years
• Shape	Round, lobular or ovoid	Irregular or star-shaped or crab-like
• Consistency	Usually firm	Firm to hard
• Discreteness	Well defined	Not clearly defined
• Number	Often single	Usually single
• Mobility	Very mobile	May be mobile or fixed to skin or underlying tissue or chest wall
• Tenderness	Non-tender	Usually non-tender
• Erythema	No erythema	Erythema may be present
• Retraction/Dimpling	Not present	Often present

Examination in standing and supine positions
(Figs. 72.3A to E and 72.4A to C)

Step 1
1. Stand in front of the mirror. Check both breasts for anything unusual. Check for any change in contour of your breasts. Check the upper and outer part of your breast (toward the armpit); this is where half of all breast cancers are found.
2. Gently squeeze the nipple to check for discharge. Check for puckering, dimpling or scaling of the skin.

Step 2
1. Clasp your hands behind your head and press your hands forward.
2. Note any change in the contour of breasts.

Step 3
1. Press your hands firmly on your hips and bow slightly toward the mirror as you pull your shoulders and elbows forward.
2. Note any change in contour of breasts in this position.

Step 4
1. Raise your left arm behind your head.
2. Use three or more fingers of your right hand to feel your left breast firmly.
3. Beginning at the outer edge, press the flat part of your fingers in small circles, moving the circles slowly around the breast.
4. Gradually work toward the nipple and examine the nipple.
5. Be sure to cover the whole breast.

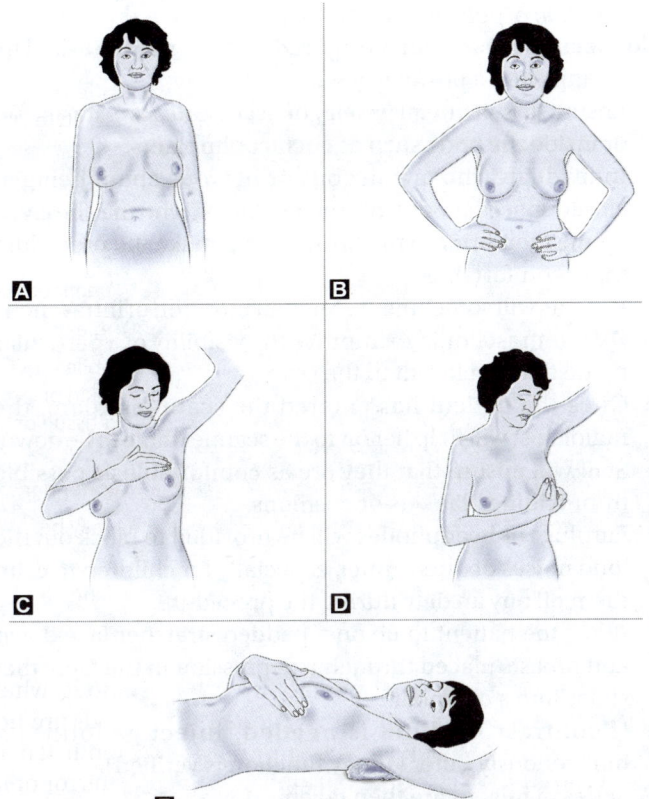

Figures 72.3A to E: Breast self-examination. (A) Standing infront of mirror; (B) Placing hands on hips; (C) Arms raised; (D) Examining nipple; (E) Examining in lying down position.

6. Pay special attention between the breasts and underarm, including the underarm itself.
7. Feel for any unusual lumps or masses under the skin.
8. Repeat the examination on the right breast.

Examination in lying down position

Step 5
1. Lie flat on your back with your left arm over your head and a pillow or folded towel under your left shoulder. This position flattens the breast and makes it easier to check.
2. Use the same circular motion described above, i.e. from periphery towards nipple. The entire surface of the breast is palpated from the outer edge of the breast to the nipple. Alternative palpation patterns are circular or clockwise, wedge and vertical strip **(Figs. 72.4A to C)**.
3. Repeat the same on right breast.

Clinical Examination

Physical assessment

When a patient presents with breast problem, the healthcare personnel conducts a general health assessment including history of cancer, obstetric history, present medications and use of hormonal contraceptives, hormonal therapy or fertility treatment.

Inspection of breasts

The breasts are inspected for size and symmetry. The skin is inspected for color, thickening or edema. Erythema (redness) may indicate benign local inflammation or a superficial lymphatic invasion by a neoplasm. To identify dimpling or retraction, the patient is instructed to raise both arms overhead as well as place her hands on her waist and push in. Changes seen during these suggest underlying mass.

Palpation

The breasts are examined with the patient sitting up (upright) and lying down (supine). The entire surface of the breast and axillary tail is systematically palpated using the pads of second, third and fourth fingers held together making small circles. The axillary lymph nodes are examined for size, location, mobility and consistency.

Mammography (Fig. 72.5)

Mammography is a breast imaging technique, which can detect non-palpable lesions and assist in diagnosing palpable masses. The breast is mechanically compressed from top to bottom (craniocaudal view) and side to side (mediolateral and oblique view) for obtaining pictures. Women may experience some fleeting discomfort because maximum compression is necessary for proper visualization. Mammography may detect a breast tumor before it is clinically palpable (i.e. smaller than 1 cm).

Ultrasonography

Ultrasonography (ultrasound) is used as a diagnostic adjunct to mammography to help distinguish fluid-filled cysts from other lesions. A thin coating of lubricating jelly is spread over the area to be imaged. A transducer is then placed on the breast. The transducer transmits high-frequency sound waves through the skin toward the area of concern. The technique diagnoses cysts with accuracy, but cannot rule out definitively the presence of malignant lesions.

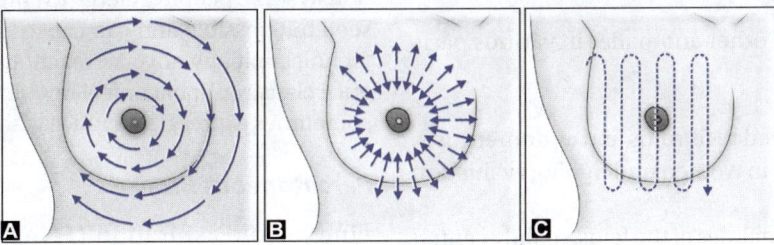

Figures 72.4A to C: Breast palpation patterns. (A) Circular; (B) Wedge; (C) Vertical strip.

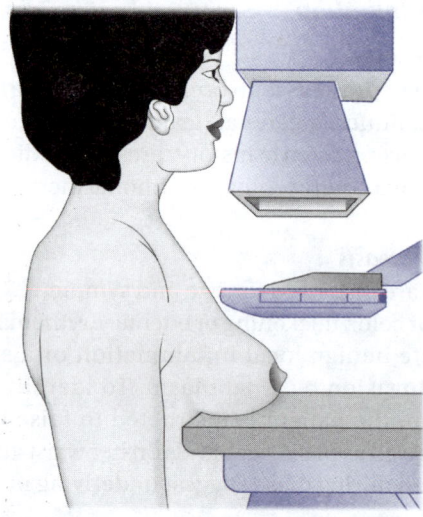

Figure 72.5: Mammography.

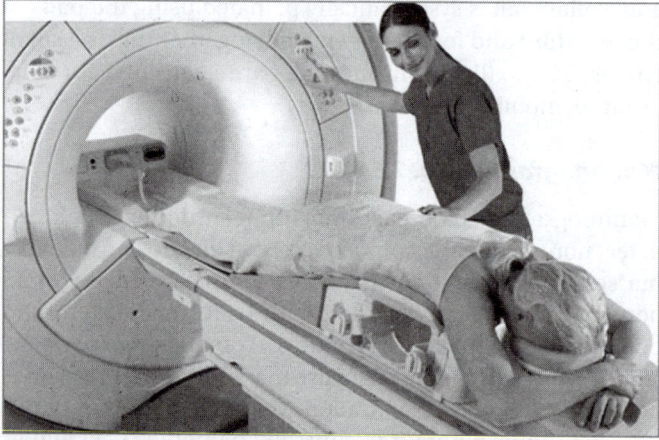

Figure 72.6: Magnetic resonance imaging (MRI) of the breast.

Magnetic Resonance Imaging (Fig. 72.6)

Definition
Magnetic resonance imaging is a non-invasive imaging technique that uses a magnetic field and computer generated radiowave to create detailed images of the organs and tissues inside of the body. It produces three-dimensional detailed anatomical images. An MRI scanner is a large tube that contains powerful magnets. The patient lies inside the tube during the scan **(Fig. 72.6)**.

Purposes
MRI scan is used to:
- Detect tumors, cysts and other anomalies in various parts of the body.
- Screen for breast cancer.
- Evaluate pelvic pain related to fibroids and endometriosis.
- Detect uterine anomalies in women undergoing evaluation for infertility.
- Detect congenital abnormalities of the fetus, mainly central nervous system anomalies.

Preparation of patient
No special preparation is required. Patient may be asked to:
- Change into a hospital gown.
- Ensure that no metal jewelry or accessories are present on or inside the body such as cochlear implants.
- Individuals who are anxious or nervous about being in closed spaces should inform the doctor, who may be given medication prior to the MRI, to help make the procedure more comfortable.
- Patients will sometimes receive an injection of intravenous (IV) contrast liquid to improve the visibility of a particular tissue that is relevant to the scan.
- Once the patient has entered the scanning room, the radiologist will help her on to the scanner table to lie down. Staff will ensure that they are as comfortable as possible by providing blankets or cushions.
- Earplugs or headphones will be provided to block out the loud noises of the scanner, especially for children to calm them off any anxiety during the procedure.
- Allow the patient to lie on a padded stretcher face down and breasts placed through a depression in the table that slides into a chamber.
- If contrast medium is needed, inject gadolinium intravenously (after kidney function is verified).
- Series of images are then taken.

During an MRI scan
Once inside the scanner, the MRI technician will communicate with the patient via the intercom to make sure that they are comfortable. They may not start the scan until the patient is ready. During the scan, it is vital to stay still. Any movement will disrupt the images much like a camera trying to take a picture of a moving object.
- Inform the patient that loud and changing noises will come from the scanner and this is perfectly normal.
- If the patient feels uncomfortable, during the procedure, they can speak to the technician via the intercom and request that the scan be stopped or press the buzzer to inform the technician, whichever facility is provided.
- After the scan, the radiologist will examine the images to check whether any more are required. If the radiologist is satisfied, the patient can go home.

Side effects
It is extremely rare that a patient will experience side effects from an MRI scan. However, the contrast dye if used, can cause nausea, headache and pain or burning at the point of injection in some people. Allergy to contrast material is also seldom seen but possible and can cause hives or itchy eyes. Notify the technician if any adverse reactions occur. People who experience claustrophobia or feel uncomfortable in enclosed spaces, sometimes express difficulties with undergoing an MRI scan.

Percutaneous Biopsy

Fine needle aspiration (FNA) is a non-invasive biopsy technique that is generally well tolerated by most women. For palpable masses, a surgeon performs this procedure. A small gauge needle (25 G or 22 G) attached to a syringe is inserted into the mass or area of nodularity. Suction is applied to the syringe and multiple passes are made through the mass. Any cellular material obtained in the hub of the needle is spread on a glass slide or placed in a preservative and sent to the laboratory for analysis.

Core Needle Biopsy

Core needle biopsy procedure is similar to FNA except a larger gauge needle is used (usually 14G). A local anesthetic is applied and tissue cores are removed via a spring loaded device. The procedure allows more definitive diagnosis than FNA, because actual tissue and not just cells are removed. It is often performed for relatively large tumors that are close to the skin. Ultrasound-guided core biopsy and MRI-guided core biopsy are newer diagnostic techniques.

Surgical Biopsy

Surgical biopsy is usually performed using local anesthesia and IV sedation. After an incision is made, the lesion is excised and sent to laboratory for pathologic examination.

Types
- *Excision biopsy:* This is the standard procedure for complete pathological assessment of a palpable breast mass. The entire mass, plus a margin of surrounding tissue is removed. This may be referred to as a lumpectomy. A frozen section analysis of the specimen may be performed at the time of biopsy by the pathologist who does an immediate reading intraoperatively and provides a provisional diagnosis for a patient who had no previous tissue analysis.
- *Incision biopsy:* This method surgically removes a portion of mass. This is done to confirm a diagnosis and to conduct special studies. This is often performed on women with locally advanced breast cancer or on women with suspected recurrence, whose treatment may depend on the results of special studies. This procedure is less common as core needle biopsy may give the same information.

Types of Breast Cancer

Ductal Carcinoma In Situ

The DCIS type of cancer is characterized by the proliferation of malignant cells inside the milk ducts without invasion into the surrounding tissues. Therefore it is a non-invasive form of cancer and is also called intraductal carcinoma. The DCIS is frequently manifested on mammogram with the appearance of calcifications and it is considered as breast cancer stage '0'. If DCIS is left untreated there is an increased likelihood that it will progress to invasive cancer. The most traditional treatment is total or simple mastectomy (removal of breast only) with a cure rate of 98–99%. Addition of the medication tamoxifen (Nolvadex) significantly reduced local recurrence rates after surgery and radiation. The medication is usually prescribed for 5 years.

Invasive Cancer

Infiltrating ductal carcinoma: This is the most common histological type of breast cancer and accounts for 75% of all cases. The tumor arise from the duct system and invade the surrounding tissues. They often form a solid irregular mass in the breast.

Infiltrating lobular carcinoma: This type of carcinoma accounts for 5–10% of all breast cancers. The tumor arise from the lobular epithelium and typically occur as an area of ill-defined thickening in the breast. They are often multicentric and can be bilateral.

Medullary carcinoma: This type of carcinoma accounts for about 5% of breast cancers and it tends to be diagnosed more often in women less than 50 years. The tumor grow in a capsule inside a duct. They can become large and may be mistaken for a fibroadenoma. The prognosis is often favorable.

Mucinous carcinoma: This type of carcinoma accounts for about 3% of breast cancer and often presents in postmenopausal women of age 75 years and older. A mucin producer and the tumor is also slow-growing and thus the prognosis is more favorable than in many other types.

Tubular ductal carcinoma: This type of carcinoma accounts for about 2% of breast cancer. Because axillary metastases are uncommon with this histology, prognosis is usually excellent.

Inflammatory carcinoma: This type of carcinoma is rear (1–2%) and aggressive type that has unique symptoms. The cancer is characterized by diffuse edema and brawny erythema of the skin, resembling an orange peel. This is due to malignant cells blocking the lymph channels in the skin. An associated mass may or may not be present. The disease can spread to other parts of the body rapidly. Chemotherapy is usually given to control the disease progression, but radiation and surgery may also be useful.

Paget's disease of breast: This disease accounts for 1% of diagnosed breast cancer cases. Symptoms typically include a scaly, erythematous, pruritic lesion of the nipple. Paget's disease often represents ductal carcinoma in situ of the nipple, but may have an invasive component.

Prognosis

The two most important factors considered while determining the prognosis of patient with breast cancer are the tumor size and whether the tumor has spread to the lymph nodes under the arm (axilla). Generally, the smaller the tumor, the better is the prognosis.

Carcinoma of the breast starts with a genetic alternation in a single cell and takes time to divide and double in size. A carcinoma may double in size (30 times) to became 1 cm or larger, at which point it becomes clinically apparent. Tumors are often present for several years before they become palpable. The most common route of regional spread is to the axillary lymph nodes. Distant metastasis can affect any organ, but the most common sites are bone, lung, liver, pleura, adrenals, skin and brain.

Treatment/Management

Surgical Management

The main goal of surgery is to obtain local control of the disease. For non-invasive breast cancers, the options are given below.

* *Breast conservation treatment:* Lumpectomy with wide excision, partial or segmental mastectomy and quadrantectomy.
* *Total mastectomy (Fig. 72.7):* The surgery involves removal of the breast and nipple- areola complex, but does not include axillary lymph node dissection. This may be performed for patients with non-invasive cancer, which does not have a tendency to spread to the lymph nodes. It may also be performed prophylactically for patients who are at high risk for breast cancer, e.g. those with BRCA mutation. For invasive cancers the surgical procedures recommended include the following.
* *Total mastectomy with sentinel lymph node dissection (SLND) or axillary lymph node dissection (ALND):* The sentinel lymph node is the first node in the lymphatic basin that receives drainage from the primary tumor in the breast. This is identified by injecting a radioisotope and/or blue dye into the breast, the radioisotope and dye then travel via lymphatic pathways to the node. The surgeon then identifies the node using a probe, excises it and sends it for pathologic analysis, i.e. frozen section analysis. If the sentinel lymph node is positive the surgeon proceeds with immediate ALND.
* *Modified radical mastectomy:* The procedure involves removal of the entire breast tissue, including the nipple-areola complex. In addition, a portion of the axillary lymph nodes are also removed (ALND). In modified radical mastectomy, the pectoralis major and pectoralis minor muscles are left intact, unlike in radical mastectomy in which the muscles are removed. Radical mastectomy is performed rarely these days.

Radiation Therapy

Radiation therapy is used to decrease the chance of local recurrence in the breast by irradiating residual microscopic cancer cells. Breast conservation treatment followed by radiation therapy for stage 1 and 2 breast cancer results in a survival rate equal to that of modified radical mastectomy.

External beam radiation is the most common type, which begins about 6 weeks after breast surgery. If systemic chemotherapy is indicated, radiation therapy usually begins after its completion. External beam radiation, which delivers high-energy photons from a linear accelerator, is administered to the entire region. Each treatment lasts only for few minutes and generally given 5 days a week for 5–6 weeks.

Another approach is intraoperative radiation therapy (IORT) in which a single intense dose of radiation is delivered to the surgical site in the operating room immediately following the lumpectomy. This method of radiation is indicated for women at high risk for cancer recurrence (i.e. chest wall involvement, four or more positive nodes and tumors larger than 5 cm).

Generally, radiation therapy is well tolerated. Acute side effects consist of mild- to-moderate erythema, breast edema and fatigue. Occasionally skin breakdown may occur. These side effects usually dissolve within few weeks to few months.

Self-care instructions for patients receiving radiation include:
* Use of mild soap with minimal rubbing
* Avoiding deodorants and perfumed soaps
* Use of hydrophilic lotions (water dissolving) such as Eucerin, Lubriderm or Aquaphor
* Avoiding tight clothes, excessive temperatures and ultraviolet light
* Use of non-drying soap if pruritus occurs.

Sun exposure to the treated area to be minimized and use of sunscreen lotion with sun protection factor (SPF) of 15 or above is advised. Momentary sharp or shooting pains of minor degrees are normal after radiation.

Chemotherapy (Systemic)

Chemotherapy as an adjuvant therapy and involves the use of anticancer agents in addition to other treatments (i.e. surgery, radiation) to delay or prevent recurrence of breast cancer. It is considered for patients who have positive lymph nodes or invasive tumors.

Chemotherapy regimens combines several agents (polychemotherapy) generally administered over a period of 3–6 months. A regimen of cyclophosphamide, methotrexate and fluorouracil is usually given to patients who are at low risk of recurrence. In combination regimen, combination of cyclophosphamide, doxorubicin (Adriamycin) and fluorouracil (CAF) is administered to higher risk patients. Common physical side effects of chemotherapy for breast

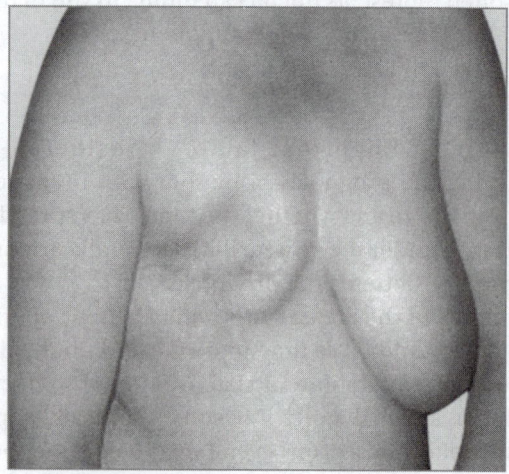

Figure 72.7: Postmastectomy (right) breast.

cancer may include nausea, vomiting, bone marrow suppression, taste changes, alopecia, mucositis, skin changes and fatigue. A weight gain of more than 5 kg occurs in about half of all patients, the cause is unknown.

Hormonal Therapy

The use of adjuvant hormonal therapy, with or without the addition of chemotherapy, is considered in women who have hormone receptor-positive tumors. Its use can be determined by the results of an estrogen and progesterone receptor assay. About two-thirds of breast cancers are found to be estrogen receptor-positive. Hormone therapy involves the use of medications that compete with estrogen by binding to the receptor sites or by blocking estrogen production [selective estrogen receptor modulators (SERMs)]. Premenopausal and perimenopausal women are more likely to have non-hormonal dependent lesions, whereas postmenopausal women are more likely to have hormone-dependent lesions.

Tamoxifen has been the primary hormonal agent used in the treatment of premenopausal and postmenopausal breast cancers. Tamoxifen has estrogen antagonistic (estrogen blocking) effects on certain tissues. Its effect in the breast prevent estrogen from binding to the receptor sites thus preventing tumor growth. Tamoxifen can also stop the growth and even shrink tumors in women with metastatic breast cancer. It can also be used to reduce the risk of developing breast cancer in women at high risk.

Side effects of adjuvant hormonal therapy include hot flashes, vaginal dryness, nausea and vomiting, risk of thromboembolic events and risk of osteoporosis. Patients need to be instructed to take measures for prevention and management of such conditions.

Breast Reconstruction after Surgery

Breast reconstruction can provide a significant psychological benefit for women who are struggling with the emotional distress of losing a breast. Consultation with a plastic surgeon can help the patient understand the procedures for which she is a candidate. Factors to consider include body size and shape, physical health and personal habits. Realistic explanation can help the patient avoid unrealistic expectations. Once reconstruction is complete, the opposite breast may require augmentation, reduction or mastopexy to achieve symmetry on both sides.

Prosthetics

Breast prosthesis is an external form, which simulates the breast and is another option for breast reconstruction. Most prosthesis is made of silicone. They can be placed inside a pocket, in a bra or can adhere directly to the chest wall. Until the surgical incision is well healed, i.e. 4–6 weeks, temporary lightweight cotton filled form can be used. Breast prosthesis can provide a psychological benefit and assist the woman in resuming proper posture, because it helps balance the weight of the remaining breast.

Prevention Strategies in the High-risk Patients

American Cancer Society (ACS) recommend following prevention strategies:
1. *Long-term surveillance:* This includes clinical breast examination twice a year starting as early as 25 years of age:
   - Mammograms from age 25
   - Breast self-examinations from age 25
   - Ultrasound and MRI of breasts in addition to screening tests. MRI is more sensitive than mammography in *BRCA1* and *BRCA2* carriers (Warner, Plews, Hill et al. 2004).
2. *Chemoprevention:* It is a primary prevention modality that aims at prevention of the disease before it starts. The drug tamoxifen was found to be an effective chemotherapeutic agent.
      Raloxifene (Evista) is another medication found effective in reducing breast cancer risk with fewer side effects.
3. *Prophylactic mastectomy:* It is an another therapeutic modality found effective in reducing the risk of cancer by 90%. Possible candidates include women with a strong family history of breast cancer, a diagnosis of atypical hyperplasia, *BRCA* gene mutation and previous cancer in one breast.

Potential Complications of Surgical Management

Possibility of developing some potential problems must be considered and these include:
- Lymph edema of the affected arm
- Hematoma or seroma formation
- Infection.

Nursing Management

The diagnosis of cancer or its recurrence causes great anxiety in patients about their future and long-term survival. Some patients are more likely than others to experience side effects of certain therapies such as vomiting after chemotherapy and edema after radiation therapy. This allows nurses to reduce their discomforts and teach about appropriate management strategies. The nurse must understand that the patients who undergo mastectomy and lymph node dissection may experience problems such as lymphedema, decreased arm mobility and seroma formation (collection of serous fluid) in the axilla, and neuropathic sensations with resulting distress. Psychological needs of the patient should also be addressed.

Nursing Assessment

Assessment for patients with breast conditions involve careful medical and gynecologic history taking with special emphasis on breast history including symptoms, especially suspected of breast conditions, laboratory test results and biopsy reports.

Preoperative Nursing Diagnoses

Based on the health history and other assessment data, major preoperative nursing diagnoses may include the following:
- Deficient knowledge about the planned surgical treatments
- Anxiety related to the diagnosis of cancer
- Fear related to specific treatments and body image changes
- Risk for ineffective coping (individual or family) related to diagnosis of breast cancer and related treatment options
- Decisional conflict related to treatment options.

Postoperative Nursing Diagnoses

Major postoperative nursing diagnoses may include the following:
- Pain and discomfort related to surgical procedure
- Disturbed sensory perception related to nerve irritation in affected arm, breast or chest wall
- Disturbed body image related to loss or alteration of the breast
- Risk for impaired adjustment related to the diagnosis of cancer and surgical treatment
- Self-care deficit related to partial immobility of upper extremity on affected side
- Risk for sexual dysfunction related to loss of body part, change in self-image and fear of partner's responses
- Deficient knowledge regarding drain management following surgery
- Deficient knowledge regarding arm exercises to regain mobility of affected extremity
- Deficient knowledge regarding hand and arm care after an ALND.

Patient Goals to be Achieved

The major goals of nursing care may include increased knowledge about the disease and its treatment, reduction of preoperative and postoperative fear, anxiety and emotional stress, improvement of decision-making ability; pain management, improvement in coping abilities, improvement of sexual function and the absence of complications. Plans for nursing interventions should include specific actions that the client completes to achieve the highest level of wellness possible or to achieve peace regarding the diagnosis.

Nursing Interventions

Nursing interventions should be planned and implemented to achieve the goals listed above in the pre- and postoperative periods. Adequate health educations to be provided to enable the patient to go home without undue fear and anxiety, when discharged from the hospital.

Interventions involve educating the clients regarding the diagnosis, consequences, specific procedures, counseling regarding expected outcomes, providing emotional support as well as reducing anxiety, fear and stress. It is important to educate about strategies for promotion of good health, disease prevention and recommendations for regular exercise, healthy eating and scheduling necessary assessments and screening (medical checkups).

Patient Education for Hand and Arm, and Care after Axillary Lymph Node Dissection

- Avoid blood pressure readings, injections and blood draws in affected extremity
- Use sunscreen (higher than SPF 15) for extended exposure to sun
- Apply insect repellent to avoid insect bites
- Wear gloves for gardening
- Use cooking mitt for removing objects from oven and pot-holding forceps for removing vessels from stove/cooktops
- Avoid cutting cuticles and nails too short
- Use electric razor for shaving arm pit
- Avoid lifting objects greater than 2–4 kg
- Perform hand exercise after mastectomy operation to maintain movements of the affected hand and to avoid/reduce lymph edema
- If a trauma or break in the skin occurs, wash the area with soap and water, and apply an antibacterial ointment (bacitracin or Neosporin). Observe the area and extremity for 24 hours; if redness, swelling or a fever occurs, contact physician.

POSTMASTECTOMY EXERCISES

Postmastectomy exercises are done by patients who have undergone mastectomy or surgical removal of one or both breasts to avoid possible movement restrictions, contractures and lymph edema.

Purposes

- To increase blood circulation.
- To increase muscle strength.
- To prevent joint stiffness and contractures.
- To restore full range of motion of arms.

Importance of Postmastectomy Exercises

Exercises after mastectomy help to:
- Regain and maintain normal movement of arms and shoulders.
- Decrease the side effects of surgery and help to get back to normal activities.
- Reduce after-surgery limitations in shoulder range of motion.
- Reduce pain in chest wall, shoulders and neck.
- Return to daily activities faster such as wearing dress, bathing, etc.
- Keeps muscles strong.
- Improves overall well-being.

Articles Needed for Different Exercises

1. A rod or broom stick.
2. A squeeze ball.

Patient Instructions

1. Begin exercises like deep breathing the day after surgery as appropriate and advised by the doctor.
2. Plan to take pain medications 20 to 30 minutes before starting exercises.
3. Do the exercises three times a day, every day, until you have regained full range of motion in your arm(s).
4. Try to do the exercises daily at the same time as far as possible, for example, before breakfast, lunch and dinner.
5. Wear comfortable, loose clothing.
6. Exercise after a warm shower, whenever possible, when the muscles are warm and relaxed.
7. Breathe deeply and often as you do each exercise.
8. Do the exercise until you feel a slight stretch and no pain?
9. Do not exercise too much in the early weeks following surgery.
10. If you have more pain or discomfort than before, you may be doing too much exercise.

General Guidelines for Exercises

Start the following exercises 3–7 days after surgery when your doctor says it is alright.

- Use the hand on your affected side to comb hair, bathe, get dressed and eat.
- With your arm raised, open and close your hand 15–20 times.
  - Bend and straighten your elbow several times.
  - Bend your elbow and touch your opposite shoulder a few times.
  - Raise your arm up to shoulder height or whatever is tolerable without putting strain on your drains. Repeat 3 to 4 times.
- Practice deep breathing exercise at least six times a day. This exercise will help maintain normal movement of chest making it easier for your lungs to work. Further exercise can be started a week or more after surgery after your doctor says it is alright.
- Wear comfortable loose clothing when doing the exercise.
- Do the exercise slowly until you feel a gentle stretch and hold each stretch till the end of the motion and slowly count to five.
- Do each exercise 5–7 times and try to do the exercise correctly.
- Do the exercise twice a day until you get back to your normal flexibility? Continuing to do some exercises during the months after surgery can help you keep good mobility of your hand.
- Be sure to take deep breaths, in and out as you do each exercise.
- The exercises are set up so that you start them lying down, move to sitting and finish them standing up.

Stage 1 Exercises

These are exercises that can be taken while the drains are still in place **(Figs. 72.8 to 72.12)**.

1. *Pump it up (Fig. 72.8):* This exercise helps reduce swelling after surgery by using the muscles as a pump to improve the circulation in the affected arm.
   - Patient to lie on the unaffected side with the affected arm straight out, resting on top of a pillow.
   - Slowly bend the elbow while making a fist at the same time.
   - Next, slowly straighten your elbow while opening the fist at the same time.
   - Repeat this pumping motion 15–25 times.

2. *Shoulder circles/shoulder rolls (Fig. 72.9):* This exercise can be done sitting or standing. This can help relieve tension in the shoulders.
   - Lift both shoulders up toward your ears, keeping the chin tucked in slightly.
   - Gently rotate both shoulders forward, arm slowly down and back making a circle.
   - Make five slow circles in one direction, then switch and make five slow circles in the opposite direction.

3. *Arm lifts (Fig. 72.10):* This exercise can be done sitting or standing, it helps improve movement in shoulders.
   - Clasp the hands together in front of chest. Point the elbows out.
   - Slowly lift the arms upwards until you feel a gentle stretch, but no pain.

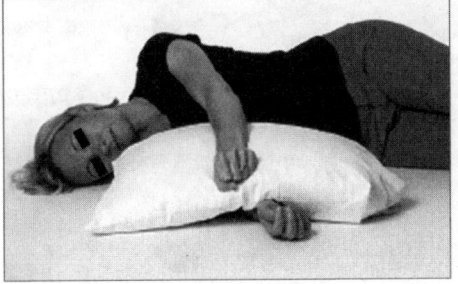 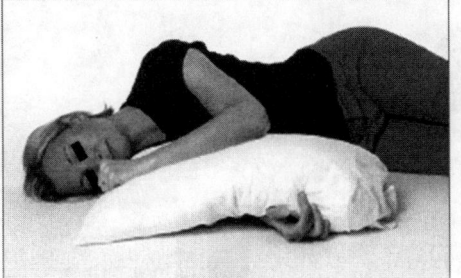 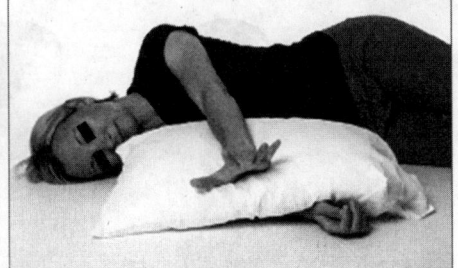

Figure 72.8: Pump it up exercise.

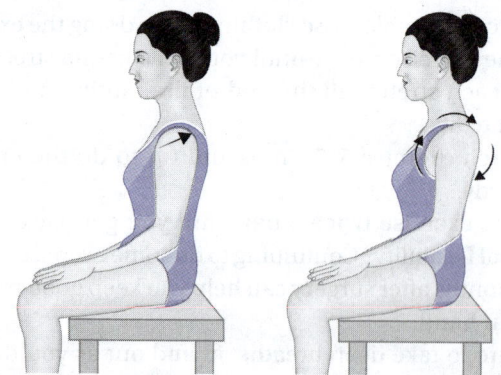

Figure 72.9: Shoulder circles or shoulder rolls exercise.

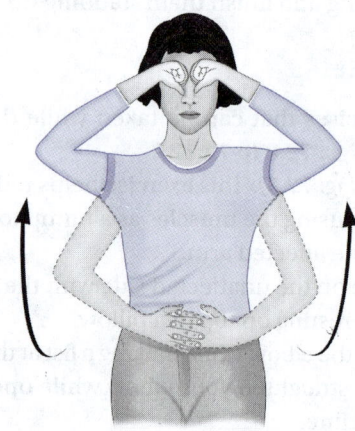

Figure 72.10: Arm lift exercise.

- Hold for 5–10 seconds and then slowly return to the start position.
- Repeat 5–10 times.

4. *Shoulder blade squeeze (Fig. 72.11):* This exercise helps increase your shoulder blade movement.

This can be done sitting (without resting the back on the chair) or standing.

- Hold the arms at the side, against body with elbows bent.
- Slowly bring the elbows straight backwards, while squeezing the shoulder blades together to feel a gentle stretch.
- Hold this position for 5–10 seconds and then slowly return to the start position.
- Relax your arm(s) and repeat 5–7 times.
- Remember to keep breathing throughout the stretch.

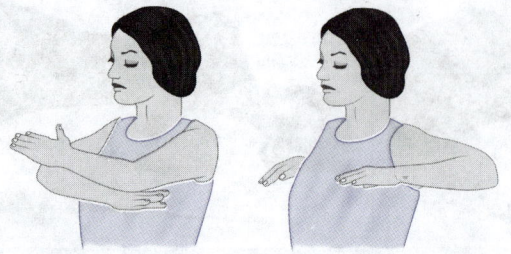

Figure 72.11: Shoulder blade squeeze exercise.

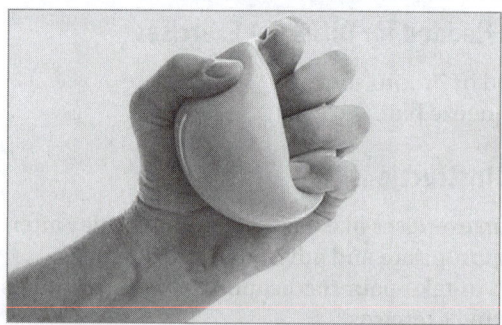

Figure 72.12: Ball squeezing exercise.

5. *Ball squeezing exercise (Fig. 72.12):* A rubber ball or a crumpled newspaper is squeezed in the hand of the involved side.
- Hold the ball and squeeze it as hard as possible with thumb and fingers.
- Squeeze for 3–5 seconds and then release.
- Perform ten repetitions before doing it with the other hand (if needed).

Stage 2 Exercises

These exercises are to be done after the drain(s) have been removed **(Figs. 72.13 to 72.20)**.

6. *Wand exercises (external rotation) (Fig. 72.13):* This exercise helps increase your ability to move your shoulders forward.

To do this exercise, a wand (cane) is required—try a broom handle, rod or stick.
- Lie on your back with knees bend. Hold the wand/rod in hands. The hands should be as wide apart as shoulders.
- Lift the wand over the head as far as you can until you feels a stretch. The unaffected arm can be used to lift the wand higher.
- Hold for five seconds, then gently lower arms.
- Repeat 5–10 times.

7. *Elbow spread exercise (winging it exercise) (Fig. 72.14):* This exercise helps to stretch the front of chest and shoulders. Do the exercise on a bed or floor.
- Lie on the back with the knees bend.
- With the fingers touch the ears with the elbows pointed to the ceiling.

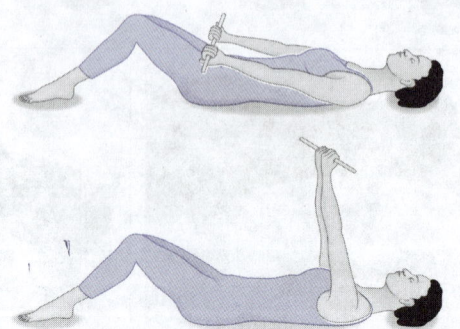

Figure 72.13: Wand exercise.

Chapter 72: **Genital Malignancies** 687

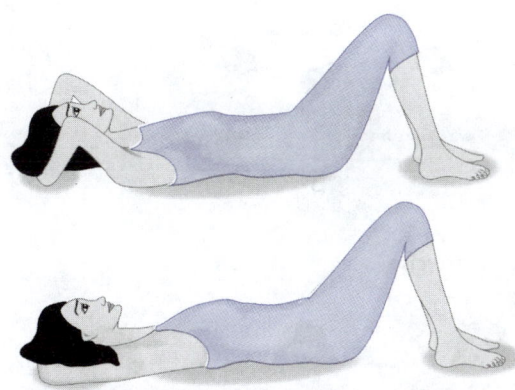

Figure 72.14: Elbow spread exercise.

- Move the elbows apart until a stretch is felt, but no pain.
- Hold this position for 5–10 seconds, and then slowly return to the start position.
- Remember to keep breathing throughout the stretch.

8. *Wall climbing (wall crawling) (Figs. 72.15A and B):* This exercise help increase movements in shoulders. Try to reach a little higher on the wall each day. This exercise is done in two positions:

i. Facing the wall **(Fig. 72.15A)**
- Stand facing the wall.
- Place the palm of the hand of affected arm flat on the wall.
- Slowly slide the hand up the wall as high as the patient can until she feels a stretch, but no pain.
- Hold for 5–10 seconds.
- Return to the start position.
- Repeat 5–10 times.

If surgery was done on both sides, repeat this exercise with the other arm.

ii. Sidewall stretch **(Fig. 72.15B)**
- Stand with your affected side to the wall.
- Place the palm of your hand flat against the wall.
- Slowly slide the hand up the wall, as high as the patient can go until she feels a stretch. Do not rotate the body toward the wall. Keep the body facing forward even if it means you cannot go up as high.
- Hold for 5–10 seconds.

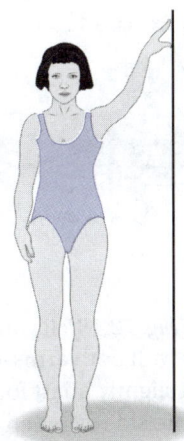

Figure 72.15B: Wall climbing exercise side wall stretch.

- Return to start position.
- Repeat 5–10 times.

9. *Side bends (Fig. 72.16):* This exercise is more advanced and can be performed once a day when the patient feels ready.
- Sit on a chair and clasp both hands together in the lap.
- Slowly lift both arms above the head.
- Bend at the waist to move the body to the right. Use the right hand to gently pull the left arm a little further to the right. Keep sitting firmly on the chair.
- Hold this position for five seconds and then slowly return to the start position.
- Repeat this stretch to the left side using the left hand to pull the right arm further.
- Repeat 5–10 times.

10. *Arm swinging/pendulum exercise (Fig. 72.17):* Pendulum exercise is to prevent shoulder joint stiffness.
- Lean over with your arm supported on a table or chair.
- Relax the arm of the affected side, letting it hang straight down.
- Slowly begin to swing the relaxed arm by moving the body.
- Let gravity gently sway the arm.
- Move the arm in a circle, then reverse the direction. Next move the arm backward and forward.
- Do this exercise three times a day, for 5–10 minutes

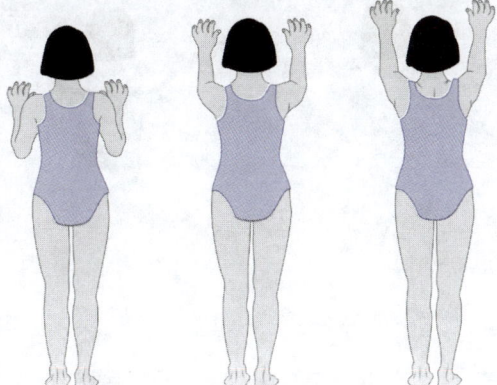

Figure 72.15A: Wall climbing facing the wall.

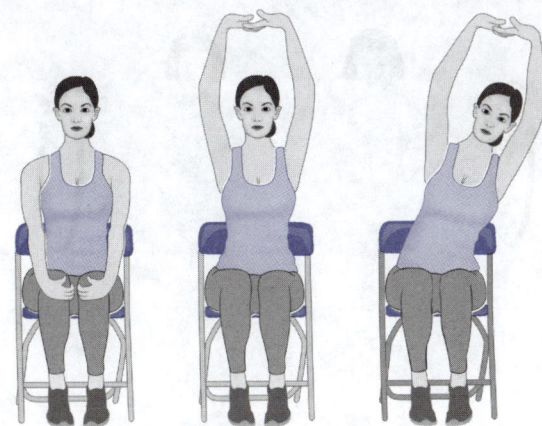

Figure 72.16: Side bends exercise.

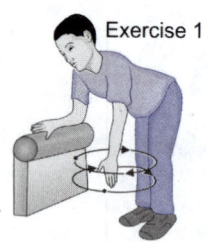 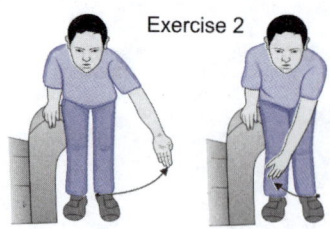 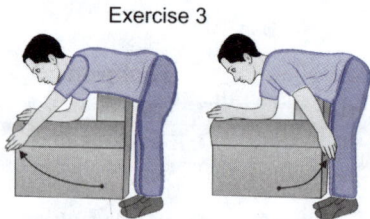

Figure 72.17: Arm swinging/pendulum exercise.

11. *Arm circle exercise (Fig. 72.18):* If you had surgery on both breasts do this exercise with both arms, one arm at a time.
   ❖ Stand with your feet slightly apart for balance. Raise your affected arm out to the side as much as you can.
   ❖ Start making slow backward circles in the air with your arm. Make sure you are moving your arm from your shoulder and not from elbow. Keep your elbow straight.
   ❖ Increase the size of circles until they are as big as you can comfortably make them. If you feel any aching of if your arm is tired, take a break. Start doing the exercise when you feel better.

12. *Hands behind head exercise (Fig. 72.19):* This exercise can be done while sitting or standing.
   ❖ The exercise can be done in sitting or standing position
   ❖ Clasp your hands together on your lap if sitting, and clasp the extended hands in front at the hip level if standing
   ❖ Slowly raise the clasped hands towards the head, up to forehead level. Do not bend your head forward
   ❖ Slide your hands behind your head until you reach well at the back of your neck. When you get to this point, spread your elbows out to the sides. Hold in this position for one minute.
   ❖ Slowly bring your elbows together and slide your hands over your head and then bring them down.
   ❖ Repeat the steps at a slower pace and perform the exercise.

13. *Figure "W" exercise (Fig. 72.20):* You can do this exercise while sitting or standing.
   ❖ Form a "W" with your arms out to the side and arms facing forwards. Try to bring your up so they are even with your face. Then bring them to the highest comfortable position.

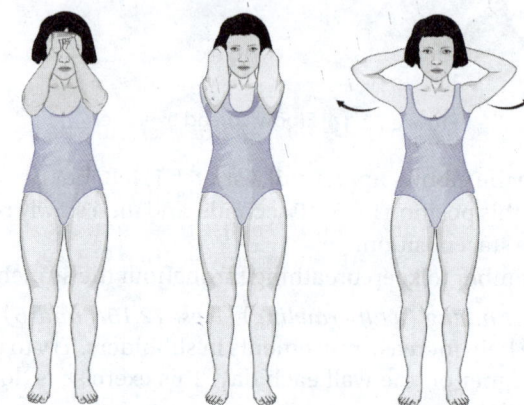

Figure 72.19: Hands behind head exercise.

   ❖ Pinch your shoulder blades together as if you are squeezing a pencil between them.
   ❖ Hold the furthest position that does not cause discomfort. Squeeze your shoulder blades together and downward for five seconds.
   ❖ Slowly bring your arms back down to the starting position. Repeat the movement 10 times.

Precautions to be Taken

❖ If any shortness of breath, pain or tightness in the chest is felt, stop exercising immediately. Inform the doctor to develop a plan of movement right for the patient.
❖ If changes are noticed in the arm, hand, trunk or shoulder including swelling stop doing upper body exercises and inform doctor.

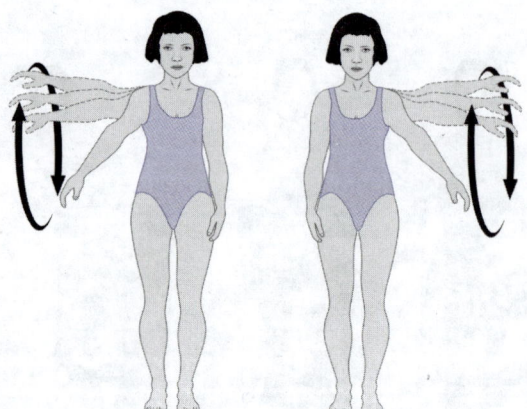

Figure 72.18: Arm circle exercise.

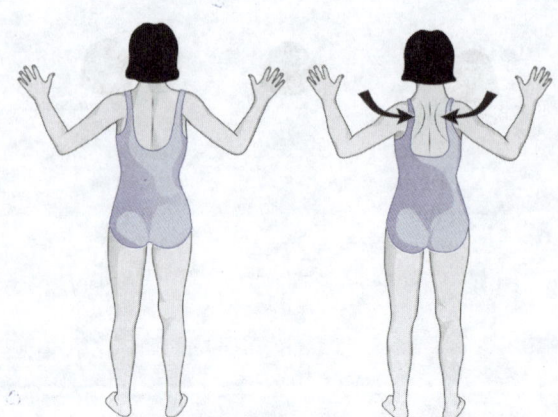

Figure 72.20: Figure "W" exercise.

Special Considerations

1. Proper assessment should be done before and after exercise to prevent complications.
2. Inform the treating physician for any untoward complications noted. Early detection can lessen the extent of damage that might happen.
3. It may take 6–8 weeks to regain full movement of arm(s). If difficulties in regaining full movement in arms after this time, the surgeon may make a referral to physiotherapy.

Support of Family Members after Breast Surgery

Family members and significant others should be included in the treatment plan and follow-up care of patients. The highest priorities in the care of patients should be alleviating pain and providing comfort measures. They also play an impotent role in providing palliative care if indicated.

NURSING MANAGEMENT OF PATIENTS WITH GENITAL MALIGNANCIES

Nursing management includes those related to the patient's treatment plan, which may include surgery, chemotherapy, radiation, palliation or combination of these. Emotional support, comfort measures and information plus attentiveness and caring are important components of nursing care for the patient and her family.

Nursing Interventions

Nursing interventions after pelvic surgery to remove the tumor are similar to those after other abdominal surgeries. Patients with pelvic organ cancer may develop ascites and pleural effusion. Nursing care may include administering intravenous (IV) fluids prescribed to alleviate fluid and electrolyte imbalance, administering parenteral nutrition to provide adequate nutrition, providing postoperative care after intestinal bypass to avoid any obstruction, controlling pain and managing drainage tubes. Comfort measures may include providing small frequent meals, decreasing fluid intake, administering diuretic agents and providing rest.

Nursing Diagnoses

The possible major nursing diagnoses include the following:

- Anxiety related to the diagnosis of cancer and surgery
- Acute pain related to the surgical incision and subsequent wound care
- Impaired skin integrity related to the wound and drainage
- Sexual dysfunction related to change in body image
- Self-care deficit related to lack of understanding of health status and care needs
- Deficient knowledge of the perioperative aspects and postoperative self-care.

STUDY QUESTIONS

Short Answer Questions

1. List the risk factors for ovarian cancer.
2. Etiology of uterine cancer.
3. Choriocarcinoma.
4. Malignant breast conditions.
5. Outline patient instructions following lymph node dissection.

Essay Questions

1. Explain cancer of cervix, its causes, signs and symptoms and diagnostic measures. Discuss the treatment of cervical cancer.
2. Discuss the nursing management of patients with genital malignancies.
3. Explain breast self-examination (BSE).
4. Explain the nursing management of client admitted for unilateral mastectomy with axillary lymph node dissection (ALND).

CHAPTER 73

Special Gynecological Conditions

Learning Objectives

Upon completion of this chapter, the learner will be able to:
- Discuss the pathological changes manifestations and management of adenomyosis, endometriosis and dyspareunia.
- Describe the physiological changes, symptoms and management of females in puberty and menopause.

ADENOMYOSIS

Adenomyosis is a condition where there is ingrowth of the endometrium directly into the myometrium. It is an ectopic occurrence of adenomatous tissue in the uterine muscle.

Pathology

The growth and tissue reaction in the endometrium depend on the response of ectopic endometrial tissue to the ovarian hormones. The response to hormones is minimal, if the basal layer only is involved and marked if the functional layer is involved. There is hyperplasia of the myometrium producing diffuse enlargement of the uterus sometimes symmetrically, but at times more on the posterior wall. The growth may be localized or diffuse. When localized, it may grow to the size of a large orange or 12–14 weeks pregnant uterus. Unlike fibroid, there is no capsule surrounding the growth **(Fig. 73.1)**.

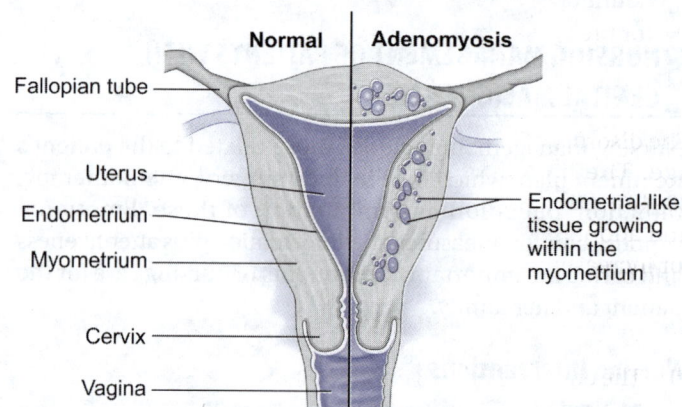

Figure 73.1: Adenomyosis of the uterus.

Clinical Features

About one-third, the condition remains asymptomatic. Patients are usually parous with age over 40:
1. Menorrhagia (70%) excessive bleeding occurs due to bigger uterine cavity associated with endometrial hyperplasia and inadequate uterine contraction.
2. Dysmenorrhea (30%) colicky, pain during menses probably due to disturbed myometrial contraction.
3. Frequency of micturition.
4. Intermenstrual bleeding.
5. Pain during defecation.
6. Dyspareunia.
7. On abdominal examination, mass may be felt in the midline arising out of the pelvis.
8. On pelvic examination, uniform uterine enlargement.
9. Ultrasound and color Doppler examination may reveal: Heterogeneous echogenicity, hypoechoic myometrium with multiple small cysts and increased vascularity within the myometrium.
10. Magnetic resonance imaging (MRI) will reveal thickened junctional zone in the myometrium.

Treatment

- Levonorgestrel into releasing intrauterine system (IUS) to improve the menorrhagia and dysmenorrhea
- Conservative surgery for partial resection of adenomyomata
- Hysterectomy for parous and aged women.

- Levonorgestrel-releasing intrauterine system (IUS) is a device that contains the female hormone levonorgestrel. It is placed in the uterus where it slowly releases the hormone to prevent pregnancy for upto 5 years

ENDOMETRIOSIS

Endometriosis is a chronic disorder resulting from the implantation of endometrial tissue (glands and stroma) outside the uterus.

Common Sites (Fig. 73.2)

1. Pelvic sites of endometrial tissue include the cervix, pouch of Douglas, ovaries, fallopian tubes, pelvic peritoneum, broad ligaments and sigmoid colon.
2. Distant sites of endometrial tissue implantation occur less commonly and can include the abdominal wall, kidneys, spleen, gallbladder, diaphragm, lungs, stomach or breasts.

Prevalence

The disorder affects nearly one in 10 women of childbearing age. The incidence is high in infertile women, about 30–40%. Delayed marriage, postponement of first conception and adoption of small family norm are contributing factors for increased prevalence.

Pathology

1. The endometrium in the ectopic sites has the potentiality to undergo changes under the action of ovarian hormones.
2. Cyclic growth and shedding continue till menopause (each of the sites will bleed during the menstrual cycle). The periodically shed blood may remain encysted or the cyst may become tense and rupture.
3. There is dense tissue reaction surrounding the lesion (where bleeding occurred) with fibrosis. If the fibrosis occurs on the pelvic peritoneum, it produces adhesions.
4. If the blood gets encysted, the cyst enlarges with cyclic bleeding and the content inside becomes chocolate colored. Those are called endometrial cysts or endometriomas. Because of the color the term 'chocolate cysts' may also be used.
5. Depending on the location, size and reaction, the lesions appear differently as:
    a. Small, black dots like 'powder burns' on uterosacral ligaments and pouch of Douglas.
    b. Red flame shaped, red polypoid or yellow brown patches on the peritoneum and surrounding tissues.
    c. Bluish lesions for endometriomas (chocolate cysts) in ovaries.

Clinical Features

1. Patients are mostly nulliparous or have had one child.
2. Age is between 30 and 45.
3. Infertility or voluntary postponement of conception till late age.
4. *Abnormal menstruation:* Short menstrual cycles (less than 28 day), increased duration of bleeding (7 day or more), excessive bleeding (for at least 5 day) and significant cramping.
5. Bladder—frequency, dysuria or hematuria.
6. Pain, inflammation or pelvic heaviness depending on the location of endometrial tissue implantation, duration of the disorder and the phase of menstrual cycle.
7. Sigmoid colon and rectum—painful defecation (dyschezia), diarrhea, rectal bleeding, dyspareunia.
8. Chronic fatigue and premenstrual syndrome.

Diagnosis

1. Classic symptoms of progressively increasing dysmenorrhea, dyspareunia and infertility.
2. Pelvic examination findings of nodules in the pouch of Douglas, uterosacral ligaments, fixed retroverted uterus and unilateral or bilateral adnexal mass.
3. *Ultrasonography:* Transvaginal and endorectal ultrasound are found better for diagnosing rectosigmoid endometriosis.
4. Laparoscopy and biopsy.

Complications

The following complications may occur:
- Infertility
- Rupture of chocolate cysts
- Infection of chocolate cyst
- Obstructive features:
    - Ureteral infection → hydroureter → hydronephrosis → renal infection
    - Intestinal obstruction.

Treatment

Therapeutic interventions are focused on stopping the progressive destruction of pelvic organs caused by endometrial implants and preserving fertility options for the woman.

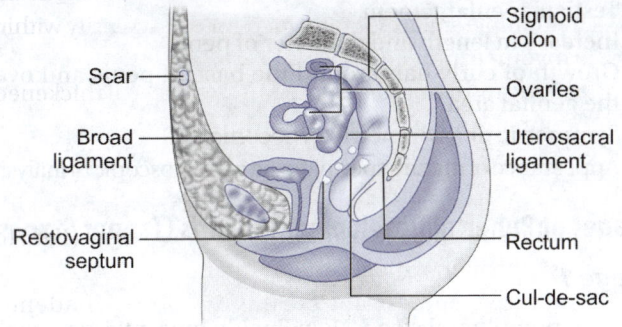

Figure 73.2: Common sites of endometriosis.

Medical

1. Encourage married women with family history of endometriosis not to delay first conception and to complete the family.
2. Nonsteroidal anti-inflammatory drugs (NSAIDs) to control pain by reducing prostaglandin production by the endometrial implants during menses.
3. Gonadotropin-releasing hormone (GnRH) to prevent release of luteinizing hormone (LH), thus causing temporary cessation of menstruation.
4. *Combined estrogen and progesterone:* Low-dose oral contraceptives help to reduce the growth and pain of endometriosis.

Surgical

Endometriosis with severe symptoms unresponsive to hormone therapy is treated surgically:

1. Endometrial ablation or removal of endometrial implants with laser or electrocautery for those who need to preserve childbearing capacity.
2. Hysterectomy with bilateral salpingo-oophorectomy along with resection of endometrial tissues as complete as possible for women who have completed the family.

DYSPAREUNIA

Dyspareunia is a sexual dysfunction characterized by difficult and painful sexual intercourse.

Causes

Male Causes

- Impotence
- Premature ejaculation
- Congenital anatomic defect of the penis
- Improper technique of coital act.

Female Causes

1. *Superficial or entrance dyspareunia:*
   - Narrow introitus
   - Tough hymen
   - Bartholin's gland cysts
   - Tender perineal scar
   - Vulval infection
   - Urethral infection
   - Vestibulitis.
2. *Vaginal causes:* This produces burning pain along the barrel of vagina either during intercourse or following intercourse. The conditions are:
   - Vaginitis
   - Vaginal septum
   - Tender scar following delivery or gynecological operation
   - Secondary vaginal atresia
   - Vaginal atrophy due to menopause
   - Growth or tumor.
3. *Deep causes:* With deep causes the patient experiences pain while the penis penetrates deep into the vagina. Deep pain usually results from pathology of paravaginal tissues or pelvic organs. Such lesions are:
   - Endometriosis on rectovaginal septum
   - Chronic cervicitis
   - Chronic pelvic inflammatory disease (PID)
   - Retroverted and fixed uterus
   - Ovary prolapsed in the pouch of Douglas.

Treatment

Treatment is given according to the cause and the measures are:
- Sex education of both partners
- Treatment of the infective lesion
- Excision of scar tissue on the perineum and vagina
- Surgical correction of retroversion of uterus or prolapsed ovary.

PUBERTY

Puberty is the period of life during which secondary sex characteristics develop and the capability of sexual reproduction are attained. It is the period, which links childhood to adulthood.

Physical Changes

In Girls

Certain important physical changes are evident during puberty. These are breast development, pubic and axillary hair growth, growth in height and starting of menstruation. Most of the changes occur gradually and only menarche can be dated. The changes follow a common order beginning with a growth spurt and the last one is menstruation.

The factors that control the onset of puberty are genetic, nutrition, body weight, psychological state, social and cultural background, and exposure to light.

Pubertal Changes

In Boys

In male, pubertal sexual maturation is based on genital size and pubic hair development. The changes are:
- Testicular enlargement
- Increase in length and diameter of penis
- Growth of curly hair around the base of penis and over the genital area
- Symmetric or asymmetric gynecomastia
- Appearance of mature spermatozoa in microscopic urinalysis.

Stages of Pubertal Development in Girls (Tanner Stages)

Stage 1

It is the prepubertal stage. No palpable breast tissue, areola generally less than 2 cm in diameter. Nipples may be inverted, flat or raised. No pubic hair.

Stage 2

Breast budding occurs with a visible and palpable mound of breast tissue. The areolae begin to enlarge and nipples develop to varying degree. Sparse long hair on either side of labia majora.

Stage 3

Further growth of entire breast tissue—darker, coarser and curly hair over the mons pubis.

Stage 4

Secondary mound of areola and papillae projecting over the breast tissue, adult type hair covering the mons pubis.

Stage 5

Areola recessed to general contour of breast. Adult hair with an inverse triangle distribution.

Endocrinology in Puberty

1. *Hypothalamopituitary gonadal axis:* As puberty approaches, the hypothalamic centers involved in the release of GnRH becomes more and more sensitive to the feedback of ovarian steroids. There is augmented GnRH pulse release. This result in gradually increasing gonadotropin secretion, increasing ovarian stimulation and increasing estrogen levels, tonic and pulsatile release of gonadotropins. This increasing level of estrogen is responsible for the growth and initiation of thelarche (breast budding) and finally menarche.
2. Thyroid gland plays an active role in the hypothalamopituitary gonadal axis.
3. Adrenal glands increase their activity of sex steroid synthesis (androstenedione). Increased sebum formation, pubic and axillary hair and change in voice are primarily due to adrenal androgen production.
4. Gonadal estrogen is responsible for the development of uterus, vagina, vulva and also the breasts in girls.
5. Testosterone secretion from testes increases in boys.
6. Growth hormone secretion increases along with gonadotropin at the onset of puberty.

Menarche

Menarche is the onset of first menstruation in life. It may occur any time between 10 and 16 years, the peak time being 13 years. The endometrium, which proliferates due to stimulation of ovarian estrogen sheds when the level (of estrogen) drops and visible bleeding occurs.

The first period is usually anovular and ovulation may be irregular for a variable period following menarche. The menses may be irregular and short to start with and it may take about 2 years for regular ovulation to occur.

Growth

Growth in height in an adolescent girl occurs mainly due to hormones. The important hormones are growth hormone, estrogen and insulin like growth factor.

Genital Organ Changes

- *Ovaries:* Shape changes from elongated to ovoid and becomes bulky due to follicular enlargement and proliferation of stromal cells.
- *Uterus:* Enlargement of the body of uterus occurs. Uterine body to cervix ratio becomes 1:1 when menarche occurs and thereafter rapid enlargement of the body occurs so that the ratio becomes 2:1.
- *Vagina:* The epithelium becomes thick with many layers. The cells become rich with glycogen. Doderlein's bacilli appear, which convert glycogen into lactic acid. The vaginal pH becomes acidic ranging between 4 and 5.
- *Vulva:* It becomes more reactive to steroid hormone.
- *Mons pubis and labia minora:* Increase in size.
- *Breast changes:* Marked proliferation of duct systems and deposition of fat occurs under the influence of estrogen. Breasts become prominent and round. Under the influence of progesterone the development of acini increases.

Disorders of Puberty

The commonly seen disorders of puberty are precocious puberty and delayed puberty.

In precocious puberty, girls exhibit secondary sex characteristics before the age of 8 or menstruate before the age of 10.

In delayed puberty, development of breast tissue and/or pubic hair does not occur by 13–14 years or menarche does not happen as late as 16 years.

These conditions need to be investigated to find the cause, which may often be hormonal and treated accordingly.

MENOPAUSE

Menopause is defined as permanent physiologic cessation of menstruation at the end of reproductive life due to loss of ovarian follicular activity. It is the point of time when last and final menstruation occurs.

Climacteric is the phase of aging process during which a woman passes from the reproductive to the non-reproductive stage. This phase covers 5–10 years on either side of menopause.

Premenopause is the part of the climacteric before menopause, when the menstrual cycle is likely to be irregular. Postmenopause is the phase that comes after the menopause.

Age of Menopause

Age of menopause is genetically predetermined. The age of menopause ranges between 45 and 55 years, average being 50 years. Cigarette smoking and severe malnutrition may cause early menopause.

Endocrinology of Climacteric and Menopause

1. Few years prior to menopause, depletion of ovarian follicles occurs and the existing follicles become resistant to gonadotropins. This results in impaired folliculogenesis and diminished estradiol production. The serum estradiol level falls from 50 to 300 pg/mL before menopause to 10–20 pg/mL after menopause. This decreases the negative feedback effect on hypothalamopituitary axis resulting in increase in follicle stimulating hormone (FSH).
2. The diminished folliculogenesis result in anovulation, oligo-ovulation and corpus luteum insufficiency. The sustained level of estrogens may cause endometrial hyperplasia and menstrual abnormalities.
3. Shortening of the follicular phase leads shorter menstrual cycles.
4. There is fall in the levels of prolactin and inhibition.
5. Ultimately, there are no more follicles responsive to gonadotropins. Estradiol production drops and endometrial growth stops resulting in absence of menstruation.

Organ Changes

1. *Genitourinary system:*
   a. *Ovaries* shrink in size, become wrinkled and white. Thinning of cortex and abundance of stroma cells occur.
   b. *Fallopian tubes* show features of atrophy. The muscle coat becomes thinner, the cilia disappear and the plicae become less prominent.
   c. *The uterus* becomes smaller, endometrium becomes thin and atrophic. The cervical secretion becomes scanty.
   d. *The vagina* becomes narrower due to gradual loss of elasticity. The rugae progressively flatten. There is no glycogen and Döderlein's bacillus. The vaginal pH becomes alkaline.
   e. *The vulva* shows features of atrophy. The labium becomes flattened and the pubic hair becomes scantier resulting in a narrow introitus.
   f. *Breast* fat gets reabsorbed and the glands atrophy. The nipples decrease in size, the breasts become flat and pendulous.
   g. In *bladder and urethra,* the epithelium becomes thin and is more prone to damage and infection.
   h. *Loss of muscle tone* leads to pelvic relaxation, uterine descend and anatomic changes in the urethra and neck of bladder.
2. *Skeletal system:* Following menopause, there is loss of bone mass by about 3–5% per year due to deficiency of estrogen leading to osteoporosis.
3. *Cardiovascular system:* Deficiency of estrogen increases the risk of cardiovascular disease because of its function of decreasing high density lipoprotein (HDL) cholesterol and antioxidant property.

Menstruation Pattern Prior to Menopause

Any of the following patterns may be observed prior to menopause:

- Abrupt cessation of menstruation
- Gradual decrease in both amount and duration
- Irregular with or without excessive bleeding.

Menopausal Symptoms

Majority of women do not experience any symptom apart from cessation of menstruation. Some women experience symptoms and health concerns:

1. *Vasomotor symptoms:* The characteristic symptom of menopause is 'hot flush'. It is characterized by sudden feeling of heat followed by profuse sweating with cutaneous vasodilatation.
2. *Genital and urinary symptoms:* Atrophy of the epithelium of vagina, urinary bladder and urethra causes dyspareunia, vaginal infections, dryness, pruritus and leukorrhea. Urinary symptoms include urgency, dysuria, stress incontinence and frequent urinary tract infections.
3. *Psychological symptoms:* Estrogen deficiency is associated with decreased sexual desire. There may be psychological changes such as increased anxiety, headache, insomnia, irritability, dysphasia and depression. Dementia, mood swings and inability to concentrate are also seen.
4. *Osteoporosis:* Osteoporosis occurs in postmenopausal women due to estrogen loss, deficiency of calcium and vitamin D or hereditary. Osteoporosis may lead to back pain, loss of height and kyphosis and fracture of bones. Fracture may involve vertebral body, femoral neck or distal forearm.
5. *Cardiovascular and cerebrovascular effects:* Risks of ischemia, heart disease, coronary artery disease and stroke are increased due to atherosclerotic changes, vasoconstriction and thrombus formation.

Diagnosis of Menopause

- Cessation of menstruation for 12 consecutive months during climacteric
- Occurrence of hot flushes and night sweats
- Features of low estrogen on vaginal cytology
- Serum estradiol is less than 20 pg/mL
- Serum FSH, LH is greater than 40 mIU/mL at 1 week interval for three times.

Management

1. *Counseling:* Adequate explanation to every woman with symptoms may help understand and accept the changes. Those who have artificial and early menopause due to bilateral oophorectomy or radiation may require more reassurance.
2. *Non-hormonal treatment:*
   a. Nutritious diet balanced with protein and calcium.
   b. Supplementary calcium: Total daily requirement of calcium is 1.5 g.
   c. *Exercise:* Walking, jogging and weight bearing exercises.

3. To follow healthy lifestyle, health promotion and regular health screening:
   a. Supplementation with vitamin D 400–800 IU/day.
   b. Cessation of smoking and alcohol.
   c. *Hormone replacement therapy (HRT):* Replacement of estrogen and progestin are prescribed for women with premature ovarian failure, gonadal dysgenesis and surgical or radiation menopause.

Abnormal Menopause

1. *Premature menopause* occurs at or below the age of 40. Treatment by substitution therapy is usually followed.
2. *Delayed menopause:* Menopause does not occur beyond 55 years of age. Detailed investigations for any pelvic pathology and appropriate treatment are indicated.
3. *Artificial menopause:* Permanent cessation of ovarian function as a result of surgical removal of ovaries or by radiation.

Nursing Implications for Menopausal Conditions

Nursing diagnoses are individualized to each woman and her specific menopausal condition. Applicable diagnoses may include:
- Pain (mild or moderate) related to specific menopausal condition
- Grief related to mid to late life losses
- Deficient knowledge related to limited experience regarding specific menopausal condition
- Ineffective coping related to lack of acceptance of prognosis (for specific menopausal condition).

Nursing Interventions

- Education regarding reduction of risk factors
- Emphasizing prevention strategies
- Explaining therapeutic interventions to ensure successful compliance
- Education to focus on health promoting nutrition, maintenance of appropriate weight for height body mass index (BMI) and exercise.

STUDY QUESTIONS

Short Answer Questions

1. Adenomyosis.
2. Endometriosis.
3. Dyspareunia.

Essay Question

1. Describe menopause, common organ changes in menopausal phase, symptoms experienced by women and measures of management.

BIBLIOGRAPHY

1. Dutta DC. Textbook of gynecology, 5th edition. Kolkata: New Central Book Agency; 2009.
2. Kumari N, Sharma S, Gupta P. A textbook of midwifery and gynecological nursing. Jalandhar City: S Vikas and Company. India; 2010.
3. Rao K. Textbook of midwifery and obstetrics for nurses. Noida: Reed Elsevier India Private Limited; 2011.
4. Adenomyosis – Stages, Symptoms and Treatment. https://www.healthdirect.gov
5. Adenomyosis. https://nhinform.scot

CHAPTER 74

Diagnostic Procedures in Gynecology

Learning Objectives

Upon completing this chapter, the learner will be able to:
- Outline the diagnostic tests performed for gynecologic and obstetric patients for identifying specific conditions.
- Explain the significance of specific tests to clients who will need to undergo the diagnostic procedure.
- Develop their knowledge of the diagnostic procedure in relation to the patients' specific difficulties manifested.
- Explain about the performance of the tests in order to prepare patients and to assist the medical personnel performing the procedures.
- Educate patients regarding the preparation for undergoing the required procedure in order to be informed and assured.
- Explain to patients about the recommended therapeutic interventions planned and aftercare to be followed or continued.

INTRODUCTION

A diagnostic procedure is an examination or test to identify an individual's specific areas of weakness and strength in order to determine a condition, disease or illness. Investigative procedures include a patient procedure where it is both diagnostic and therapeutic. Biopsies computerized tomography and ultrasound examination are examples of diagnostic procedures.

PAPANICOLAOU TEST/PAP SMEAR/CERVICAL SMEAR

Definition

Papanicolaou test also known as Pap smear or cervical smear is a screening test in which a sample of cells taken from the endocervical canal is smeared and screened under the microscope to detect potentially cancerous or precancerous cells.

Principles

- Follow aseptic technique.
- Screening should be done after 10–20 days of the first day of menstruation.

Purpose

To evaluate the condition of the internal female structures and to obtain specimens for cytological screening.

Indications

- As part of routine health check-up after the age of 21 years.
- To screen for cancer.
- To detect abnormal cells or precancerous cells.
- To diagnose inflammation and infection.

Articles Needed (Figs. 74.1 to 74.3)

A tray containing:
1. A drape sheet to expose the particular or needed area.
2. A bowl for antimicrobial solution.

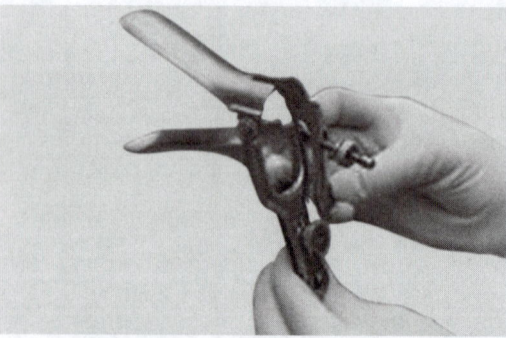

Figure 74.1: Vaginal speculum.

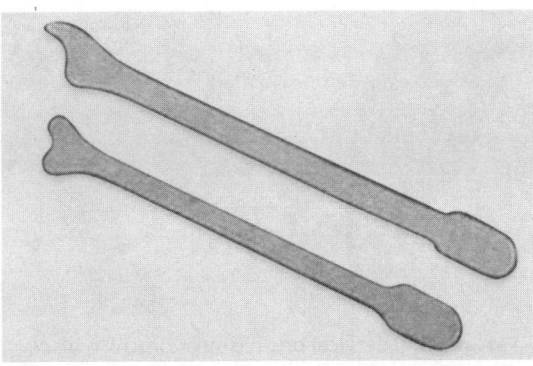

Figure 74.2: Ayer spatula (Pap smear sampling device).

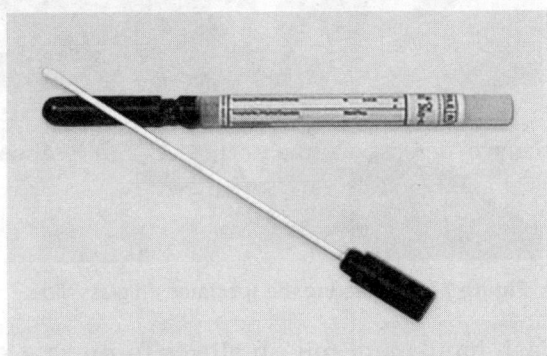

Figure 74.3: Cotton-tipped applicator and tube for collecting specimen.

3. A sponge holding forceps.
4. A Cusco's speculum to retract posterior vaginal wall.
5. A Vulsellum to catch hold of the anterior lip of the cervix.
6. A pair of sterile gloves.
7. Cotton swabs for cleaning excess discharge.
8. An Ayer spatula to swab around the cervix.
9. Cotton tipped applicators to swab the endocervix by rotating it 180°.
10. Glass slides to prepare the smear.
11. Spray fixative/methanol spray
12. Ether/95% alcohol solution (1:1)
13. A graphite pencil.

Preparation of the Patient

- Explain the Pap cytology test to the patient.
- Reassure and provide psychological support.
- Ask the mother to empty her bladder and bowel to avoid discomfort during the procedure.
- Explain to patient not to use vaginal medications or vaginal contraceptive for 48 hours before the test. Intercourse should be avoided the night before the test.

Procedure

1. Ask the patient to undress from waist down.
2. Position her in supine position with knees flexed and legs abducted and drape the area with sterile sheet.
3. Wash hands and wear the sterile gloves.
4. Spread the labia and clean the vulva with antiseptic solution.
5. Insert the speculum gently into the vagina. Blades should be closed until inserted fully and slowly open the blades and lock them.
6. a. *For endocervical smear:*
   Insert a sterile cotton tipped applicator into the cervical os and rotate it 360°. Leave the swab in place for 10–20 seconds.
   Remove the swab gently and smear on to a glass slide and apply fixative. (Fixative must be applied immediately, before the specimen dries).
   b. *For ectocervical scraping:*
   Insert the Ayre's spatula into the cervical os, rotate or scrape the squamocolumnar junction. Remove the spatula and smear on to a glass slide and fix it immediately.
   c. *For cervical scraping:*
   Insert the pointed edge of a wooden Ayre's spatula into the cervical os and rotate the spatula by 360°. Spread the cervical scrapings on a glass slide, fix it with an ether/95% ethyl alcohol solution, and dry the slide. A cervix-brush sampling device may be used, and it is recommended to rotate it a full 180° to improve the sampling for abnormal cervical cells. Remove the speculum gently.
7. Give the patient a perineal pad after the procedure, to absorb any bleeding or drainage.
8. Watch for any bleeding for 15 minutes.
9. Make the mother comfortable and tell her to rest for 10–15 minutes.
10. Document the date, time smear obtained and any needed details about the procedure.

Aftercare

- Replace all the articles.
- Send the microscopic slide and cotton applicator for cytology.
- Inform the mother that she may have some mild bleeding or discomfort which is normal.
- Check the vital signs and general condition of the mother for the periods she is asked to rest.

Special Considerations

- Smears that dry before fixative is applied cannot be properly interpreted.
- Do not lubricate the speculum as it may distort the cells.
- A smear taken any time other than the mid-menstrual cycle can result in abnormal findings.
- Tetracycline or digitalis preparations can affect the appearance of squamous epithelium.
- Blood, mucus or pus on the slide makes interpretation difficult.

VAGINAL SMEAR/VAGINAL WET MOUNT

Description

A vaginal smear or vaginal wet mount is a gynecological test wherein a sample of vaginal discharge is observed by wet mount microscopy by placing the specimen on a glass slide and mixing it with salt solution (saline). It is used to find vaginal thrush, bacterial vaginosis and Trichomoniasis (a sexually transmitted infection caused by *Trichomonas vaginalis*, a parasitic protozoan which is a group of single celled microorganisms).

Purpose of the test is to find the cause of vaginitis or vulvitis.

Principles

- Follow aseptic precautions.
- Avoid contamination of swab in the lower perineum.
- Should not be done during menstruation

Indications

- Vaginitis
- Yeast infection
- Trichomonas infection
- Bacterial vaginosis
- Infections such as chlamydia, genital warts, syphilis, herpes simplex and gonorrhea
- It may also be done as rape investigation to detect the presence of semen.

Contraindications

- Acute human papillomavirus (HPV) herpes
- Abnormal Pap smear
- Active vaginal infection
- Undiagnosed vaginal bleeding
- Uncontrolled diabetes
- Rectal or vaginal injury
- Any active bleeding including menses.

Articles Needed (Figs. 74.4 and 74.5)

A tray containing:
1. A vaginal speculum to visualize the vagina.
2. Sterile gloves to maintain asepsis.
3. Lubricant to avoid friction
4. A smear brush/vaginal smear kit/cotton tipped applicator for collecting sample.
5. A sterile drape
6. Methanol spray for fixation
7. An apron to avoid contamination/sepsis
8. Fixative.

Procedure

1. Place the woman on the examination table in lithotomy position for clear visualization.
2. Drape the area and expose only the needed part.

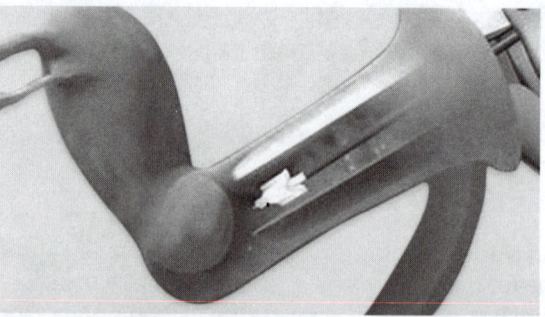

Figure 74.4: Cervical brush (smear brush) in place.

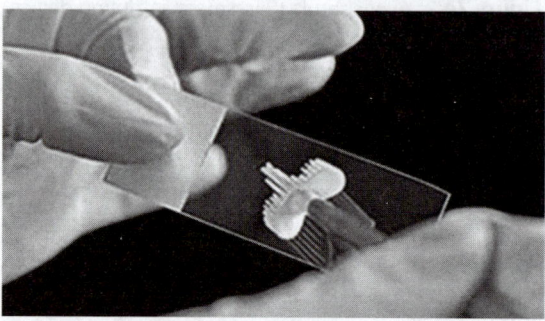

Figure 74.5: Smearing the specimen on glass slide.

3. Wash hands and put on gloves to prevent cross contamination.
4. Apply lubricant jelly on the speculum for easy insertion.
5. Separate the labia and insert the speculum in sideways direction gently and rotate it so that the clamp is at 12-O' clock position. Gently open the speculum and view the inside to inspect the vagina.
6. Clean the vagina with plain gauze.
7. Insert the long bristles of the cervical brush into the endocervical canal deep enough to allow the shorter bristles to fully contact the endocervix. Push gently and rotate the broom in a clockwise direction, about 5 times to clear the cervical mucus.
8. Insert the specimen collection applicator or cervical brush into the cervical canal and gently rotate clockwise for 10–30 seconds.
9. Withdraw the brush/applicator carefully avoiding contact with the vaginal mucosa to prevent contamination
10. Gently smear the collected sample on a glass slide and apply fixative
11. Remove the speculum gently, watch for any bleeding
12. Remove gloves, label the specimen and send it to the laboratory.
13. Reposition the mother, making her comfortable and ask her to take rest for 10 minutes.
14. Document the time of swab collection and needed details and any complications if identified.

Aftercare

- Replace articles
- Clean or soak the speculum immediately to dislodge secretions

- Wash hands
- Explain to the woman about follow up care.

HIGH VAGINAL SWAB COLLECTION

Definition

Collection of vaginal mucus secretion by swabbing the vagina for histopathological examination for the presence of candidiasis, bacterial vaginosis and trichomonas vaginalis.

The test is done for cytohormonal study or as a screening procedure.

Principles

- Follow aseptic precaution
- During insertion do not contaminate the swab in the perineum.

Contraindications

- Vaginal bleeding
- Vaginal tear.

Articles Needed

1. Vagina speculum (Cusco's speculum) for clear visualization and inspection
2. Sterile gloves
3. Lubricant to avoid friction
4. Drape sheet.
5. Smear brush/cotton tipped applicator
6. Slide for placing the sample

Preparation of the Patient

- Provide adequate information about the procedure
- Reassure and provide psychological support
- Ask the mother to empty the bladder

Procedure

1. Position the mother in lithotomy position
2. Drape the woman and expose the needed part
3. Wash and put on gloves
4. Apply lubricant jelly on the speculum for easy insertion
5. Separate the labia and insert the speculum sideways slowly and then rotate so that the clamp is at 12-o' clock position and gently open the speculum and lock it.
6. Insert the long bristles of the cervical brush into the endocervical canal deep enough to allow the shorter bristles to fully contact the endocervix. Push gently and rotate the broom in a clockwise direction 5 times.
7. Insert the specimen collection swab in to the endocervical canal and slowly rotate clockwise for 10-30 seconds.
8. Withdraw carefully avoiding the vaginal mucosa to prevent contamination
9. Smear the sample collected on the slide.
10. Remove gloves, label the specimen and send it to the laboratory.
11. Reposition the mother
12. Document the date and time of the sample collection, complications identified if any for further planning of care.

Aftercare

- Replace articles.
- Clean or soak the speculum immediately to dislodge secretions
- Wash hands
- Explain to the patient about the follow-up care

CULDOSCOPY

Description

Culdoscopy is a technique of endoscopic visualization and/or minor operative procedure performed on the female pelvic organs in which the instrument is introduced through a puncture in the wall of the pouch of Douglas, an extension of peritoneal cavity, between the rectum and back wall (posterior wall) of the uterus. The word Culdoscopy is derived from the term cul-de-sac and refers to the rectouterine pouch. Purpose of the procedure is to examine the retrouterine pouch and pelvic viscera. Diagnostic value of the procedure is to diagnose pathologic conditions of the female pelvis and pelvic organs.

Indications

- Ectopic pregnancy.
- Salpingitis.
- Tubal ligation.
- Tubal adhesions.
- Assessment of diethylstilbestrol exposure in uterus.

Contraindications

- Chronic pelvic inflammatory disease (PID).
- Vaginitis and acute cervicitis.
- Vaginal atresia.
- Acute pelvic inflammation.
- Ruptured ectopic pregnancy.
- Inability to assume knee-chest position due to cardiac or respiratory disease

Articles Needed

A sterile tray containing:
1. A bowl with antiseptic solution and cotton swabs
2. A Vulsellum to hold the cervix
3. A perineal retractor to hold the targeted tissue
4. A 10 mL syringe and sterile container to aspirate the fluid and collect the specimen

5. A draping sheet to expose the procedural site
6. A vaginal speculum to visualize the vagina and cervix
7. Catgut to suture the vaginal wound
8. Sterile trocar and culdoscope with lens to visualize the pelvic organs.

Preparation of the Environment

- Arrange all the articles
- Provide privacy.
- Ensure adequate lighting
- Ensure aseptic environment.

Preparation of the Patient

- Explain the procedure and get informed consent
- Do a pregnancy test prior to the test
- Administer enema for emptying the bowel
- Patent should be kept in 'nil per oral' status for 8 hours prior to the test
- Catheterize the bladder
- Administer premedication half hour before the procedure
- Perineum and vagina to be cleaned with antiseptic solution.

Procedure (Fig. 74.6)

1. Culdoscopy is performed with the patient in knee-chest position under local or general anesthesia.
2. Retract the perineum using a retractor.
3. Grasp the posterior lip of the cervix with a Vulsellum.
4. Insert the sterile torcher of the culdoscope into the posterior fornix and then into the pelvis between two uterosacral ligaments.
5. Withdraw the torcher from the sheath, insert the sterile culdoscope through the sheath without touching the vaginal mucous membrane and view the uterus, tubes, broad ligaments uterosacral ligaments, rectal wall, sigmoid and small intestine by manipulating the scope.
6. Remove the culdoscope after the examination and leave the sheath in position.
7. Suture the virginal wound and then remove the sheath, suture the wound and clean the perineum.
8. Document the indication for the procedure, date, time and any difficulties encountered.

Aftercare

- Monitor the vital signs for about 1 to 2 hours.
- Send the patient home after 4 to 6 hours if the procedure was done as out-patient.
- Instruct the patient not to have sexual intercourse for 6-weeks, but can start normal activities as soon as she feels comfortable and fit.
- Observe for any possible complications such as injuries, hydrosalpinx, bleeding.

DIAGNOSTIC LAPAROSCOPY

Definition

Laparoscopy is a surgical procedure in which a fiber optic instrument is inserted through a small incision (about 0.5 to 1.5 cm) on the abdominal wall to visualize the abdominal or pelvic organs.

Purposes

- To reduce hemorrhage.
- To allow access to the inside of abdomen and pelvis without having to make a large incision in the skin.
- To keep the procedure as a key-hole surgery or minimally invasive surgery.
- To shorten the hospital stay nearby allowing faster recovery and return to day-to-day activities.
- To reduce the exposure of internal organs to possible external contaminants reducing the risk of acquiring infections.

Indications

To rule out the cause of the following:

- Infertility—site of tubal block, hydrosalpinx, pyosalpinx, tuboovarian mass, tubal kinks and peritubal adhesions, genital tuberculosis, polycystic ovarian disease and pelvic endometritis.
- *Amenorrhea:* Müllerian agenesis, genital tuberculosis.
- *Acute pelvic pain:*
  - Ectopic pregnancy.
  - Acute salpingo-oophoritis.
  - Corpus luteum hematoma.
  - Twisted ovarian cyst.
  - Acute appendicitis.
- *Chronic pelvic pain:*
  - Chronic PID
  - Endometriosis
  - Pelvic congestion syndrome

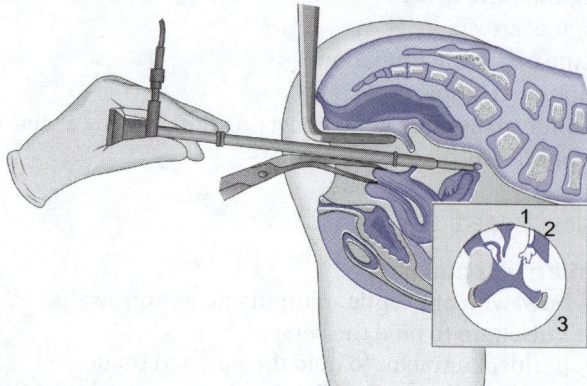

Figure 74.6: Culdoscope in rectouterine pouch.

- Small pelvic masses:
  - Ovarian cyst.
  - Tuboovarian mass
  - Broad ligament cyst or tumor.

Contraindications

- Severe cardiorespiratory disease.
- Generalized peritonitis.
- Bowel obstruction, ileus.
- Diaphragmatic or abdominal hernia.
- Second or third trimester pregnancy.
- Tuberculosis peritonitis with adhesions.
- Large pelvic mass.

Articles Needed (Figs. 74.7 to 74.9)

A sterile tray containing:
1. Toothed thumb forceps to hold the tissues
2. Needle holder to hold the suturing needle
3. Dissection hook to dissect the tissues
4. Curved dissector
5. Scissors for cutting the tissues and suturing material
6. Trocar and cannula
7. Suction catheter to suck out the blood and body fluids
8. Clip applicators with suitable clips to hold the surgical towels.

Other instruments:
9. A telescope usually 10 mm diameter and 25 cm long rod lens to visualize the abdominal/pelvic organs
10. Inflation cannula (Rubin's cannula)
11. Telescope for viewing
12. Laparoscope
13. A laparoscopic camera to use as a guide for procedure
14. Halogen or xenon light source
15. TV or video monitor to monitor the procedure
16. Suction—irrigation apparatus to collect the body fluids
17. Cautery machine with cables and foot control to cauterize the bleeding sites.

Preparation of the Patient

- Explain the procedure to patient and get informed consent
- Perform skin preparation
- Enquire about any kind of allergy to medication
- Administer enema several hours before the procedure
- Advise to empty the bladder prior to the procedure
- Advise to be NPO for 8 hours prior to the procedure
- Administer premedication as per prescription
- Remove jewelry
- Remove eye glass/contact lenses, dentures and removable bridge before surgery.

Procedure (Fig. 74.10)

- Position the mother in supine position.
- Anesthetize the mother.
- Cleanse the abdominal wall with antiseptic.
- Drape the mother.
- A small incision is made in the para umbilical region.
- Insufflate the abdomen using CO_2 gas.
- Gently push the laparoscope through the incision.
- Visualize the internal organs in the TV monitor connected to the laparoscope.

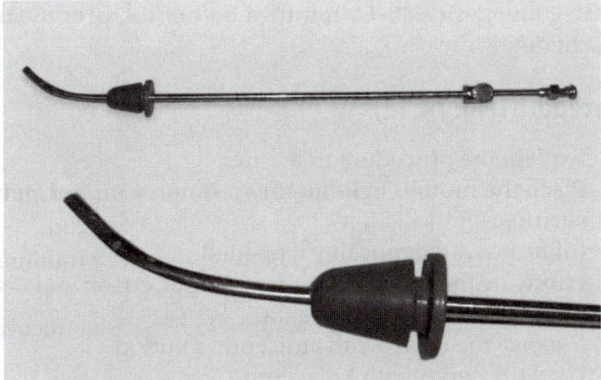

Figure 74.7: Rubin's cannula/Insufflation cannula.

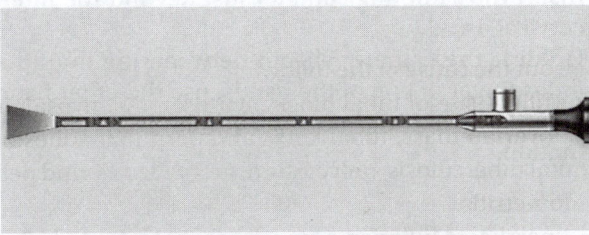

Figure 74.8: Telescope for viewing:

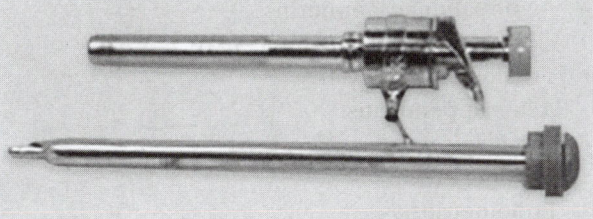

Figure 74.9: Trocar and cannula.

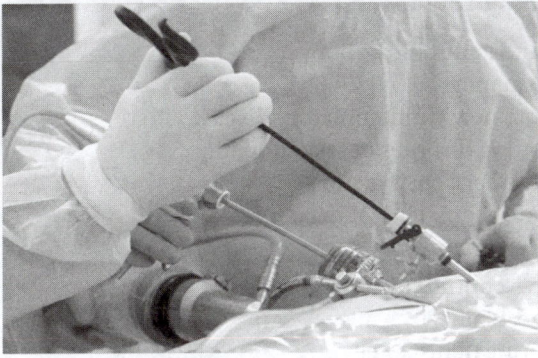

Figure 74.10: Laparoscopy procedure.

- ❖ Remove the laparoscope.
- ❖ Suture the incised area and apply dressing.
- ❖ Position the patient and make her comfortable.
- ❖ Check vital signs.
- ❖ Document the date, time, type of anesthesia and surgery and complications if any is noticed.

Aftercare

- ❖ Monitor vital signs for 2–3 hours
- ❖ Check the dressing for any oozing of blood.
- ❖ Administer analgesics and antibiotics as prescribed
- ❖ Tell the mother that she may experience sore throat which is due to the tube in throat applied during anesthesia.

ENDOMETRIAL BIOPSY

Definition

The endometrial biopsy is a gynecological procedure that involves taking a tissue sample from the inner lining of the uterus.

Purposes

- ❖ To determine the cause of abnormal uterine bleeding
- ❖ To evaluate infertility
- ❖ To test for uterine infection
- ❖ To monitor the response of endometrium with hormonal therapy.

Principles

- ❖ Strict aseptic technique to be followed
- ❖ The test should be done with the help of ultrasonography.

Indications

- ❖ Abnormal uterine bleeding
- ❖ Postmenstrual bleeding
- ❖ Screening for endometrial cancer after finding atypical cells
- ❖ Testing the response to hormonal therapy
- ❖ Abnormal Pap smear.

Contraindications

Absolute contraindications:
- ❖ Pregnancy
- ❖ Acute pelvic inflammatory disease (PID)
- ❖ Clotting disorder or coagulopathy
- ❖ Acute cervical infection
- ❖ Acute vaginal infection
- ❖ Cervical cancer.

Relative contraindications:
- ❖ Morbid obesity
- ❖ Uterine dehiscence
- ❖ Severe cervical stenosis.

Articles Needed (Fig. 74.11)

A sterile tray containing:
1. Sponge holding forceps
2. Bowl with povidone iodine solution
3. Draping sheet
4. Vaginal speculum to visualize vagina and cervix
5. Uterine sound to measure the length of uterine cavity
6. Endometrial suction catheter to aspirate the sample tissue
7. Cervical dilators to dilate the cervix
8. Scissors to cut the tip of catheter

A clean tray containing:
1. Sterile gloves
2. Sterile sample container with formalin solution
3. Anesthetic gel or spray to use as local anesthetic agent

Preparation of Patient

- ❖ Get informed consent from the patient
- ❖ Check whether she is taking any medications
- ❖ Check whether she is allergic to any medication
- ❖ Advise the patient to empty her bladder
- ❖ Give analgesics 30–60 minutes before the procedure is scheduled.

Procedure (Fig. 74.12)

1. Explain the procedure to mother.
2. Place the mother in lithotomy position with her feet on stirrups.
3. Infiltrate with lignocaine if needed.
4. Lubricate the speculum with antiseptic cream and insert the speculum into the vagina.
5. Cleanse the cervix with antiseptic solution.
6. Hold the cervix with Vulsellum.
7. Insert the uterine sound till you feel resistance which indicates fundus.
8. Insert the sampling catheter just beyond the internal cervical os.
9. Holding the catheter sheath between the thumb and index finger of one of the hands, use the other hand to draw the internal piston out of the tube in one continuous motion.

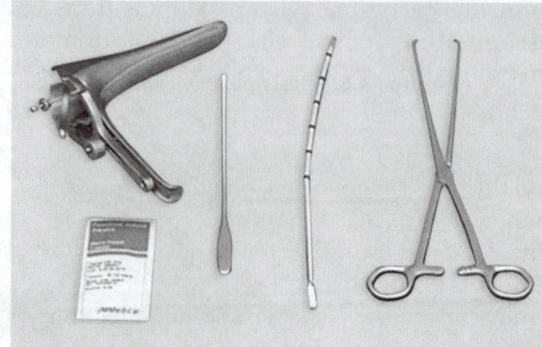

Figure 74.11: Instruments for endometrial biopsy (vaginal speculum, cervical dilator, uterine sound and sponge holding forceps).

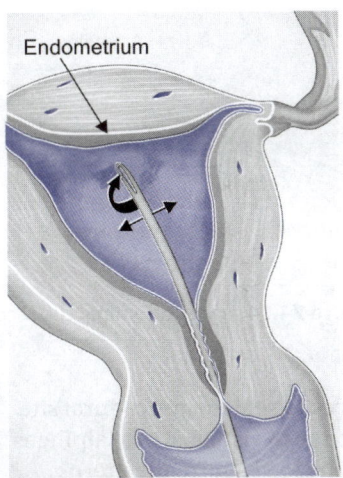

Figure 74.12: Site of endometrial biopsy showing biopsy catheter in place.

10. Hold the catheter sheath between the thumb and index finger and insert the tube up as far into the fundus as possible until resistance is felt (without perforating the uterine wall).
11. Slowly withdraw the tube using both hands in a spiral or swirling movement from the fundus toward the cervix while simultaneously moving the catheter back and forth within the uterine cavity between the fundus and internal os. Have the lumen of the sampling tube fill up with endometrial tissue.
12. Place the removed tissue in formalin solution for preservation.
13. Send the tissue to the laboratory.
14. Remove the Vulsellum and speculum and reposition the woman in supine or lateral position. Allow her to rest for some time.
15. Document in patient's chart the date and time of the procedure, type of anesthesia used and biopsy done.

HYSTEROSCOPY

Definition

Hysteroscopy is a gynecological procedure that allows the doctor to look inside the uterus in order to diagnose and treat abnormal bleeding. Hysteroscopy is done using a hysteroscope, a thin lighted tube that is inserted into the vagina to examine the cervix and inside of the uterus.

Purposes

- To find the cause of abnormal bleeding.
- To find out the cause of infertility.
- To obtain a tissue sample/biopsy.
- To remove polyps or small fibroids.
- To remove adhesions caused by earlier infections or past surgery.
- To detect the cause of repeated miscarriages.
- To locate and remove an intrauterine device.
- To perform tubal ligation.
- To stop bleeding using electric current, freezing, heat or chemicals.

Indications

- Asherman's syndrome/intrauterine adhesions.
- Endometrial polyp.
- Endometrial ablation/removal of layer of tissue (endometrium).
- Evaluation of retained products of conception.
- Removal of embedded intrauterine contraceptive devices (IUCDs)
- Congenital uterine malformations.
- Postmenopausal bleeding.
- Abnormal Pap test results.

Contraindications

- During menstruation.
- Pelvic inflammatory disease
- Cervical cancer.
- Vaginal or cervical infection.

Preparation of Patient

- Explain the procedure and obtain informed consent.
- Keep the patient on 'nil per oral' status.
- Advise mother to empty her bladder before the procedure.
- Perform skin preparation.
- Advise not to douche, use tampons or vaginal medications 24 hours prior to hysteroscopy.
- An IV line may be placed.

Procedure (Fig. 74.13)

- Position the patient on operating table supine with feet in stirrups.
- Vagina is cleaned with antiseptic solution.
- Cervix is then dilated and hysteroscope is inserted through the cervix into the uterus.
- The uterus is then expanded by injecting liquid or gas through the hysteroscope.
- The uterine cavity is then examined and required procedure is performed.

Aftercare

- Observe the mother for 2–4 hours
- Tell the patient that she may have cramping or mild sore throat due to anesthesia. This will get relieved after few days and salt water gargles help relieve throat symptoms
- Inform her that it is normal to have small amount of bleeding for a day
- Advise mother to avoid sexual intercourse and using tampons for a day after hysteroscopy
- Analgesics may be given to relieve pain

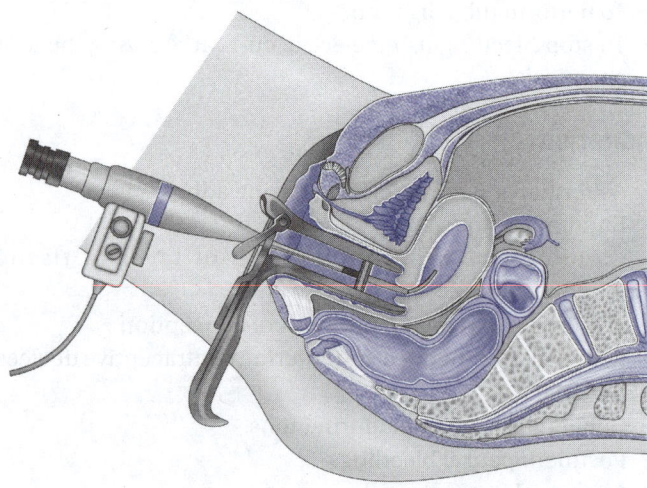

Figure 74.13: Hysteroscope in place inside the uterus.

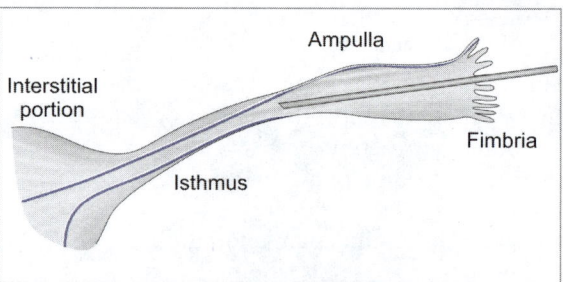

Figure 74.14: Transabdominal tuboscopy.

- Advise the mother to report to the hospital if she develops:
  - Heavy bleeding or discharge
  - Fever
  - Severe abdominal or pelvic pain.

TUBOSCOPY/SALPINGOSCOPY

Definition
Tuboscopy is a procedure in which a thin fiber-optic telescope is passed into the fallopian tubes to evaluate the inner structure.

Purpose
- Diagnostic
- Therapeutic

Indications
- Proximal tube disease
- Pelvic inflammatory disease (PID) affecting the distal tubal segments
- Endometriosis
- Ectopic pregnancy
- Unexplained infertility
- Prior to assisted fertilization

Types/Approach (Fig. 74.14)
- Transvaginal
- Transabdominal

Articles Needed
A sterile tray containing:
1. A bowl with antiseptic solution to paint the procedural site
2. Disposable syringe 5 cc for irrigation
3. Sterile gloves
4. Lignocaine 2% local anesthetic
5. Gauze pieces to seal the procedural site
6. Salpingoscope to visualize the salpinges
7. Hysteroscope to visualize the uterus
8. Flexible guidewire 0.3–0.8 mm to rule out adhesions and blocks
9. Teflon cannula (outside diameter) up to 1.3 mm over the guidewire
10. Ringer lactate solution/saline for irrigation
11. The inner eversion catheter system to remove the adhesions
12. Automatic tube-holding forceps to grasp and hold the fallopian tube

Accessory Instruments
1. Light source
2. Fiber-optic cables and camera
3. Automatic laparoflator (inflator)
4. Electrosurgical generator and laser

Preparation of Patient
1. Explain the procedure to patient
2. Position the mother in lithotomy position
3. Administer anesthesia to decrease pain

Procedure for Transvaginal Salpingoscopy
- Paint the perineum with antiseptic solution
- Insert vaginal speculum
- Dilate the cervix using cervical dilators
- Insert the hysteroscope/salpingoscope transvaginally into the fallopian tubes (depending on the procedure and mother's condition, either fluids or CO_2 gas is introduced to expand the cavity)
- Introduce hysteroscope and Teflon cannula
- Obtain a tissue sample if needed for histopathological examination
- Withdraw the scope and speculum
- Document the date, time, procedure, findings and vital signs
- Make the patient comfortable and allow to rest for 2 hours

Aftercare
- Observe the patient for 2–4 hours
- For mild sore throat she may use salt water gargles

- She may have small amount of vaginal bleeding for a day or two
- Pain medication may be used as prescribed
- Advise patient to report to hospital if she finds:
  - Problem urinating
  - Heavy bleeding or discharge
  - Vomiting
  - Severe abdominal pain or cramping
  - Fever.

HYSTEROSALPINGOGRAPHY

Description

Hysterosalpingography (HSG), also known as uterosalpingography, is a radiologic procedure to investigate the shape of the uterine cavity and the shape and patency of the fallopian tubes. This is a special X-ray using a dye to look at the uterus and fallopian tubes. This type of X-ray used is called a fluoroscopy, which creates a video image rather than a still picture.

The radiologist can watch the dye as it moves through the reproductive system. He will then be able to see if there is any blockage in the fallopian tubes or other structural abnormalities in the uterus.

Indications

- Infertility.
- Suspected structural abnormalities in the uterus which may be congenital or required.
- Blockage of the fallopian tubes.
- Scar tissue in the uterus.
- Uterine polyps, tumors or fibroids.
- Post-tubal pregnancy.

Patient Preparation

- Pain medication is given about an hour before the scheduled test.
- A sedative may be prescribed to help the patient relax, if she is nervous.
- The test will take few minute only and patient can go home after 2–3 hours.
- An antibiotic may be prescribed to take before or after the test to help prevent infection.
- The test will be scheduled a few days to a week after menstrual period.
- The patient will be asked to remove any mental or her body, such as jewelry and the metal can interfere with the X-ray machine.
- Explain to patient that a contrast dye will be used as instillation into the uterus to help highlight the uterine cavity and fallopian tubes. The dye will either dissolve or leave the body through urine. It is important to let your doctor know if you have had an allergic reaction to barium or contrast dye.

During the Test (Figs. 74.15 and 74.16)

- The patient will need to put on a hospital gown and lie on her back with knees bent and feet spread, as would for a pelvic examination.
- The radiologist or doctor will then insert a speculum into the vagina. This is done to visualize the cervix, which is located at the back of the vagina.
- The cervix will then be cleaned and a local anesthetic injected to reduce discomfort.
- Next, a cannula will be inserted into the cervix and the speculum will be removed. The dye will be instilled through the cannula which will flow into the uterus and fallopian tubes.
- The patient will then be placed under the X-ray machine and X-rays will be taken. The patient will feel some cramping and pain as the dye will move through the fallopian tubes.
- After the X-rays are taken, the cannula will be removed.
- Medications for pain and a prevent infection are usually prescribed.

Complications

Complications from a hysterosalpingography is rare. Possible risks include:
- Allergic reaction to contrast dye.
- Endometrial or fallopian tube infection.
- Injury to the uterus, such as perforation.
- Vaginal bleeding.

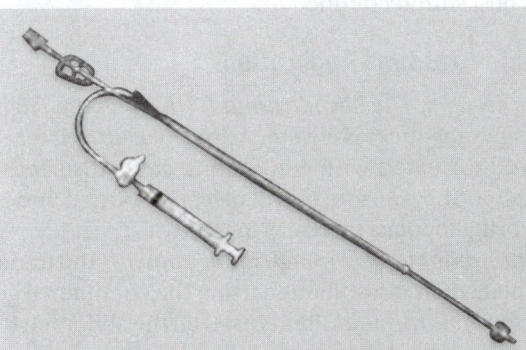

Figure 74.15: Syringe and catheter for injecting dye.

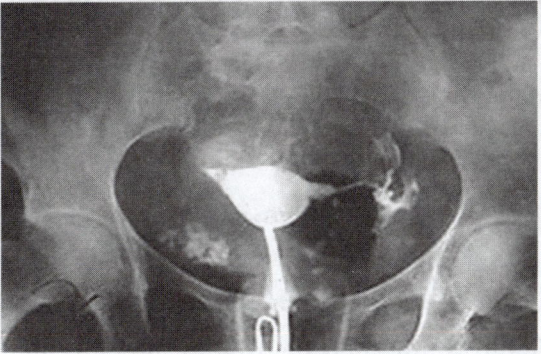

Figure 74.16: X-ray image of uterus and fallopian tubes.

Aftercare

- Tell the patient that small amount of spotting may be present following the procedure which is normal.
- There may also be leakage of the contrast dye.
- Wearing a sanitary pad for the rest of the day and for few days will protect her clothing.

ULTRASONOGRAPHIC EXAMINATION

Introduction

Gynecologic ultrasonography refers to the application of medical ultrasonography to the female pelvic organs, especially the uterus, ovaries, fallopian tubes as well as bladder, the adnexa and the rectouterine pouch. The test is often referred to simply as an ultrasound or as a sonogram.

How is ultrasonography performed?

Sonography uses a device called a transducer to send out ultrasound waves at a frequency too high to be heard. The transducer is placed on the skin and the ultrasound waves move through the body to the organs and structures within. The organs like an echo return the waves to the transducer. The sound waves bounce through the organs like an echo and return to the transducer. The transducer processes the reflected waves, which are then converted by a computer into an image of the organs or tissues being examined.

An ultrasound gel is placed on the transducer and on the skin to allow for smooth movement of the transducer over the skin and to eliminate air between the skin and the transducer for the best sound conduction.

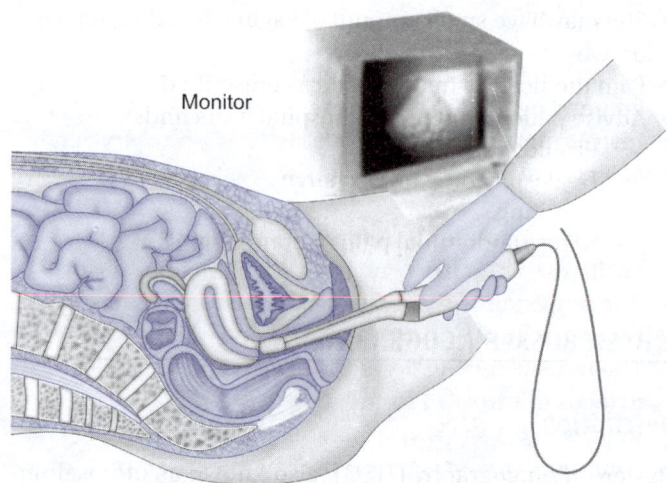

Figure 74.17: Pelvic ultrasound.

Types of Ultrasound Application

1. *Transvaginal/pelvic ultrasound (through the vagina):* A long, transducer is covered with a plastic or latex sheath and lubricated with conducting gel is inserted in the vagina. The transducer will be gently turned and angled to bring to focus the areas for study.
2. *Transabdominal (through the abdomen):* The transducer is placed on the abdomen using the conductive gel.
3. *Doppler ultrasound:* This is used on the abdomen to show the speed and direction of blood flow in certain pelvic organs. Unlike a standard ultrasound, some sound waves during the Doppler examination are audible. This is used in obstetrics to assess placental blood flow and fetal heart sounds.

This type of ultrasound procedure is performed on the reason for the test. Only one method may be used or both methods may be needed to provide information needed for the diagnosis or treatment.

Pelvic Ultrasound/Transvaginal Ultrasound Examination (Fig. 71.17)

Reasons for Pelvic Ultrasound

Pelvic ultrasound may be used for measurement and evaluation of female pelvic organs and include:

- Size, shape and position of the uterus and ovaries.
- Thickness, echogenicity (darkness or lightness of the image related to the density of the tissue) and presence of fluid or masses in the endometrium, myometrium, fallopian tubes or in or near the bladder.
- Length and thickness of the cervix.
- Changes in bladder shape.
- Blood flow through pelvic organs.
- Abnormalities in the anatomic structure of the uterus.
- Fibroid tumors, masses, cysts and other types of tumors within the pelvis.
- Presence and position of an intrauterine contraceptive device (IUCD).
- Pelvic inflammatory disease (PID).
- Postmenopausal bleeding.
- Monitoring of ovarian follicle size for infertility evaluation.
- Aspiration of follicle fluid and eggs from ovaries for in-vitro fertilization.
- Ectopic pregnancy.
- It may also be used to assist with procedures such as endometrial biopsy.

Risks of Pelvic Ultrasound

- There is no radiation used and generally no discomfort from the application of ultrasound transducer to skin during transabdominal ultrasound. Slight discomfort with the insertion of transvaginal transducer into the vagina.
- Some women may have allergic reaction to the plastic or latex sheath used as covering for the ultrasound transducer.
- During a transabdominal ultrasound some women experience discomfort from having a full bladder or lying on the examination table.
- Severe obesity.
- Barium within the intestines from a recent barium procedure.
- Intestinal gas.

Procedure of Pelvic (Vaginal) Ultrasound

- For vaginal ultrasound examination, bladder needs to be emptied before the procedure.
- Instruct patient to remove any clothing or jewelry or other objects that may interfere with the scan and wear a hospital gown.
- Help patient to lie on the examination table with feet and legs positioned as for pelvic examination (lithotomy position).
- The physician will introduce the transvaginal transducer covered with a plastic or latex sheath and lubricated.
- The transducer will be gently turned and angled to bring to focus the areas of study.
- Images of organs and structures will be displayed on the computer screen. Images may be recorded on various media for healthcare record.
- Once the procedure has been completed, the transducer will be removed.
- Assist patient to get down from the examination table and instruct to change to her own clothes.

Aftercare of the Patient

No special type care is required after pelvic ultrasound. Patient may resume normal diet and activities.

Abdominal Ultrasound Examination (Fig. 74.18)

Preparation of Patient

Generally no fasting or sedation is required for abdominal ultrasound.

- Drink a minimum of 750 mL of clear fluid at least one hour before procedure. Do not empty the bladder until after the examination.
- For vaginal ultrasound, bladder to be emptied before the procedure.

Explain to the patient:

- To remove any clothing, jewelry or other objects that may interfere with the scan and wear a hospital gown.
- To lie on her back on an examination table.

The physician will:

- Apply ultrasound gel on abdomen.

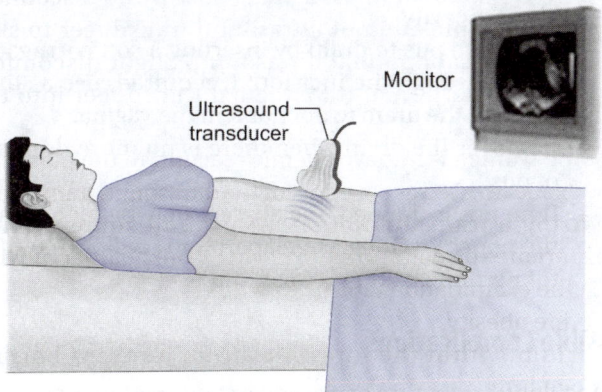

Figure 74.18: Abdominal ultrasound.

- Press the transducer against the skin and moved around over the area to be studied.
- If blood flow is being assessed, a 'whoosh' sound will be heard.
- Images will be displayed on the computer screen and recorded on various media for health record.
- Once the procedure is completed, the gel on abdomen will be removed.

Patient will be asked to empty her bladder.

CULDOCENTESIS

Introduction

Culdocentesis is a procedure in which peritoneal fluid is obtained and/or drained from the cul-de-sac (pouch of Douglas) of a female patient. It involves the introduction of a spinal needle through the posterior vaginal wall into the peritoneal space of the pouch of Douglas.

Prior to the wide availability of ultrasonography, culdocentesis was considered a valuable procedure in the diagnosis of ectopic pregnancy, at which time, 97% of ectopic pregnancies ruptured before diagnosis. Recently, the frequency of tubal rupture has decreased and thus the incidence of hemoperitoneum has declined and the use of culdocentesis has decreased. Further, the ultrasonography with its increased resolution has virtually replaced culdocentesis as the test of choice. Because of its sensitivity and specificity of echogenic fluid found in the ultrasound for establishing hemoperitoneum is 100% compared with 66% for culdocentesis. Additional advantage is its noninvasive nature and provision of additional information about the pelvis. However, the procedure (culdocentesis) is still widely used in some of the developing countries that may not have access to sonography where it is the most common aid for the diagnosis of ruptured ectopic pregnancy.

Use of Culdocentesis

The procedure can aid in the diagnosis of:

- Acute salpingitis.
- Pelvic inflammatory disease (PID).
- Ruptured ectopic/tubal pregnancy.
- Hemoperitoneum related to other pathologic conditions.

Indications

Clinical suspicion of ruptured ectopic pregnancy and hemoperitoneum with signs of:

- Positive pregnancy test.
- Elevated human chorionic gonadotropin (hCG).
- Abdominal pain and vaginal bleeding.
- Peritoneal signs such as rigidity and rebound tenderness of abdomen.
- Rectal pressure.
- Hemodynamic instability such as tachycardia and hypotension.

Contraindications

- Known pelvic mass.
- Retroverted uterus that occupies the pouch of Douglas.

Articles Needed (Fig. 74.19)

A sterile tray containing:
- Vaginal speculum.
- Sponge holding forceps.
- Sterile gauze pieces.
- Tenaculum or Vulsellum forceps
- 18 gauge spinal needle of 5 cm length.
- 10 mL syringe with 3- finger control.
- Sterile gloves.

A clean tray containing:
- Lubricant jelly.
- Iodine solution (Povidone iodine).
- Lidocaine.
- Receptacle for used material.

Procedure (Fig. 74.20)

- Explain the procedure to patient and reassure her.
- Have her empty the bladder.
- Help the patient to assume lithotomy position with legs in stirrups.
- Assist the physician (gynecologist) to:
  - Cleanse cervix and posterior fornix with iodine.
  - Perform a speculum examination.
  - Hold cervix with Vulsellum and move it toward and upward.
  - Anesthetize the mucosa about 1 cm below the posterior rim of cervix.
  - Insert the spinal needle 1 cm below where the cervix ends in the posterior fornix and advance it 3–4 cm and inject 2–3 mL saline or air.
  - Aspirate the fluid from posterior fornix.

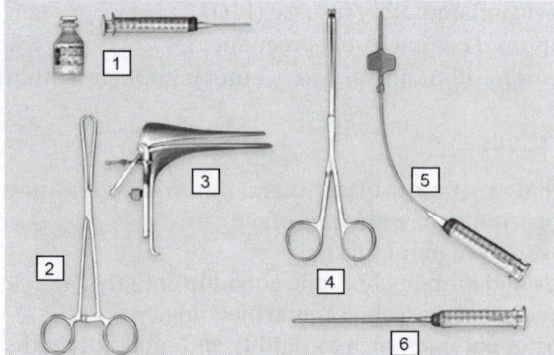

Figure 74.19: Instruments for culdocentesis: (1) Lidocaine with epinephrine; (2) Uterine cervical tenaculum; (3) Bivalve vaginal speculum; (4) Ring forceps; (5) 19 gauge butterfly needle; (6) 18 gauge spinal needle.

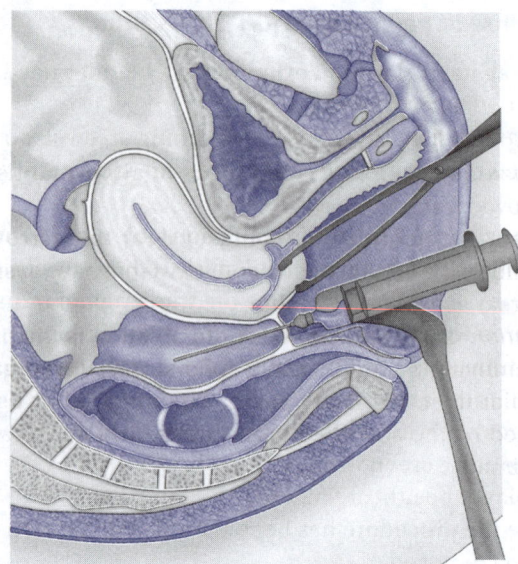

Figure 74.20: Aspiration of fluid from pouch of Douglas.

- Fluid may be sent to the laboratory for testing.
- Make the patient comfortable and transfer to her bed after checking vital signs.
- Clean and replace articles used as appropriate.
- Record the procedure and patient's condition in the chart.

Nature of Aspirate

- If non-clotting blood is obtained, suspect ectopic pregnancy.
- If clotting blood is obtained, a vein or artery must have been aspirated (remove the needle, reinsert and aspirate again).
- If clear or yellow fluid is obtained, there is no blood in the peritoneum. Further observation and test may be required as the woman may still have an unruptured ectopic pregnancy.
- If pus is obtained, keep the needle in place, and proceed with colpotomy. For colpotomy, the physician will:
  - Remove the needle and insert a blunt forceps or a finger through the incision to break the loculi in the abscess cavity.
  - Allow the pus to drain by inserting a soft corrugated drain through the incision. If required, use a stitch through the drain to anchor it in the vagina.
  - Remover the drain when there is no more drainage of pus.
  - If no pus is drained, the abscess may be higher than the pouch of Douglas. A laparotomy will be required for peritoneal lavage (wash-out).

Possible Complications

- Accidental puncture of visceral organs, rectum or uterus.
- Puncture of blood vessels, cysts or tumors.

LASER PROCEDURES/SURGERIES FOR GYNECOLOGICAL CONDITIONS

Important Terms

- *Conization:* A cone-shaped piece of abnormal tissue is removed from the cervix.
- *Laser vaporization:* Use of laser heat to destroy cells usually of the cervix, vagina and vulva that have dysplastic (premalignant) cells in them.
- *Ablation:* Laser ablation or photo ablation is the process of removing material from a solid surface (an organ) by irradiating it with laser beam. The material or tissue is heated by the absorbed laser energy and evaporated or sublimated.

Introduction

Laser surgery is the use of a type of energy that uses special light beams instead of instruments for surgical procedures. Laser stands for "Light Amplification by Stimulated Emission of Radiation". Lasers were first developed in 1960. In gynecological surgeries CO_2 (carbon dioxide) and iridium Lasers are used for the treatment of many female genital tract diseases with applications in colposcopy, laparoscopy and hysteroscopy, obtaining many advantages against more traditional techniques or open surgeries. CO_2 laser coupled with colposcope has become an indispensable tool for ablation and excision of numerous lesions of the lower genital tract especially when it is necessary to minimize tissue removal.

Indications for Laser Surgery

In gynecology, laser surgery is recommended for the treatment of:

- Condylomata accuminata (warts) in the anogenital region.
- Dysplasia (abnormal cells within the tissue or organ) of the vulva, vagina and cervix which were treated with colposcopy.
- Intrauterine and endometrial pathologies which were treated with hysteroscopy or laparoscopy depending on the location of the lesion.

Contraindications

- Active vaginal or vulvar lesions such as herpes, candida, STDs
- Pregnancy or within three months postpartum.
- History of radiation to vaginal or colorectal tissue.
- History of reconstructive pelvic surgery.
- History of impaired wound healing and keloid formation.
- Known anticoagulant therapy or thromboembolic condition.
- Vaginal prolapse of uterus beyond the hymen.

Specific laser equipment and instruments are used with colposcopy, laparoscopy or hysteroscopy (Figs. 74.21 and 74.22)

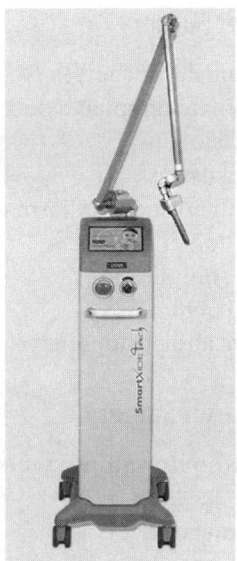

Figure 74.21: CO_2 laser machine.

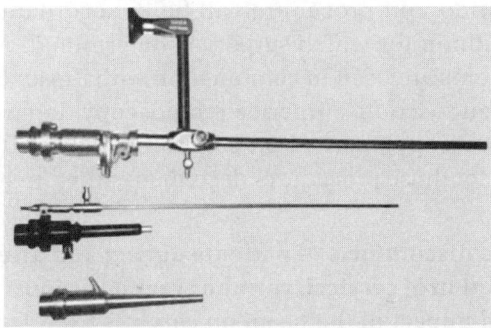

Figure 74.22: Laser instruments: Head piece and coupler, laser wave guides.

- Laser machine
- Laser wave guides
- Hand pieces
- Couplers.

Gynecological Conditions for which Laser Surgery is Used

- Cervical intraepithelial neoplasia (CIN) and vulvar-vaginal intraepithelial neoplasia (VIN).
- Condyloma of cervical, vulvar or perineal tissue.
- Leukoplakia (vulvar dystrophies).
- Incision and drainage of Bartholin's and Nabothian (mucus filled) cysts located on the surface of the cervix or cervical canal).
- Urethral caruncle.
- Cervical dysplasia.
- Benign or malignant lesions of external genitalia.
- Erythroplasia
- Uterine tumors (myomas) and cysts.
- Endometriosis
- Adhesions

Advantages of Laser Surgery

- High degree of clinical efficacy.
- Bloodless field by sealing small blood vessels.
- Microscopic precision.
- Sparing of normal tissue.
- Rapid healing with normal scar formation.
- Significant reduction of pain.
- Small number of complications.
- Accurate removal of tumors.
- Low perioperative and postoperative morbidly.

Disadvantages of Laser Surgery

- Absence of histologic sample when vaporization is performed.
- Expense of laser machine.

Patient Preparation and Procedure

Preparation and procedure will be in accordance with the condition for which surgery is determined. As laser instruments are used in combination with those required for the endoscopic surgeries (colposcopy, laparoscopy or hysteroscopy), patient preparation and procedure are same as for those procedures described earlier in the same chapter.

Possible discomforts of patients during and after laser vaporization of cervical, vulvar or vaginal lesions:

- Initial impact of the beam on cervix is experienced as a pinch similar to that experienced with applying a tenaculum or taking a punch biopsy.
- As vaporization progresses, many women complain of uncomfortable warmth. Stopping the treatment for a moment usually gives relief.
- Menstrual like cramping due to liberation of prostaglandin like substances. This can be relieved by administration of prostaglandin synthetase inhibitor (Motrin) 30 minutes prior to laser vaporization.

Possible Complications

Complication rates are very low:
- Cervical stenosis occurs in 1.3% of cases.
- Cervical incompetence in 0.05%.
- Major bleeding in less than 1% of all patients.

CRYOSURGERY/ CRYOTHERAPY

Description

Cryotherapy also termed cryoablation or cryosurgery is a type of therapy that involves the use of extreme cold to destroy abnormal tissues, such as tumors, warts and polys.

The surgery most often involves the use of liquid nitrogen or argon. When liquid nitrogen has a temperature between -65°C and -75°C, it instantly freezes nearly anything that is in contact with it.

Mechanism of Action of Cold

- Ice formation with in the cell occurs approximately at 40° C or less Intracellular lethal ice crystals begin to for and will destroy almost any cell.
- Nursing from swelling caused by ice expansion inside the cell or shrinking caused by water existing the cell.
- Loss of blood supply occurs and cells die when their blood supply is choked off by ice forming within the small tumor blood vessels causing clotting.
- In order to achieve cell death, tumors are repeatedly frozen and thawed (two or more freeze—thaw cycles. Once the cells die, the white blood cells of the immune system work to clear out the dead tissue.

Indications

- Cervical, vaginal, endometrial and vulvar lesions.
- Confirmed premalignant cervical lesions.
- Recurrent cervicitis and cervical erosion.
- Cervical dysplasia.
- Condyloma (warts) caused by human papillomavirus (HPV).
- Cervical intraepithelial neoplasm (CIN).

Contraindications

- Undiagnosed cervical lesions.
- Pregnancy
- Menstruation
- Unsatisfactory colposcopy
- High grade CIN or persistent CIN after previous cryosurgery.
- Lesions that extend more than 5 cm into endocervical canal.

Cryotherapy Instruments (Fig. 74.23)

- Liquid nitrogen or argon gas or liquid nitrogen oxide machine to create the required temperature of -40°C--45°C.
- Cryoprobe (needle-like applicator)

Procedure (Fig. 74.24)

Preparation of Patient

Patient has to stop taking criteria medications such as aspirin or blood thinners a few days prior to internal cryotherapy.

Performance

For external cryotherapy, the cryoprobe is inserted through vagina and into the cervix using ultrasound imaging guide.

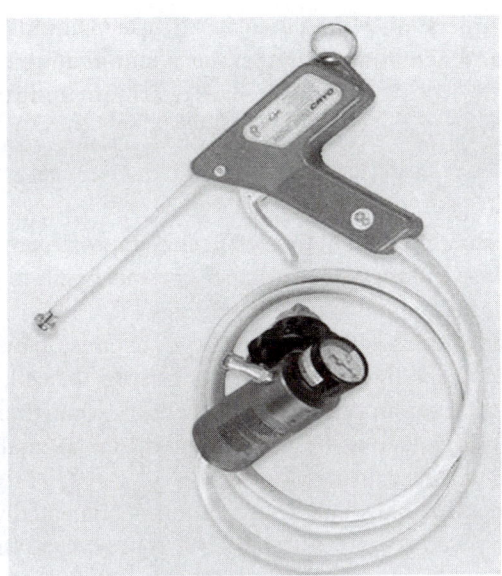

Figure 74.23: Cryotherapy machine and probe.

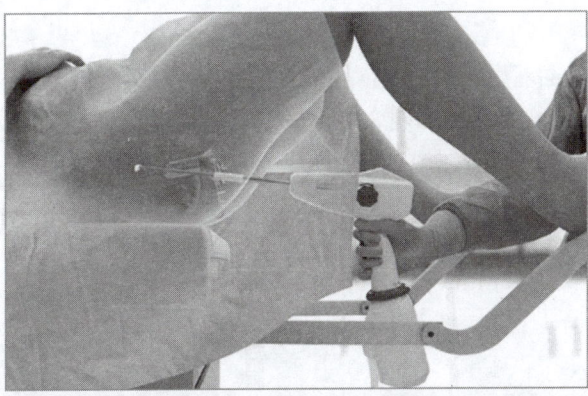

Figure 74.24: Applying cryotherapy probe.

For other parts of the body, the probe is inserted through a small incision in the skin. Ultrasound imaging is used to guide the cryoprobe to the tissue to the frozen. Depending on the location os the abnormal cells, you may be given either local anesthesia or general anesthesia.

After Cryotherapy

Following cryotherapy for an external skin condition, the treated area will turn red and possible and possibly a blister after treatment. Mild pain may subside after about three months. The treated area will form a scab which usually heels in one to three weeks.

Advantages

* Cryosurgery is a minimally invasive treatment compared to traditional surgery.
* It usually has less pain and bleeding and a lower risk of damaging healthy tissues near the abnormal cells.

Risks

Risks are small but complications may include:
* Bleeding, cramping or pain after cryosurgery around the cervix.
* Nerve damage resulting in loss of feeling.
* Swelling, scarring and skin infection.

BIBLIOGRAPHY

1. Hacker N, Gombone J, Hobel C. Hacker & Moore's Essentials of Obstetrics and Gynecology. Philadelphia, PA: Elsevier; 2016.
2. James D. Evidence based Obstetrics. London: WB Saunders; 2004.
3. Lucas C, Hassim AM. Place of culdocentesis in the diagnosis of ectopic pregnancy. Br Med J. 1970;1:200-02.
4. Mac Donald S, Johnson G, Warwick C. Mayes' Midwifery: A textbook for midwives, 14th edition. Philadelphia: Elsevier; 2011.
5. Norwitz E, Schorge J. Obstetrics and Gynecology at a glance. Chichester, West Sussex; John Wiley & Sons; 2013.
6. Seshadri. Essentials of Gynecology. New Delhi: Wolter Kluwer; 2011.
7. Vera M. Nursing Diagnosis guide for 2022. https://nurselabs.com
8. Webster HD, Barclay DL, Fischer CK. Ectopic pregnancy: a seventeen year review. Am J Obstet Gynecol. 1965; 92: 23-4.

Bibliography

Common bibliography for Chapters 63 to 74

1. American College of Obstetrics and Gynecology. [online]. Available from www.acog.org
2. American Society of Reproductive Medicine. [online]. Available from www.asrm
3. Dutta DC. Textbook of Gynecology, 5th edition. Kolkata: New Central Book Agency; 2008.
4. Dutta DC. Textbook of Obstetrics, 5th edition. Kolkata: New Central Book Agency; 2001.
5. Government of India, Ministry of Health and Family Welfare. Annual Report 2005–2006. New Delhi; 2006.
6. Government of India, Rural Health Division Bulletin for Rural Health Statistics in India. New Delhi; 2002.
7. Kozier R, Erb G, Berman A, et al. Fundamentals of nursing, 3rd edition. New Delhi: Dorling Kindersley (P) Ltd; 2007. pp. 1010-20.
8. Littleton LY, Engebretson JC. Maternity nursing care. Thomson Delmar Learning, Australia. 1st Indian reprint. Haryana: Sanat Printers; 2007. pp. 191-238.
9. Mitchel H. Vaginal discharge—causes, diagnosis, and treatment. British Medical Journal. 2004;328(7451):1306-8.
10. Park K. Park's Textbook of Preventive and Social Medicine, 21st edition. Jabalpur: M/s Banarsidas Bhanot Publishers; 2011. pp. 408-526.
11. Pilliteri A. Maternal and Child Health Nursing, 5th edition. Philadelphia: Lippincott Williams & Wilkins; 2007.
12. Sharma KN, Gupta P. Textbook of Midwifery and Gynecological Nursing. Jalandhar City: S Vikas and Company; 2010.
13. Skidmore RL. Mosby's Nursing Drug Reference. Noida: Reed Elsevier India (P) Ltd; 2009.
14. Smeltzer SC, Bare BG, Hinkle LJ, et al. Textbook of medical-surgical nursing, 11th edition. New Delhi: Wolters Kluwer Health (P) Ltd; 2008. pp. 1610-98.
15. Yadav A, Arora VS. Synopsis of Medical Instruments and Procedures. New Delhi: Jaypee Brothers Medical Publishers (P) Ltd; 2003.

APPENDIX: Maternal Newborn Nursing Care Plans

NURSING DIAGNOSES FOR PRENATAL CLIENTS

Deficient Knowledge Related to Self-care Activities during Pregnancy

Definition
Inadequate understanding of information needed to practice health-related behaviors during pregnancy.

Assessments
- Age of patient
- Psychosocial aspects such as health beliefs, knowledge regarding pregnancy and learning ability
- Previous obstetric history, support system and coping pattern
- Mental status and orientation, and memory.

Defining Characteristics
- Inability to follow through instructions
- Inappropriate or exaggerated behaviors such as hostility, apathy and agitation
- Inadequate knowledge of care to be taken during pregnancy
- Verbalization of problems.

Expected Outcomes
- Patient will communicate whenever need more information
- Patient will demonstrate understanding of information taught
- Patient will demonstrate ability to perform new behaviors learned
- Patient will continue to practice appropriate health-related behaviors after pregnancy.

Nursing Interventions
1. Establish a trusting relationship and respect, so that patient will be relaxed and be receptive to learning.
2. Communicate and negotiate realistic learning goals with the patient.
3. Assess patient's knowledge of pregnancy to establish a basis for nursing care plans.
4. Provide information or teach the content to suit the patient's level of understanding.
5. Provide instructions to seek appropriate resource persons for obtaining comprehensive care during pregnancy.
6. Review exercise routines designed for pregnant women to enhance well-being and improve muscle tone in preparation for childbirth.
7. Review dietary intake during pregnancy based on physician's recommendations. Explain to patient that she needs an extra 300 calories per day, for a total of 2,100–2,400 calories per day.
8. Instruct patient to avoid wearing constrictive clothing, using high-heeled shoes and taking non-prescription drugs. Constrictive clothing can decrease venous circulation and high-heeled shoes can increase the likelihood of back strain.
9. Discuss dangers of exposure to toxic chemicals or gases to avoid possible teratogenic effects on fetus.
10. Instruct the woman to contact physician or go to hospital, if she experiences any danger signs or symptoms like:
    - Severe vomiting
    - Frequent and severe headache
    - Epigastric pain
    - Vision disturbances
    - Swelling of fingers and face
    - Altered or absent fetal movements after quickening
    - Signs of vaginal tract or urinary infection
    - Unusual or severe abdominal pain

- Fluid discharge from vagina
- Vaginal bleeding.

Evaluation of Expected Outcomes

- Patient expresses need for more information about self-care
- Patient establishes realistic goals
- Patient demonstrates understanding of matters taught:
  - Follows appropriate exercises
  - Limits or stops smoking and/or consumption of alcohol if indicated
  - Obtains sufficient rest
  - Avoids areas that may contain toxic chemicals or gases
  - Stops wearing constrictive clothing and high-heeled shoes
  - Reports danger signals to physician promptly
  - Takes prenatal vitamins as prescribed.
- Patient demonstrates ability to perform health-related behaviors learned
- Patient continues to practice health-related behaviors after pregnancy.

Documentation

- Patient's knowledge of self-care activities
- Expressions indicating motivation to learn
- Teaching carried out and methods of teaching used
- Dietary intake reported or observed
- Demonstration or return demonstration skills
- Response to teaching observed.

Nausea and Vomiting Related to Physiological Changes of Pregnancy

Definition

A minor disorder of pregnancy is experienced by pregnant woman between 4th and 16th week of gestation.

Assessments

- Characteristics and patterns of occurrence of nausea and vomiting
- Types of food and smell to which patient has intolerance
- Physical health status
- Patient's understanding of the physiological changes of pregnancy
- Support system available.

Defining Characteristics

- Change in appetite and pattern of eating
- Vomiting in the morning and/or later in the day
- Increased salivation
- Inability to retain food and fluids
- Fatigue and signs of dehydration.

Expected Outcomes

- Patient will identify the factors that aggravate vomiting
- Patient will appreciate the physiological changes of pregnancy that cause vomiting
- Patient will modify her eating habits
- Patient will adopt appropriate measures to obtain relief
- Patient will experience cessation of vomiting and improvement of general health.

Nursing Interventions

1. Assess and document the extent of nausea and vomiting to have a database.
2. Reassure patient that nausea will usually subside by the 4th month of pregnancy in order to reduce her anxiety.
3. Instruct patient to eat dry, unsalted crackers before rising in the morning to prevent nausea from an empty stomach.
4. Instruct the patient to avoid greasy or spicy food, which irritates the stomach. Fats with meals depress gastric motility and secretion of digestive enzymes and slow intestinal peristalsis causing gastroesophageal reflux.
5. Advise patient to avoid cooking odors that precipitate nausea.
6. Advise pregnant woman to eat six small meals instead of three large ones to avoid overloading the stomach.
7. Advise pregnant woman to eat foods, which high in carbohydrates as they are easier to digest.
8. Instruct pregnant woman to take iron pills and vitamins after meals to avoid irritating the stomach.
9. Advise to take frequent walks outside, as fresh air reduces nausea and helps reinforce a positive outlook.
10. Instruct to separate food and fluid intake by half-an-hour. Drinking excessive fluids with food distends stomach, predisposing to nausea.
11. Advise pregnant woman to avoid very cold food and fluids at meal times as they may cause nausea and abdominal cramping.
12. Instruct pregnant woman to consult physician before taking over-the-counter medications for nausea and vomiting to avoid harmful effects on fetus.

Evaluation of Expected Outcomes

- Patient identifies factors and food habits that aggravate nausea and vomiting
- Patient modifies her eating habits
- Patient adopts measures to obtain relief from nausea
- Patient experiences reduction in nausea and cessation of vomiting
- Patient experiences improvement of general health.

Documentation

- Patient's description of nausea, vomiting and aggravating factors

- Patient's general health observed
- Instructions given to patient and her response to teaching
- Change in eating and drinking habits observed and reported by patient
- Expected outcomes evaluated.

Acute Pain: Backache Related to Physiological Changes of Pregnancy

Definition

Discomfort experienced by some pregnant women during pregnancy in the lower back region.

Assessments

- Patient's posture, lifting techniques and footwear
- Lifestyle and exercise pattern
- Type and duration of pain
- Relief measures.

Defining Characteristics

- Strain of muscles in the lower back
- Difficulty in changing position and lifting objects
- The anxiety due to disruption of normal activities
- The anxiety due to inability to continue exercises.

Expected Outcomes

- Patient identifies characteristics of pain
- Patient verbalizes factors that intensify the pain and modify behaviors, accordingly
- Patient will carry out appropriate interventions for pain relief.

Nursing Interventions

- Instruct patient to maintain good posture, hold her shoulders back and to wear low-heeled shoes to decrease spinal curvature, which may reduce backache
- Instruct the patient about proper body mechanics to help her avoid stress to her lower back
- Advise patient to rest in recumbent position or with her legs bent and elevated on a bed, or chair to relieve strain in the lower back
- Instruct the patient to perform moderate daily exercises to tone and maintain muscle strength in the lower back
- Explain the benefits of massaging and applying warm, moist heat to the lower back to relax and soothe tight muscles.

Evaluation of Expected Outcomes

- Patient identifies characteristics of back pain
- Patient lists factors that intensify pain and modifies behavior accordingly
- Patient carries out appropriate interventions for pain relief.

Documentation

- Patient's description of pain and expression of feelings about pain
- Observations about patient's responses to pain
- Comfort measures and medications provided to reduce pain
- Effectiveness of interventions for pain relief
- Patient teaching carried out about pain relief measures
- Expected outcomes observed and reported by patient.

Urinary Frequency and Dysuria Related to Physiological Changes of Pregnancy

Definition

Frequency, urgency and pain on urination experienced by some women during pregnancy.

Assessments

- Nature and duration of urinary frequency
- Daily fluid intake
- Symptoms of urinary tract infection (UTI) such as pain on micturition and fever
- Patient's understanding of the physiological changes in pregnancy.

Defining Characteristics

- Frequency and urgency of urination
- Dysuria, if associated infection present
- Sleep disturbance due to urinary frequency
- Occurrence of complaints in the early and late months of pregnancy.

Expected Outcomes

- Patient will experience relief from frequency of urination and dysuria
- Patient will increase her fluid intake during day time
- Patient will practice measures to prevent bladder distention and urinary stasis
- Patient will learn to report signs of developing UTI.

Nursing Interventions

- Reassure patient that urinary frequency is normal in the early and late months of pregnancy because the enlarging uterus places pressure on the bladder
- Instruct patient to avoid drinking large amounts of fluids within 2–3 hours of bedtime to prevent nocturnal urination and sleep loss
- Instruct client to ingest the required amount of fluid early in the day to reduce the need for evening liquids
- Instruct client to void whenever the urge occurs, to prevent bladder distention and urinary stasis, which may predispose to UTI
- Teach patient, signs and symptoms of UTI

- Teach patient to report signs and symptoms of UTI promptly
- Early detection of UTI allows early treatment and helps to prevent complications such as pyelonephritis.

Evaluation of Expected Outcomes

- Patient develops knowledge of the causes of urinary frequency
- Patient adapts and adjusts to the change in urinary elimination
- Patient modifies her fluid intake pattern
- Patient learns to identify and report signs of UTI, if she develops it
- Patient experiences more rest during night and relaxation during day time.

Documentation

- Patient's description of urinary frequency and dysuria
- Measures of relief explained and response of patient
- Relief measures observed and reported
- Health instructions given.

Acute Pain: Leg Cramps Related to Physiological Changes of Pregnancy

Definition

A minor disorder of pregnancy experienced as sudden severe pain in leg muscles.

Assessment

- Dietary pattern
- Pain status such as location, time and duration
- Activity and rest pattern
- Relief measures
- Body mechanics and exercise practices.

Defining Characteristics

- Contraction of muscle and severe pain
- Inability to change position
- Anxiety due to the acute pain
- Fear of recurrence of pain
- Lack of knowledge of measures for relief of cramps.

Expected Outcomes

- Patient will identify factors that cause leg cramps
- Patient will discuss the measures to deal with episodes of leg cramps
- Patient will increase her intake of calcium containing foods and decrease the consumption of phosphorus
- Patient will practice exercises to increase general circulation
- Patient will stop getting cramps.

Nursing Interventions

- Reassure patient that leg cramps are normal during pregnancy to help reduce her anxiety
- Assess dietary pattern for inadequate dietary protein and excessive soft drink intake as alteration of calcium-phosphorus ratio can lead to leg cramps
- Instruct patient to increase the intake of milk and other sources of calcium rich food items
- Instruct patient to elevate her legs periodically and to avoid lying with toes pointed; lying prone with toes pointed predisposes to blood vessel occlusion and subsequent cramping
- Instruct patient to exercise and use good body mechanics to prevent leg cramping by increasing general circulation
- Advise patient to take warm bath at bedtime to relax muscle fibers and increase blood flow to muscles
- Teach patient, what she needs to do when cramping occurs; straighten the affected leg and dorsiflexion of the foot; these measures pull the contracted muscles taut, thus relieving a cramp caused by contraction
- Caution the mother not to rub the affected calf to avoid the risk of dislodging any undetected thrombus.

Evaluation of Expected Outcomes

- Patient expresses understanding of factors that cause leg cramps
- Patient verbalizes the measures and practice to reduce the occurrence of leg cramps
- Patient discusses the measures to practice when cramping occurs
- Patient reports changes in dietary pattern and exercises
- Patient reports relief from occurrence of leg cramps.

Documentation

- Patient's knowledge of causes and measures to deal with leg cramps
- Instructions given and patient's response
- Patient's report of lifestyle changes to avoid leg cramps
- Changes reported by patient regarding reduction of the problem of leg cramps.

Acute Pain: Heartburn Related to Physiological Changes of Pregnancy

Definition

Uncomfortable sensation in the abdomen experienced in relation to food intake during pregnancy.

Assessments

- Dietary patterns
- Intake of greasy and spicy foods

- Pattern of fluid intake
- Occurrence of heartburn in relation to food intake.

Defining Characteristics

- Onset of heartburn after eating heavy meals
- Onset after greasy and spicy food
- Discomfort in supine position
- Discomfort after consuming cold foods.

Expected Outcomes

- Patient will change eating pattern to small, frequent meals
- Patient will avoid high-fat content in food
- Patient will avoid unhealthy posture after meals
- Patient will avoid drinking very cold fluids and fluids with meals.

Nursing Interventions

- Assess patient's nutritional habits for selection of appropriate interventions
- Reassure patient that normal changes in pregnancy can cause heartburn to reduce her anxiety
- Instruct patient to eliminate greasy and spicy foods, and to avoid fats as such foods decrease stomach motility and increase gastric acidity
- Instruct patient to reduce fluid intake with meals as it tends to inhibit gastric juices
- Instruct pregnant woman to avoid very cold foods as they may cause gastric reflux
- Instruct pregnant woman to drink low-fat or skimmed milk rather than whole milk
- Instruct pregnant woman to avoid assuming supine position after eating to provide more space in stomach for function
- Instruct patient to take small, frequent meals to avoid overloading the stomach
- Instruct to avoid over bending, which doing housekeeping activity
- Instruct patient to remain upright for 3–4 hours after each meal to decrease the possibility of reflux
- Instruct patient to take antacids, if prescribed by physician for relief of discomfort.

Evaluation of Expected Outcomes

- Patient expresses understanding of the physiological changes in pregnancy that cause heartburn
- Patient expresses measures that she will adapt for reducing heartburn
- Patient reports decreased discomfort from heartburn
- Patient demonstrates signs of reduced anxiety.

Documentation

- Patient's description of discomfort due to heartburn
- Patient's description of relief measures she uses

- Change in eating and drinking habits reported and observed
- Expected outcomes evaluated.

NURSING DIAGNOSES FOR LABOR AND DELIVERY CLIENTS

Acute Pain: Related to Physiological Response of Labor

Definition

An unpleasant sensory and emotional experience arising from actual or potential tissue damage; pain may be sudden or slow in onset, vary in intensity from mild to severe and constant, or recurring.

Assessments

- Characteristics of pain including location, intensity and source of relief
- Physiological variables including age and pain tolerance
- Psychological variables including personality, previous experience with pain and anxiety
- Sociocultural variables such as cognitive style, culture, attitudes and values
- Knowledge and expectations of labor, and delivery.

Defining Characteristics

- Alteration is muscle tone such as listless to rigid
- Autonomic response such as diaphoresis, change in blood pressure and respiratory rate, dilated pupils
- Change in appetite
- Communication of pain
- Behavior such as pacing and seeking out other people
- Expressions of pain such as moaning and crying
- Grimacing and other facial expressions
- Guarding or protective behavior
- Narrowed focus such as altered perception, impaired thought process and withdrawal from people
- Self-focusing
- Sleep disturbance.

Expected Outcomes

- Patient will identify characteristics of pain
- Patient will describe factors that intensify pain
- Patient will modify behavior to decrease pain
- Patient will express decrease in intensity of pain
- Patient will express satisfaction of her performance during labor and delivery.

Nursing Interventions

- Orient patient to labor and delivery rooms on admission
- Explain admission protocol and labor process
- Show patient her room, bed and facilities such as call bell, toilet, television, etc. to allay her fear and anxiety

- Assess patient's knowledge of labor process to plan nursing interventions
- Explain availability of analgesics and/or anesthesia (epidural) to patient and family for reducing anxiety
- Encourage support person or family member to remain with patient, if hospital policy permits
- Instruct patient and support person in techniques to decrease the discomfort of labor:
  - Discuss techniques of conscious relaxation
  - Instruct to concentrate on an internal or external focal point
  - Instruct in deep chest breathing during contractions
  - Instruct in shallow chest breathing and slow panting-like breathing, which will avoid hyperventilations
  - Instruct patient in effleurage.
- In early labor, provide patient with diversional activities such as watching television, if possible to reduce anxiety
- As labor progresses to active phase, modify environment to reduce distractions and promote concentration, e.g. close curtains and door, turn off television
- Apply sacral pressure if needed to decrease back pain
- Assist to change position and provide additional pillow to reduce stiffness, and promoter comfort
- Assess bladder for distention and encourage to void every 2 hours to reduce discomfort during contractions, and facilitate fetal descend
- Provide frequent mouth care; provide ice chips or wet gauze for dry lips caused by breathing techniques and nil by mouth
- Apply cool, damp washcloth to forehead to relieve diaphoresis
- Provide clean gown and bed linen as needed, diaphoresis and vaginal discharge can dampen bed lines and gown
- Encourage patient to rest and relax between contractions to decrease discomfort
- Discuss with patient and support person that pain medications are available, if alternate pain control methods provide inadequate relief
- When required, administer prescribed analgesics to cope with labor process.

Evaluation of Expected Outcomes

- Patient identifies characteristics of pain and describes factors that intensify it
- Patient modifies behaviors to decrease pain and discomfort such as using breathing techniques, asking for analgesia and assuming comfortable position
- Patient reports decrease in discomfort
- Patient expresses satisfaction with her performance during childbirth.

Documentation

- Patient's childbirth preparation
- Patient's description of pain and discomfort
- Observation of patient's response to labor
- Nursing interventions carried out to decrease discomfort
- Patient's response to nursing interventions.

Deficient Knowledge Related to Information about Birth Process

Definition

Inadequate understanding of or inability to perform skills needed to cope effectively with the process of labor.

Assessments

- Age of patient
- Psychosocial status such as expectations of the birth process and interest in learning
- Current knowledge about pregnancy, birth and recovery
- Ability to learn and attention span
- Support system including presence of support person interested in helping the patient.

Defining Characteristics

- Inability to follow through with instructions
- Inappropriate or exaggerated behaviors such as hysteria, hostility, agitation and apathy
- Verbalization of problems.

Expected Outcomes

- Patient will recognize that increased knowledge and skill will help her cope better with birth process
- Patient will demonstrate understanding of what is taught
- Patient will demonstrate ability to perform skills needed for coping with labor
- Patient will express realistic expectations about birth process
- Patient will express satisfaction with her increased knowledge.

Nursing Interventions

- Find a quite private place to teach the patient
- Establish a trusting relationship with the patient and develop mutual goals for learning
- Select appropriate teaching methods and materials such as discussions and demonstrations using audiovisual aids
- Teach information and skills needed for understanding, and coping during birth to increase the patient's sense of competence.

Evaluation of Expected Outcomes

- Patient expresses desire to put knowledge into practice during labor
- Patient describes birth process in her own words
- Patient responds to labor without undue anxiety and uses breathing, relaxation, and position changes

- Patient voices satisfaction with newly acquired knowledge and skills.

Documentation

- Patient understands about birth process
- Patient's expression of need for better understanding
- Learning goals established with the patient
- Information and skills taught to patient
- Teaching methods used
- Patient's response to teaching
- Patient's mastery of knowledge and skills demonstrated
- Evaluation of expected outcomes are observed.

Ineffective Coping Individual Related to Labor and Delivery

Definition

Inability to use adaptive behaviors in response to labor and delivery.

Assessments

- Age, health beliefs, feelings about pregnancy, decision-making ability motivation to learn and obstacles to learning
- Pain threshold, perception of pain and response to analgesia
- Stage and length of labor, complications, ability to concentrate, and use techniques, presence and effectiveness of support person
- Mode of delivery
- Previous experience with pregnancy, labor and deliver, and knowledge of birth process
- Pre-existing pregnancy induced or medical conditions.

Defining Characteristics

- Expressed inability to cope
- Fatigue
- Inability to meet basic needs and role expectations
- Poor concentration and problem-solving abilities
- Destructive behavior toward self or others.

Expected Outcomes

- Patient will express need to develop better coping behaviors
- Patient will set realistic learning goals
- Patient will use learned coping skills
- Patient will communicate feelings about pregnancy, labor and delivery
- Patient will maintain appropriate sense of control throughout the course of labor and delivery
- Patient will demonstrate ability to cope with unexpected changes.

Nursing Interventions

- Establish a relationship of mutual trust and respect to enhance patient's learning
- Develop learning goals with the patient to foster a sense of control
- Select appropriate teaching strategies to encourage compliance
- Teach skills that the patient can use during labor and delivery, and give her a return demonstration of each skill
- During the latent phase of labor (dilation 1–4 cm):
    - Encourage patient to participate in her own care
    - Encourage breathing techniques that she can use during labor
    - Involve support person in care and comfort measures
    - Provide continuous or frequent monitoring to identify any deviation from normal.
- During the active phase of labor (dilation 4–8 cm):
    - Encourage patient to assume comfortable position to promote relaxation between contractions
    - Assist patient with breathing techniques to reduce anxiety and prevent hyperventilation
    - Encourage the support person to participate in patient care such as changing soiled linen, providing sacral pressure, back rub and offering ice chips to moisten lips
    - Administer analgesia as ordered to reduce pain
    - Reassure patient about fetal status.
- During the transitional phase of labor (dilation 8–10 cm):
    - Assist patient with breathing during contractions
    - Encourage rest between contractions
    - Explain all procedures and treatments and answer patient's questions to allay fears.
- During delivery of the placenta:
    - Encourage patient to maintain her position to facilitate delivery of placenta
    - Show the neonate to the patient and reassure about the neonate's condition to provide emotional support
    - Allow the patient to hold the neonate, if permitted
    - Allow her to breastfeed the neonate, if she desires to promote bonding.
- In a delivery, allow the patient to express her feelings and explain to her the care being provided to enable her cope with the task of motherhood.

Evaluation of Expected Outcomes

- Patient participates in establishing learning goals
- Patient successfully uses breathing and relaxation techniques during labor, and delivery
- Patient maintains appreciable sense of control during labor and delivery
- Nurses and support persons provide effective comfort to patient during labor and delivery
- Patient demonstrates ability to cope with unexpected changes.

Documentation

- Patient's knowledge of labor and delivery
- Patient's expressions of motivation to learn
- Methods used to teach patient
- Information taught and skills demonstrated
- Patient's level of satisfaction with delivery
- Evaluation of expected outcomes.

Anxiety Related to Hospitalization and Birth Process

Definition

Feeling of threat or danger to self-related to pregnancy or delivery.

Assessments

- Expressed worries, fears and concerns
- Expectations of labor experience
- Reactions to uterine activity, fetal movement and interactions with nurse, and significant others
- Ability to concentrate, learn and remember
- Physiological status
- Usual coping methods
- Mood and personality
- Progress of labor.

Defining Characteristics

- Excessive attention to uterine activity and fetal movements
- Excessive reaction to uterine contractions
- Expressed concern about childbirth
- Expressed fear of unspecified negative outcomes
- Expressed feelings of helplessness
- Fear and apprehension
- Inability to concentrate and remember
- Increased muscle tension in body
- Increased perspiration
- Rapid pulse rate
- Restlessness, shakiness and trembling.

Expected Outcomes

- Patient will express feelings of anxiety
- Patient will identify causes of anxiety
- Patient will make use of available emotional support
- Patient will show fewer signs of anxiety
- Patient will identify positive aspects of her efforts to cope during childbirth
- Patient will acquire increased knowledge about childbirth
- Patient will be better prepared to cope with future births.

Nursing Interventions

- Assess the patient's knowledge and expectations of labor to identify the precise source of anxiety
- Discuss normal labor progression with patient and explain, what to expect during labor to help her to understand her own experience
- Involve the patient in making decisions about care to reduce the sense of powerlessness
- Share information about progress of labor and neonate's condition with patient to provide reassurance, and to increase her sense of participation
- Interpret to patient, sights and sounds in labor room such as fetal heart sounds, fetal monitor strip, and activities to reduce anxiety and increase confidence
- Attend to the patient's comfort needs to increase her trust
- Encourage patient to use coping skills such as breathing relaxation and positioning to increase her sense of power, and control
- Provide adequate explanation regarding all procedures performed on her in the labor room
- Spend as much time as possible with the patient to provide comfort and assistance, thereby promoting the patient's sense of security
- Allow family member to participate in care to promote comfort and help patient cope with labor.

Evaluation of Expected Outcomes

- Patient expresses feelings of anxiety about pregnancy and childbirth
- Patient identifies causes of anxiety
- Patient communicates with nurse and family members to gain reassurance, and emotional support
- Patient's physiologic and behavioral signs return to normal
- Patient express satisfaction with her behavior, while giving birth.

Documentation

- Patient's expression of anxiety
- Patient's statement of reason for anxiety
- Observations of physical and behavioral signs of anxiety
- Interventions to assist patient with coping
- Patient's response to interventions
- Evaluation of expected outcomes observed.

Risk for Infection Related to Labor and Delivery

Definition

Presence of internal or external hazards that threaten maternal and neonatal well-being.

Assessments

- Maternal vital signs
- Fetal heart rate
- Health history including previous infection

- Detail regarding rupture of membranes such as time of rupture and characteristics of amniotic fluid (amount, color and odor)
- Laboratory findings such as white blood cell (WBC) count, platelet count, clotting factors, hemoglobin, hematocrit and culture of blood, and urine
- Signs and symptoms of chorioamnionitis such as maternal pulse rate over 160 beats per minute, foul smelling amniotic fluid, increasing uterine tenderness and fetal tachycardia.

Associated Medical Conditions

- Early rupture of membranes
- Peritonitis
- Pyelonephritis
- Urinary tract infection.

Expected Outcomes

- Patient will maintain good hygiene
- Patient will remain free from infection
- Patient's temperature will remain within normal range.

Nursing Interventions

- Monitor and record the patient's temperature every 4 hours before rupture of membranes and every 2 hours after they rupture to detect early signs of infections
- Monitor fetal heart rate continuously, if a monitor is used and every 30 minutes, otherwise; report rates over 160 beats per minute and variability under 3–5 beats per minute as these are signs of maternal fever
- Wash hands thoroughly before and after providing care to mother to prevent spread of infection
- Wear gloves when contact with patient's blood and body fluids is expected for prevention of spread of infection
- Use strict sterile technique for procedures such as applying scalp electrode, inserting urinary catheter and inserting intravenous (IV) lines to reduce the likelihood of nosocomial infection
- Minimize vaginal examinations after rupture of membranes and always use sterile gloves to reduce the risk of chorioamnionitis
- Clean perineal area and maintain good hygiene, clean from front to back to reduce the risk of infection
- Monitor intake and output to assess for dehydration.

Evaluation of Expected Outcome

- Patient maintains good hygiene
- Patient remains free from infection as evidenced by clear, odorless, sediment-free urine, WBC count within normal limits and cultures free from pathogens
- Patient's temperature stays between 97°F and 99°F (36.1°C and 37.2°C).

Documentation

- Maternal vital signs
- Fetal heart rate and variability
- Date, time and sites of catheter insertions
- Nursing interventions performed to reduce risk of infection
- Evaluation of expected outcomes.

Risk for Injury Related to Induction of Labor

Definition

Increased risk to maternal or fetal well-being resulting from oxytocin stimulation.

Assessments

- History of previous pregnancies
- Prenatal history of present pregnancy (including laboratory findings, pelvic measurements, allergies, weight gain, last menses and estimated date of confinement)
- Physical examination including vital signs, Leopold's maneuvers, uterine contractions, vaginal examination and fetal heart rate
- Diagnostic studies such as ultrasonography test (to determine gestational age and fetal size, and non-stress or contraction stress test to assess fetal placental function)
- Laboratory studies including complete blood count, blood type and Rh factor, platelets, and urine test for protein and glucose levels
- Contraindications such as cephalopelvic disproportion, fetal distress, grand multiparity, overdistention of uterus from multiple gestation or polyhydramnios, vaginal bleeding and unfavorable fetal presentation, or position.

Risk Factor

- Dysfunctional labor
- Hypotonic contractions
- Postmaturity
- Previous precipitous delivery
- Prolonged rupture of membranes.

Expected Outcomes

- Patient will have effective uterine contractions, i.e. every 2–3 minutes for 30–40 seconds or with intensity of 40–60 mm Hg by electronic monitor
- Continuous fetal monitoring will show fetal heart rate variability of 6–10 beats per minute with reassuring pattern
- Patient will achieve good labor pattern and neonate will be delivered without complications
- Patient and fetus will maintain optimal well-being.

Nursing Interventions

- Explain oxytocin protocol to the patient and her support person (explain that oxytocin induced contractions may peak more quickly and last longer than spontaneous

contractions to reduce apprehension and encourage patient participation)
- Encourage patient to void before applying fetal monitor and administering oxytocin (palpate bladder for distention every 2 hours to avoid discomfort during induction period)
- Monitor intake and output, and measure urine specific gravity to detect urine retention, which may delay descend
- Place patient in comfortable position as possible and in left lateral (as it relieves pressure of gravid uterus on the inferior vena cava, and promotes blood flow to the placenta)
- Apply the fetal monitor and obtain a 15-20 minutes baseline strip
- Start a primary IV line with an 18G or 20G catheter
- Prepare oxytocin as ordered; add the drug to a 5% dextrose or normal saline solution (10 units to 1,000 mL solution initially); label the bottle with the patient's name, amount of oxytocin, date and time prepared, and the nurse's name
- Piggyback the oxytocin solution to the primary IV line; use an IV infusion pump to control the flow rate; the infusion pump guarantees exact dose administration for accurate assessment of uterine response
- Begin infusion at the rate of 0.5-1 mg/min and remain with the patient during the first 20 minutes to evaluate the patient's response to uterine stimulation
- Increase the oxytocin infusion as ordered, by increments of 1-2 mU/min as ordered, every 30-60 minutes until the desired contraction pattern is achieved and cervix is dilated 5-6 cm; monitor blood pressure before and after each increase
- Monitor the contraction pattern and fetal rate every 15 minutes; document the fetal heart rate, variability and any fetal strip changes
- If the patient responds poorly to oxytocin infusion, check the IV mixture and IV lines for patency; increase the flow rate according to agency policy and physician's order
- Observe for hypertonicity; contractions lasting longer than 90 seconds and occurring less than 2 minutes apart, and a reaching (on minor strip) greater than 75 mm Hg; if detected discontinue infusion immediately check maternal vital signs and notify physician; increase the flow rate of primary IV solution and position the patient on her left side; these measures help arrest hypertonicity
- Monitor continuously for loss of variability, late decelerations or persistent bradycardia to detect fetal distress resulting from impaired uteroplacental perfusion caused by increased tonicity of contractions
- If signs of fetal distress are noted, take the following steps:
  – Discontinue oxytocin infusion, administer oxygen using a rebreathing mask at 8-12 breaths per minute to increase the oxygen supply to fetus
  – Increase the flow rate of primary IV line to increase fluids
  – Reposition patient on her left or opposite side to increase placental blood flow.
- Assess the patient's intake and output, and monitor the amount of oxytocin administered. Total fluid intake should not exceed 125 mL/h (the antidiuretic effect of oxytocin and large volume of electrolyte free solution can lead to water intoxication).

Evaluation of Expected Outcome

- Patient has contractions at every 2-3 minutes that last for 30-60 seconds and are of moderate intensity with adequate resting tonus
- Continuous fetal monitoring shows reassuring fetal heart pattern with variability of 6-10 beats
- Patient achieves good labor pattern and delivers neonate without complications
- Patient maintains fluid balance
- Patient and fetus maintain optimal well-begin during labor, and delivery.

Documentation

- Vital signs on admission and at every 15-30 minutes according to facility policy
- Baseline assessment of uterine activity (frequency, intensity, interval, duration and tonus) before oxytocin stimulation and at every 30 minutes, thereafter via continuous electronic fetal monitoring
- Assessment of fetal heart rate including baseline rate, long-term variability, short-term variability, accelerations and periodic changes using internal or external monitoring
- Patient's physical and emotional response to induction or augmentation, or labor.

Deficient Knowledge Related to Premature Labor

Definition

Inadequate understanding of, or inability to perform, skills needed to cope with premature labor.

Assessments

- Age of patient
- Health beliefs
- Knowledge regarding pregnancy and birth process
- Previous experience with premature labor
- Financial resources
- Learning ability
- Support system.

Defining Characteristics

- Inappropriate or exaggerated behaviors, e.g. hysteria, hostility, agitation
- Inability to follow instructions
- Inadequate knowledge of the condition
- Verbalization of the problems.

Expected Outcomes

- Patient will express desire to learn about premature labor
- Patient will express understanding of causes, signs and symptoms, and management of premature labor

- Patient will identify and report danger signals without delay
- Patient will use available support systems
- Patient will cope successfully with premature labor
- Pregnancy will result in positive outcome.

Nursing Interventions

- Provide measures to reduce anxiety such as:
  - Introducing staff members to patient and family
  - Providing orientation to surroundings and routine.
- Establish mutual trust and respect, which will calm the patient
- Assist patient to develop realistic goals
- Assess patient's understanding of pregnancy and premature labor using appropriate teaching strategies
- Remain with patient for uninterrupted period of time and project a warm, and caring attitude
- Include patient in decision-making when possible to give her a sense of participation and control
- Provide information related to health status and condition of fetus to relieve her anxiety
- Teach patient the danger signs and symptoms to be reported immediately such as:
  - Contractions occurring at every 10 minutes or less for 1 hour
  - Fluid leaking from vagina
  - Reduced or lack of or fetal movements.
- Prompt reporting helps avoid premature labor
- Review discharge instructions if patient are discharged for home before delivery
- Emphasize taking prescribed medications limiting activities and reporting danger signs.

Evaluation of Expected Outcomes

- Patient express desire to learn about premature labor
- Patient demonstrates ability to identify causes and signs, and symptoms of premature labor
- Patient expresses understanding of methods of management of premature labor
- Patient reports promptly danger signals and receive appropriate interventions
- Patient uses available support systems
- Patient successfully copes with premature labor as demonstrated by verbal and non-verbal behaviors
- Pregnancy results in positive outcome.

Documentation

- Patient's understanding of premature labor expressed in her own words
- Methods used to teach patient and family support person
- Response to teaching demonstrated by patient and family
- Maternal and fetal physical status
- Evaluation of expected outcomes.

Deficient Fluid Volume Related to Altered Intake during Labor

Definition

Inadequate hydration resulting from reduced intake or excessive loss of body fluids.

Assessments

- Vital signs such as temperature, pulse rate, respiration and blood pressure
- Fluid and electrolyte status including weight, intake and output, urine specific gravity, skin turgor, mucous membranes, electrolytes and blood urea levels.

Defining Characteristics

- Change in mental status
- Decreased pulse volume and pressure
- Decreased urine output
- Decreased venous filling
- Dry skin and mucous membranes
- Increased body temperature
- Increased hematocrit
- Increased pulse rate
- Increased urine concentration
- Low blood pressure
- Poor skin turgor
- Sudden loss of weight
- Increased weakness.

Associated Medical Conditions

- Diabetes mellitus
- Hemorrhage
- Pregnancy-induced hypertension (PIH)
- Premature rupture of membranes
- Shock.

Expected Outcomes

- Patient will maintain fluid balance
- Patient will demonstrate optimal hydration
- Patient will show no sign of dehydration.

Nursing Interventions

- Monitor vital signs at frequency intervals according to the policy of the institution
- Assess skin turgor and examine oral mucous membrane for dryness periodically
- Monitor intake and output according to protocol
- Administer and monitor parental fluids (usually 125–175 mL/h). Output should approximate to intake in order to help ensure adequate hydration
- Monitor electrolyte values and report abnormal values
- Provide patient with ice chips and cold compress to increase comfort, and decrease mouth dryness
- Measure the amount and character of vomitus, and assess the need for an antiemetic [when labor begins gastrointestinal (GI) motility and absorption decreases as

blood is rerouted to meet the energy needs of contracting uterus causing food to remain in the stomach for up to 12 hours; this predisposes to nausea and vomiting especially during the transition phase of labor]
- Administer antiemetics as ordered
- Keep patient cool and comfortable by changing soiled linen, and applying cold compress to face and body to reduce discomfort caused by diaphoresis
- Position patient on her left side to aid kidney perfusion and increase cardiac, and urine output.

Evaluation of Expected Outcomes

- Patient maintains fluid balance with intake approximately equaling output
- Patient maintains optimal hydration
- Patient has no signs of dehydration:
  - Mucous membranes remain pink and moist
  - Skin turgor remains optimal
  - Vital signs stay within normal limits
  - Urine output is at least 30 mL/h or 100 mL in 4 hours.

Documentation

- Vital signs
- Observation of fluid volume status
- Fluid intake and output
- Nursing interventions and patient's response
- Evaluation of expected outcomes.

NURSING DIAGNOSES FOR POSTPARTUM CLIENTS

Deficient Knowledge Related to Postpartum Care

Definition

Inadequate understanding of the postpartum self-care activities or inability to perform skills needed to practice health-related behaviors.

Assessments

- Age and learning ability
- Decision-making ability
- Interest in learning
- Knowledge and skill regarding postpartum self-care
- Obstacles to learning
- Support systems and usual coping pattern
- Physical abilities to perform the self-care activities.

Defining Characteristics

- Inability to follow through with the instructions
- Inappropriate or exaggerated behaviors such as hostility, agitation or apathy
- Poor knowledge level
- Verbalization of problem.

Expected Outcomes

- Patient will express desire to learn, how to care for herself after delivery
- Patient will verbalize or demonstrate understanding of what she has learned about self-care
- Patient will incorporate newly learned skills into daily routine
- Patient will make changes in postpartum routine
- Patient will seek help from healthcare professional if required.

Nursing Interventions

- Establish mutual trust and respect to enhance patient's learning
- Assess patient's level of understanding of postpartum self-care activities to establish a baseline for learning
- Assist patient in making decisions regarding target dates for mastering postpartum self-care skills
- Select teaching strategies best suited for patient's individual learning style to enhance learning
- Teach skills, which the patient can incorporate into her daily life such as perineal care, sitz bath, application and removal of perineal pads and breast care
- Teach patient about the process of involution that help her to understand postpartum changes
- Teach the patient about importance of adequate nutrition and hydration to ensure proper urinary, and bowel elimination
- Discuss the importance of adequate rest to promote emotional and physical stability
- Help the patient to incorporate learned skills into her daily routine during hospitalization
- Encourage patient to continue hygienic practices even after discharge from the hospital.

Evaluation of Expected Outcomes

- Patient expresses motivation to learn
- Patient establishes realistic learning goals
- Patient demonstrates understanding of what she has learned
- Patient incorporates what she has learned into her daily routine such as breast care, perineal care and obtaining adequate rest, and sleep
- Patient states intention of making changes in daily routine
- Patient expresses intention to seek help from health professional, if required.

Documentation

- Patient's understanding and skill in post-partum self-care
- Patient's expressions, which indicate her motivation to learn

- Methods used to teach patient
- Information taught to patient
- Skills demonstrated to patient
- Patient's response to teaching
- Evaluation of expected outcomes.

Pain Related to Postpartum Physiological Changes

Definition

An unpleasant sensory and emotional experience that arises from actual or potential tissue damage.

Assessments

- Patient's description of pain
- Patient's age, parity and pain tolerance
- Previous experience with pain in postdelivery period
- Presence of physical factors such as breast engorgement, cracked nipples and hemorrhoids.

Defining Characteristics

- Alteration in vital signs, diaphoresis, etc.
- Communication of pain in verbal and non-verbal forms
- Behavior changes such as pacing and repetitive actions
- Expressions of pain such as crying, groaning and grimacing
- Sleep disturbance.

Expected Outcomes

- Patient will identify characteristics of pain and describe the factors that intensify it
- Patient will carry out appropriate interventions for pain relief
- Patient will express relief from pain and comfort.

Nursing Interventions

- Assess patient's pain symptoms
- Discuss the reasons for pain and its expected duration to reduce the patient's anxiety
- Inspect the presence of hemorrhoids and provide instructions for hemorrhoid care, if indicated
- Assess for uterine tenderness and presence, and frequency for afterbirth pains at every 4 hours for first 24 hours and every shift thereafter as indicated; oxytocin administration, multiparity and breastfeeding are factors that may intensify uterine contractions
- Instruct breastfeeding mother to wear supportive bra to increase comfort
- If breastfeeding mother is engorged, instruct her to use warm compress or take warm shower to simulate the flow of milk and help relieve stasis, and discomfort
- If nipples become sore, instruct mother to air dry the nipples for 20–30 minutes after feeding to roughen the nipples
- Apply breast cream as ordered to soften nipples and relieve pain
- Instruct non-breastfeeding mother to wear tight, supportive bra or breast binder and apply ice packs as needed to prevent or reduce lactation.

Evaluation of Expected Outcomes

- Patient describes pain and factors that intensify it
- Patient carries out appropriate interventions for pain relief as instructed
- Patient expresses relief of pain and discomfort
- Patient's breasts remain soft and lactation continues to be adequate
- Patient expresses understanding of instructions and follows through.

Documentation

- Patient's description of pain and discomfort
- Observations of pain manifestations
- Comfort measures and medications provided for pain relief
- Effectiveness of interventions carried out
- Instructions provided to patient about pain and pain relief measures
- Evaluation of expected outcome.

Deficient Fluid Volume Related to Postpartum Hemorrhage

Definition

Excessive fluid and electrolyte loss resulting from excessive postpartum bleeding.

Assessments

- History of problems that can cause fluid loss such as hemorrhage, vomiting and diarrhea
- Vaginal signs such as visible bleeding and lacerations
- Fluid and electrolyte status including weight, intake and output, urine specific gravity, skin turgor, mucous membranes, and serum electrolytes and blood urea nitrogen levels
- Laboratory values such as hemoglobin (Hb) level and hematocrit (Ht) value
- Risk factors such as grand multiparty, overdistended uterus, prolonged labor, previous history of postpartum hemorrhage, traumatic delivery, uterine fibroids, and bleeding disorders.

Defining Characteristics

- Decreased pulse volume and pressure
- Decreased urine output and increased concentration
- Dry skin and mucus membranes
- Increased hematocrit
- Increased pulse rate
- Low blood pressure
- Poor skin turgor

- Thirst
- Weakness
- Change in mental status.

Expected Outcomes

- Patient's vital signs will remain stable
- Patient's hematology values will be within normal range
- Patient's uterus will remain firm and contracted
- Signs of shock will be identified quickly and treatment initiated immediately by medical personnel
- Patient's blood volume will return to normal
- Patient's urinary output will return to normal.

Nursing Interventions

- Following delivery, monitor the color, amount and consistency of lochia every 15 minutes for 1 hour, at every 4 hours for 24 hours and then every shift until discharge
- Count or weigh sanitary pads, if lochia is excessive
- Monitor and record vital signs at every 15 minutes for 1 hour, every hour for 4 hours and at every 4 hours for 24 hours to detect signs of hemorrhage, and shock
- Immediately after delivery, palpate the fundus at every 15 minutes for 1 hour, at every hour for 4 hours, at every 4 hours for 24 hours and then every shift until discharge to note its location and muscle tone; lack of uterine muscle tone or strength (atony) is the most common cause of postpartum hemorrhage
- Gently massage a boggy fundus, to make it become firm (overstimulation can cause relaxation)
- Teach patient to assess and gently massage the fundus, and notify if bogginess persists
- Explain to patient about the process of involution and the need to palpate the fundus to decrease her anxiety, and increase cooperation
- Evaluate postpartum hematology studies and report abnormal values to plan required interventions
- Administer fluids, blood or blood products or plasma expanders as ordered to replace lost blood volume
- Monitor patient's intake and output every shift
- Note bladder distention and catheterize as ordered as distended bladder interferes with involution of uterus
- Administer oxytocic agents such as ergometrine as ordered as distended bladder interferes with involution of uterus
- Assess patient regularly for signs and symptoms of shock such as rapid thready pulse, increased respiratory rate, decreased blood pressure and urine output, and cold, clammy, pale skin.

Evaluation of Expected Outcomes

- Patient's vital signs remain stable
- Results of hematology studies are within normal range
- Patient's uterus remains firm
- Patient does not develop distended bladder
- Patient's blood loss after delivery is less than 500 mL

- Patient's blood volume is replenished
- Quick identification and prompt treatment are provided, if patient develops shock.

Documentation

- Estimation of blood loss
- Location and tone of fundus
- Laboratory results
- Replacement of lost fluid
- Nursing interventions to control active blood loss
- Vital signs, intake and output
- Patient's response to nursing interventions.

Risk for Infection Related to Altered Primary Defenses during Postpartum Period

Definition

Presence of internal or external hazards, which threaten maternal well-being during postpartum period.

Assessments

- Laboratory values including WBC and platelet count, hemoglobin level, hematocrit, blood and body fluid culture
- History of labor and delivery such as episiotomy, and premature rupture of membranes
- Presence of medical conditions such as diabetes mellitus that increase the likelihood of infection
- Signs and symptoms of infection such as pallor, fatigue, malaise, anorexia, fever with hills, foul-smelling lochia, calf tenderness, dysuria, abdominal tenderness and tender, reddened breasts.

Risk Factors

- Chronic illness
- Exposure to pathogens during and prior to labor
- Inadequate primary defenses such as broken skin
- Invasive procedure
- Lack of knowledge about causes of infection
- Malnutrition
- Premature rupture of membranes
- Tissue destruction and trauma.

Expected Outcomes

- Patient's vital signs will remain within normal range
- Results of laboratory studies will not indicate infection
- Patient's urine and body secretions such as lochia will not show evidence of infection
- Patient's episiotomy or abdominal incision site will remain free from infection
- Patient's IV site will not become inflamed
- Patient will maintain good personal hygiene
- Patient will state risk factors that can lead to infection

- Patient will remain free from signs and symptoms of infection.

Nursing Interventions

- Minimize the patient's risk of infection by:
  - Washing hands before and after providing care
  - Wearing gloves to maintain asepsis when giving direct care and when in contact with blood and body fluids.
- After delivery, monitor vital signs: Every 15 minutes for 1 hour, then every 4 hours for 24 hours and then every shift until discharge, and report any abnormal change.
- Elevated vital signs indicate infection
- A temperature greater than 100.4°F (38°C) on two consecutive readings after the first 24 hours postdelivery may indicate endometriosis, mastitis or other infection
- Monitor WBC count as ordered and report abnormal values as it indicates increased production of leukocytes in response to bacterial pathogens
- Culture urine, wound drainage, lochia or blood as ordered to identify pathogens for antibiotic therapy
- Instruct patient in proper personal hygiene such as perineal wash, sitz bath, handwashing and breast care to reduce risk of infection
- Teach patient, how to apply perineal pads front to back and how to remove them back to front, and to clean perineum from front to back after elimination; these measures reduce bacterial concentrations and help prevent genitourinary tract infection
- Follow universal precautions to prevent nosocomial infections
- Use strict sterile technique, while performing invasive procedures such as IV line insertion or urinary catheterization to minimize the risk of infection
- Assess IV site every shift for redness or warmth and change IV tubing, and site every 72 hours, or according to hospital policy
- Instruct the postoperative patient to deep breathe and cough to help remove secretions, and prevent respiratory complications
- Assess the patient for generalized signs of infection such as pallor, fatigue, malaise and anorexia, and chills every shift and instruct her to report danger signs immediately.

Evaluation of Expected Outcomes

- Patient's vital signs remain within normal limits
- Patient's WBC count and differential count remain within normal range
- Patient's respiratory secretions are clear and odorless; urine is clear, yellow and odorless, and sediment free
- Patient's IV site does not become inflamed
- Patient's lochia discharge remains normal in color, consistency and odor
- Patient performs personal hygiene correctly at regular intervals
- Patient discusses risk factors that can cause infection
- Patient remains free from infection.

Documentation

- Vital signs
- Appearance of episiotomy or abdominal incision site
- Date, time and sites of culture if done
- Appearance of IV site
- Patient teaching about infection control
- Interventions performed to reduce risk of infection
- Patient's response to nursing interventions
- Evaluation for expected outcome.

Pain Related to Episiotomy or Cesarean Incision

Definition

An unpleasant sensory and emotional experiences arising from tissue damage, which vary in intensity from mild to severe, and be constant or recurring.

Assessments

- Patient's description of pain including quality and intensity
- Patient's age and pain tolerance
- Patient's anxiety level and any symptoms of secondary gain.

Defining Characteristics

- Alteration in vital signs, diaphoresis or dilated pupils
- Change in appetite and eating
- Communication of pain in verbal and non-verbal forms
- Expressions of pain such as crying, moaning and grimacing
- Guarding or protective activities
- Sleep disturbance.

Expected Outcomes

- Patient will describe nature of pain and intensity
- Patient will understand and carry out appropriate interventions for pain relief
- Patient will express comfort and relief from pain.

Nursing Interventions

- Examine the episiotomy site for redness, edema, ecchymosis, drainage and approximation to detect trauma to perineal tissues or developing complications
- Discuss reasons for pain and discomfort, and measures to be carried out for relief
- Apply ice pack to the episiotomy site for the first 24 hours to increase vasoconstriction and reduce edema and discomfort
- Provide warm sitz bath [temperature 100–105°F (37.8–40.6°C)] from 2nd postpartum day; instruct patient to take sitz baths three times a day with each lasting for 20 minutes; sitz bath increases circulation, reduces edema, and promotes healing

- Provide infrared light to perineum if ordered to reduce discomfort
- Apply any prescribed sprays, creams or ointments for reduction of swelling and discomfort
- Instruct patient to tighten buttocks before sitting and to sit on flat firm surface; this reduces stress and direct pressure on the perineum
- Administer prescribed pain medications to provide pain relief
- For post cesarean patients, provide an additional pillow and teach to splint the incision site when moving or coughing to provide support for abdominal muscles.

Evaluation of Expected Outcomes
- Patient reports characteristics and intensity of pain
- Patient carries out appropriate interventions for pain relief as instructed
- Patient expresses relief of pain and discomfort
- Episiotomy or cesarean incision heals normally
- Patient expresses the understanding of instructions given and implements care activities.

Documentation
- Patient's description of pain and pain relief experienced
- Nurse's observation of patient's response to interventions for pain relief
- Comfort measures and medications provided for pain relief
- Instructions provided to patient for self-care activities.

Impaired Skin Integrity Related to Episiotomy or Abdominal Incision

Definition
Interruption in skin integrity resulting from surgical incision in the perineum or abdomen made for delivering the fetus.

Assessments
- Vital signs
- Integumentary status such as color, hygiene, drainage and texture
- Extent of interruption of skin integrity because of delivery
- Health history including past skin problems, trauma and surgery
- Dietary intake, appetite, hydration and weight
- Laboratory data such as hemoglobin, hematocrit and WBC levels
- Patient's understanding of her condition and readiness to learn
- Presence of any medical condition that may interfere with healing.

Defining Characteristics
- Destruction of skin layers surrounding episiotomy or abdominal incision
- Disruption of skin surfaces
- Signs of infection (invasion by pathogens) such as elevation of temperature local inflammation, discharge, etc.

Expected Outcomes
- Patient will demonstrate understanding of self-care activities
- Patient will perform skin care routine
- Patient will identify possible danger signs and report immediately
- Patient will regain skin integrity
- Patient's episiotomy or abdominal incision will heal without infection.

Nursing Interventions
- Inspect the incision every shift for redness, edema, ecchymosis, discharge and approximation (REEDA) to detect signs of possible infection
- Instruct and assist the patient with hygienic practices such as handwashing, and toileting practices to prevent wound contamination
- Carry out prescribed treatment such as cleaning and applying medications, and dressing changes to decrease bacterial contamination
- Instruct and assist the patient in performing perineal wash/perineal care, and sitz baths three to four times a day to maintain cleanliness and promote healing
- Teach patient, how to apply and remove perineal pad; clean pad to be applied front to back, and soiled pad to be removed from back to front to reduce the risk of contaminating the vaginal area
- Maintain infection control standards to reduce the risk of nosocomial infections
- Instruct patient to report possible danger signs and symptoms such as temperature above 100.4°F (38°C), incision drainage, increased discomfort at the episiotomy or incision site and reddened, warm skin surrounding the incision site.

Evaluation of Expected Outcomes
- Patient demonstrates correct self-care practices
- Patient performs skin care or episiotomy care routine
- Patient identifies and reports to physician possible danger signs
- Patient regains skin integrity
- Patient's episiotomy or abdominal incision shows no sign of infection.

Documentation
- Patient's expressed concerns about change in skin integrity
- Patient's ability to perform self-care practices
- Observations of episiotomy or abdominal incision site

- Response to treatment and nursing care
- Instructions regarding treatment and self-care
- Prescribed treatment carried out
- Nursing interventions and supportive care carried out and patient's response
- Self-care practices performed by patient
- Expected outcomes evaluated.

NURSING DIAGNOSES FOR NEONATES

Risk for Aspiration Related to Immature Cough or Gag Reflex

Definition

Entry of oropharyngeal and GI secretions or exogenous fluids into neonate's tracheobronchial passages.

Assessments

- Gestational age of neonate
- Weight of neonate in relation to gestational age
- Maternal sedation during labor (before delivery)
- Neonate's health status including pre-existing conditions, intrauterine environment, cardiovascular status, respiratory status, GI status and anomalies
- Laboratory values of the neonate such as fluid, electrolyte and blood gas levels
- Vital signs of the neonate
- Nutritional status of the neonate.

Risk Factors

- Decreased GI mobility and delayed gastric emptying
- Depressed cough and gag reflexes
- Impaired swallowing
- Incompetent lower esophageal sphincter
- Increased gastric residual contents
- Conditions contraindicating elevation of upper body
- Surgery or trauma to face, mouth or neck
- Tracheostomy or endotracheal tube
- GI tubes.

Expected Outcomes

- Neonate will maintain clear airway (through suctioning as needed)
- Neonate will not exhibit gastric distention
- Neonate will demonstrate minimal quantity of nasopharyngeal and oropharyngeal secretion
- Neonate will tolerate initial feeding
- Neonate will demonstrate appropriate suck and swallow reflex
- Neonate will not exhibit signs and symptoms of aspiration
- Neonate will have no abnormal breath sounds.

Nursing Interventions

- Assess the neonate's respiratory status until stable afterbirth, to evaluate the respiratory system during transition to extrauterine life
- Monitor vital signs according to agency protocol to determine the neonate's adjustment to extrauterine existence
- Suction as needed to keep the upper and lower airway clear; in the labor room, suction the oropharynx and nasopharynx with a bulb syringe, DeLee catheter or suction catheter attached to wall suction
- Assist physician with laryngoscopy to suction below vocal cord, if the neonate aspirates meconium
- Perform a head-to-toe physical assessment to detect abnormalities in other systems that may affect respiratory effort
- Withhold oral feedings and provide IV fluids, if signs of respiratory distress occur
- Observe for sucking and swallowing reflex, gag and cough reflex, and color changes when offering the initial feeding
- Keep the head of bed elevated during and after gavage feeding, if not contraindicated
- Monitor residual gastric contents and follow parameters for withholding feedings
- Measure abdominal girth every shift to check for distention and stop feeding immediately if aspiration is suspected; perform suctioning as needed
- Explain to parents the reasons for these interventions
- Instruct mother in feeding techniques that will help to prevent a distended abdomen leading to aspiration:
  - Instruct mother to avoid overfeeding and to burp the neonate at frequent intervals (after intake of 15–30 mL)
  - Instruct mother to position the neonate on his right side with the head of the bed elevated for 30–60 minutes after feeding.

Evaluation of Expected Outcomes

- Neonate receives suctioning as needed and maintains patent airway
- Neonate does not have gastric distention
- Neonate tolerates initial feeding
- Neonate does not manifest color changes during feeding
- Neonate has appropriate suckling and swallowing reflex
- Neonate has no adventitious (abnormal) breath sounds
- Neonate shows no signs and symptoms of aspiration.

Documentation

- Neonate's tolerance of initial feeding and gavage feedings
- Residual gastric contents after gavage feeding
- Episodes of vomiting, aspiration or both
- Breath sounds

- Observations of physical findings including heart rate and respirations
- Interventions performed to prevent aspiration
- Expected outcomes evaluated.

Ineffective Breastfeeding Related to Difficulty with Breastfeeding Process

Definition

State in which mother or neonate experiences dissatisfaction or difficulty with breastfeeding process.

Assessments

- Maternal status such as age, parity, previous bonding history and breastfeeding preparation in prenatal period
- Adequacy of milk supply, nipple shape and perceptions about breastfeeding
- Neonate's growth rate and age-weight relationship.

Defining Characteristics

- Inadequate milk supply
- Arching and crying when at breast
- Evidence of inadequate milk intake
- Fussiness and crying within an hour of breastfeeding
- Inability to latch on to nipple correctly
- Lack of sustained sucking at breast
- Insufficient emptying of breasts
- Lack of response to other comfort measures
- Sore nipples for mother after 1st week of breastfeeding.

Expected Outcomes

- Mother will express satisfaction with breastfeeding techniques and practice
- Mother will show decreased anxiety and apprehension
- Neonate will feed well on both breasts and appear satisfied for at least 2 hours after feeding
- Neonate will grow and thrive.

Nursing Interventions

- Educate mother in breast care and breastfeeding techniques
- Be available and encourage mother during initial breastfeeding episodes
- Teach techniques for encouraging the let-down reflex such as warm shower before feeding, breast massage and holding the neonate close to the breasts
- Provide quiet, private, comfortable, environment for mother and baby to promote successful breastfeeding
- Encourage mother to clarify questions regarding successful breastfeeding.

Evaluation of Expected Outcomes

- Mother expresses satisfaction with breastfeeding practices
- Mother will exhibit decreased anxiety and apprehension
- Neonate feeds successfully on both breasts and appears satisfied for at least 2 hours after feeding
- Neonate grows and thrives.

Documentation

- Mother's expressions of satisfaction and comfort with breastfeeding ability
- Observations of bonding and breastfeeding processes
- Teaching and instructions given
- Neonates weight and growth
- Expected outcomes evaluated.

Interrupted Breastfeeding Related to Contraindicating Conditions

Definition

Break in the continuity of breastfeeding resulting from inability or inadvisability to feed the baby from breasts.

Assessments

- Maternal status such as nipple anomaly, psychological stress, presence of infection and use of medication
- Neonatal status such as age-weight relationship, respiratory status, suck reflex, prematurity, hyperbilirubinemia and anomalies that interfere with proper sucking (e.g. cleft lip or palate).

Expected Outcomes

- Mother will express her understanding of factors that necessitate interruption of breastfeeding
- Mother will express understanding that she may resume breastfeeding
- Mother will express and store breast milk appropriately
- Mother will resume breastfeeding when interfering factors cease
- Mother will have adequate milk supply when breastfeeding resumes
- Mother will experience relief from discomfort associated with engorgement
- Neonate's nutritional needs will be met.

Nursing Interventions

- Assess the mother's understanding of the reasons for interrupting breastfeeding
- Teach mother about alternate methods to meet the nutritional needs of the baby
- Assess mother's desire to resume breastfeeding
- Instruct mother in techniques of expressing and storing breast milk to ensure adequate milk supply

- Teach the use of breast pump to empty the breasts
- Educate mother to save her breast milk in a sterile container and store it in the refrigerator for future feedings
- Instruct her the ways to relieve breast engorgement
- Instruct mother in use of devices such as nipple shield in case of flat or inverted nipple
- If the mother does not wish to resume breastfeeding, instruct her to wear supportive bra/binder, apply ice and take mild analgesic to alleviate discomfort related to engorgement.

Evaluation of Expected Outcomes

- Mother describes factors that necessitate interruption in breastfeeding
- Mother explains her decision about whether to resume breastfeeding
- Mother demonstrates proper milk expression and storage techniques
- Mother resumes breastfeeding when interrupting factors are eliminated
- Mother has adequate milk supply when breastfeeding resumes
- Mother obtains relied from discomfort associated with engorgement
- Infant's nutritional needs are met as evidenced by appropriate weight gain (e.g. 1 oz per day for first 6 months of life).

Documentation

- Factors that necessitate interruption of breastfeeding
- Mother's feeling expressed about need to interrupt breastfeeding
- Mother's decision whether to continue breastfeeding when possible
- Mother's efforts to ensure adequate milk supply
- Mother's response to nursing interventions
- Neonate's weight and growth
- Expected outcomes evaluated.

Ineffective Breathing Pattern Related to Adjustment to Extrauterine Existence

Definition

State in which a neonate's initial breathing pattern does not provide adequate lung expansion for successful transition to extrauterine life.

Assessments

- Gestational age
- Weight in relation to gestational age
- Maternal sedation before delivery
- Pre-existing conditions such as anomalies, adverse intrauterine environment and prematurity
- Assessment of cardiovascular, respiratory and GI status and fluid, and electrolyte balance
- History of meconium aspiration or neonatal asphyxia.

Defining Characteristics

- Use of accessory muscles for breathing
- Altered chest excursion (increased chest movement)
- Altered respiratory rate or depth, or both
- Dyspnea
- Nasal flaring
- Retractions of chest wall
- Shortness of breath.

Expected Outcomes

- Neonate will establish normal respiratory rate (40–60 breaths per minute) within 1 hour of birth
- Neonate will have no signs of respiratory distress 1 hour after birth
- Neonate will not require assisted ventilation or supplemental oxygen
- Neonate will have Apgar score of 8 to 10 at 1 and 5 minutes of age
- Neonate will make successful transition to extrauterine life with adequate respiratory function.

Nursing Interventions

- Carry out the following immediately after delivery:
  - Dry the baby and place the body under a radiant warmer
  - Suction the oropharynx and nasopharynx as needed with a bulb syringe, DeLee catheter or suction catheter connected to wall suction
  - Obtain 1 minute and 5 minutes Apgar scores
  - Provide oxygen, if indicated
  - Remove wet blankets and replace them with dry ones
  - Observe for signs of respiratory distress such as nasal flaring, tachypnea, retractions, grunting and use of accessory muscles for breathing
  - Provide or assist with resuscitative measures as indicated including bag and mask ventilation, administration of Narcan (naloxone), intubations and suctioning below the vocal cords.
- Transfer the neonate to nursery when condition is stable or if the neonate needs more extensive resuscitative measures
- On admission to the nursery carry out the following:
  - Obtain vital signs
  - Observe central and peripheral color
  - Note signs of respiratory distress
  - Perform a physical assessment noting anomalies or abnormal findings
  - Maintain a neutral thermal environment
  - Obtain a brief history of labor and delivery, and condition of the neonate before arrival in nursery to identify the risk factors
  - Obtain laboratory studies as ordered
  - Provide resuscitative measures if needed
  - Monitor vital signs until stable and then routinely.
- Continually assess the need to repeat suctioning to maintain a patent airway.

Evaluation of Expected Outcome

- Neonate establishes respiratory rate of 40–60 breaths per minute within 1 hour of birth
- Neonate has no signs of respiratory distress 1 hour after birth; neonate does not require assisted ventilation or supplemental oxygen
- Neonate has Apgar score of 8 to 10 at 1 and 5 minutes of age
- Neonate makes successful transition to extrauterine life.

Documentation

- Vital signs
- Physical findings
- Interventions performed to enhance neonate's ability to breathe effectively
- Neonate's response to nursing interventions
- Expected outcomes evaluated.

Ineffective Breastfeeding Related to Limited Maternal Experience

Definition

State in which mother or neonate experiences dissatisfaction or difficulty with breastfeeding process.

Assessments

- Age and maturity of mother
- Previous bonding history—parity
- Level of prenatal breastfeeding preparation
- Previous breastfeeding experience
- Actual or perceived inadequate milk supply
- Nipple shape such as inverted nipple
- Stressors such as family and career
- Views on breastfeeding
- Support from spouse and family members
- Satisfaction and contentment of neonate.

Defining Characteristics

Mother
- Actual or perceived inadequate supply of milk
- Insufficient emptying of each breast
- Lack of observable signs of oxytocin release
- Sore nipples after 1st week of breastfeeding.

Baby
- Arching and crying when at breast
- Evidence of inadequate intake of milk
- Fussing and crying within 1 hour after feeding
- Inability to latch on to nipple correctly
- Lack of response to comfort measures and efforts at pacifying
- Lack of sustained sucking at breast
- Resistance to latch on to breast
- Unsatisfactory breastfeeding process.

Expected Outcomes

- Mother will express understanding of breastfeeding techniques and practice
- Mother will display decreased anxiety and apprehension
- Mother and baby will experience successful breastfeeding
- Neonate's initial weight loss will be within accepted norms
- Neonate's nutritional needs will be met adequately.

Nursing Interventions

- Assess mother's knowledge of breastfeeding
- Educate mother in breast care and breast-feeding techniques
- Provide written materials and audiovisual aids, which illustrate the proper feeding techniques
- Teach techniques for encouraging the let-down reflex such as warm shower, breast massage, relaxation, holding neonate close to the breasts and initiating sucking
- Stay with mother during feeding and encourage asking questions to increase her understanding
- Evaluate nipple position in neonate's mouth and sucking motion
- Ensure that the neonate is awake and alert when feeding, unwrap as needed
- Evaluate neonate for anomalies that may interfere with breastfeeding ability such as cleft lip or palate
- When ready to start feeding, let a drop or two of breast milk fall on baby's lips; the neonate may open his mouth on tasting the milk
- Instruct the mother in breast care techniques such as wearing supportive bra, washing and air drying nipples to prevent cracking, soreness and bleeding, which interfere with feeding
- Teach mother on ways to prevent breast engorgement
- Teach mother the factors that enhance mild production as well as those that can alter production and quality of milk
- Provide positive reinforcement for the mother's efforts in order to decrease her anxiety and increase her confidence, and self-esteem.

Evaluation of Expected Outcomes

- Mother properly positions baby during breastfeeding
- Uses appropriate techniques to encourage attachment to nipple
- Mother expresses decreased anxiety and increased enthusiasm for breastfeeding
- Neonate feeds successfully on both breasts and appears satisfied for at least 2 hours after feeding
- Neonate's nutritional needs are met
- Neonate's initial weight loss remains within accepted norms.

Documentation

- Mother's level of knowledge related to breastfeeding
- Mother's expression of dissatisfaction with breastfeeding ability

- Mother's breast care practices
- Maternal conditions that interfere with breastfeeding such as inverted nipples
- Mother's and neonate's behavior during, and after breastfeeding such as positioning on breasts and baby's level of satisfaction
- Frequency and duration of breastfeeding
- Teaching and instructions given and mother's response to teaching
- Neonate's weight and growth
- Mother's and neonate's response to nursing interventions.

Risk for Infection Related to Neonate's Immature Immune System

Definition
Presence of internal or external hazards that threaten neonate's health.

Assessments
- Gestational age of neonate
- Temperature, heart rate and respirations
- Labor and delivery record including maternal fever, premature rupture of membranes, and foul-smelling amniotic fluid
- Recent or current maternal infections
- Signs of infection of umbilical cord and skin at base of cord such as redness, odor, and discharge
- Signs and symptoms of developing infections such as lethargy, jaundice, skin lesions, thrush, unstable body temperature, hypoglycemia, diarrhea, vomiting, poor feeding patterns, cyanosis and mottling of skin
- Signs of respiratory distress such as grunting, retractions, nasal flaring and cyanosis
- Evidence of chronic intrauterine infections such as growth retardation and hepatosplenomegaly.

Risk Factors
- Early rupture of amniotic membranes
- Environmental exposure to pathogens during birth process
- Inadequate primary responses such as broken skin
- Invasive procedures
- Poor feeding pattern
- Tissue destruction
- Trauma
- Medication use.

Expected Outcomes
- Neonate's vital signs will remain within normal range
- Neonate will be alert and active
- Neonate will remain free from signs and symptoms of infection
- Neonate's umbilical cord will remain free of infection and heal properly
- Mother and family members will practice good handwashing technique before handling neonate.

Nursing Interventions
- Review the maternal chart and delivery record to detect risk factors that predispose the neonate to infection
- Assess the neonate's gestational age (as passive immunity via the placenta increases significantly in last trimester, premature neonates are more susceptible to infection)
- Follow sterile techniques, remove rings, wrist watch and bracelet before handling the neonate
- Scrub hands and arms with antimicrobial preparation before entering nursery and after contact with contaminated material
- Wash hands after handling the neonate and instruct parents in handwashing techniques
- Perform umbilical cord care with each diaper change or as facility policy dictates in order to promote healing
- Assess respirations, heart rate and temperature every 15 minutes for 1 hour, then every hour for 4 hours, then every 4 hours for 24 hours, then every shift or as indicated (unstable vital signs, persistent elevations in temperature or hypothermia may indicate neonatal infection)
- Observe neonate for signs and symptoms of infection and notify physician, if signs and symptoms of infection appear
- Observe standard precautions, wear gloves for neonate's first bath and when in contact with blood and body secretions (these actions prevent cross-contamination and transmission of pathogens)
- Encourage mother to begin breastfeeding early; colostrum and breast milk provide passive immunity, and helps reduce infection.

Evaluation of Expected Outcomes
- Neonate's vital signs remain within normal range
- Neonate remains alert and active
- Neonate is free from signs and symptoms of infection
- Umbilical cord is clean, dry and healing
- Mother and family members demonstrate proper handwashing technique before handling neonate.

Documentation
- Vital signs
- Appearance of umbilical cord
- Feeding pattern and weight gain
- Condition of oral mucosa
- Skin color and rashes
- Elimination pattern
- Activity pattern
- Interventions performed to reduce risk of infection
- Neonates response to nursing interventions
- Evaluation of outcomes observed.

Imbalanced Nutrition Less than Body Requirement Related to Ineffective Suck Reflex

Definition

Inability to ingest sufficient fluids and nutrients resulting from ineffective sucking reflex.

Assessments

- Gestational age
- Perinatal history
- Apgar score
- Suck and swallow reflex
- Gastrointestinal assessment including vomiting, regurgitation and stool characteristics
- Examination of abdomen including inspecting auscultation of bowel sounds, percussion and palpation for abnormalities
- Nutritional status including intake and output, weight changes, skin turgor, and urine characteristics, signs of dehydration and feeding pattern
- Laboratory studies such as urine glucose levels, urine bilirubin levels and urine specific gravity
- Adequacy of breastfeeding techniques (practices) of mother such as condition of nipple and positioning of neonate.

Defining Characteristics

- Lack of interest in feeding
- Weight loss more than expected normal for the neonatal period
- Diarrhea
- Inadequate intake
- Pale conjunctiva and mucous membranes
- Signs of abdominal pain or cramping.

Expected Outcomes

- Mother will demonstrate effective feeding technique
- Neonate will not lose more than 10% of birth weight
- Neonate will retain entire feeding without vomiting or regurgitating
- Neonate will establish effective sucking and swallowing reflexes allowing for adequate nutritional intake
- Neonate will maintain good skin turgor, moist mucous membranes, adequate urine output and flat soft fontanels.

Nursing Interventions

- Check neonate's weight at the same time each day
- Record feedings accurately, if breastfeeding—number of minutes at each feeding and if bottle feeding, amount ingested at each feeding
- Teach mother on how to position the neonate during and after feeding, and how to burp the neonate
- Regularly assess the neonate's suckling pattern and provide teaching as needed
- Instruct mother to make sure that the neonate is awake before feeding; unwrap the blanket and tap the soles of the feet
- Record the number of stools and amount of urine voided in each shift
- Monitor the neonate for signs of dehydration such as poor skin turgor, dry mucous membranes, decreased or concentrated urine and sunken fontanels and eyeballs
- Assess the need for gavage feeding.

Evaluation of Expected Outcomes

- Mother demonstrates competence when feeding neonate
- Neonate retains entire feeding
- Neonate establishes effective suckling and swallowing reflexes
- Neonate maintains good skin turgor, moist mucous membranes, adequate urine output and soft fontanels
- Neonate regains the birth weight by 10 days after birth.

Documentation

- Frequency, fluid amount and type of feeds taken
- Incidence of regurgitation and vomiting
- Frequency of the bowel elimination and urination
- Effectiveness of suckling reflex
- Neonate's daily weight
- Care given and bonding pattern by mother/parents
- Signs of dehydration
- Nursing interventions carried out and neonate's response
- Expected outcomes evaluated.

Hypothermia Related to Cold Stress or Sepsis

Definition

State in which neonate's body temperature is below normal range.

Assessments

- Gestational age
- Intrapartal history
- Presence of maternal risk factors such as fever, diabetes mellitus dystocia and perinatal asphyxia
- Vital signs including core temperature, heart rate respiration and blood pressure
- Laboratory values such as arterial blood gas values, serum glucose and electrolytes
- Skin color: Central and peripheral
- Birth weight.

Defining Characteristics

- Body temperature below normal level
- Cool, pale skin
- Cyanotic nail beds
- Increased heart rate and blood pressure

- Piloerection
- Shivering
- Slow capillary refill.

Expected Outcomes

- Neonate will exhibit the normal body temperature
- Neonate will have warm, dry skin and normal capillary refill
- Neonate will not develop complications of hypothermia
- Neonate will not shiver
- Neonate will maintain the normal body temperature
- Mother will verbalize knowledge of how hypothermia develops and will state measures to prevent recurrence of hypothermia.

Nursing Interventions

- Monitor body temperature every hour by axillary route, if using a radiant warmer, monitor the device's temperature reading hourly and compare it with the neonate's body temperature
- Monitor and record vital signs every 1–4 hours, perform continuous electronic cardiorespiratory monitoring as appropriate
- For *mild hypothermia*, dress the baby with a shirt, diaper, stockinette cap or knitted hat and wrap in double blankets
- Avoid overheating and wet diaper
- Perform all procedures under a radiant warmer, if possible
- Postpone bathing
- For severe hypothermia, place the neonate in an Isolette or overhead radiant warmer bed and provide supportive measures:
  - Keep the neonate undressed
  - Set the Isolette temperature at 36– 36.6°C (96.8–97.8°F)
  - Attach a skin probe to the right upper quadrant of the neonate's abdomen
  - Monitor carefully for evaporative and insensible fluid loss.
- Carry out prescribed treatment regimen such as administering IV fluids and small frequent feeding
- Discuss precipitating factors with mother and family members to prevent recurrence
- Instruct family members in preventive measures such as dressing the neonate appropriately and providing adequate nutrition for neonate's growth needs.

Evaluation of Expected Outcomes

- Neonate's temperature returns to normal
- Neonate exhibits warm, dry skin and normal capillary refill time
- Neonate does not develop complications of hypothermia
- Neonate does not demonstrate signs of hyperthermia related to radiant heat source
- Neonate is successfully weaned from Isolette or radiant warmer
- Parents verbalize understanding of causes of hypothermia and preventive measures
- Mother demonstrates proper temperature measurement technique.

Documentation

- Neonate's physical findings such as cardiovascular status and temperature
- Nursing interventions carried out
- Neonate's response to interventions
- Mother's and family members' willingness and ability to provide adequate care at home
- Expected outcomes evaluated.

ANNEXURES

Section Outline

1. Common Abbreviations used in Obstetrics
2. Common Signs in Obstetrics
3. Maneuvers used in Obstetrics

ANNEXURE 1

Common Abbreviations used in Obstetrics

Sl. No.	Abbreviations	Description
1.	AFB	Alpha fetoprotein
2.	AFI	Amniotic fluid index
3.	APH	Antepartum hemorrhage
4.	AFB	Acid-fast bacilli
5.	AGA	Appropriate for gestational age
6.	BBT	Basal body temperature
7.	BPP	Biophysical profile
8.	BUS	Bartholin's glands, urethra, Skene's gland
9.	BUBBLE HE	• Breasts • Uterine fundus • Bowel • Bladder • Lochia • Episiotomy • Homan's sign • Emotional status
10.	BSO	Bilateral salpingo-oophorectomy
11.	BTL/BPS	Bilateral tubal ligation/bilateral salpingectomy
12.	Bx	Biopsy
13.	CS	Cesarean section
14.	CST	Contraction stress test
15.	CT scan	Computerized tomography scan
16.	CMV	Cytomegalovirus
17.	CVS	Chorionic villus sampling
18.	CTG	Cardiotocography
19.	CCT	Controlled cord traction
20.	CSF	Cerebrospinal fluid
21.	D&C	Dilatation and curettage
22.	DES	Diethylstilbestrol
23.	DMPA	Depo medroxy progesterone acetate
24.	DIC	Disseminated intravascular coagulation
25.	EFW	Estimated fetal weight

Sl. No.	Abbreviations	Description
26.	EAB	Elective abortion
27.	EDC	Expected date of confinement
28.	ERT	Estrogen replacement therapy
29.	EFM	Electronic fetal monitoring
30.	EPF	Early pregnancy factor
31.	EUA	Examination under anesthesia
32.	FHS	Fetal-heart sound
33.	FHR	Fetal-heart rate
34.	FTN	Full term nursery
35.	FTND	Full term normal delivery
36.	FSE	Fetal scalp electrode
37.	FSH	Follicle stimulating hormone
38.	FHT	Fetal heart tone
39.	FISH	Fluorescence in situ hybridization
40.	FDIU	Fetal death in utero/Intrauterine fetal demise
41.	GBS	Group B streptococci
42.	GTD	Gestational trophoblastic disease
43.	GTT	Glucose tolerance test
44.	GDM	Gestational diabetes mellitus
45.	G6PD	Glucose-6-phosphate dehydrogenase deficiency
46.	GTN	Gestational trophoblastic neoplasm
47.	GPA	• G gravida (number of pregnancies) • P para (number of births of viable offspring) • A abortion
48.	hCG (hcg)	Human chorionic gonadotropin hormone
49.	HRT	Hormone replacement therapy
50.	HPL	Human placental lactogen
51.	HELLP	Hamolysis, elevated liver enzymes, low platelets
52.	Hbg/Hb	Hemoglobin
53.	H/H	Hemoglobin, hematocrit
54.	HIB	*Haemophilus influenzae* bacteria
55.	HIV	Human immune deficiency virus
56.	IUFD	Intrauterine fetal death
57.	IUD/IUCD	Intrauterine contraceptive device
58.	IUGR	Intrauterine growth retardation
59.	IUP	Intrauterine pregnancy
60.	IDDM	Insulin-dependent diabetes mellitus
61.	JODM	Juvenile onset of diabetes mellitus
62.	LOA	Left occipitoanterior
63.	LTCS	Low transverse cesarean section
64.	LSCS	Lower segment cesarean section
65.	LOP	Left occipitoposterior
66.	MAS	Meconium aspiration syndrome
67.	MH	Menstrual history
68.	MMR	Measles, mumps, rubella

ANNEXURE 1: Common Abbreviations used in Obstetrics

Sl. No.	Abbreviations	Description
69.	MOM	Milk of magnesia
70.	NTG	Nitroglycerin
71.	NST	Nonstress test
72.	NSVD	Normal spontaneous vaginal delivery
73.	OCT	Oxytocin challenge test
74.	OPV	Oral polio vaccine
75.	OB	Obstetrics
76.	PROM	Premature rupture of membranes
77.	PG oral	Prostaglandin oral
78.	PG gel	Prostaglandin gel
79.	PICU	Pediatric intensive care unit
80.	PID	Pelvic inflammatory disease
81.	PIH	Pregnancy-induced hypertension
82.	PKU	Phenylketonuria
83.	PP	Postpartum
84.	PMS	Premenstrual syndrome
85.	PMH	Past medical history
86.	Q6H	Every 6 hours (L) quaque six hora
87.	QID	Four times a day (L) quaque four hora
88.	RBC	Red blood cells/corpuscles
89.	RBS	Random blood sugar
90.	RDA	Recommended daily allowance
91.	RDS	Respiratory distress syndrome
92.	RFA	Radiofrequency ablation
93.	REEDA	Redness, erythematous/ecchymosis, edema, discharge and approximation of wound
94.	Rh	Rhesus factor in blood
95.	RIA	Radioimmunoassay
96.	RMA	Right mentum anterior
97.	RMP	Right mentum posterior
98.	RMT	Right mentum transverse
99.	R/O	Rule out
100.	ROA	Right occipitoanterior
101.	ROP	Right occipitoposterior
102.	ROT	Right occipitotransverse
103.	ROM	Rupture of membranes/Range of motion
104.	SAB	Spontaneous abortion
105.	SaO_2	Oxygen saturation
106.	SROM	Spontaneous rupture of membranes
107.	SGA	Small for gestational age
108.	SVE	Sterile vaginal examination
109.	STD	Sexually transmitted disease
110.	SFH	Symphysis fundus height
111.	TAH	Total abdominal hysterectomy
112.	TVH	Total vaginal hysterectomy
113.	TTP	Thrombotic thrombocytopenic purpura

Sl. No.	Abbreviations	Description
114.	TTS	Twin to twin transfusion syndrome
115.	TORCH	Toxoplasmosis, other, rubella, cytomegalovirus, herpes simplex virus
116.	TPAL	Term births, preterm births, abortions, living children
117.	UTI	Urinary tract infection
118.	V/V	Vulva/vagina
119.	VBAC	Vaginal birth after cesarean
120.	VTOP	Voluntary termination of pregnancy
121.	VAS	Vibroacoustic stimulation
122.	VE	Vaginal examination
123.	WNL	Within normal limits

ANNEXURE 2

Common Signs in Obstetrics

Sl. No.	Name of the sign	Description
1.	Ball sign	Radiological sign of intrauterine fetal death. X-ray shows crumpled-up spine of the fetus
2.	Banana sign	Ultrasound sign in open spina bifida of fetus. Shows abnormal anterior curvature of cerebellum
3.	Buddha sign	"Buddha" attitude due to abdominal distension and edematous fetus in hydrops fetalis. Seen in ultrasonography
4.	Cullen sign	Bluish discoloration of skin around umbilicus. Occurs due to intraperitoneal hemorrhage. Seen in ruptured ectopic pregnancy
5.	Chadwick's sign/ Jacquemier's sign	Bluish or purple hue of the vestibule and anterior vaginal wall. Seen in first trimester of pregnancy due to increased blood flow to the pelvic organs
6.	Double bubble sign	Seen in the presence of duodenal atresia of fetus. Usually presents with polyhydramnios and produces dilation of stomach and first part of duodenum
7.	Double decidual sac sign	Normal ultrasonography appearance of gestational sac. Seen as two concentric echogenic rings separated by a hyperechoic space
8.	Goodel's sign	Marked softening of the cervix in contrast to non-pregnant state and occurs due to increased blood flow
9.	Halo sign	Elevation of the subcutaneous fat layer over the fetal skull in a dead or dying fetus. The most common radiologic sign of fetal death (edema of the scalp in Rh incompatibly of the fetus)
10.	Homan's sign	Pain in the calf muscle when ankle is slowly and gently dorsiflexed, with the knee bent. This is indicative of incipient or established thrombosis in leg vein
11.	Jacquemier's sign	This is one of the early signs of pregnancy. Bluish discoloration of the vagina during pregnancy as a result of increased blood supply
12.	Kustner's sign	A sign of placental separation. On pushing the uterus upwards the cord does not move with it due to separation
13.	Ladin's sign	Softening in the midline of the uterus anteriorly at the junction of the uterus and cervix. It occurs at about 6 weeks of gestation
14.	Lambda sign	Ultrasonic sign seen in dichorionic pregnancies. Due to the presence of chorionic tissue between the two layers of the membrane between the twins
15.	Lemon sign	Ultrasound sign in open spina bifida, shows abnormal anterior curvature of cerebellum. Occurs due to associated Arnold-Chiari malformation in which brain tissue extends into the spinal canal
16.	Osiander's sign	Pulsations in the lateral fornix due to the increased vascularity
17.	Palmer's sign	Regular rhythmic contractions of uterus felt as early as 6–8 weeks. It is a sign of pregnancy
18.	Piskacek's sign	Asymmetric growth occurs to the uterus in initial stages of pregnancy due to the lateral implantation of the blastocyst. The area of implantation feels soft compared to the other parts
19.	Robert's sign	Radiological sign of intrauterine fetal death. X-ray shows presence of gas in the fetal great vessels. This is the earliest radiological sign of intrauterine fetal death

Sl. No.	Name of the sign	Description
20.	Schroder's sign	A sign of placental separation. Uterus rises up when the separated placenta is passed downwards
21.	Stallworthy sign	Slowing of fetal heart rate on pressing the head down into the pelvis and prompt recovery on release of pressure. This is a sign suggestive of posterior placenta previa
22.	Spalding's sign	A sign of intrauterine death. Overlapping of skull bones after fetal demise and observed by ultrasonogram
23.	Sure sign	Passage of vesicles through vagina in hydatidiform mole (molar pregnancy)
24.	Stuck Twin sign	Seen in twin-to-twin transfusion syndrome. Due to severe oligohydramnios, smaller twin is held in a fixed position along the uterine wall. It is called stuck twin sign
25.	"T" sign	Ultrasonic sign seen in monochorionic twins. As the intertwined membrane does not have chorionic tissue it gives a 'T' sign in ultrasound
26.	Turtle sign	Failure of restitution seen in shoulder dystocia is called turtle sign
27.	Von Braun-Fernwald's sign	A clinical sign in which there is an irregular softening and enlargement of the uterine fundus during early pregnancy. It occurs at 5–8 weeks of gestation
28.	Danger signs of pregnancy	• Vaginal bleeding • Pelvic or abdominal pain • Persistent back pain • Gush of fluid from vagina • Swelling of hands and face • Severe headache and blurry vision • Regular uterine contractions prior to 37 weeks • No fetal movements
29.	Snowstorm sign	This is present in hydatidiform molar pregnancy. Classic sonographic appearance of a complete mole is as "snowstorm" or "granular". There is central heterogeneous mass with numerous anechoic (cystic) spaces

ANNEXURE 3

Maneuvers used in Obstetrics

Sl. No.	Name of maneuver	Condition	Description
1.	Ritgen maneuver	Delivery of fetal head	This aids the mechanism of extension as the fetal head comes under the symphysis pubis. Pressure is applied to the fetal chin through the perineum, at the same time pressure is applied to the occiput
2.	Burns-Marshall maneuver	Breech delivery	For delivery of the after-coming head by promoting flexion of the head. For this maneuver, the baby is allowed to hang by its own weight for a minute or so. The assistant gives suprapubic, downward pressure to promote flexion of the head. Once the nape of the neck is visible, identified by the hairline, the baby's trunk is lifted and swung towards mother's abdomen holding the baby just above the ankle through an arc of 180° left hand guards and slips the perineum over fetal mouth. As the mouth is born, air passage is cleared of mucus and now by depressing the trunk the head is allowed to be born
3.	Mauriceau-Smellie-Veit maneuver	Breech delivery (delivery of the after-coming head)	This is the classical method of assisted breech delivery. The after-coming head is delivered with the child resting on the physician's forearm. The baby is placed supinated on the left forearm with the limbs hanging on either side. The middle finger and the index finger of the left hand are placed over the malar bones on either side. This is modification of the original method in which the index finger is placed inside the mouth. The ring and little fingers of the right hand are placed on the right shoulder of the baby, the index finger is placed on the sub-occipital region. Traction is given in downward and backward direction till the nape of the neck is visible under the public arch. The assistant gives suprapubic pressure to maintain the flexion. Traction is applied to draw the head out of the vagina and when the occipital region appears, the body is lifted to assist the head pivot around the symphysis pubis. The fetus is delivered in an upward movement towards the mother's abdomen releasing the face, brow and the trunk is depressed to release the occiput and vertex
4.	Pinard's maneuver	Breech delivery	The maneuver is used in breech with extended legs. Once the groin is visible gentle pressure can be applied to abduct the thigh and reach the knee. The knee can be flexed with pressure in the popliteal fossa and the leg delivered. The middle and index fingers are inserted up to the popliteal fossa. It is then pressed and abducted to get the legs flexed. The fetal feet are grasped at the ankle and breech extraction is done
5.	Lovset maneuver	For delivery of shoulders in breech	This maneuver involves rotation of the trunk of the fetus during a breech delivery to facilitate delivery of the arms and shoulders. The body is lifted to cause lateral flexion. The trunk is rotated through 180° keeping the back anterior and maintaining a downward traction. This will bring the posterior arm to merge under the pubic arch which is hooked out. The trunk is rotated in the reverse direction keeping the back anterior to deliver anterior shoulder under the symphysis pubis
6.	Zavanelli's maneuver	Shoulder dystocia (baby's head is born but the shoulders are stuck)	This maneuver is used for internal cephalic replacement. It involves pushing back the delivered fetal head in to the birth canal while holding continuous upward pressure until cesarean delivery is accomplished. This maneuver is performed only after other maneuvers have failed as it is associated with high risk to both mother and baby

Sl. No.	Name of maneuver	Condition	Description
7.	Robert maneuver	Shoulder dystocia	• This maneuver involves hyperflexion of the maternal thighs against the abdomen, usually involving two assistants. The maneuver straightens the sacrum relative to the lumbar spine allowing cephalic rotation of the symphysis pubis sliding over the fetal shoulder • It is often done with the application of suprapubic pressure which involves an assistant other than the primary ones to apply pressure to the anterior shoulder of the fetus just cephalad to the symphysis pubis so that the shoulder is pushed anteriorly relative to the fetus • Due to the possibility of complications to mother and fetus these maneuvers are not practiced in the present day obstetrics
8.	Rubin I & Rubin II maneuvers	Shoulder dystocia	• Rubin I (suprapubic pressure) attempts dislodge the anterior shoulder from behind the pubic symphysis, thereby reducing the bisacromial diameter • Rubin II maneuver consists of inserting of the fingers of one hand vaginally behind the posterior aspect of the anterior shoulder of the fetus and rotating the shoulder toward the fetal chest. This motion will abduct the fetal shoulder girdle reducing the diameter • Insertion of left index and middle fingers anteriorly to access the posterior aspect of anterior (left) shoulder. Pressure by the fingers can sometimes rotate fetal trunk into the (wider) oblique plane • If Rubin's rotation can be accomplished, the anterior shoulder should emerge from below the symphysis with little or no additional traction.
9.	Modified Brandt Andrew's method (controlled cord traction)	Placental delivery	This maneuver is used when the uterus is hard and contracted as it helps more uterine contraction which facilitates expulsion of placenta. The palmar surface of the fingers of the left hand is placed above the symphysis pubis. The body of the uterus is pushed upwards and backwards using the non-dominant hand towards the umbilicus. The dominant hand gives a steady traction in downward and backward direction holding the clamp, until the placenta comes out the vagina
10.	Crede's maneuver	Placental delivery	A method of expressing the placenta after the infant had been delivered by kneading the body of the uterus to produce placental separation. Because this procedure usually traumatizes the placental site, it is not recommended
11.	Leopold's maneuver	Abdominal palpation	• Leopold's maneuver is used for palpating the abdomen in order to determine the lie, presentation and position of the fetus. There are four specific steps • Step-1: The top of the uterus (fundus is felt and palpated to establish which end of the fetus (fetal pole) is in the upper part of the uterus. If either the head or breech of the fetus is in the fundus then the fetus is in vertical lie. Otherwise the fetus is most probably transverse lies • Step-2: Firm pressure is applied to the sides of the abdomen to establish the location of the spine and extremities (small parts) • Step-3: Using the thumb and fingers of one hand, the lower abdomen is grasped just above the symphysis pubis to establish if the part is engaged. If not engaged a movable body part will be felt. The presenting part is the part of the fetus that is felt to be in closest proximity to the birth canal • Step-4: Facing the maternal feet, the tips of the fingers of each hand are used to apply deep pressure in the direction of the axis of the pelvic outlet. If the head presents, one hand is arrested sooner than the other by a rounded body (the cephalic prominence) while the other hand descends deeply into the pelvis. If the cephalic prominence is on the same side as the small parts, then the fetus is in vertex presentation. If the cephalic prominence is on the same side as the back, then the head is extended and the fetus is in face presentation
12.	Gaskin's maneuver	Shoulder dystocia	The maneuver is also called as "all fours" to deal with shoulder dystocia. It is the first medical maneuver named after a midwife. Named after Ina May Gaskin, an American Midwife. In this maneuver, the mother supports herself on her hands and knees to resolve the shoulder dystocia. Since this maneuver requires a significant movement from the standard lithotomy position, it can be substantially more difficult to perform while under epidural anesthesia, but still possible and can be performed by an experienced delivery room team.
13.	Wood's screw maneuver	Shoulder dystocia	This maneuver is used to achieve at least a 180 degree rotation of the fetal trunk using pressure on the dorsal aspect of the posterior shoulder to help adduct the shoulders. In this, the anterior shoulder is pushed towards the baby's chest, and the posterior shoulder is pushed towards the baby's back, making the baby's head somewhat face the mother's rectum. This maneuver is tried only after the McRobert's maneuver and application of suprapubic (lower abdomen) pressure have been tried.

Sl. No.	Name of maneuver	Condition	Description
14.	Jacquemier's maneuver (Barnum's maneuver)		• This is used to deliver the posterior shoulder first, in which the forearm and hand are identified in the birth canal and gently pulled • The physicians hand (including the thumb) is inserted in the birth canal in an effort to deliver the posterior arm (not just the shoulder) first. (When the left shoulder is anterior, the operator's right hand is used; if the right shoulder is anterior, the operator's left hand is used) • Sliding the hand along the dorsal aspect of the humerus and pressing it against the fetal chest, the clinician then palpates the elbow. If the elbow is already flexed, the operator's hand grasps the fetal forearm and wrist and sweeps the forearm over the chest and across the infant's face, extending the arm at the elbow and shoulder, to deliver it first. Movements should be directed only medially toward and then across the fetal chest, supporting and continually pressing the humerus against the chest to avoid possible humeral fracture from attempting to flex it laterally against resistance from the vaginal wall • If the elbow is extended, making the forearm difficult to reach and deliver, the operator should attempt to flex it by applying finger pressure to the dorsal aspect of the forearm, and if needed, simultaneously pressing on the ventral aspect of the elbow crease to cause it to bend. After flexion of the elbow, the operator grasps and sweeps the forearm and wrist as described above. If the elbow will not flex, the operator should continue directly woods screw maneuver (once the posterior arm is delivered, the fetal trunk almost always follows because of the additional 20 mm of clearance). If not the delivered arm can be used to help rotate the trunk; so that the remaining anterior shoulder is brought to occupy the oblique plane of the pelvis, anterior to the pubic symphysis
15.	McRobert's maneuver	Shoulder dystocia	McRobert's maneuver is an obstetric maneuver used to assist in childbirth. It is named after William A McRobert Jr. It is employed in case of shoulder dystocia during childbirth and involves hyper flexing the mother's legs tightly to her abdomen

Glossary

ABO incompatibility: A condition that may lead to neonatal hemolytic disease. The mother who has type 'O', red cells has antibodies to type 'A' and type 'B'. These antibodies are transferred to the fetus and cause destruction of fetal red blood cells (RBCs). The hemolytic disease resulting from ABO incompatibility is usually less severe than the disease caused by Rhesus (Rh) incompatibility. Unlike Rh incompatibility, ABO incompatibility cannot be prevented by giving the mother Rh immune globulin.

Abortion: The termination of pregnancy by expulsion of the products of conception prior to viability (the ability to survive, if born), which is less than 28th week of gestation. The international acceptance is either 20th week or fetus weighing 500 g.

Abruptio placentae: Premature separation or detachment from the wall of the uterus of a normally situated placenta; can be partial or complete separation.

Acceleration: *Refer*s to a periodic rise in fetal heart rate from the baseline in response to stress of lowered oxygen availability or fetal movement.

Acidosis: A decrease in the pH of the blood. The range of pH in a neonate is between 7.30 and 7.40. A blood pH of 7.20 or lower is considered severe acidosis. If a baby is gasping, the pH is probably 7.0 or less.

Acrocyanosis: The slightly bluish, grayish discoloration of a newborn's hands and feet within the first 24 hours of birth.

AGA: Abbreviation for 'appropriate for gestational age', when a newborn's birth weight is within the 10th to 90th percentile expected for that length gestation.

Albumin: The major protein in blood. In 5% concentration, it is used as an emergency blood volume expander in the treatment of shock.

Alkalosis: An increase in the pH of blood. Alkalosis may result from a high (pH above 7.40) serum bicarbonate or more commonly if the carbon dioxide concentration in the baby's blood is lowered by hyperventilation (assisting the baby's breathing at an excessively fast rate).

Alpha-fetoprotein: A glycoprotein and a major component of fetal blood; small amounts are found in the amniotic fluid of normal fetuses. Elevated levels may indicate neural tube malformations.

Amniocentesis: A procedure for removing amniotic fluid from the amniotic sac by inserting a needle through the abdominal wall, usually to assess fetal health or maturity.

Amniotomy: The artificial rupture of amniotic membranes when an Amnihook or other rupturing device is introduced into the vagina and a small tear is made in the membranes.

Anencephaly: A congenital anomaly in which there is partial or complete absence of the skull and brain.

Anomaly: An abnormal occurrence or malformation, e.g. a cleft lip is an anomaly.

Anoxia: Absence or deficiency of oxygen as reduction of oxygen in body tissues below physiological levels.

Antenatal period: The time of pregnancy from the 1st day of last menstrual period (LMP) to the start of true labor.

Anterior fontanel: Diamond-shaped fontanel located at the juncture of the coronal, frontal and sagittal sutures.

Antibody titers: A test used to indicate the relative concentration of a particular antibody present in a person's blood. For example, a high rubella titer indicates a person has been exposed to rubella (German measles) and has formed a significant amount of antibody against the rubella virus and therefore will most likely be able to ward off another attack of the virus without becoming ill.

Apgar: A five part scoring system to assess newborn's at 1–5 minutes after birth regarding heart rate, respiratory effort, muscle tone, reflex irritability and color.

Appropriate for gestational age: When a newborn's birth weight is within the 10th to 90th percentile expected for that length gestation (*refer* AGA).

Asphyxia: A decrease in the amount of oxygen and an increased amount of carbon dioxide in the body because of some interference with respiration.

Attachment: The establishment of a reciprocal relationship between the parents and the newborn after a period of bonding; development of a deeper intimacy, which grows overtime.

Attitude: The relationship of the fetal head and limbs to its trunk.

Autosomes: The chromosomes in the body other than the sex (X and Y) chromosomes.

Azoospermia: A condition in which sperm is absent in the semen.

Baby blues: A common transient mild depression or emotional disturbance affecting the mother after delivery due to hormonal changes, sleep deprivation and emotional let-down.

Ballottement: When palpated, the fetus floats away then returns to touch the examiners fingers.

Bicornuate uterus: A double uterus.

Bilirubin: The orange or yellow-colored pigment in bile produced by the breakdown of hemoglobin and excreted by the liver cells.

Biophysical profile (BPP): A combination of measures used to evaluate fetal well-being; each of the five components (non-stress test, ultrasound evaluation of amniotic fluid volume, fetal body movements, muscle tone and respirations) are scored. These scores are added together for the final BPP score.

Bishop's score: A prelabor scoring system with five components (cervical dilatation, effacement, consistency, position and fetal station), which help to determine, if induction of labor will be effective.

Bloody show: Rupture of the small cervical capillaries when the cervix begins to dilate and efface; when the mucus plug is lost, the resultant cervical drainage is pink tinged.

Bonding: The initial attraction and period of exploration between the parents and newborn becoming acquainted.

Bradycardia (slow heart rate):
1. *Fetal*: A sustained heart rate less than 100 beats per minute (bpm) (a heart rate less than 120 bpm may also be abnormal depending upon the clinical situation).
2. *Neonatal*: A sustained heart rate less than 100 bpm.

Braxton-Hicks: The intermittent, irregular painless uterine contractions, which occur during pregnancy; they do not dilate and efface the cervix (*refer* true labor).

Breech presentation: The feet-first or buttocks-first presentation of the fetus; the position is termed breech whether one foot, both feet or the buttocks are born first; frank breech is the buttocks-first presentation.

Brown fat: Fat tissue, which has a rich blood and nerve supply. Babies have proportionately more brown fat than do adults and metabolize or 'burn' it as their main source of heat production, while adults produce heat by shivering. Extra oxygen and calories are used when brown fat is metabolized.

Bubble: An acronym standing for the five most important assessment areas of a postpartum woman; breasts, uterus, bowels, bladder, lochia, episiotomy and extremities.

Cesarean delivery: Surgical delivery of the fetus through an abdominal incision; the uterine incision may be classical (vertical cutting through both the contractile and/or non-contractile segments) confined to the non-contractile lower uterine segment (either vertical or transverse incision).

Caput succedaneum: Localized edema occurring just under the presenting part of the fetal scalp during labor; disappears within 36–48 hours of life.

Cardinal movements: The predictable sequence of movements through the birth canal that the fetus will go through during labor and birth; descent, flexion, internal rotation, extension, external rotation and expulsion.

Cephalohematoma: A collection of blood between the newborn's skull bone and periosteum resulting from pressure or trauma during labor or delivery; does not cross suture lines.

Cephalic presentation: When the head of the fetus is the presenting part; may be vertex, face, sinciput or brow presentation.

Cervical dilatation: The opening or enlargement of the external cervical os from a few millimeter to 10 centimeter when completely dilated.

Cervical effacement: The thinning or shortening of the cervix during labor from 0% to 100% when completely effaced.

Chadwick's sign: The bluish or purple coloration of the vagina and cervix when pregnancy is presumed.

Chest compressions: Artificial pumping of the blood through the heart by a bellows effect created from intermittent compression of the sternum over the heart during resuscitation.

Chloasma: Irregular, brownish discolorations of the forehead, nose, cheeks and neck during pregnancy (the mask of pregnancy).

Choanal atresia: Congenital obstruction of the posterior nares (between the nose and throat). Since, baby's breath mainly through their noses, a baby with choanal atresia will have severe respiratory distress at birth. The immediate treatment is insertion of an oral airway.

Chromosome: The microscopic, rod-shaped bodies (46 in man), which develop from cell nucleus material that contain the genes.

Chorionic villus sampling: A procedure to obtain a sample of the chorionic villi from the placenta via aspiration; tests for chromosomal and biochemical disorders during early pregnancy.

Coach: A person who assumes the role of advocate and support person for the laboring woman; assists with conditioned techniques for relaxation and breathing.

Colostrum: The 'first milk' secreted from the lactiferous glands.

Conceptional age: Age of the fetus calculated from the day of fertilization.

Congenital: *Refer*s to conditions that are present at birth, regardless of cause. Congenital defects may result from a variety of causes including genetic factors, chromosomal factors and diseases affecting the mother or drugs taken by the mother. The cause of most congenital defects is unknown.

Conjugation of bilirubin: Process that occurs in the liver and combines bilirubin with another chemical so it may be removed from the blood and pass out of the body in the feces. Failure of bilirubin conjugation is one of the causes of jaundice.

Continuous positive airway pressure (CPAP): A steady pressure delivered to the baby's lungs by means of a special apparatus or mechanical ventilator. CPAP may be used for babies with respiratory distress syndrome to prevent alveoli from collapsing during expiration.

Contraction stress test (CST): A procedure, which help to measure fetal well-being by stimulating the uterus to contract with oxytocin administration or nipple stimulation and measuring the response of the fetus to the contractions that can be interpreted as positive, negative or equivocal (suspicious) (*refer* oxytocin challenge test).

Coombs' test: Test to determine the presence of antibodies in blood or red cells. It is used to detect antibodies against the red cells of Rh-positive babies born to Rh-negative sensitized mothers.

Couplet care: A system in which one nurse cares for the postpartum mother and her newborn as a single unit also known as mother-baby dyad.

Denominator: The name of the presenting part, which is used when *refer*ring to fetal position.

Diaphragmatic hernia: A condition when the diaphragm does not close completely and the abdominal contents slip into the thoracic cavity causes respiratory distress in the newborn.

Dilatation of cervix: The enlargement of the external os from an orifice, a few millimeters in size to an opening large enough to allow the passage of the infant and a cervical opening approximately 10 cm in diameter is usually considered complete dilatation.

Doppler monitor: Uses ultrasound to detect audible fetal heart sounds; an intermittent and simple monitoring technique.

Down syndrome: A chromosomal abnormality resulting in a typical facial appearance, mental retardation and sometimes other congenital defects—it is also called mongolism or trisomy 21. Down syndrome individuals have 47 instead of the normal 46 chromosomes.

Ductus arteriosus: A connection between the main pulmonary artery and the aorta of the fetus; closes after birth and becomes a ligament.

Ductus venosus: A fetal blood vessel that connects the umbilical vein and the inferior vena cava.

Dysfunctional labor: Occurs when there is a problem with the frequency, duration and intensity of uterine contractions and/or the resting tone of the uterus between contractions.

Dyspareunia: Painful sexual intercourse experienced by females'.

Dystocia: Abnormal or difficult labor, or delivery. Used to *refer* to weak or ineffective uterine contractions; may also be used to describe the situation in which the shoulders of a baby in vertex presentation become trapped after delivery of the head (shoulder dystocia).

Early deceleration: A transitory decrease in the fetal heart rate caused by head compression, which stimulates the vagus nerve to slow down the heart rate.

Eclampsia: It is a pregnancy-induced hypertensive (PIH) disease associated with hypertension, proteinuria, edema, tonic and clonic seizures and coma.

Effacement: A thinning and shortening of the cervix, which occurs during pregnancy and/or labor.

Effleurage: A stroke used in massage.

Electronic fetal monitoring: A type of monitoring in which information about the fetal heart rate and the laboring woman's uterine contraction pattern is continually assessed; can be either direct (invasive or internal) or indirect (noninvasive or external).

Embryo: The term used for the conceptus from 4 to 8 weeks following conception.

Encephalocele: Protrusion of the brain through a cranial fissure generally in the occipital area.

Engagement: Also *refer*red to as lightening, when the widest fetal presenting diameter has passed through the brim of the pelvis, engagement is said to have occurred.

Engorgement: The swelling and distention of the breasts, usually during the early days of initiation of lactation due to vascular dilatation as well as the arrival of the early milk.

Epicanthus: A fold of skin extending from the root of the nose to the median end of the eyebrow and covering the inner canthus and caruncle.

Epidural block: A type of regional anesthesia used to produce relief from pain during labor and delivery.

Epinephrine: A natural body hormone that is released into the blood during stressful activity; it may also be used as a drug during resuscitation to constrict the blood vessels, increase the blood pressure and to increase the heart rate, and volume of blood pumped.

Episiotomy: An incision in the perineum to facilitate delivery.

Erythema toxicum neonatorum: An urticarial condition affecting newborns in the first few days of life, the lesions consist of dead white papules, grainy to the touch, with or without surrounding areas of redness.

Erythroblastosis fetalis: A blood dyscrasia of the newborn characterized by agglutination and hemolysis of erythrocytes; usually caused by incompatibility between the infant's blood and the mother's.

Esophageal atresia: A condition in which the esophagus ends in a blind pouch or narrows into a thin cord; usually occurs between the upper and mid third of the esophagus.

Expected data of delivery (EDD): The estimated date of delivery based on Naegele's rule or ultrasound.

Epstein's pearls: Small, white epithelial cysts along both sides of the median raphe of the hard palate; commonly found in newborn infants.

False labor: Characterized by irregular Braxton-Hicks contractions, which do not change the cervix and do not increase in intensity, duration or frequency (*refer* true labor).

Facies: The expression or appearance of the face; certain congenital syndromes present with a specific facial appearance.

Family-centered care: The maternity delivery system that emphasizes professional quality health care of the total family unit; utilizes a combined nursery and postpartum nursing staff to form one mother-baby dyad (*refer* couplet care).

Fetal bradycardia: The fetal heart rate is less than 120 bpm during at least a 10 minutes period of continuous monitoring.

Fetal distress: A compromise in fetal well-being; can be either acute or chronic.

Fetal heart rate acceleration: An increase in the fetal heart rate that occurs during a uterine contraction with the fetal heart rate decreasing to its previous rate as the contraction subsides.

Fetal heart rate baseline: Average fetal heart rate between periodic rate changes (accelerations or decelerations). The baseline fetal heart rate is the average fetal heart rate during any 10 minutes period. The normal baseline range is between 120 and 160 bpm.

Fetal heart rate deceleration: A decrease in the fetal heart rate that occurs in response to a uterine contraction. There are three types of decelerations (early, late and variable).

Fetal heart rate variability: The beat-to-beat changes that occur in the baseline fetal heart rate.

Fetal monitoring, external: *Refer*s to continuous electronic monitoring using leads strapped to the mother's abdomen to detect the fetal heart rate, periodic rate changes and the timing of the uterine contraction.

Fetal monitoring, internal: *Refer*s to continuous electronic monitoring using a wire placed on the fetal presenting part to detect the fetal heart rate, variability and periodic rate changes and a tube placed inside the uterus to detect the onset, and intensity of the uterine contractions.

Fetal lie: The relationship of the body of the fetus to the body of the mother, which is either longitudinal or transverse.

Fetal position: The relationship of the landmark on the presenting fetal part to the front, sides or back of the maternal pelvis.

Fetal presentation: The lowest part of the fetus that comes first through the maternal pelvis and birth canal; either vertex (cephalic), shoulders or breech.

Fetal station: *Refer*s to the relationship of the fetus presenting part to an imaginary line drawn between the maternal ischial spines and the pelvic outlet.

Fetal surveillance: Methods to assess and monitor the well-being of the fetus during pregnancy, labor and birth includes fetal biophysical profile, biochemical assessments, amniocentesis, genetic studies, antenatal testing, fetal movement counting, non-stress testing, contraction stress testing and clinical assessments.

Fetal tachycardia: When the fetal heart rate is greater than 160 bpm during at least for a 10 minutes period of continuous monitoring.

Fetus: The term applied to the conceptus from 9th week until birth.

Floating: When the presenting part is entirely out of the maternal pelvis and can be moved by the examiner, not engaged.

Fontanel: An unossified space or 'soft spot' lying between the cranial bones of the skull of a fetus.

Foramen ovale: The septal opening between the atria of the fetal heart that closes soon after birth.

Four P's: The four forces of labor including passage, passenger, power and psyche.

Freidman curve: A method of evaluating the relationship of three factors to help and determine normal or abnormal labor patterns overtime; these three factors are uterine activity, cervical dilatation and fetal descent can be plotted on a graph.

Gastroschisis: Congenital opening of the abdominal wall allowing the abdominal organs to protrude.

Gene: A factor responsible for the transmission of hereditary characteristics of offspring.

Generative: Capable of reproducing.

Genotype: The hereditary combination of genes, which makes up a person.

Gestational age: The number of completed weeks of fetal development calculated from the 1st day of the last menstrual cycle.

Gestational diabetes mellitus (GDM): Glucose or carbohydrate intolerance of variable severity, which develops or is discovered during the present pregnancy; the condition subsides at the completion of the pregnancy.

Gestational period: The number of completed weeks of pregnancy calculated from the 1st day of the LMP.

Grand multipara: A woman who has given birth five times or more.

Gravida: The number of times a woman has been pregnant or a pregnant woman.

Gravidity: *Refer*s to the total number of a woman's pregnancies regardless of their duration.

Grunting: Audible sound made by the newborn on expiration often indicating respiratory distress.

Hematoma: Occurs when blood escapes into the connective tissue of a traumatized area; can be life-threatening; may or may not cause severe pain.

Hemoconcentration: An increase in the number of RBCs resulting from a decrease in the volume of plasma.

Hemorrhage: Blood volume loss of more than 500 cc or blood loss of more than 15% of the total estimated blood volume.

Hegar's sign: Softness and compressibility of the uterine isthmus during the 2nd and 3rd month of pregnancy.

HELLP syndrome: This syndrome *refer*s to a severe and potentially fatal complication of pregnancy-induced hypertension involving hemolysis of RBCs, elevated liver enzyme levels and a low-platelet count.

Homans' sign: A method for detecting thrombophlebitis in which the leg is held straight and the foot flexed back; if the maneuver produces pain upon dorsiflexion of the foot, the test is positive and thrombophlebitis should be suspected.

Hydatidiform mole: Cystic proliferation of chorionic villi resembling a cluster of grapes.

Hydrocephalus: The increased accumulation of cerebrospinal fluid within the ventricles of the brain; may result from congenital anomalies, infection and injury or brain tumor.

Hyperbilirubinemia: A condition when there is an excessive amount of bilirubin in the blood; excessive levels can lead to brain damage.

Hyperemesis gravidarum: Excessive vomiting during pregnancy.

Hypospadias: A condition in which the urethral orifice is at some point between the scrotal raphe and the base of the glans penis.

Hypertonic uterus: Labor contractions lasting longer than 90 seconds, caused by too much stimulation of the uterus.

Hypotonic labor: Occurs during the active phase of labor causing ineffectual contractions and a lack of progression of labor.

Hypoxia: A broad term meaning diminished availability of oxygen to the body tissues.

Idiopathic respiratory distress syndrome (hyaline membrane disease): A severe respiratory condition found almost exclusively in preterm infants.

Inborn error of metabolism: A hereditary disease caused by a deficiency of a specific enzyme.

Incompetent cervix: A condition in which the cervix dilates prematurely causing a spontaneous abortion or preterm delivery.

Intrapartum period: The time from the onset of labor to the delivery of the newborn and the placenta.

In utero *(Latin)*: Inside the uterus.

Jacquemier's sign: The violet-blue discoloration of the vulva and vaginal mucosa including the vaginal portion of the cervix.

Jaundice: A condition characterized by a yellow color of the skin, the whites of the eyes, the mucous membranes and body fluids that is due to deposition of bile pigment resulting from excess bilirubin in the blood.

Kernicterus: A clinical syndrome in newborn infants manifested by pathological changes in the central nervous system resulting from deposition of unconjugated bilirubin in certain nuclei of the brain.

Labor: A process that involves a series of integrated uterine contractions that occur overtime and work to propel the fetus from the birth canal, relies on the uterine muscles and cervical compliance.

Labor delivery recovery and postpartum (LDRP) care: A system of healthcare delivery in which a woman labors, delivers, recovers and is discharged for home from the same room, and cared for by a primary care nurse; in home-like environment within a hospital setting.

Lactation: The process of preparing for and maintaining the production and secretion of milk including mammogenesis, lactogenesis, and galactopoiesis.

Lamaze method: An approach to childbirth emphasizing relaxation and breathing techniques to allow for a 'painless childbirth' also known as psychoprophylaxis method.

Lanugo: A fine, downy hair covering the fetus between the 17th week of gestation and soon after birth.

Late deceleration: A periodic decrease in the fetal heart rate below baseline occurring after the peak of the contraction; due to uteroplacental insufficiency and a sign of fetal distress.

Lecithin: One of the surfactant substances produced in the lungs; the amount of lecithin produced increases with increasing gestational age of the fetus. Therefore, the ratio of lecithin to sphingomyelin (LS ratio) in the amniotic fluid is used to estimate the lung maturity of the fetus.

Leopold's maneuvers: A system of evaluating the position and presentation of the fetus by palpating the maternal abdomen in four distinct locations.

Lie: The relationship of the long axis of the fetus to the long axis of the mother.

Lightening: The movement of the fetus and uterus downward into the pelvic cavity, an early sign of impending labor (*refer* engagement). A reduction in fundal height due to the fetus sinking into the lower uterine segment, which may occur at the end of pregnancy.

Lochia: The discharge from the uterus of blood, mucus and tissue during the postpartum period; changes from rubra to serosa and alba.

Lochia alba: The thin, colorless discharge, which follows lochia serosa.

Lochia rubra: The color description of the red, sanguineous vaginal flow, which follows delivery and lasts 2–4 days postpartum.

Lochia serosa: The serous, pinkish brown watery discharge, which follows lochia rubra.

Low birth weight (LBW): Infant weighing less than 2,500 g.

Low forceps: Application of forceps when the leading point of the fetal skull is at +2 station or lower with further specification as to whether the rotation of the fetal head is less than 45° or more than 45°.

Lysozyme: An enzyme with antiseptic qualities, which destroys foreign protein.

Macrosomia: Large body size; newborn at term weighing more than 4,000 g or is large for her gestational age.

Mastitis: Breast infection because of milk in the ducts.

Maternity care: Complete care of the pregnant, laboring and newly delivered woman and her newborn; also includes pre-pregnancy counseling, infertility counseling, and parenting education.

Meconium: The first stool passed by the newborn; dark-green or black material passed from the large intestine from the term or near-term fetus.

Midforceps: Application of forceps when the head is engaged, but the leading part of the fetal head is above +2 station.

Milia: Distended sebaceous glands, which produce tiny pinpoint papules on the skin of newborn infants, commonly found over the bridge of the nose, chin and cheeks.

Molding: Normal overlapping of the skull bones of the baby to allow the fetal head to fit through the pelvis during labor.

Mongolian spots: Benign bluish pigmentation over the lower back, buttocks or occasionally over the extensor surfaces may be present at birth, particularly in dark-skinned races.

Morbidity: Any form of permanent damage those results from an illness or accident.

Mucus trap suction apparatus: A type of suction apparatus used in aspirating the nasopharynx and trachea of a newborn infant. It consists of a catheter with a mucus trap, which prevents mucus from the baby from being drawn into the operator's mouth.

Multigravida: A woman who has been pregnant two or more times.

Multipara: A woman who has given birth to two or more babies live or still excluding abortions.

Multiple gestation: Pregnancy with more than one fetus, e.g. twins.

Naegele's rule: Used to determine the EDD or delivery date by subtracting 3 months from the 1st day of the LMP, then adding 7 days.

Nasal flaring: A sign of respiratory distress; the edges of the nostrils fan outward as the baby inhales.

Necrotizing enterocolitis: A serious disease in which sections of the intestines die and must be surgically removed; it occurs more often in preterm infants, but the cause is unclear.

Newborn period: From birth through the first 28 days of life.

Neonatal period: From birth to 28 days.

Neonatologist: A pediatrician who specializes in caring for newborn infants, particularly at risk and sick babies.

Neural tube defect: Any congenital defect in the brain or spinal cord (neural tube of the embryo) including anencephaly, encephalocele and meningomyelocele.

Neutral thermal environment (thermoneutral environment): The very narrow environmental temperature range that keeps a baby's body temperature normal with the baby having to use the least amount of calories and oxygen to produce heat.

Non-stress test (NST): A non-invasive test used to determine fetal well-being involves external fetal monitoring of the fetal heart rate and observing the response of the heart rate to fetal movement; interpreted as reactive or nonreactive.

Nuchal cord: The presence of one or more loops of the umbilical cord around the neck of the newborn.

Nullipara: A woman who has not carried a pregnancy to the point of viability.

Nursing process: Perceiving, assessing, planning, implementing and evaluation.

Omphalocele: A defect resulting from failure of closure of the abdominal wall or muscles, whereby abdominal viscera covered by a thin membrane protrudes and forms a sac outside the abdominal cavity.

Operculum: The thickened mucus that forms a cervical plug during pregnancy.

Ophthalmia neonatorum purulent: Infection of the eyes of the newborn, usually caused by gonococcus.

Ortolani's sign: A technique for determining the presence of a congenital dislocation of the hip, performed as part of the newborn examination.

Osiander sign: Increased pulsation felt in the lateral vaginal fornices.

Outlet forceps: Application of forceps when the fetal head is visible at the introitus without separating the vulva, the fetal skull has reached the pelvic floor, the sagittal suture is in the anteroposterior diameter, the fetal head is at or on the perineum and rotation of the head does not exceed 45°.

Ovulation: The release of an egg, ready for fertilization from an ovary.

Oxytocin: A hormone occurring naturally in the body and also used to induce labor, to enhance weak labor contractions and to cause contraction of the uterus after delivery of the placenta.

Oxytocin challenge test (OCT): A test to assess fetal well-being by administering oxytocin via intravenous (IV) infusion to induce uterine contractions and assessing the fetus response; can be interpreted as positive (abnormal), negative (normal) or suspicious (inconclusive) (*refer* contraction stress test).

Palmar erythema: Reddening of the palms seen in pregnant women.

Parity: *Refers* to the number of viable infants live or dead that a woman has delivered regardless of the number of children involved (e.g. the birth of triplets increases the parity by only one).

Parturient: A woman in labor.

Perinatal: The time surrounding the baby's birth; denotes a period from 20 weeks of gestational age to 28 days after birth.

Phenylketonuria: A congenital disease caused by a defect in the metabolism of the amino acid phenylalanine. The condition is hereditary and results from lack of an enzyme, phenylalanine hydroxylase and necessary for the conversion of the amino acid phenylalanine into tyrosine.

Phosphatidylglycerol (PG): A chemical substance produced by the mature fetal lung, which passes into the amniotic fluid with fetal breathing. Its presence in the amniotic fluid is associated with a better than 99% chance that the baby will not develop respiratory distress syndrome (RDS).

Phototherapy: Use of fluorescent lights to treat hyperbilirubinemia in neonates by breaking down bilirubin accumulated in the skin; the color of phototherapy lights ranges from nearly white to deep blue, depending upon the brand of lights.

Pica: Craving to eat bizarre substances like coal, wall plaster, mothballs, etc. in pregnancy.

Placenta: The oval or discoid spongy structure attached to the uterus through which the fetus derives its nourishment and through which waste products from the fetus pass into the mother's blood.

Placental abruption: A premature separation of a normally implanted placenta.

Placental dysfunction: A placenta that is failing to meet fetal requirements.

Placenta previa: A placenta, which is abnormally implanted in the lower uterine segment, so that it partially or fully covers the internal os of the cervix.

Polyhydramnios: Excessive volume of amniotic fluid usually greater than 1.2 L.

Position: The relationship between the denominator and the six points on the pelvic brim.

Positive pressure ventilation (PPV): Artificial breathing for a person by forcing air and/or oxygen into the lungs under pressure, either by bag and mask, bag and endotracheal tube or with a mechanical respirator.

Postpartum depression: Delayed emotional disturbance affecting the new mother sometimes 1–3 weeks postpartum; less commonly experienced; more intense and serious than the postpartum 'baby blues'.

Postpartum period: Period after a woman gives birth until her recovery 6 weeks later, when all of the reproductive changes, which occur over a 9 month pregnancy, return to the pre-pregnant state.

Post-term pregnancy: When the pregnancy continues past 42 weeks gestation.

Precipitate delivery: When labor lasts for less than 2 hours before spontaneous delivery; unexpected, sudden and often unattended.

Preeclampsia: Also *refer*red to as toxemia or PIH; a hypertensive disorder of pregnancy usually occurring after the 20th week gestation; characterized by high-blood pressure, proteinuria and edema (*refer* eclampsia).

Pregnancy-induced hypertension (PIH): A hypertensive disorder during pregnancy including conditions preeclampsia and eclampsia; characterized by hypertension, proteinuria and edema (*refer* eclampsia and preeclampsia).

Premature infant: A live born infant of less than 38 weeks gestation (37th completed week).

Prenatal period: The time of pregnancy from the 1st day of LMP to the start of true labor.

Presentation: *Refers* to the part of the fetus, which lies at the pelvic brim or in the lower pole of the uterus.

Preterm labor: When labor begins before the 37th completed week of gestation from the 1st day of the LMP.

Primigravida: A woman pregnant for the first time.

Primipara: A woman who has given birth to a fetus or fetuses that has reached the point of viability.

Prolapsed cord: An emergent event, when the umbilical cord slips in front of the presenting part and protrudes from the cervix into the vagina, the presenting part may press against the mother's pelvis cutting off the blood and oxygen to the fetus.

Prolonged labor: The latent phase of labor lasts longer than 24 hours without spontaneous delivery.

Pseudocyesis: False pregnancy.

Psychoprophylaxis: Term first applied to the Lamaze childbirth method, which emphasizes relaxation, breathing and positioning to help obtain a 'painless childbirth' (*refer* Lamaze method).

Ptyalism: Increased salvation in pregnancy.

Quickening: Sensation of the first fetal movement usually felt by the mother around the 16th week of pregnancy; a presumptive sign of pregnancy.

Regional anesthesia: A nerve block with an anesthetic agent, which ranges from local infiltration to spinal block anesthesia, the most commonly used regional anesthesia in childbirth is the epidural.

Resuscitation: Restoration of life or consciousness of one, apparently dead, or whose respiration has ceased.

Retractions: A sign of respiratory distress; occur each time the baby breathe as the skin is pulled inward between the ribs as the baby tries to expand stiff lungs.

Retinopathy of prematurity (previously called retrolental fibroplasia): Partial or complete blindness that results from abnormal blood vessel growth in the eye and may lead to detachment of the retina. The blood vessel changes may result from many factors including excessively high arterial blood oxygen levels for a period of time that can be as short as a few hours. The more preterm the baby, the more likely the baby is to develop retinopathy of prematurity (ROP).

Rooming-in concept: Healthy newborns are allowed to stay in their mothers' rooms, where they are cared for instead of remaining in the nursery.

Rupture of the membranes (ROM): *Refers* to the breaking of the amniotic membranes and the leaking of the amniotic fluid; may happen spontaneously as an early sign of the onset of labor or artificially ruptured with a device (*refer* amniotomy).

Scaphoid abdomen: Sunken or hollow-looking abdomen occurring when there is a diaphragmatic hernia, which allows the intestines to slip out of the abdomen through a hole in the diaphragm and into the chest cavity.

Shake test (also called bubble test): A bedside test of amniotic fluid formerly used for rapid estimation of fetal lung maturity and now largely replaced by more refined tests.

Shirodkar procedure: A suturing operative procedure carried out during pregnancy for correcting an incompetent cervix.

Single room maternity care: A system of caring for a woman and family during labor, delivery and recovery in one room from her admission to the hospital until her discharge for home [*refer* labor delivery recovery and postpartum (LDRP)].

Small for gestational age (SGA): A classification for infants based on weight and gestational age at birth; *refers* to an infant whose birth weight is below the 10th percentile expected for that length of gestation.

Sniffing position: Proper position of the baby's head during bag and mask ventilation or endotracheal intubation. The baby's head and back are in straight alignment and the baby's chin is pulled as if sniffing. The neck is not hyperextended.

Spermatogenesis: The process by which mature spermatozoa are formed and during which the diploid chromosome number is reduced to the haploid.

Sphingomyelin: One of the chemical substances in the lungs; the amount of sphingomyelin remains fairly constant throughout gestation. Using amniocentesis, a sample of amniotic fluid is obtained and the L/S ratio is compared in order to estimate the pulmonary maturity of the fetus.

Spina bifida occulta: A congenital defect of the walls of the spinal canal caused by the lack of union between the laminae of the vertebrae.

Stillborn: Born without life.

Striae gravidarum: The bluish or pink streaks occurring on the abdomen, thighs and breasts during pregnancy due to the stretching of the abdomen as the uterus grows; the streaks turn silvertone in time.

Surfactant: A group of substances including lecithin that contributes to the compliance (elasticity) of the lungs by coating the alveoli and allowing them to stay open during exhalation without surfactant the alveoli collapse during expiration and are difficult to open with the next breath.

Telangiectasia: The presence of small, red focal lesions usually in the skin or mucous membrane caused by dilation of capillaries, arterioles or venules.

Teratogenic agent: Virus, irradiation or drugs, the exposure to which can damage the fetus in a pregnant woman.

Term infant: A live born infant of between 38 and 42 weeks completed gestation.

Thermoregulation: The regulation of body temperature; prevention of heat loss by regulating the newborn's environment.

Tetralogy of Fallot: A common congenital cardiac malformation consisting of pulmonary stenosis, ventricular septal defect, dextroposed aorta and hypertrophy of the right ventricle.

Thrombocytopenic purpura: A hematological disorder in the newborn in which the bleeding time is prolonged, platelets is greatly decreased and there is cell fragility.

Thromboembolus: A blood clot in a vein.

Thrombophlebitis: Inflammation of a vein developing before the formation of a thrombus.

Thrush: Infection of the oral membrane by a fungus usually *Candida albicans*; it is characterized by white patches on a red, moist, inflamed surface and may occur anywhere in the mouth; commonly seen on the tongue.

Tocolytic therapy: Medication to quiet or inhibit the smooth muscle activity of the contracting uterus.

Tonus: The amount of continuous contraction of muscle. Uterine tonus *refer*s to how tightly the muscle of the uterus is contracted between labor contractions. Hypertonus *refer*s to a uterus that remains excessively tense and does not relax normally between labor contractions.

TORCH syndrome: An acronym for a group of infections, which are particularly damaging to the fetus or newborn includes toxoplasmosis, rubella, cytomegalovirus and herpes virus type 2.

Torticollis: Wryneck; stiff neck caused by spasmodic contraction of neck muscles drawing the head to one side with the chin pointing to the other side; congenital or acquired.

Toxemia: Disorders occurring during pregnancy or early puerperium, which are characterized by one or all of the following such as hypertension, edema, albuminuria and in severe cases, convulsions and coma.

Tracheoesophageal fistula: A congenital anomaly in which there is an abnormal tube-like passage between the trachea and the esophagus.

True labor: When uterine contractions are regular with increasing intensity and occur with greater frequency; contractions that effect a change in the dilatation and effacement of the cervix (*refer* false labor).

Turner's syndrome: A chromosomal defect in which there are 45 chromosomes instead of the usual 46 with the sex chromosomes identified as XO instead of XX (female) or XY (male) and may be accompanied by physical abnormalities including webbed neck, low hairline and certain skeletal, urinary tract and cardiac abnormalities. The baby will have female external genitalia, but the ovaries may be completely absent and sexual development will be severely retarded.

Ultrasound: Also called sonogram; used to visualize the uterine environment by using sound waves that pass through soft tissue until an interface between the structures of different tissue densities is reached. When this occurs, some of the energy is reflected back to the transducer, which creates an image on the screen.

Vacuum extraction: Used to assist in the delivery of the infant instead of applying forceps; after a vacuum cup is applied to the fetal scalp, a negative pressure is exerted to help draw the fetus head through the birth canal.

Vaginal birth after cesarean (VBAC): Permits patients the opportunity of a trial of labor and possibly a vaginal delivery after previously delivering by cesarean section.

Variability: The change in the baseline fetal heart rate caused by the interplay of the sympathetic and parasympathetic nervous systems; may vary from 5 to 10 bpm with contractions and fetal or maternal movement.

Variable deceleration: A periodic slowing of the fetal heart rate either with a contraction or between contractions due to umbilical cord compression; variable in duration, intensity and timing of the deceleration.

Vernix caseosa: A protective cheese-like substance found on the newborn to protect the skin from the drying effect of the amniotic fluid.

Vertex presentation: The fetal head or cranium is the presenting part with the head flexed on the chest and the chin in contact with the thorax also called cephalic presentation.

Very low-birth-weight (VLBW) infant: When an infant weighs from 500 to 1,499 g.

Zygote: The term used for a fertilized ovum for the first 3 weeks following conception.

Index

Page numbers followed by *f* refer to figure and *t* refer to table

A

Abdomen 198, 394
   girth of 310
   incision on 345
   inspection of 103, 104*t*
   lower 127
   predominate, acute 252
   rebound tenderness of 707
   X-ray of 311
Abdominal palpation 103, 105*f*, 105*t*, 299, 310, 320, 327, 332, 613, 614, 748
   preparation for 104*t*
Ablation 709
ABO blood group 101, 474
ABO incompatibility 231, 477, 751
Abortion 216, 221, 226, 289, 293, 557, 580, 581, 751
   classification of 221, 222*f*
   complete 222, 223*f*
   elective 742
   first trimester 336
   habitual 223
   incomplete 222, 223*f*, 573
   induced 223
   inevitable 222, 222*f*
   legal 223
   medical method of 595
   missed 223, 336
   recurrent 272
   septic 225, 239
   spontaneous 216, 221, 252, 743
   threatened 221, 222*f*
   tubal 227, 227*f*
Abruptio placentae 248, 249*f*, 573, 751
Acanthosis nigricans 638
Acardiac formation 300
Acceleration 751
Accredited Social Health Activist 514
   job functions of 521
   responsibilities of 596
   roles of 596
   selection of 521, 596
Aches, posture for relief of 539
Achondroplasia 465
Acid-fast bacilli 741
Acidosis 158, 399, 476, 751
   correction of 355
Acne 638
Acquired immunodeficiency syndrome 7, 273, 479, 501, 509, 589
Acrocyanosis 390, 390*f*, 751
Acupressure 529
Acupuncture 529
Acyanotic cardiac defects 459
Adenocarcinoma 669, 672
Adenomyosis 690
   endometrial 624
Adhesions 709
Adipose tissue 388
Adnexal fullness 633
Adoption 656, 662
   Laws in India 662
   procedure 663
Adrenal 332
   disease 621
   hyperplasia, congenital 648
Adrenaline 354, 399, 400
Adriamycin 682
Airborne infection 491
Airway 354, 357
   obstruction 345
   support 357*f*
Albumin 751
   binding capacity 473
   solution 397
Alcohol 558, 654, 659
Aldactone 552
Aldomet 261
Aldosterone 354
   production of 191
Alimentary tract 72
Alkalosis 751
All India Postpartum Services 502
Allergic disorders 419
Allergic reaction 204, 705
Allergy 654
Allis forceps 337, 600, 600*f*
Alpha-fetoprotein 352, 741, 751
   testing 116
Alpha-thalassemia 282
   major 282
   minor 282
Alveolar air-water interface 443
Amenorrhea 227, 621, 624, 700
   lactational 205

primary 621, 647
   secondary 621
American Cancer Society 683
American Institute of Architecture Guidelines 491
American Joint Committee on Breast Cancer TNM System 678
American Nurses Association 11
   Model for Quality Assurance and Implementation of Standards 610
Amikacin 558
Aminoglycosides 558
Ammonium dermatitis 409
Amniocentesis 114, 115*f*, 118, 751
   midtrimester 470
   reasons for 115
   risk of 114
   technique of 114, 115
Amniography 572
Amnioscopy 116
Amniotic fluid 65, 66, 114, 115, 143, 353, 477, 633
   disorders of 252
   embolism 251, 352, 353
   index 741
   large amount of 66
   measurement 311
   observation of 143
   reduced amount of 614
   studies 114
   transfer of 353
   volume of 66
Amniotomy 315, 751
   beneficial effects of 315
   hazards of 315
Amphetamines 558
Ampicillin, intravenous 307
Ampulla 413
Anal sphincter, external 40
Analgesia 158, 269, 317, 324, 345
   patient-controlled 526
   types of 187
Analgesics 526, 556
   drugs 527
Androgen excess 660
Android 37
   Android pelvis 38
Anemia 172, 269, 276, 290, 297, 425, 434, 504, 511, 562, 669,

causes of 434
classification of 276
congenital 477
effects of 278
hemolytic 277, 284
hemorrhagic 277
increased prevalence of 277
megaloblastic 280
pathological 276
physiological 84, 276, 277
previous 278
routine screening for 278
severe 307
Anencephaly 352, 460, 460*f*, 572, 751
Anesthesia 158, 345, 527
   balanced 529
   epidural 341, 371, 527
   general 227, 340, 360, 528, 529
   inhalation 136
   peridural 527
   perineal block 270
   regional 527, 758
   spinal 178, 527
   types of 187
Anesthetic agents 558
Anganwadi workers 514
Anger 567
Anorexia 271, 623
   nervosa 621
Anovulation 621, 623, 638, 657
Anovulatory bleeding, cyclic progesterone for 623
Anoxia 751
Antenatal care 268, 271, 273, 276, 285, 499, 507, 562
   component of 508
Anterior vaginal wall retractor 602, 602*f*
Anthropoid 37
   pelvis 38
Antibiotics 355, 476, 558
   intravenous 225
   prophylactic 269
Antibody
   gestation for 509
   titers 751
Anticoagulants 455, 555, 558
Anticonvulsants 455, 553, 558

therapy 262
    prophylactic 261
Anti-deoxyribonucleic acid 558
Antidepressant therapy 291
Antidiabetic drugs, oral 558
Antifibrinolytics 625, 637
Antihistamines 558
Antihypertensive 263
Antihypertensive drugs 547, 558
Antihypertensive therapy 259
Antimetabolites 558
Antinuclear antibodies 284
Antiprogesterone 623, 637
Antisperm antibodies 657, 661
Antithyroid drugs 276, 558
Anuria 263, 355
Anus 394
    gaping of 152
    imperforate 438, 457
Anxiety 419, 525, 623, 722
    disorder 290, 291
    phase of 568
Anxiolytics 291
Aorta 460f
    coarctation of 267, 459
Aortic valve incompetence 268
Apgar score 311, 389f, 390, 494, 512, 752
Apnea 444, 558
    primary 395
    secondary 395
Appendicitis, acute 700
Appetite
    disturbance 290
    loss of 667
Areola 88f, 417f
Arm 394
    circle exercise 688, 688f
    lift exercise 686f
    recoil 407
    swinging 687
Arterial oxygen pressure 388
Artery 73
    forceps 598, 599f
    pulmonary 460f
    umbilical 72, 73
Arthritis 239
Artificial caput succedaneum 342
Artificial feeding 421
    indications for 421
Artificial insemination
    donor 660
    husband 660, 661
Aseptic delivery kits, provision of 592
Asherman's syndrome 670, 703
Asphyxia 274, 298, 341, 425, 752
    clinical features of 395t
    neonatorum 395
    perinatal 395
    severe 436
Aspiration 263, 441
Aspirin 558
    low-dose 258
Assisted breech delivery 330
Assisted reproductive technology 660
    different techniques of 660
Asthenozoospermia 657
Asthma 99
Athenospermia 660

Atresia 456, 658
    duodenal 438, 457, 457f
    esophageal 456, 456f, 754
    pulmonary 459, 460f
Atrial septal defect 267
Atrophy, vaginal 635, 692
Attitude 76, 108, 568, 752
Auscultation 103, 328, 641
Authorized Foreign Adoption Agency 662
Autoimmune diseases 284
Autoimmunity 275
Automated external defibrillator 356
Automatic laparoflator 704
Autonomy 582
Autosomal recessive disorders 466
Autosomes 752
    numerical abnormalities of 467
Auvard's weighted vaginal speculum 603, 603f
Auxiliary Nurse Midwives Program 10
Axillary lymph node dissection 682, 684
Axis traction
    device 338, 606f
    forceps 606, 606f
Ayer spatula 697f
AYUSH 596
Azoospermia 659, 752

B

Babcock's tissue forceps 609, 609f
Babinski's reflex 404
Baby-friendly hospital initiative 420
Bacille Calmette-Guérin 594
    vaccine 271
Back pain 539, 667
Back rub 145
    types of 145
Backache 95, 543, 717
Bacteriuria
    asymptomatic 282
    risk of 191
Bacteroides fragilis 381
Bag and mask
    equipment 397
    ventilation 398, 398f
Bag and midwifery kit 503
Bakri balloon 364, 364f, 365f
    parts of 364f
    place of 364
Ball squeezing exercise 686, 686f
Ballard score, new 407f
Balloon
    mechanisms of action of 364
    use, indications for 364
Banana sign 745
Bandl's ring 319, 320f
Barlow's sign 406f
Barlow's test 406
Barnum's maneuver 749
Barrier methods 202
Bartholin's gland 42, 741
    abscess 635
    cancer 675
    cysts 635, 692
    openings of 42, 633
Bartholinitis 635

Basal body temperature 658, 741
Basal cell carcinoma 674
Basal metabolic rate 92
Basic Nursing Education Programs 577
Battledore placenta 67
B-cell lymphomas 236
Bednar's aphthae 409
Below poverty line 596
Beneath epithelium lies 42
Benign ovarian tumors 637
    complications of 637
Beta-blockers 558
Betamethasone 442
Beta-thalassemia 282
    major 282
    minor 282
Betnesol 305
Bilirubin 752
    conjugation of 753
    excretion of 472
    formation of 472
    levels, estimation of 475
    toxicity 472
Binocular twins, prevalence of 295
Binovular twins 295, 296
    placenta of 296f
Biomedical waste management 580
Biophysical profile 114, 311, 741, 752
Biopsy 675, 741
    cervical 643
    endometrial 623, 624, 643, 659, 702
    excision 681
    percutaneous 680
    procedures 655
    surgical 681
Biparietal diameter 76, 311, 573
Bipolar disorder 291, 291
Birth
    asphyxia 395
    canal 370
    control 202
        postconception methods of 216
    injury 274, 331, 447f
    premature 298
    rate, reduction of 592
    register 565
    registration 511
    trauma 446
    weight 423f, 513
Bisacromial diameter 77
Bishop's score 313, 313t, 752
    measurement, indications for 313
Bitrochanteric diameter 77
Bivalve vaginal speculum 708f
Bladder 191, 289, 373, 649, 691, 694, 741
    care of 138, 139, 157, 188, 531
    changes 289
    displaces 175
    dysfunction 673
    hypotonicity 178
    injury 321, 374, 630
    inspection of 178
    palpable 191
Blastomeres 59

Bleeding 207
    abnormal 621, 623
    acyclic 625
    control of 364
    disorders 190
    extraplacental 246
    heavy 705
    intermenstrual 625, 690
    irregular premenopausal 669
    management of 190
    ovular 625
    placental 246
    postmenopausal 703
    postmenstrual 702
    secondary 437
    severe 135
    vaginal 111, 135, 373, 669, 698, 699, 705, 707
Blighted ovum 573
Blindness, control of 592
Blood 72, 258, 654
    clots 168
    coagulation disorders 173, 308, 360
    examination 669
    flow 83
    glucose 669
        estimation 274
        level 272, 622
    group, dominant 296
    investigations 641
    loss 209, 222, 278, 346
    pressure 101, 126, 131, 137, 152, 186, 259, 264, 400
        aortic 388
        consistent 265
        maintenance of 355
    stained discharge 635
    sugar, random 743
    tests 101, 623
    tinged mucus discharge 127
    transfusion 279
    uterine discharge of 191
    vessels 171
        clamping of 176f
        maternal 63
    volume 83
Body reflex 405
Bone
    innominate 33
    marrow toxicity 558
    trauma 448
Bony pelvis 35f
Bottle feeding 427
Bowel 191, 741
    care of 188
    malignancy of 652
    movement 634
    obstruction 701
    symptoms 630
Brachial palsy 447
Bradley method 534
Bradycardia 558, 752
    baseline 142
    fetal 754
Brandt-Andrews maneuver 168
Brandt-Andrews method 169f
    modified 169, 748
Braxton-Hicks contractions 91, 126, 752

Index

Breast 46, 100, 184, 189, 190, 198, 394, 408, 413, 417f, 422, 694, 741
  abscess 380
  ailments 419
  cancer 676-678
    diagnosis of 678
    invasive 677
    metastatic 677
    risk factors of 677
    staging of 678
    treatment 669
    types of 681
  care of 188, 197, 417
  changes 87, 693
  complications 378, 379f
  conditions, malignant 677
  conservation treatment 682
  disease, benign 211
  engorged 418f
  engorgement 195, 378, 419
    prevention of 379
    treatment for 379
  female 47f
  inspection of 679
  lymphatic system of 677
  magnetic resonance imaging of 680f
  malignancy 224
  massage 196
  masses, characteristics of 678t
  milk 241, 413
    components of 413
    properties of 413
  normal 677
  ovarian cancer syndrome, hereditary 666
  Paget's disease of 681
  palpation patterns 679f
  poor attachment of 419
  postmastectomy 682f
  reconstruction 683
  self-examination 678, 679f
  tenderness 623
  tissue 677f
Breastfeeding 190, 195, 196, 205, 270, 302, 419, 420, 504, 511, 512, 518, 557, 558
  beneficial effects of 418
  commencement of 415
  difficulties 196, 419
  effective 18
  interrupted 732
  management of 196, 414
  preparation for 298
  process 732
  technique of 417f
Breathing 161, 357
  abdominal 541, 541f
  difficulties 444
  exercise 540
Breech
  complete 328, 328f
  delivery 442, 747
    spontaneous 330
    types of 330
    vaginal 452
  extraction 330
  hook 607, 607f
  impacted 331
  presentation 108, 327, 331f, 752

    complications of 331
    positions of 327
    six positions in 328f
    types of 327, 328f
Brenner cell 666
Brenner tumor 637
Brim 35f, 38
  different diameters of 36f
  landmarks of 35
Broad ligament
  cyst 701
  tumor 701
Bromides 558
Bromocriptine 185, 309, 558, 660
Brow presentation 77, 327, 327f
Brown fat 752
Bubble test 758
Buddha position 352
Buddha sign 745
Budin's cannula 346f
Bulb syringe 605, 605f
Bullous impetigo 435, 435f
Burns-Marshall maneuver 747
Burns-Marshall method 331
Burping positions 418f
Butorphanol 526
Butterfly needle 708f
Buttocks, internal rotation of 329

C

Cabergoline 660
Caffeine 559
Calcium 622
  gluconate 263
Cancer 208, 665, 672, 674, 676
  cervical 625, 673, 702, 703
  cervix 288
  endometrial 625, 702
  preinvasive 288
  vaginal 675
  vulval 674
Candida 237, 480
  albicans 83, 236, 237f, 273, 375, 477, 480, 635, 759
  infections 480
  tropicalis 236
Candidiasis, cutaneous 481
Cannula 701f
Caput succedaneum 393, 446, 447f, 449f, 454, 752
Carbamazepine 559
Carbimazole 276
Carbohydrate
  excessive 486
  metabolism 272
Carcinoid tumor 666
Carcinoma 669
  adenosquamous 673
  cervical 243
  cervix 625, 641
  endometrial 670t
  inflammatory 681
  medullary 681
  mucinous 681
  neuroendocrine 673
  papillary serous 669
  vaginal 675t
  vulval 675t
Carcinosarcoma 669
Cardiac arrest 356
Cardiac defects

  congenital 459
  detection of 459
Cardiac disease 267
Cardiac failure 263
Cardiopathy 558
Cardiorespiratory disease, severe 701
Cardiorespiratory system 100
Cardiotocography 140, 311, 741
Cardiovascular disease 500
Cardiovascular system 401, 436, 694
  changes in 83
Care, principles of 426
Carotid pulse 357f
Carpal tunnel syndrome 97
Carunculae myrtiformes 42, 184
Carus curve 154, 169
Catheter
  insertion of 364
  test 650
Causative organisms 632, 634, 635
Cavity 44
Cells, endometrial 59
Cellulitis, pelvic 376
Central Adoption Resource Authority 662
Central nervous system 72, 100, 139, 236, 437
  abnormalities 460
  disorders 443
  hemorrhage of 485
  signs 478
Cephalhematoma 341
Cephalic curve 338
Cephalohematoma 391, 393, , 447f, 449, 449f, 752
Cephalopagus 300
Cephalopelvic disproportion 344, 502
Cephalotribe 607, 608f
Cerebrospinal fluid 479, 741
Cervical
  brush 698f
  canal 44, 337f, 709
    occlusion of 658
  cancer 625, 673, 702, 703
    staging of 673t
  carcinoma 243
  dilatation 124, 129, 148, 313, 752
    rate of 317
  discharge 641
  effacement 128, 313, 752
  erosion 710
  factors 657
  friability 633
  hoods 557
  hostility 661
  incompetence 306
  infection 702, 703
  intracellular neoplasia 242
  intraepithelial neoplasia 288, 709
  laceration 190, 191
    extension of 372
  lesions 710
    premalignant 710
  motion tenderness 633
  mucus 661
    character of 210
    study 658

  scraping 697
  smear 641
  stenosis 630, 660
    severe 702
  tears 371
    minor degrees of 371
  tissue, condyloma of 709
  vascularity 83
Cervicitis 239, 634
  acute 699
  chronic 657, 692
  recurrent 710
Cervicopexy 630
Cervidil 314
Cervix 44, 82, 133, 158, 184, 221, 239, 311, 316, 376, 534, 709
  assessment of 313
  cancer of 672
  congenital elongation of 657
  dilatation of 129,, 129t, 148, 753
  edematous 635
  effacement of 129t
  incompetent 755
  inspection of 176
  malignancy of 652
  mucous polyp of 625
  position of 132
  ripeness of 313
Cesarean birth preparation 535
Cesarean delivery 752
  emergency 373
Cesarean incision 729
Cesarean ligation 215
Cesarean section 4, 274, 299, 308, 343, 442, 542, 741
  classical 344
  complications of 346
  elective 343, 399
  emergency 344
  indications for 260, 299, 343
  low transverse 742
  lower segment 742
  place of 270
  previous history of 341
  procedures in 345
Chadwick's sign 91, 745, 752
Chancroid 234
Chemicals 204
Chemoprevention 683
Chemotherapy 668, 671, 673, 682
  regimens 682
Chest 393
  compressions 357, 357f, 398, 752
  X-ray 654, 669
Child Health Services Program in India 506
Child Survival and Safe Motherhood Project 592
Childbirth Preparation Program 532
Chlamydia 101, 487
  infection 234, 238f, 480
  trachomatis 235, 238, 632, 634
Chloasma 752
  gravidarum 87f
Chloramphenicol 558
Chloroquine 558, 596
Chlorpromazine 487
Chlorpromide 558

Chlorthiazide 558
Choanal atresia 458, 459f, 752
Chocolate cyst
　infections of 691
　rupture of 691
Chordee 464
Chorioamnionitis 239
Choriocarcinoma 228, 230, 666, 670
Chorionic villus 63, 64f
　sampling 470, 741, 753
Chromosomal abnormality 455, 468, 558, 563, 621
Chromosome 752
　instability syndrome 469
Chromotubation, laparoscopic 659
Circulatory diseases 210
Circulatory system 96
Circumoral cyanosis 393
Circumvallate placenta 67, 67f
Civil law 578
Clavicle fracture 448
Clear airway 389, 395
Clear cell
　carcinoma 675
　endometrial carcinoma 669
Cleft
　lip 458, 458f
　palate 419, 458, 458f
Cleidotomy 348
Clitoral abnormalities 647
Clitoris 41
Clomiphene citrate 295
Clostridium
　perfringens 308
　welchii 375
Clotrimazole 237
Clots, expression of 177
Clotting disorder 702
Cluster testing 236
CO_2 laser machine 709f
Coagulopathy 172, 450, 702
Cocaine 559
Coccydynia 543
Coccyx 34
Coital act, improper technique of 692
Coitus interruptus 205
Cold
　mechanism of action of 710
　stress 736
Color Doppler 623
Colorectal cancer, hereditary non-polyposis 666
Colostrum 184, 185, 413, 753
Colpoperineorrhaphy 630
Colporrhaphy, anterior 630
Colporrhexis 371
Colposcopy 642, 709, 710
Colpotomy 215
Coma, stage of 262
Community 520
　Health Center Level 507
　health nurse 503
　level 596
　midwife 499, 615
Complete blood count 191, 669
Compression, bimanual 173, 363, 363f
Computed tomography 642, 652, 667
　scan 637, 642, 652, 667, 675, 741

Condom 202, 270, 596
　distribution 565, 593
　female 203, 203f
　male 203, 203f
　use of 203
Condyloma 709, 710
Condylomata accuminata 709
Confusion 623
Congenital anomalies 201, 253, 429, 563
　diagnosis of 572
Conjoined twins 300, 300f, 352
　types of 300
Conjugation, defective 473
Conjunctivitis 239, 409, 435, 435f
Consciousness, level of 655
Conservative therapy 366
Constipation 95, 187, 196, 276, 287, 634, 667
Constriction ring 320, 320f, 360
Consumer Protection Act 579
Continuous positive airway pressure 445, 753
Contraception 194, 202, 244, 272, 275
　barrier method of 275
　conventional methods of 205
　method of 202, 205, 270
　natural 204
　postcoital 211
　temporary methods of 202
Contraceptives 209, 236, 565, 593
　hormonal 209
　injectable 211
　methods, failure rates of 205t
　oral 622, 623, 625
　steroidal 209
　vaginal 202, 204
Contraction 128, 128f, 151
　duration of 124, 130
　frequency of 124, 130
　intensity of 124, 130
　pain 161
　painful 151
　ring 320
　stress test 117, 741, 753
Controlled cord traction 169, 169f, 741, 748
Convulsions 446, 452, 453
　causes of 453
　control of 453
　eclamptic 262
　myoclonic 452
　neonatal 452
　subtle 452
　tonic 452
Coombs' test 753
　direct 475
　indirect 474
Copper T 209
Copper T-200 206, 206f
Copper T-380a 206, 206t, 209
Cord 311
　blood 168
　breaking of 363
　care of 512
　clamp 605
　compression 311
　hemorrhage 451
　insertion of 171

　knotting 68
　length 171
　looping 68
　presentation 349, 350, 350f
　　management of 351
　prolapse 299, 301, 327, 331, 339, 344, 349, 350, 350f
　　incidence of 349
　　management of 351
　umbilical 66, 66f, 164, 176, 410
Cordocentesis 116, 116f
Core needle biopsy 681
Corneal reflex 404
Cornua 44
Coronal suture 75
Coronary heart disease 267
Corpus 44
　cancer syndrome 669
　luteum 48
　hematoma 700
Corticosteroids 355, 558
Cotton-tipped applicator 697f
Cough 217, 404
　chronic 287
　immature 731
Couple protection rate 588, 592
Cow's milk
　components of 421
　modification of 421
Cramps 95, 540
Cranioclast 607, 607f, 608f
Craniotomy 346
　instruments for 346f
C-reactive protein 633
Creatinine 669
Crede's maneuver 748
Criminal law 578
Crohn's disease 652
Crown-rump length 311, 574f
Crude birth rate 588, 592
Cryosurgery 710
Cryotherapy 710, 711
　instruments 710
　machine 711f
Cryptorchidism 464, 464f
Crystalloid solution 262
Cul-de-sac aspiration 667
Culdocentesis 643, 707
　instruments for 708f
　use of 707
Culdoscopy 643, 699
Cullen sign 745
Curved artery forceps 599f
Cusco's bivalved speculum 603, 603f
Cyanosis 269, 270, 434, 442
Cyanotic cardiac defects 459
Cyclic progesterone therapy 622
Cyclophosphamide 682
Cystadenoma
　mucinous 637
　serous 637
Cystectomy, ovarian 638
Cystic fibrosis 457, 466, 484
Cystitis 630
　pyelonephritis 673
Cystocele 628, 628f, 630
　correction of 630
Cystography 650
Cystoscopy 643, 652
Cysts 637, 709

　dermoid 637
　ovarian 701
Cytology 637
　smear test for 675
Cytomegalovirus 241, 741
　infection 235, 479
Cytotoxic drugs 557
Cytotrophoblast 61

D

Danazol 637
Das' cervical dilators 603, 603f
Das' long curved obstetric forceps 605
Deafness 500, 501
Deaths
　antepartum 564
　intrapartum 564
　intrauterine 273, 312, 558, 572, 573
　leading causes of 519
　perinatal 302
　prevention of 594
Decapitation 347
　hook 607f
Decidua 82
　basalis 60
　capsularis 60
　defective 246
　parietalis 60
Deep sedation, complications of 263
Deep vein thrombosis 381
Deficient fluid volume 20, 725, 727
Dehydration 319, 487
　signs of 140
Delayed cord clamping 399
Delivery
　location of 162
　management of 274, 299, 330
　placental 748
　position for 162
　postcesarean 365
　preparation for 162
　second stage of 370
Demerol 526
Denominator 108, 753
Deoxyribonucleic acid 455
Depo medroxy progesterone acetate 741
Depression 290, 623
　major 290, 291
　maternal 290
Dermatitis, perianal 409
Dexamethasone 660
Dextrose 397
Diabetes mellitus 224, 272, 273, 307, 669
　detection of 272
　effects of 273
　gestational 272, 290, 742, 755
　insulin-dependent 742
　juvenile onset of 742
　maternal 256, 563
　neonatal 485
Diagonal conjugate 36
Diaphragm 203, 203f
　insertion of 203f
　position of 203f
Diarrhea 437, 438, 486, 623, 667
　dietetic causes of 486

infective 486
protracted 243
severe 487
Diastasis
　recti 543
　symphysis 542
Diazepam 554, 558
Diazoxide 549
Diethylstilbestrol 557, 741
　exposure, assessment of 699
Digestive system 94
Dilantin 554
Dilatation
　and curettage 525, 655, 741
　dangers of 337
Diphtheria 594, 597
Dislocation, congenital 463f
Disposable
　cord clamp 605f
　delivery kit 503, 596
　use of 492
Disseminated intravascular coagulation 251, 261, 451, 741
Distal tubal segments 704
Distress 528
　maternal 317, 318, 339
District Child Protection Unit 662
Diuretics 263, 550, 558
Diverticulitis 652
Dizziness 191, 279
　feelings of 83
Doll's eye reflex 404
Domiciliary care 502, 510
　advantages 510
　disadvantages 510
Domiciliary midwifery service 502
Donor egg 660
Donovanosis 234
Dopamine 400
　agonist 660
Doppler ultrasound 574, 706
Double bubble sign 745
Double decidual sac sign 745
Douglas pouch 658, 691, 692, 708f
Down syndrome 116, 201, 455, 509, 753
Doxorubicin 682
Doyen's retractor 602, 602f
Doyen's towel clip 601, 602f
Drew Smythe catheter 604, 604f
Dropper feeding 427
Dropping down theory 246
Drowsy state 406
Drugs 148, 179, 621
　use of 508
Dryness 635
Duchenne's muscular dystrophy 467
Ductal carcinoma in situ 678, 681
Ductus arteriosus 73, 753
　closure of 74, 388
Ductus venosus 753
　closure of 74, 388
Dye test 650, 652
Dysgenesis 648
Dysgerminoma 666
Dysmenorrhea 210, 621, 622, 624, 633, 646, 690
　primary 622
　secondary 622

Dyspareunia 237, 630, 633, 635, 658, 690, 692, 753
　entrance 692
　superficial 692
Dysplasia 709
　bronchopulmonary 443
　cervical 319, 709, 710
Dyspnea 252, 459
Dystocia 351, 563, 753
　types of 319
Dysuria 191, 239, 633, 647, 717

E

Ear 100, 393, 408
Early pregnancy 113
　abnormalities of 221
　factor 742
Ecchymosis 192, 743
Eclampsia 251, 256, 261, 339, 341, 344, 502, 753
　complications of 263
　diagnosis of 262
Ectocervical scraping 697
Ectoderm 61
　embryonic 69
Ectopic pregnancy, secondary abdominal 227
Edema 96, 100, 192, 264, 743
　leg 667
　pulmonary 257, 263
　vulva 667
Edwards' syndrome 455, 467, 468
Ehlers-Danlos syndrome 466
Eisenmenger's syndrome 269
Ejaculation
　premature 661, 692
　retrograde 661
Ejaculatory defects 657
Ejaculatory ducts 55
Elbow spread exercise 686, 687f
Electrical nerve stimulation 529
Electrocardiogram 669
Electroencephalogram 453
Electrolyte 669
　imbalance 486
　risk for 14
　intravenous 355
Electronic fetal monitoring 7, 141t, 742, 753
Embolism, pulmonary 263, 380, 381
Embryo 61, 753
　determination of 61f
　implantation of 60
　transfer 660, 661
Embryonal cell carcinoma 666
Embryotomy 346, 347f
　scissors 607, 607f
Empathy 568
Encephalocele 753
Endocarditis 270, 376
　bacterial 268, 269
Endocervical canal 710
Endocrine 65
　disorders 483, 484, 625
　factors 657
　imbalance 563
　system, changes in 87
Endoderm 61
　embryonic 69
Endodermal sinus tumor 666

Endometrial ablation 623, 625, 692, 703
Endometrial biopsy 623, 624, 643, 659, 702
　site of 703f
Endometriosis 210, 623, 661, 691, 692, 700, 704, 709
　cervical 625
　common sites of 691f
　pelvic 622
　peritoneal 657
　tubal 657
Endometritis 190, 633, 657
　acute 632
　atrophic 632
　chronic 632
　tuberculous 625
Endometrium 44, 59, 228, 703
　carcinoma of 211
Endosalpingeal damage 657
Endoscopic procedures 655
Endotracheal intubation 399
Enema 135
　purposes of 135
　set 503
Energy spurt 127
Enterocele 628f, 629, 641
Entonox 529
Enzyme 257, 466
　beta-hexosaminidase 467
　deficiency 473
Epicanthus 55, 753
Epidural block 753
Epilepsy 99, 285
Epimenorrhea 625
Epinephrine 397, 400, 708f, 754
Epiphyses 402
Episiotomy 159, 159f, 192, 729, 730, 741, 754
　mediolateral 160
　scissors 504, 604f
　types of 159, 159f
　wound 367
Epispadias 464, 464f
Epithelium 59
Epstein pearls 393, 409, 754
Erb's palsy 331, 332, 447, 448f, 454
Erectile dysfunction 657
Ergometrine 162, 170, 177, 179, 260, 361
Ergot derivatives 546
Erythema 678
　toxicum 410f, 435
　neonatorum 754
　vaginal 635
Erythroblastosis fetalis 116, 477, 754
Erythrocyte sedimentation rate 187, 633, 641
Erythromycin 238
Erythroplasia 709
Erythropoiesis 277
Erythropoietin 277
Escherichia coli 282, 375, 477, 481, 486, 632
Estradiol serous 659
Estriol level determination 116
Estrogen 50, 413, 559, 622, 625, 669, 692
　high level of 669
　replacement therapy 621, 669, 742

stimulation theory 127
synthetic 209
Ethacridine 224
Ethinyl estradiol 185
European Union United Kingdom Central Council 10
Euthanasia 586
　passive 586
Exchange transfusion 475, 476
　complications of 476
Excretion 65
　failure 473
Excretory urography 652
Exercises 194, 539, 542, 685, 686
　abdominal 541
　general guidelines for 685
　postmastectomy 684
　postnatal 511, 541
　postpartum 189
Exomphalos 456, 456f
Expulsion 208
External beam therapy 668
External genitalia 41, 513
　abnormalities of 647
　benign lesions of 709
　malignant lesions of 709
Extremities 192, 391
　assessment of 192
　edema of 131
　swelling of 623
Eyes 100, 393, 408
　care of 475, 512
　ptosis of 393
　reflexes of 404

F

Face 76, 391
　presentation 77, 325, 327f
　　diagnosis of 325
　　midwifery management of 326
　　six positions in 325f
　　to-pubis delivery 324f
Facial nerve palsy 393, 447, 447, 454
Facies 754
Fainting 96
Fallopian tube 48, 82, 632, 656, 694
　blockage of 705
　cancer 676
　　primary 676
　　secondary 676
　Falope ring on 215f
　Hulka clip on 214f
　infection 705
　sperm perfusion 660
　X-ray of 705f
Fallot's tetralogy 267, 459, 460f, 759
Falope ring 214, 215f
False labor 127, 754
　management of 135
Family planning 7, 200, 202, 502, 504, 508, 509, 511, 518
　health aspects of 201
　information 9, 501
　modern concept of 201
　program 201
　services 593
Family Welfare Programs 588
Fascia 39, 187

Fat 187, 414
  excessive 486
  proportion 421
  subcutaneous 70
Fatigue 138, 270, 525, 623, 667, 691
Fear 525
Feeding 424, 443
  behaviors 417
  fequency of 417
  infant 505
  methods 427
  positions 415f
  status 410
  timing of 417
Felony 578
Female breast, structure of 47f
Female health
  assistant 520
  worker 503, 506, 519
Female infertility
  causes of 657
  management of 660
Female metal catheter 608, 608f
Female sterilization 213, 215
Femidom 203f
Femoral artery lines 451
Femshield 203
Femur fracture 448
Fentanyl 556
Fertility
  and Family Welfare 593
  factors required for 656
  rate, total 588, 592
Fertilization 59, 60f, 70, 661, 704
Fertilized ovum 59
  determination of 59, 60, 60f, 61f
  transportation of 656
Fetal alcohol syndrome 488
Fetal anomalies 114, 252, 298, 351
Fetal blood sampling 116, 142
Fetal cells, transfer of 114
Fetal circulation 73, 73f
  persistent 444
Fetal complications 253, 335
Fetal cortisol theory 128
Fetal death 114
  in utero 742
    intrauterine 251, 304, 307, 309, 742
Fetal distress 140, 143, 342, 754
  management of 144
  signs of 144
Fetal head 75f, 108, 614
  attitude of 76
  delivery of 747
  descend of 148
  engagement of 110f
  manual rotation of 340
Fetal heart 70
  rate 139, 144f, 160, 641, 742
    acceleration of 143f, 754
    accurate detection of 107
    baseline 142, 754
    deceleration 754
    normal 141f
    pattern 139t
    periodic 155
    variability 754
  response of 142
  sound 319, 742
    auscultation of 106f

tone 92, 131, 742
  location of 107t
  maximum intensity of 107f
Fetal hemolytic disease, severity of 116
Fetal lie 108f, 754
Fetal liver 72
Fetal macrosomia 351
Fetal maturity 113, 572
  determination of 115
Fetal monitoring 7, 754
Fetal movement 116
Fetal scalp 142
  electrode 140, 742
Fetal skull 75, 76f
  diameters of 76, 77f
  molding of 78f
  position of 155f
  regions of 76
Fetal tachycardia 754
Fetal weight 131
  estimate 741
Fetal well-being
  evaluation of 140, 160
  indicators of 111
  monitoring of 138
Feticide, selective 302
Fetofetal transfusion syndrome 300
Fetoscope 608f
Fetotoxic drugs 558
Fetus 754
  acardiacus 296
  compressus 296
  congenital malformation of 312
  determination of 63, 68
  effects on 258, 273, 298, 321, 353
  in fetu 300
  intrauterine death of 572
  papyraceus 296
  positions of 109f
  size of 350
  ultrasound of 574f
Fever 633, 634, 705
  low-grade 242
Fiberoptic blankets 475
Fiberoptic light systems 475
Fibrin degradation products 451
Fibroid 286, 625, 657, 705
  effects of 286
  growth of 636
  interstitial 636
  intramural 636
  majority of 636
  polyp 638
  submucosal 624, 625, 636
  subperitoneal 636
  subserous 636
  tumor 627, 636
  types of 636
  uterus 190, 211, 285
Fibroplasia, retrolental 425, 443, 758
Figure W exercise 688, 688f
Filshie clip 214
Fimbrioplasty 660
Fine needle aspiration 680
Fingernails 70, 73
First response pregnancy test 93f
Fistula
  diagnosis of 650

genital 649
urethrovaginal 651
Fits 262
Flagella 237
Floppiness 437
Fluid 178
  aspiration of 708f
  balance 260, 262, 318, 655
  excretion 186
  loss 187, 486
    shock 353
  pressure, general 129
  replacement 20
  ultrasound evidence of 633
Fluorescence in situ hybridization 742
Fluorescent treponemal antibody 240
Fluorouracil 682
Fluothane 529
Flushing curette 604, 604f
Foam tablet 202
Foley's catheter 263
Folic acid 280
  administration of 285
  deficiency 277
    anemia 280
  tablets 596
Follicle-stimulating hormone 48, 49, 49f, 192, 210, 638, 648, 657, 694, 742
Follicular growth, monitoring of 661
Fontanels 75, 754
Foot exercises 540
Footling breech 328
Foramen ovale 73, 754
  closure of 74, 388
Forceps
  application, steps of 340f
  basic construction of 337
  blades, identification of 340f
  delivery 331, 337, 342
    prerequisites for 339
  marks 393f
  measurements 338
  operation
    complications of 341
    difficulties in 340
    indications for 339
  over ventouse, advantages of 342
Fossa ovalis 74
Fothergill's operation 630
Fragile X syndrome 469
Frank breech 327, 328f, 331
Freidman curve 754
Fresh-frozen plasma 450
Fundal
  descends 188
  development 92f
  dominance 128
  height 102, 102t, 103, 103f, 131, 170, 170f, 184f
    measurements of 102
  palpation 105f
  pressure 169
  weight 102
Fundus 44
  approximate height of 102f
  assessment of 190

expression of 177
measurement of 177
palpation of 363
Furadantin 558
Furosemide 551

G

Gag 404
  reflex 731
Galactokinesis 185
Galactopoiesis 185
Galactosemia 484
Galant reflex 405
Gamete intrafallopian transfer 642, 660, 661
Gartner's cyst 650
Gaskin's maneuver 748
Gastroenteritis 481, 487
  diarrhea of 486
Gastrointestinal infections 481
Gastrointestinal system 100, 191, 198, 402
  changes in 85
  defects of 573
Gastrointestinal tract 354, 437
  syndromes of 456
Gastroschisis 456, 456f, 754
Gate control theory 529
Gene disorder
  multiple 465
  single 465
  types of 465f
General anesthesia 227, 340, 360, 528, 529
  types of 529
Genetic counseling 455, 470, 563
  prenatal diagnosis for 470
Genetic disorders 455, 465
  diagnosis of 115
  timings of 469
Genetic screening 455, 469
  prenatal 502, 509
Genital crisis 409
Genital organs
  female 644
  internal 42
Genital tract 317, 649
  female 644
  infections, antibiotics for 660
  injuries 173
Genitalia 391, 394, 408, 446
  ambiguous 465, 465f, 647
  external 41, 41f, 513
Genitourinary abnormalities 621
Genitourinary fistula 649
  types of 649f
Genitourinary system 96, 100, 437, 694
  abnormalities of 464
Germ cell 665
  tumors 665, 666
German measles 242, 501, 509
Gestation
  ectopic 226
  multiple 66, 114, 756
  period of 310
Gestational age 107, 113, 423, 423f, 424f, 755
  appropriate for 423, 741, 751, 752
  assessment of 406, 433

estimate 614
   large for 429
   small for 743, 758
Gestational trophoblastic neoplasia 670
   clinical features of 671
   management of 671
   spread of 671
Giant vulsellum 347, 347f
Glands
   adrenal 88, 693
   sebaceous 70
Glomerular filtration rate 272
Glomerulonephritis 224, 283
Glottis 161
Glucocorticoids 559
   therapy 305
Glucose
   6-phosphate dehydrogenase deficiency 467, 476, 484, 742
   tolerance test 742
Glycerin 145
Glyceryl trinitrate 315
Glycogen storage disease 485
Glycosuria 272
   causes of 272
   persistent 272
   renal 272
Goiter 558
Gonadal estrogen 693
Gonadal steroids 209
Gonadoblastoma 666
Gonadotropin 295
   releasing hormone 49, 622, 637, 657, 692
      agonists 623, 625
   suppression 657
Gonococcal infection 237, 238, 480
   effects of 239
   manifestations of 239
Gonorrhea 234, 239, 487
   infection 239f
Goodell's sign 91, 745
Graafian follicle 48, 46, 49f
   and ovulation, determination of 48
   lifecycle of 48f
Grand multipara 99, 293, 500, 503, 508, 755
Granulosa cell tumor 624, 666
Grasp reflex 403
Gravid uterus, retroversion of 232
Gray baby syndrome 558
Great arteries, transposition of 459
Green-Armytage's forceps 600, 600f
Green-Armytage's hemostatic clamps 345
Grief 566
   situations 567
Growth 17, 406, 692, 693
   bacterial 192
   hormone secretion 693
   monitoring 519
   promotion of 428
Guilt 567
Gut, malrotation of 438
Gynecoid 37
   pelvis 38
Gynecological disorders 267, 285
Gynecology, diagnostic procedures in 696

H

Haemophilus influenzae 742
Hair 100
   growth 70
Halo sign 745
Halothane 529
Hamolysis, elevated liver enzymes, low platelets 742
Hand
   hygiene 491
   rubs, alcohol-based 491
   washing
      station 491
      steps 491f
Hands behind head exercise 688, 688f
Head 100, 391, 393, 410
   and shoulder raising exercise 541, 541f
   birth of 326f
   box oxygen 444
   circumference 513
   external rotation of 154, 326
   growth 70
   internal rotation of 154, 324, 329
   lag 405
   tilt-chin lift maneuver 357, 357f
Headache 279, 623, 633
Health
   care 506, 507, 590
      levels of 506
         primary 506, 514, 519
         quality of 518
   center 520
   education 236, 505, 570, 597
   facility 618
   promotion 14, 16
   seeking behavior 8, 228, 570
   workers, levels of 562
Hearing 405
Heart 83, 393
   defects, structural 444
   disease 339, 341, 344
      congenital 268, 501
      rheumatic 268
   failure 269
      previous 267
   murmurs 270
   muscle 83
   normal 267
   rate 396, 400, 401
      assessment of 399
      slow 752
Heartburn 94, 95, 718
Heat loss 397
   prevention of 390
Heavy discharge 705
Hegar's sign 91, 91f, 755
HELLP syndrome 261, 755
Hematemesis 451
Hematocele, pelvic 227
Hematocolpos 647
Hematocrit 101, 654, 742
Hematoma 372, 683, 755
   formation 174
   risk of 192
   infralevator 372
   pelvic 372
   small 372
   supralevator 372

Hematometra 630, 646, 647
Hematopoietic system 100
Hematuria 451
Hemoconcentration 755
Hemoglobin 101, 193, 273, 278, 281, 654, 669, 742
   abnormal 281
   estimation 511, 641
   fetal 72
   glycosylated 273, 274
   low 278
   S 467
Hemoglobinopathies 281
Hemolysis 261
Hemolytic crisis 281
Hemolytic diseases 476
Hemoperitoneum 670, 707
Hemophilia 451, 467
Hemorrhage 176, 190, 318, 334, 362, 366, 437, 446, 449, 450, 451, 562, 673, 755
   antepartum 246, 298, 307, 315, , 502, 562, 617, 741
   cerebral 263, 265, 327, 425
   control of 354
   intracranial 159
   intracystic 637
   intraventricular 443, 450
   periventricular 450
   postpartal 139
   postpartum 171-173, 177, 301, 359, 362, 365, 574, 646, , 317, 346, 359, 363, 503, 727
   pulmonary 443
   retinal 257
   risk of 168
   secondary 510
   subaponeurotic 449, 450f
   subarachnoid 450
   subcapsular 261
   subconjunctival 393
   subdural 449
   third stage of 359
   traumatic 360
   true postpartum 359
   umbilical 451
Hemorrhagic disease 450
Hemorrhagic disorder 451
Hemorrhoids 96, 196
Hemostasis 167, 175
Heparin therapy 381
Hepatic disease, chronic 621
Hepatitis
   B
      infection 241, 487
      virus 480
   infective 562
Hepatotoxicity 558
Hermaphroditism
   female 648
   true 648
Hernia
   abdominal 701
   diaphragmatic 458, 458f, 701, 753
Herpes infection, genital 234, 241, 241f
Herpes simplex virus 240, 435, 435f, 477, 479, 673
High vaginal swab collection 699
High-density lipoprotein cholesterol 694

Hilar cell tumor 666
Hip
   dysplasia, congenital 463, 463f
   hitching 542, 542f
Hirschsprung's disease 438, 457
Hirsutism 211, 638
Hodge-Smith pessary 609, 609f
Homans' sign 192, 192f, 199, 741, 745, 755
   assessment of 192
Home delivery, preparation for 503
Hookworm 278
Hormonal contraceptives 209
   classification of 209
Hormonal fluctuations, natural 209
Hormonal pregnancy tests 92
Hormonal therapy 683
Hormone
   estimation 658
   levels 192
   luteinizing 48, 49f, 55, 192, 210, 638, 648, 658
   male 55
   ovarian 50
   pituitary 87
   placental 87
   replacement therapy 695, 742
   therapy 625
Hostile cervical mucus 660
Hot intrauterine douche 363
Hour-glass contraction 344, 366
Hulka clip 214, 214f
Human chorionic gonadotropin 61, 65, 660, 707
   hormone 742
   test, immunologic assays of 93
Human immunodeficiency virus 243, 477, 487, 501, 654, 672, 742
   infection 243, 501, 509
      diagnosis of 243
      end stage of 243
   test 101
Human menopausal gonadotropin 660
Human organs, transplantation of 580
Human papillomavirus 675, 710
   acute 698
   infection 672
   genital 234
Human placental lactogen 65, 272, 671, 742
Humerus, fracture of 332, 448
Hunter syndrome 466
Hurler syndrome 466
Hyaline membrane disease 442, 755
   complications of 443
Hydatidiform mole 113, 228, 229f, 230, 256, 336, 573, 755
   complete 229
   diagnosis of 572
Hydralazine 261, 549
Hydramnios 502, 508, 572
   minor degree 253
   severe degree 252
Hydration 138, 140, 158, 445, 475
Hydrocele, congenital 409
Hydrocephalus 351, 461, 755

Hydrochlorothiazide 551
Hydronephrosis 691
Hydrops fetalis 477
Hydroureter 691
Hydroxyprogesterone 557
Hydroxyzine 136
Hymen
    abnormalities 646, 647
    imperforate 647
Hyperactive reflexes 192
Hyperandrogenism 638
Hyperbilirubinemia 273, 477, 558, 755
    complications of 472
    neonatal 14
Hypercalcemia 486, 558
    neonatal 486
Hypercholesterolemia, familial 466
Hyperemesis 231, 671
    gravidarum 230, 755
    intractable 224
Hyperglycemia 485
Hyperinsulinemia 660
Hypernatremia 486
Hyperplasia
    adrenal 465
    endometrial 624, 669
Hyperprolactinemia 660
Hyperpyrexia 307
Hypersomnia 623
Hyperstimulation 118, 315
Hypertension 111, 256, 269, 669
    chronic 265, 307
    classification of 256
    essential 265
    gestational 256, 264
    malignant 224
    persistent pulmonary 444
    residual 258
Hypertensive disorders 562
Hyperthermia 436
Hyperthyroidism 275, 621, 624
    treatment for 276
Hypertonic glucose infusions, cessation of 485
Hypertrophy 647
Hypoactive bowel sounds 633
Hypocalcemia 273, 388, 453, 475, 486
    signs of 486
Hypogastric ligaments 388
Hypoglycemia 273, 274, 388, 453, 485
    clinical signs of 485
    management of 485
Hypomagnesemia 273, 453
Hypomenorrhea 621, 624, 625, 658
Hyponatremia 486
Hypopituitarism, selective 363
Hypoplasia 646
    diagnosis of 647
Hypoprolactinemia 657
Hypospadias 464, 464f, 657, 660, 661, 755
Hypotension 707
    orthostatic 191
Hypothalamopituitary-gonadal axis 693
Hypothalamopituitary-ovarian axis 657
Hypothermia 425, 558, 736

Hypothyroidism 276, 621, 622, 624
    congenital 484, 513
    routine neonatal screening for 485
Hypotonia 399, 437
Hypoxia 312, 317, 403, 450, 755
    fetal 158, 161, 332
Hysterectomy 363, 367, 623, 637, 690, 692
    cesarean 346
    radical 673
    total abdominal 743
    vaginal 630
Hysterosalpingography 642, 659, 705
Hysteroscope 704f
Hysteroscopy 624, 643, 703, 709
Hysterotomy 225

I

I-can test kit 93f
Icterus neonatorum 473, 473f
Iliac artery, internal 43
Iliac crest 33, 330
Ilium 33
Imferon 279
Immune system 194
    immature 735
Immunity 84
    acquired 477
    innate 477
    natural 477
Immunization 188, 594, 597
Immunoglobulins 185, 194
Immunotherapy 668
Impaired glucose tolerance 272
Implantation 59, 60
Impotence 692
In vitro fertilization 295, 660, 661
Incision
    abdominal 730
    biopsy 681
Incomplete rupture 356, 373
    signs of 356
Incontinence 543
Indian Medical Association 591
Indian Nursing Council 585, 591, 615
Induction
    dangers of 312
    drugs used for 315
    indications for 312
    methods of 313
Infections 286, 308, 425, 441, 453, 472, 479, 480, 625, 630, 638, 657, 683, 698
    acquired after birth 481
    alimentary 563
    asymptomatic 237, 238
    bacterial 238
    chlamydial 237, 238
    control 490
        protocols 493
    fungal 236
    intrapartum 239
    intrauterine 129, 251, 317, 321
    management of 478
    neonatal 477, 479
    pelvic 208, 635
    placental 65
    prevention of 426, 518

    protozoal 237
    puerperal 239
    pyogenic 632
    recurrent 241
    respiratory 481, 563
    severe 376
    syphilitic 501
    transmission of 477
    treatment of 442, 478
    types of 632
    urethral 692
    vaginal 237, 274, 634, 703
    viral 240
    vulval 634, 635, 692
Infertility 630, 634, 638, 656, 669, 691, 705
    causes of 656
    female 657
    management of 659, 662
    primary 656
    secondary 563, 656
    treatments 295
    unexplained 660, 661, 704
    work-up 642
Infusion, intravenous 136
Injury 370, 373, 374, 446, 578
    intracranial 487
    risk for 723
    urethral 374
    vaginal 698
    visceral 373, 449
Inlet 38
Inner cell mass 61
Insemination 660
    intrauterine 660
Insomnia 14, 97, 623
Insufflation test 659
Integrated Child Development Scheme 589
Integrated Child Development Services 515, 593, 597
    team 597
Integumentary system 97, 100, 193, 434
Intensive care unit 514
Intensive neonatal care unit 442
Intermittent positive pressure ventilation 445
International Confederation of Midwives 9
International Conference on Population Development 593
International Council of Nurses Code of Ethics 583
International Federation of Gynecology and Obstetrics 9, 673
Intersex disorders 647
Interstitial fluid 186
Interval tubal ligation 215
Intestinal obstruction 691
Intestines 227
Intra-amniotic instillation 224
Intracytoplasmic sperm injection 660, 661
Intramuscular ergometrine 222
Intranatal care 502, 509
Intrapartum care 269, 271, 284, 285
Intrathoracic pressure 269
Intrauterine balloon tamponade 364

Intrauterine devices 205, 270, 275, 511, 593, 622, 625, 633, 642, 703, 742
    complications 207
    first generation 205, 206f
    indications for removal of 208
    mode of action of 206
    register for 565
    second generation 205, 206f
    side effects 207
    third generation 205, 206, 209
    types of 205
    use of 632, 658
Intrauterine growth
    restriction 117, 284, 344, 479
    retardation 118, 273, 292, 293, 573, 742
    causes of 424
Intravaginal device 203
Intravenous fluids 283, 355
    therapy 427
Intravenous indigo carmine test 651
Introitus 42
Intubation equipment 397
Invasive cancer 681
    cervix 288
Invasive carcinoma 289
    cervix, effects of 288
Invasive mole 670
Inversion
    classification of 367
    complete 631
    incomplete 631
    types of 631
Iodide 558
    containing drugs 500
Iron
    deficiency 277
        anemia 210, 278, 279
    intramuscular 279
    loss 277
    metabolism 84
    oral 279
    parenteral 279
    requirements 278
    therapy 279
        supplementary 279
Irritability 623
Ischial spines 38, 130
Ischial tuberosities 34
Ischiopagus 300
Ischium 33
Isolation
    room 491
    techniques 617
Isoniazid 558
Isosorbide mononitrate 315
Isoxsuprine 552
Isthmus 44
Itching 635

J

Jacquemier's maneuver 749
Jacquemier's sign 91, 745, 755
Janani Suraksha Yojana 593, 595
Jardine's decapitation hook 607
Jaundice 425, 434, 472, 671, 755
    management of 474
    neonatal 474
    pathological 473

Index

physiological 473, 473f
types of 473
Jaw flexion 331
Jaw-thrust maneuver 357
Jitteriness 437
Joints 513
    pelvic 34
Justo minor pelvis 38

K

Kangaroo care 428
Kaposi's sarcoma 243
Kegel exercise 189, 540, 541
Kelly's deep retractor 602, 602f
Kernicterus 472, 558, 755
Ketoacidosis 319
Ketones 101
Kidney 354, 402
    absence of 253
    disease 500
    function 136
Kielland's forceps 338, 338f, 606, 606f, 649
Klinefelter's syndrome 657
Klumpke's palsy 448
Knee
    chest position 650
    presentation 328, 328f
    rolling exercises 542
Kocher's forceps 498, 599f
Krukenberg tumors 666
Kustner's sign 745

L

Labetalol 261, 548
Labia majora 41
    abnormalities 647
Labia minora 41, 693
    abnormalities 647
Labial tears, anterior 160
Labor 123, 286-288, 293, 311, 361, 755
    abnormalities of 219
    assessment 527
    character of 525
    course of 323, 324
    delivery recovery and postpartum care 8, 755
    diagnosis of 135
    duration of 124
    dysfunctional 753
    early stage of 530
    evaluation of progress of 142, 161
    fetal intolerance of 143
    first stage of 123, 124, 124f, 128, 135, 136, 146, 149, 269, 317, 533, 534, 540
    fourth stage of 126, 175, 179
    induction of 310, 312, 313, 723
    management of 260, 274
    mechanisms of 153f, 324, 325, 329
    normal 123
    obstructed 139, 320, 326, 646
    physiological response of 719
    precipitate 172, 318, 360
    premature 111, 135, 646, 724
    preparation for 111
    prolonged 301, 310, 316, 360, 758
    second stage of 125, 125f, 151, 157, 164, 269, 318, 446, 533, 534
    stages 123, 268
        average length of 124t
    status, evaluation of 130
    stress of 175
    third stage of 125, 126f, 166, 167, 172, 270, 359, 360
    true 759
Lacerations 370
Lactating breast, cross-section of 414f
Lactation 413, 621, 755
    maintenance of 185
    stimulation of 185
    suppression of 185, 420
Lactiferous tubule 413
Lactobacillus bifidus 403
Lactose 414
Ladd's bands 438
Ladin's sign 745
Lamaze method 533, 755
    modified 534
Lambda sign 745
Lambdoidal suture 75
Laminaria tent 337f, 601, 601f
Lanugo 73, 408, 755
Laparoscopy 622, 623, 637, 638, 643, 659, 700, 709
    diagnostic 700
    procedure 701f
Laparotomy method 215
Laryngomalacia 459f
Laryngoscope 397
Laser 643
    instruments 709f
    machine 709
    procedures 709
    surgery
        advantages of 710
        disadvantages of 710
        indications for 709
    vaporization 660, 709
    wave guides 709
Last menstrual period 69
Laws, knowledge of 576
Laxative 259
Lead, delivery of 331, 345
Leave against medical advice 618
Lecithin 115, 756
Leg
    cramps 718
        alleviation of 146
    exercises 540
    position of 176
    raising 541
        exercise 542f
Lemon sign 745
Leopold's maneuvers 103, 105f, 105t, 106, 748, 756
Lesch-Nyhan syndrome 467
Lesions
    endometrial 710
    infectious 435, 435f
    precancerous 672
Leukemia 624
Leukocytes 414
Leukopenia 284
Leukoplakia 709
Leukorrhea 83, 96
Levator ani muscles 151
Levonorgestrel-releasing intrauterine system 206, 207f, 690, 691
Libido
    change in 623
    loss of 658
Lidocaine 708f
Lids, ptosis of 393
Lie 107, 756
Ligament
    sacrospinous 34
    sacrotuberous 34
Ligamentum
    arteriosum 74, 388
    teres 74, 388
    venosum 74
    venosus 388
Light amplification by stimulated emission of radiation 643
Lignocaine hydrochloride 371
Limb 513
    defects 558
        diagnosis of 572
    reduction anomalies 462
Linea nigra 87f
    observation of 101
Lippes loop 206f
Lips
    cyanosis of 270
    examination of 406
Liquor amnii 311
Listeria monocytogenes 482
Lithium 557, 559
Lithotomy position 530
Liver
    diseases of 210
    function
        impaired 14
        tests 670
Lochia 184, 191, 198, 199, 741, 756
    alba 184, 191, 756
    amount of 189, 191
    rubra 184, 756
    serosa 184, 191, 756
Long curved obstetric forceps 338, 338f, 605f
Loop electrical excision procedure 673
Løvset maneuver 330f, 747
Low forceps operation 339
    procedure of 339
Low-birth weight 339, 341, 419, 423, 513, 756
    incidence of 423
Lower uterine segment 167f, 170, 175
    formation of 128
Lumbar epidural block 159
Lumen 657
Lung 72, 354
    abscess 376
    immaturity 442
Lymph edema 683
Lymph nodes 677f
    internal iliac 42
Lymphangiography 642
Lymphatic drainage 42, 44
Lymphatic system 100
Lymphogranuloma venereum 652
Lynch syndrome 666
Lysergic acid diethylamide 558, 559
Lysozyme 414, 756

M

Macrophages 414
Macrosomia 311, 756
Magnesia, milk of 743
Magnesium sulfate 263, 553
    administration of 262
Magnetic resonance imaging 572, 642, 667, 675, 680, 680f, 690
    uses of 642
Makesure test kit 93f
Mala D 210, 210f
Mala N 210, 210f
Malaise 634
Malaria 307
Male reproductive system 53, 53f
    parts of 53
Malformation, congenital 307, 312, 501, 644, 657
Malignancy 638, 650, 652
    cervical 224
    genetic 666
    genital 665, 689
    ovarian 665, 666
Malnutrition 621, 626
Malpresentation 111, 301, 323, 646
Malrotation 438, 457
Mammary glands 183, 185
    protuberant 70
Mammography 679, 680f
Manchester operation 630
Manipulative procedures 334
Manual vacuum aspiration 595
Marfan's syndrome 466
Mass
    abdominal 669
    peritoneal 638
    tubo-ovarian 701
Mastectomy
    prophylactic 683
    total 682
Mastitis 380, 419, 756
Maternal and Child Health 508
    Program in India 499
    Services 507
Maternal deaths
    causes of 515, 562, 564
    classification of 561
    indirect 561
Maternal infection 242
Maternal medications, effects of 557
Maternal mortality 263
    causes of 222
    rate 515, 561, 591, 592
Maternal newborn nursing care plans 715
Maternal nutrition 413
    improvement of 564
Maternal trauma 327, 332
Maternal vital statistics 560
Maternal well-being 148
    evaluation of 138, 157
Maternity care 756
    object of 7
Matthew Duncan method 167f
Maturity, determination of 573
Mauriceau-Smellie-Veit
    grip 331f
    maneuver 331, 747

Mayer-Rokitansky-Küster-Hauser syndrome 647
McRoberts maneuver 334, 749
Mean corpuscular hemoglobin 282
Measles 742
Meconium 402, 756
    aspiration syndrome 311, 441, 742
    ileus 438
    passage of 185
    stained amniotic fluid 118
Medical termination pregnancy Act 223, 595
Medicine, integrate Indian systems of 589
Meditation 530
Megaloblastic anemia 280
    effects of 280
Melanin pigmentation 392
Melanoma 674
Melena 451
Membranes
    artificial rupture of 299, 315
    delivery of 168
    examination of 171, 171f, 296
    high rupture of 316
    low rupture of 311, 315
    premature rupture of 127, 301, 304, 306, 743
    rupture of 129, 151, 152, 315, 329, 743, 758
    spontaneous rupture of 306, 743
    stripping of 313, 316
Menarche 51, 693
    early 669
Mendelson's syndrome 353
Meningitis 482
Meningocele 460, 461f
Meningomyelocele 461, 461f
Menometrorrhagia 624, 625
Menopause 51, 692-694
    abnormal 695
    age of 693
    artificial 695
    clinical aspects of 48
    delayed 695
    diagnosis of 694
    late 669
    premature 695
Menorrhagia 210, 623, 624, 690
    polymenorrhea 621
Menstrual cycle 50, 209
    disorders 621, 624
    normal 52
    overview of 51f
    regulation 623
Menstrual induction 216
Menstrual period 99
Menstrual regulation 216, 224
Menstruation 50f, 187, 694, 710
    abnormal 691
    clinical aspects of 48, 51
    different phases of 48
    frequent 623
    hormonal control of 49f
    infrequent 623
    normal 209
Mental
    confusion 354
    Mental preparation 502, 509

Mental retardation 403, 558
Mental status 654
Meperidine 136, 556
    hydrochloride 526
Meptazinol 526
Mercy killing 586
Mesoderm 61
Metabolic disorders 438, 483
    acquired 485
Metabolic imbalance syndrome, risk for 14
Metabolism 152
    changes in 85
    inborn error of 483, 755
Metal suction cups 606f
Metastatic disease 672
Metformin 660
Methergine 162, 170, 177, 179, 299, 337, 345, 347, 363
    dose of 224
Methimazole 276
Methotrexate 224, 558
Methoxyflurane 529
Methyldopa 547
Methylene blue 650f
Methylergonovine 179
Metoclopramide 345
Metronidazole 237, 238, 558, 559
Metrorrhagia 621, 624, 625
Miconazole pessaries 237
Microcephaly 461, 461f, 501
Microsurgical epididymal sperm aspiration 661
Micturition, frequency of 96, 283, 690
Mid forceps operation 339, 340
Midstream urine 283
Midwife 9
    management 487
    responsibility 9, 10
        regarding prenatal screening 574
    role of 9, 202, 263, 383
    skills of 9, 10
Midwifery 614
    education 5
        determination of 10
    practice, development process of 5
    standards, format of 613
    trained personnel 614, 615
Mifepristone 224
Milia 409, 434, 756
Miliaria 434
Milk
    allergy 487
    concentration 558
    inadequate supply of 419
    pressure 185
    production 185
    secretion 185
Minerals 277, 414
Minilaparotomy 215
Minipill 209
Miscarriage, late 646
Misoprostol 315
Mitral stenosis 268
Mittelschmerz's syndrome 210, 621, 622

Mixogen 185
Molding 77, 78f, 756
Mole
    partial 229
    tubal 227, 227f
    types of 229
Molecular weight 558
Mongolian spots 390, 392, 392f, 409, 756
Mons
    pubis 41, 693
    veneris 41
Montgomery tubercles, determination of 88f
Mood
    disorders 290
    swings 623
Morbidity, permanent causes of 563
Moro reflex 403, 403f
Morphine 320
Morquio syndrome 466
Mortality 208, 263, 756
    neonatal 516, 564
    rate, infant 517, 564, 591, 592
Morula 59
Moulding 148
Mouth 100, 393, 410
    care 145
    reflexes of 404
    to-mouth respiration 357f
Mouthwash 145
Mucopolysaccharidosis 466
Mucus
    rhythm, users of 204
    sucker 605, 605f
    trap suction apparatus 756
Müllerian duct 644, 647
    anomalies 644
Multifocal clonic convulsions 452
Multigravida 99, 332, 756
Multiload Cu-250 206, 207f
Multiload Cu-375 206, 206f
Multipara 274, 756
Multiparity 350
Mumps 742
Muscle 39, 345
    abdominal 153
    bulbocavernosus 40
    fibers 176f
    ischiocavernosus 40
    layers 82, 82f
    skeletal 152
    subcostal 442
    tone, loss of 694
    trauma 447
Muscular systems 100
Muscular tone 177
Musculoskeletal deformities 462
Musculoskeletal system 95, 193, 402
Mushroom cap 204
Mycoplasma hominis 632
Myoepithelial cells 413
Myomas 709
Myomectomy 637
    hysteroscopic 625
Myometrium 45, 82
Myrtiform caruncles 184
Myxoma 638

N

Naegele's pelvis 39
Naegele's rule 99, 756
Naloxone 400
    hydrochloride 397
Napkin rash 409
Narcotic 558
    analgesics 137, 526
    handling of 617
    medicines 580
Narrow introitus 646, 647, 658, 692
Nasal cannula 444
Nasopharyngitis 481
National Commission on Population 589
National Family Welfare Program 588, 591
National Population Policy 588
National Rural Health Mission 593, 595
Nausea 94, 95, 279, 623, 633, 667, 716
Neck 100, 391, 393
Necrotizing enterocolitis 437, 438, 476, 481, 756
Neonatal abstinence syndrome 487
Neonatal intensive care unit 7, 489, 490, 493
Neonatal mortality 516, 564
    causes of 516
    rate 564, 592
Neoplasia, gestational trophoblastic 670
Neoplasms 623
Nephritis, chronic 307
Nephrotic syndrome 283
Nerve trauma 447
Nervous system 97
    changes in 88
Neural tube defect 352, 756
Neurofibromatosis 466
Neurological disorders 437
Neurological system 403
Neuromuscular maturity, assessment of 407
Neutrophils 414
Nevus flammeus 409
Nifedipine 549
Night sweats 271
Nipple 88f, 100
    blistered 419
    care of 185
    cracked 379, 419
    depressed 419
    flat 419
    inverted 419
    preparation for 185
    retracted 379
    short 419
    stimulation test 118
    supernumerary 394
Nitric oxide 257, 315
Nitrofurantoin 558
Nitroglycerin 743
Nitrous oxide 529
Non-metastatic disease 672
Non-particulate antacid 345
Nonsteroidal anti-inflammatory drugs 284, 622, 623, 692
Non-stress test 117, 311, 743, 756
Normal puerperium 181

management of 183
physiology of 183
No-scalpel vasectomy 213
Nose 100, 393
Nova ring 212
Nuchal cord 163f, 756
management of 163
Nuchal translucency 470
Nulligravida 99
Nullipara 99, 756
Nurse
legal roles of 577
registration 576
responsibilities of 494, 577
rights of 577
role of 662
Nursing Manpower Committee 615
Nutrition 14, 16, 65, 445, 511
education 597
Nutritional deficiencies 501, 509
Nystatin pessaries 237

O

Obesity 625, 669
morbid 702
Obsessive compulsive disorder 291
Obstetrics 614, 743, 745
audit 614
complications 563
diagnostic uses in 113
emergency 349, 381
forceps 337
invention of 337
types of 338f
management 261, 321
operations 336
Obstructed labor 139, 320, 326, 646
management of 321
signs of 321
Occlusion method 214
Occult prolapse 349, 350
Oldham's perforator 346f
Oligohydramnios 253
Oligomenorrhea 621, 623, 624, 625, 658
Oligo-ovulation 657
Oligospermia 659-661
Oliguria 354
Omentum 227
Omphalitis 481
Omphalocele 456, 757
Omphalopagus 300
Oncogenicity 572
Oophoritis 632
Operculum 757
Ophthalmia neonatorum 480, 757
Opiates 558
Oral polio vaccine 594, 743
Oral rehydration
solutions 487
therapy 592
Oral thrush 409, 410f, 435, 435f
Organ
changes 694
generative 33, 41
Orogastric tube 456
Oropharynx 396
Ortolani's sign 406f, 757
Ortolani's test 406
Osiander's sign 91, 745, 757
Osteogenesis imperfecta 466

Osteoporosis 211, 694
Ovarian agenesis 648
Ovarian arteries 46
Ovarian cancer 665, 667, 669
borderline 668
classification of 666
epithelial 665, 666, 668
risk factors of 666
surgical stages of 668t
Ovarian cycle 48
Ovarian cyst
functional 211
twisted 700
Ovarian drilling, laparoscopic 660
Ovarian failure 661
Ovarian pathology 622
Ovarian tumor 287, 288, 669
benign 637
effects of 288
Ovary 45f, 46, 46f, 632, 693, 694
accessory 648
anomalies of 648
carcinoma of 211
cysts of 637
granulosa cell tumor of 624
supernumerary 648
Ovulation 48, 49f, 50f, 187, 656, 757
hormonal control of 48, 49f
inhibition of 210
Ovulatory dub 624
Ovulatory dysfunction 660
Ovum
forceps 599, 599f
retrieval 661
Oxygen 396
administration, supplementary 399
saturation 655, 743
supply of 490
Oxygenation 444
assessment of 399
Oxytocic 545
agent 162
use of 170
drug 301, 345
use of 179
Oxytocin 148, 170, 190, 225, , 308, 315, 360, 367, 413, 545, 757
administration of 170, 317
challenge test 118, 743, 757
contraction test 118
dose of 314t
drip 299
induction 313, 314
infusion 308
side effects of 314
stimulation theory 127

P

Paget's disease 678, 681
Pain 207, 525, 539, 690, 691, 727, 729
abdominal 373, 707
acute 717-719
lower abdominal 227
bilateral lower abdominal 633
causes of 526
epigastric 671
false 310
lower abdominal 208, 634
management 194

ovular 622
pelvic 539, 633, 634, 667
perception of 525
perineal 196
relief 260, 525
nonpharmaceutical methods of 529
severe abdominal 705
tearing 373
Pallor 434, 667
causes of 434
Palmar
erythema 757
reflex 403, 403f
surface 408
Palmer sign 91, 745
Palpation 323, 363, 641, 679
abdominal 103, 105f, 105t, 299, 310, 320, 327, 332, 613, 614, 748
Papanicolaou smear 624
abnormal 698, 702, 703
sampling device 697f
Papanicolaou test 696
Papilledema 257
Papilloma, laryngeal 242
Parametritis 376
Parietal bones 75
Partograph 146, 147f
components of 148
Patau syndrome 455, 468
Patent ductus arteriosus 267, 443
Pathological jaundice 473
causes of 473
features of 473
Pawlik's grip 105f, 106
Pawlik's maneuver 106
Pediatric intensive care unit 743
Pedicle, torsion of 637
Pelvic
adhesions 622, 627
arch 38
brim 35
canal, measurements of 37f
cavity 36
lower 323
congestion syndrome 700
contraction 342
curve 338
examination 110, 130, 131, 320, 624, 641
floor 39
exercise 540, 541
ligaments of 35f
muscles 40f
organs 40
supports 40
grip 105f, 106
inclination 37, 37f
infection, chronic 622
inflammatory disease 208, 211, 623, 632, 633, 658, 703, 704, 707, 743
acute 702
chronic 692, 699, 700
inlet 325
laboratory tests 101
ligaments 34
mass
large 701
small 701

organs, infectious conditions of 632
outlet 36
diameters of 37f
measurements of 36
pain
acute 700
chronic 633, 700
palpation 105f, 110f
radiation therapy 669
relaxation 629
support system, stretching of 629
tilt 189, 542
exercises 542f
ultrasound 670, 706, 706f
procedure of 707
reasons for 706
risk of 706
scan 624
variations 39
Pelvimeter 103f, 608, 608f
Pelvis 33
brim of 35f
clinical evaluation of 41
contracted 299, 325, 332
deformed 39
evaluation of 41
false 35f, 36
female 33
four types of 37f
high assimilation 39
maternal 110t
normal 33f
sagittal section of 44f
segments of 109f
true 34, 35f
types of 37
Pemphigus neonatorum 481
Pendulum exercise 687
Penis 55
congenital anatomic defect of 692
Pentazocine 526
Penthrane 529
Pentothal 529
Perez reflex 405
Pericarditis 376
Perimetrium 45
Perinatal loss 566
nature of 567
Perinatal mortality 283, 479, 516, 563
causes of 516, 563
Perinatal period 516, 567
Perineal body 41
Perineal bulging 152
Perineal discomfort 199
Perineal infiltration 371
Perineal laceration 190
Perineal muscles
repair of 371
transverse 40
Perineal pad
change of 178
inspection of 178
Perineal scar 692
Perineal shave 135
Perineal tear 160, 160f, 370
complete 652
third degree 371

Perineal tissue, condyloma of 709
Perineal trauma, posterior 160
Perineorrhaphy 630
Perineum 40f, 184, 376, 504
   inspection of 178
   lacerations of 370
   painful 543
   relaxed 629
Periodic lower abdominal pain 647
Peripheral vascular collapse 558
Peripheral venous infusion sites 451
Peritoneal signs 707
Peritoneum 187
   abdominal 345
   pelvic 208, 207
Peritonitis 376
   generalized 701
   pelvic 376, 634
Peritubal adhesions 657, 658
Pertussis 594, 597
Petechiae 434
Pethidine 556
Phagocytosis 65
Pharyngitis 240
Phenergan 557
Phenobarbital 555
Phenobarbitone 285, 476, 558, 559
Phenylalanine hydroxylase deficiency 466
Phenylketonuria 466, 484, 513, 743, 757
Phenytoin 554, 558, 559
Phlebothrombosis 380
Phlegmasia alba dolens 381
Phosphatidylglycerol 757
Phototherapy 474, 474f, 475, 757
   fiberoptic 475
   indications for 474
   types of 475
Physiological jaundice 473, 473f
   causes of 473
   management of 473
Pierre Robin syndrome 458
Pigmented nevi 392
Pills 209
   curve 209
   long-acting 211
   oral 209, 558, 565, 596
   postcoital 209, 211
   types of 210
   use, length of 210
Pinard's fetoscope 608
Pinard's maneuver 747
Pinard's stethoscope 106f, 608
Pinocytosis 65
Piskacek's sign 745
Pitocin 170, 177
   injection 179
Placenta 66, 167, 167f, 169, 170, 190, 208, 272, 311, 323, 362, 757
   abnormalities of 66
   accreta 367
   anomalies of 66
   assessment of 171
   circumvallata 67
   delivery of 168, 170, 175
   descend of 167
   determination of 63, 63f
   edema of 66
   evaluation of 176
   examination of 171, 296
   expulsion of 167
   extrachorial 67
   fetal surface of 64f
   functions of 65
   incomplete separation of 360
   inspection of 176
   localization of 573
   manual removal of 361, 362f
   marginata 67
   maternal surface of 64f
   mature 64
   premature
      expulsion of 301
      separation of 332
   previa 172, 175, 246, 247f, 299, , 308, 315, 332, 344, 360, 375, 573, 574f, 757
      degrees of 246
      diagnosis of 247
      signs of 247
      types of 247f
   receiver 503
   removal of 345
   retained 190, 366, 367
   retention of 172
   separation of 329
   succenturiate 67, 67f
   syphilitic 66
   variations of 66
   weight of 171
Placental abruption 251, 259, , 353, 360, 757
   grading of 249
   types of 249
Placental expulsion 174
   Duncan mechanism of 167
   method of 167f
   Schultz mechanism of 167
Placental separation 166, 168, 168f
   mechanism of 166f
   signs of 125, 174
Placental site 363
   trophoblastic tumor 670, 671
Placental tissue 367
Plantar reflex 403, 404f
Plasma protein 84
Plastic applicators 204
Platelet
   adhesiveness 187
   count 641
Platypelloid 37
   pelvis 38
Plethora 434
Pneumonia 594
   acquired 441
   chlamydial 238
   congenital 441
   neonatal 481
   septic 263
Pneumothorax 443
   clinical signs of 443
Poliomyelitis 597
Polychemotherapy 682
Polycystic kidney disease 283, 466
Polycystic ovarian
   disease 669
   syndrome 621, 622, 624, 625, 636, 638, 660, 669
Polycythemia 273
Polydactyly 462, 462f
Polyethylene frame 206
Polyhydramnios 114, 172, 252, 300, 306, 325, 332, 350, 757
   acute 252
   chronic 252
   maternal 456
   signs of 252
   symptoms of 252
   types of 252
Polymenorrhea 625, 625
Polyps 638, 657, 658
   endometrial 622, 624, 669, 703
   mucoid 625, 638
Pomeroy method 214f
Ponder's index 114
Port-wine stain 392f, 409
Positive pressure ventilation 396, 398, 757
Positron emission tomography 642, 667
Postnatal care 271, 274, 282, 284, 504, 510
   psychological aspect of 504
Postnatal period, management of 301
Postpartum depression 382, 757
   symptoms of 382
Postpartum hemorrhage 171-173, 177, 301, 646, , 317, 346, 359, 363, 503, 727
   signs of 360
Post-term pregnancy 310, 312, 757
   dangers of 311
   management of 311
Potassium chloride 487
Potent synthetic steroid 206
Potter syndrome 467, 468
Prednisolone 558, 559
Pre-eclampsia 186, 251, 256, 258, 261, 265, 276, 293, 298, 307, 339, 757
   acute fulminant 260
   clinical classification of 257
   mild 257
   severe 136, 257, 299
   tests in 258
   treatment for 259
Pregnancy 95, 96, 98, 99, 113f, 208, 239, 243, 256f, 265, 267, 272, 278, 285, 288-290, 297, 311, 355, 539, 562, 570, 621, 702, 710
   abdominal 227
   abnormalities of 219
   adolescent 291
   cervical 228
   complications 307
   continuation of 312
   danger signs of 746
   diagnosis of 90, 92, 570, 572, 573
   disorders of 246
   duration of 297
   early 113
      registration of 515
   ectopic 208, 226, 226, 228, 573, 633, 699, 700, 704
   effects of 265, 273, 281, 284, 286, 287, 289, 297
   first half of 352
   hypertensive disorders of 118, 256
   induced hypertension 99, 229, 256, 284, 344, 502, 743, 757
   intrauterine 742
   length of 102
   loss 221
   maternal disease in 425
   medical termination of 222f, 223, 581
   minor disorders in 94
   multiple 107, 172, 246, 252, 269, 295, 300, 306, 332, 350, 425, 502, 508, 572, 614
   natural protection of 205
   normal 79
   physiological changes of 81, 716-718
   post-term 310, 312, 757
   post-tubal 705
   preterm 332
   previous 304
   prolonged 500, 508
   rapidity of 187
   ruptured ectopic 699, 707
   services, medical termination of 593
   signs of 92
   spacing 511
   special exercises for 538
   termination of 216, 259, 274, 281, 308, 469
   test
      kits 93, 93f
      placental 707
   tubal 226, 227f
   voluntary termination of 744
Pregnant uterus, displacement of 289
Premature births 298
   occurrence of 208
Prematurity 503
   apnea of 444
   causes of 425
   retinopathy of 425, 758
Premenstrual syndrome 621, 623, 691, 743
Premenstrual tension syndrome 210
Prenatal card 504
Pre-Natal Diagnostic Technique Act and Rules 580
Prepidil gel 314
Pressure dilatation 647
Preterm labor 298, 304, 758
   management of 305
Primigravida 82, 99, 257, 274, 311, 323, 758
Primipara 99, 758
Pritchard regimen 262
Probe test 652
Procaine penicillin, single dose of 239
Proctitis 239
Proctoscopy 643
Progestasert 206, 207f
Progesterone 50, 65, 413, 692
   releasing intrauterine system 625
   serous 658
   withdrawal theory 127
Progestogen 559, 625
   only pill 209, 211
   synthetic 209
Prolactin 50, 413
   excess 660

Prolapse
　degrees of 629
　recurrence of 630
Prolonged labor 301, 310, 316, 360, 758
　causes of 316
　dangers of 317
Promethazine 136, 557
Prophylactic forceps application 341
Prophylaxis 172, 279, 361
Propranolol 548
Propylthiouracil 276
Prostaglandin 225, 308, 313, 315, 316, 546
　gel 260, 743
　induction 314
　oral 743
　stimulation theory 128
　synthetic inhibitors 637
Prostate gland 55
Prosthetics 683
Protein 101, 277, 414, 669
　binding, degree of 558
　deficiency 277
　diarrhea 486
　energy malnutrition 513
　types of 281
Proteinuria 140, 257, 264
　non-pathologic 186
Prothrombin 401
Proximal tube disease 704
Pseudocyesis 758
Pseudohermaphroditism 647
Pseudomyxoma peritonei 638
Psychiatric disorders 99, 267, 290
　treatment of 291
Psychoprophylaxis 533, 758
Psychosis, puerperal 382, 383
Psychotherapies 291
Psychotic disorders 291
Ptosis 393
Ptyalism 758
Pubertal development, stages of 692
Puberty 51, 692
　delayed 693
　disorders of 693
　endocrinology in 693
　precocious 693
Pubic arch 38
Pubic bones 33
　upper margin of 34
Pubic ligaments 34
Pudendal arteries, external 42
Pudendal block 158, 527
Pudendal nerve 42
　perineal branch of 40
Puerperal sepsis 263, 375, 377, 510
　predisposing factors of 375
Puerperium 183, 186f, 198, 258, 260, 280, 287, 293, 298, 382, 538
　abnormalities of 219
　anatomical changes of 183
　complications of 375
　discomforts of 195
　normal 181
　physiological changes of 183
Pulmonary disease, chronic 287
Pulse 354
　irregular 270
　oximetry 263
　rate 126, 152
Pulselessness 356
Purandare's operation 630
Purpuric rash 434
Purulent sputum 271
Pus
　cells 669
　collection of 632, 633
Pushing technique 162
Putrid endometritis 376
Pyelography
　intravenous 647, 667
　retrograde 650
Pyelonephritis
　acute 282
　chronic 283
Pyemia 376
Pyloric stenosis 457, 458f
Pyoderma 435, 435
Pyometra 632
Pyrexia 381
　puerperal 375

Q

Quality assurance 610, 618
　goals of 610
　plan, components of 610
Quinine 307

R

Rachipagus 300
Radial artery lines 451
Radiant warmer 390f
Radiation 501, 650, 652, 668, 671
　therapy 682
　intraoperative 682
Radical mastectomy, modified 682
Radioactive iodine 558
Radiofrequency ablation 743
Radioimmunoassay 743
Radiotherapy 676
　primary 673
Raised intracranial tension 453
Raloxifene 683
Rapid surfactant test 115
Rectal atresia 457, 457f
Rectal examination 624, 641
Rectal fistulas 438
Rectal injury 630, 698
Rectal mucosa 371
Rectal pressure 707
Rectal sheath 345
Rectocele 629, 629f, 630, 641
Rectouterine pouch 700f
Rectovaginal examination 641
Rectovaginal fistula 348, 563, 630, 647, 652, 673
Rectovaginal septum 692
Rectum 374, 691
Rectus abdominis 345
Red blood cell 72, 187, 225, 391, 743
Red cell
　breakdown 473
　enzyme 476
　fragility 476
Reflex, embracing 403
Regional anesthesia 527, 758
　advantages of 528
　disadvantages of 528
Regurgitation 345
Renal abscess 376
Renal blood flow 83
Renal calculi 283
Renal disease 283
　chronic 283, 621
Renal function tests 283, 670
Renal infection 691
Renal system 138, 402
　changes 186
Renal tubular damage 272
Renal ultrasound 652
Reproductive methods, artificial 662
Reproductive mortality 561
Reproductive organs
　accessory 46
　female internal 44f
Reproductive system 402
　changes in 81
　female 43f
　male 53, 53f
Reproductive tract infections 234
　management of 589
Respiration 65, 393
Respiratory arrest 356
Respiratory disorders 271
Respiratory distress syndrome 115, 273, 436, 442, 563, 667, 743, 757
　idiopathic 755
　mild 490
　risk of 346
Respiratory infections, acute 592
Respiratory problems 440
　causes of 441
　clinical signs of 441
Respiratory rate, assessment of 399
Respiratory support 426
Respiratory system 387, 401, 435, 458
　anatomy of 440
　changes in 84
　physiology of 440
Resuscitation 395, 396f, 758
　cardiopulmonary 356
　degrees of 396
　neonatal 399, 400
　rationale for 395
Retained placenta 190, 366, 367
　removal of 173
　signs of 366
Retention 191, 647
Retinopathy 224
Retraction 128, 678, 758
　ring 128
　　formation of 128f
　　pathogenesis of 320f
Retrospective diagnosis, clinical presentation for 311
Retroversion 289
Retroverted gravid uterus 289
　incarceration of 232
Rhesus 389
　factor 743
　incompatibility 476
　status 509
Rheumatic valvular lesion 267
Rheumatoid arthritis 211
Rhinitis 481
Rhythm method 204
Rhythmic breathing, control of 70
Ring forceps 708f
Ring pessary 608, 609f
Ringer's lactate 262, 397
Ritgen maneuver 747
Ritodrine hydrochloride 553
Robert's maneuver 748
Robert's sign 745
Rooting reflex 404
Rubella 242, 479, 742
　immune status 101
　infection 501
　vaccination 202
Rubin's cannula 701f
Rubin's maneuver 334, 748
Rubin's test 659
Rupture, incomplete 356, 373

S

Sacral nerve 40
Sacral promontory 36, 39
Sacrococcygeal joint 34
Sacrococcygeal ligaments 34
Sacroiliac joint 34, 323
Sacroiliac ligaments 34
Sacrosciatic notch 38
Sacrum 34, 38, 108
Safe abortion services 593, 595
Saline, normal 397
Saliva 241
　pooling of 393
Salivation, excessive 95
Salmonella 481
Salpingectomy
　bilateral 741
　partial 214, 214f
Salpingitis 376, 657, 699
　acute 632, 707
　chronic 632
Salpingo-oophorectomy 638
　bilateral 741
Salpingo-oophoritis, acute 700
Salpingoscopy 643, 704
　transient 704
Sanfilippo syndrome 466
Sarcoma 669
Scalp 100
Scanty vaginal mucus 658
Scaphoid abdomen 758
Scar
　inspect abdomen for 614
　lower segment 373
　rupture 355, 372
　tissue 705
Scarf sign 408
Schroder's sign 746
Schultz method 167f
Sciatic notch
　greater 33
　lesser 34
Scrotal hematoma 213
Scrotum 53, 214f
　cross-sectional overview of 54f
　external view of 54f
Sebum, mixture of 70
Secundigravida 99
Sedatives 259
Seizures 437
Selective estrogen receptor modulators 683

Semen
  collection 661
  parameters 657
  values, normal 657t
Semi-Fowler's position 530
Seminal fluid, errors in 657
Seminiferous tubules 53
Sensory deprivation 475
Sentinel lymph node dissection 682
Sepsis 346, 367, 476, 562, 736
  development of 375
  umbilical 435, 435f
Septicemia 376, 377, 634
Septum 658
Seroma formation 683
Serosanguineous fluid 446
Sertoli-Leydig cell tumor 666
Severe anemia 307
  treatment of 279
Sex
  chromosomes, numerical abnormalities of 468
  hormone-binding globulin 638
Sexual dysfunction 15
Sexually transmitted
  diseases 7, 234, 433, 501, 593, 633, 658, 673, 743
    control of 236
    prevention of 292
  infection 589
    diagnosis of 235
  oncogenes 673
  organisms 632
Shake test 758
Sheehan's syndrome 563
Shigella 481
Shirodkar procedure 758
Shock 346, 353, 368
  cardiogenic 353
  classification of 353
  endotoxic 353
  hemorrhagic 353
  hypovolemic 353, 354
  neurogenic 353
  septic 353, 354, 634
  treatment of 372
Shoulder
  birth of 154, 326
  blade squeeze exercise 686, 686f
  circles 685
  delivery of 163, 330
  dystocia 159, 311, 333, 334, 351, 747-749
  internal rotation of 154, 324, 326
  posterior 331f
  presentation 332, 332f
  rolls 685
  traction 331
Sickle cell
  anemia 281
  disease 118, 281, 467
  disorders 281
  trait 281
Sickle hemoglobin 281
Side bends exercise 687, 687f
Sigmoid colon 691
Silastic
  rubber cup 343, 343f
  vacuum cup 606f

Silicone 343, 343f
  rubber cup 343
Simpson's perforator 607, 607f
Sims' double-bladed vaginal speculum 602, 602f
Sims' double-ended uterine curette 603
Sims' position 530, 650
Single fertilized ovum 295
Sinuses, lactiferous 185
Skeletal system 100, 694
Skene's glands 42, 741
Skin 73, 354, 390, 392, 408
  care 424, 427, 475, 512
  changes 86
  color 655
  infections 481
  integrity, impaired 730
  rashes 434, 434f
Skull
  collapse 347
  fracture 448
  landmarks of 76
Sleep 188
  deprivation 14
  disturbance 290
Small cell carcinoma 673
Smell 405
Smellie lock 337
Sneeze reflexes 404
Snowstorm sign 746
Sodium
  bicarbonate 397, 400
  chloride 487
  citrate 487
Soft tissue
  displacement 151
  obstructions 321
Sonography 308, 637, 638, 659
  transabdominal 642
  transient 642
Sonosalpingography 659
Sore throat 242
Soreness 635
Spalding's sign 114f, 746
Sparse pubic hair 635
Specialized Adoption Agency 662, 663
Speculum examination 658
Sperm 660
  cell 204
    parts of 55f
  motility, loss of 657
Spermatic cord 55
Spermatogenesis 758
  defective 656
Spermatozoa, formation of 55
Spherocytosis, congenital 476
Sphingomyelin 115, 758
Spina bifida 572
  aperta 460
  occulta 461, 758
Spinal needle 708f
Spiritual distress 570
Spironolactone 552
Sponge holding forceps 598, 598f, 702f
Spoon feeding 427
Squamous cell carcinoma 672, 674, 675
Squamous epithelium 42
Stallworthy sign 746

Staphylococcus
  albus 375
  aureus 375, 481
  epidermidis 441
State Adoption Resource Agency 662
Static endometrial hypoplasia, production of 210
Stenosis, pulmonary 267
Stepping reflex 404, 404f
Sterile vaginal examination 743
Sterilization 212, 657
  female 213
  male 212
  register 565
  services 593
Steroids 442, 559
  androgenic 557
Sticky eyes 409
Stillbirths 564
  causes 564
Stomach
  overdistention of 419
  tube 345
Stool 391
Stork beak mark 392f
Straight artery forceps 599f
Straight Mayo scissors 604f
Strawberry mark 392f
Streak ovaries 648
Streeter's dysplasia 464, 464f
Strengthening referral system 595
Streptomycin 271, 500, 558, 559
Stress 290, 419
  emotional 567
  intracranial 318
  physical 567
  tolerance 17
Striae gravidarum 758
Stridor, laryngeal 459
Stromal cell
  cancers 665, 666
  tumors 666
Stuck twin sign 746
Stuffy nose 409
Subdermal implant 212, 212f
Subfertility 656
Subinvolution disorders 190
Sugar 669
Sulfonamides, long-acting 558
Sulphonilamide 559
Superfecundation 296
Superficial vein thrombosis 380
Supernumerary digits 462
Supine hypotensive syndrome 353
Supportive therapy 365
Suprapubic pressure 334
Sure sign 746
Surgery 668, 671, 675
  abdominal 658
  conservative 690
  pelvic 658
  primary 673
  types of 653
Surgical management, potential complications of 683
Swaddle wrapping 416f
Swallowing reflex 404, 404f
Swelling
  abdominal 634
  suprapubic 647
Swim-up methods 661

Symphysis
  fundus height 743
  pubis 34, 102, 170f, 178, 326f
  upper border of 614
Syncytiotrophoblast 61
Syndactyly 462, 462f
Syntocinon 177, 314
  injection 179
Syntometrine 162
Syphilis 234, 239, 239f, 307, 480, 501, 509
  congenital 240
  latent 240
  tested for 501
  Treponema pallidum of 65
Systemic lupus erythematosus 284

T

T sign 746
Tachycardia 270, 381, 707
  baseline 142
Tachypnea 442, 459
  transient 443
Talipes
  calcaneovalgus 463, 463f
  equinovarus 462, 462f
Tamoxifen 669, 683
  use of 669
Tamponade, intrauterine 364
Tanner stages 692
Taste 405
Taxonomy 13, 16
Tay-Sachs disease 467
Tearfulness 623
Tears, spontaneous 370
Teenage pregnancy 291
  causes of 292
  prevention, programs for 292
Teflon graft 457
Telangiectasia 758
Telangiectic nevi 409
Telescope 701f
Temperature rhythm, users of 204
Tenaculum forceps 601, 601f
Tenderness 633, 678
Tension 623
Teratogenesis 208
Teratogenic agent 758
Teratoma
  immature 666
  mature 666
Testicular sperm extraction 661
Testis 53
  anatomy of 55f
  structure of 54f
Testosterone secretion 693
Tetanus 509, 594, 597
  protection 501
Tetracycline 558, 559
Thalassemia 281
  syndromes 282
Thalidomide 559
Theca cell tumor 666
Thermal regulation 388, 402, 759
Thermoneutral environment 756
Thiopental sodium 529
Thoracopagus 300
Three swab test 650, 650f, 650t, 651
Throat 100
Thrombocytopenia 284, 450
  neonatal 434

Thrombocytopenic purpura 759
　idiopathic 284
Thromboembolism 562
Thromboembolus 759
Thrombophlebitis 376, 380, 381, 510, 759
　pelvic 381
　postpartum 381
　prevention of 192
Thromboplastin time, partial 450
Thrombosis, superficial 380
Thrombotic thrombocytopenic purpura 743
Thromboxane A2 256
Thrush 759
Thumb technique 399f
Thyroid
　dysfunction 275, 290, 625
　function 88
　　tests 622
　gland 693
　hormone replacement 622
　problems 484
Thyroiditis, postpartum 276
Thyroxine 276
Tiredness 623, 633
Tissue
　integrity, impaired 16
　superficial 446
Tocolytic
　agents 305, 552
　therapy 759
Tolbutamide 559
Tonic neck reflex 403, 403f
Tonic uterine contraction 319, 320
Tonus 759
TORCH syndrome 759
Torsion 286
Tort law 578
Torticollis 447, 454, 759
Torulopsis glabrata 236
Total brachial plexus palsy 448
Tough hymen 692
Toxemia 118, 759
Toxoplasma 455
　gondii 478
Toxoplasmosis 478
　other, rubella, cytomegalovirus, herpes simplex virus 744
Trace elements 414
Trachelectomy 673
Tracheoesophageal fistula 759
Traditional birth attendants 502
　training of 592
Transabdominal placement 365
Transcutaneous electrical nerve stimulation 530
Transvaginal color Doppler sonography 642
Transvaginal ultrasound 668, 706
　examination 706
Trauma 321, 373, 393, 449
　prevention of 452
Traumatic delivery, effects of 321
Treponema pallidum 239, 480
Trichomonas
　infection 698
　vaginalis 237, 237f, 698
Trichomoniasis 698
Tricuspid
　atresia 459
　valve 460f

Trimethoprim 559
Trisomy 455, 468
　profile test 470
Trocar 701f
Trophoblast 60
Trophoblastic disease
　gestational 670, 742
　persistent 670, 671
Trunk 391
　delivery of 345
　incurvation of 405
Tubal adhesions 699
Tubal disease 661
Tubal ligation 213, 356, 699
　bilateral 741
　laparoscopic 215
　method of 214, 215
　puerperal 215
　timing for 215
Tubal rupture 227, 227f
Tubal surgery, previous 657
Tube feeding 427
Tubectomy 213
Tubercular cervicitis 625
Tuberculosis 633, 658
　endometrial 625
　mycobacterium of 65
　peritonitis 701
　pulmonary 271
Tuboscopy 704
　transabdominal 704f
Tubotubal anastomosis 660
Tubular ductal carcinoma 681
Tumor 289, 666, 692, 705
　androgen producing 625
　gestational trophoblastic 671t
　malignant
　　epithelial 666
　　trophoblastic 228
　marker 667
　ovarian 287, 288, 669
Tunica
　vaginalis 53
　vasculosa 53
Turner's syndrome 648, 759
Turtle sign 333, 746
Twins 500
　diagnosis of 573
　dizygotic 295
　genesis of 295
　locked 301, 301f
　monoamniotic 301
　monozygotic 300
　placentae 296f
　pregnancy 295, 297, 297f
　　diagnosis of 296
　to twin transfusion syndrome 744
　uniovular 296
　vanishing 296
　varieties of 295
Two-finger technique 399f

U

Ultrasonic Doppler device 107f
Ultrasonography
　high-resolution 470
　intravaginal 470
Ultrasound 113f, 622, 623, 759
　abdominal 707, 707f
　application, types of 706

examinations 642
　use of 642
Umbilical arteries 72, 73
　closure of 74
Umbilical cord 66, 66f, 164, 176, 410
　abnormalities of 67
　anomalies of 67
　prolapse of 349
　variations of 67
Umbilical ligaments, lateral 74
Umbilical vein 73
　closure of 74
Umbilical vessels 171
Umbilicus 170f
Uniovular twins 296
　placenta of 296f
United Nations International Children's Emergency Fund 420
Upper respiratory infection, maternal 528
Upper uterine segments, formation of 128
Upper vaginal vault, inspection of 176
Urea 669
Ureter 649
Ureteral ligation 652
Ureteral sheath denudation 652
Ureteric injury, complications following repair of 652
Ureteric obstruction 652
Urethra 189, 289, 374, 649, 694, 741
　membranous sphincter of 40
Urethral caruncle 625, 709
Urethral catheter 503
Urethral meatus 239, 633
Urethrocele 629, 630
Urge urinary incontinence, risk for 14
Uridine diphosphate glucuronyltransferase, levels of 473
Urinalysis 101
Urinary frequency 191, 647, 667, 717
Urinary incontinence 192, 667
Urinary system
　changes in 84
　defects of 573
Urinary tract infection 98, 186, 274, 283, 481, 717, 744
　monitor for 275
Urine 241, 258, 391, 654
　drainage of 188
　elimination 198, 641, 669
　reflux of 652
　retention of 630
　sample 241
　testing 138, 140
Urography, intravenous 650, 652
Urticaria neonatorum 435
Uterine 46
　abnormality 332
　　congenital 644
　abscess formation 634
　action 128, 151, 172
　　abnormal 563
　　disorders of 310, 318
　activity 143f
　agenesis 646, 646f

　anomalies 425, 646
　　congenital 644
　　determination of 644
　　types of 644
　atony 139, 190
　bleeding
　　abnormal 624t, 669, 702
　　dysfunctional 621, 622, 624, 625
　blood flow, regulation of 83
　body drains 45
　cancer 668
　cavity 60, 337, 345, 632
　cervical tenaculum 708f
　contractions 83, 141f, 142, 148, 221
　　abnormal 299
　　intensity of 525
　curette 603f
　dehiscence 702
　dressing forceps 600
　enlargement 91, 252
　　combination of 92
　factors 657
　fibroids 172, 293, 622, 636f
　fluid thrill, elicitation of 252
　fundus 188, 741
　hemostasis 175
　hyperplasia 657
　hyperstimulation, interventions for 315
　hypoplasia 557
　inertia 172, 308
　infection 376
　involution 184f
　lining, benign growths of 669
　malformations, congenital 703
　massage 372
　muscle 166, 332, 345
　　fibers, retraction of 128f
　over distension 172
　packing forceps 600, 600f
　pain, assessment of 190
　perforation 208, 670
　polyp 625, 705
　prolapse 287, 563, 628, 628f, 629f
　　degrees of 628f
　　management of 630
　　second-degree 657
　relaxant anesthetic agents 172
　rupture 344, 373f, 646
　shape 81
　souffle 92
　sound 604, 604f, 702f
　synechiae 625, 657
　tetany 319
　tube 45, 226
　　normal function of 226
　tumor 287, 709
　wall 166f
　wound, suturing of 345
Uterovaginal prolapse 628f
Uterus 44, 173, 175, 176, 183, 188, 190, 198, 222, 236, 289, 364, 365f, 376, 504, 627, 632, 693, 694, 699, 705
　acute
　　inversion of 367f
　　retroversion of 657
　arcuate 644, 645f
　atonic 172, 346, 359

bicornuate 645, 645f, 752
bimanual compression of 363f
body of 81
chronic inversion of 630
congenital anomalies of 644
didelphys 644, 645f
displacement of 627
distension of 360
enlarged 131, 172
evaluation of 175
exploration of 363
fixed 692
fundus of 177, 177f
hypertonic 755
intrapartum rupture of 355
inversion of 367
massage of 177
muscle layers of 82f
perforation of 670
retraction of 359
retroflexion of 628f
retroversion of 627, 628f
rupture of 334, 355, 372
septate 646, 646f
subinvolution of 253, 348, 378
top portion of 190
tubes 45f
unicornuate 644, 645f
X-ray of 705f

V

Vacuum extraction 341, 342f, 606, 759
Vagina 42, 83, 184, 189, 321, 376, 504, 647, 693, 694, 744
    condition of 132
    local infections of 236
    malignancy of 652
    tuberculosis of 652
Vaginal agenesis 646
    diagnosis of 647
Vaginal atresia 641, 646, 647, 699
    secondary 692
Vaginal bacteria, normal 633
Vaginal birth
    after cesarean 744, 759
    essential for 154
Vaginal bleeding 111, 135, 373, 669, 698, 699, 705, 707
    abnormal 634, 667
    absence of 131
    excessive 633
    irregular 633, 671
    presence of 131
Vaginal cancer, primary 675
Vaginal delivery 194, 242, 327
    assessment for 329
    normal spontaneous 743

Vaginal discharge 633, 641
    abnormal 634
Vaginal examination 130, 131, 142, 299, 317, 319, 323, 327, 328, 332, 337, 641, 744
    painful 641
Vaginal hysterectomy, total 743
Vaginal infection
    active 698
    acute 702
Vaginal introitus 169
Vaginal laceration 191
Vaginal lesions 710
Vaginal malformations 646
Vaginal mucus discharge 659
Vaginal orifice 42
Vaginal ring 212
Vaginal secretion 126
Vaginal septum 646, 647, 692
Vaginal smear 698
Vaginal speculum 696f, 702f
Vaginal stenosis 557
Vaginal tear 371, 699
Vaginal tubal ligation 215
Vaginal ultrasound 707
Vaginal wet mount 698
Vaginitis 635, 692, 698, 699
Vaginoplasty 647
Vaginosis, bacterial 238, 698
Valium 554
Valporic acid 559
Valproate 558
Vande Mataram Scheme 593, 595
Varicella zoster
    immune globulin 480
    virus 480
Varicose veins 96
Varicosities 96
Vasa previa 68, 315, 349
Vascular nevi 392
Vascular systems 100
Vasectomy 212
    open-ended 213
    operation 214f
    site of 214f
Vasodilator prostaglandin, production of 83
Vault
    bones of 75
    cellulitis 630
Vein, umbilical 73
Velocit eazy test device 93f
Venereal disease research laboratory 222, 501
    test 101, 641
Veno-occlusive diseases, pulmonary 269

Ventilation, mechanical 444
Ventouse
    contraindications for 342
    cup 606, 606f
    delivery 341
    extractor 342f
    over forceps, advantages of 342
Ventral suspension 405, 405f
Ventricular septal defect 267
Vernix caseosa 70, 73, 114, 759
Vertex 76
    positions of 109f
    presentation 77, 759
Very low-birth-weight 759
Vesicovaginal fistula 348, 563, 630, 647, 649, 654, 673
Vessels, umbilical 171
Vestibular glands, greater 42
Vestibule 41, 42f
Vestibulitis 692
Vibroacoustic stimulation 744
Vigorous exercise 625
Vigorous uterine contraction 175
Viremia, maternal 241
Vision 405
Vital signs 131, 137-139, 157, 176, 198, 260, 408, 504, 655
    continuous monitoring of 528
    temperature 511
Vitamin 277
    A 594
    B12 280
        deficiency 277, 280
        supplements 281
    C 258
    D 558
    E 258
    fat-soluble 414
    K 285, 391, 558
    K1 390
    water-soluble 414
Volvulus 438
Vomiting 94, 95, 279, 437, 487, 633, 705, 716
    causes of 487
von Braun-Fernwald's sign 746
von Willebrand's disease 624
Vulsellum forceps 599, 599f
Vulva 41, 301, 370, 693, 694, 744
    cancer of 674
    congestion of 152
    examination of 674
    inspection of 641
    local infections of 236
Vulval intraepithelial neoplasia 675
Vulvar atrophy 635
Vulvar dystrophies 709
Vulvar erythema 635

Vulvar lesions 710
Vulvar tissue, condyloma of 709
Vulvar vaginal intraepithelial neoplasia 709
Vulvovaginitis 635
    atrophic 635

W

Walking reflex 404
Wall climbing
    exercise side wall stretch 687, 687f
    facing wall 687f
Wand exercise 686, 686f
Warfarin sodium 555
Warts 710
    genital 242
Waste, segregation of 492f
Weight
    gain 264, 623
    loss 187, 271, 310
    sudden loss of 667
Wharton's jelly 68, 311
White blood cells counts 84, 641
Wolf clip 214
Wood's screw maneuver 334, 748
Wound
    approximation of 743
    complications 346
    sepsis 630
Wrigley's forceps 338, 345, 605, 605f

X

Xiphisternum 82, 107
X-linked disorders 467

Y

Yeast
    fungus 480
    infection 698
Yoga 530
Yoon ring 214

Z

Zavanelli's maneuver 334, 747
Zuspan regimen 262
Zygosity, determination of 296
Zygote 59, 759
    intrafallopian transfer 660, 661